Psychopharmacological Agents

VOLUME II

MEDICINAL CHEMISTRY
A Series of Monographs

EDITED BY

GEORGE DESTEVENS

*CIBA Pharmaceutical Company
A Division of CIBA Corporation
Summit, New Jersey*

Volume 1. GEORGE DESTEVENS. Diuretics: Chemistry and Pharmacology. 1963

Volume 2. RUDOLFO PAOLETTI (ED.). Lipid Pharmacology. 1964

Volume 3. E. J. ARIËNS (ED.). Molecular Pharmacology: The Mode of Action of Biologically Active Compounds. (In two volumes.) 1964

Volume 4. MAXWELL GORDON (ED.). Psychopharmacological Agents. Volume I. 1964. Volume II. 1967.

Volume 5. GEORGE DESTEVENS (ED.). Analgetics. 1965

Volume 6. ROLAND H. THORP AND LEONARD B. COBBIN. Cardiac Stimulant Substances. 1967

Volume 7. EMIL SCHLITTLER (ED.). Antihypertensive Agents. 1967

Volume 8. U. S. VON EULER AND RUNE ELIASSON. Prostaglandins. 1967

Volume 9. G. D. CAMPBELL (ED.). Oral Hypoglycaemic Agents: Pharmacology and Therapeutics. 1969

Volume 10. LEMONT B. KIER. Molecular Orbital Theory in Drug Research. 1971

In Preparation

E. J. ARIËNS (ED.). Drug Design (in three volumes).

PSYCHOPHARMACOLOGICAL AGENTS

∽∽∽

Edited by
MAXWELL GORDON

SMITH KLINE & FRENCH LABORATORIES
Philadelphia, Pennsylvania

VOLUME II

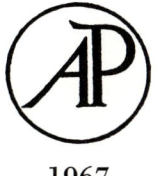

1967

ACADEMIC PRESS • New York and London

COPYRIGHT © 1967, BY ACADEMIC PRESS INC.
ALL RIGHTS RESERVED.
NO PART OF THIS BOOK MAY BE REPRODUCED IN ANY FORM,
BY PHOTOSTAT, MICROFILM, OR ANY OTHER MEANS, WITHOUT
WRITTEN PERMISSION FROM THE PUBLISHERS.

ACADEMIC PRESS INC.
111 Fifth Avenue, New York, New York 10003

United Kingdom Edition published by
ACADEMIC PRESS INC. (LONDON) LTD.
Berkeley Square House, London W.1

LIBRARY OF CONGRESS CATALOG CARD NUMBER: 64–17794

Second Printing, 1971

PRINTED IN THE UNITED STATES OF AMERICA

TO MY WIFE

List of Contributors

Numbers in parentheses indicate the pages on which the authors' contributions begin.

JOHN H. BIEL *Aldrich Company, Inc., Milwaukee, Wisconsin* (519)

LOUISE H. GREENBERG *Smith Kline & French Laboratories, Philadelphia, Pennsylvania* (249)

MAXWELL GORDON *Smith Kline & French Laboratories, Philadelphia, Pennsylvania* (1, 249, 283)

A. HORITA *Department of Pharmacology, University of Washington School of Medicine, Seattle, Washington* (523)

PAUL A. J. JANSSEN *Janssen Pharmaceutica, Research Laboratories, Beerse, Belgium* (199)

R. J. F. MCCANDLESS *Smith Kline & French Laboratories, Philadelphia, Pennsylvania* (249)

Foreword

The many advances made in medicinal chemistry within the past quarter-century have done much to further our knowledge of the relationship between chemical structure and biological activity. This relationship has led to a tremendous collaborative effort between chemists and biologists, and this has been evidenced further by the considerable number of reviews which have appeared on various aspects of medicinal chemistry. For the most part, these have been confined to single chapters on selected topics. Of necessity, in such a format, it has been difficult to cover a particular area very broadly.

The purpose of this series is to present a series of monographs, each dealing with a specific field in medicinal chemistry. Thus, these edited or authored volumes will make available to the medicinal chemist and biologist an opportunity to review critically a topic; consequently, a broader perspective of a subject can be realized.

GEORGE DESTEVENS

Preface to Volume I

The multidisciplinary nature of research on psychopharmacological agents, coupled with the rapid rate of growth of research in this area, has prompted us to make available a review on this topic. This book is written primarily for medicinal chemists and pharmacologists, but researchers in other disciplines such as clinical investigation, biochemistry, analytical chemistry, etc., may also find material of interest here.

The organization of this book is generally based on a treatment of the major classes of psychopharmacological agents in separate chapters. To the extent allowed by the diverse nature of the subject matter, each chapter covers the history, synthesis, pharmacological activity, *in vivo* distribution and metabolic fate, analytical methods, and, briefly, the clinical uses of each class of psychopharmacological agents. We feel that, by having these chapters written, in the main, by the discoverers or developers of each class of compounds, we have achieved an authoritative treatment of this complex subject. We hope that we have attained a successful balance in respect to the scientific disciplines involved, and we shall be grateful to our readers for pointing out any errors in fact or interpretation.

The disproportionate length of the phenothiazine review, relative to the other chapters, has resulted in this topic being put into a separate second volume. This arrangement was also deemed advisable because of the over-all size of the treatise; publication in a single volume would have resulted in too large a book. Volume I covers the literature up to 1963, with supplementary material made available in the appendix of Volume II.

It is our pleasure to acknowledge the valuable aid of many people in the preparation of these volumes. We are grateful to Dr. Charles E. Berkoff and Mr. R. F. McCandless for editorial assistance and to Mrs. Hilda Kihm and Miss Rita De Sanctis for excellent clerical assistance. We would like to thank Drs. S. Archer, A. Burger, L. Cook, P. N. Craig, R. B. Doughty, B. Douglas, M. Finkelstein, H. Green, C. Kaiser, J. Laubach, B. Loev, R. McLean,

R. F. Raffauf, L. J. Sternbach, G. deStevens, C. W. Scull, D. H. Tedeschi, R. E. Tedeschi, J. A. Weisbach, and C. L. Zirkle for reading various chapters.

We greatly appreciate the assistance of Mr. Paul Ackley of Smith Kline & French Laboratories in alphabetizing and tabulating the subject index by means of electronically sorted punched cards.

Philadelphia, Pennsylvania MAXWELL GORDON
June 1964

Preface to Volume II

The motivation for the publication of the reviews in Volume I carries even greater force in this volume. The literature of the phenothiazines is very large and is growing very rapidly. Thus we hope that by putting the significant published reports in context, and by providing a convenient source book for much of the rest, we will have performed a service. We have not been able to review the chemistry of the phenothiazines in depth in this volume, and this will have to be done elsewhere.

In this volume we have also included a chapter on the butyrophenones, one on miscellaneous psychopharmacological agents, and a chapter on the biochemical basis of mental disease. The last named chapter is not exhaustive, but is merely meant to be illustrative of the currents of research that one finds in this field. We can certainly expect that these biochemical researches will play a large role in uncovering future psychopharmacological agents.

The appendixes have been used as a vehicle for collecting part of the flood of reports that could not be included in either of the two volumes. It is hoped that the subject index will make this otherwise amorphous section of value to the user.

Some progress in systematizing the nomenclature of psychopharmacological agents in clinical practice has been made since the first volume was written, and the major terms now favored are given below:

1. Antipsychotic drugs. This term is employed for drugs useful in psychoses (other than depressions). It is often used in place of the terms tranquilizer, psychotropic drug, neuroleptic, etc. The major phenothiazines and the butyrophenones are examples of antipsychotic drugs.

2. Anti-anxiety drugs. This term is used for drugs applied in neuroses (other than depressions). It is used in place of tranquilizer, neuroleptic, etc. Examples of anti-anxiety drugs include meprobamate, chlordiazepoxide, and low dose phenothiazines.

3. Antidepressant drugs. This term is used to describe compounds useful in psychotic or neurotic depressions.

Many people have helped us in the preparation of this volume—almost too many to name. But I do want to single out, first of all, Dr. Roscoe B.

Doughty, to whom I would like to express my appreciation for his constructive review of Chapter 1. I am also grateful to Drs. E. F. Domino, C. Jelleffe Carr, and M. Finkelstein for their review of the phenothiazine chapter.

In writing Chapter 3 the suggestions of Drs. Bernard B. Brodie and Seymour Kety were very helpful. I would also like to acknowledge the assistance of many colleagues throughout the industry in the accumulation of references for the appendixes.

I am indebted to Mr. John Balthaser for assistance with the section on rating scales in Chapter 1, "Phenothiazines," and to Mr. Alan Gordon for valuable proofreading assistance

Finally, I would like to express my thanks to Dr. L. Cook for useful discussions on operant conditioning, to Dr. C. L. Zirkle for reviewing various sections, and to many other colleagues at Smith Kline & French Laboratories whose assistance was invaluable.

Philadelphia, Pennsylvania MAXWELL GORDON
April, 1967

Contents

List of Contributors vii
Foreword ix
Preface to Volume I xi
Preface to Volume II xiii
Contents of Volume I xviii

1. Phenothiazines
    Maxwell Gordon

      I. Introduction 2
     II. Synthesis of the Phenothiazines 3
   III. Some Procedures for the Pharmacological Evaluation of
         Psychopharmacological Agents 33
   IV. Pharmacology of Chlorpromazine 37
    V. Structure-Activity Relationships in the Phenothiazines . . . 119
   VI. *In Vivo* Distribution and Metabolism of Phenothiazines . . . 132
 VII. Analytical Methods for Phenothiazines 146
VIII. Miscellaneous Properties of Phenothiazines 150
  IX. Summary of Clinical Applications 150
      References 161

2. Haloperidol and Related Butyrophenones
    Paul A. J. Janssen

    I. Origin 199
   II. Structure-Activity Relationships 206
  III. Pharmacological Activity of the Butyrophenones 209
  IV. Clinical Uses 217
     References 231

3. Biochemical Basis of Mental Disease
    Louise H. Greenberg, R. F. J. McCandless, and Maxwell
      Gordon

   I. Introduction 249
  II. Theories of Mental Disease 251
    References 277

4. Miscellaneous Psychotherapeutic Agents
    Maxwell Gordon

   Text 283
   References 300

Appendix A. Phenothiazine Bibliographies

Compiled by Maxwell Gordon

A.1 Acetophenazine	305
A.2 Carphenazine	308
A.3 Fluphenazine	311
A.4 Mepazine	323
A.5 Methdilazone	330
A.6 Methoxypromazine	332
A.7 Perphenazine	335
A.8 Pipamazine	363
A.9 Prochlorperazine	365
A.10 Promazine	389
A.11 Propiomazine	406
A.12 Prothipendyl	408
A.13 Thiethylperazine	414
A.14 Thiopropazate	416
A.15 Thioridazine	421
A.16 Trifluoperazine	435
A.17 Triflupromazine	460
A.18 Trimeprazine	469

Appendix B. Meprobamate-like Agents Bibliographies

Compiled by Maxwell Gordon

B.1 Phenaglycodol	477
B.2 Mephenoxalone	479
B.3 Promoxalone	481
B.4 Emylcamate	482
B.5 Hydroxyphenamate	483
B.6 Phenylpropanolcarbamate	484
B.7 Metaxalone	485
B.8 Methocarbamol	486
B.9 Oxanamide	490
B.10 Ectylurea	491
B.11 Methyprylone	492
B.12 Ethchlorvynol	497

Appendix C. Addenda to Volume I

C.1 Chlorprothixene 501
C.2 Clinical Applications of the Monoamine Oxidase Inhibitors (Hydrazines): Addendum

John H. Biel

I. Mental Depression	519
II. Angina Pectoris	519
III. Hypertension	520
IV. Epilepsy	520
V. Diabetes	521
VI. Side Effects and Toxicity	521
References	521

C.3 Biochemistry and Pharmacology of the Monoamine Oxidase Inhibitors (Hydrazines): Addendum

A. HORITA

I. Biochemical Properties of MAO and MAO Inhibitors. . . . 523
II. Factors Influencing MAO Inhibitors 525
III. MAO Inhibitors and Tissue Amines 526
IV. Other Biochemical Actions of the Hydrazine Inhibitors . . . 526
V. Pharmacological Properties of MAO Inhibitors 527
VI. Interaction of MAO Inhibitors with Other Substances . . . 528
VII. Miscellaneous Actions 530
References 530

Author Index 533
Subject Index 575

Contents of Volume I

Introduction
Maxwell Gordon

Tranquilizing Drugs from Rauwolfia
Emil Schlittler and Albert J. Plummer

Iminodibenzyl and Related Compounds
Franz Häfliger and Verena Burckhardt

Meprobamate and Related Compounds
F. M. Berger and B. J. Ludwig

1,4-Benzodiazepines (Chlordiazepoxide and Related Compounds)
Leo H. Sternbach, Lowell O. Randall, and Sarah R. Gustafson

2-Benzylpiperidines and Related Compounds
G. L. Krueger and W. R. McGrath

Piperazine Derivatives (except Phenothiazines)
H. G. Morren, V. Bienfet, and A. M. Reyntjens

Benactyzine
Erik Jacobsen

Thiaxanthene Derivatives
P. V. Petersen and I. Møller Nielsen

Benzoxazoles, Benzothiazoles, and Benzimidazoles
C. K. Cain and A. P. Roszkowski

Monoamine Oxidase Inhibitors (Hydrazines)
J. H. Biel, A. Horita, and A. E. Drukker

Monamine Oxidase Inhibitors (Nonhydrazines)
C. L. Zirkle and C. Kaiser

Psychotomimetic Compounds
D. F. Downing

AUTHOR INDEX—SUBJECT INDEX

~1~
Phenothiazines

MAXWELL GORDON

Smith Kline & French Laboratories, Philadelphia, Pennsylvania

I. Introduction	2
A. Table of Phenothiazines Used Clinically	3
II. Synthesis of the Phenothiazines	3
A. Introduction	3
B. Nomenclature	24
C. Synthetic Methods	24
D. Alkylation Procedures	26
E. Synthesis of Clinically Useful Phenothiazines	28
F. Synthesis of Miscellaneous Phenothiazines of Research Interest	30
III. Some Procedures for the Pharmacological Evaluation of Psychopharmacological Agents	33
IV. Pharmacology of Chlorpromazine	37
A. Introduction	37
B. Effects on the Central Nervous System (CNS)	40
C. Antiemetic Effects	57
D. Effects on Activity of Other Drugs	60
E. Effects on Body Temperature	68
F. Metabolic Effects of Chlorpromazine	70
G. Autonomic Nervous System	84
H. Cardiovascular Effects	91
I. Endocrine Effects	95
J. Gastrointestinal and Hepatic Effects	104
K. Neuromuscular Effects (Muscle Relaxation)	106
L. Miscellaneous Effects	108
M. Toxicity of Chlorpromazine	112
V. Structure-Activity Relationships in the Phenothiazines	119
A. Side Chain Modifications	121
B. Ring Substituents	128
VI. *In Vivo* Distribution and Metabolism of Phenothiazines	132
A. Tissue Distribution	134
B. Metabolic Fate	139
C. Distribution and Metabolism of Phenothiazines in Man	143

VII. Analytical Methods for Phenothiazines 146
VIII. Miscellaneous Properties of Phenothiazines 150
IX. Summary of Clinical Applications 150
    A. CNS Activity 150
    B. Use of Rating Scales or Psychometric Techniques . . . 153
    C. Pediatric Applications 154
    D. Vascular and Respiratory Effects 155
    E. Miscellaneous Effects 155
    F. Side Effects 156
    G. Phenothiazine Overdosage 160
    H. Veterinary Use 161
    References 161

I. Introduction

The first two phenothiazines employed in medicine did not have psychopharmacological applications. The first was unsubstituted phenothiazine, which was employed as an anthelmintic in animal infestations. The second was the dye, methylene blue, which has been used as an antidote in certain types of poisoning, and to some extent as an antibacterial agent.

The development of the alkylated phenothiazines as psychopharmacological agents occurred about the same time as the introduction of reserpine. The former development stemmed from the observation that certain antihistaminic compounds had sedative side effects. In attempts to enhance the sedative effects of these phenothiazines, notably promethazine, chlorpromazine was synthesized. An indication of the qualitative differences between promethazine and the psychopharmacological phenothiazines like chlorpromazine is seen in the fact that promethazine is characterized by pronounced

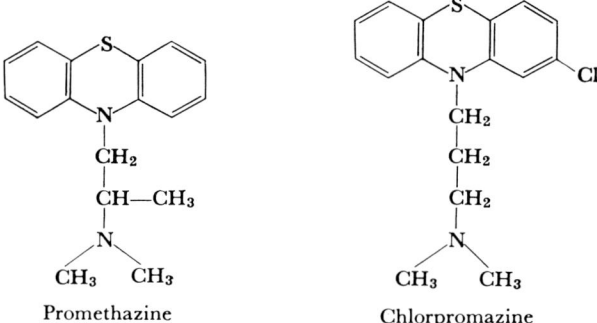

Promethazine   Chlorpromazine

antihistaminic activity and a relative lack of blockade of the conditioned escape response (see Section III), whereas chlorpromazine is a weak antihistaminic but shows pronounced antiemetic and conditioned response blocking activity. It is thus remarkable that small differences in chemical structure produce marked *qualitative* changes in pharmacological effects (Gordon, 1962a,c,d; Gordon *et al.*, 1963).

It is perhaps characteristic that in the development of the psychopharmacological agents new pharmacological tests had to be devised to uncover the novel activity of these compounds. Many of the effects are so subtle that they might be missed entirely in a classical pharmacological evaluation. The subtlety of these actions has led to various sophisticated test methods including operant conditioning, implanted brain electrodes, electroencephalography, and many other complex procedures. An introduction to some of these procedures is given in this chapter, and other methods are cited in Volume I.

A. Table of Phenothiazines Used Clinically

Most of the clinically used phenothiazines are listed in Table I in molecular formula order (cf. Negwer, 1961).

II. Synthesis of the Phenothiazines

A. Introduction

Although a great deal of synthetic work has been published on the phenothiazines, we will not attempt to review this subject in detail for this chapter. More than 3000 different phenothiazines have been synthesized to date, and a detailed review of these has been published by Schenker and Herbst (1963). An excellent review of the early chemistry of phenothiazines was prepared by Massie (1954).

The first synthesis of phenothiazine was by Bernthsen (1883) in the course of some chemical work related to methylene blue (I) and Lauth's violet (II). The latter compounds led to a whole family of phenothiazine dyes (Venkataraman, 1952).

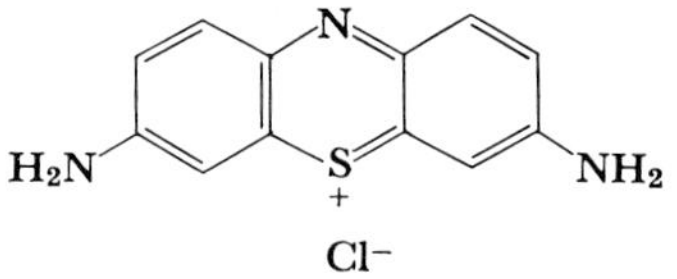

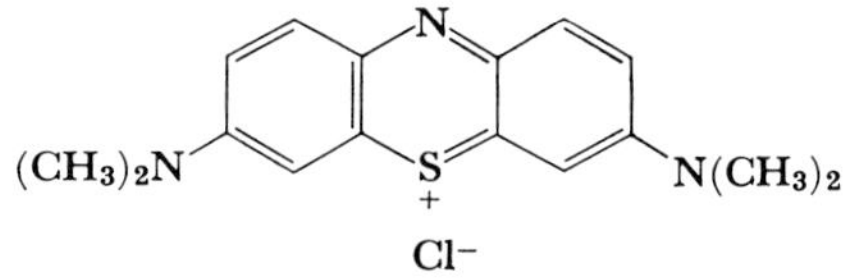

Apart from the anthelmintic (Findlay, 1950; Craig and Tate, 1961) and antihistaminic uses (Halpern, 1946; Halpern and Ducrot, 1946; Vanderbrook *et al.*, 1948), a number of other early medicinal applications have been reported. These include the activity of phenothiazine as a urinary antiseptic (De Eds and Thomas, 1942) and the application of alkylated phenothiazines

TABLE I

TABLE OF PHENOTHIAZINES USED CLINICALLY[a]

Structure and chemical name	Molecular formula	Nonproprietary name	Proprietary name and company
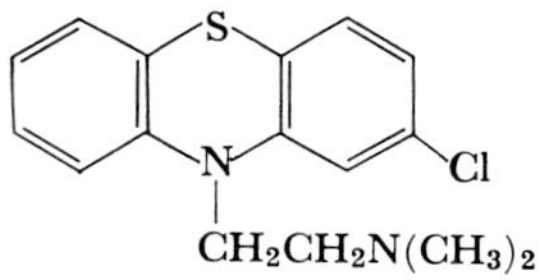 2-Chloro-10-(2'-dimethylaminoethyl)phenothiazine	$C_{16}H_{17}ClN_2S$	Chlorphenethazin	Marophen
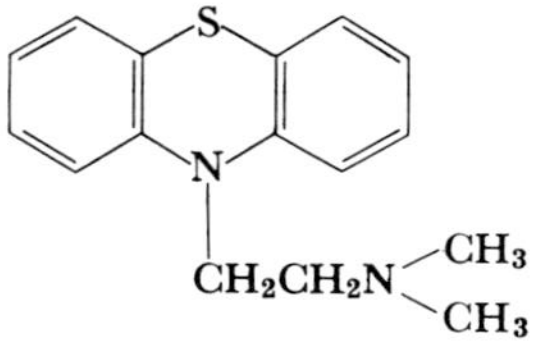 10-(2'-Dimethylaminoethyl)phenothiazine	$C_{16}H_{18}N_2S$	Fenethiazin Phenetazin	Lisergan (Specia) Rutergan (Lab. Dousse) RP 3015
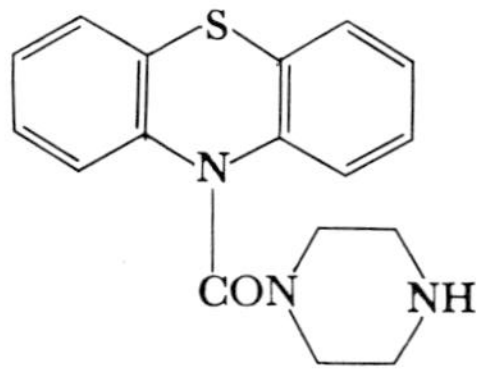 10-(1'Piperazinocarbonyl)phenothiazine	$C_{17}H_{17}N_3OS$	—	MD 5501

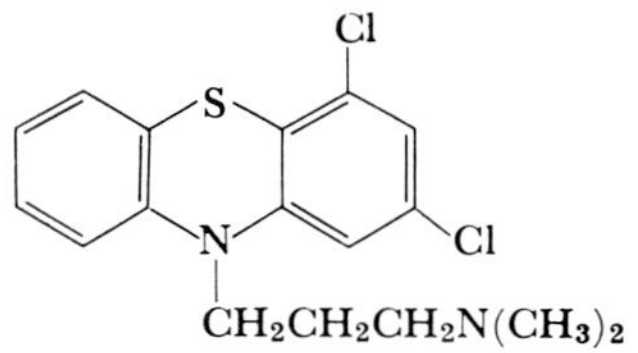

[structure: 2,4-dichloro phenothiazine with CH₂CH₂CH₂N(CH₃)₂ side chain]	$C_{17}H_{18}Cl_2N_2S$	Dichlorpromazine	RP 8030 Vinar et al., 1965

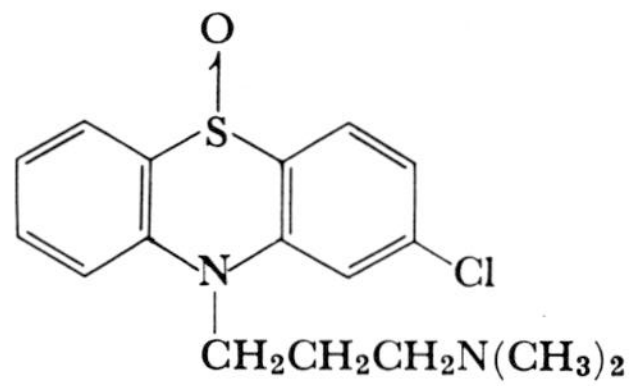

2,4-Dichloro-10-(3′-dimethylamino-1′-propyl)phenothiazine

[structure: 2-chloro phenothiazine-5-oxide with CH₂CH₂CH₂N(CH₃)₂ side chain]	$C_{17}H_{19}ClN_2OS$	—	Secotil (La Sintetica S.A.)

2-Chloro-10-(3′-dimethylamino-1′-propyl)phenothiazine-5-oxide

[a] Compounds showing only antihistaminic, antitussive, adrenolytic, anthelmintic, or spasmolytic properties have generally been omitted from this table [i.e. ahistan (Blazek and Stejskal, 1955), aprobith (Negwer, 1961), chlorazisin (Negwer, 1961), diaspasmyl (Negwer, 1961), dimethoxanate (Merck Index, 1960), diphazin (Negwer, 1961), fenethazin (Merck Index, 1960), isophenergan (Blazek, 1963a,b), mephazine (Negwer, 1961), multezin (Blazek, 1963a,b), P 784 (Nieschultz et al., 1956, Blazek, 1963a,b, Protiva, 1955), secergan and transergan (Negwer, 1961), multergan (Neuman, 1960)] (cf. Blazek, 1963a).

TABLE I—continued

Structure and chemical name	Molecular formula	Nonproprietary name	Proprietary name and company
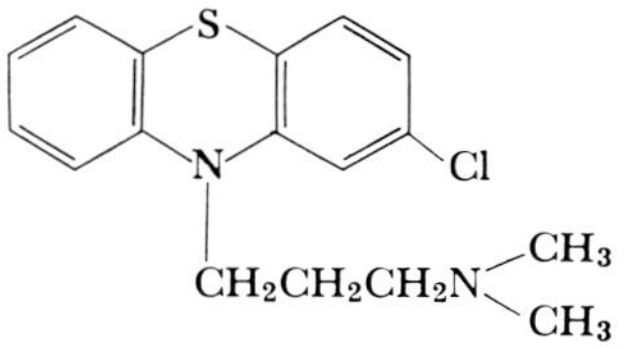 ![structure] 2-Chloro-10-(3'-dimethylamino-1'-propyl)phenothiazine	$C_{17}H_{19}ClN_2S$	Chlorpromazine	Aminazin (Rhodia) Amphactil Ampliactil (Rhodia) Amplictil Chlorderazin Cloropromazina (Doctomex) Contomin Fenactil Hebanil Hibanil (Specia) Hibernal (Leo) Klorpromex (Dumex) Largactil (Rhône-Poulenc) Largaktyl (Rhône-Poulenc) Megaphen (Bayer) Novomazina Plegomazin Promactil Promazil (Sanitas) Promazol Propaphenin (Rodieben) Prozil Sanopron Thorazine (SK&F) Torazina Winterain RP 4560 SK&F 2601

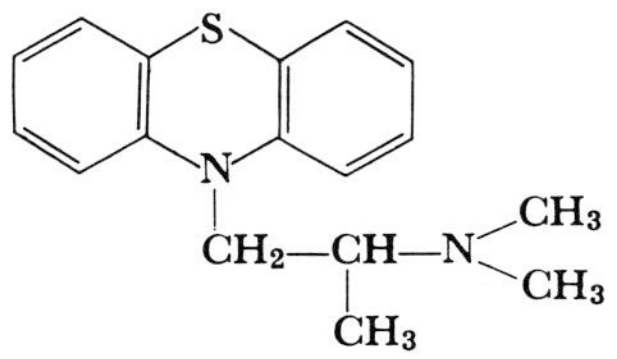

Promethazine C₁₇H₂₀N₂S

Allergan
Atosil (Bayer)
Avomine[b] (May and Baker)
Dimapp
Diprazin (Russian)
Diprozin
Fargan (Farmitalia)
Fenazil (Sella)
Fenergan (Specia)
Hiberna
Lergigan (Recip)
Phargan
Phenergan (Wyeth) (RP)
Pipolphen
Proazamin
Promazinamid
Prothazin (Heyden)
Pyrethia
Tanidil
Thiergan (Astra)
Vallergin
RP 3277

10-(2'-Dimethylamino-1'-propyl)phenothiazine

[b] 8-Chlorotheophylline salt.

TABLE I—continued

Structure and chemical name	Molecular formula	Nonproprietary name	Proprietary name and company
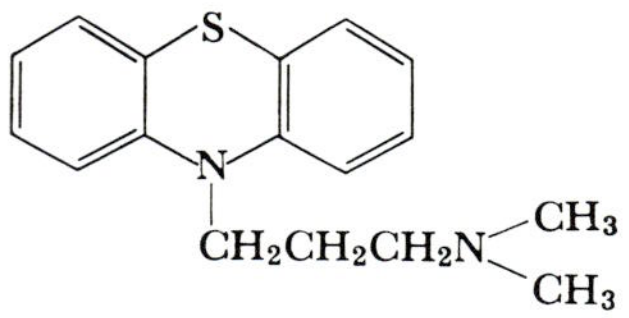 ![structure] CH₂CH₂CH₂N(CH₃)(CH₃) phenothiazine 10-(3'-Dimethylamino-1'-propyl)phenothiazine	$C_{17}H_{20}N_2S$	Promazine	Ampazine Centractil Centractyl (Astra) Delazin Esparin Liranol (Wyeth) Medeprozin Neo-Hibernex Prazine (Dutch Wyeth) Promazionon Promilene Promwill Propazin (Pharmacologico, Venezolano) Protactyl (Asche, Hamburg) Sedistor Sinophenin Sparine (Wyeth) Starazin Sterazin Talofen (Pierrel) Verofen (Bayer) Verophen (Bayer) RP 3276

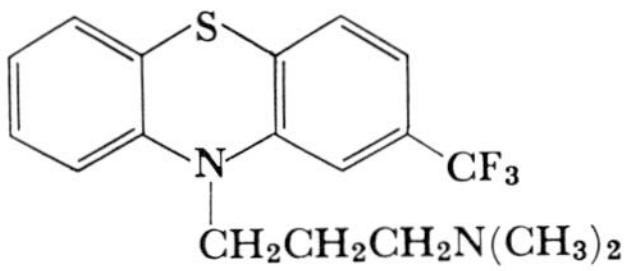

![structure]	Triflupromazine	$C_{18}H_{19}F_3N_2S$	Adazine (Upjohn) Fluomazina Fluorofen (Savio) Fluopromazine Nivoman (Heyden, Squibb) Psyquil (Heyden) Siquil (Squibb) Vespral (Squibb) Vespril Vesprin (Squibb) Me 4703 SK&F 4648

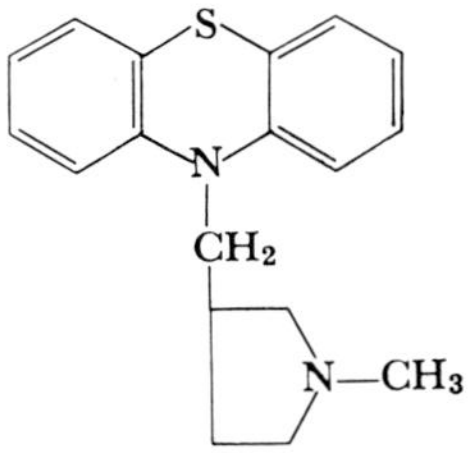

2-Trifluoromethyl-10-(3'-dimethylamino-1'-propyl)-phenothiazine

![structure]	Methdilazine	$C_{18}H_{20}N_2S$	Dilosyn (Brit. Drug Houses) Disyncran (Lab. Allard) Tacaryl (Mead Johnson) Tacryl

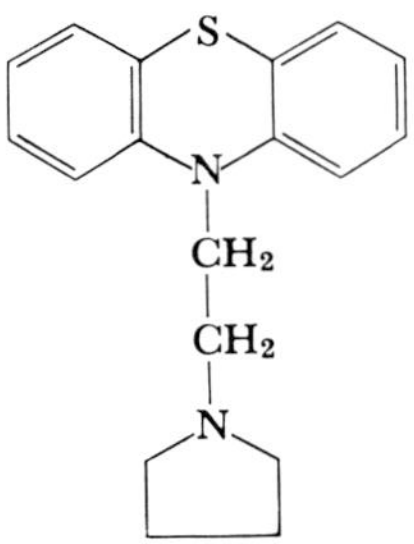

10-(1'-Methyl-3'-pyrrolidinomethyl)phenothiazine

![structure]	Pyrathiazine	$C_{18}H_{20}N_2S$	Médiamer[b] Parathiazin Pyrrolazote (Upjohn) Rolazote RP 4270

10-(N,2'-Pyrrolidino-1'-ethyl)phenothiazine

TABLE I—continued

Structure and chemical name	Molecular formula	Nonproprietary name	Proprietary name and company
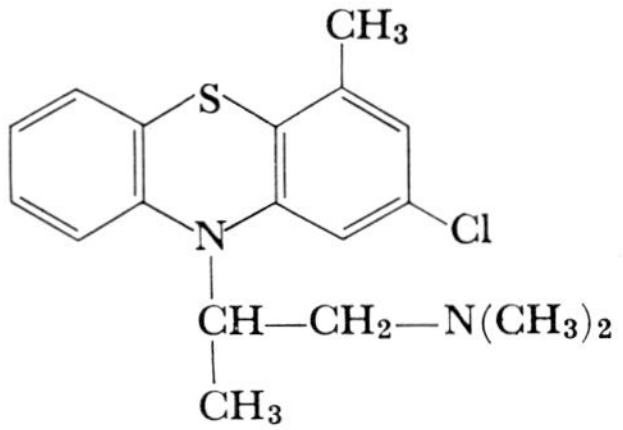 2-Chloro-4-methyl-10-(3'-dimethylamino-2'-propyl)phenothiazine	$C_{18}H_{21}ClN_2S$	Methylchlorisophenergan	
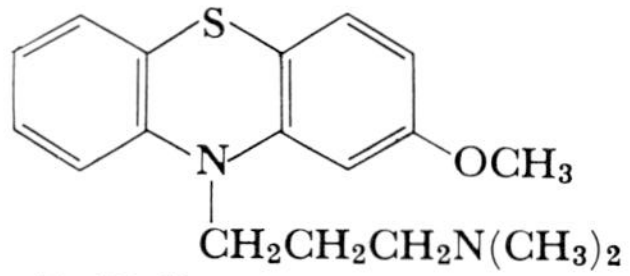 2-Methoxy-10-(3'-dimethylamino-1'-propyl)phenothiazine	$C_{18}H_{22}N_2OS$	Methoxypromazine Methopromazin	Methopromazin Metoxypromazin Mopazine (Specia) Neoproma Tentone (Lederle) Vetomazin RP 4632
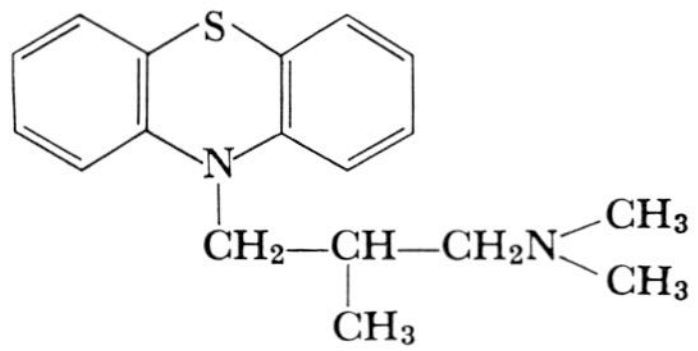 10-(3'-Dimethylamino-2'-methyl-1'-propyl)-phenothiazine	$C_{18}H_{22}N_2S$	Trimeprazine	Alimemazin Alimenazine Methylpromazine Panectyl (Specia) Repeltin (Bayer) Temaril (SK&F) Teralen Théralène (Rhône-Poulenc) Vallergal Vallergan (May and Baker) RP 6549

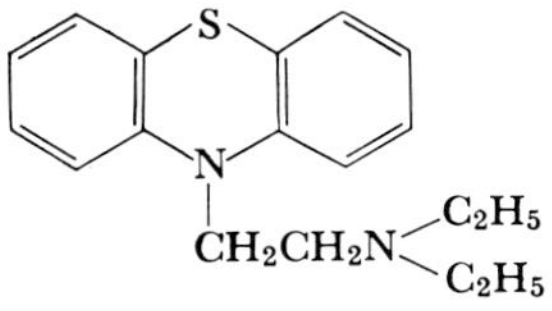 [structure: phenothiazine with N–CH₂CH₂N(C₂H₅)₂]	Diethazine $C_{18}H_{22}N_2S$	Antipar (Farmitalia) Casantin (Casella) Deparkin Dinezin Diparcol (Specia) Dolisina Eazaminum (Casella) Ethylemin (Bayer) Latibon (Bayer) Parkazin Parkezin Parkinofen (Rhône-Poulenc) RP 2987 Thiantan Thiantettin Thiontan (May and Baker) Thionthan (VEB Deutsche Hydrierwerke)

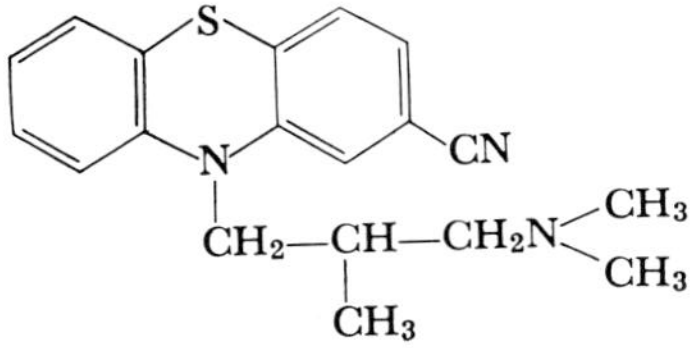

10-(2'-Diethylaminoethyl)phenothiazine

[structure: 2-cyano phenothiazine with N–CH₂–CH(CH₃)–CH₂N(CH₃)₂]	Cyamepromazine $C_{19}H_{21}N_3S$	Cianatil (Rhône-Poulenc) RP 7204

2-Cyano-10-(3'-dimethylamino-2'-methyl-1'-propyl)-phenothiazine

TABLE I—continued

Structure and chemical name	Molecular formula	Nonproprietary name	Proprietary name and company
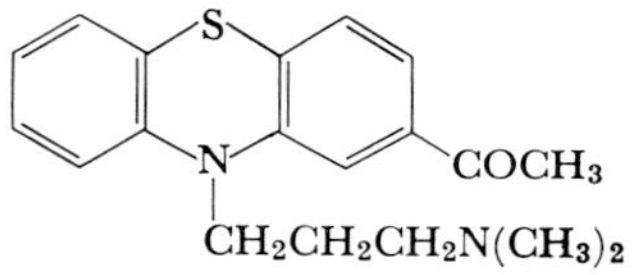 [structure] 2-Acetyl-10-(3′-dimethylamino-1′-propyl)phenothiazine	$C_{19}H_{22}N_2OS$	Acepromazin	Acetazin Acethylpromazin Acetopromazin Acetylpromazin Anatran CB 1522 Notenquil Notensil (Benger) Notesil Plegicil (Labfarmi) Plegicin (Clin Byla) Plegicyl Soprintir (Knoll) Soprontin (Knoll) CB 1522
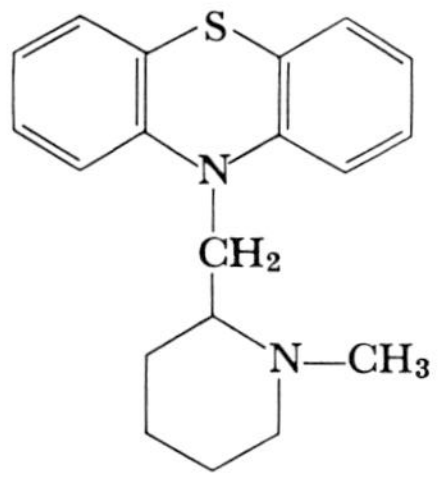 [structure] 10-(1′-Methyl-2′-piperidinylmethyl)phenothiazine	$C_{19}H_{22}N_2S$	Mepazine	Lacumin (Lundbeck) Mepasin MPMP Nothiazine Pacatal (Warner-Chilcott, Promonta) Pacatol Paxital Pecazin

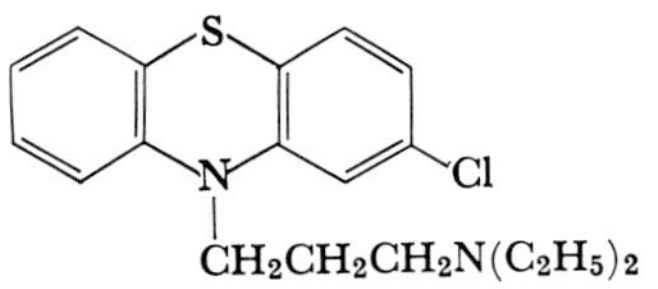

Chlorproethazin C₁₉H₂₃ClN₂S Neuriplége (Rhône-Poulenc)
RP 4909

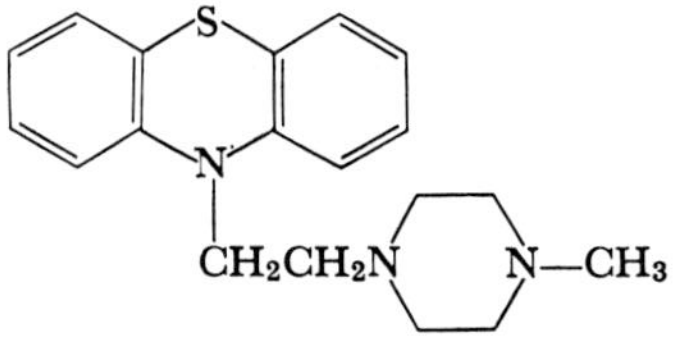

2-Chloro-10-(3'-diethylamino-1'-propyl)-phenothiazine

Phenazin C₁₉H₂₃N₃S

10-(1"-Methyl-4"-piperazinyl-2'-ethyl)-phenothiazine

Levomepromazine (1-isomer) C₁₉H₂₄N₂OS Hirnamin
Methotrimeprazine   Minozinan (Specia)
    Neozin
    Neuractil (May and Baker)
    Neurocil (Bayer)
    Nirvan
    Nozinan (Rhône-Poulenc)
    Sinogan (Specia)
    Veractil (May and Baker)
    Veractyl
    RP 7044
    Levoprome (Lederle)

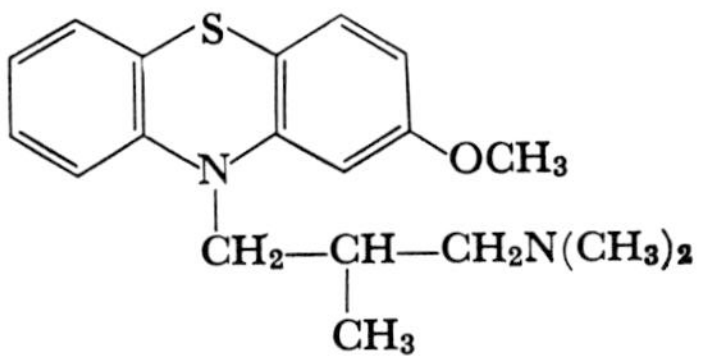

2-Methoxy-10-(3'-dimethylamino-2'-methyl-1'-propyl)-phenothiazine

TABLE I—continued

Structure and chemical name	Molecular formula	Nonproprietary name	Proprietary name and company
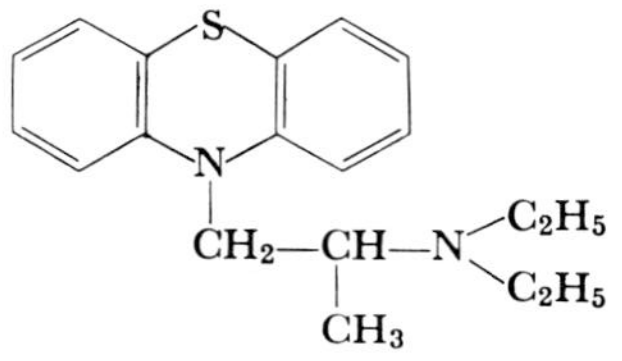 10-(2'-Diethylamino-1'-propyl)-phenothiazine	$C_{19}H_{24}N_2S$	Ethopropazine Isothiazin Prophenamin	Dibutil (Bayer) Isotazin Isothazine Isothiazin Lysivane (May and Baker) Parcidol Pardidol Parfezin Parphezein Parphezin Parsidol (Warner-Chilcott) Parsitan Parsotil Phenopropazin Prodictazin Profenamin Rochipel (Specia) Rodipal RP 3356
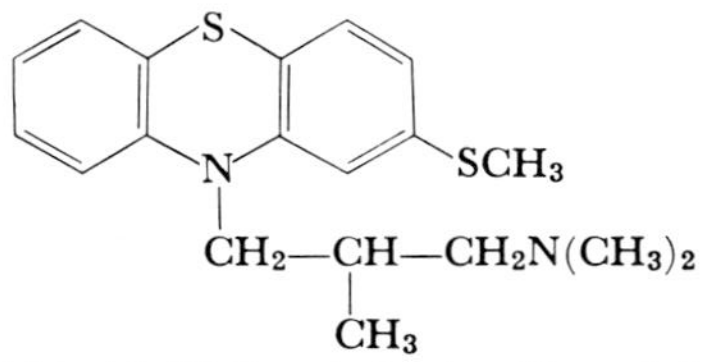 2-Methylthio-10-(3'-dimethylamino-2'-methyl-1'-propyl)-phenothiazine	$C_{19}H_{24}N_2S_2$	Methiomeprazin	SK&F 6270

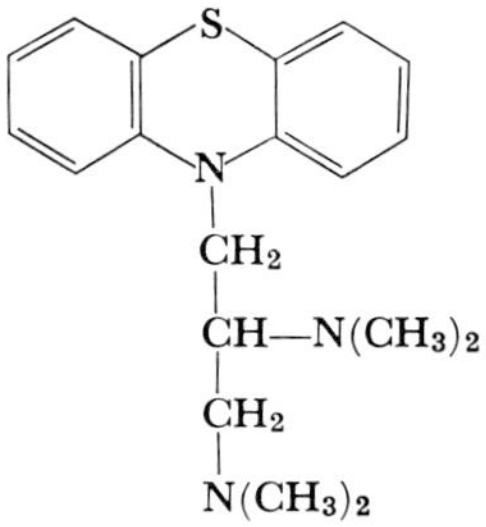 Aminopromazin	$C_{19}H_{25}N_3S$		Jenotone Lispamol (Rhône-Poulenc) Lorusil (Bayer) Proquamezin Spamol Tetrameprozine (Rhône-Poulenc) Tetraprozin RP 3828

10-(2′,3′-bis-dimethylamino-1′-propyl)-phenothiazine

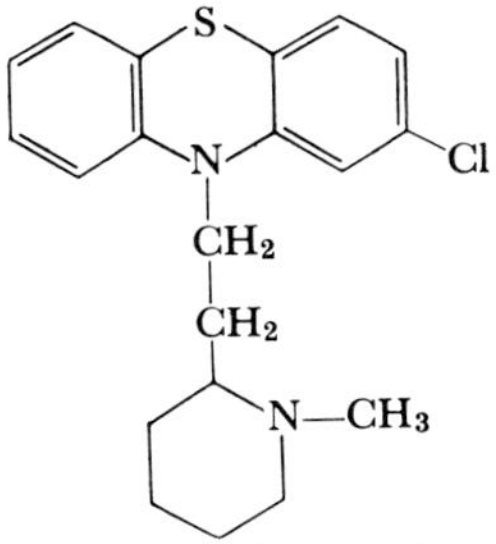 Piperidinochlorphenothiazin	$C_{20}H_{23}ClN_2S$		Ridazin (Sandoz) NP-207

2-Chloro-10-(1′-methyl-2′,2″-piperidinylethyl)-phenothiazine

Prochlorperazine Prochlorpemazin	$C_{20}H_{24}ClN_3S$		Capazine Chlormeprazine Compazine (SK&F) Meterazin (Russian) Nipodal (Bayer) Novamin Prochlorpemazine Stémétil (Rhône-Poulenc) Stemmetil Tematil Tementil (Specia) RP 6140 SK&F 4657

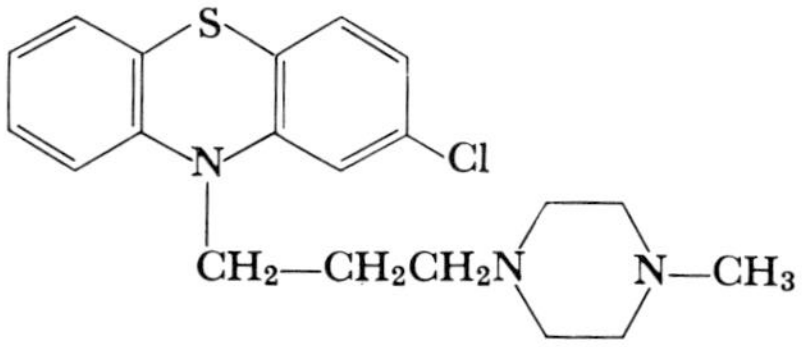

2-Chloro-10-(1″-methyl-4″-piperazinyl-3′-propyl-1′)-phenothiazine

TABLE I—continued

Structure and chemical name	Molecular formula	Nonproprietary name	Proprietary name and company
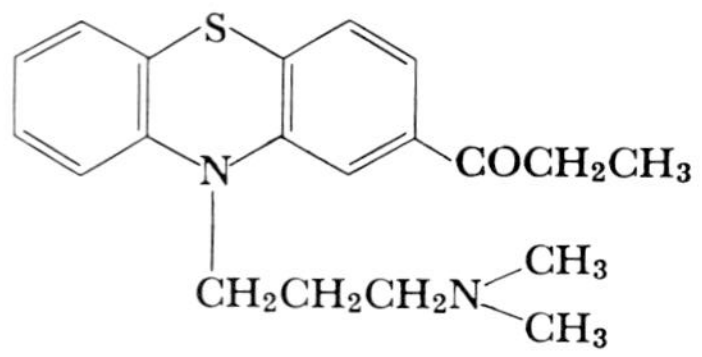 2-Propionyl-10-(3′-dimethylamino-1′-propyl)-phenothiazine	$C_{20}H_{24}N_2OS$	Propionylpromazine	Combelen
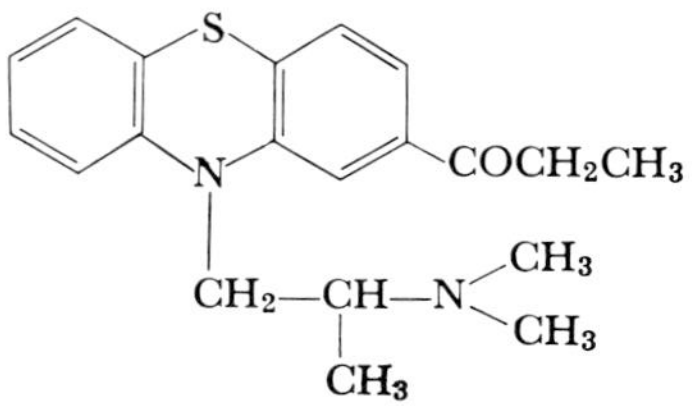 2-Propionyl-10-(2′-dimethylamino-1′-propyl)phenothiazine	$C_{20}H_{24}N_2OS$	Propiomazine	Dorevan (Clin-Byla) Indorm (Wyeth) Largon (Wyeth) Phenoctyl (Clin-Byla) Propavan (Pharmacia) CB 1678 Wy 1359
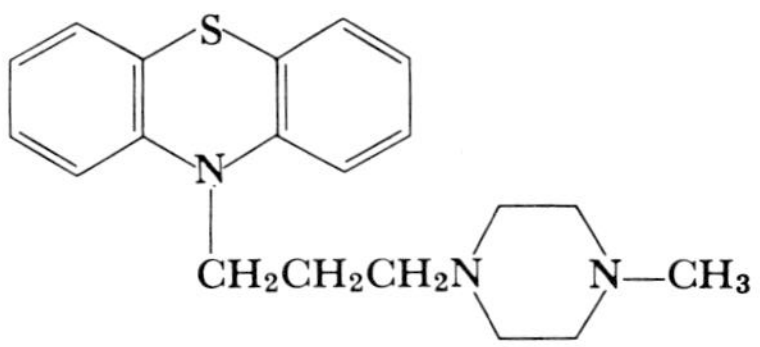 10-(1″-Methyl-4″-piperazineyl-3′-propyl-1′)phenothiazine	$C_{20}H_{25}N_3S$	Perazin	Taxilan (Promonta)

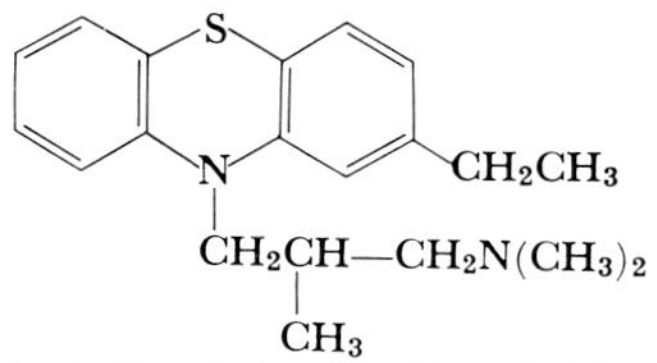

Ethylisobutrazine	$C_{20}H_{26}N_2S$	Diquel (Jensen) Sergetyl (Vailland-Defresne) RP 6484

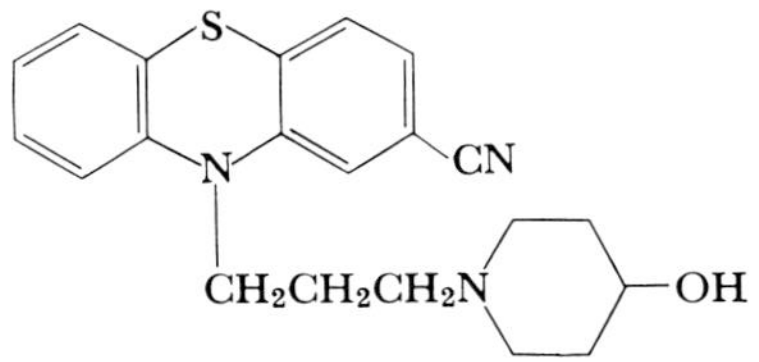

2-Ethyl-10-(3'-dimethylamino-2'-methyl-1'-propyl)-phenothiazine

Propericiazine	$C_{21}H_{23}N_3OS$	(Rhône-Poulenc) RP 8909

2-Cyano-10-(4''-hydroxy-N,3'-piperidinopropyl-1')-phenothiazine

Pipamazine	$C_{21}H_{24}ClN_3OS$	Mornidine (Searle) Nométine RP 9153

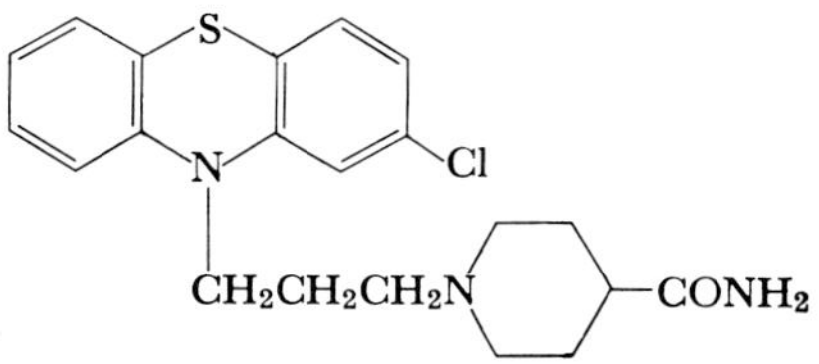

2-Chloro-10-(4''-carboxamido-N,3'-piperidino-1'-propyl)phenothiazine

TABLE I—continued

Structure and chemical name	Molecular formula	Nonproprietary name	Proprietary name and company
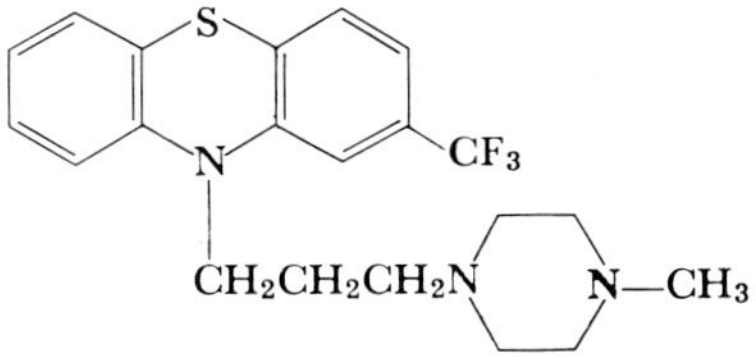 $C_{21}H_{24}F_3N_3S$ 2-Trifluoromethyl-10-(4″-methyl-1″,3′-piperazinyl-1′-propyl)phenothiazine	$C_{21}H_{24}F_3N_3S$	Trifluoperazine	Eskazinyl (SK&F) Jatroneural (Röhm & Haas) Stelazine (SK&F)[c] Terfluzin (Theraplix) Trifluorperazine SK&F 5019
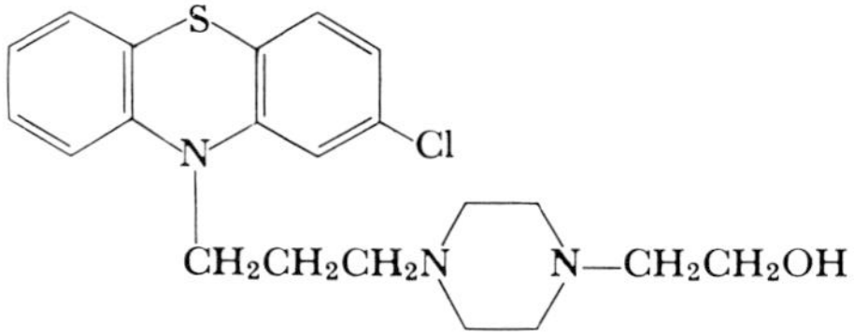 2-Chloro-10-(2″,N^1-hydroxyethyl-N^2,3′-piperazinyl-1′-propyl)phenothiazine	$C_{21}H_{26}ClN_3OS$	Perphenazine	Chlorpiperazin Clorpiprozin Decentan (Merck AG) Etaperazin Ethaperazin (Russian) Fentazin (Allen & Hanbury) Perfenacin Perphenan Trilafon (Schering)
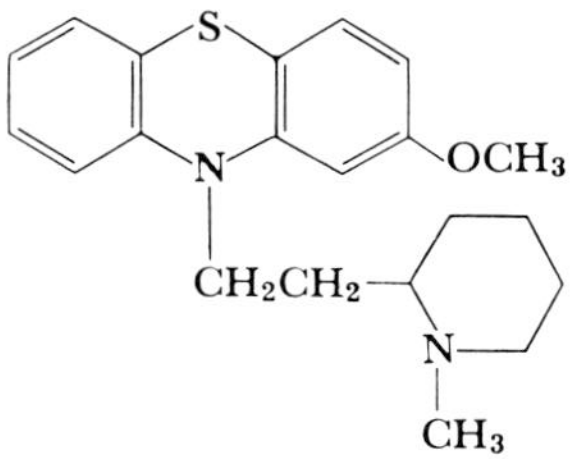 2-Methoxy-10-[2′-(1-methyl-2-piperidinyl)ethyl]phenothiazine	$C_{21}H_{26}N_2OS$	—	Ks 33

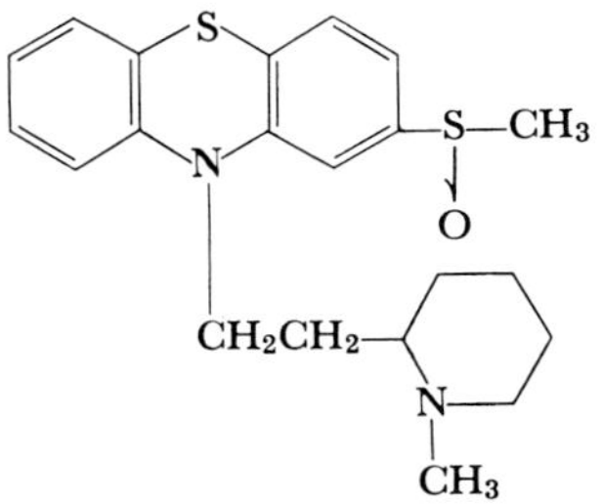

[structure: 2-methylsulfinyl phenothiazine with 1-methyl-2-piperidinyl ethyl side chain]	$C_{21}H_{26}N_2OS_2$	TPS-23 (Sandoz)	Gallant (1965)
2-Methylsulfinyl-10-[2'-(1-methyl-2-piperidinyl)ethyl]phenothiazine			
[structure: 2-methylthio phenothiazine with 1-methyl-2-piperidinyl ethyl side chain]	$C_{21}H_{26}N_2S_2$	Thioridazine	Mallorol (Sandoz) Malloryl Meleril (Sandoz) Mellaril (Sandoz) Melleretten (Sandoz) Melleril (Sandoz)
2-Methylthio-10-[2',1-(1-methyl-2-piperidinyl)ethyl]phenothiazine			
[structure: phenothiazine with propyl-piperazinyl-hydroxyethyl side chain]	$C_{21}H_{27}N_3OS$	—	Phenazin
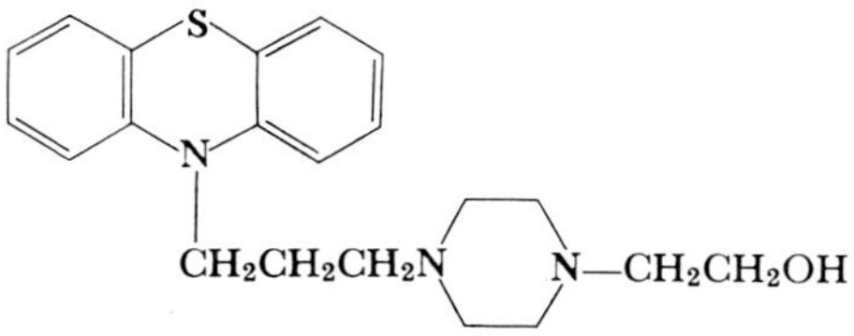 10-{3'-[4-(2-Hydroxyethyl)-1-piperazinyl]propyl}phenothiazine			

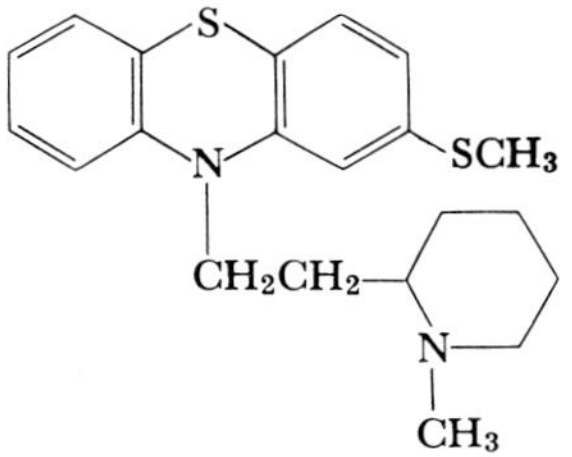

_{*e*} "Parstelin" (SK&F) is a combination of trifluoperazine and tranylcypromine.

TABLE I—continued

Structure and chemical name	Molecular formula	Nonproprietary name	Proprietary name and company
$C_{22}H_{26}F_3N_3OS$ — structure with CF_3 and $CH_2CH_2CH_2$–N(piperazinyl)–CH_2CH_2OH	$C_{22}H_{26}F_3N_3OS$	Fluphenazine	Anatensol (Squibb) Fulmezine Lyogen (Byk-Gulden) Moditen (Squibb) Omca (Heyden) Pacinol Permitil (White) Prolixin (Squibb) Sevinol (Schering) Sevinon (Schering) Siqualine Tensofin Trancin (Schering)
2-Trifluoromethyl-10-{3′-[4-(2-hydroxyethyl)-1-piperazinyl]propyl}phenothiazine			
structure with $S-CH_2CH_3$ and piperazinyl-$N-CH_3$	$C_{22}H_{29}N_3S_2$	Thiethylperazine	Torecan (Sandoz)
2-Ethylthio-10-[3′-(4-methyl-1-piperazinyl)propyl]phenothiazine			
structure with $SO_2N(CH_3)_2$ and piperazinyl-$N-CH_3$	$C_{22}H_{30}N_4O_2S_2$	Thioproperazine Thioperazine	Majeptil (May and Baker) (Rhône-Poulenc) Vontil RP 7843
2-(N,N-Dimethylsulfamoyl)-10-[3′-(4-methyl-1-piperazinyl)propyl]phenothiazine			

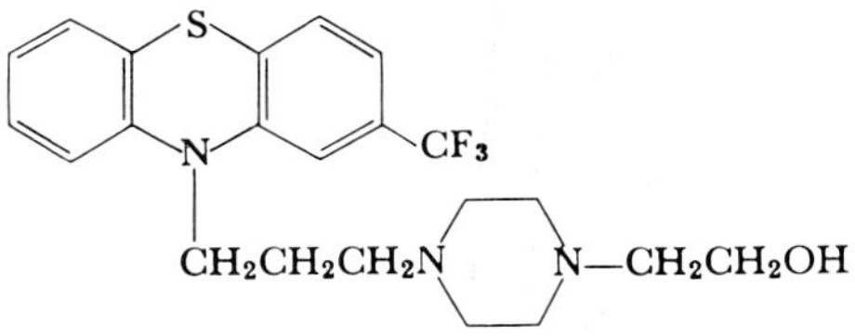

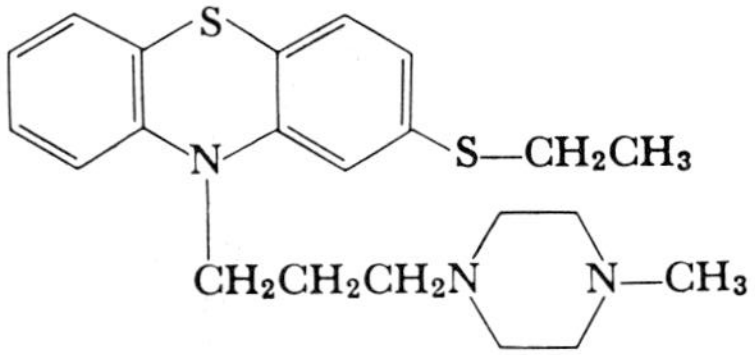

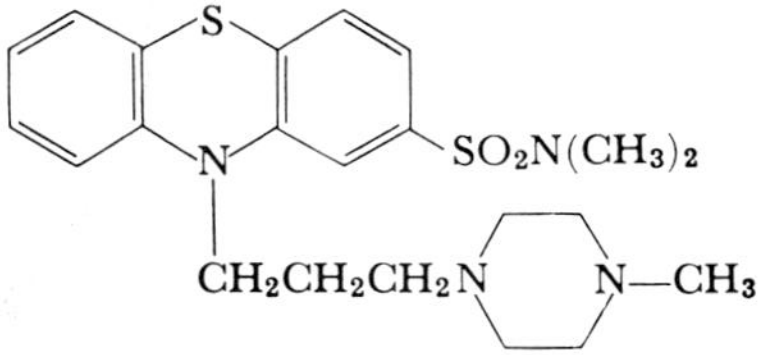

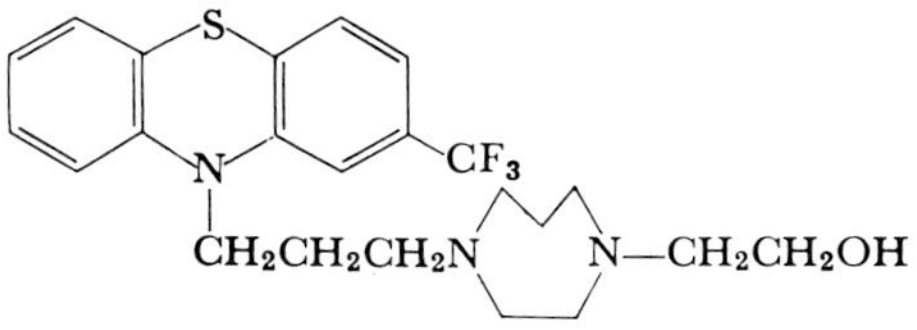

$C_{22}H_{28}F_3N_3OS$ D-775 Pasaden (Homburg)

1-(2-Hydroxyethyl)-4-[10-(2-trifluoromethylthiazinyl)-3-propyl]-homopiperazine

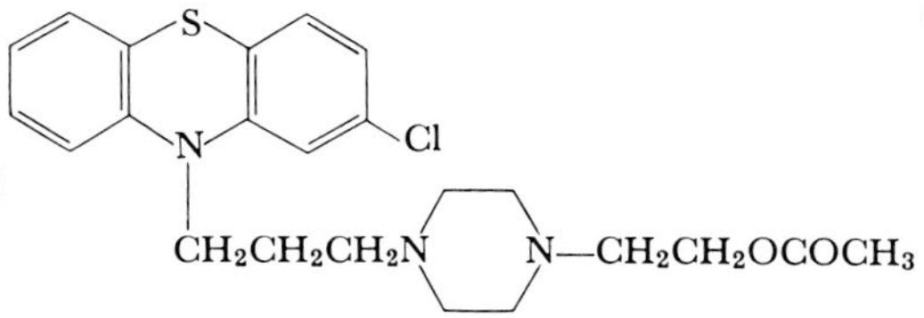

$C_{23}H_{28}ClN_3O_2S$ Thiopropazote Dartal (Searle)
Dartalan
Dartan (Searle)
Dartilan

2-Chloro-10-{3'-[4-(2-acetoxyethyl)-1-piperazinyl]propyl}phenothiazine

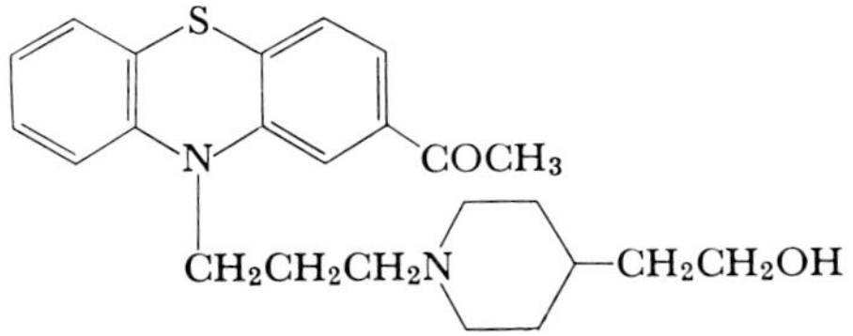

$C_{23}H_{29}N_3O_2S$ Acetophenazine Tindal (Schering)

2-Acetyl-10-{3'-[4-(2-hydroxyethyl)-1-piperazinyl]propyl}phenothiazine

TABLE I—continued

Structure and chemical name	Molecular formula	Nonproprietary name	Proprietary name and company
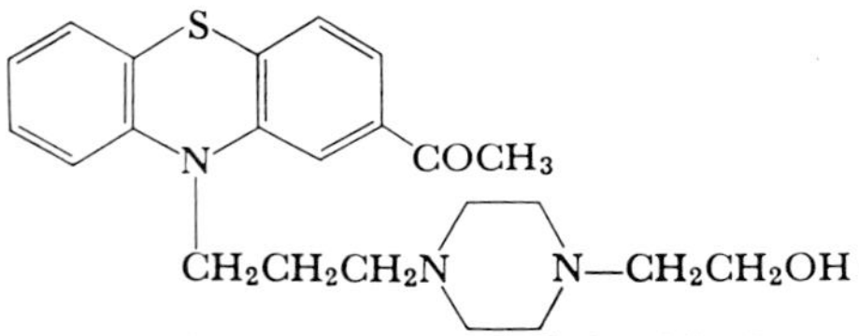 2-Acetyl-10-{3′-[4-(2-hydroxyethyl)piperidino]propyl}phenothiazine	$C_{24}H_{30}N_2O_2S$	Piperacetazine	Quide (Pitman-Moore)
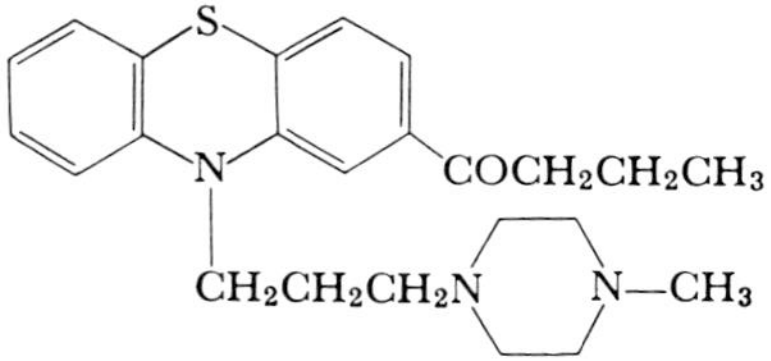 2-Butyryl-10-[3′-(4-methyl-1-piperazinyl)propyl]phenothiazine	$C_{24}H_{31}N_3OS$	Butyrylperazine	Randolectil (Bayer)
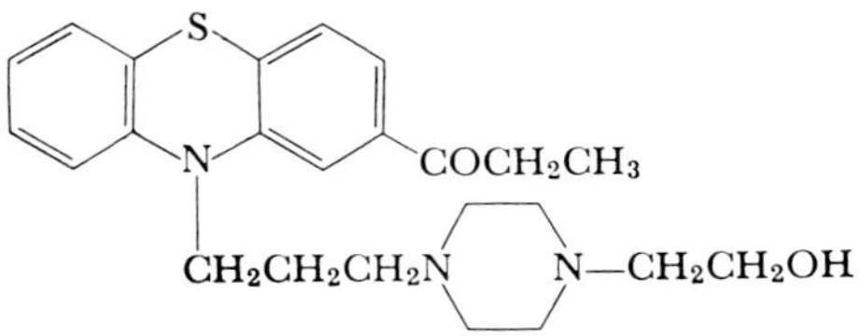 2-Propionyl-10-{3′-[4-(2-hydroxyethyl)-1-piperazinyl]propyl}phenothiazine	$C_{24}H_{31}N_3O_2S$	Carphenazine	Proketazine (Wyeth)

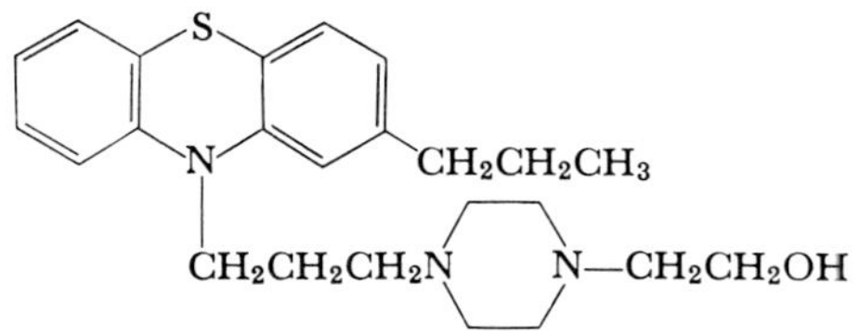

$C_{24}H_{33}N_3OS$　　Proketazin

2-Propyl-10-{3'-[4-(2-hydroxyethyl)-1-piperazinyl]propyl}phenothiazine

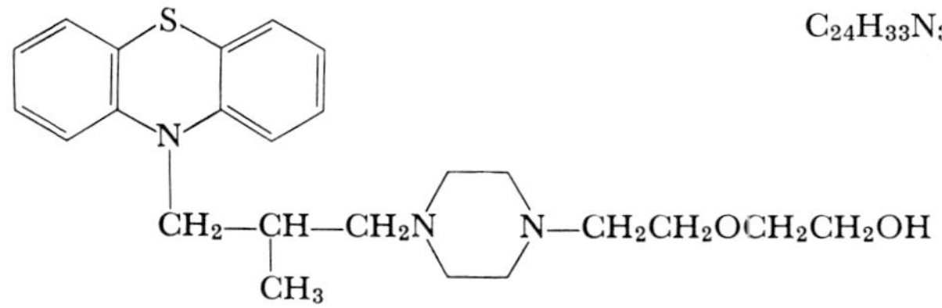

$C_{24}H_{33}N_3O_2S$　　Dixyrazine

10-{2'-Methyl-3'-[4-(2-hydroxyethoxyethyl)-1-piperazinyl]propyl}phenothiazine

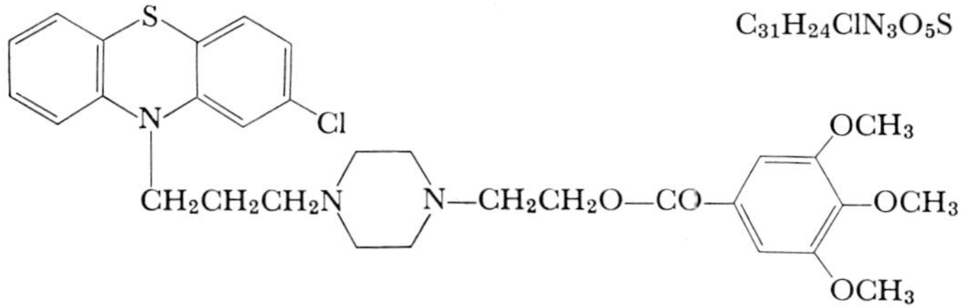

$C_{31}H_{34}ClN_3O_5S$　　Methophenazin

2-Chloro-10-{3'-[4-(3,4,5-trimethoxybenzoyloxyethyl)-1-piperazinyl]propyl}phenothiazine

Esucos (UCB)

Frenolone (Richter)

in the treatment of Parkinson's disease (Burger, 1960). There has also been a great deal of work on the application of phenothiazines as antioxidants and the subject has been reviewed by Murphy *et al.* (1950). Phenothiazine has been reported to be more active than rotenone in killing culicine mosquito larvae (Campbell *et al.*, 1934).

With respect to the early work, Meyer and Jacobsen (1920) have summarized the chemistry of the phenothiazines up to that date. Other reviews have appeared by Nelson (1951), Shirley (1943), and Van Ess (1936) in Professor Gilman's department at Iowa State. Additional reviews on phenothiazines have been written by Metcalf (1948), Beeler (1942), Findlay (1950), and Lewis (1964).

Some discussion of the chemistry of the phenothiazines has been published by Gordon and Ullyot (1957), by Gordon (1960d), and some additional pertinent references are cited by Gordon and McCandless (1959).

B. Nomenclature

Phenothiazine, first called thiodiphenylamine by Bernthsen (1883), has had several numbering systems employed, the most frequently used being the Beilstein system (A) and the Chemical Abstracts system (B). The former is found in the European literature and the latter is preferred in this country and will be used in this chapter.

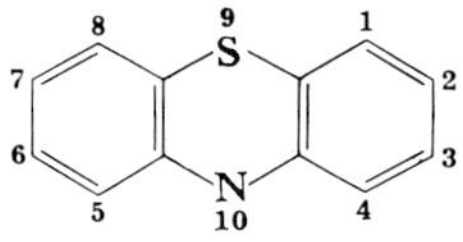

(A) 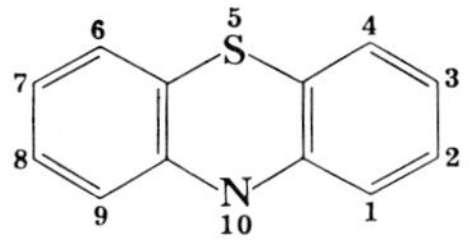　　　　　　　　　　(B)

C. Synthetic Methods

1. Thionation (Bernthsen, 1883)

Thionation was the first synthetic method employed and it is still useful for the synthesis of certain phenothiazines. In those cases in which it works, it offers the simplest method of making phenothiazines (III → IV).

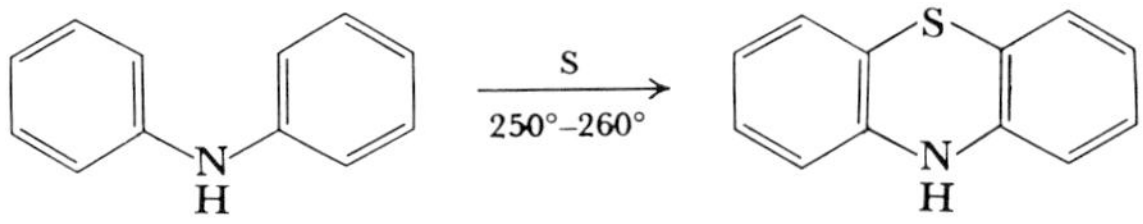

(III) → (IV)　S, 250°–260°

Obviously starting with *meta*-substituted diphenylamines, a mixture of isomers is possible. In this instance the 2-isomer predominates, as illustrated in the 2-chlorophenothiazine (VI) synthesis where 4-chlorophenothiazine (VII) is obtained as a by-product (Baltzly et al., 1946; Gilman and Shirley, 1944a,b), from m-chlorodiphenylamine (V).

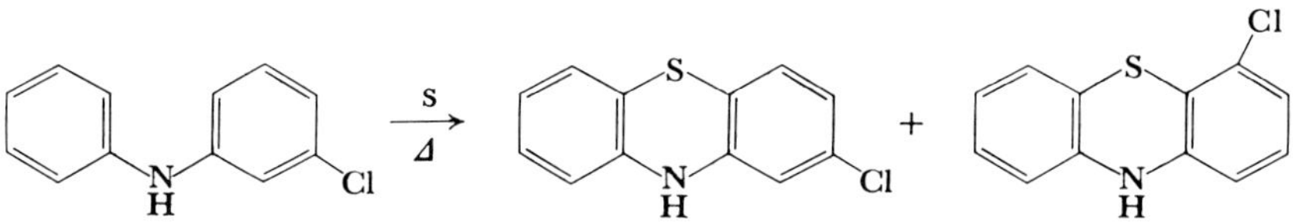

(V)   (VI)   (VII)

Sulfuryl chloride has been used as the thionating agent in place of sulfur (Holzmann, 1888). A variation of this theme involves the use of a sulfinyl diphenylamine (VIII) as an intermediate (Krishna and Jain, 1931) as shown in the conversion of VIII to 3-nitrophenothiazine sulfoxide (IX).

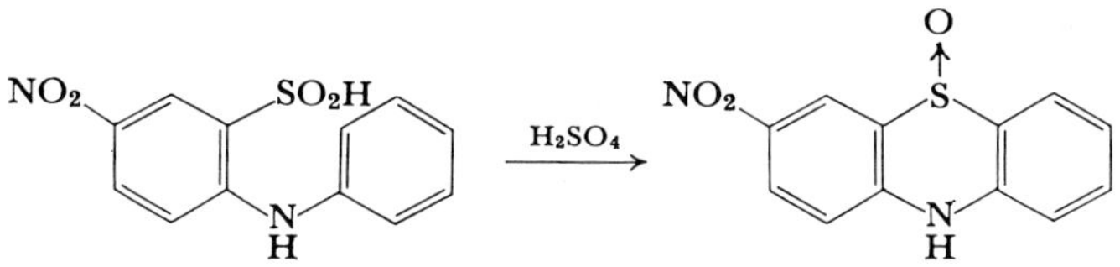

(VIII)   (IX)

2. Smiles Rearrangement

This method is useful in certain selected cases and it involves an inversion of the ring bearing the nitro group (Bennett, 1953; Evans and Smiles, 1935a,b; Wight and Smiles, 1935). In this reaction, the nitro group is displaced and the thio-ring bond migrates to the position formerly occupied by the leaving group, perhaps in a concerted reaction (X → XI).

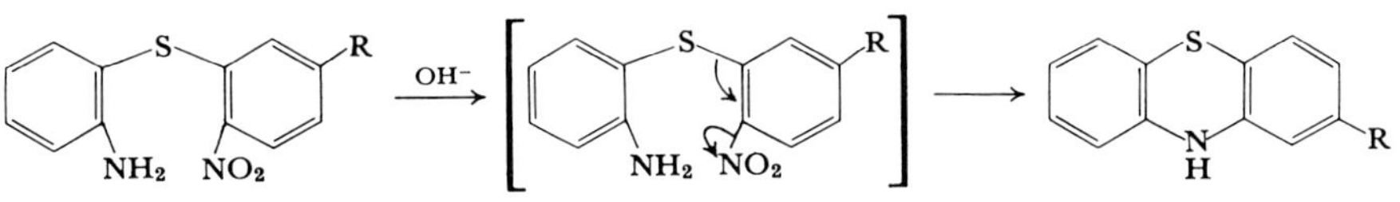

(X)   (XI)

Anomalous cases have recently been discovered where a Smiles-type inversion of the ring bearing a halogen *ortho* to the sulfur takes place under Ullmann conditions (Nodiff and Hausman, 1964) or in the presence of sodamide (Bonvicino et al., 1962). In the example that will be given (XII → XIII) any rearrangement of the halogen-bearing ring would not be apparent since the rearrangement product would be identical with the normal reaction product, there being no third substituent present.

3. Ullmann Reaction

Probably the most general reaction for phenothiazine syntheses is the Ullmann reaction, involving copper-catalyzed dehydrohalogenation of substituted 2-amino-2'-halodiphenylsulfides (XII) (Buisson et al., 1956; Nodiff et al., 1960). It must be kept in mind, however, that the halogen-bearing ring may invert, so starting materials must be selected to avoid anomalous consequences.

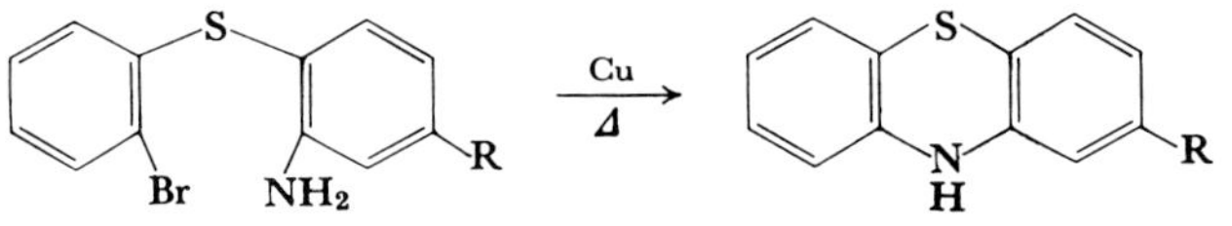

D. Alkylation Procedures

Inasmuch as all centrally acting phenothiazines have substituents in the 10-position, it is necessary to alkylate the phenothiazines whose syntheses were described in the previous section. In most cases, it is possible to alkylate directly using a basic catalyst (Charpentier, 1953) as shown in the synthesis of chlorpromazine (XIV).

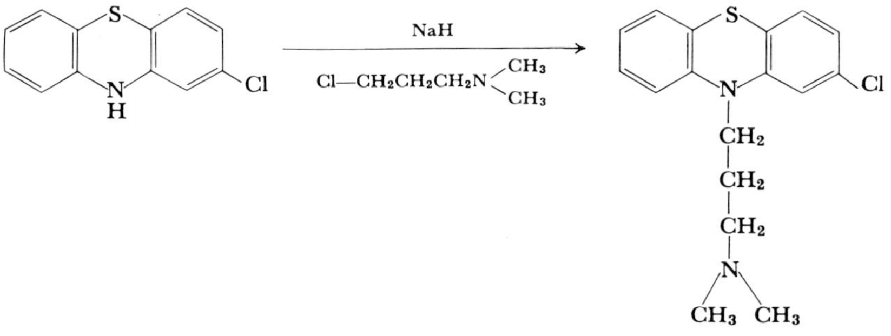

In a few cases, the phenothiazine intermediate will not withstand alkaline treatment and indirect methods employing the carbamate (XV) must be employed (Schmitt et al., 1957), to give (XVI).

Other alternative alkylation procedures that have been employed include addition of ethylene oxide to give hydroxyethyl derivatives (XVIa) (Dahlbom, 1951) and the cyanoethylation procedure (N. L. Smith, 1950, 1951) which gives a product (XVIb) that can be reductively alkylated to chlorpromazine (Fujii, 1956b).

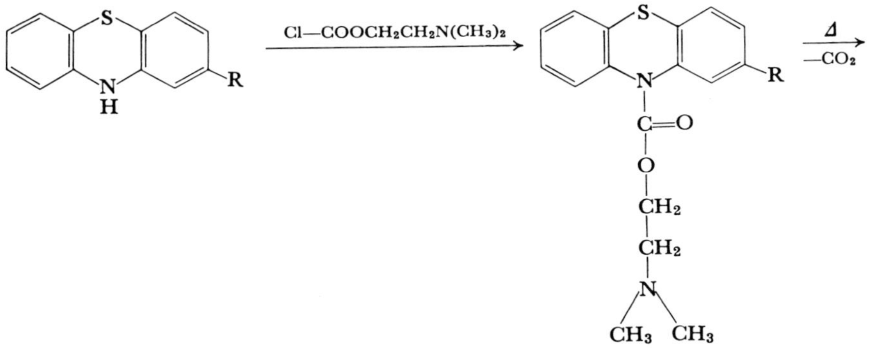

1. PHENOTHIAZINES

(XV)

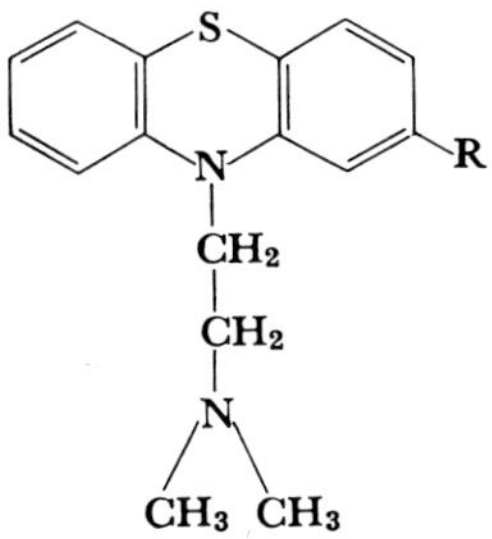

(XVI)

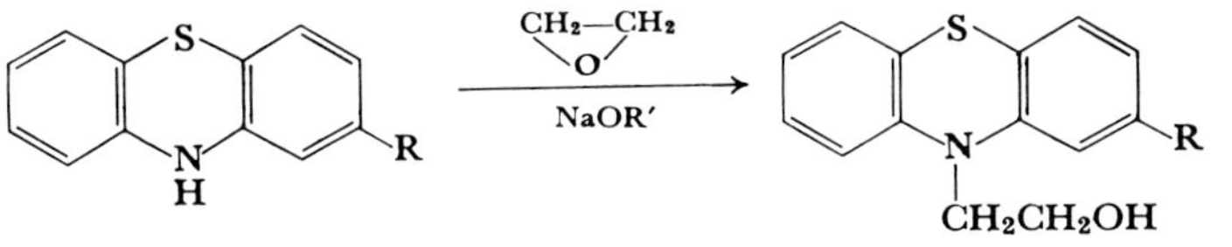

(XVIa)

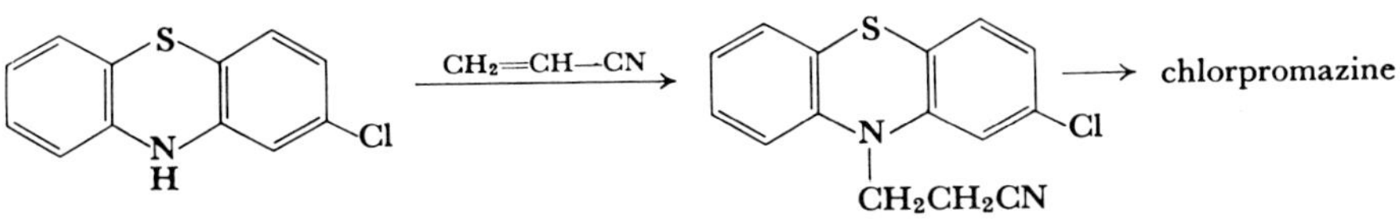

(XVIb) → chlorpromazine

Reduction of the cyanoethyl derivative can also be carried out in the presence of dimethylamine or piperidine to give the corresponding dimethylaminopropyl or *N*-piperidinopropylphenothiazines (Fujii, 1956c).

Still another alkylation procedure (Fujii, 1956a) makes use of tosylate derivatives for alkylation.

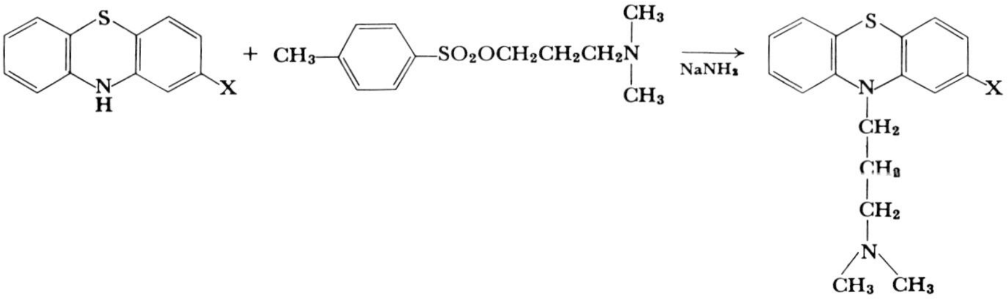

E. Synthesis of Clinically Useful Phenothiazines

Prochlorperazine (XVIII) was synthesized in a manner analogous to that used for chlorpromazine (XIV), employing the piperazinopropyl side chain (XVII) (Horclois, 1959).

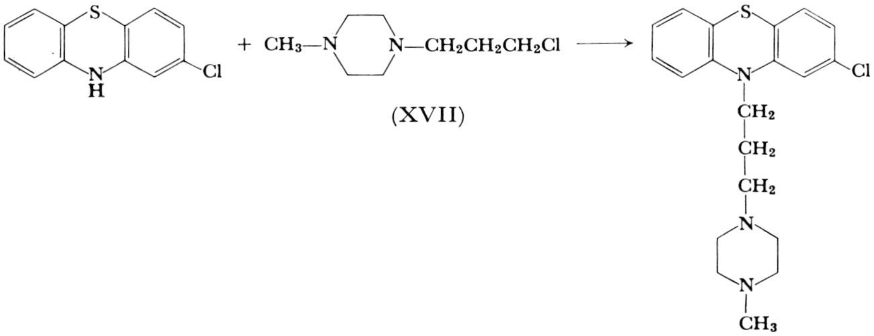

(XVII) (XVIII)

The side chain can be prepared as follows:

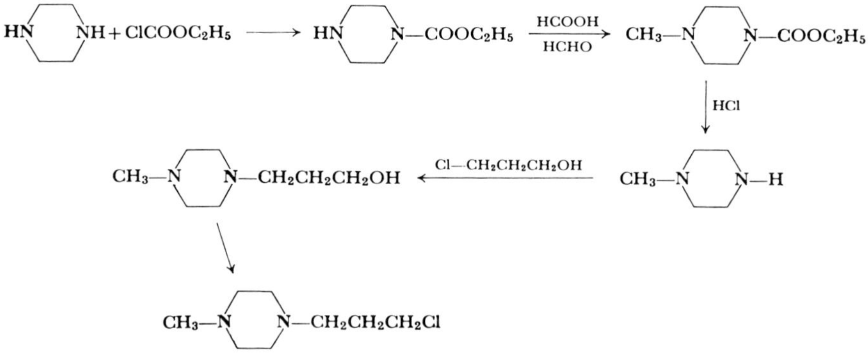

(XVII)

Promethazine (XIX) (Charpentier, 1950b) and promazine (XX) (Charpentier, 1950a) were prepared in the same way from phenothiazine using 2-dimethylaminopropyl chloride and 3-dimethylaminopropyl chloride, respectively, as the alkylating agents. In the preparation of XIX, a mixture of isomers (XIX and XIXa) was obtained due to rearrangement of the cation from 2-dimethylaminopropyl chloride.

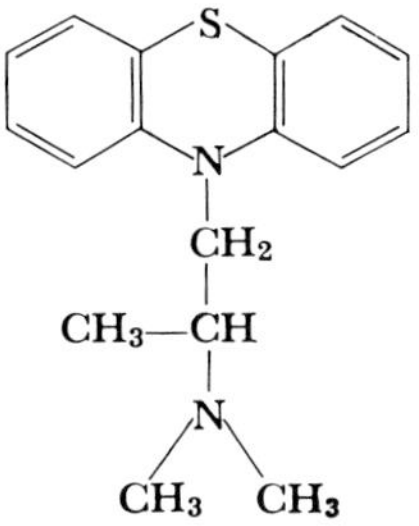

(XIX) 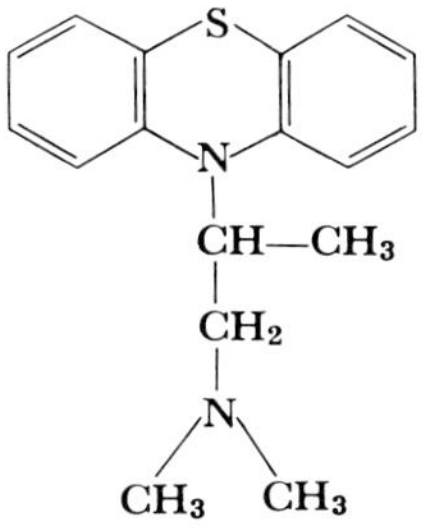 (XIXa) 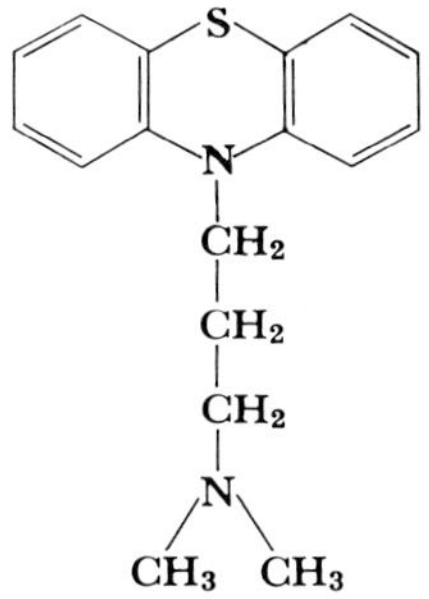 (XX)

Mepazine (XXI) was prepared in the same way using N-methyl-3-bromomethylpiperidine as the alkylating agent (Schuler, 1959). Triflupromazine (XXII) (Craig et al., 1957; Yale et al., 1957) and trifluoperazine (XXIII) (Craig et al., 1957; Ullyot, 1962) were prepared by appropriate alkylation of 2-trifluoromethylphenothiazine (N. L. Smith, 1950).

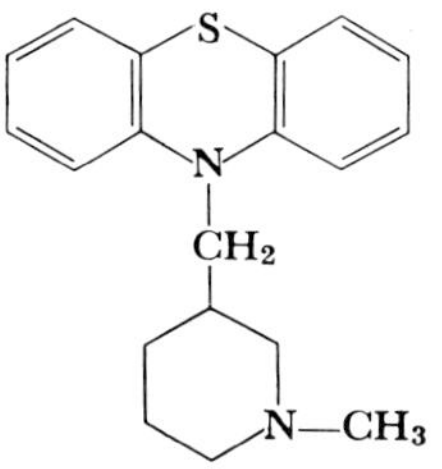

(XXI) 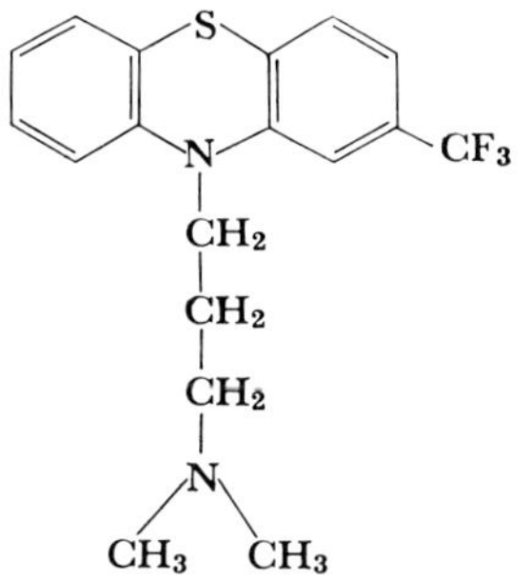 (XXII) 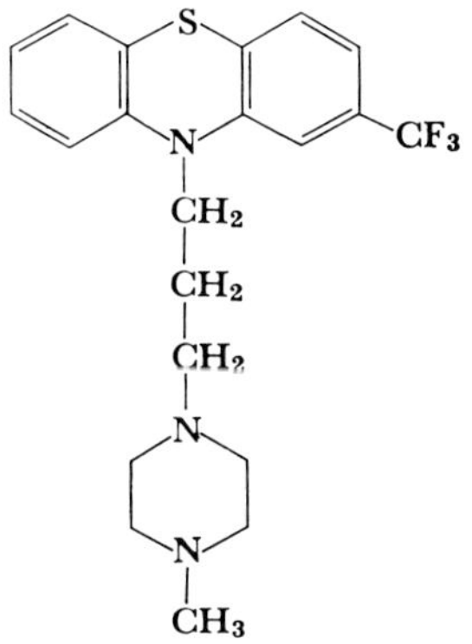 (XXIII)

Diethazine (XXV) has been prepared (Berg and Nicholson, 1952) by forming the Grignard adduct (XXIV) of phenothiazine, followed by reaction with the appropriate halide.

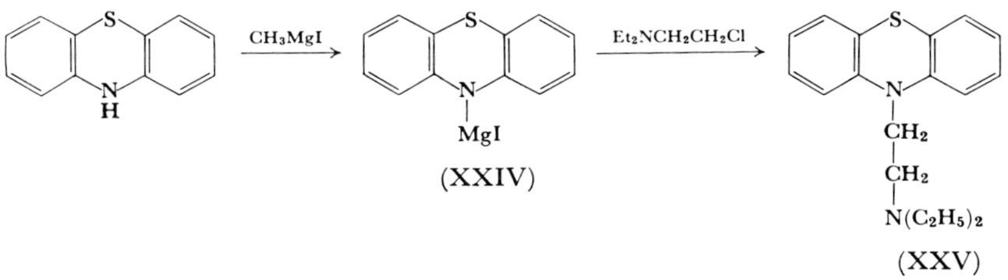

(XXIV)

(XXV)

Pyrathiazine (XXVI) (Reid et al., 1948) and trimeprazine (XXVII) (Jacob and Jacques, 1958) were prepared by appropriate alkylation with *N*-pyrrolidylethyl chloride and 3-dimethylaminoisobutyl chloride, respectively.

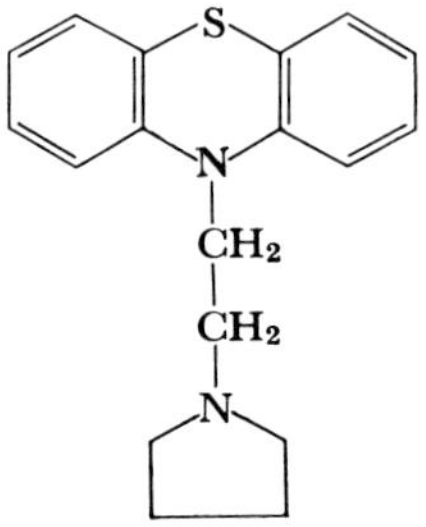

(XXVI)

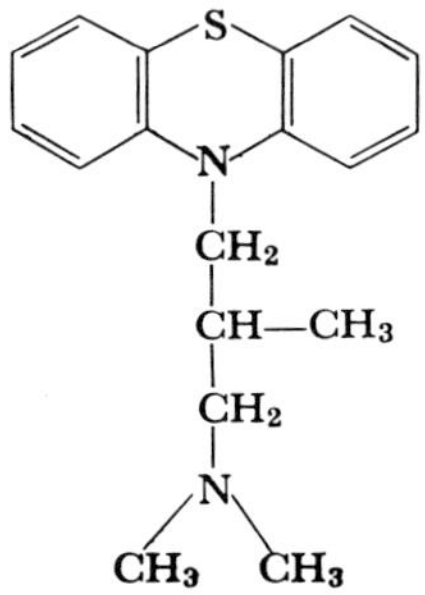

(XXVII)

The close relatives, perphenazine (XXIX) (Cusic and Hamilton, 1958) and thiopropazate (XXX) (Cusic and Hamilton, 1956) may have their side chains elaborated in a variety of ways, but obviously the free hydroxy group in perphenazine must be protected during alkylation.

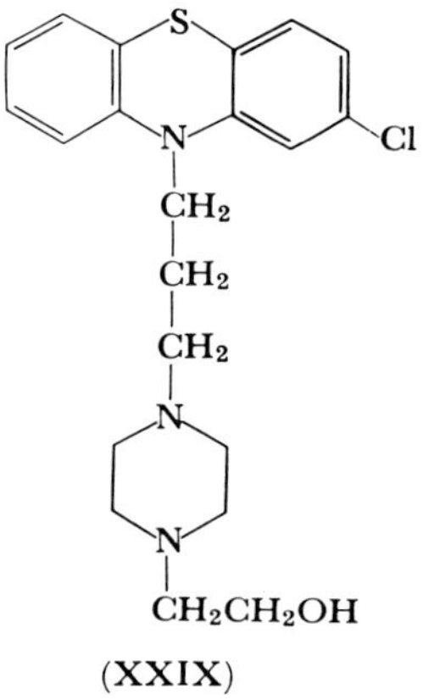

(XXIX)

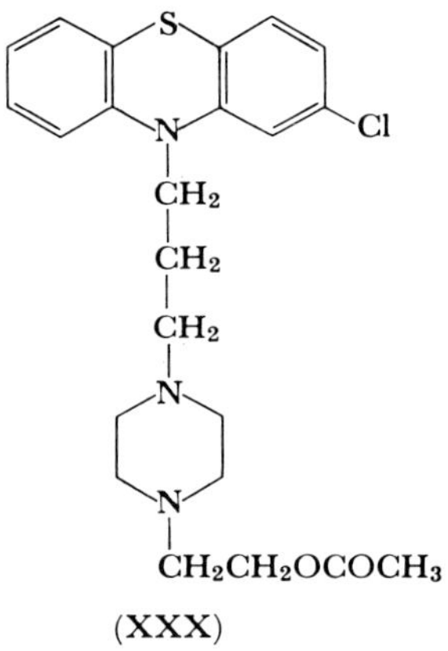

(XXX)

F. Synthesis of Miscellaneous Phenothiazines of Research Interest

As a result of the clinical importance of chlorpromazine, a great deal of synthetic work on analogs has been undertaken—so much so that more than three thousand phenothiazines have been prepared for pharmacological testing. These syntheses have stemmed from the application of a variety of structure-function principles (cf. Schenker and Herbst, 1963; Gordon, 1962a–e; Gordon et al., 1958; Craig et al., 1960).

1. Aromatic Ring Substituents

The synthesis of 2-trifluoromethylsulfonylphenothiazine (XXXI) started with *p*-bromobenzenesulfonic acid (Nodiff *et al.*, 1960).

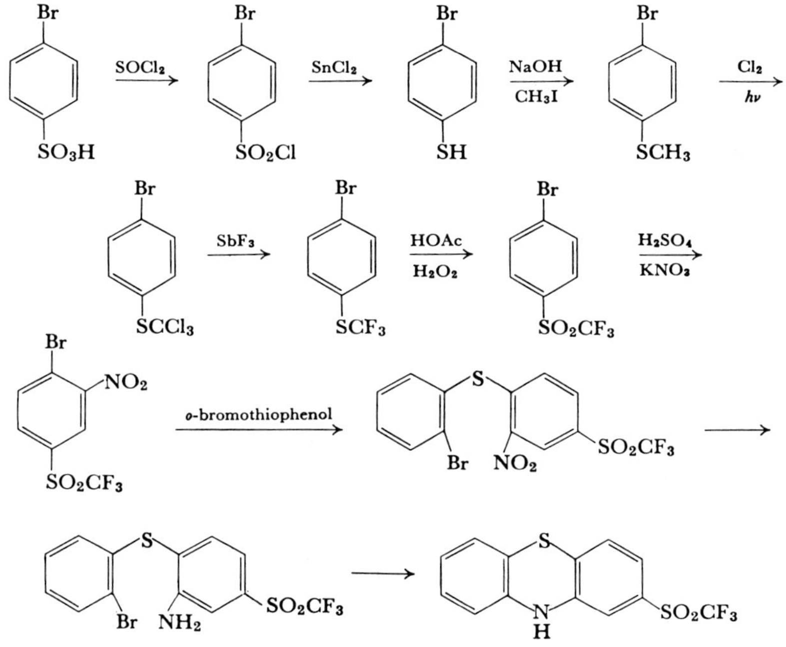

(XXXI)

Alkylation of XLI was described by Craig *et al.* (1960).

The synthesis of 2,3-methylenedioxyphenothiazine (XXXII) was carried out in an analogous fashion (Craig *et al.*, 1961; Gordon, 1960b).

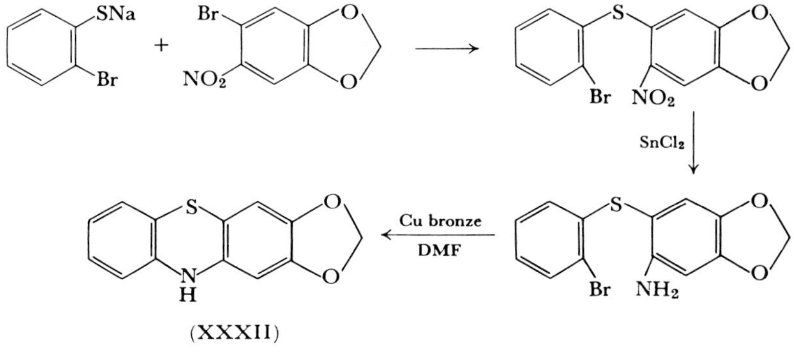

(XXXII)

Other substituents in the 2-position were also investigated (cf. Section V) as illustrated below (Craig *et al.*, 1961).

X = OH (Nodiff et al., 1960)
 = SCH₃
 = SO₂CH₃
 = SCF₃
 = SO₂CF₃
 = OCH₂C₆H₅
 = CN
 = N(CH₃)₂
 = CON(CH₃)₂

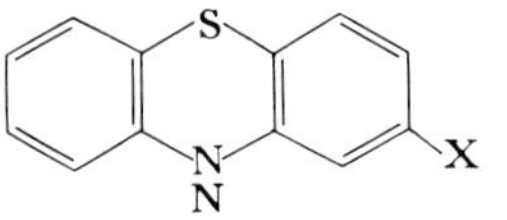

$$X = COCH_3 \text{ (Schmitt et al., 1957)}$$
$$-\underset{\parallel}{C}-CH_3$$
$$NOH$$
$$-C\begin{array}{c}CH_3\\ \diagdown\\ CH_3\end{array}$$
$$\mid$$
$$OH$$

Alkylation of these phenothiazines was carried out in the usual way, except that the acetyl compound had to be protected by means of the ethylene ketal derivative (Schmitt et al., 1957).

2. Nitrogen Substituents

A large variety of N-10 alkyl derivatives have been prepared in the usual ways, and some of these follow (Anderson et al., 1962):

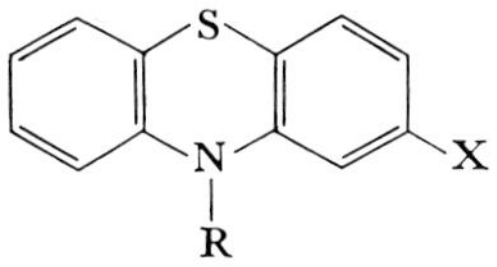

X = Cl, CF₃

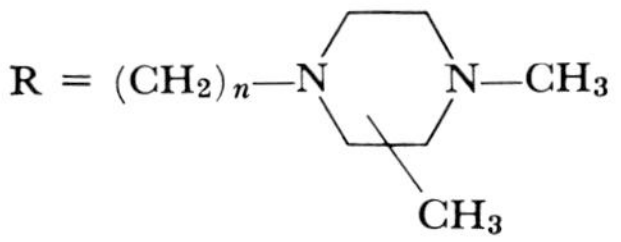

R = (CH₂)ₙ—N⟨ ⟩N—CH₃
            │
           CH₃

n = 1–3

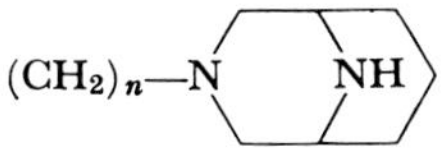

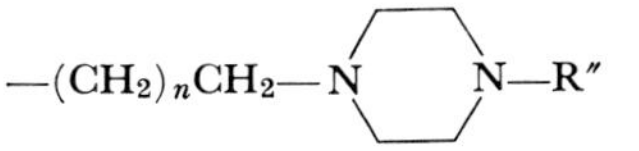

(CH₂)ₙ—N⟨ ⟩NH

—(CH₂)ₙCH₂—N⟨ ⟩N—R″

n = 1–2

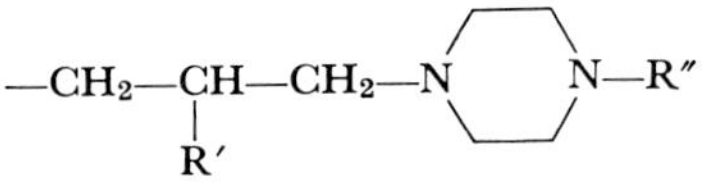

—CH₂—CH—CH₂—N⟨ ⟩N—R″
        │
        R′

R′ = H, OH, CH₃

—CH₂CH₂CON⟨ ⟩N—R″

—CO—CH₂CH₂N⟨ ⟩N—R″

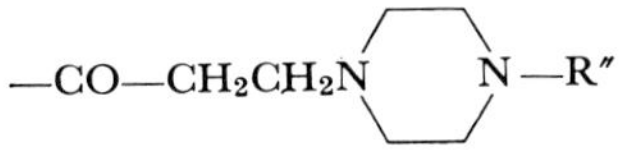

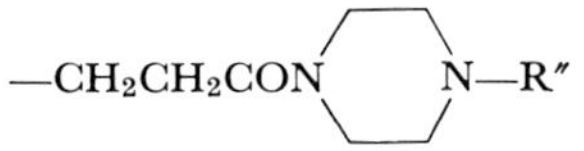

R″ = H
 CHO
 COOC₂H₅
 CH₂CH₂OH
 CH₂CH₂OCOCH₃
 COCH₂C₆H₅
 COCH₃
 COC₆H₅
 CON(CH₃)₂ (Ullyot, 1962)
 SO₂N(CH₃)₂
 CH₂CH₃
 CH₂CH₂CH₃

A number of other nitrogen substituents follow:

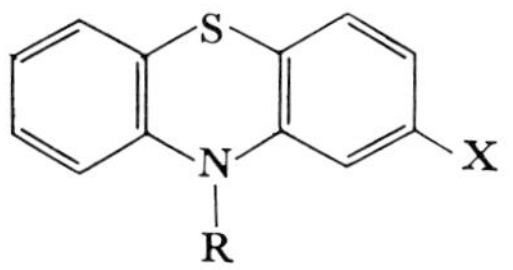

$X = Cl, CF_3$

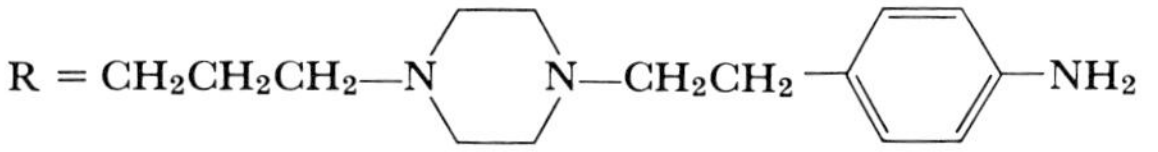

R = CH₂CH₂CH₂—N⌐⌐N—CH₂CH₂—⟨⟩—NH₂ (Gordon, 1961, 1960a, 1962c)

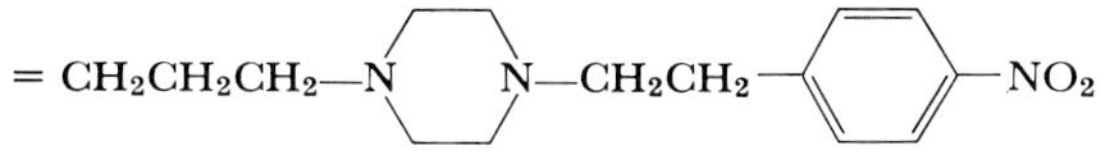

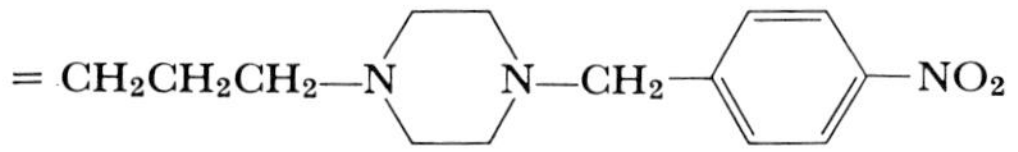

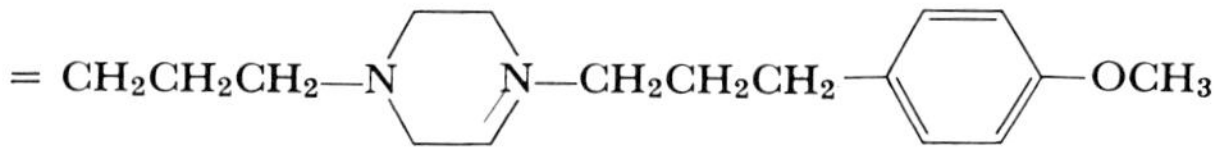

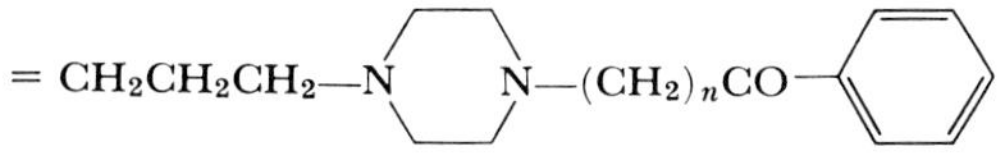

= CH₂CH₂CH₂—N⌐⌐N—CH₂CH₂—⟨⟩—NO₂

= CH₂CH₂CH₂—N⌐⌐N—CH₂—⟨⟩—NO₂

= CH₂CH₂CH₂—N⌐⌐N—CH₂CH₂CH₂—⟨⟩—OCH₃

= CH₂CH₂CH₂—N⌐⌐N—(CH₂)$_n$CO—⟨⟩   (Edgerton et al., 1961)

$n = 1-3$

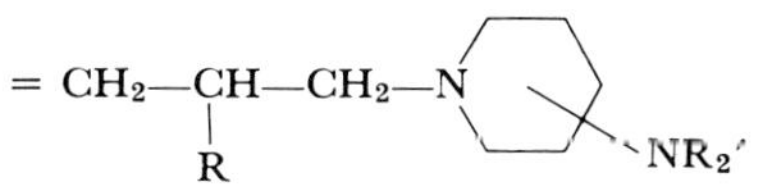

= CH₂—CH—CH₂—N⌐⌐—NR₂'   R″ = H, CH₃ (Gordon, 1962b)
           | R' = CH₃, C₂H₅
           R

Azaphenothiazines (Rodig et al., 1964; Saggiomo et al., 1958; Schuler et al., 1964), phenoxazines (Olmstead et al., 1961), phenoselenazines and other phenothiazine-related ring systems are not included in this chapter. Some related ring systems have been reviewed in Volume I (thiaxanthenes, iminodibenzyl, dibenzocycloheptatriene, etc.), and others are listed in Chapter 4.

III. Some Procedures for the Pharmacological Evaluation of Psychopharmacological Agents

It is well known that the testing of any new drug for human application is a long and complex process. If, as in the case of many infectious diseases, the effectiveness of drugs can be measured by standard clinical and laboratory methods, indications of potential usefulness can be obtained relatively easily. Similarly, when the nature of the malfunction responsible for an illness is well established, simple animal, or even *in vitro*, tests may be used to determine the likely usefulness of the new drug. Finally, in many diseases, therapy is required for only a short period of time, and this reduces the burden of prolonged testing for efficacy and possible toxic effects.

The investigation of psychopharmacological agents enjoys none of these relative advantages. Although methods of measuring the effects of drugs on the complex symptomatology of psychoses and psychoneuroses have been greatly refined from the early days, they are still quite imprecise. Furthermore, since psychopharmacological agents are often used over extended periods of time, any new agents must be put through very prolonged and thorough laboratory and clinical tests before being made generally available.

Obviously, in the development of psychopharmacological agents, as indeed in the development of other therapeutic agents, the ideal approach would be to design antagonists or simulators of naturally occurring substances which produce mental disturbances when present in excess or in insufficient amounts. However, until the nature of these substances is precisely known, this is not likely to be a very rewarding approach. Thus, the hope that a solution to these problems might be found in the study of psychotomimetic drugs such as LSD (lysergic acid diethylamide) and mescaline has not been realized. Furthermore, the extensive studies of central nervous system (CNS) components, e.g., acetylcholine, serotonin, and catecholamines have not contributed materially to the development of new psychopharmacological agents as yet (see Chapter 3).

Obviously one of the first tests employed in screening is the dose range in mice or rats, where depressant or stimulant properties may be uncovered.

One of the early procedures employed in the evaluation of tranquilizing agents was a modification of the dose range and involved measurement of behavior (aggression) in monkeys. The sedative effects produced by reserpine or chlorpromazine are different from those produced by barbiturates or other hypnotics in that the animals are readily aroused from a somnolent state and are capable of performing essential functions such as eating and drinking. In the case of the classical sedatives or hypnotics, one finds that either the action of the drug is insufficient to permit easy handling of the animals if the dose is low, or the sedation is so complete that the animals sleep deeply and cannot be readily aroused with higher doses.

As mentioned earlier, medicinal research in the psychopharmacological area is more difficult than the more classical areas like chemotherapy because the biochemistry and physiology of behavior are so incompletely understood. Thus, assay procedures must often measure some indirect effect of a tranquilizing drug. For example, one may measure the production of ptosis in mice, as seen with reserpine, or one may investigate the protection that drugs may confer against electric shock or convulsant shock produced by pentylenetetrazole, as observed with meprobamate, or chloridazepoxide. Other procedures used in the evaluation of psychopharmacological agents include studies of muscle relaxant activity, inhibition of apomorphine induced vomiting, motor activity depression or antagonism to amphetamine or mescaline.

Among the most important of the pharmacological procedures used in testing psychopharmacological agents is the conditioned response blocking test. This experimental technique, developed from Pavlov's experiments, involves conditioning a test animal to respond to a certain sound or other signal which accompanies an unpleasant stimulus like an electric shock. The response of the animal may be seen through some escape maneuver like climbing a pole to avoid shock applied through the grid on which it rests. When the animal has been adequately trained by paired applications of the sound stimulus and the shock, the animal will respond to the sound alone without the shock. The animal is then ready for the introduction of drugs which are tested for their ability to block response to the sound in an animal which has been trained to produce an avoidance response in this situation. These tests may be made more complex so that one may investigate the effects of drugs on anxieties produced by the environmental situation itself.

The operant behavior technique pioneered by Skinner (1955) has been used to study changes in the functioning of the central nervous system which are not grossly observable. Here the training technique involves bringing a simple response of the animal under the control of the experimenter in one of two ways, either by positive reinforcement (reward) or by negative reinforcement (punishment). A positive reinforcement (food, water, sexual contact, etc.) is defined as a stimulus for which an animal will perform his response, assuming that he has been appropriately deprived of these stimuli. A negative reinforcement on the other hand is a stimulus which will cause the animal to perform a response to avoid or escape the noxious stimulus. Examples of this type of stimulus include electric shock, noise, or a very bright light. Once the animal has been trained appropriately to respond to positive or negative reinforcement of his working behavior, and is thus brought under the control of the experimenter, the relationship between reinforcement schedule and the frequency with which the response is made can be studied.

The apparatus generally used in this procedure is the "Skinner box." The animal, usually a pigeon, rat, or a monkey, stands on a grid floor which is suitably wired to permit the introduction of electric shock. On the wall of the box is mounted a lever or a key at the appropriate position for the species. Thus, for example, in pigeon experiments a key on the wall can be pecked by the animal, and in rat or monkey experiments there is a lever or button that the animal may press. Food or water reinforcement is presented to the animal by means of a tray that is automatically raised into an accessible position by operation of the lever or key. The entire unit is placed in a sound-proof and light-proof chamber to avoid outside distractions. The animal's behavior may be observed through a one-way mirror, through a window opening in a darkened room, or by closed-circuit television. Usually, an electronic programming device controls the reinforcement schedule, namely the relationship between the reinforcement period and the response rate. A recording device keeps track of the number of lever presses per unit of time. Also recorded are the number of reinforcements, avoidance stimuli, and the onset and duration of visual or auditory cues.

Two basic types of reinforcement schedules are usually employed. In the first, the interval reinforcement schedule, the reinforcement depends on the passage of a time interval under the control of the experimenter, and this interval may be either fixed or variable. It is significant that the behavior of the animal is quite different for the two schedules. In the variable interval schedule, with which the animal cannot anticipate when he will be rewarded, the response rate is at a moderate level. The behavior under this schedule is quite stable and is useful in studying the effects of other variables. In the fixed interval schedule, the animal will learn not to press the lever during the early stages of the time interval since these early responses are never reinforced. However, as the time of reinforcement approaches, the response rate increases sharply. Therefore, this technique essentially measures the animal's ability to discriminate time passage. If the animal receives one reward every 30 seconds, for example (regardless of how often the lever is pressed), he will respond rapidly only a few seconds before the 30-second interval expires. On the other hand, in the variable interval the animal is rewarded at irregular intervals and cannot anticipate when a reward is to come; therefore, he works steadily in anticipation of reward.

In the ratio reinforcement schedule, a fixed number of responses must be made by the animal in order to obtain reinforcement, i.e., for every five lever presses he obtains food. On this schedule a very high response rate is generated. It is also possible to study combined schedules by training an animal to respond appropriately to a visual or auditory cue which indicates he will be rewarded on a certain schedule of reinforcement. By associating different cues with different schedules of reinforcement as described, it is possible to train an animal to show combinations of different types of responses. For example, the animal may be trained to recognize that on a green light he will be on a variable interval reinforcement and on a red light he will be on a fixed ratio reinforcement, and he will respond appropriately to these visual cues. Furthermore, it is possible to use the various reinforcement schedules to study the conditioned emotional response. It has been shown, for example, that a cue like a buzzer which has been associated with electric shock provokes the stereotyped anxiety reaction in trained rats. If a cue is presented after such an experience while the animal is lever pressing for food reinforcement, the animal typically responds with a complete cessation of lever pressing during the period of presentation of the cue. Upon termination of the cue, the animal will return to lever pressing for food reinforcement. It must be emphasized throughout this discussion that exact clinical correlations for drugs active in mixed schedules, or in the intracranial electrode experiments described below, are not yet available.

In other modifications, intracranial electrodes may be used for self stimulation as a positive reinforcement of lever pressing activity. In this procedure, electrodes are sealed into specific areas of the brain, and pressing the lever causes stimulation in this area with resulting very pleasurable sensation to the animal. Rates of response to the intracranial stimulation may exceed those obtained from food and water reinforcement and are stable during the single session and over a period of many months.

Attempts have been made over the years to find indirect methods for the screening of phenothiazines. Thus the methods of Kátó and Göszy (1961a,b) and Kátó et al. (1962) attempt to classify psychotropic drugs based on their affinity for mucopolysaccharides in vivo. The test is based on the fact that dextran seems to have two reactive sites, one producing maximal edema (at 0.7 mg/100 gm i.v.) and the other inhibiting edema (at 18 mg/100 gm i.v.). The active phenothiazines appear to act in vivo with both sites on the mucopolysaccharide, as evidenced by both inhibition and provocation of the dextran edema. An exact explanation of these correlations, or an extension to other series, is not yet available.

Injection of 5-hydroxytryptophan into mice produces a characteristic head twitch, presumably due to the central action of the drug. Using a quantal response, this head-twitch reaction can be used to screen centrally active drugs. Thus the response is potentiated by MAO (monoamine oxidase) inhibitors and antagonized by major tranquilizers, analgetics, sympathomimetic amines, and some antihistamines. Drugs without effect include barbiturates and minor tranquilizers (Corne et al., 1963).

IV. Pharmacology of Chlorpromazine

A. Introduction

The literature on the pharmacology of the phenothiazines is quite extensive, and it has never been thoroughly reviewed. In view of the fact that there are more than 2000 papers on chlorpromazine alone, it is not possible to review here the pharmacology of all of the phenothiazines, or even of chlorpromazine itself. However, inasmuch as the pharmacology of chlorpromazine is fairly typical, it will be reviewed in some detail.

In order not to provide too lengthy a treatment, yet be reasonably comprehensive, we have decided to review the chlorpromazine pharmacology which has been published in the major journals through 1963, with some 1964 material being included. Hence, we hope that all of the pertinent observations are at least exemplified here. Many of the papers in the minor journals are not cited here since it has not been practicable to review these sources for this chapter.

In this chapter, we have felt it to be of value to collect in one place the entire spectrum of pharmacological and biochemical experiments that have been performed with chlorpromazine. Perhaps future reviewers will be able to put these observations into perspective.

The phenothiazines are almost unique in the variety of the pharmacological responses which they evoke (Moyer, 1955; Piala *et al.*, 1959). Chlorpromazine, for example, has activities, depending on dose, ranging from antibacterial and possibly antitumor activity to antihistaminic and tranquilizing properties. Chlorpromazine tends to influence virtually all organs or organ systems at sufficiently high doses, and this explains the extraordinary complexity of its pharmacology (Bruecke, 1956). Furthermore, the central and peripheral effects of chlorpromazine cannot always be plainly differentiated. A review of the variability seen in drug responses has been published by Irwin (1964).

The first pharmacological investigations of chlorpromazine were carried out by Courvoisier and colleagues (1953). In the development of chlorpromazine from the antihistaminic (Neuman, 1960) phenothiazines, Laborit and collaborators (1952a,b; Laborit and Huguenard, 1951), using the pharmacological insights of Courvoisier *et al.*, introduced the use of chlorpromazine in anesthesia and developed its use as an anesthetic potentiator and in producing the state of "artificial hibernation." The French psychiatrists, Delay and Deniker (1952a,b) and Delay *et al.* (1952a,b), recognized the centrally acting properties of this compound and its therapeutic value in psychoses. More recently, speculations on the mechanism of action of psychotropic drugs have been published by Laborit (1964).

The most important central effect of chlorpromazine is its singular sedative effect (Summerfield, 1964). Animals become quiet and sleepy, remain in unnatural positions (so-called catalepsy), and at higher doses fall asleep. However, they are always readily awakened. Aggressive animals like rhesus monkeys and fighting fish become calm. Anxious animals like rabbits lose their fear. In the brain, chlorpromazine is said to influence the hypothalamus and the limbic system. The reticular apparatus of the brain stem is depressed with small doses of chlorpromazine; large doses cause a stimulation of the reticular formation. This stimulation results in the appearance of extrapyramidal symptoms, resembling the tremors of Parkinsonism in man. Chlorpromazine also inhibits the "arousal reaction," a response of the electrical activity of the brain, recorded in the electroencephalogram (Serbinenko, 1960; Chin, 1964).

Chlorpromazine is a potent local anesthetic. It blocks epinephrine and is a potent serotonin antagonist. Chlorpromazine is a potent antiemetic, and a weak antihistaminic and ganglionic blocking agent. It has anticonvulsant properties against nicotine and nikethamide convulsions, but not against pextylenetetrazole, strychnine, or electroshock. Chlorpromazine has some antipyretic properties; it reduces edema, is spasmolytic and antifibrillatory, dilates blood vessels, and reduces blood pressure, but these pharmacological properties do not have clinical applications. Respiration is increased with small doses of chlorpromazine; with higher doses there is some depression. Vasomotor centers of the brain are depressed by chlorpromazine, and it potentiates the action of narcotics and analgetics at doses which are not in themselves hypnotic or analgetic. High concentrations of chlorpromazine decrease the conductivity of isolated nerve fibers.

A review on some aspects of the pharmacology of the phenothiazines has been published by Marconi (1961), Mashkovsky (1956), and most recently by Carr (1963), Lewis (1964), and Harper and Tait (1964).

1. Mechanism and Site of Action

The site and mechanism of action of chlorpromazine have been the objects of a good many investigations, but no definitive decisions can be reached. Chlorpromazine is said to uncouple oxidative phosphorylation and to inhibit the activity of adenosinetriphosphatase, but it is difficult to say whether these actions are causes or consequences of its central nervous system activity.

The effects of chlorpromazine on the reticular formation are often studied through the influence of the drug on mono- and polysynaptic reflexes. Inasmuch as the latter are usually studied under anesthesia, one has to consider the interaction of chlorpromazine and the anesthetic, so conclusions are difficult to reach.

If membranes are involved in chlorpromazine's activity then its specific effects might be due to the differential concentration of chlorpromazine in different areas of the brain, or certain membranes may be unusually sensitive to the effect of the drug (Guth and Spirtes, 1961; Zografi, 1964). Mitochondria may be particularly sensitive in this regard (Spirtes and Guth, 1961, cf. pp. 117, 119).

Blocking of pinnal and corneal reflexes in animals has been used in the evaluation of drug effects. Thus chlorpromazine blocks the pinnal reflex at doses that leave the corneal reflex intact. Hypnotics, on the other hand, block the corneal reflex at lower doses than those that block the pinnal reflex (Witkin et al., 1959). Drug effects on mono- and polysynaptic motor reflexes have been studied (Silvestrini and Maffii, 1959). Chlorpromazine caused a drop in survival time of the corneal reflex in rabbits during stagnant anoxia (Boeles and Blok, 1956).

The effect of chlorpromazine on septal hyperactivity in the rat has been studied (Raitt et al., 1961). Chlorpromazine (8 mg/kg i.p.) markedly reduced overt emotional activity, as measured by an "emotional rating scale."

The effects of chloridazepoxide, chlorpromazine, and other drugs on the limbic system of the brain were studied by Schallek (1962). Chlorpromazine, chlordiazepoxide, and meprobamate, but not scopolamine, depressed vicious behavior in cats with induced septal lesions. Electroencephalographic determinations of spontaneous limbic activity showed depression by chlorpromazine, chlordiazepoxide, and meprobamate (cf. Horovitz and Chow, 1962; Anokhina-Itskova, 1961).

It has been reported by Herman and Barnes (1964) in studies in decerebrate cats that chlorpromazine has a direct action on the spinal cord in addition to its supraspinal activity.

The central cholinolytic action of chlorpromazine was described by Steiner and Himwich (1962). Chlorpromazine antagonized EEG alerting produced by cholinergic agents, especially eserine salicylate and acetylcholine in rabbits. Thus chlorpromazine, in addition to its adrenolytic actions, apparently also has central cholinolytic effect.

Disturbances of the central nervous system may be due in part to a deficiency of nutrient substances (Quadbeck, 1962). This deficiency may be due to a diminished utilization of food by the brain or by an enhanced requirement of energy in consequence of stress phenomena (cf. Chapter 3). Furthermore, it has been known for many years that a marked reduction in blood sugar, reduced oxygen pressure in the air, or diminished cerebral blood flow can produce psychotic symptoms. In addition, it is known that a latent psychosis can be activated by sleep deprivation or by certain central stimulants.

D. H. Tedeschi (1966, personal communication) has recently found that there is a good correlation between the potency of neuroleptics in causing ptosis and their clinical tranquilizing activity. The ptosis caused by neuroleptics, and part of their mechanism of action in tranquilization is associated with a reduction in central sympathetic outflow. Thus Tedeschi concludes that an action critical for neuroleptic activity may be a reduction in the interaction of sympathetic centers with other levels of integration in the CNS.

B. Effects on the Central Nervous System (CNS)

One of the most interesting aspects of the pharmacology of chlorpromazine relates to its effects on the central nervous system. Chlorpromazine causes a reduction in motor activity, without inducing sleep or anesthesia except at high doses. Electroencephalographic records of animals given chlorpromazine resemble those observed in a normal state of sleep, with a rapid and normal-appearing "arousal response" following stimuli. Chlorpromazine blocks conditioned responses more than responses to unconditioned stimuli such as electric shock. In addition to the decrease in motor activity, there is a dose-related loss of aggressive behavior in intact animals. In animals displaying sham rage, the intensity of the rage is depressed by chlorpromazine.

1. Effects on Activity and Behavior in Intact Animals

Intravenous administration of chlorpromazine to monkeys in doses of 0.7 to 2.0 mg/kg produced drastic changes in behavior (Das *et al.*, 1954). The animals were peaceful and easily handled, and could be kept unrestrained outside of their cages. They reacted to stimuli by withdrawal of the stimulated arm or leg, but remained in any position in which they were placed by the investigators.

In spite of this state of akinesia and somnolence, their eyes were open and their tendon and postural reflexes were normal. After larger doses the monkeys would sleep, but would awaken and show some spontaneous activity if irritated. The effects of chlorpromazine lasted 3 to 8 hours, followed by a gradual return to a normal behavioral pattern.

Administration of 0.83 mg/kg of chlorpromazine to monkeys intramuscularly produced a physiological-appearing sleep (Baruk *et al.*, 1955a,b). At doses of about 5 mg/kg the monkeys were in a state of catalepsy. At doses of 13 mg/kg the monkeys suffered paralysis and general prostration, with effects differing from those of bulbocapnine in the absence of hyperkinesia and epilepsy. Cats showed similar effects at these doses, while guinea pigs required doses 15 to 20 times as large for the production of catalepsy and paralysis. Pigeons showed only a reduction in motor activity and reduced response to stimulation after 100 mg/kg. Hence they were less than 1/100 as sensitive to chlorpromazine as monkeys.

In mice 1–5 mg/kg of chlorpromazine orally or subcutaneously produced a reduction in spontaneous motor activity proportional to the dose (Cook *et al.*, 1955). Activity in mice was reduced about 50% for the first hour after a dose of 2 mg/kg subcutaneously, and completely suppressed at 5 mg/kg. Even at the latter dose, however, the mice showed no ataxia or prostration and responded readily to stimuli with coordinated activity. This behavior is in marked contrast to the effects of barbiturates, which caused reduction in spontaneous motor activity only at doses which produced ataxia or hypnosis. Some of the chlorpromazine effect was still evident 5 hours after small doses and it was partially antagonized by large doses of pipradrol (Feldman and Brown, 1955). Other studies on motor behavior were published by Taeschler and Cerletti (1959), Irwin *et al.* (1958), Jannsen *et al.* (1960a, b), Boyd and Miller (1954), Kaufmann (1955), Haley (1957), Kaelber and Joynt (1956), Herr *et al.* (1961), Liberson (1964), and Kinnard and Carr (1957).

In addition to the conditional response blocking tests described earlier, a number of other procedures have been described that are said to correlate with the clinical activity of chlorpromazine. Thus, spiders given solutions containing chlorpromazine practically ceased spinning webs for 1 to 3 days, but any webs made were normal in structure indicating a decrease in drive but not in motor ability (Witt, 1955).

Another screening test for tranquilizers consisted of placing a mouse head-first in a horizontal tube, marked off 20 cm from the base (Boissier et al., 1960). When the animal has reached the end, the tube is turned vertically and the mouse must climb backward 20 cm in less than 30 seconds. The ED_{50} for chlorpromazine in this test was 4.5–4.8 mg/kg i.p.

A method for measuring visible differences between chlorpromazine-treated and untreated animals using an ordinal scale for ranking judgment of two unbiased and independent observers has been described by Janssen (1961a). Binomial and sequential analysis were used for evaluating reliability and significance of drug effects.

A combination of a spontaneous motor activity test [Kinnard and Carr, 1957—activity cages] and a rolling roller performance test was used to evaluate chlorpromazine, promazine, hydroxyzine, ectylurea, and meprobamate in mice (Weaver and Miya, 1961). This method could detect compounds which have differential effects on two areas of the brain, namely those which control spontaneous movements, and those which control muscular coordination. This procedure is reported to be particularly suitable for screening drugs used in daytime sedation (see also Rutledge and Doty, 1957; Read et al., 1960; Kinnard and Carr, 1957).

Investigators have speculated whether chlorpromazine, by reducing motivational strength, would eliminate stereotyped behavior caused by pretrial submersion of rats swimming in a water T-maze. However, chlorpromazine produced severe behavioral disorganization and decreased learning and retention of both stereotyped and nonstereotyped responses. The results suggested that chlorpromazine may affect sensory input and effective integration of sensory data rather than motor incoordination or motivational strength (Mitchell and King, 1960; Grandjean and Bättig, 1962).

The classification of a wide variety of CNS drugs, including chlorpromazine, d-amphetamine, and iproniazid, by two different tests in mice has been studied. The first test involves grading the sequence of disappearance of motor response in an isolated situation and the second, measuring spontaneous coordinated activity in group situation (Brown, 1960). Chlorpromazine and reserpine were characterized by absence of excitant phase, absence of hypnosis at less than the LD_{50} dose, a low level activity over wide dose ranges, and parallel depressant effects in both isolation and group situations.

A "scale-jiggling" test in animals has been carried out using both chlorpromazine and amphetamine sulfate as reference compounds. Simple movements, for instance those of the head, could be recorded on a kymograph. Chlorpromazine depressed equally both spontaneous activity and forced motor activity in mice (Cho, 1961). Pentobarbital depressed mainly forced activity (Furgiuele et al., 1961). The effect of some centrally acting drugs on disjunctive reaction time was studied by Evans and Jewett (1962), the transfer of drug-trained responses, to other drugs, was studied by Stewart (1962).

Footshock-induced fighting behavior in mice was suppressed by chlorpromazine and reserpine, but not by meprobamate, barbiturates, or chloral hydrate (Chen, 1963). Other behavioral effects of chlorpromazine have been reported by Torres (1963) and by Delphaut (1963).

In a study of the effect of reserpine, chlorpromazine, and meprobamate on learning in the newborn, the drugs were given to gravid rats and the offspring were measured for learning activity. Only the offspring of the meprobamate-treated mothers required significantly more trials to reach a control level of learning (Werboff and Kesner, 1963; cf. Murphree and Peters, 1956; Doty and Doty, 1963).

The sexual behavior of male rats under the influence of chlorpromazine has been reported by Zimbardo and Barry (1958) and by Gillett (1960). A reduction in rate of copulation, the number of copulations, and the latency period was observed, but there was a wide range of individual variation.

2. Effects on Activity of Decerebrate Animals

Decerebrate and diencephalic cats were much more sensitive to the depressant effects of chlorpromazine than normal animals (Dasgupta et al., 1954). Sham rage reactions were completely suppressed by 100–250 μg/kg intravenously, less than one-tenth of the dose required for reduction of spontaneous motor activity and loss of response in intact cats. Muscle tone and decerabrate rigidity were also abolished at these doses.

Another report by the same group described the effects of chlorpromazine on responses to electrical stimulation of various areas of the brain in intact and decerebrate cats, in an attempt to determine the site of action of the drug (Dasgupta and Werner, 1955). Chlorpromazine at doses of 0.5 mg/kg in cats decreased motor responses to stimulation of the pericruciate area of the cortex in intact animals, abolished flexor or extensor responses to cerebellar stimulation in decerebrate animals, decreased the head-turning response to lateral reticular stimulation in decerebrate-decerebellate animals and the motor response stimulation of descending medullary tracts in decerebrate animals, and abolished the crossed-extensor reflex in decerebrate cats. Chlorpromazine was 20 to 40 times as effective as mephenesin in all of these preparations. In spinal cats, however, chlorpromazine had little effect on the crossed-extensor reflex, while mephenesin had an inhibitory effect. Thus, chlorpromazine appeared to interfere with motor activity primarily by its depressant action on the brain stem reticular formation.

Intravenous injection of chlorpromazine in doses of 0.5–0.75 mg/kg produced transient rapid breathing in decerebrate cats, with the degree of response depending on the rate of injection (De Risio and Manghi, 1954). Muscular hypertonia gradually decreased and was replaced by flaccidity in 8 to 10 minutes.

The amplitude of the patellar reflex tended to increase as muscle tone decreased but reflexes of spinal automatism were not affected, and muscle tone gradually returned after about 2 hours (cf. Krivoy, 1957).

Serbinenko (1960) reported that the inhibitory effect of chlorpromazine on motor reflexes of decerebrate cats may have a double mechanism of action. Thus chlorpromazine blocks the activity of the reticular formation of the midbrain and pons varolii, and small doses show primary stimulatory effects on the inhibitory parts of the reticular formation of brain stem and cerebellum.

In dogs with a mid-collicular brain stem transection, extensor hypertonicity and hyperreflexia were completely blocked by chlorpromazine in doses of 3.3–5.0 mg/kg intravenously (Sheatz and Fazekas, 1955).

In several human subjects with "decorticate hypertonicity" due to irreversible brain damage, intramuscular injection of 100 mg of chlorpromazine produced marked relaxation and sedation. Intravenous chlorpromazine produced electromyographic evidence of a marked reduction or elimination of spasticity in patients with upper motor neuronal lesions (Basmajian and Szatmari, 1955).

3. Miscellaneous CNS Effects

Injections of high doses of chlorpromazine into the arterial cephalic circulation of the isolated perfused head of the dog had no influence on the responses of the cardio-inhibitory center provoked reflexly by blood pressure increase or by electrical stimulation of the carotid sinus nerves (De Vleeschhouwer *et al.*, 1957).

4. Effects on Conditioned Reflex Response

a. *Without Operant Conditioning.* The conditioned escape response test was one of the first pharmacological procedures used to characterize the phenothiazine class of central nervous system depressants. Chlorpromazine has the unusual ability to suppress responses to auditory or visual conditioned stimuli in doses which do not markedly alter responses to unconditioned stimuli. In rats conditioned to climb a pole at the sound of a bell, pretreatment with 2 mg/kg of chlorpromazine subcutaneously blocked response to the bell in about 40% of the trials (Cook *et al.*, 1955; Altschule *et al.*, 1955; Fink and Swinyard, 1962; Aston *et al.*, 1962). Chlorpromazine doses of 10 mg/kg blocked the conditioned response in about 85% of the rats, although the animals were capable of responding to an unconditioned stimulus—namely an electric shock to the feet. Although morphine also selectively blocked conditioned escape responses, barbiturates were ineffective except at doses which also blocked response to the unconditioned stimulus. In a similar situation, 0.5 mg/kg of chlorpromazine reduced the response of rats to an auditory stimulus and higher doses abolished the response, without loss of muscular coordination (Courvoisier et al., 1953).

In rats trained to jump through a hole in the wall to obtain food at the sound of a buzzer, chlorpromazine in doses of 3–9 mg/kg intraperitoneally markedly decreased the proportion of responses, without interfering with spontaneous motor activity (Guha et al., 1954). Chlorpromazine also interfered with maze performance in fasted rats at 3 mg/kg i.p. (Archer, 1954).

The evaluation of alcohol and chlorpromazine as fear-reducing drugs was reported by Grossman and Miller (1961). A variable-length "telescope alley" apparatus was used, and the procedure involved approach training and avoidance training with and without drugs. Two testing conditions were measured, i.e. fear and fear-plus-pain (electroshock). Hungry rats tested under alcohol ran reliably faster and farther toward food than did controls in both fear and fear-plus-pain tests. Chlorpromazine-treated rats ran consistently farther and faster than controls in fear-plus-pain test but ran significantly slower than controls in fear only test (cf. Barry and Miller, 1962).

In the study of the correlation in rats between the locomotor and avoidance suppressant potencies of eight phenothiazines, including chlorpromazine, Irwin (1961) reported that most of the drugs produced similar suppression of both locomotor and avoidance suppression.

Observations on conditioned and unconditioned on- and off-behavioral responses to a buzzer were made by Izquierdo (1962). Chlorpromazine (2–2.5 mg/kg i.p.), extinguished both on- and off-conditioned reflexes in acutely, but not in chronically, stimulated rats.

Acquisition of a fear-motivated response to chlorpromazine was studied by Davis et al. (1961). In their procedure, basically similar to the classical conditioned avoidance response experiments, training was sequential so that drug effects on the conditioning process could be partially analyzed. Chlorpromazine inhibited establishment of an association between conditioned stimulus and internal fear-motivated behavior and its drive and cue function. The data indicated that chlorpromazine might prevent progressive extension of psychoneurotic symptoms. Chlorpromazine also promoted persistent extinction of fear-conditioned response (cf. Otis, 1964).

Tolerance development to drugs in conditioned rats was investigated by Mercier et al. (1962). Thirsty male rats were conditioned to drink only green-colored water; consumption of red-colored water was prevented by electric shock. When the animals gave 100% positive response they were injected with various drugs in amounts which significantly reduced performance either partially (30–70%) or completely (70–100%). Partial tolerance developed to chlorpromazine (4 mg/kg/day), but only after 60 days. When the drug was stopped, there were no behavioral or autonomic symptoms suggestive of abstinence syndrome.

A study in rats, Irwin (1963) showed that tolerance development to chlorpromazine was considerably accelerated by increasing the intensity of the conditioned (buzzer) or the unconditioned (shock) stimulus.

In a comparison of chlorpromazine and chlordiazepoxide in conflict-induced fixations in rats, it was concluded that the latter was more effective than the former (Feldman, 1962).

In studying the effect of drugs upon defensive behavior of rats Kelemen and Bovet (1961) employed an electric stimulator and a hot plate apparatus; a bell was used as the conditioned stimulus. Defensive reactions to unconditioned stimuli were examined in two phases. In the first phase, the animal discovered the escape pathway (jumping on top of cylinder in case of electric shock). In the second phase (heat stimulus), the adequate response became stereotyped and the activity more economical. The second phase was useful for investigating drug effects on automatization of formerly found solutions, and it was facilitated by strychnine and amphetamine, and inhibited by chlorpromazine.

In cats conditioned to lift a foreleg in response to stimulation of the cerebral cortex through implanted electrodes, chlorpromazine in doses of 4–7 mg/kg had no effect on the response (Rutledge and Doty, 1955). Response to auditory or visual stimuli in some of these animals was abolished by these doses and higher doses also blocked response to the cortical stimulus. Their results caused the authors to believe that chlorpromazine acts on afferent mechanisms. Other experiments in cats have indicated that drugs which decreased free catecholamines or increased serotonin decreased performance, while drugs which decreased serotonin and increased catecholamines improved performance. These data suggest that the mechanisms for behavioral sedation or excitation are not identical with those of either inhibition or facilitation of the conditioned avoidance response (Wada, 1963).

The effect of drugs on conditioning and habituation to arousal stimuli in animals was studied by Key and Bradley (1960). Chlorpromazine increased threshold for both conditioned (behavior) and unconditioned (EEG) arousal response to auditory stimuli in cats and eventually blocked arousal response completely.

In determining the effect of drugs on discrimination and on sensory generalization of auditory stimuli in cats, Key (1961a) found that LSD (15 μg/kg i.p.) produced an increased amount of generalization without modifying the discriminatory ability of the animal in terms of physical parameters of stimulation. Chlorpromazine produced opposite effects; i.e., rapid extinction of conditioned and generalized responses without affecting gradient of generalization.

A dose of 0.5 mg/kg chlorpromazine decreased, while 1–1.5 mg/kg completely suppressed food- and respiratory-conditioned reflexes in dogs. Higher doses (1–25 mg/kg) decreased the magnitude and completely suppressed secretory-digestive reflexes. Depending on doses administered, conditioned reflexes were reestablished within 2 to 6 days (Aganyants, 1960).

The effect of chlorpromazine on the relationship between the motor and autonomic components of a defensive conditioned reaction in animals during early development was studied by Nikitina (1961). Chlorpromazine inhibited motor, respiratory, and cardiac components of a conditioned reflex in young rabbits. Levels of inhibition depended on the dose and age of the animal. High doses inhibited both motor and respiratory components; low doses inhibited only motor. Apparently reticular formation is involved in integration of a conditioned reflex at an early age and the involvement increases with age.

It has been reported that, based on thirteen phenothiazines, activity in the conditioned escape response test correlates well with *in vitro* effects on oxidative phosphorylation and adenosinetriphosphatase activity in the brain (Décsi, 1961). It is questionable, however, whether these relationships would be maintained for a larger series of compounds.

The effects of drugs on the conditioned psychogalvanic reflex in man were studied by Alexander and Horner (1961). Chlorpromazine, in normal and in psychiatric patients, lowered the magnitude of responses to inhibitory and excitatory conditioned stimuli. The data confirmed the hypothesis that chlorpromazine inhibits orienting behavior and unlearned reactivity to a greater degree than specific learned reactivity. There was correlation between psychogalvanic reflex and clinical improvement.

Other avoidance conditioning experiments have been carried out by Ader and Clink (1957), Miller *et al.* (1957a, b), Smith *et al.* (1957), Gliedman and Gantt (1956), Taeschler and Cerletti (1959), Sines and Sines (1958), Kopmann and Hughes (1958), Shaklee (1958), Blumberg and Dayton (1959), Denenberg *et al.* (1959), Huntzinger *et al.* (1959), Gowdey *et al.* (1960), Gonzalez and Ross (1961), Bhargava and Chandra (1964), Halasz and Marrazzi (1964), Jackson (1964), and Fowler *et al.* (1964).

b. *With Operant Conditioning.* Some specific experiments will be cited here in regard to the effects on conditioned reflex response with operant conditioning. Pigeons trained to respond to a red light with a fixed ratio response (rewards given after a given number of pecks) and to a blue light with a fixed interval response (reward after 5 minutes), still differentiated between the colored lights after 1.7 or 3 mg/kg of chlorpromazine i.m. (Dews, 1956). There was no interference with fixed rate performance, but long pauses developed during fixed interval periods. Phenobarbital in doses producing a general decrease in activity appeared to interfere with discrimination, since the birds often pecked steadily through the fixed interval period.

The relative potencies of some phenothiazines as pecking syndrome inhibitors in pigeons were determined by Burkman (1961a,b; 1962a,b). The behavioral data were said to correlate with the antiemetic activity, and identical receptors may be involved (Dhawan *et al.*, 1961).

The effect of drugs on a fixed-ratio performance of pigeons was suppressed by a pre-time-out stimulus in a study by Ferster *et al.* (1962). Pecking was reinforced in a fixed-ratio (FR) schedule with food; responses during a red light produced time-out. If the bird did not respond during red light, it terminated and the bird could complete a FR schedule of positive reinforcement uninterrupted. The bird stopped responding during red light sufficiently to avoid most of the possible time-outs. In general, the pre-time-out stimulus suppressed responding more when the FR schedule was large than when it was small. Amobarbital, pentobarbital, chlorpromazine, and d-amphetamine, given when FR performance was trained by a pre-time-out stimulus, produced marked increases in responding. Drug administration lowered the rate of responding only at higher doses.

Pigeons were trained by Kelleher *et al.* (1962) in an observing-response procedure in which periods of variable ratio (VR 100) and extinction alternated unpredictably during white light (mixed stimulus). Responses on the food-producing key were intermittently reinforced. Responses on the observing key produced a green light (positive stimulus) when the variable ratio was in effect and a red light (negative stimulus) for extinction. The birds did not respond on either key during negative stimulus; they responded on food-producing key when positive stimulus appeared. When observing responses produced positive or negative stimulus on the fixed ratio schedule, observing responses were maintained until the fixed ratio reached a maximum; beyond this, only food-producing responses occurred. When observing responses did not produce either stimulus, observing-response rates fell to zero. Chlorpromazine decreased total response output but markedly increased observing-response rates except when it was given before sessions of observing response extinction.

In a study of temporal discrimination in pigeons (Reynolds and Catania, 1962), birds were trained to peck a lighted key and were presented with the key alternately dark and lighted. The key was dark for intervals of 3–30 seconds. Pecking of the lighted key was reinforced only after the shortest or, in a second experiment, longest interval that the key was dark. The pigeons were able to estimate the duration of dark interval. Chlorpromazine attenuated discrimination of duration of a stimulus but did not abolish pecking.

Various behavioral tests in the classification of psychopharmacological agents were reviewed by Cook and Kelleher (1962, 1963). The relationship of the autonomic nervous system to behavior, as well as the relationship of behavioral studies to clinical syndromes was discussed.

In a study of the effects of chronically administered chlorpromazine on multiple-schedule performance Waller (1961) administered chlorpromazine to dogs 2 hours prior to the start of session. Low doses increased the rates of response on all components of multiple schedule used. At higher doses, the rates were not depressed to the extent one would expect in the interval components. It was also noted that tolerance could occur after chronic administration and some indication of withdrawal effect was observed.

The effects of chlorpromazine on "aggressive" responding in rats trained in lever pressing on a regular water-reinforcement schedule were studied by Thompson (1961). The results showed that chlorpromazine-treated animals made fewer responses both before and after onset of extinction but exhibited relatively greater acceleration in rate of responding immediately after onset of extinction as compared with a saline control group.

An operant conditioning and extinction technique (bar press) was used by Aceto et al. (1961) to compare effects of various drugs, including chlorpromazine and d-amphetamine in the rat. In general, only those drugs which interfered with normal motor activity and those with anorexic properties had significant effects when compared with controls (cf. Sidley and Schoenfeld, 1963).

Chlorpromazine effects on instrumental learning based on conditioned fear, were studied by Gonzalez and Shepp (1962) in rats. During training, a motivationally neutral stimulus was paired with shock repeatedly in a situation in which no response that was instrumental in terminating shock was possible. Then the conditioned response was presented alone and the effect of chlorpromazine on learning a new response (cf. Chamberlain et al., 1963), instrumental in escaping the conditioned stimulus, was tested. When chlorpromazine was given from the very beginning it completely inhibited learning. When given after "fear conditioning" chlorpromazine also inhibited learning, but if given during conditioning and withdrawn during testing, effects were less pronounced.

The effects of chlorpromazine and perphenazine on bar-pressing performance in an approach-avoidance conflict were measured by Grossman (1961). Differential effects of high and low doses of chlorpromazine (2 and 4 mg/kg i.p.) and perphenazine (0.125 and 0.250 mg/kg i.p.) on acquired fear were studied in an approach-avoidance (hunger-fear) conflict situation, using increasing levels of avoidance motivation (shock). Both drugs exerted equally strong depressant effects on bar-pressing performance under nonavoidance conditions; effects were greater with high doses. Increasing levels of avoidance motivation reduced performance of control rats but had relatively little effect on performance of drug animals (cf. Kelleher et al., 1961; Waller and Waller, 1962).

In human subjects conditioned to experience a galvanic skin response upon being stimulated by a light flash, chlorpromazine did not interfere with extinction of the unconditioned response, but did inhibit the reestablishment of the response the next day (Schneider and Costiloe, 1956). Response of the subjects to an unconditioned stimulus, namely an electric shock, was not affected.

Additional operant conditioning experiments were carried out by Maffii (1959), Verhave *et al.* (1958), Stone *et al.* (1958), Heistad (1958), Blough (1958), Barry *et al.* (1963), Sines and Sines (1958), Fuller *et al.* (1960), Fry *et al.* (1960), Hughes and Kopmann (1960), Kelleher and Cook (1959), Holliday and Dille (1958), Dews (1958), Leary and Stynes (1959), Terrace (1963), Clark *et al.* (1962), Laties and Weiss (1964), Hanson (1964), Boyd *et al.* (1963), Weiss and Laties (1964).

5. Electroencephalographic (EEG) Effects

In intact monkeys, cats, and dogs, and animals subjected to surgical section at various levels of the central nervous system, and in normal, psychotic, neurotic, or epileptic and brain-damaged human subjects, the effects of chlorpromazine have been studied on electroencephalographic patterns. (See Killam and Killam, 1956; Setekleiv *et al.*, 1960; Carreras and Angeleri, 1957; White and Boyajy, 1959; Costa and Rinaldi, 1958; Kaelber and Correll, 1958; Ladinskaya, 1958; Kimura, 1957; Yagi *et al.*, 1960a,b; Goldring *et al.*, 1959; DeMaar *et al.*, 1958; Bradley and Key, 1958; Tokizane *et al.*, 1957; McIlwain and Greengard, 1957; Ingvar and Söderberg, 1957; Marrazzi and Hart, 1956; Bradley and Hance, 1955, 1956, 1957; Preston, 1956; Baker *et al.*, 1956; Kreindler *et al.*, 1959; Martin *et al.*, 1958; Gunn *et al.*, 1955; Monnier and Krupp, 1959; Gangloff and Monnier, 1957; Selbach, 1956; Sedivec, 1964.)

a. *Intact Animals.* Intravenous chlorpromazine administered to restrained normal monkeys produced an immediate increase in voltage of the alpha waves, followed by bursts of delta waves, particularly in leads from the frontal areas (Das *et al.*, 1954). With doses of chlorpromazine above 3 mg/kg occasional sleep spindles appeared, alternating with bursts of high voltage delta waves. In monkeys with implanted cortical and subcortical electrodes, chlorpromazine produced a record resembling that of drowsiness and light sleep (Monroe *et al.*, 1955). Essig and Carter (1957) have reported that chronic administration of high doses of chlorpromazine (44–77 mg/kg i.m.) produced major convulsions and behavior suggestive of hallucinations in monkeys (*Macaca mulatta*).

Administration of small doses of chlorpromazine to conscious cats and dogs immobilized with a curarizing agent produced a progressive disappearance of rapid EEG activity and the appearance of irregular slow waves, not typical of either normal sleep or barbiturate narcosis due to the absence of spindles (Hiebel *et al.*, 1954). Auditory or olfactory stimulation caused transient waking activity. Electrical stimulation of the reticular formation produced activation and sympathetic discharge, but only at higher voltages than in normals. After prebulbar section the activation response to adrenaline was completely blocked. With slightly higher doses of chlorpromazine (1–15 mg/kg) there was a marked decrease in frequency in cats and an increase in amplitude of spontaneous cortical activity, inhibition of the arousal response to stimulation of the reticular substance, and a lesser inhibition of arousal response to stimulation of the sciatic nerve, with no change in the cortical auditory response (Balestrieri and Fadiga, 1954). Key and Bradley (1958) have studied the effects of drugs on conditioning and habituation to arousal stimuli in animals.

Implanting electrodes in conscious unrestrained cats and administering chlorpromazine intravenously, there was a production of slow wave activity in all areas, or bursts of rhythmic 5–8 times per second activity (Bradley and Hance, 1955). No change in the slow wave activity was produced by sensory stimuli. The effects of amphetamine and lysergic acid diethylamide (production of fast, low voltage wave activity in the corticogram) were blocked, but not those of physostigmine. Slow wave activity produced by atropine was potentiated. Another study, devoted to the investigation of pressor thresholds in the mesencephalic and bulbar reticular formations in curarized cats, revealed a barbiturate-like action of chlorpromazine (Gunn *et al.*, 1955). With small doses, thresholds were unchanged or decreased with cortical arousal. Larger doses produced sleep-like EEG activity, an increase in reticular threshold, and a decrease in afferent evoked potentials in the reticular formation.

b. *Encephal Isolé and Cerveau Isolé Animals.* In one rabbit *encephal isolé* preparation (spinal cord transected at C_1, leaving cortical reticular connections intact) the control EEG resembled that of the normal rabbit, so long as shock was prevented by slow intravenous infusion of epinephrine (Longo *et al.*, 1954). The effects of chlorpromazine also resembled those in normals, with increased slow wave activity and superimposed spindle bursts. The arousal response to external stimuli was diminished or abolished by chlorpromazine, as was the activation response to stimulation of the reticular formation. Chlorpromazine also blocked seizure responses to nicotine, but not to pentylenetetrazole or strychnine.

A characteristic EEG pattern of short bursts of spindling alternating with slow high-voltage activity was found in the cat *cerveau isolé* in which the mesencephalic section at the collicular level had separated the cortex and reticular formation (Das *et al.*, 1955). Administration of small doses of chlorpromazine (0.2–0.5 mg/kg) resulted in immediate disappearance of slow high-voltage activity and gradual decline of spindling, leaving slow low-voltage waves. In a few of the animals, chlorpromazine produced a bilateral synchronous three-per-second spike and wave discharge resembling that seen in petit mal or after stimulation of the "thalamic reticular system," whereas convulsions occurred in two cats with an intact pyramidal system. A similar blocking of spindling and slow activity in *cerveau isolé* cats was found in another study only when the collicular section was incomplete or large doses of chlorpromazine were used (Bradley and Hance, 1955). With complete section and doses of 0.5–0.1 mg/kg, no change in activity occurred, although blood pressure fluctuated briefly. In the cat *encephal isolé*, temporary blocking of the characteristic spindle and slow wave activity occurred 1 or 2 minutes after injection of chlorpromazine. Martin and Eades (1960) have reported a decrease in excitability of both the ascending activating system and the descending vasomotor system.

c. *Humans.* Electroencephalographic studies in normal human subjects after intravenous or intramuscular administration of chlorpromazine have shown patterns associated with fatigue, drowsiness, or sleep, depending on the doses used (Terzian, 1952; Dobkin *et al.*, 1954a,b,c; Bente and Itil, 1954; Goldman, 1955). In patients given chlorpromazine, the changes induced by intravenous hexobarbital were intensified and occurred sooner. Tolerance to the potentiating effects of chlorpromazine were noticed after 3 weeks (Bente and Itil, 1954). In epileptic patients with normal resting EEG records, the administration of chlorpromazine usually showed an activation of paroxysmal discharge, while those with abnormal resting EEGs showed intensification of abnormal patterns (Terzian, 1952; Bente and Itil, 1954; Turner *et al.*, 1955; Fabisch, 1955). Several patients, mostly schizophrenics, with implanted subcortical electrodes showed records associated with relaxation with short bursts of EEG activity like the patterns of normal drowsiness or light sleep (Monroe *et al.*, 1955).

Quantitative electroencephalography and human psychopharmacology studies were carried out by Fink (1961). He described the application of EEG frequency analysis to a study of the mode of action of imipramine (300 mg), chlorpromazine (1200 mg) and procyclidine (15 mg) in psychiatric patients. Chlorpromazine increased total activity and shifted some peak frequencies. Possibly this technique might provide a basis for developing a screening method for studying new psychotropic compounds in man.

6. Effects on Convulsive Thresholds

The intensity of convulsions resulting from intravenous injections of nicotine or nikethamide was markedly reduced by pretreatment of the rabbits and mice with 1.25 or 5.0 mg/kg of chlorpromazine (i.v.) (Courvoisier *et al.*, 1953). Similar effects were seen in cats (Marquardt *et al.*, 1955). The EEG activation was also blocked (Longo *et al.*, 1954).

Anticonvulsant studies with chlorpromazine have been carried out in rats using electroshock and convulsants like strychnine, pentylenetetrazole, and picrotoxin (Virtue and Jones, 1956; Meidinger, 1956; Brown *et al.*, 1957; Dobkin *et al.*, 1954a,b,c; Fink and Swinyard, 1960). No significant protective effects were seen (cf. Raevsky, 1961).

On the other hand, chlorpromazine does provide protection in some species against audiogenic seizures (Plotnikoff, 1958, 1960; Plotnikoff and Green, 1957), and tolerance to this protective effect may develop due to inbreeding (Plotnikoff, 1961).

In pigeons, chlorpromazine appeared to increase the convulsive and lethal effects of picrotoxin (Madjerek and Stern, 1956). The injection of chlorpromazine in monkeys, made epileptic by the application of alumina cream to the surface of the cortex or by the injection of the irritant into the occipital or temporal areas, caused increased EEG abnormalities and sometimes increased the incidence of spontaneous seizures and the convulsive effects of pentylenetetrazole or of prodding (Kopeloff *et al.*, 1955). Epilepsy caused by section of the sciatic nerve in guinea pigs (Brown-Sequard epilepsy) was not affected by chlorpromazine (Mercier, 1955). The duration of discharge resulting from transcranial electrical stimulation in dogs was decreased by doses of chlorpromazine above 1 mg/kg. After 20 mg/kg, there was only a brief localized response to four times the normal threshold stimulus (Mercier, 1955).

The electroshock threshold in rats was unchanged or questionably decreased after single doses of 10–25 mg/kg of chlorpromazine. Repeated daily doses of 20 mg/kg of chlorpromazine definitely lowered shock threshold in intact but not in adrenalectomized rats. The increase in shock threshold resulting from deoxycorticosterone at 2 mg/kg/day was less in both intact and adrenalectomized rats when chlorpromazine was also given. The decrease in threshold caused by hydrocortisone was less in adrenalectomized animals, but greater in intact animals. The combination of chlorpromazine and phenacemide (phenacetylurea), each in doses which raised shock threshold 50% in mice, was reported to be less effective than either drug alone (Feller, 1955a,b).

The effects of drugs on secondary epileptogenic lesions were studied by Morrell and Baker (1961). Previous data had shown that early surgical excision of a primary focus could prevent secondary lesions. However, since most patients are treated by drugs rather than surgery, it was of interest to determine whether chronic administration of drugs in experimental animals would delay or prevent development of these lesions. Chlorpromazine was ineffective, but phenobarbital prevented development of the lesions.

Chlorpromazine, levomepromazine, and imipramine only slightly altered cardiovascular effects and did not prolong apnea or respiratory arrest in rabbits given electroconvulsive therapy (ECT). Thus, these drugs can be used concomitantly with ECT (Piette, 1961).

The effect of chlorpromazine, along or with other agents, in human epileptics appears to be variable, some patients respond with fewer seizures, some with more, and some with no change (Meyer and Meyer-Burg, 1964; David *et al.*, 1953; Caussade *et al.*, 1954; Bonafede, 1955; Robb, 1955; Pozdnyakov, 1963).

7. Effects on Vasomotor and Respiratory Centers

Intracisternal injection of (0.2–0.5 mg/kg) of chlorpromazine in monkeys caused a fall in blood pressure and a complete suppression of the pressor reflex to carotid occlusion, although the pressor effect of epinephrine was not blocked (Dasgupta et al., 1954; Dasgupta and Werner, 1954).

A dose of 0.5 mg/kg of chlorpromazine given i.v. to anesthetized cats blocked the pressor response to sciatic nerve stimulation or to stimulation of the hypothalamic and medullary pressor areas in about half the animals. In decorticate cats, both responses were completely blocked by 50–100 μg/kg. Injection of 2 mg/kg of chlorpromazine into the lateral cerebral ventricles in dogs rapidly produced narcosis, complete muscle relaxation, loss of corneal reflex, decrease in respiratory rate and increase in amplitude, and blocking of the central vagal and carotid occlusion pressor reflexes (Cathala and Pocidalo, 1952). When 1 mg/kg of chlorpromazine was injected into the fourth ventricle, blood pressure fell progessively and respiratory arrest occurred in 3 minutes (Donnet et al., 1954).

Smaller amounts of chlorpromazine given intravenously to rabbits and dogs reduced the respiratory rate, but had only a slight effect on blood pressure. Carotid occlusion and central vagal pressor reflexes were blocked. Local application of the drug to the floor of the fourth ventricle with a cotton tampon produced similar effects of lesser intensity. Injection of 0.5 mg/kg into the vertebral artery of anesthetized dogs led to a marked transient fall in blood pressure, followed by a prolonged secondary decrease (Jourdan et al., 1955).

Chlorpromazine in intravenous doses of 0.5 mg/kg partially protected rabbits against the hypotension and respiratory arrest caused by rhinencephalic stimulation (Meidinger, 1955). Larger doses of chlorpromazine seemed to increase the lethal effects of this procedure. The decrease in hypothalamic noradrenaline resulting from injection of morphine in cats was not prevented by 25 mg/kg of chlorpromazine (Holzbauer and Vogt, 1954).

Human subjects with normal central sympathetic reactivity (Funkenstein test) showed decreased activity after 100 mg of chlorpromazine orally (Schneider, 1955). Patients who were considered to have decreased activity in control tests responded to chlorpromazine with an increase in activity. In this test, an injection of methacholine causes a drop in blood pressure which reflexly invokes a central sympathetic discharge from the hypothalamus which returns the blood pressure to its base line value.

Chlorpromazine (2 mg/kg i.m. in rabbits or cats) significantly increased cardiac contractions, decreased arterial pressure, and either increased or decreased respiratory rate (Korneva and Yakovleva, 1962). In decerebrate animals, cardiac contractions and blood pressure decreased markedly and severe respiratory depression occurred.

The mechanism of reflex respiratory arrest following intravenous administration of chlorpromazine was studied by Wellhöner et al. (1960). Intravenous administration of chlorpromazine caused a transient respiratory arrest in cats. The effect depended upon the site of administration and the dose of chlorpromazine. It was most pronounced after injection into the pulmonary artery, less pronounced after injection into the jugular or femoral artery, and no effect was noted after injection into the left pulmonary artery or bulbus aortae. Respiratory arrest was abolished by vagotomy and by cooling both vagi to 0° but not 6°C. Possible reflex action was discussed with the conclusion that pulmonary vascular chemoreceptors are involved in the reflex respiratory arrest after chlorpromazine. Similar results were also obtained with promethazine and diethazine.

Respiratory output (tidal volume) in anesthetized rabbits increased 20 to 40% after intravenous injection of chlorpromazine in doses of 0.05–2 mg/kg (Courvoisier et al., 1953). Higher doses caused temporary apnea followed by increased respiratory activity, and doses over 10 mg/kg resulted in death due to respiratory arrest.

Unanesthetized rabbits previously acclimatized to restraints showed a fall in respiratory rate from 350 to 36 per minute during 1.5 hours after 1–2 mg/kg intravenously; much of the effect was probably due to the general quieting action of the chlorpromazine (Dasgupta and Hausler, 1955a,b,c). Anesthetized and decerebrate cats responded to similar doses with transient increases in respiratory rate corresponding in time to the decreases observed in blood pressure. In anesthetized dogs, respiratory rate decreased and tidal volume increased after intravenous injection of 2–5 mg/kg of chlorpromazine (Bourgeois-Gavardin et al., 1955). The increase in respiratory volume in dogs exposed to cold was prevented by 2 or 10 mg/kg of chlorpromazine intravenously (Filk and Loeser, 1954).

Normal human subjects given approximately 1.5 mg/kg of chlorpromazine by intravenous infusion showed a slight increase in respiratory rate, a decrease in tidal volume, and occasional dyspnea (Dobkin and Gilbert, 1956; Dobkin et al., 1954a,b,c). In surgical patients premedicated with chlorpromazine, respiratory rate was unchanged and minute and tidal volumes were decreased. When chlorpromazine was given to potentiate the analgesic effect of morphine or meperidine, respiratory depression due to the narcotic was reported to be reversed; depression due to thiopental was reported to be inhibited (Reckless and Hopkin, 1954).

8. Electrode Implant Experiments

A biphasic effect of chlorpromazine after electrical stimulation of the mesodiencephalon has been reported by Bergmann and Gutman (1962).

In a study of the effects of chlorpromazine and related compounds on synaptic transmission in the dorsal hippocampus, the hippocampus was stimulated by paired brief stimuli and the amplitude of the recorded potential was determined (Liberson et al., 1962). The hippocampal-evoked potentials were increased by the drug in three cases and decreased in the other two when using LSD (cf. Olds, 1964).

9. Other Central Nervous System Effects

The release of acetylcholine from the cortex was almost completely suppressed in rabbits by 30 mg/kg of chlorpromazine and slightly depressed in human subjects by 20 mg intramuscularly (Dobkin and Gilbert, 1956). "Jumping fits" induced in mice by subcutaneous injection of cevine (sebadinine) were prevented by chlorpromazine at 5 mg/kg. Tremor and struggling after veratramine or retching movements due to proveratrine were not prevented (Tanaka, 1955).

Intra-arterial injection of 0.5–1 mg/kg of chlorpromazine caused a transient increase in action potential in the saphenous nerve in cats, followed by complete suppression of activity (Budde and Witzleb, 1955). Responses to intra-arterial acetylcholine or potassium chloride and to touching the skin were completely blocked or markedly decreased.

After administration of 2–5 mg/kg doses of chlorpromazine, complete block of all activity occurred which lasted 60 minutes. When isolated guinea pigs' accessory saphenous and sciatic nerves were exposed to solutions of chlorpromazine, the threshold for excitability was increased and amplitude of maximum response was decreased (Coraboeuf et al., 1955). Effects on the sciatic nerve were slower in appearing at pH 6.2 than at pH 7.2, while inhibition of the saphenous nerve was not affected by change in pH. Chronaxie of peripheral motor nerves of the rat was increased by chlorpromazine and chronaxie of the corresponding motor areas of the cortex was decreased (Chauchard and Chauchard, 1952a,b,c).

Spontaneous oscillations in the electrode dermagrams of neurotic human subjects were abolished after chlorpromazine, as were the responses to various stimuli (Turner et al., 1955; Clerc et al., 1955). Involuntary electromyographic activity associated with muscular tension, generalized tic, or Parkinsonian tremor were reduced or abolished. Parkinsonian tremor and rigidity and choreic hyperkinesia were reduced by chlorpromazine (Manghi, 1954).

The effects of chlorpromazine (5 mg/kg) on the electrical response of the cochlea and the electrical potential of 8th cranial nerve were observed by recording from the round window membranes of guinea pigs (Schuette and Gulick, 1961). Chlorpromazine did not produce significant losses in the cochlear or N_1 responses in anesthetized animals as long as normal body temperature was maintained, but marked losses in cochlear and N_1 responses occurred when hypothermia was produced. Recovery depended on the duration and severity of the hypothermia, and decrements in these responses were more severe when hypothermia was produced by chlorpromazine than by cold pack.

Chlorpromazine (4 mg/kg i.v.) produced an initial brief period of enhancement of positive intermediary potential of cat spinal cord. This was followed by prolonged depression. The former effect is probably associated with changes in blood pressure. The latter effect is probably due to direct action of chlorpromazine on the spinal cord (Krivoy and Kroeger, 1962).

In a study of comparative physiological features of an extinguishing inhibitor, the intensity of external inhibition (stimulation of cortex at one point leading to development of inhibition of other points) varied in animal species, increasing with degree of nervous system complexity; i.e., hens < rats < guinea pigs < dogs (Shlyafer, 1961).

Chlorpromazine-induced tremor was abolished in cats by intraventricular perfusion or injection of epinephrine, norepinephrine, chloralose, calcium, and magnesium chloride, but not by amphetamine, ephedrine, phenylephrine, or anti-parkinsonian drugs (atropine, hyoscine). Since chlorpromazine depresses body temperature, its mode of action in producing tremor is thought by the authors cited to be similar to that of pentobarbitone and cold. Both types of tremor were refractory to anti-parkinsonian drugs, which may indicate that a different mechanism is responsible for Parkinson's tremor (Domer and Feldberg, 1960).

Electrical stimulation of areas of the brain in a midline system running from the midbrain through the hypothalamus and midline thalamus and into the subcortical and cortical groups of the rhinencephalon gives rise to very pleasurable sensations in animals, exceeding those of sexual or hunger gratification. These preparations have been used to measure drug effects, and these effects vary widely with the positioning of the electrodes (Olds, 1958; Olds et al., 1956).

C. Antiemetic Effects

Chlorpromazine antagonizes the emetic effects of certain drugs, irradiation, and motion sickness in animals. Consideration of relative effectiveness against various agents and the known sites of emetic action of these agents suggests that the antiemetic effect of chlorpromazine is due primarily to depression or inhibition of the medullary chemoreceptor trigger zone. However, there appears to be some inhibitory activity on the vomiting center as well at elevated dosages.

1. Drug Induced Emesis[1]

a. *Apomorphine* (Bourgeois-Gavardin et al., 1955; Courvoisier et al., 1953; Boyd et al., 1954; Staniszewski, 1960; Freedman and Giarman, 1956).

[1]Brand et al., 1954; Cook and Toner, 1954; Glaviano and Wang, 1954.

Experiments using various combinations of doses and routes of administration have all demonstrated an excellent protective effect of chlorpromazine against apomorphine-induced emesis in dogs. Given 1 hour before 0.1 mg/kg of apomorphine subcutaneously, 1 or 2 mg/kg of chlorpromazine by the same route decreased the frequency of emesis by 82–92%, and higher doses gave complete protection.

A dose of 2–5 mg/kg of chlorpromazine orally reduced the frequency of emesis by 40 to 100%. With 0.05 mg/kg of apomorphine (i.m.) oral doses of 5 mg/kg of chlorpromazine completely prevented emesis in 87% of the dogs, and 20 mg/kg of chlorpromazine gave protection in 100%. Smaller doses of apomorphine were antagonized by proportionately smaller doses of chlorpromazine with protection lasting 3 to 72 hours, depending on the dose of chlorpromazine. The frequency of emesis was also markedly reduced when chlorpromazine was given intramuscularly after the onset of emesis.

When apomorphine was given intravenously, 3 mg/kg of chlorpromazine subcutaneously protected 77% of the dogs against 0.05 mg/kg and 23% against 0.1 mg/kg. Chlorpromazine given at a dose of 1.5 mg/kg (s.c.) raised the threshold dose of apomorphine 2 to 4 times and delayed the onset of emesis after large doses (cf. Bhargava and Chandra, 1963).

Pigeons given 25 mg/kg of apomorphine (i.m.) did not regurgitate but were ataxic and restless. When 5 mg/kg of chlorpromazine had been given 90 minutes or 3 hours previously, apomorphine produced emesis in several of the birds and ataxia was less evident (Madjerek and Stern, 1956). The antagonism of apomorphine-induced emesis in pigeons was also reported by Burkman (1961a,b; 1962a,b). Phenothiazines also inhibited the apomorphine-induced pecking syndrome in pigeons (Burkman, 1961a,b).

A method for evaluating apomorphine antagonism in rats based on prevention or inhibition of "chewing movements" has been reported by Janssen et al. (1960a). Low dose neuroleptics liable to produce Parkinson-like effects (haloperidol, thiopropazate, perphenazine, trifluperazine, prochlorperazine) had strong anti-apomorphine effects in rats, whereas moderate dose neuroleptics (triflupromazine, chlorpromazine, pipamazine, acepromazine) were reported to inhibit apomorphine-induced chewing only at dose levels producing loss of righting reflex.

A 50 mg dose of chlorpromazine gave almost complete protection to a group of human subjects against the emetic effects of 1 mg of apomorphine administered subcutaneously (Isaacs and MacArthur, 1954).

b. *Morphine.* Pretreatment with 1.5 mg/kg of chlorpromazine (s.c.) prevented emesis from 1 mg/kg of morphine sulfate (i.m.) in five of six dogs (Brand et al., 1954). On the other hand, another group (Glaviano and Wang, 1954) reported that chlorpromazine in doses of 3 mg/kg gave only slight protection against 0.5–5.0 mg/kg of morphine by the same routes of administration.

Morphine-mania in cats was partially antagonized by chlorpromazine and reserpine (Sturtevant and Drill, 1957).

c. *Other Alkaloids*. Emesis was prevented in 6 out of 6 dogs when 1.5 mg/kg of chlorpromazine was given subcutaneously before administration of 12 μg/kg of Hydergin®. Almost complete protection against 0.03 mg/kg of Hydergine was given by 3 mg/kg of chlorpromazine (s.c.).

The emetic effect of veratrum alkaloids, which have been shown to act via nodose ganglia rather than the chemoreceptor trigger zone, was not prevented by chlorpromazine, although the emetic threshold dose was slightly increased by 10 mg/kg (s.c.). A dose of 50 mg (i.m.) did not prevent emesis induced by 2 mg of veratrum alkaloids in human subjects (Isaacs and MacArthur, 1954). Emesis induced in dogs by intravenous lanatoside C was not prevented by chlorpromazine in doses up to 10 mg/kg (s.c.). The emetic effect of digitalis tincture was not prevented in pigeons (Madjerek and Stern, 1956). Emesis produced by 5-hydroxytryptophan was antagonized by 0.5 mg/kg of chlorpromazine (Cahen, 1964).

d. *Copper Sulfate*. Doses of 1.5 or 3 mg/kg of chlorpromazine (s.c.) failed to protect dogs against the emetic effect of oral or intravenous copper sulfate. Higher doses of chlorpromazine do protect against this emetic agent, indicating some activity of chlorpromazine on the vomiting center.

2. Radiation Sickness

In cats subjected to whole-body radiation to a total dose of 5500 r in about 30 minutes, chlorpromazine in doses of 3–12 mg/kg (route not specified) gave only slight protection against the resulting emesis (Borison et al., 1955). Chronic vagotomy and medullary C-T zone ablation protected only 2 of 5 animals. Similarly, chlorpromazine gave only slight protection against emesis induced by whole-body irradiation in dogs, although the onset of emesis was delayed (Chinn and Sheldon, 1954).

Bloch *et al.* (1961) report that increased response to X-irradiation occurred in 14 patients with cerebral glioblastoma multiforme, placed under mild hypothermia (31–32°C) with pethidine, promethazine, and chlorpromazine. Data from experiments in mice suggest that cerebral tissues become more sensitive to X-rays under hypothermia and that differential sensitivity, favorable to treatment, may exist between tumor and normal tissue cells.

3. Motion Sickness

Emesis resulting from motion sickness in dogs in swinging cages occurred in only 23% of those pretreated with 3 mg/kg of chlorpromazine (s.c.) and 37% of those given 5 mg/kg orally compared with 91 to 94% in untreated control groups. In contrast, diphenhydramine at 10 mg/kg orally protected only 16%, and hyoscine had no effect. Handford *et al.* (1954) reported no significant protection against human seasickness by use of chlorpromazine at 50 mg three times a day orally.

Chlorpromazine only affected the central phase of nystagmus and did not influence the slow vestibular phase of nystagmus nor compensatory eye movements in parallel swing tests in rabbits (Jongkees and Philipszoon, 1960).

D. Effects on Activity of Other Drugs

1. Central Nervous System Depressants

a. *Barbiturates.* Sleeping time of mice treated with hexobarbital was significantly prolonged by chlorpromazine in doses of 1.25 mg/kg (s.c.) and in oral doses of 2.5 mg/kg. Chlorpromazine will not only prolong the sleeping time of a hypnotic dose of hexobarbital, but it will also convert a subhypnotic dose of hexobarbital to a hypnotic dose, depending on the amount of chlorpromazine employed. The duration of hypnosis is prolonged in proportion to the dose of chlorpromazine. Maximum effects are obtained when the chlorpromazine is given 1 hour before the hexobarbital, although significant prolongation can be observed when the two agents are given simultaneously.

Although the duration of hypnosis after hexobarbital was more than doubled by 5 mg/kg of chlorpromazine (i.p.), no alteration in the rate of metabolism of the barbiturate or its concentration in brain tissue could be demonstrated (Brodie *et al.*, 1955). When chlorpromazine was given subcutaneously a $\frac{1}{2}$ hour before intravenous hexobarbital, a combination of 30 mg/kg of barbiturate and 15 mg/kg of chlorpromazine had an effect equivalent to 150 mg of hexobarbital alone in rats (Courvoisier *et al.*, 1953). Similar potentiation has also been observed in guinea pigs and dogs, as well as rabbits (Sadove *et al.*, 1956). Other investigators have reported potentiation of hexobarbital hypnosis in mice (Zipf and Alstaedter, 1954; Fink and Swinyard, 1962; Gujral *et al.*, 1956; Frommel and Fleury, 1959a,b; Aston and Cullumbine, 1960) and rats (Streicher and Garbus, 1955). The lethal dose of hexobarbital for mice was not significantly changed by pretreatment with 20 mg/kg of chlorpromazine (s.c.).

The potentiating effect of chlorpromazine appears to extend to all sedative barbiturates, as well as ethinamate (McGrath and Jenkins, 1958). In mice, doses of 2.5–5 mg/kg of chlorpromazine prolonged sleeping time after pentobarbital (van Proosdij-Hartzema, 1955; Kopera and Armitage, 1954), phenobarbital (Zipf and Alstaedter, 1954), butabarbital (Courvoisier *et al.*, 1953), barbital, thiamylal, and thiopental. In rats, doses of 10–50 mg/kg were effective in combination with thiopental, pentobarbital, and amobarbital, and 100 mg/kg of chlorpromazine moderately prolonged secobarbital sleeping time (Smith Kline and French Laboratories, 1956; Herr *et al.*, 1961).

The potentiating effect of chlorpromazine and other phenothiazines on the sedative effects of subhypnotic doses of barbiturates has been used to evaluate the behavioral effects of the former drugs (Cohen and Nelson, 1964).

There have been many speculations about the interaction of phenothiazines and barbiturates in the central nervous system. Thus, Child et al. (1960) find that pretreatment with chlorpromazine decreases the induction time of barbital anesthesia without increasing the rate of brain penetration. The data suggest that reduced induction time does not necessarily imply increased permeability of blood-brain barrier; it may have resulted from increased sensitivity of brain cells to barbital or hypothermia produced by these drugs.

On the other hand, Kátó and Chiesara (1962) reported an *increase* of pentobarbital metabolism induced in rats by chlorpromazine and other drugs, with a decrease in sleeping time. These effects occurred 24 hours after treatment and reached a maximum at 48 hours (Kato, 1960). Increased pentobarbital metabolism was also noted *in vitro*. The data suggest that the ability of these drugs to increase pentobarbital metabolism is related to their ability to act directly on liver microsomal enzymes.

Structure-activity relationships of phenothiazines in pentobarbital anesthesia in mice were related to effects of these compounds on saline-induced diuresis in rats. The release of antidiuretic hormone may be involved (Jindal et al., 1960).

b. *Anesthetics.* The subcutaneous administration of chlorpromazine in mice, rats, and guinea pigs shortened the time of onset of ether anesthesia, and its duration was considerably increased at doses of 1.25–20 mg/kg (Courvoisier et al., 1953). On the other hand, pigeons did not show this effect (Madjerek and Stern, 1956). The incidence of anesthesia in rats exposed to 80% nitrous oxide was increased by chlorpromazine at 20 mg/kg. In rats exposed to 70% nitrous oxide the incidence of anesthesia was increased by 50 mg/kg of chlorpromazine (s.c.) (cf. Carson and Domino, 1962).

c. *Ethyl Alcohol.* Chlorpromazine in doses of 0.25–10 mg/kg (s.c.) eliminated the excitement stage and significantly prolonged the hypnotic effect of intraperitoneal or oral alcohol in rats (Courvoisier et al., 1953). A similar effect was seen in mice, although the rate of alcohol metabolism was not affected (Brodie et al., 1955). The toxicity of alcohol in mice was slightly but significantly increased by doses of 0.5 mg/kg of chlorpromazine. The effects of chlorpromazine on alcohol blood levels of patients were studied by Le Breton et al. (1962; cf. Herr et al., 1961).

Chlorpromazine increased blood alcohol level above that expected after ethanol, either p.o. or i.v. in rabbits. The effect of chlorpromazine probably was related to inhibition of ethanol metabolism and only partly due to increased absorption. The hazards of alcohol ingestion together with phenothiazines have been reported (Tipton et al., 1961; Burbridge et al., 1958).

The influence of alcohol-tranquilizer combinations on choice discrimination was studied in rats. In animals trained on a choice-discrimination apparatus, it was found that alcohol is not a tranquilizer since reaction to anticipated punishment (anxiety) is effectively decreased only with corresponding decrease in performance. Pentobarbital is also not a tranquilizer for the same reason. Reserpine, meprobamate, hydroxyzine, and chlorpromazine decreased anxiety while having only minimal effect on performance, while pentobarbital with alcohol resulted in generalized depression in behavior, not tranquilization. Small quantities of alcohol with chlorpromazine did not decrease performance to as great an extent as alcohol with reserpine, meprobamate, or hydroxyzine, and alcohol decreased the capacity of tranquilizers to lower anxiety (Hughes and Rountree, 1961).

d. *Analgesics*. In mice pretreated with chlorpromazine there was a marked increase in the analgesic effects of morphine, meperidine, aspirin, salicylamide, and phenacetin (Courvoisier *et al*., 1953; Frommel and Fleury, 1959a,b; Barkov, 1961). The rate of tolerance development to morphine was not retarded by chlorpromazine in rats (Mazurkiewicz and Lu, 1960). On the other hand, Carter and David (1960) report that chlorpromazine in rats significantly decreased the rate of development of tolerance to narcotic analgetics and hastened recovery during withdrawal. With aminopyrine and chlorpromazine, similar increases in analgetic effects were noted (Kent *et al*., 1954a,b; Friebel and Reichle, 1955).

The threshold doses of morphine, meperidine, and levorphan were reduced to one-half or one-third of the control values in rats and guinea pigs (Wirth, 1954), but the toxicity of the analgetics was not altered. In determining potentiation of analgesia, methods using electrical or mechanical stimulation were more satisfactory than those using heat (Friebel and Reichle, 1955; Wirth, 1954). The duration of action of the maximally effective dose of morphine (10 mg/kg) was markedly prolonged by 10 mg/kg of chlorpromazine (Schneider, 1954). On the other hand, a different group reported that a minimally effective morphine dose (1.5 mg/kg) plus chlorpromazine at 10 mg/kg gave a lower incidence of analgesia than chlorpromazine alone (Kopera and Armitage, 1954).

In view of the variability of chlorpromazine's analgetic activity in animals, depending on the tests, these results must be viewed with reservations. In general, it may be said that chlorpromazine and related phenothiazines do not produce analgesia by the tail-pinch procedure, but seem to be uniformly effective by the hot plate technique (Eddy, 1963; Friebel and Kastner, 1955).

The clinical implications of these observations are still obscure, although there are several reports of the analgetic effects of methotrimeprazine in man by the parenteral route (Lasagna *et al*., 1963; Bloomfield, 1964). The lack of analgetic effect of methotrimeprazine in man by the oral route tends to put these results in doubt, since it is known that the phenothiazines are well absorbed orally.

The effect of chlorpromazine and reserpine on the central actions of morphine in the cat have been described by Quinn and Brodie (1961; see also Sturtevant and Drill, 1956; Loewe, 1956). Morphine-treated cats (25 mg/kg) showed CNS stimulation and a fall in brain norepinephrine; serotonin was unchanged. Chlorpromazine pretreatment (25 mg/kg in two divided doses) prevented both CNS stimulation and the fall in norepinephrine. Cats were sedated and showed miosis, ptosis, and relaxation of nictitating membrane. Morphine had no effect on brain epinephrine in rabbits. Reserpine-pretreated cats, however, behaved differently. The effects of reserpine were reversed almost immediately by morphine, and animals showed spontaneous motor activity instead of sedation and muscular rigidity. The authors concluded that the CNS action of morphine is not mediated through norepinephrine liberated in brain.

2. Sympathomimetic Amines

The centrally acting phenothiazines like chlorpromazine were found by Fink and Swinyard (1962) to decrease amphetamine toxicity (cf. Hardinge, 1964; Taylor and Winters, 1964). The pressor amine nylidrin (Arlidin®) has been reported to potentiate the activity of chlorpromazine (Lehmann, 1964). The weight reducing properties of phenmetrazine were reported to be antagonized by chlorpromazine (Reid, 1964).

A study was done in rats by Stein and Seifter (1961) to support the theory that drugs which are effective against agitation inhibit, whereas those effective in depression enhance, reward (self-stimulation) activity. Imipramine, 5–15 mg/kg, augmented and prolonged d-methamphetamine-induced self stimulation; in contrast, chlorpromazine antagonized both methamphetamine-induced self stimulation and also the augmenting effect of imipramine on the same stimulation. The authors concluded that imipramine has a sensitizing effect on central adrenergic synapses. It should be noted, however, that chlorpromazine seemed to act in some indirect manner (since amphetamine was required for the action), rather than through direct stimulation.

Phenoxybenzamine, chlorpromazine, and guanethidine inhibited the action of butyrylcholine and tyramine on the isolated atrium, and they potentiated the action of norepinephrine on isolated guinea pig atrium. Phenoxybenzamine and cocaine abolished parasympathetic and potentiated the sympathetic effects of vagus stimulation in the same preparation (Benfey and Greeff, 1961).

Chlorpromazine reversed the hypertensive effect of epinephrine in anesthetized dogs. This effect was counteracted by vasopressin and purified oxytocin (Hazard *et al.*, 1961). Raevsky (1957) has reported that chlorpromazine inhibits the development of experimental toxic edema of the lungs produced by adrenaline.

3. Hallucinogenic Agents

Chlorpromazine has been found by Elder and Dille (1962) and by Schwarz *et al.* (1955) to antagonize the behavioral effects of LSD, although it inhibits the metabolism of it (Axelrod *et al.*, 1956). Ray and Marrazzi (1961) have studied quantitative relationships of LSD and chlorpromazine effects. LSD-25, in doses (0.10 mg/kg) small enough to be devoid of gross effect, increased response latency in rats to a tone indicating the availability of water reward. This effect was greatly reduced by chlorpromazine in doses (0.30 mg/kg) that *per se* did not affect performance. On the other hand, larger but nondepressant doses (1 mg/kg i.p.) of chlorpromazine increased rather than reduced LSD-25 inhibition, whereas still larger doses produced depression of approach behaviour.

Doses of LSD sufficient to dilate pupils, but producing no other physiological effect (25 μg) could be recognized by human subjects (Murphree, 1962). Recognition of the threshold dose could be blocked by 25 mg of chlorpromazine or 10 mg of phenoxybenzamine if given 30 minutes before the LSD.

The effects of chlorpromazine and lysergic acid diethylamide on the arousal response were reported by Key (1961a,b, 1965). Chloropromazine (5 or 10 mg/kg i.p.) increased the intensity of stimulation necessary to elicit arousal response in cats with permanently implanted electrodes. After LSD (10–15 μg/kg i.p.), presentation of an auditory stimulus was followed by abrupt arousal and long-lasting periods of alerting. The data with chlorpromazine suggest that the effect on sensory-induced arousal is not produced solely by an increased rate of negative learning; there appears to be a decrease in significance attached to novel tone.

An extensive study of the effects of mescaline on total amino acids, cholesterol blood glucose, leukocytes, differential count, eosinophils, sedimentation rate, cephalin cholesterol flocculation, bilirubin, and thymol turbidity was made by Denber (1961) in acute and chronic psychotic females. Mescaline decreased total amino acids and eosinophils and increased blood glucose and leukocytes within 1 hour. Chlorpromazine or trifluoperazine reversed the effect on blood glucose but did not affect the fall in amino acids or eosinophils. However, chlorpromazine and trifluoperazine caused a sharp increase in amino acids in patients who received saline instead of mescaline. The data suggest a positive correlation between biochemical changes and behavioral improvement. Delay *et al.* (1956) and Sturtevant and Drill (1956) reported that chlorpromazine considerably reduced the hypertension and hyperpnea produced by mescaline. The catatonia produced by bulbocapnine is potentiated by chlorpromazine (Sergio and Alemà, 1957; Zetler and Moog, 1958).

4. OTHER DRUGS

Chlorpromazine antagonized the EEG alerting produced by cholinergic agents, especially eserine salicylate and acetylcholine in rabbits (Steiner and Himwich, 1962). Cholinesterase inhibitors potentiated the behavioral effects of chlorpromazine (Goldberg and Johnson, 1964).

Chlorpromazine has been used to reverse the effects of iproniazid in patients (Clement and Benazon, 1962; see also Franco-Browder et al., 1958; Chessin et al., 1957; Ehringer et al., 1960; Axelrod, 1961; Axelrod et al., 1961a,b).

A decrease in the hypoglycemic action of antidiabetic compounds by neuroleptics was observed by Opitz and Loeser (1962). Both chlorpromazine and chlorprothixene reduced the hypoglycemic action of sulfonylureas and insulin in rats. Costa et al. (1960) and Camanni et al. (1959) have reported on the antagonism of reserpine effects by chlorpromazine in the rat. Chlorpromazine antagonized the accumulation of brain serotonin produced by tranylcypromine (Morpurgo, 1962). Pletscher and Gey (1962) found that imipramine and amitriptylene were less potent than chlorpromazine or chlordiazepoxide in antagonizing the serotonin increase produced by iproniazid, or the serotonin increase produced by reserpine (cf. Gey and Pletscher, 1962).

A study of the interaction of nicotinamide with chlorpromazine in the mouse showed that nicotinamide alone reduced spontaneous motor activity in mice, whereas chlorpromazine (10 mg/kg) reduced, and chlorpromazine plus nicotinamide completely inhibited, activity. Nicotinamide alone had little effect on pentobarbital anesthesia but did potentiate the effect of chlorpromazine and reserpine on pentobarbital anesthesia (Burton et al., 1960b).

The DNP (diphosphopyridine nucleotide) content in murine liver, elevated by nicotinamide administration, usually returns to control values quickly. However, reserpine or tranquilizing phenothiazines (chlorpromazine, prochlorperazine, etc.) maintained and further increased the DPN levels. Non-tranquilizing phenothiazines (promethazine) and sedatives (meprobamate, phenobarbital) did not have this effect. The data are said to indicate a positive correlation between tranquilizing ability and maintenance of increased DPN levels. Chlorpromazine may interfere with the formation of nicotinamide metabolites (Burton et al., 1960a).

Yohimbine (0.1 mg/kg/min) for 5 minutes i.v., produced psychic and autonomic changes resembling anxiety in man. Both reserpine and amobarbital reduced psychic and autonomic effects, while atropine decreased pressor response to yohimbine. Chlorpromazine acted paradoxically, i.e., it potentiated both psychic and autonomic effects of yohimbine. This suggests that in the combination, yohimbine does not exert its usual alpha-adrenergic blocking action, but it may produce these reactions by central stimulation of the autonomic nervous system (Ingram, 1962).

Tremors induced by tremorine (1,4-di-1-pyrrolidinyl-2-butyne) were effectively antagonized by various agents including scopolamine, atropine, benactyzine, chlorpromazine, and caramiphen. Benactyzine, atropine, and scopolamine antagonized a decrease in skin and rectal temperature induced by tremorine, whereas physostigmine had no effect and chlorpromazine had slightly additive effect. Chlorpromazine inhibited tremorine-induced analgesia in mice. The data indicate that the analgesic mechanism of tremorine differs from that of morphine (Keranen et al., 1961; Lenke, 1961).

The effects of tranquilizing drugs on the pharmacological actions of diethyltryptamine were described by Pfeiffer et al. (1961). Diethyltryptamine increased the latency time of pain reaction, as measured by the hot plate method in mice. This reaction time was inhibited by reserpine, decreased by meprobamate, and unaffected by chlorpromazine. It was increased by iproniazid and azacyclonol. Diethyltryptamine decreased both spontaneous motor activity and mescaline-induced excitation. The effects were reversed by amphetamine (5 mg/kg) and combined administration resulted in sedative action. The diethyltryptamine-induced decrease in spontaneous activity was inhibited by reserpine, chlorpromazine, and iproniazid.

Chlorpromazine was reported not to enhance the renal toxicity of edathamil disodium (a chelating agent, ethylenediaminetetracetic acid calcium disodium salt) in rats (Altman et al., 1962).

The antagonism of chlorpromazine by β-melanocyte stimulating hormone (β-MSH) has been reported (Krivoy and Guillemin, 1962). Chlorpromazine (4–10 mg/kg) inhibited the positive intermediary potential of the spinal cord in decerebrate and decerebrate-spinal cats. β-MSH (0.14–0.25 mg/kg) antagonized chlorpromazine and restored the positive intermediary potential to normal. There were no changes in blood pressure or respiration.

Histamine catabolism during treatment with chlorpromazine was studied by Johansson et al. (1961). Chlorpromazine (600 and 750 mg) did not affect catabolism of labeled histamine in two psychiatric patients. These doses were twice those required for therapeutic improvement.

Chlorpromazine decreased the Indoklon® (hexafluorodiethyl ether) threshold for clonic, but not tonic, convulsions in rats. Prior treatment with iproniazid markedly increased the clonic threshold. The data suggest that iproniazid, by increasing brain concentrations of serotonin and other amines, may stabilize the cortex against seizures (Truitt and Ebersberger, 1960).

Von Ledebur et al. (1962) and Frommel et al. (1963) have reported that nalorphine antagonized some of the CNS effects of chlorpromazine, meprobamate, and chlordiazepoxide. This antagonism by nalorphine of compounds which bear no structural or pharmacological resemblance to morphine may require some revision of analgetic-antagonist theories.

Levine and Klein (1959) have reported that cyanide intoxication is antagonized by chlorpromazine in rodents. The protective effect is thought to be due to the hypothermia induced.

The duration of paralysis produced by mephenesin in mice and rats was markedly prolonged by chlorpromazine in doses of 5–10 mg/kg (s.c.). The LD_{50} of mephenesin was slightly decreased by the same dose of chlorpromazine (Courvoisier et al., 1953).

In rats subjected to supramaximal electroshock, the anticonvulsant effect of diphenylhydantoin was increased by pretreatment with chlorpromazine at 20 mg/kg (s.c.) (Bertrand et al., 1954). The anticonvulsant ED_{50} for diphenylhydantoin alone was approximately 35.5 mg/kg; after chlorpromazine it was approximately 22 mg/kg.

The average lethal dose of digitalis tincture in guinea pigs was reduced from 1.31 ml/kg to 1.01 ml/kg by administration of 6–10 mg/kg of chlorpromazine 2 hours before testing (Madjerek and Stern, 1956).

The addition of chlorpromazine potentiated the effect of dihydroergotamine in the isolated virgin guinea pig uterus (Torres-Acero Fernandez and De La Pena Regidor, 1955).

Aronsen et al. (1957) have shown that in the isolated phrenic-nerve-diaphragm preparation of the golden hamster, chlorpromazine had a prolonging effect on the action of succinyl choline (see Section IV, K and cf. Kotkin et al., 1956).

Preoperative administration of chlorpromazine has been reported to increase the effectiveness of the preoperative sedatives, reduce the amount of anesthetic and relaxant agents required, and decrease the need for postoperative analgesics (Vandewater and Gordon, 1955; Lear et al., 1955; Boulton, 1955; Stephen et al., 1955, and others).

The duration of spinal and local anesthesia was increased by chlorpromazine (Lipton and Hershey, 1955; Elo and Turunen, 1955). The amount of narcotic and anesthetic agents required during labor was decreased (Handford et al., 1954; Browne and Mannion, 1955; Arnold, 1955; Davies, 1955; Brodie, 1955); best results were obtained if chlorpromazine was not started until labor was well established.

In the control of severe pain from terminal cancer, chlorpromazine increased the effectiveness of narcotics and permitted reduction of doses (Sadove et al., 1954; Sadove and Balagot, 1955; Litteral, 1955). The effectiveness of mephenesin in controlling the spasms of tetanus was increased and prolonged by administration of chlorpromazine (Houde and Wallenstein, 1955); required doses varied greatly from patient to patient. No definite increase in the anticonvulsant action of phenobarbital was noted in epileptics when chlorpromazine was given (Bonafede, 1955). With chlorpromazine and reduced dosage of phenobarbital, some patients responded with increased seizure frequency and some with no change; it is possible that in the latter group the previous doses of the barbiturate had been higher than necessary to control seizures.

E. Effects on Body Temperature

Chlorpromazine lowers body temperature in various laboratory animals, the extent of the change depending on room temperature and chlorpromazine dose. This hypothermic action was initially attributed to inhibition of central thermoregulation, with resulting increased heat loss, and muscular relaxation, with decreased heat production. Later speculation involved effects on catecholamines (Johnson, 1964). In mice kept at 25°C, 2 mg/kg of chlorpromazine subcutaneously produced an average minimum temperature of 32.8°C, 5 mg/kg a minimum of 31.9°C, and 10 mg/kg a minimum of 30.2°C (Courvoisier *et al.*, 1953; Laborit and Huguenard, 1951; Laborit *et al.*, 1952a,b). With the higher doses, temperatures remained below normal for over 24 hours. The hypothermic effect in dogs was less marked.

In another study in mice, the average maximum decrease in body temperature after 1 mg/kg was 3°C; after 3 mg/kg it was 5.7° (Kopera and Armitage, 1954). When the high dose of 50 mg/kg was given intraperitoneally to mice kept at a room temperature of 27°C, body temperature fell to a low of 23.1°C within an hour and then gradually rose to normal (Dawson and Hiestand, 1955). The same dose given to mice kept at 3°C reduced body temperature to an average of 11.7°C in $1\frac{1}{2}$ hours. As noted elsewhere, the beneficial effect of chloropromazine in mice infected with *Trypanosoma* was attributed to the decrease in body temperature (Friebel and Kastner, 1955). With doses of 20 or 30 mg/kg, body temperature depended on ambient temperature, increasing slightly in a warm room and falling to 17.6°C after 6 hours exposure to 10°C. After single doses of chlorpromazine, body temperature effects in rats were about the same as those in mice, again depending on room temperature (Dawson and Hiestand, 1955; Giaja and Markovic-Giaja, 1954). Doses of 2.5 mg. every 5 hours maintained body temperature at 25°C in small rats and 32°C in large ones; small animals showed a further decrease if exposed to cold (Schaumkell, 1955a,b,c). With 5 mg every 24 hours, temperature fell after each dose and returned to near normal before the next one (Maier *et al.*, 1955a,b). (Compare Sharma and Arora, 1961.)

When exposed to air temperatures of 45° or 55°C, chlorpromazine-treated rats reached a lethal temperature of 45° more rapidly than did untreated controls (Binet and Decaud, 1954). In a cold room, if body temperature was maintained at 23° by means of a rectal thermostat controlling a heat lamp, rats treated with chlorpromazine survived more than twice as long as did controls (Maier *et al.*, 1955a,b).

Mice at 4°C given chlorpromazine (2 or 5 mg/kg) had a considerably higher mortality rate than untreated mice at the same temperature (van Proosdij-Hartzema, 1955). When exposed to 39°C for 30 minutes, mice given 2 mg/kg had a lower 24-hour mortality than controls, but with 5 or 10 mg/kg, mortality rates were higher both at 30 minutes and at 24 hours.

In anesthetized dogs covered with ice bags, 2 mg/kg of chlorpromazine intramuscularly prevented shivering and lowered body temperature by 10°C, compared to 5.4° in dogs not given chlorpromazine (Dundee et al., 1954). Hypothermia was potentiated by barbiturates (Tanche and Klepping, 1955). Pigeons given 7.8–10 mg/kg showed little change in cloacal temperature; double doses produced a maximum fall of 1.4°C (Madjerek and Stern, 1956). In rabbits, 1.2 or 2.5 mg/kg decreased temperatures about 2°C, and 5 mg/kg approximately 3°C (Cheymol and Levassort, 1955). Pyrexia caused by dinitrophenol (Cheymol and Levassort, 1955) was not prevented by chlorpromazine.

Hypothermia was induced by chlorpromazine in rats, hamsters, etc. by Hoffman and Zarrow (1958; cf. Söderberg, 1956; LeBlanc, 1958a–d; Hoffman, 1959; Jackson et al., 1959; Shemano and Nickerson, 1958; Witherspoon et al., 1957; Lessin and Parkes, 1957; Moyer et al., 1957; Terzioğlu and Özer, 1956; Brendel and L'Allemand, 1955; Castaigne, 1954).

Fenters and Jeter (1961) reported on the effect of variation in body temperature on antibody production in rabbits and mice. Chlorpromazine, 5 mg/kg i.m. at 12-hour intervals or intra-abdominally, alone or with refrigeration, depressed body temperature of control rabbits and those immunized with bovine serum albumin or mice immunized with *Diplococcus pneumoniae* vaccine. Pyrogen treatment increased temperature. However, alterations in body temperature had no effect on antibody production in immunized animals.

Hypothermia, induced by 48/80 (a histamine releaser) in rats, appears to be due to liberation of histamine and serotonin from ruptured mast cells; it is antagonized by mepyramine and LSD without preventing rupture of mast cells (Jamieson and Van Den Brenk, 1961). However, hypothermia produced by phenothiazines, including chlorpromazine, trifluoperazine, and trimeprazine, is associated with release of serotonin in the CNS. Because hypothermia is not antagonized by mepyramine, hypothermia can be dissociated from histamine release. The hypothermic, but not the mast cell-disrupting, activity of chlorpromazine can be abolished by LSD. The peripheral serotonin antagonists, BOL (bromolysergic acid diethylamide) and UML 491 (1-methyl-*d*-lysergic acid butanolamide tartrate), do not reduce chlorpromazine-induced hypothermia.

Human subjects given ordinary doses of chlorpromazine show inconsistent temperature effects. When lightly anesthetized patients were given 50 mg intravenously and 100 mg intramuscularly, reinforced by doses of 50 mg intramuscularly every hour or two, body temperature was maintained at 92–94° F for long periods (Ripstein et al., 1954).

The antagonistic effect of cold acclimatization on chlorpromazine hypothermia is reported to be associated with increased sensitization of tissues to adrenaline and noradrenaline (LeBlanc, 1958a–d). The acute toxicity of chlorpromazine in mice has been found to be eighteen times higher at a room temperature of 4° than at 30°C (Dandiya et al., 1960). This may be due to vasodilatation and associated phenomena.

LeBlanc and Rosenberg (1958) found that N-(2-chloroethyl)dibenzylamine and tripelennamine markedly potentiated the hypothermic effects of chlorpromazine (cf. Maickel et al., 1964). Kollias and Bullard (1964) concluded that chlorpromazine affected mechanisms of temperature regulation under conditions of both hyperthermia and hypothermia.

F. Metabolic Effects of Chlorpromazine

There are many components of the body whose levels are influenced by the administration of phenothiazines. Some of these, like serotonin, and catecholamines, are discussed in Chapter 3 of this volume. Many of these chemical changes have been postulated as being responsible for tranquilizing actions, including depletion of epinephrine and its precursors, increased oxidation of epinephrine, chelation of epinephrine, combination with indoles, and competitive inhibition of indoles (Altschule, 1960).

The metabolic effects of psychotropic drugs were studied by Opitz (1962a,b,c). In these studies, the compounds employed were chlorpromazine, chlorpromazine sulfoxide, chlorprothixene, chlorprothixene sulfoxide, promazine, N-N-dimethylaminopropylphenoxazine, prothipendyl, imipramine, captodiamine, reserpine, and meprobamate. The normal increase in respiratory rate following a rapid lowering of room temperature from 29° to 19°C was inhibited by chlorpromazine and other drugs.

Experiments performed on rats kept without food and subsequently fed with glucose showed a considerable increase of hepatic glycogen production following chlorpromazine and other drugs. These were also found to stimulate production of glucose. Rats under the influence of drugs showed marked hyperglycemic effects, and these effects were also evident following removal of the adrenal cortex. Marked stimulation of the adrenal cortical hormone production was observed after chlorpromazine. The glucose uptake of epididymal fat tissue *in vitro* was considerably reduced by chlorpromazine.

1. Effects on Oxygen Consumption in Intact Animals

Rats given single subcutaneous or oral doses of chlorpromazine from 10–50 mg/kg usually showed little change or a slight decrease in oxygen consumption (Courvoisier et al., 1953; Giaja and Markovic-Giaja, 1954; Filk et al., 1954; Boyd et al., 1955; Filk and Loeser, 1954; Feller, 1955a,b; Hadnagy et al.,

1958), which appeared to be in proportion to the decrease in body temperature. After administration of 20 mg/kg/day for 25 or 36 days, or of doses gradually increased to 180 mg/kg/day, this metabolic effect had disappeared. No antagonism to the metabolic effects of thyroxine was found (Feller, 1955a,b; Filk et al., 1954; Boyd et al., 1955; Filk and Loeser, 1954) when the differences due to change in body temperature were taken into consideration, nor were the effects of dinitrophenol (Feller, 1955a,b; Popovic, 1954) or adrenaline (Popovic, 1954) antagonized even at low body temperatures. Further evidence that the changes in oxygen consumption were due to changes in body temperature is found in cold-room studies (Courvoisier et al., 1953; Giaja and Markovic-Giaja, 1954; Popovic, 1954). When chlorpromazine-treated rats were placed in room temperatures between 0° and 17°C, oxygen consumption increased nearly as much as in untreated animals for the first hour or so, and then decreased as body temperatures fell, reaching control levels or below at the time of maximum temperature decreases. Dogs have shown similar effects, namely, little change in metabolic rate at normal room temperatures, and an increase equal to that of untreated animals when exposed to cold (Bourgeois-Gavardin et al., 1955; Giaja and Markovic-Giaja, 1954).

In human subjects, basal metabolic rate changed little after chlorpromazine doses up to 2 mg/kg (Dobkin et al., 1954a,b,c; Dobkin and Gilbert, 1956).

Similarly, cerebral oxygen consumption was not changed by chlorpromazine in intravenous or intramuscular doses of 50–300 mg, unless the blood pressure dropped considerably (Morris et al., 1955; Fazekas et al., 1955). Anesthetized dogs also showed no change in cerebral oxygen consumption after 2–10 mg/kg of chlorpromazine parenterally. Resistance to hypoxia or anoxia may be increased or decreased by chlorpromazine. Survival time of mice exposed to atmospheric pressure of 180 mm Hg was increased by pretreatment with chlorpromazine or other agents which decreased body temperature (Flacke et al., 1953); use of a warm chamber prevented this increase. Mice submerged in water at 37.5°C survived nearly twice as long if pretreated with chlorpromazine 50 mg/kg (Dawson and Hiestand, 1955). Heyck (1962) has reported on the effect of long therapy with high doses of phenothiazines on brain metabolism in various age groups.

A study was made of prolonged administration of high doses of phenothiazines (chlorpromazine, chlorprothixene, levomepromazine, and others) in mental patients of various ages without organic brain disease. Neither cerebral circulation nor metabolism were affected by phenothiazines in young patients. In older patients (over 50 years), significant changes were noted. There was marked decrease in oxygen consumption and less pronounced decrease in glucose uptake. There was only a slight decrease in cerebral circulation. The authors concluded that age-dependent response was due to different adaptive ability of brain to the chemical effects of phenothiazines.

2. Blood Sugar, Electrolytes, etc.

Mice given 5 mg/kg of chlorpromazine intraperitoneally showed a progressive rise in blood sugar which reached approximately twice the control level at 3 hours and then gradually fell to near normal at 5 hours after injection (Norman and Hiestand, 1955a,b). The hyperglycemic effect was considerably less in hamsters and absent in rats. In alloxan-diabetic mice, chlorpromazine increased the severity of diabetes and markedly shortened survival time. Normal mice were protected against the lethal effect of insulin (one-sixth unit/18 gm) and partially protected against its convulsant effect. In rabbits, 2.5–5 mg caused some increase in blood sugar and did not block the hyperglycemic effect of epinephrine (Courvoisier et al., 1953). Dogs showed little change in blood sugar after chlorpromazine 20 mg/kg intravenously, this dose given 15 minutes before alloxan prevented the development of diabetes (Simoes and Osswald, 1955).

Insulin potentiates the hypothermia and prolonged hexobarbital sleeping time normally caused by chlorpromazine; chlorpromazine does not potentiate the hypoglycemic effects of insulin (LeBlanc, 1960a).

Human subjects given 25–50 mg of chlorpromazine intramuscularly or 1.5 mg/kg intravenously showed a slight tendency to increased blood sugar 1 hour later (Dobkin et al., 1954a,b,c; Celice et al., 1955; Gupta et al., 1960). When 50 mg was given intravenously immediately after 50 gm of glucose orally there was a prolonged delay in return to normal blood sugar levels (Chartan and Bartlett, 1955). No change was noted in the response to intravenous insulin of patients pretreated with chlorpromazine (Lancaster and Jones, 1954), and no change in the hyperglycemic response to surgical stress was observed (Azima and Richman, 1956). Little change was observed in plasma electrolytes in human subjects given single or repeated doses of chlorpromazine (Dobkin et al., 1954a,b,c; Bruscha, 1954). Patients who developed extrapyramidal symptoms showed a progressive increase in plasma copper levels; other patients showed a lesser tendency to increased levels (Azima and Richman, 1956).

Serum total proteins were unchanged in patients undergoing chlorpromazine therapy (Rizzo and Russo, 1953; Mars and Morpurgo, 1955; Trigos and McCullough, 1955; Conqvist et al., 1955); serum globulin tended to be increased and albumin decreased. Electrophoretic study of serum proteins in nine patients showed a double β-globulin peak in all of them (Trigos and McCullough, 1955). Such a "beta-split" has been reported in various states involving tissue damage (infectious disease, acute rheumatism); its significance in relation to chlorpromazine is uncertain.

There is one report that administration of chlorpromazine to two patients with essential hyperlipemia caused marked clearing of serum and a decrease in total blood lipids and most lipid fractions (Hollister and Kanter, 1955).

It was suggested that this effect may be related to changes in liver function, especially since one of the patients developed jaundice during therapy.

3. Effect on Isolated Tissues

a. *Brain*. Chlorpromazine, in mouse brain homogenates, protected them against autooxidation and aging of tissues. On the other hand, compounds devoid of antioxidant action, such as barbiturates, facilitate mitochondrial shrinking and autooxidation (Eberhard *et al*., 1961).

The effect of chlorpromazine, ether, and phenobarbital on the active-phosphate level of rat brain was studied by Minard and Davis (1962). Using an improved extraction technique which prevents degradation of nucleotides during isolation, the authors report, in contrast to published data, that chlorpromazine, ether, and phenobarbital do not increase ATP (adenosine triphosphate) in rat brain. Phosphocreatine was increased slightly by ether and decreased slightly by chlorpromazine and phenobarbital. The reason for the slower degradation of ATP is unknown but is probably owing to, in fact, the depressed body temperature. Chlorpromazine (10–60 mg/kg) increased incorporation of acetate-C^{14} into the brain ATP of rats; reserpine at 2.5 mg/kg decreased it. The data indicate that chlorpromazine and reserpine influence the rate of synthesis of the purine skeleton from simpler precursors, such as acetate (Albaum and Milch, 1962).

A comparison of the action of triethyltin with other drugs on creatine phosphate levels in rat brain and diaphragm preparations was made by Cremer (1961). In presence of triethyltin and chlorpromazine, creatine phosphate synthesis was inhibited to greater extent than oxygen uptake, and creatine leaked from the brain slice into the medium. Chlorpromazine, but not triethyltin, inhibited creatine phosphate synthesis, but did not cause creatine leakage in diaphragm segments. Thus, chlorpromazine does not share the selective effect on nervous tissue shown by triethyltin.

Jóhannesson and Lausen (1961) studied the *in vitro* effect of chlorpromazine on brain cholinesterase. They found that chlorpromazine at 200 μg/g inhibited cholinesterase activity in brain tissue from an infant. The authors concluded that excitation seen as side effect of chlorpromazine (parodoxical action) is due to its inhibition of cholinesterase.

Oxygen uptake by slices of rat brain cortex showed no change during the first $\frac{1}{2}$ hour after the addition of 20–250 mg/l of chlorpromazine, remained steady for the next $\frac{1}{2}$ hour and then decreased in proportion to the concentration of chlorpromazine (Peruzzo and Forni, 1953a,b). Brains from rats given 5 mg of chlorpromazine 90 minutes before sacrifice also showed a decrease in respiratory rate. Slices incubated at 37°C had a respiratory rate about 57% less than slices from untreated controls tested at the same temperature, or about the same as slices from untreated animals incubated at

30°C. Respiration of guinea pig brain slices was reduced about 21% by 175 mg/l of chlorpromazine and about 63% by 700 mg/l (Courvoisier et al., 1953). Slices from the frontal lobe of mouse brains showed a significant decrease in oxygen consumption when incubated in 10^{-7} M chlorpromazine at 37.5°C, and whole brain homogenates in 10^{-6} M solution at concentrations considerably lower than those used in the experiments mentioned previously (Ganshirt and Brilmayer, 1954). At lower temperatures, the depressant effects of chlorpromazine and temperature appeared to be additive. The oxygen uptake of cat heart and brain slices was significantly decreased by chlorpromazine in a concentration of 10–20 mg/100 ml (Finkelstein et al., 1954a,b).

Rat brain mitochondria showed a decrease in oxygen uptake and phosphorylation when incubated in a solution containing chlorpromazine at 2×10^{-5} M, and complete inhibition of both at 2×10^{-4} (Abood, 1955). Cytochrome oxidase activity was reduced by 50% at a concentration of 5×10^{-5} M, and ATPase activity was decreased 31% at 10^{-4} M. In rats treated with high doses of chlorpromazine, the greatest effect was noted in the region of the basal ganglia. Brain tissue from rats given 10 or 50 mg/kg of chlorpromazine 30 minutes before sacrifice showed accumulation of ATP during incubation, which was greatest in the midbrain (Grenell et al., 1955). A concentration of 10^{-3} M completely inhibited aerobic and anaerobic glycolysis, oxygen and phosphate uptake, and pyruvate oxidation, partially inhibited succinate oxidation, and had no effect on citrate synthesis in brain homogenates (Bernsohn et al., 1955; Quastel, 1962; Laborit et al., 1962).

Chlorpromazine inhibited cytochrome oxidase in rat brain homogenates, liver mitochondria, and other tissue preparations (Yamamoto et al., 1960). This inhibition was reversed by dialysis of chlorpromazine with the enzyme preparation; it was decreased by ferric chloride but not glutathione. Chlorpromazine inhibited catalase but not homogentisic acid oxidase or ascorbic acid oxidase.

The oxidative activity of the rat cerebrum was enhanced by LSD, MAO inhibitors, phenothiazines, and reserpine. It was decreased by meprobamate. Chlorpromazine had slight decreasing effect (Siva Sankar, 1961). The oxidative activity of rat cerebellum was decreased by LSD, meprobamate, chlorpromazine, and reserpine. It was enhanced by MAO inhibitors. LSD enhanced the effect of tranquilizers but decreased the effects of MAO inhibitors (cf. Aghajanian, 1963).

Glende and Cornatzer (1963) found that chlorpromazine and other phenothiazines inhibited the uptake of S^{35} into the sulfolipids of rat brain. The incorporation of galactose-1-C^{14} was also inhibited, as was the incorporation of P^{32} into the phospholipids (Magee and Rossiter, 1963). Histamine levels in the brain were reported to be increased by chlorpromazine (Adam and Hye, 1964). Brain transaminases are also reported to be increased (Suva, 1964).

b. *Liver.* Histochemical examination of livers from rats given 15 mg/kg of chlorpromazine subcutaneously and fasted for 24 hours showed little difference in glycogen content and distribution from control-fasted animals (Cosnier and Drouin, 1954). In control animals, fat was abundant in some cells, not localized within the cells, and showed little change with time. In treated rats, fat was localized at the vascular pole of cells, mostly in the periportal zones. After egg white feeding, livers of chlorpromazine-treated animals showed an abundance of fat droplets marginally distributed in all cells, while livers of untreated rats had little fat. After a fat meal, the picture in treated rats was similar to protein-fed chlorpromazine rats; untreated controls showed more fat than on other diets but still less than treated animals. Liver non-protein sulfhydryl was decreased in rats lightly anesthetized with chlorpromazine and other agents; barbiturate-anesthetized rats, but not chlorpromazine treated, showed a further decrease when exposed to cold (Bartlett and Register, 1955).

It has been reported that prolonged administration of chlorpromazine decreased biliary excretion of bromosulfophthalein, probably by direct effect on secretory function of the liver cell (Clodi and Schnack, 1960). The metabolic effects of tranquilizers and hypophysectomy was studied by Greengard and Quinn (1962). Nicotinamide (500 mg/kg) increased DPN levels in liver of normal, hypophysectomized, or adrenalectomized rats. The increase in hypophysectomized rats was greater than that in adrenalectomized rats and was ten times higher than that in normal rats. The increase in DPN levels in nicotinamide-treated rats was prolonged by prior administration of chlorpromazine (50 mg/kg) or reserpine (10 mg/kg). Cold-stress (4°C) abolished sedation and elevated DPN levels in reserpine-treated but not in chlorpromazine-treated rats.

Chlorpromazine significantly inhibited various types of mitochondrial swelling in rat brain and liver preparations. The effects were noted at concentrations as low as 10^{-6} M for brain using Triton® as the swelling agent, or at 10^{-7} M for liver with thyroxine as the swelling agent. The concentrations of chlorpromazine were less than those necessary to produce changes in enzyme activities or oxidative phosphorylation; thus, chlorpromazine changes membrane permeability (Spirtes and Guth, 1961, 1963; Smith, 1964).

Chlorpromazine has been found to reduce the rate of cholesterol turnover in pigeon liver, and to diminish cholesterol levels considerably (Yakubovskaya and Kiseleva, 1961). The action of antihistamine drugs *in vitro* on mitochondrial swelling has been studied by Judah (1961). Chlorpromazine, 10^{-4} M, in the presence of calcium ions, markedly reduced mitochondrial swelling. All antihistaminics inhibited water movements in mitochondria but did not alter respiratory metabolism; agents which reduced mitochondrial swelling preserved levels of phosphoprotein, those which inhibited reversal of swelling prevented protein phosphorylation.

Prolonged treatment with chlorpromazine was reported to cause weight gains and an increase in C^{14} incorporation from acetate in the fatty acids, especially in the liver (Christensen and Wase, 1960).

Chlorpromazine was reported to inhibit endogenous respiration of mouse and hamster liver slices, whereas no inhibition was seen in rat and guinea pig liver slices at the same levels of the drug (10^{-3} M) (Moraczewski and DuBois, 1959).

The effects of chlorpromazine on liver hemodynamics have been studied by a number of investigators (Plaa et al., 1960; Bianchi and Craig, 1960; Freund and Levine, 1958; Hadnagy et al., 1958; Hall and Ryman, 1958; Danhof, 1958; Scholz and Kretzschmar, 1956, 1958; Peters, 1956; Popper et al., 1957). The general conclusions were that chlorpromazine caused a decrease in hepatic blood flow and an increase in biliary viscosity and intrabiliary pressure. There was an absence of cellular damage, and choleretics may have been protective. In cats, there was no effect on the rate of secretion of bile or on the biliary sphincter mechanism (Hall and Ryman, 1958). There is no increased sensitivity to hepatotoxic substances or infectious hepatitis (Peters, 1956) except in the case of ethionine damage (Popper et al., 1957). Thioctic acid has been reported to exert a protective effect against chlorpromazine effects on the liver (Ritschel, 1959).

c. *Blood.* The effect of some phenothiazine derivatives on the hemolysis of red blood cells *in vitro* was studied by Freeman and Spirtes (1963). The compounds studied in human and dog erythrocytes were chlorpromazine, chlorpromazine sulfoxide, promazine, prochlorperazine, and promethazine. Chlorpromazine caused the greatest increase in hemolysis time; prochlorperazine was effective at the lowest concentration. The data suggest that phenothiazines decrease permeability of erythrocytes to water by altering cell membrane structure (Freeman and Spirtes, 1962).

Burton et al. (1962) studied the effect of chlorpromazine, nicotinamide, and nicotinic acid on pyridine nucleotide levels of human blood. Nicotinic acid (0.5–0.8 g/day p.o.) increased blood pyridine nucleotide four- to sixfold in human subjects, whereas nicotinamide (0.5–1.1 g/day p.o.) did not. Chlorpromazine (50 mg/day p.o.) did not alter nicotinic acid-induced increase in blood pyridine nucleotide levels.

Chlorpromazine has weak inhibitory action against serum cholinesterase and pseudocholinesterase (Delay et al., 1952a,b; Morand and Gay, 1953; Usdin et al., 1961).

Human serum procaine esterase activity was reduced 70% by a concentration of 500 mg/l (Visentini, 1954), and subcutaneous injection of 5–100 mg/kg protected mice against the convulsant action of procaine. Transfer of cholinesterase from red cells to plasma in stored blood was prevented or markedly slowed by chlorpromazine in 5.5×10^{-5} M concentration (Greig and Gibbons, 1955). Hemolysis of red cells by lysolecithin was also inhibited. Venous blood carbonic anhydrase activity was decreased for 2 hours in dogs given chlorpromazine (4 mg/kg intravenously) (Bianco et al., 1955). Histochemical study of tissues from rats given 2.5 mg of chlorpromazine intraperitoneally every 4 hours for a total of twelve doses showed a significant decrease in peroxidase activity in all organs; the decrease was more or less proportional to the fall in body temperature during the period of chlorpromazine administration (Schaumkell, 1955a,b,c).

A drop in hematocrit of sheep after chlorpromazine administration was reported by Turner and Hodgetts (1960) B. M. Kóvacs et al. (1956), and K. Kóvacs et al. (1956) reported a lipemia clearing effect. LeBlanc (1958a–d) has reported that a single dose of chlorpromazine (10 mg/kg, i.p.) in rats causes a large drop in eosinophiles, leucocytes, and platelets in the blood and mast cells in the mesentery. He has also found (LeBlanc, 1959) that chlorpromazine destroys mast cells *in vivo*, and this effect is reversed by cyanide. The latter also partially prevents the hypothermic effects of chlorpromazine, and it is postulated that these effects may be related to mast cell disruption. Vinegar and Berger (1959) have found that large doses of chlorpromazine and other drugs decreased the phagocytic activity of the reticulo-endothelial system. Chlorpromazine was found to inhibit the hemostatic effect of serotinin (Laporte, 1964).

d. *Tumors*. In mice inoculated with ascites tumor cells, chlorpromazine seemed to increase the effectiveness of either radium or colchicine treatment (Peters et al., 1955; Peters, 1955). Survival time was slightly increased in mice given chlorpromazine and radiation, and decreased in those given chlorpromazine and colchicine, compared to groups not receiving chlorpromazine.

Chlorpromazine has been reported by Belkin and Hardy (1957) and by Gottlieb et al. (1960) to show tumor-inhibiting properties in rodents at high doses. Whether this is a specific effect or a consequence of generalized metabolic depression is not known. Chorazy (1959), Cranston (1958a,b), and Lacassagne (1959) were not able to substantiate the anti-tumor effect of chlorpromazine.

The action of chlorpromazine and imipramine on respiration and anaerobic glycolysis of mastocytoma P-815 and Ehrlich ascites tumor was studied by Schellenberg (1961a). The effect of chlorpromazine and imipramine was studied *in vitro* after tumors had been removed from mice. Chlorpromazine (50 μg/ml) produced a 73% inhibition of respiration in Ehrlich's tumor and a 75% inhibition of respiration in mastocytoma P-815 after 4 hours. Imipramine had similar effect but was only one-half as potent. Glycolytic activity of these tumors was not affected by either drug at concentrations of 10–100 μg/ml.

Schellenberg (1961b) also compared the action of chlorpromazine and imipramine on cultures of some malignant and normal tissues. Mastocytoma P-815 (a serotonin-synthesizing tumor) was chosen to determine whether anticancer activity of chlorpromazine might be due to its anti-serotonin action.

Chlorpromazine (10–50 μg/ml) inhibited growth and caused cell destruction in 24 hours *in vitro*; however, there was no selective action because chlorpromazine had the same effect on chick fibroblasts, amniotic cells, and HeLa cell cultures. Imipramine had a similar but smaller effect. In general, 10 μg of chlorpromazine was equipotent with 25 μg of imipramine. The author concluded that the inhibitory effects of chlorpromazine and imipramine are not due to anti-serotonin action.

Several phenothiazine and iminodibenzyl compounds, including chlorpromazine and imipramine, were studied by Wilhelmi (1961) in growth processes. The compounds significantly decreased the cell division of fertilized eggs of sea urchin and frog (*Rana temporia*). They inhibited regeneration in planarians and axolotl and decreased granulation and exudation of rat granuloma. They also inhibited the liquid form of ascites tumor in mice. In all tests, chlorpromazine was much more effective than imipramine.

Chlorpromazine (5 or 40 mg/kg s.c.) produced a 13–19% increase in survival time of leukemic mice (Kruger *et al.*, 1960). However, doses of 17 or 33 mg/kg had no effect. Concomitant administration of CNS stimulants (amphetamine) with reserpine did not increase survival time. Addition of other substances, including LSD, JB-516 (β-phenylisopropylhydrazine hydrochloride), yohimbine, and phenoxybenzamine, completely abolished antileukemic effects.

It is known that 2-acetaminofluorene causes cancer in male but very seldom in female rats. However, the addition of chlorpromazine (0.25 mg/kg/day, s.c.) to the carcinogen caused female rats to develop liver tumors at the same rate as the males (Theret, 1962c). It is postulated by the above author that chlorpromazine, by blocking the hypothalamo-pituitary function, decreased the levels of follicle stimulating hormone and lactogenic hormone, thus inhibiting the protective effects of estrogens (Theret, 1962a,b). Fujita *et al.* (1958) have reported that chlorpromazine delays the formation of hepatic neoplasia induced by 4-dimethylaminoazobenzene.

e. *Effects of Chlorpromazine on Membrane Permeability.* There have been several studies reported on the effect of chlorpromazine on membrane permeability. Thus, Quadbeck (1962) reported that chlorpromazine and related compounds were effective in the activation of passive transport of phosphorus across the blood-brain barrier, and the effect of these drugs resembled that of electric shock treatments. The chlorpromazine derivatives also reduced sodium exchange at the blood-brain barrier. Similar effects are seen with narcotics at high doses.

It has been suggested that chlorpromazine alters the permeability of various membranes to substances like norepinephrine and serotonin, and the antipsychotic activity of chlorpromazine has been attributed to its membrane effects (Jenkins and Samborski, 1964). Schanker *et al.* (1963) showed that the rate of passive diffusion of norepinephrine through red cell membranes was not altered by 10 µg/ml of chlorpromazine (cf. Winters and Husa, 1960). In studies with serotonin (C^{14}), which enters platelets by both passive diffusion and active transport, chlorpromazine inhibited the diffusion process but not active transport (see p. 39).

4. Other Effects

a. *Tryptamines.* Tedeschi et al. (1961a,b) reported on the central serotonin antagonist activity of a number of phenothiazines. Comparative potencies of phenothiazines were studied in rats by conditioned response, unconditioned response, catalepsy, locomotor activity depression, serotonin antagonism, and tryptamine antagonism test procedures. In general, rank order of potency as conditioned response blockers agreed favorably with rank order of potency as tranquilizers in man. In addition, it was shown that tranquilizing activity is not always associated with serotonin antagonizing activity and vice versa (cf. Pidevich, 1961; Paasonen, 1964; Telkka, 1964).

Chlorpromazine, imipramine, chlorprothixene, amitriptyline, and reserpine decreased the serotonin content in rabbit and human thrombocytes *in vitro* (Bartholini et al., 1961). The effect was less pronounced in human thrombocytes.

Gey and Pletscher (1961) have reported on the influence of chlorpromazine on decarboxylases of aromatic amino acids. *In vitro*, chlorpromazine, ($10^{-4}\,M$) did not affect decarboxylation of 5-HTP (5-hydroxytryptophan) or DOPA (3,4-dihydroxyphenylalanine) in a supernatant of rat brain or kidney suspension. A concentration of $10^{-3}\,M$ inhibited DOPA decarboxylation in brain supernatant to which no pyridoxal-5′-phosphate had been added. *In vivo*, pretreatment of rats with high doses of chlorpromazine had no significant effect on decarboxylation of DOPA or 5-HTP in total homogenates or in supernatants of brain. However, there was 30–70% increase in decarboxylation of DOPA and 5-HTP in the supernatant of the kidney, provided no pyridoxal phosphate had been added.

Chlorpromazine, chlorprothixene, imipramine, cocaine, ibogaine, α-methyltryptamine, harmaline, amphetamine, benzylhydrazine, and phenylisopropylhydrazine competitively and reversibly inhibited uptake of serotonin by ox-blood platelets *in vitro* (Long and Lessin, 1962). Chlorpromazine at higher concentrations, interfered with a colorimetric method for estimation of serotonin uptake in platelets.

Chlorpromazine (30 mg i.v.) increased serotonin in the spleen, decreased serotonin in the heart, and had little effect on serotonin in the visceral tissues of rabbits previously given 5-hydroxytryptophan-3-C^{14} (10 µg i.v.); LSD and BOL (bromolysergic acid diethylamide) (500 µg i.v.) increased serotonin levels in visceral tissues of the same rabbits; LSD increased serotonin levels in heart and BOL decreased them. Chlorpromazine and BOL decreased serotonin in all parts of brain (Sankar et al., 1962).

In a study of drug-induced alterations in the subcellular distribution of 5-hydroxytryptamine in rat's brain, Schanberg and Giarman (1962) reported that CNS depressants (chlorpromazine, reserpine, phenobarbital, α-methyl-DOPA, and methylparafynol) significantly increased the proportion of free 5-HT, regardless of whether they increased, decreased or had no effect on total 5-HT. LSD-25, imipramine, and β-phenylisopropylhydrazine increased the total 5-HT, accounted for by greater increase in bound than in free 5-HT.

b. *Carbohydrates.* The effect of chlorpromazine on carbohydrate metabolism of rat brain was reported by Máthé et al. (1961). Chlorpromazine (0.35 mg/100 g i.p.) significantly increased the reducing substances but had no effect on glycogen content. After 4 weeks' treatment, the reducing substances decreased significantly and the glycogen content increased significantly above control values (cf. Opitz, 1962c).

Chlorpromazine (60–75 mg i.v.) was given to goats, and various parts of brain were incubated with labeled glucose 15 minutes later. Respiratory exchange and lactic acid-C^{14} and amino acid formation from endogenous glucose was depressed in the hypothalamus and posterior pituitary. The cerebellar and cerebral cortex were not affected (Larsson, 1961; Estler, 1961).

The action of phenothiazine derivatives on carbohydrate uptake of isolated rat diaphragm and isolated rat spinal cord was studied by Rafaelsen (1959, 1961). Chlorpromazine and prochlorperazine reduced glucose uptake of the isolated rat diaphragm and isolated rat spinal cord by about 25%. Insulin prevented the effects of chlorpromazine.

c. *Amino Acids.* The effect of drugs on amino acid levels in rat brain was studied by De Ropp and Snedeker (1961). Convulsive agents and CNS stimulants, including amphetamine, significantly increased free alanine in brain. Chlorpromazine and methoxypromazine significantly increased brain glutamine and alanine. The authors concluded that there is correlation between the rise in brain alanine and convulsant or excitant activity.

The interference of chlorpromazine with the metabolism of aromatic amino acids in rat brain was described by Gey and Pletscher (1962). Studies in rats showed that chlorpromazine inhibited uptake of DOPA and 5-HTP, primarily by reducing permeability of membranes responsible for their uptake. It is improbable that this effect of chlorpromazine is due to hypothermia.

A report on the influence of chlorpromazine on nuclear and cytoplasmic uptake of methionine-S^{35} was published by Carneiro and Cardoso (1962). Chlorpromazine inhibited nuclear and cytoplasmic uptake of methionine-S^{35}. The authors suggested that this reduced uptake is probably due to a decrease in protein synthesis induced by chlorpromazine.

In a study by Mennear et al. (1962) rat brain non-protein sulfhydryl (NPSH) levels were increased by electrical stimulation of sciatic nerve. Pretreatment with morphine (15 mg/kg), meperidine (20 mg/kg), chlorpromazine (10 mg/kg), or meprobamate (275 mg/kg), blocked the rise in cerebral levels of NPSH in curarized rats. These compounds themselves did not affect nonstimulated cerebral NPSH levels. The results suggest that increased cerebral NPSH levels may reflect increased glutathione indicating accelerated cerebral metabolism following electrical stimulation of the sciatic nerve.

d. *Catecholamines.* Hornykiewicz et al. (1961) have studied the effect of chlorpromazine on the brain catecholamine and 5-HT response to iproniazid in rats. Chlorpromazine (20 mg/kg i.p.), simultaneously with or 17 hours after iproniazid, inhibited or reversed the effects of iproniazid on catecholamines and serotonin in rat brain. The authors concluded that the effects of chlorpromazine may either be due to a hypothermic or a direct-specific effect (cf. Bulle, 1957a,b; Ariens and Simonis, 1964; Martin et al. 1960).

Chlorpromazine, imipramine, and dichlorisoproterenol reduced the concentration of tritium-labeled norepinephrine in the rat heart given before, but not after, labeled compound. Thus, this group of drugs blocks entry of labeled norepinephrine into storage sites, but does not cause its release (Axelrod et al., 1962; Gey and Pletscher, 1964).

On the other hand, chlorpromazine does not influence serotonin levels in the brain, and causes an acceleration of metabolism of epinephrine in the whole animal (Pletscher and Gey, 1960). Millar and Benfey (1959), in studying hemorrhagic shock, found that adrenalin and noradrenalin levels were not appreciably altered by chlorpromazine (cf. Hsi-Jui, 1961).

Chlorpromazine consistently increased epinephrine content of various areas of dog brain, whereas small doses increased and higher doses decreased norepinephrine levels (Malhotra and Prasad, 1962; cf. Masse and Chollot, 1962; Deshpande and Tiwaskar, 1960; Greenberg and Sabelli, 1964; Hapke, 1964). Data from Andén (1964) indicate that chlorpromazine delays the elimination of acid metabolites of dihydroxyphenylalanine (i.e., homovanillic and dihydroxyphenylacetic acids) in rabbit brain.

e. *Enzyme Effects.* Chlorpromazine was found by Burton and Salvador (1962) to be bound to nicotinamide-methylpherase *in vivo* in mice, and *in vitro*. In the presence of this drug, enzyme activity was increased but the affinity for substrate (nicotonamide) was reduced. Competitive inhibition between chlorpromazine and nicotinamide may also be a factor. The relationship between the drug-enzyme complex and psychophysiology was speculated on.

The mechanism of dehydrogenase inhibition by phenothiazines was studied by Wollemann and Keleti (1962). *In vitro* data were given on chlorpromazine and its oxidation products, i.e., the sulfoxide and the "red chlorpromazine" which results through photooxidation of chlorpromazine. The red chlorpromazine inhibits dehydrogenase immediately, whereas chlorpromazine and its sulfoxide inhibit it slowly during the course of incubation.

Other phenothiazines have been reported to inhibit glucose-6-phosphate dehydrogenase, 6-phosphogluconate dehydrogenase (Carver, 1963), and glyceraldehyde-3-phosphate dehydrogenase (Wollemann and Elödi, 1961).

Chlorpromazine, like 2,4-dinitrophenol, has been shown to produce uncoupling of oxidative phosphorylation in various preparations of liver and brain (Berger et al., 1956; Andrejew et al., 1956a,b; Bernsohn et al., 1956a,b; Kok, 1956; Yamamoto et al., 1957; Sinigaglia, 1955; Décsi and Méhes, 1957, 1958; Dawkins et al., 1958, 1959a,b,c; Andrejew and Rosenberg, 1956, 1958; Berger, 1957; Kirpekar and Lewis, 1960; cf. Kozák et al., 1958; Century and Horwitt, 1956). Like dinitrophenol, chlorpromazine also inhibits adenosine-triphosphatase activity (Andrejew et al., 1956a,b; Low, 1959; Dawkins et al., 1960). It is also said to resemble 2,4-dinitro-o-cresol in its effects (Garner and Skude, 1956).

Chlorpromazine has been reported to inhibit the aerobic "old yellow enzyme" system prepared from yeast (Kistner, 1960). Chlorpromazine decreases the activity of acetylcholinesterase (daCruz, 1955; Bonomolo and Mariani, 1955; Dasgupta and Mukherjee, 1956; Kivalo et al., 1958; Erdos et al., 1958; Kozák et al., 1960) acid phosphatase (daCruz, 1955; Kivalo et al., 1958) and succinic dehydrogenase (Kivalo et al., 1958; Bose et al., 1959; Bernsohn et al., 1956b).

Chlorpromazine does not significantly alter the α-keto acid levels of rabbit blood (Bernsohn et al., 1958), but low doses do increase the synthesis of glutamine (Messer, 1958). Ernsting et al. (1960) found that chlorpromazine influenced the distribution of glutamic acid and γ-aminobutyric acid between brain slices and incubation fluid. Greenberg et al. (1959) reported that chlorpromazine had little effect on glutamic acid decarboxylase, but did inhibit pyridoxal kinase activity in both normal and B_6-deficient rat brain homogenates.

Chlorpromazine has been shown to produce a marked inhibition of oxygen uptake by rat brain homogenates (Starbuck and Heim, 1959; Hoskin, 1960). It brings about a reduction in the uptake of glycine-1-C^{14} into rat brain protein (Lindan et al., 1957; Zoller et al., 1958).

Chlorpromazine has been found to inhibit cytochrome oxidase in mitochondria isolated from both brain and liver (Dawkins et al., 1959a,b,c). The drug was reported to inhibit D-amino acid oxidase as a result of competition with flavin adenine dinucleotide (Yagi et al., 1956, 1959, 1960a,b; cf. Lessin, 1959; Løvtrup, 1964).

Chlorpromazine produced an increase in carbonic anhydrase activity in growing rats (Ashby et al., 1957) and produced a decrease in brain alkaline phosphatase (Clark el al., 1956; Das Gupta et al., 1956). Chlorpromazine reduced phospholipid turnover in brain according to Ansell and Dohmen (1957) but Magee et al. (1956) and Grossi et al. (1960) reported an increase for low levels of the drug.

Chlorpromazine has been reported to produce a decrease in aconitase in kidney particle preparations due to complexing of the drug and enzyme (Peters, 1959). In an interesting study, Khouw et al. (1960) reported that chlorpromazine increases blood levels of alcohol by inhibition of the conversion of ethanol to acetaldehyde. Rat brain hexokinase activity was reported to be markedly inhibited by chlorpromazine (Buzard, 1960), as was lipid peroxidase (Bernheim, 1959).

On the other hand, chlorpromazine, according to Masurat et al. (1960), in concentrations from 8.5×10^{-6} M to 6.8×10^{-5} M, either greatly activated or inhibited hexokinase activity, determined by measuring spectrophotometrically the reduction of TPN (triphosphopyridine nucleotide). The biphasic action of chlorpromazine was a function of the relative concentration of drug and Mg-ATP substrate. The data suggested that chlorpromazine may function as metabolic regulator, primarily by interfering with utilization of ATP.

A study of the effects of chlorpromazine and other drugs on choline oxidase activity showed no causal relationship between choline oxidase inhibition and psychotherapeutic effect (Göschke, 1963).

f. *Miscellaneous.* Harris and Teodoru (1961) studied the effect of chlorpromazine on calcification *in vitro*.

The effect of chlorpromazine on the synthesis of cholesterol in pigeon liver was studied by Yakubovskaya and Kiseleva (1961). Pigeons were given chlorpromazine (25 mg/kg s.c.) and acetate-2-C^{14} (50 μc/kg i.p.). After 3 hours, the animals were killed and cholesterol was determined. Chlorpromazine reduced cholesterol synthesis by 70% and its concentration by about 19%. The authors conclude that the inhibitory action of chlorpromazine on cholesterol synthesis may be related to its toxic effect on coenzyme A, since chlorpromazine is known to block SH-groups of tissues. Similar results were obtained in rabbits (Wilens and Gallo, 1957; Wilens et al., 1956).

Chlorpromazine-induced water inhibition of frog gastrocnemius muscle is unrelated to tranquilizing activity and seems to be related to loss of sodium and potassium from the muscle (Eckhardt and Govier, 1958; cf. Peterson et al., 1960; Jindal and Deshpande, 1961; Mandell, 1963).

Sapeika (1959) reported that chlorpromazine administered orally in single doses to rats produced a decrease in ascorbic acid content of the adrenal glands, but not of the liver (cf. Sevy et al., 1957). Rupp and Paschkis (1957) reported that chlorpromazine caused a significant increase in urinary nitrogen excretion in rats. Furthermore, the catabolic effects of cortisone were potentiated by chlorpromazine.

Chlorpromazine has been reported to cause a decrease in food (Schmidt and Van Meter, 1958; Edgren, 1956; Reynolds and Carlisle, 1961; Ross and Rhoades, 1961) and water intake (Schmidt, 1958) in experimental animals, even though it sometimes causes a weight gain in humans.

Chlorpromazine inhibited the incorporation of leucine-C^{14} into rat brain protein. Swimming tended to overcome this inhibition (Glasky, 1963). White (1961) showed that chlorpromazine inhibited methylation of labeled histamine in cat brain, and Axelrod et al. (1961a,b,c) showed that chlorpromazine inhibited the uptake of norepinephrine-H^3 in various other tissues of cats. Studies on the effect of chlorpromazine on the incorporation of tritium-labeled thymidine into DNA were carried out by Pisciotta and Hinz (1964).

G. Autonomic Nervous System

Early investigators attributed many of the effects of chlorpromazine to autonomic activity. Further work has shown that most of its peripheral effects are the result of a moderate adrenolytic activity.

1. Blocking Action Against Adrenergic Agents

a. *Blood Pressure.* A number of investigators have reported that the pressor effect of epinephrine can be reduced, blocked, or reversed by appropriate doses of chlorpromazine, while the pressor effect of norepinephrine is only partially blocked. Table II lists these results. It will be seen that chlorpromazine has a moderate adrenolytic action, producing a blockade which may be complete for small doses of epinephrine, but is only partial for norepinephrine or larger doses of epinephrine. Pressor responses to other sympathomimetic amines, like ephedrine, methamphetamine, methoxamine, mephentermine, and amphetamine, are also blocked by chlorpromazine in doses of 0.05–5 mg/kg intravenously (Bourgeois-Gavardin et al., 1955; Kaufmann, 1955; Marquardt et al., 1955; Stephen et al., 1955; Huidobro, 1954; Martin et al., 1960; Eggers et al., 1959; Bradshaw et al., 1958; Feldman and Eliakim, 1958; Melville, 1958; Archdeacon and Giles, 1956). The only exception seems to be phenylephrine, which is only partially blocked at these doses. Chlorpromazine does not block pressor responses to isoproterenol. Supek et al. (1959) on the other hand, report that chlorpromazine markedly augments the vascular effects of vasopressin, angiotonin, and ergotamine.

It has been suggested by Hudson and Domino (1964) that, based on experiments on rabbits, effects on blood pressure and depression of the patellar reflex are unrelated phenomena.

Several clinical reports have noted that surgical patients premedicated with chlorpromazine sometimes responded poorly to pressor drugs (Stephen et al., 1955; Lipton and Hershey, 1955; Dripps et al., 1955). As would be expected from the results of animal studies, adequate pressor effect could usually be obtained from larger doses or continuous infusion, particularly of norepinephrine or phenylephrine. Dripps et al. (1955) also found that the use of epinephrine packs in the course of mastoidectomies and fenestration operations, which usually caused an increase in blood pressure, had much less effect in chlorpromazine-treated patients.

b. *Cardiac*. The inotropic effects of epinephrine and similar amines were decreased by chlorpromazine in the cat papillary muscle (Finkelstein *et al.*, 1954a,b), the isolated perfused rabbit heart (Melville, 1954), and the dog heart *in situ* (Witzleb and Budde, 1955). Epinephrine-induced arrhythmias were prevented in unanesthetized rabbits by doses of 2.5–5 mg/kg (Courvoisier *et al.*, 1953; cf. Sharma and Arora, 1961), and electrocardiographic abnormalities resulting from intravenous injection of a number of amines in anesthetized dogs were blocked by similar doses (Bourgeois-Gavardin *et al.*, 1955). In cats or dogs sensitized by inhalation of petroleum ether (Di Palma and Catenacci, 1955), chloroform (Melville, 1954), trichlorethylene (Bourgeois-Gavardin *et al.*, 1955), or cyclopropane (Dobkin and Gilbert, 1956), premedication with chlorpromazine at doses of 0.5–5 mg/kg completely prevented the development of arrhythmias usually occurring after injection of epinephrine or other similar amines. The coronary dilator response to epinephrine and norepinephrine was not blocked by chlorpromazine (Ngai and Wang, 1955) nor was the cardioaccelerator action (Chauchard and Chauchard, 1952a,b,c; Melville, 1954).

Moran and Perkins (1961) reported as a result of measuring the positive inotropic effect of adrenergic stimuli in cat hearts, that chlorpromazine and phenoxybenzamine did not have selective cardiac adrenergic blocking activity.

On the other hand, Moe *et al.* (1962) working with dogs, reported that the direct effects of chlorpromazine and chlordiazepoxide appeared to be a transitory adrenergic blockade in the myocardium and associated vasculature. The drug concentrations were above those expected to be used therapeutically.

In anesthetized and unanesthetized animals, chlorpromazine (2 mg/kg i.m. or i.v.) significantly increased cardiac contractions, decreased arterial pressure, and either decreased or increased respiratory rate. In decerebrate animals, cardiac contractions decreased significantly from 150 to 70 in cats, blood pressure decreased (48–53%), and severe respiratory depression occurred. In spinal cats, no significant effect on cardiac contractions was seen. In cats with complete CNS destruction, changes were similar to those of spinal animals. In vagotomized cats, no appreciable effect on cardiovascular or respiratory system was seen (Korneva and Yakovleva, 1962).

c. *Other Effects*. The local vasoconstrictor effect of 1–2 μg of epinephrine injected into the femoral artery was blocked or reversed by chlorpromazine (0.03–1.0 mg/kg intravenously) but the effect of norepinephrine was only partially blocked by the same doses (Ngai and Wang, 1955). Chlorpromazine also blocked the vasoconstrictor effect of epinephrine in the perfused rabbit ear (Kopera and Armitage, 1954). The delay in absorption of intramuscular strychnine caused by the addition of epinephrine to the injected solution was markedly reduced when the rats were pretreated with chlorpromazine (25 or 50 mg/kg subcutaneously) (Courvoisier *et al.*, 1953). The time of appearance of convulsions was used as an indicator of the rate of absorption of the strychnine. Delay in absorption due to posterior pituitary hormone was also reduced by chlorpromazine. In anesthetized human subjects, intra-arterial chlorpromazine decreased and intravenous chlorpromazine reversed the vasoconstrictor response in the hand to intra-arterial infusion of epinephrine (0.1 μg/minute for 5 minutes) (Foster and O'Mullane, 1954). The constrictor effect of norepinephrine was only slightly decreased. Sweating, induced by intradermal epinephrine, was blocked by pretreatment with 50 mg chlorpromazine intravenously (Clerc et al., 1955).

In the rabbit uterus, chlorpromazine has been reported to block the contractions produced by epinephrine (Kopera and Armitage, 1954). Courvoisier et al. (1953) reported that in vitro a concentration of 1 mg/l blocked the effect of 1–20 mg adrenaline per liter, making chlorpromazine as effective as ergotomine. Huidobro (1954) found no blockage in the anesthetized cat of the inhibitory action of adrenaline in the nonpregnant uterus, the urinary bladder, or intestine by doses of chlorpromazine up to 6.3 mg/kg.

Chlorpromazine also protects against the lethal effects of epinephrine. Rats were completely protected against 5 mg/kg of epinephrine (i.p.) intraperitoneally by chlorpromazine 5 mg/kg given subcutaneously 1 hour before the epinephrine (Smith Kline and French, 1956). A dose of 1.0 mg/kg intravenously 1 minute before testing gave complete protection against 3.6 mg/kg epinephrine intravenously (six times the lethal dose) in mice; 15 mg/kg epinephrine (25 LD) had to be given before the mortality equalled that of 0.6 mg/kg in unprotected mice (Courvoisier et al., 1953). The lethal effect of norepinephrine was also markedly reduced by chlorpromazine. Rats pretreated with thyroxine 0.1 mg/kg/day for 3 days were protected against epinephrine 5 mg/kg intraperitoneally by chlorpromazine given orally at a dose of 20 mg/kg/day for 4 days before testing (Smith Kline and French, 1956).

The hyperglycemic effect of subcutaneous epinephrine (0.5 mg/kg) in rabbits was not blocked by pretreatment with chlorpromazine 2.5–25 mg/kg subcutaneously (Courvoisier et al., 1953). Pulmonary edema in rabbits resulting from injected epinephrine was prevented by chlorpromazine (Danese and Cesare, 1955).

2. Blocking Action Against Sympathetic Stimulation

The pressor effect of stimulation of the splanchnic nerve was reduced by 1–5 mg/kg of chlorpromazine intravenously in intact or adrenalectomized dogs (Jourdan et al., 1955; Pocidalo et al., 1953; Kalkoff, 1955) or spinal cats (Kopera and Armitage, 1954) while the inhibitory effect on the gut in cats was not altered by doses up to 6.3 mg/kg (Huidobro, 1954). One dissenting author (Chauchard and Chauchard, 1952a,b,c; see also Chardon, 1955) reported that the pressor effect and acceleration of the denervated heart were not blocked and renal vasoconstriction was only slightly decreased in dogs by 5 mg/kg intravenously. Another found, however, that vasoconstriction resulting from stimulation of the renal plexus was completely blocked for up to 2 hours by doses over 0.25 mg/kg (Bubnoff et al., 1955).

In crossed-circulation experiments, in which adrenal venous blood from a treated dog was diverted to the jugular vein of an untreated recipient, the pressor response of the recipient to splanchnic stimulation in the donor was reduced or prevented by pretreatment of the donor dog with 2–18 mg/kg of chlorpromazine indicating that adrenaline secretion had been reduced or prevented (Vanlerenverghe et al., 1954; Brunaud et al., 1953; Malmejac et al., 1954). The pressor effect in the recipient of nicotine injection in the donor (believed to act directly on the adrenaline-secreting cells) was progressively inhibited by increasing doses of chlorpromazine (donor) (Brunaud et al., 1953). These effects have been attributed by the various authors to adrenolytic action, ganglionic blockade, or a "narcobiotic" effect on chromaffin cells or nerve fibers.

Chlorpromazine appears to be a less potent blocking agent against the effects of preganglionic sympathetic stimulation than against splanchnic stimulation. Intravenous doses of 4.5 or 5 mg/kg did not block the ocular effects of stimulation of the cephalic and of the cervical sympathetic ganglia in dogs (Jourdan et al., 1955; Holzbauer and Vogt, 1954). Doses of 0.05 to 1.0 mg/kg in the cat reduced the contraction of the nictitating membrane caused by adrenaline but not that produced by preganglionic stimulation (Krause and Schmidtke-Ruhnau, 1955). Doses from 2.5 to 4.0 mg/kg had no effect on contraction of the nictitating membrane following preganglionic stimulation while 9–18 mg/kg reduced it slightly. Whether this was a sympatholytic or adrenolytic action cannot be determined from the data presented. The cats were under pentobarbital anesthesia and the chlorpromazine is presumed to have been administered intravenously (Bourgeois-Gavardin et al., 1955). In cats under pentobarbital anesthesia, the nictitating membrane was brought to a steady state of contraction by stimulation of the pre- and postganglionic fibers. Intra-arterial injection of chlorpromazine 0.8–1.65 mg/kg caused the membrane to relax. When similar contractions were produced by acetylcholine or adrenaline (via the carotid artery), the administration of 1.0 mg chlorpromazine by the same route relaxed the membrane (Huidobro, 1954). Secretory and vasodilator effects on the submaxillary gland resulting from cervical sympathetic stimulation in the cat were completely blocked by 0.1–0.2 mg chlorpromazine/kg i.v.; the vasoconstrictor effect was blocked by 2–5 mg/kg (Emmelin, 1955; Sherif et al., 1958).

3. Blocking Effect on Vascular Reflexes

The pressor response to carotid occlusion was blocked in dogs pretreated with chlorpromazine in doses of 0.5–5 mg/kg (Smith Kline and French,

TABLE II

BLOCKING ACTION OF CHLORPROMAZINE AGAINST EPINEPHRINE AND NOREPINEPHRINE

Species	Chlorpromazine dose[a] (mg/kg)	Effect	Epinephrine dose[a] (μg/kg)	Chlorpromazine dose[a] (mg/kg)	Effect	Norepinephrine dose[a] (μg/kg)	Reference
Cat	5	No block reversed	12.5				Smith Kline and French (1956)
	10	No block	>12.5				
	1–10	Reduced (spinal cat)	10	1–10	Slightly reduced	10	Kopera and Armitage (1954)
	0.01–0.5	Reversed	10/min	0.01–0.5	Reversed	10/min	Melville (1954)
	14	Reversed	2	14	Slightly reduced, duration increased	1	Marquardt (1953)
	8.5	Reversed	5–100	8.5	No effect	?	Huidobro (1954)
	2.5–30 1.6–58	Reduced Reversed	?				Marquardt et al. (1955)
Dog and cat	0.05–1	Reduced, blocked, or occasionally reversed	1.5–4	0.05–1	Reduced	1–2	Krause and Schmidtke-Ruhnau (1955)

Species							Reference
	5–60	Variable, no relation to chlorpromazine dose	15	12–60	Reduced	2	Bourgois-Gavardin et al. (1955)
Dog	0.5–5	Reversed, reduced	"Therapeutic" to 400	0.5–5	No effect	2–20	Dobkin and Gilbert (1956)
	5	Blocked, occasionally reversed	50–100	5	Little effect	?	Jourdan et al. (1955)
	1.5	Reduced	5	5	Reduced	5	Stephen et al. (1955)
	0.03–0.3	Reduced or blocked	0.5–3	to 2.2	Reduced	0.5–3	Ngai and Wang (1955)
	0.3	Reversed					
	1.5	Reversed	4	1.5	Reduced	4	Holzbauer and Vogt (1954)
	0.5–1	Reduced, blocked or reversed	2–5				Courvoisier et al. (1953)
	5	Reversed	2–5	1	Reduced	5	
	1	Blocked	5				Pocidalo et al. (1953)
Rat	1.5–3 i.p.	Blocked	0.5–2 mg	1.5–3	Reduced	2 mg	Smith Kline and French (1956)

[a] All doses given i.v. unless otherwise stated.

1956; Courvoisier *et al.*, 1953; Krause and Schmidtke-Ruhnau, 1955; Pocidalo *et al.*, 1953; Kalkoff, 1955). Early reports (Courvoisier *et al.*, 1953; Pocidalo *et al.*, 1953) stated that the pressor response to central vagal stimulation was blocked by similar doses, but closer investigation revealed that these doses block only the first phase, due to epinephrine release. The true central vagal pressor response was decreased somewhat by considerably higher doses of chlorpromazine (15 mg/kg).

Reference to Table II suggests that most of the inhibitory effect of chlorpromazine on these reflexes is due to peripheral adrenergic blockade, rather than to ganglionic or central effects. This was confirmed by experiments (Smith Kline and French, 1956) showing that in individual animals the carotid occlusion reflex and the pressor response to dimethylphenylpiperazinium iodide (a ganglion stimulant) were inhibited only by chlorpromazine doses which also blocked or reversed epinephrine. That other effects may be involved when high doses are used is suggested by some experiments involving local application of chlorpromazine. Applied to the isolated perfused cat superior cervical ganglion, 10–100 μg of chlorpromazine slightly reduced the response of the nictitating membrane to preganglionic stimulation or application of acetylcholine to the ganglion; 200 μg produced a complete reversible block of preganglionic stimulation and a lasting inhibition of the acetylcholine effect (Madjerek and Stern, 1956). Intracarotid injection of 500–1000 μg produced a marked prolonged reduction in action potential of the carotid sinus nerve, a complete block of the effects of acetylcholine or lobeline, and a partial block of the pressor effect of hypoxia (Madjerek and Stern, 1956). Injection of 2–5 mg completely suppressed both chemo- and pressoreceptor activity. The authors suggest that a local anesthetic action may be involved here. Direct application of a 2.5% solution of chlorpromazine to nerve fibers produced a sharp increase in chronaxie of preganglionic vagal fibers with eventual block of conduction, a slow moderate increase in chronaxie in sympathetic fibers, and little change in postganglionic fibers (Chauchard and Chauchard, 1952a,b,c).

4. Effects on the Parasympathetic Nervous System

Blocking effects of chlorpromazine on the parasympathetic nervous system are weak and variable. The decrease in pulse rate resulting from stimulation of the central vagus has been reported to be slightly reduced by 5 mg/kg (Holzbauer and Vogt, 1954), reduced by 1–2 mg/kg, and blocked by 10 mg/kg (Courvoisier *et al.*, 1953) in dogs, and unaffected by up to 18 mg/kg in cats (Bourgeois-Gavardin *et al.*, 1955); all chlorpromazine doses were given intravenously. The effects of vagal stimulation on blood pressure and on intestinal motility were not blocked by doses up to 1 mg/kg (Krause and Schmidtke-Ruhnau, 1955), but the hypotensive response was blocked by doses varying from 2.5 to 18 mg/kg in individual cats (Bourgeois-Gavardin *et al.*, 1955). Salivary secretion in response to stimulation of the chorda tympani was reduced but not prevented by large doses of chlorpromazine, 15–20 mg/kg, but not by lower doses (Holzbauer and Vogt, 1954; Emmelin, 1955; Decourt *et al.*, 1953b). This low degree of activity is further evidence that chlorpromazine is not a ganglionic blocking agent, at least in ordinary doses.

Chlorpromazine, in contrast to reserpine, does not increase parasympathetic tone, nor does it induce an enhanced light reflex (Bogdanski *et al.*, 1961).

Chlorpromazine is moderately effective against acetylcholine spasm in the isolated gut preparation. Given intravenously to dogs and rabbits, it did not block the blood pressure or pulse rate response to acetylcholine (Chauchard and Chauchard, 1952a,b,c). Intradermal injection did not inhibit the sweating provoked by intradermal carbachol in human subjects (Clerc *et al.*, 1955). In mice, the pupillary dilation produced by 63 μmoles/kg of chlorpromazine (approximately 20 mg/kg) intravenously was somewhat greater and lasted longer than that following atropine 0.1 μmole/kg (van Proosdij-Hartzema, 1955).

Chlorpromazine has produced a drop in intraocular pressure in the rabbit (Paul and Leopold, 1956a,b; Constant and Becker, 1956).

H. Cardiovascular Effects

1. Major Vessels

Chlorpromazine in intravenous or intraperitoneal doses of 1–10 mg/kg produces a fall in blood pressure in anesthetized dogs (Jourdan *et al.*, 1955; Courvoisier *et al.*, 1953; Moyer *et al.*, 1954a,b; Spurr *et al.*, 1956a,b), cats (Huidobro, 1954; Ahrens and Witzleb, 1955; Dasgupta and Werner, 1954), or rabbits (Jourdan *et al.*, 1955). The degree and duration of the effect vary with the dose, with 8–10 mg/kg required for more than a slight transient change. One report (Bourgeois-Gavardin *et al.*, 1955) stated that, with progressively increasing intravenous doses, the hypotensive dose was quite variable from animal to animal; rabbits required 4–12 mg/kg, dogs 30–60 mg/kg, and cats 10–15 mg/kg. In unanesthetized rats (Smith Kline and French, 1956), 1.5–3 mg/kg intraperitoneally produced a significant fall in blood pressure lasting at least 1 to 3 hours. The hypotensive effect was partially antagonized by phenylephrine, norepinephrine, ephedrine, and Pitressin® given 1 hour after chlorpromazine, but not by epinephrine (see pages 84–86). When rats were given oral doses of 0.2–10 mg/kg/day for 4 days, blood pressure measured on the fifth day was decreased in proportion to the dose administered (see Stevenson and Sjoerdsma, 1954; Lehmann and Hanrahan, 1954; Delay and Deniker, 1952b; Rea *et al.*, 1954; Marquardt, 1953; Karp *et al.*, 1955; Cliche and Fortin, 1953).

Injected into the intact rabbit ear, chlorpromazine (1 ml of 1.25% solution) produced a rise in skin temperature, followed by edema (Courvoisier *et al.*, 1953); histological examination showed capillary dilatation and exudation but no evidence of vascular damage. In the perfused ear, 0.1–1 gm/l of perfusion fluid increased the rate of flow by 50–100%, suggesting a direct effect on vascular muscle.

In anesthetized cats, 2–5 mg/kg of chlorpromazine intravenously produced increased blood flow in the mesenteric, renal, and carotid arteries (Ahrens and Witzleb, 1955). The effect was maximal 30 seconds after injection and declined gradually after that time. Injected into the femoral artery, 0.2–2 mg/kg caused a marked increase in blood flow lasting up to 10 minutes. Spinal cats showed similar effects from intravenous injection and longer lasting effects after intra-arterial administration.

In guinea pigs, 10–20 mg/kg of chlorpromazine intraperitoneally had no effect on capillary permeability as measured by the amount of vacuum which had to be applied to the skin to produce bleeding (Courvoisier *et al.*, 1953). However, pretreatment of rats with 12.5 mg/kg subcutaneously slowed, and 50 mg/kg prevented, the accumulation of trypan blue (given intravenously) in skin areas irritated by application of xylene or chloroform. Rabbits required 50–100 mg/kg for partial inhibition of this phenomenon.

Studies of peripheral blood flow in humans have shown that chlorpromazine causes an increase in both blood flow and skin temperature in the extremities (Duff *et al.*, 1956). Blood flow in hands and feet of normal subjects increased approximately 300% after intravenous injection of 10–50 mg of chlorpromazine and to a considerably lesser degree after intra-arterial infusion (Foster and O'Mullane, 1954). Skin temperatures increased in the extremities and dropped slightly in more proximal areas (Dobkin, *et al.*, 1954a,b,c; Clerc *et al.*, 1955). Patients with vascular spasm showed a gradual increase in skin temperature, while those with occlusive vascular disease showed little or no effect (Dobkin *et al.*, 1954a,b,c; Dobkin and Gilbert, 1956). Cerebral oxygen consumption was not altered by 50–300 mg of chlorpromazine intravenously or 50 mg intramuscularly, although cerebral blood flow decreased somewhat when systemic blood pressure dropped to relatively low levels (Morris *et al.*, 1955; Fazekas *et al.*, 1955).

Warecka (1960) studied the influence of chlorpromazine and reserpine on the pia mater blood vessels of cats and rabbits. Chlorpromazine (0.5–25 mg/kg i.v. or into carotid artery) dilated cerebral blood vessels in most cats; pia mater blood vessels in rabbits showed either no changes or contracted. After a transient fall in blood pressure, there was a gradual return to normal. There was no correlation between dilatation or contraction of pia mater blood vessels and systemic blood pressure. There was no consistent change with reserpine.

Internal carotid injection of chlorpromazine invariably increased blood brain flow promptly and sustained it for some time, with or without an attendant decrease in blood pressure. Chlorpromazine also provided protection against the toxicity of oxygen at high pressure, but the mechanism of this protective effect is obscure (Bean and Wagemaker, 1960).

The vasopressor effect of serotonin 0.5–0.25 mg/kg intravenously was reversed by chlorpromazine 0.5 or 2.0 mg/kg in atropinized vagotomized cats (Smith Kline and French, 1956); in spinal cats the pressor effect of 20–40 μg/kg of serotonin was almost completely prevented by 1 mg/kg chlorpromazine (Gyermek, 1955). The effect of serotonin on the isolated rat uterus (Gyermek, 1955; Costa, 1956) and rat colon strip (Benditt and Rowley, 1956) were also decreased or prevented by chlorpromazine, as was the edema formation resulting from subcutaneous injection of serotonin in the rat (Benditt and Rowley, 1956).

2. Heart

In isolated heart preparations, chlorpromazine usually produces a negative inotropic effect and an increase in coronary blood flow. In the cat papillary muscle, for example, 0.1–0.5 mg/100 ml decreased amplitude of contraction by 40–60% and increased the threshold for electrical stimulation by 100 to 300% (Finkelstein et al., 1954a,b); automaticity was also depressed and the inotropic effects of epinephrine, norepinephrine, and isoproterenol were decreased. No chronotropic, inotropic, or tonotropic effects were noted in the Straub frog heart preparation or isolated rabbit auricle (Courvoisier et al., 1953), while coronary flow in the Langendorff rabbit heart was increased 60 to 100% by 0.05–1 mg/kg chlorpromazine. Cardiac depression, heart block, and increased coronary blood flow were noted in isolated perfused rabbit hearts (Melville, 1954).

Unanesthetized rabbits showed no electrocardiographic changes after intravenous doses of chlorpromazine up to 10 mg/kg; repeated doses caused progressive slowing of pulse rate, delay in conduction, and finally heart block and asystole or auricular fibrillation (Bourgeois-Gavardin et al., 1955; Courvoisier et al., 1953). Small doses (2.5–5 mg/kg) partially inhibited the fibrillatory action of aconitine, prevented epinephrine arrhythmias, and temporarily reduced or prevented A-V block following intravenous adenosine monophosphate (Courvoisier et al., 1953; see Section G,1 for further references).

Cats given repeated intravenous injections of chlorpromazine showed ECG changes similar to those described only at near-lethal total doses, while such changes were never observed in dogs (Bourgeois-Gavardin et al., 1955). In the denervated dog heart (Starling heart-lung preparation), doses of 5–20 mg intravenously caused a marked increase in coronary flow lasting several minutes, with little or no change in minute volume, rate, oxygen uptake, or cardiac work and efficiency (Witzleb and Budde, 1955). In the innervated heart in situ, the increase in coronary flow was less but of longer duration, cardiac rate increased moderately, and other functions were unchanged; doses of chlorpromazine were 0.5–2 mg/kg.

When chlorpromazine was given intravenously to dogs in progressively increasing doses at 10- or 20-minute intervals, pulse rate increased sharply at 1–5 mg/kg and cardiac output showed no change or some decrease at high doses; an occasional animal showed slight flattening of T-waves and delayed conduction at 10 mg/kg while marked tachycardia and intraventricular block were evident at high doses (Moyer et al., 1954a,b). Another study using 5 mg/kg every 5 minutes showed little change in ECG except a decrease in rate up to 120 mg/kg; at 125 mg/kg ectopic foci appeared, along with marked conduction disturbances (Gadermann and Donat, 1955). Feller and Staib (1964) reported primarily a bradycardic effect of chlorpromazine i.v. in dogs.

When chlorpromazine was injected through a pericardial catheter, the heart rate increased up to 50%; the increase in dogs pretreated with intravenous digitoxin or strophanthin reached a maximum of over 100% with the same dose of chlorpromazine (2.5 mg/kg) (Busse and Loennecken, 1953; cf. Sharma and Arora, 1961).

The only significant change in cardiac function seen in human subjects given oral or parenteral chlorpromazine is usually some degree of tachycardia. The tachycardia, which occurs in some cases, is considered to be compensatory for orthostatic hypotension. In normal subjects given 0.3–2.0 mg/kg intravenously, pulse rate was variable and ECG showed sinus arrhythmias with abrupt rate changes and minor T-wave changes at the higher doses (Jourdan et al., 1955; Moyer et al., 1954a,b; Boer, 1955; Bensoussan and Klein, 1953; Donnadieu et al., 1955; Delay and Deniker, 1952a; Baruk et al., 1955a,b; Arnold et al., 1952). Some reports (Lewis et al., 1955; Winbury et al., 1958; Weinberg and Haley, 1956; Arora and Das, 1956; Bourgeois-Gavardin et al., 1957) noted that chlorpromazine appeared to reduce or prevent the occurrence of arrhythmias during electroshock therapy. Yoshitani (1963) has also commented on the antiarrhythmic action of chlorpromazine in man and experimental animals. On the other hand, chlorpromazine had no effect on fibrillation in dogs induced by deep hypothermia (Riley et al., 1957).

Chlorpromazine had no effect on the hypertension resulting from implantation of DCA (deoxycortisone acetate) pellets in uni-nephrectomized rats given saline to drink (Masson et al., 1955). Blood pressure and histological changes in blood vessels, heart, and kidneys were not altered by 1 mg/day subcutaneously. The sharp rise in blood pressure on rapid cooling or warming of rats, guinea pigs, and hamsters was prevented by chlorpromazine in doses of 2 mg/kg (Breuninger and Schmid, 1955); it was also blocked by meperidine hydrochloride and high doses of aminopyrine and by adrenolytic agents, but not by morphine or hexamethonium.

Hypotension, produced by chlorpromazine, persists in spinal or reserpinized animals and is related to a peripheral factor. Chlorpromazine decreases blood pressure when injected intracisternally only at high doses, and is more effective when injected into the third ventricle. In addition, chlorpromazine reduces excitability of hypothalamic and bulbar vasomotor centers. The data support the complementary ideas of independence of the efferent hypothalamic pathways and the bulbar centers, tonic action of the hypothalamus, integration of vasomotor reflexes at suprabulbar level, and the autonomic action of vasopressor and vasodepressor centers (Schmitt and Schmitt, 1961).

3. Miscellaneous Cardiovascular Effects

Supek *et al.* (1962) studied the effect of adrenergic blocking agents and of chlorpromazine on the blood pressure increase by vasopressin and angiotensin. Chlorpromazine potentiated the pressor effect of vasopressin and angiotensin in anesthetized dogs. Potentiation was not due to the blood pressure lowering effect of adrenergic blockade of chlorpromazine.

Chlorpromazine and chlorprothixene (1 mg/kg i.v.), increased respiratory amplitude, whereas the sulfoxides did not. The respiratory rate was reduced by chlorprothixene only. Prompt and prolonged hypotensive response was observed after chlorprothixene, chlorpromazine, triflupromazine, and promazine. None of the compounds tested inhibited or potentiated noradrenaline-induced hypertension (Schültz, 1960).

Giao and Rico (1961) have reported on the effect of some phenothiazine derivatives on capillary permeability in studies with radioactive isotopes. Pretreatment of rats with promazine, promethazine, chlorpromazine, perphenazine, or pyrathiazine, s.c., inhibited capillary permeability to albumin-I^{132} with hyaluronidase. Chlorpromazine was the most effective. The antiinflammatory action seems to be direct and unrelated to systemic effects of these drugs.

Chlorpromazine (i.v.) at large doses caused a drop in blood pressure and a rise in cerebrospinal fluid. The latter rise does not occur at clinically used doses (Feldman and Kidron, 1957).

LeBlanc (1960a,b) has found no difference in the blood pressure effects of chlorpromazine in normal and cold-adapted animals. Eliakim and Feldman (1958) report that chlorpromazine (3 mg/kg i.v. then 3 mg/kg i.a.) has a direct cardiac effect on the cat.

Cardiovascular effects of chlorpromazine have been studied in horses (Hall, 1960) and dogs (Hall and Stevenson, 1960).

I. Endocrine Effects

1. Antishock and Stress Effects

a. *Shock Effects.* Dogs were completely protected against the lethal effects of hemorrhagic shock by 2 mg/kg of chlorpromazine given intravenously before or immediately after hemorrhage (Courvoisier *et al.*, 1953; Fournel, 1952; Jaulmes *et al.*, 1952; Laborit *etal.*, 1952a,b). Protected dogs showed none of the usual signs of shock. Excellent protection was also obtained in intact or eviscerated rodents subjected to hemorrhage (cf. Janssens, 1954; Hershey *et al.*, 1955; Inglis *et al.*, 1959; Roth *et al.*, 1958; Wendel and Charkey, 1958; Millican and Rhodes, 1958a,b; Kajikuri *et al.*, 1957; Gujral and Dhawan, 1957; Jones and Ripstein, 1957; Hunder and Spink, 1957; Zapata-Ortiz and Stastny, 1956; Beck and Redick, 1956; Spurr *et al.*, 1956a,b; Horvath *et al.*, 1956; Carruthers and Gowdey, 1956; Overton and DeBakey, 1956; Mahfouz and Ezz, 1958; Savlov, 1959).

Injection of 2.5–5 mg/kg of chlorpromazine subcutaneously before tumbling in a Noble-Collip drum significantly reduced the resulting mortality in rats; 20 mg/kg after tumbling gave no protection (Fournel, 1952). These effects are similar to those reported for other adrenergic blocking agents such as Dibenzyline®.

Mice were protected against the effects of intravenous or intraperitoneal injection of *Brucella melitensis* toxin by 10 mg/kg of chlorpromazine intramuscularly during the first 2 hours after administration of the toxin; lower or higher doses were less effective (Abernathy and Halbert, 1955). Suboptimal doses of chlorpromazine increased the protective effect of fluorocortisone. Chlorpromazine also prolonged survival time of adrenalectomized mice given *Brucella* toxin. Similarly, chlorpromazine markedly reduced the mortality rate in mice given typhoid or paratyphoid endotoxin (Reilly and Tournier, 1953). Chlorpromazine also protected mice against the lethal effects of the endotoxin from *Hemophilus pertussis* and other endotoxins (Chedid, 1954; Lillehei, 1963).

Survival time of mice exposed to lethal doses of X-radiation was increased by 5 mg/kg of chlorpromazine $\frac{1}{2}$ hour before radiation; higher doses increased mortality (Haley *et al.*, 1955). The state of shock resulting from injection of irritants into the cerebral peduncles of dogs was modified and mortality was greatly reduced by intravenous infusion of chlorpromazine 5 mg/kg before and 5 mg/kg after the procedure (Pocidalo and Tardieu, 1954).

Khrabrova (1961) studied chlorpromazine (5 mg/kg i.m.) in three phases of electric shock in cats: (*a*) erectile phase, characterized by increased blood pressure, excitation, and decreased respiration; (*b*) torpid phase I characterized by animal indifference, decreased blood pressure, and decrease in cardiac contractions; (*c*) torpid phase II, characterized by marked decrease in blood pressure, pulse rate, and respiration. Chlorpromazine had a protective effect in the erectile and torpid phase I, but not in torpid phase II. Torpid phase II was aggravated by chlorpromazine due to its hypotensive action. On the other hand, the combination of chlorpromazine with vasopressors had good therapeutic effect in all phases of experimental shock.

Chlorpromazine (5 mg/kg i.m.) when given 1 hour before burn shock prolonged survival time in rats (Triner and Mráz, 1962). It had no protective effect when given during or after shock. On the other hand, pentamethonium had a protective effect in all experimental conditions (cf. Mráz, 1963; Horn and Converse, 1963; Millican and Rhodes, 1958).

In a controlled study, Collins (1962) showed that chlorpromazine (10–100 mg) was able to control severe hemorrhagic shock occurring during or after surgery in 385 patients. Postoperative renal depression, anuria, or oliguria did not occur. Better results were obtained with chlorpromazine than with classical methods of shock treatment (cf. Collins, 1964).

Orgel (1962) has reviewed the present status of shock treatment, including the use of chlorpromazine and meprobamate.

b. *Stress Effects.* Ogasawara and Yasue (1959) studied intestinal hemorrhage caused by Newcastle disease virus (NDV) in mice. Intestinal hemorrhage and death caused by NDV in mice could be prevented by a prior injection of an adequate dose of chlorpromazine, prednisolone, or hydrocortisone.

The sympathogenic origin and antiadrenergic prevention of stress-induced myocardial lesions were reported on by Raab *et al.* (1961). Restraint-induced myocardial lesions in fluorocortisol-pretreated rats were moderately to markedly prevented by reserpine, chlorpromazine, phenoxybenzamine, and other drugs.

Chlorpromazine, reserpine, or ascorbic acid did not fully prevent a decrease in adrenal ascorbic acid or a compensatory increase of adrenal weight in rats exposed to heat (43°C). The survival rate was highest in the chlorpromazine groups (Juszkiewicz, 1961).

The effects of chlorpromazine and ascorbic acid in rats during simulated transportation conditions at normal and elevated temperatures were studied by Juszkiewicz and Jones (1961a). The study confirmed experimentally the beneficial effects of chlorpromazine and ascorbic acid in allaying the stress of transportation. Under simulated transport conditions, chlorpromazine protected rats against excessive weight losses, excessive depletion of adrenal ascorbic acid, and excessive mortality experienced at high temperature. Simultaneous administration of ascorbic acid seemed to promote anti-stress effects. The same authors (Juszkiewicz and Jones, 1961b) also found that chlorpromazine in pigs increased the survivor rate at 40°C and decreased body weight loss (cf. DeBias *et al.*, 1958; Hormia, 1959; LeBlanc, 1958a,b,c,d).

The effect of hypothermia on dextran and egg-white edema was studied by Szilágyi *et al.* (1961). Hypothermia of 18° and 20°C inhibited both types of edema in rats. The effect is probably based on inhibition of histamine and serotonin liberation. Chlorpromazine (3 mg/100 g i.m.) was less potent than physical hypothermia; cortisone had no effect, and phenobarbital promoted development of edema.

The effects of tranquilizers on bacterial toxemias were reported by Greenberg and Ingalls (1962). Pretreatment with chlorpromazine (25 mg/kg i.p.) but not hydroxyzine or chlordiazepoxide prolonged survival time in mice given large doses of bacterial endotoxins or exotoxins. Reserpine gave no protective effect against bacterial endotoxins. The authors concluded that the antitoxic effect of chlorpromazine is not related to its serotonin-releasing effect (cf. Noyes et al., 1956; Chatonnet and Tanche, 1955; Thomas; 1956; Abernathy et al., 1957; Grosz and Norton, 1959; Abernathy and Spink, 1957).

The effect of stress and tranquilization on plasma free fatty acid levels in the rat was reported by Mallov and Witt (1961). Plasma free fatty acids rose 32, 51, and 126% after 2, 4, and 7 hours, respectively, of stress induced by irregular unavoidable electric shocking in female rats. Chlorpromazine (4 or 8 mg/kg s.c.) 5 minutes before stress began, significantly reduced these levels in rats subjected to 4-hour shock. When 8 mg/kg s.c. of chlorpromazine was given 1 hour prior to stress, there was no increase in free fatty acid level. Meprobamate, 200 mg/kg s.c., had a similar effect. It should be noted that neither chlorpromazine nor meprobamate had any effect on free fatty acids in normal, nonstressed rats.

Intraperitoneal injection of 10 mg/kg or oral administration of 20 mg/kg of chlorpromazine in rats resulted in depletion of eosinophils by approximately 70%, equivalent to that resulting from 0.25 mg/kg of epinephrine (Smith Kline and French, 1956). The response to 15 mg/kg subcutaneously was about the same as that of 75 mg/kg of ephedrine orally (average fall in eosinophil count was 48% 4 hours after injection). Adrenalectomized rats showed very little change in eosinophil count after chlorpromazine. A steep drop in both total white cell and lymphocyte counts was observed within 2 hours after subcutaneous injection of chlorpromazine 20 mg/kg in rats (Kuchler and Koch, 1955, 1954); values returned to normal within 48 hours. Adrenalectomized rats given similar doses showed somewhat smaller but significant decreases which were less prolonged than in intact animals. In parenteral doses of 5 mg/kg and over, chlorpromazine also decreased adrenal ascorbic acid content significantly (Holzbauer and Vogt, 1954; Hamburger, 1955; Nasmyth, 1955).

Early reports indicated that chlorpromazine blocked the pituitary-adrenal response to stress in rats. Later studies have not confirmed this; the disagreement is probably due to a marked difference in doses. In the Sayers test, chlorpromazine in doses of 10–50 mg/kg (Castaigne, 1954; Aron et al., 1953; Aron, 1954) or 100–200 mg/kg (Hamburger, 1955) completely blocked the depletion of adrenal ascorbic acid resulting from the stress of unilateral adrenalectomy. Treated animals still responded to ACTH (adrenocorticotropin), and the authors suggested that chlorpromazine could replace hypophysectomy in the standard assay of this hormone (cf. Fotherby, 1959;

Saarima, 1963). Another group reported that 10–50 mg/kg decreased but did not block the adrenal ascorbic acid response to formaldehyde injection (Cheymol et al., 1954), and they were unable to establish a dose-response relationship for ACTH in chlorpromazine-treated animals.

Doses of 10 or 15 mg/kg 30 minutes or 3 hours before surgical stress did not prevent the resulting fall in adrenal ascorbic acid; the higher dose of chlorpromazine alone produced a response equivalent to that of surgery (Holzbauer and Vogt, 1954). A dose of 10 mg/kg produced a significant depletion of adrenal ascorbic acid; 2.5 mg/kg did not (Nasmyth, 1955). The latter dose did not block the effect of surgery, adrenaline 25 μg/kg, or histamine 100 mg/kg. The effects of 50 μg/kg adrenaline seemed to be increased by chlorpromazine; there was a moderate reduction of the effect of histamine (10 mg/kg) in intact and 100 mg/kg in adrenal-demedullated animals.

Single parenteral doses of 1–20 mg/kg or repeated oral doses of chlorpromazine did not prevent the eosinopenic response to surgical trauma or to the injection of epinephrine or histamine in rats. The fall in lymphocytes, eosinophils, and total white cells in an anesthetized dog cooled to 28°C was not prevented but rather increased and prolonged by 5 mg/kg of chlorpromazine intravenously (Miletzky et al., 1955). Administration of 25–50 mg intravenously or intramuscularly to surgical patients before or during anesthesia caused no significant alteration in the response to stress, as measured by eosinophil count and urinary 17-ketosteroid or corticoid excretion (Vandewater and Gordon, 1955). Doses of 50–100 mg intramuscularly 2 hours preoperatively seemed to reduce the fall in eosinophils during operation (Keating, 1954). In severely burned dogs given repeated injections of chlorpromazine 2.5 mg/kg, blood 17-hydroxysteroids and eosinophils remained unchanged, serum ADH (antidiuretic hormone) did not increase, and pituitary oxytocin content was not decreased (Shibusawa et al., 1955). Since responses to exogenous ACTH, vasopressin, and oxytocin were intact, the author concluded that chlorpromazine acted by suppressing hypothalamic-neurohypophyseal neurosecretion.

Administration of chlorpromazine in doses of 10 or 20 mg/kg/day subcutaneously to intact or adrenalectomized rats caused no change in thymus weight compared to controls and did not prevent atrophy resulting from hydrocortisone 8 mg/kg/day. Adrenal weight was significantly increased in chlorpromazine-treated animals; adrenal atrophy in hydrocortisone-treated rats was significantly reduced by chlorpromazine (10 mg/kg/day). Single doses of 100 mg/kg produced no change in adrenal weight (Hamburger, 1955). In rats kept at a temperature of 4°C, the progressive changes in adrenal histology were halted but not reversed by chlorpromazine (Schaumkell, 1955a,b,c); when treatment was started during the third hour of a prolonged period of cooling, the adrenals resembled those of controls killed after 3 hours.

Adrenalectomized rats maintained with saline died within 24 hours after chlorpromazine (20 mg/kg) administered subcutaneously (Kuchler and Koch, 1954, 1955), but they survived several days longer if epinephrine or norepinephrine was also given. When adrenalectomized mice were maintained at a temperature of 4°C, survival time was markedly decreased by subcutaneous administration of 10–25 mg/kg of chlorpromazine and the protective effect of hydrocortisone was completely abolished (Smith Kline and French, 1956). Mean survival times were: untreated mice, 5 hours, chlorpromazine-treated, 3 hours; hydrocortisone-treated, over 8 hours; hydrocortisone plus chlorpromazine, 3 hours.

Rats given a single subcutaneous injection of 19–20 mg/kg of chlorpromazine showed little change in electroshock threshold but a marked slowing and decrease in the number of body movements during seizures (Smith Kline and French, 1956). Pretreatment with 10 mg/kg/day by the same route decreased shock threshold in intact rats but had no effect in adrenalectomized animals.

The inflammatory reaction in mice to subcutaneous injection of gelatin in saline-alcohol solution was moderately decreased by intraperitoneal injection of chlorpromazine in doses of 10 mg/kg 35 minutes before the irritant, or by oral administration of 1.25 ml of a 1% solution. Mice which had been given chlorpromazine in their food for 3 days, adrenalectomized, and then tested also showed some reduction in inflammatory reaction. In all cases, the effect was much less than that of cortisone. Simultaneous subcutaneous injection of the inflammatory agent and chlorpromazine resulted in an increased reaction. The arthritic response to intra-articular injection of mustard or kaolin was not modified by chlorpromazine; the latter with phenylbutazone and aminopyrine had an effect equal to that of cortisone, in either intact or adrenalectomized rats (Ducommun, 1952).

The effects of chlorpromazine on the pituitary adrenal axis are not well defined, some authors reporting a stimulating effect (Harwood and Mason, 1957; Egdahl and Richards, 1956; Harwood, 1956; B. M. Kovács et al., 1956; K. Kovács et al., 1956) and others reporting a depressant action (Shibusawa, et al., 1956; Sulman and Winnik, 1956a,b; Olling and de Wied, 1956a,b; Ohler et al., 1956).

2. Miscellaneous Endocrine Effects

Groups of rats received thyroxine (1 mg/kg s.c.) for 3 days; on the fourth day a neuroplegic drug was added and the rise in O_2 consumption was measured. Chlorpromazine (5 mg/kg s.c.) increased O_2 consumption 201% above that of control animals given thyroxine only. Reserpine had less effect, phenobarbital decreased thyroxine effect, and meprobamate caused no change. Chlorpromazine (5 mg/kg s.c.) increased O_2 consumption 222% in thyroidectomized rats (Vogel and Tervooren, 1961). The authors suggest that thyroxine-metabolizing enzymes may be inhibited by chlorpromazine and reserpine.

On the other hand, chlorpromazine was compared with antithyroid substances by Theret (1962a,b,c). It was reported to produce lesions like those produced by 6-benzylthiouracil in certain hypothalamic cells of Wistar rats. Árvay et al. (1960) report that the effect of severe nervous traumatization on thyroid function is inhibited by chlorpromazine. Mayer et al. (1956) reported on the direct antithyroid activity of chlorpromazine and other drugs. Similar results were reported by Taterka-Seiler (1958), by Milcou et al. (1957), and by Sámel (1958).

Nine phenothiazines caused melanophore dispersion in intact frogs (Scott and Nading, 1961). The most active drugs contain a trifluomethyl group and piperazine ring. All phenothiazines were ineffective in hypophysectomized animals. The authors conclude that phenothiazines effect release of melanocyte stimulating hormone by direct action on hypophysis or indirectly via brain centers. A parallel between the minimum effective dose, therapeutic ratio and structure was drawn.

Low levels of chlorpromazine in the diet have been reported to have a favorable effect on the growth and metabolism of vitamin B_6-deficient rats. The growth enhancing effect may be similar to that seen with antibiotic feed supplements (Mathues et al., 1959).

In guinea pigs given 50 mg/kg of chlorpromazine simultaneously with 5 μc of I^{131}, uptake of the isotope by the thyroid was slowed during the first 24 hours (Marocco and Brena, 1953). After this time, release of the stored material was also slower, so that after 48 hours thyroids of treated animals contained more isotope than those of untreated animals. Maximum uptake in chlorpromazine-treated animals was less than controls. The effect of TSH (thyrotropin) on uptake was not blocked.

The decrease in I^{131} uptake resulting from surgical shock (evisceration) in guinea pigs was partially antagonized by chlorpromazine 50 mg/kg (Brena and Marocco, 1953). Chlorpromazine administration (2.5 mg intraperitoneally every 5 hours) apparently halted progressive changes in rat thyroid histology during exposure to cold (cf. similar effects on adrenals, Schaumkell, 1955a,b,c). Effects of TSH or thyroxine were also halted. (Effects of chlorpromazine on basal metabolism and oxygen consumption are discussed on pages 70 and 71.)

Chlorpromazine may also decrease growth hormone secretion in rats (Sulman and Winnik, 1956a,b).

Chlorpromazine has a rather complex effect on diuresis, depending on the dose used (Basu, 1956). Thus chlorpromazine enhanced the antidiuretic effect of nicotine and posterior pituitary extract (antidiuretic hormone), while the chloruretic effect of both drugs was diminished (Supek et al., 1960a; Kovács et al., 1957). Chlorpromazine itself was reported to have an antidiuretic effect in hydrated rats (Supek *et al.*, 1960b). This effect was at its peak early in the test, perhaps explaining the failure of Dasgupta and Hausler (1955a,b,c) to obtain an antidiuretic effect with chlorpromazine.

De Wied and Jinks (1958) reported that chlorpromazine inhibited the antidiuretic response of rats to painful stimuli, but were not able to find any effect on the antidiuretic responses to histamine or nicotine. Chlorpromazine is reported to antagonize the antidiuretic effect of serotonin (Dasgupta, 1957).

Chlorpromazine has been reported to inhibit vasopressin release in the rat (Moses, 1964).

3. Pituitary-Gonadal Effects

When prepubertal female rats were given chlorpromazine in doses of 1 or 5 mg/kg/day subcutaneously, no changes were observed in response to estrogen (Courvoisier and Ducrot, 1954; Courvoisier *et al.*, 1953). Virgin adult rats given similar doses showed no significant change in estrus cycle length. Doses of 5 mg/kg/day for 3 weeks to male guinea pigs produced no change in morphology, motility, or number of sperm (cf. Foote and Gray, 1960).

In female rats given 1 or 5 mg/kg/day for 3 weeks and then mated to treated or untreated males, or in females treated only after mating, for the duration of gestation and lactation, there were no adverse effects on duration of gestation, number of litters weaned, number of young per litter, or weight of young at birth or at weaning. Doses of 10 mg/kg/day subcutaneously intraperitoneally for 3 weeks prevented occurrence of estrus in virgin female rats (Krais *et al.*, 1954; Dasgupta, 1955). Normal cycles reappeared at varying intervals after chlorpromazine was withdrawn. However, continuous estrus induced by estradiol benzoate was not suppressed by chlorpromazine, even at 40 mg/kg (Dasgupta, 1955; Dasgupta and Hausler, 1955a,b,c), indicating that the effect of chlorpromazine is central, probably on the hypothalamus, rather than peripheral.

Another report states that intraperitoneal injection of 10 mg/kg produced continuous anestrus in normal rats, while the same dose subcutaneously prolonged both estrus and anestrus phases of the cycle (Sulman and Winnik, 1956a,b). Immature rabbits primed with estrogen and given progesterone 0.5 mg/day and chlorpromazine 10 mg/kg/day both subcutaneously maintained the progestational changes in the uterus as long as chlorpromazine was given, while those given no chlorpromazine reverted to normal after about 2 weeks.

Several clinical reports noted the irregularity of menstrual cycles or amenorrhea, increased excretion of FSH (follicle-stimulating hormone), and breast engorgement of galactorrhea in female patients treated with chlorpromazine (Donnadieu et al., 1955; Sulman and Winnik, 1956a,b; Kinross-Wright, 1954; Polishuk and Kulcsar, 1956).

Induced ovulation in the mouse and the measurement of its inhibition was studied by Purshottam et al. (1961; Purshottam, 1962). Superovulation was induced in mice by pregnant mare serum gonadotropin (2 I.U. i.p.) followed in 42 hours by human chorionic gonadotropin (1 I.U. i.p.). Inhibitory effects of various tranquilizers, sedatives, narcotics, antispasmodics, steroids, and antihistamines were studied. Fairly consistent inhibition of ovulation occurred with reserpine (0.01 mg), chlorpromazine (0.125–0.25 mg) (cf. Bhargava and Jaitly, 1964), prochlorperazine (1 mg/kg), perphenazine (0.1 mg), and promazine (0.5 mg). Other tranquilizers, including trifluoperazine, inhibited ovulation to some degree. Of eight steroids tested, only progesterone and 17α-ethynyl-estra-$\Delta^{5,10}$-enolone were inhibitory. The assay procedure offers a tool for screening of drugs affecting ovulation.

Cranston (1961), examined the effects of antiestrus drugs on subestrus of ovariectomized C3H mice. Chlorpromazine, perphenazine, and meprobamate had an antiestrus effect on intact mice (cf. Jarrett, 1963), but did not alter frequency of subestrus nor development of subestrus in ovariectomized C3H mice.

Chlorpromazine (15 mg/kg s.c.) induced lobulo-alveolar growth in mammary glands and initiated milk secretion in rats initially primed with estradiol (10 μg/day for 10 days). This dose also maintained mammary lobulo-alveolar structure and secretion in postpartum rats for 10 days after litter removal. Chlorpromazine also significantly increased adrenal weight and decreased thymus weight, indicating adrenal stimulation (Talwalker et al., 1960).

Mammotropic effects of tranquilizing drugs in rats, pigeons, guinea pigs, and rabbits were reported by Khazan et al. (1962). Reserpine, trifluoperazine, prochlorperazine, perphenazine, and triflupromazine were the most effective mammotropic agents. Chlorpromazine and chlordiazepoxide were moderately effective, levomepromazine, methopromazine, aminopromazine, prothipendyl, meprobamate, hydroxyzine, ethinamate, phenobarbital, and benactyzine were ineffective. In humans, 33/650 patients given chlorpromazine showed galactorrhea. Five cases were noted among 43 patients given reserpine and 30 given reserpine with chlorpromazine (cf. Grönroos et al., 1959; Benson, 1960; Barraclough and Sawyer, 1957, 1959; Brillhart, 1959; Cranston, 1958a,b; Chambon, 1957; Alloiteau, 1957).

Chaudhury et al. (1961) reported on stress-induced block of milk ejection. Chlorpromazine, reserpine, or meprobamate, administered to lactating guinea pigs at various periods before suckling, reduced block in milk ejection caused by stress. Phenoxybenzamine had no effect. The data suggest that stress-induced block in milk ejection is probably nervous in origin and not mediated via adrenalin.

J. Gastrointestinal and Hepatic Effects

1. Gastric Effects

Parenteral administration of chlorpromazine to pyloric ligated (Shay) rats decreased the volume of gastric secretion and lowered incidence of ulcers with little effect on acid secretion. Single injections of 20 mg/kg decreased secretion and lowered the incidence of ulcers by about 40%; lesions which did develop were smaller than those in control animals (Courvoisier et al., 1953; Sun and Shay, 1956, 1959; Shay et al., 1959). A similar dose given 2 hours before operation and repeated every 6 hours during the 24-hour survival period completely prevented the development of ulcers and hemorrhages (Aron, 1954; Aron et al., 1954); the volume of secretion was decreased about 80% although acid concentration was higher than in untreated controls. The good results were believed due to inhibition of reflex disturbances of circulation and capillary permeability resulting from pyloric irritation. When chlorpromazine was given orally after ligation, allowed to remain in the stomach for ½ to 2 hours, and then washed out, volume and acidity of secretion were both reduced during subsequent observation periods; this was probably due to a local inhibitory effect on enzymes of the gastric mucosa. Acid secretion by isolated rat gastric membrane was inhibited 50% by a 10^{-4} M solution of chlorpromazine and 85% by a 10^{-3} M solution. Bornmann (1961) reported that chlorpromazine and chlorprothixene were superior to meprobamate and chlordiazepoxide in their protective effects against Shay ulcers in rats (cf. Pfeiffer et al., 1963).

In human subjects free of active gastrointestinal disease, intramuscular injection of 50 mg of chlorpromazine markedly decreased the volume of gastric secretion without change in free acidity (Haverback et al., 1955). The response to insulin was not blocked (Dobkin et al., 1954a,b,c). Ulcer patients given the drug by infusion at rates of 2–100 mg/hour responded with significant decreases in volume, acid (total and free acid concentration), total pepsin, and total cathepsin secretion in the basal state, but had a normal response to histamine (Haverback et al., 1955).

Zimmerman (1962) reported that megacolon resulted from large doses of chlorpromazine. Forty-one of 99 rats developed megacolon after i.p. administration of one or more doses of chlorpromazine at high levels of 46 mg/kg.

Chlorpromazine inhibited the absorption of sugar from the intestine of rats. This phenomenon was said to be due to depression of the motility of intestinal villi (Gati et al., 1958).

2. Smooth Muscle

In anesthetized cats, intravenous doses of 1.7–6.3 mg/kg of chlorpromazine relaxed the tone of the small intestine, bladder, and uterus (Huidobro, 1954).

As noted previously, chlorpromazine did not block the effects of epinephrine or of pre- or postganglionic stimulation of the hypogastric or splanchnic nerves. Doses of 1–3 mg/kg temporarily blocked the effects of eserine 1 mg/kg subcutaneously on intestinal tone and peristalsis (Courvoisier et al., 1953), an effect equivalent to that of 0.5 mg/kg of atropine intravenously. In isolated rabbit and rat intestine preparations, tone and amplitude of spontaneous contractions were reduced by concentrations of 10^{-6} molar (Lamarche and Arnould, 1954) and 5 mg/liter (approximately 1.4×10^{-5} molar), and activity was completely abolished by 10 mg/liter (Courvoisier et al., 1953). Acetylcholine-induced spasm was prevented or relaxed by similar concentrations. In addition, spasm produced by barium chloride was prevented by chlorpromazine in concentrations of 1.5–5 mg/liter (Courvoisier et al., 1953). Other spasmolytic studies on phenothiazine were carried out by Vivoli (1960).

The effect of some phenothiazine derivatives on isolated gall bladder of the guinea pig was studied by Vanlerenverghe et al. (1960). Promazine, methopromazine, chlorpromazine, and acetylpromazine antagonized acetylcholine-induced contractions of the gall bladder in guinea pigs. Substitution of methoxy, chlorine, or acetyl groups had no effect on spasmolytic activity.

Cholecystokinin and histamine normally provoke prompt contraction of isolated guinea pig gall bladder perfused with Tyrode glucose solution (Giro, 1960). Chlorpromazine (12.5 mg/l) completely inhibited cholecystokinin activity. Chlorpromazine probably has no specific effect on cholecystokinin, since it also inhibited histamine. The data may be significant for the interpretation of chlorpromazine jaundice.

Chlorpromazine has been shown to reduce or abolish the twitch in guinea pig ileum induced by electrical stimulation (Dandiya, 1963).

3. Liver

As yet, no one has been able to reproduce the chlorpromazine-jaundice syndrome in animals, and there is very little published experimental data that might give a clue as to its mechanism. One study was carried out in dogs with a tube in the common duct and a second tube for recording duodenal motility (Menguy et al., 1955). After 10 mg/kg of chlorpromazine intravenously, duodenal motility increased in all animals. Pressure in the common duct increased markedly in cholecystectomized dogs; intact animals showed no change in common duct pressure but a great increase in resistance of the biliary sphincter to saline perfusion through the inlying tube (cf. Stefko and Zbinden, 1963). All these changes occurred simultaneously, about 30 to 60 minutes after chlorpromazine injection. These effects were similar to those of morphine, but of longer duration. They were more intense in fasted animals. The authors conclude that, particularly in poorly nourished patients with some biliary dysfunction, chlorpromazine might cause back-pressure in the biliary tree and eventually an obstructive type of jaundice.

Gall bladder X-ray studies have been done in a small group of human subjects given 25–50 mg of chlorpromazine intramuscularly (Celice et al., 1955). Over half the group showed delayed evacuation after chlorpromazine and most of them also showed colonic distention. These authors suggest that, in patients with subclinical liver or gall bladder disease, such effects might eventually lead to retention jaundice. Several papers (Moyer et al., 1954a,b; Cohen and Archer, 1955; Stacey et al., 1955) report repeated liver function tests on groups of patients while taking chlorpromazine; all indicate that patients who do not develop jaundice show no significant alteration in any of the tests. In jaundiced patients, blood studies revealed a picture resembling that of obstructive jaundice; histological examination of liver biopsy specimens showed changes resembling those seen in jaundice due to methyltestosterone. Kelsey et al. (1955) have published tables of data on a number of patients and Gibbons et al. (1955) discussed possible mechanisms. It seems generally agreed that jaundice is probably an idiosyncratic or allergic-like reaction occurring in a small proportion of patients. The fact that it is often accompanied or preceded by an increase in blood eosinophils tends to confirm this.

Acute experiments in rats showed that chlorpromazine (2.4 mg/kg i.v.) decreased biliary excretion of exogenous bromsulfophthalein from the control value of 67 to 54% within the first 45 minutes. Since chlorpromazine had no effect on bromsulfophthalein in the blood, Clodi and Schnack (1961) concluded that chlorpromazine has a direct effect on bromsulfophthalein secretion by liver cells. In an addendum, Wolf reported that chlorpromazine (50 mg i.v.) had no effect on circulation in liver or excretory function of liver cells in ten normal subjects.

Penetration of lipid films by compounds preventing liver necrosis in rats has been studied by Bangham et al. (1962). A correlation between protective activity of a given compound and its interaction at both air/water and lipid/water interfaces was observed. Protection was shown by promazine, promethazine, Nupercaine® hydrochloride, chlorpromazine, cetyltrimethylammonium bromide, docosanylpyridinium bromide, and stearylamine. Sodium hexadecyl sulfate and sodium dodecyl sulfate were ineffective. The data suggest that restoration of lipid membrane to normal is achieved either by presence of nonpolar portions of amphipathic molecules or by strategic positioning of their positive groups of membrane interface. Amphipathic molecules have both hydrophobic and polar groups.

K. Neuromuscular Effects (Muscle Relaxation)

Intra-arterial injection of chlorpromazine in doses of 3.1 and 4.6 mg/kg caused a gradual but marked decrease in response to stimulation of the cat sciatic nerve-gastrocnemius muscle preparation (Kopera and Armitage, 1954; Burns, 1954). The effect was not altered by blood pressure increase or by nalorphine. A dose of 1.3 mg/kg prolonged the action of d-tubocurarine. Smaller doses, up to 1.35 mg/cat, injected into the terminal aorta did not modify the intensity of the quadriceps muscle response to nerve stimulation, and neither increased nor decreased the effect of d-tubocurarine (Huidobro, 1954). The effect of the curarizing agent, gallamine triethiodide, in rabbits was increased and prolonged by 10 mg/kg s.c. of chlorpromazine (Courvoisier et al., 1953).

In the isolated, rat, phrenic-nerve-diaphragm preparation, 200 mg of chlorpromazine/50 mg of bath solution caused a rapid decrease in responsiveness to electrical stimulation (Kopera and Armitage, 1954). Concentrations of 4×10^{-6} to 4×10^{-4} M produced contracture of the isolated frog rectus abdominis muscle after a latent period which decreased with increasing concentration of chlorpromazine (Boriani, 1955; see also Su and Lee, 1960; Wislicki, 1958; Mashkovsky and Medvedev, 1956). Electromyographic records in rabbits which had received intra-muscular injections of tetanus toxin showed complete disappearance of action potentials after intravenous injection of 0.75–1.25 mg/kg of chlorpromazine (Hougs and Andersen, 1954; Kelly and Laurence, 1956). The maximal effect lasted about 2 hours, followed by a gradual return to the original spastic state. Several clinical papers report relief of muscular spasm and convulsions in patients suffering from tetanus when chlorpromazine was given intramuscularly or intravenously (Kelly and Laurence, 1956; Gelfand, 1955; Cole and Robertson, 1955; Adriani and Kerr, 1955).

An experimental basis for chlorpromazine therapy in tetanus has been suggested by Gromova et al. (1962). In normal rabbits, stimulation of reticular formation by implanted electrodes produced marked EEG changes but no electromyographic (EMG) changes. Following injection of tetanus toxin, similar stimulation altered both EEG and EMG. Chlorpromazine (5–10 mg/kg i.v.) produced muscle relaxation and reduced EMG activity in tetanus-intoxicated rabbits. Electroencencephalographic changes following chlorpromazine varied with the stage of illness. Chlorpromazine apparently acts by inhibiting effects of both cerebral cortex and reticular formation on tetanus intoxication.

The effects of some central nervous system depressants on the phasic and tonic stretch reflex have been reported by Chin and Smith (1962). The effects of cumulative i.v. doses of various drugs were studied on phasic and tonic components of the stretch reflex of ankle extensor muscles of decerebrate cats. All compounds produced more depression of the tonic than the phasic component. A difference in degree of depression of phasic and tonic reflex components was most marked with mephenesin and least with pentobarbital. The ascending order of potency of 75% depression of tonic component was:

zoxazolamine, carisoprodol, mephenesin, caramiphen, scopolamine, pentobarbital, and chlorpromazine. Chlorpromazine was 16 times as potent as zoxazolamine.

The site of action of chlorpromazine and mephenesin in experimental tetanus was studied by Webster (1961, 1962). Both compounds were studied quantitatively in intact, spinal and decerebrate rabbits with local tetanus. The effect of chlorpromazine in spinal animals differed from that in intact and decerebrate animals and depended on the level of brain-stem section. Mephenesin was equally effective in all preparations. It was concluded that mephenesin suppressed tetanus by blocking transmission in motor pathways in spinal cord, while the action of chlorpromazine was probably entirely on the reticular system.

Laurence and Webster (1961) studied tachyphylaxis to the antitetanus activity of some phenothiazine compounds. Chlorpromazine and acepromazine were the most potent inhibitors of experimental tetanus produced by *Clostridium tetani* toxin in rabbits. However, tachyphylaxis and sometimes muscle stimulation occurred. These effects were attributed to the action of the drugs on brain-stem reticular formation, since they did not occur in spinal animals. Methotrimeprazine was more potent than chlorpromazine in experimental tetanus and the data indicate its possible superiority to chlorpromazine in treatment of clinical tetanus; it induced less stimulation and had an antiepinephrine activity equal to that of chlorpromazine (cf. Kelly and Laurence, 1956; Laurence and Webster, 1958).

L. Miscellaneous Effects

1. Antihistaminic, Anti-Serotonin, and Anti-Inflammatory Activity

Although chlorpromazine is related chemically to such potent antihistaminic drugs as promethazine, it has only weak antihistaminic activity. Subcutaneous administration of 10 mg/kg gave no protection against histamine aerosol in guinea pigs, and 20 mg/kg protected for less than an hour, compared to protection for 10 hours after 1 mg/kg of promethazine (Courvoisier *et al.*, 1953). With 10 mg/kg of chlorpromazine intraperitoneally, two of three guinea pigs were protected. Given in aerosol form, chlorpromazine had about one-twentieth the effectiveness of promethazine against histamine aerosol (Kent *et al.*, 1954a,b). Chlorpromazine had about one one-hundredth the activity of promethazine against bronchospasm induced by intravenous histamine (Kopera and Armitage, 1954; Masson *et al.*, 1958); a subcutaneous dose of 20 mg/kg protected guinea pigs against five lethal doses of histamine subcutaneously (Kopeloff *et al.*, 1955). In isolated guinea pig ileum preparations, chlorpromazine was about one-third as effective as promethazine and about one-fourth as effective as pyrilamine in preventing histamine spasm (van Proosdij-Hartzema, 1955).

Although the depressor effect of histamine was decreased by chlorpromazine in both dogs and pigs, the effects of peptone and polyvinylpyrrolidone, both of which are believed to act by releasing histamine in the body, were not altered (Decortis and Lecomte, 1953; Besse and Patay, 1953).

Rajapurkar and Panjwani (1960) reported on restoration by antihistamine drugs of the pressor response to adrenaline following adrenergic blockade. The effects of mepyramine and antazoline were studied on adrenergic blockade and the depressor response produced by benzylimidazoline, dihydroergotamine or chlorpromazine in dogs. Mepyramine was more consistently effective in negating depressor response and restoring pressor response to epinephrine. Antazoline did not abolish chlorpromazine-induced blockade and 50% of the time did not restore pressor response to epinephrine after benzylimidazoline block.

Other reports on the antihistaminic/antiinflammatory/anti-serotonin activity of chlorpromazine have been published by Saxena (1960), Ryall (1956), Sackler *et al.* (1959), Ogasawara and Nakayama (1958), Herxheimer (1956), Gyermek *et al.* (1956), Harris *et al.* (1960), Jasmin and Bois (1960), Rosenberg and Savarie (1963), and by Bulle (1957a,b). Stucki and Thompson (1958) and Kátó and Gözsy (1960) have reported on the inhibition of dextran edema in the rat by phenothiazine derivatives.

Twenty-three phenothiazines were studied in rats for anti-inflammatory effects (Gözsy and Kátó, 1960). Only promethazine, chlorpromazine, trimeprazine, levomepromazine, and 2'-methyl-3"-piperidine-10-propyl-phenothiazine both prevented dextran-induced edema and the inflammatory reaction of the skin to histamine or 48/80 and were effective neuroleptics or antihistamines. The data do not exclude the hypothesis that neuroleptic action is partially due to action on capillary permeability and regulation of the blood supply in the CNS.

Rocha e Silva and Antonio (1960) reported on release of bradykinin and the mechanism of production of "thermic edema (45°C)" in the rat's paw. Heating a rat paw for 20–25 minutes in a water bath at 44–45°C produced edema very similar to that produced by egg white, dextran, or passive cutaneous anaphylaxis. The role of histamine in this edema was excluded because histamine inhibitors had no effect on intensity of edema. On the other hand, bradykinin was demonstrated to be the mediator of this type of edema. This was shown by a new technique of coaxial perfusion. The edema was reduced by chlorpromazine, reserpine, and phenoxybenzamine.

The effect of CNS depressants on experimental models of inflammation were studied by Vogel (1961). A study was made of phenobarbital, chlorpromazine, reserpine, and *Voacanaga africana* alkaloids in ovalbumin-, dextran-, and kaolin-induced edema of the rat paw. Phenobarbital was ineffective. Chlorpromazine and other compounds inhibited ovalbumin and dextran but not kaolin edema. It was concluded that the activity is not due to CNS action, but rather to a direct peripheral effect resulting in an increase in capillary resistance.

A combination of antiviral and anti-inflammatory agents in the treatment of influenzal infections in mice was studied by Berti (1961). Chlorpromazine, ABOB-X (abitylguanide), and cortisone were tested alone and in combination with P8 (bismuth and sodium pyrocatechol disulfonates) on influenza infection in mice. The drugs were given (s.c.) 24 hours before intranasal infection and repeated daily for 7 days. Chlorpromazine and ABOB-X had slight protective effect, cortisone aggravated infection, P8 alone had a favorable effect, simultaneous administration of P8 and chlorpromazine or ABOB-X significantly reduced severity of infection and was considered true potentiation. It was concluded that an antiviral drug can be potentiated by an anti-inflammatory agent.

2. Local Anesthetic Activity

Injected around the sciatic nerve in guinea pigs, a 0.1% solution of chlorpromazine was as effective in producing local anesthesia as 0.75% procaine or 0.2% cocaine (Courvoisier et al., 1953). Subcutaneous injection of 5 mg/kg doubled the effectiveness of procaine injected along the sciatic nerve, and 20 mg/kg increased the local anesthetic effect of procaine on the rabbit cornea about ten times. Concentrations of 0.1–0.2% produced plexus anesthesia in the frog and dermal anesthesia in the guinea pig (Kopera and Armitage, 1954; Burns, 1954).

Ritchie and Greengard (1961) speculated on the active structure of local anesthetics. A study was made of chlorpromazine, dibucaine, tetracaine, imipramine, and procaine in mammalian nonmyelinated fibers of the rabbit vagus nerve. The data showed that the positively charged form, rather than the uncharged form, is responsible for blocking impulse conduction.

3. Renal Effects

Tiwari et al. (1960a,b) reported on the effect of tranquilizing agents on water and saline-induced diuresis in rats. In water-hydrated rats, chlorpromazine has an antidiuretic effect in the first 120 minutes but after 180 minutes urine output equals that of controls. Chlorpromazine potentiates and preserves circulating endogenous ADH. Removal of the chlorine atom, branching of the propyl chain or substitution of the propyl group diminishes antidiuretic effect and enhances diuresis. Phenothiazines with more potent anticholinergic action have low antidiuretic action; those with anticholinesterase action show marked antidiuretic action. In saline-hydrated rats, prochlorperazine had definite diuretic action, whereas chlorpromazine had definite antidiuretic action.

Intravenous chlorpromazine, 10 mg in humans and 50 mg in dogs, produced no consistent changes in renal function except for a moderate increase in urine volume and sodium excretion noted in the dogs (Moyer *et al.*, 1954a,b). In rats given a water load by stomach tube, subcutaneous chlorpromazine increased water retention, but when they were given 0.9% saline, chlorpromazine had a diuretic effect; these effects resembled those of Pitressin (Meier *et al.*, 1955). Renal plasma flow and glomerular filtration rate decreased immediately after 25 mg of chlorpromazine intravenously in human subjects, while filtration fraction and urine flow increased (Parrish and Levine, 1956). This parodixical effect may be due to inhibition of antidiuretic hormone in the presence of renal vasoconstriction.

4. Analgesia (see page 62)

Leme and Rocha e Silva (1961) reported on the analgesic action of chlorpromazine and reserpine in relation to that of morphine. The analgesic action of reserpine reaches maximal intensity in 48–72 hours and decreases gradually until 144 hours in mice tested by the hot-plate method. The action of chlorpromazine is quicker in onset but disappears within a few hours. Both drugs potentiate the analgesic action of morphine.

Weitzman and Ross (1962) reported on a behavioral method for the study of pain perception in the monkey. The method is based on application of increasing intensities of shock to the gasserian ganglion of alert monkeys by means of implanted electrodes. The monkeys reduced the intensity of painful shock by pressing a lever and thereby regulating and maintaining level of tolerated intensity. Morphine (0.125–0.5 mg/kg i.m.) increased the level of tolerable shock. Chlorpromazine, 0.3 mg/kg, and pentobarbital, 5 mg/kg, i.v., produced large fluctuations in intensity of tolerable shock, thereby interfering with the monkeys' abilities to maintain constant levels of tolerance. Methamphetamine and procaine decreased variability and increased level of tolerable shock.

5. Decompression

Sautet *et al.* (1960) report that chlorpromazine (5 mg/kg parenterally) enabled rabbits to survive acute changes in decompression much more easily than did controls. Only minimal changes were noted with heparin. Although the exact mechanism of chlorpromazine action is unknown, it may act on the enzymatic chain which produces coagulation. Also, it probably inhibits the stress which accompanies decompression. Similar results were obtained in mice (Sautet *et al.*, 1961). Chlorpromazine gave some protection against the toxic effects of oxygen at high pressure (Bean, 1956).

6. Other Effects

A paper by Block (1961) reports that experiments in mice suggest that cerebral tissues become more sensitive to X-rays under hypothermia as seen with chlorpromazine therapy, and that a differential sensitivity, favorable to treatment, may exist between tumor and normal tissue cells.

Systemically administered chlorpromazine reduced intraocular pressure in man and in experimental animals (Paul and Leopold, 1956a,b).

M. Toxicity of Chlorpromazine

1. Acute Toxicity

The approximate 14-day LD_{50}'s in rats by various routes are (Smith Kline and French, 1956):

Intraperitoneal—75–100 mg/kg
Subcutaneous—540 mg/kg
Oral—492 mg/kg
Intravenous—25 mg/kg

The approximate LD_{50}'s in mice by various routes are:

Intravenous (14-day)—27 mg/kg
Intravenous (3-day)—26 mg/kg (van Proosdij-Hartzema, 1955)
Intraperitoneal—(24-hour) 225–250 mg/kg (Kent *et al.*, 1954a,b)
Subcutaneous—160–200 mg/kg (on mixed natural diet)
Subcutaneous—400–465 mg/kg (on balanced synthetic diet) (Courvoisier and Cosar, 1955)

One investigator found that the subcutaneous LD_{50} of chlorpromazine was somewhat higher in mice kept at 25.6° to 30.5°C than in animals kept at either lower or higher temperatures (Berti and Cima, 1954a,b,c).

It is known that aggregation of mice increases the acute toxicity of amphetamine. It is of interest that the administration of chlorpromazine reduces the aggregate toxicity of amphetamine to the level seen with single animals (Lasagna and McCann, 1957).

Chlorpromazine at 125 mg/kg i.m. produced death within 6 hours in guinea pigs (Mackiewicz and Gershon, 1954).

2. Chronic Toxicity

In general, chronic toxicity studies have revealed no ill effects with chlorpromazine except for some depression of growth (due to lower food intake) at relatively high doses. A lethal dose for humans has not been established; the variety of side effects that have been reported are mainly the result of pharmacological actions of the drug.

Chlorpromazine was given daily for 90 days to rats and dogs at a dosage of 10 mg/kg orally and to guinea pigs at a dose of 10 mg/kg subcutaneously. In another series, rats and dogs were given chlorpromazine at 20 mg/kg and 30 mg/kg orally for 3 months. The animals showed a slight depression of motor activity after each dose. The treated rats showed a slight slowing of growth rate during the second half of the test period, probably due to decreased food intake as a result of the depressant action of chlorpromazine. The guinea pigs and dogs gained weight normally throughout the test. Hematological examination every 2 weeks showed no significant variations from normal. No pathological changes in any organs that could be attributed to chlorpromazine could be seen after histological studies. The testicular and adrenal weights were increased in the treated rats, and liver weights were slightly decreased. No change was found in testicular weights in goats (Hafs and Williams, 1964).

In guinea pigs, all organs and glands were unaffected by the drug, except that the male guinea pig thymus glands showed a decrease in weight (Morocutti, 1957; Wilke and Iizuka, 1960; Koeze and Telford, 1958; Roizin et al., 1959, 1960; Camba, 1955).

Rabbits showed no abnormality of liver or kidney function after having been given chlorpromazine at a level of 25 mg/kg orally, or 4 mg/kg intramuscularly every day for 3 months (Bourgeois-Gavardin et al., 1955). After autopsy, rabbit tissues did not show any histological evidence of toxicity. In another study (Altman et al., 1962), no toxic renal effects were seen in rats on chlorpromazine.

3. In Pregnancy

Administration of 5 mg/kg of chlorpromazine per day subcutaneously to pregnant rabbits caused no significant difference from control animals in size or viability of litters. Likewise, administration of 10 mg/kg per day of chlorpromazine, in food, to female rats produced no ill effects on the mothers or litters; second generation studies showed no adverse effects.

In female rats given 1 or 5 mg/kg per day of chlorpromazine subcutaneously for 3 weeks and then mated to treated or untreated males, there were no ill effects in the litters. Likewise, females treated after mating as above showed no ill effects on duration of gestation, number of litters weaned, number of young per litter, or of weight of young at birth or at weaning (Courvoisier and Ducrot, 1954). Young rats weaned from these treated mothers were given 1–10 mg/kg subcutaneously for another month without evidence of toxicity. Puppies given 5 mg/kg/day by mouth for 6 weeks likewise showed no ill effects.

Administration of chlorpromazine, prochlorperazine, trifluoperazine, and trimeprazine singly to second and third generations of pregnant rats has resulted in no adverse effects in either pregnant animals or in offspring (Smith Kline and French, 1956). No teratogenic effects for chlorpromazine have been reported in the literature.

In several studies in rats, administration of chlorpromazine at 5 mg/kg/day subcutaneously produced no effect on gestation period, litter size, or the condition of the young (Murphree et al., 1962; Krais et al., 1954b; Palazzetti and Torsello, 1955; Torsello and Palazzetti, 1955; Werboff and Kesner, 1963). Large doses of up to 12.5 mg/kg/day (s.c.) delayed gestation, and possibly increased cannibalism (Krais et al., 1954; Roizin, 1959; Werboff and Dembicki, 1962). By the intravenous route, 12.5 mg/kg/day of chlorpromazine produced only delay in impregnation (Lesinski and Podlewska, 1957). At high doses of 30 mg/kg/day (s.c.), for specific 3-day periods (starting for 8 days post-conception), chlorpromazine resulted in resorption of ova, abortions, and stillbirths. These effects were attributed to inhibition of the pituitary (Chambon, 1955, 1957). A dose of 30 mg/kg/day (s.c.) in the rat is equivalent to about a 10-gm oral dose in a 70-kg man.

Failure to demonstrate clear-cut fetal effects of the phenothiazines cannot be attributed to failure to pass placental barrier, since this passage has been demonstrated in rabbits (Franchi and Gianni, 1957), guinea pigs (Creze, 1955), and dogs and humans (Behn et al., 1956; Glowinski et al., 1960; Lacomme and LeLorier, 1955; Hussey, 1963).

Many studies with chlorpromazine in pregnant women and many investigations of the use of chlorpromazine in the treatment of nausea and vomiting of pregnancy have failed to reveal any increase of fetal damage or wastage over that established in untreated women (Cohen, 1955; Friend and Cummins, 1953; Kent et al., 1954a,b; Kistner and Duncan, 1956; Stewart and Redeker, 1954; Swinehart, 1955; Moyer et al., 1954a,b; Sullivan, 1957; Benaron, 1955; Krais, 1955; Hall, 1960; Ayd, 1963; Kris, 1962; Kris and Carmichael, 1957; Sobel, 1960a,b; Singleton and Witt, 1956; Winkelbauer and Kimsey, 1956; Suzuki et al., 1956; Moriarity and Nance, 1963; Schrire, 1963; Moriarity, 1963; Noack, 1963).

A recent study by Blacker et al. (1962) showed that babies of mothers receiving large doses of chlorpromazine can be safely breast fed. The amount of chlorpromazine in breast milk of lactating psychotic women who received a single oral dose of 1200 mg was barely above the detectable level. Calculations indicate that a 7-pound child of a mother receiving a single dose of 1200 mg might have received 3 μg/kg of chlorpromazine. The drug was not detectable in blood or breast milk after 600 mg twice a day for 7 days.

The authors concluded that a large single dose is needed to give detectable milk levels and they suggested that an increased margin of safety could be obtained by prescribing chlorpromazine in sustained release form for the mother.

4. Tissue Culture

In hanging drop cultures of chick embryonic spinal cord, the minimal toxic concentrations of chlorpromazine were about the same as those of procaine hydrochloride (Pomerat et al., 1955). The heart tissues were about one-fourth as sensitive, and spleen tissue about one-fifteenth as sensitive as spinal cord tissue.

5. Effect on Lower Organisms

Chlorpromazine has been reported to have weak or moderate inhibitory activity *in vitro* against growth of tubercle bacilli (Geiger and Finkelstein, 1954; Raffel et al., 1960), *Coccidioides imitis* (Chinn et al., 1954), and some strains of yeast (Dimmling and Staib, 1955). Low doses shortened but high doses (60 mg/kg) increased survival time of mice infected with *Trypanosoma cruzii* or *Trypanosoma evansi* (Friebel and Kastner, 1955); the effect seemed to be due to inhibition of multiplication of the organism by low body temperature in the hosts. The effectiveness of penicillin against streptococci *in vitro* or in infected mice was increased by chlorpromazine (Lutzenkirchen and Schoog, 1954). Cellular activity of sea eggs, Infusoria, and various microorganisms, and gross activity of ascidians and small fish (cf. Rahman and Engels, 1964) were decreased by chlorpromazine at concentrations ranging from 1 : 160,000 to 1 : 600,000 (Decourt et al., 1953a,b; Decourt and Anguera, 1953; Decourt, 1953, 1955). These observations are the basis for the "narcobiotic" theory (Decourt, 1953, 1955), which states that chlorpromazine is a general depressant of cellular metabolism. According to this theory, the cumulative effect of narcobiotic agents on multiple-cell pathways accounts for selective action of low doses on the central nervous system, particularly the multisynaptic reticular formation. As doses are increased, simpler units would be affected until finally the whole organism reached a state of narcobiosis and hypometabolism (cf. Faguet et al., 1963).

McLaughlan et al. (1961) have reported on some apparent drug-vitamin interrelationships in *Lactobacillus leichmannii* and *Tetrahymena pyriformis*. Forty-four drugs were screened for possible antivitamin effects using *L. leichmannii* and *T. pyriformis* as tests. Chlorpromazine, promazine, chloroquine phosphate, methapyrilene HCl, and methantheline bromide had probable antipyridoxal activity for *T. pyriformis*. Phenformin had probable antifolic activity for *L. leichmannii*. Propylthiouracil, tolbutamide, metahexamide, and chlorpropamide had probable antipantothenate activity for *T. pyriformis*.

Chlorpromazine has demonstrated some inhibition of *Candida* (Dimmling and Staib, 1955) and *in vitro* activity against *Mycobacterium tuberculosis* (Raffel et al., 1960). It had no *in vivo* activity. Popper and Lorian (1959) have reported antibacterial properties for chlorpromazine at concentrations of 15 to 60 μg/ml.

TABLE III

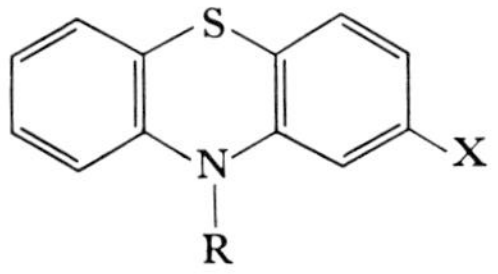

EFFECTS OF STRUCTURAL VARIATIONS OF PHENOTHIAZINE DERIVATIVES ON BIOLOGICAL RESPONSES

Compound	Motor activity 50% depression DD_{50} in mice[a] (mg/kg) (p.o.)	Conditioned response 50% block in rats (mg/kg) (s.c.) (p.o.)		Apomorphine vomiting 50% reduction of frequency in dogs (mg/kg) (s.c.) (p.o.)		Toxicity LD_{50} in mice (mg/kg) (p.o.)	Safety margin LD_{50}/DD_{50}
Chlorpromazine $R = CH_2CH_2CH_2N(CH_3)_2$ $X = Cl$	4.4 (1)[b]	2.4 (1)	10.5	0.3 (1)	2.1 (1)	336 (1)	76
Promazine $R = CH_2CH_2CH_2N(CH_3)_2$ $X = H$	17.8 (1/4)	6.2 (1/2.5)		5.8 (1/20)		420 (1/1.2)	23
Promethazine $R = CH_2-CH-N(CH_3)_2$ | CH_3 $X = H$	83.3 (1/19)	12.0 (1/5)		17.0 (1/55)		792 (1/2.3)	7

X = 2-chloro
R = CH$_2$—CH—N(CH$_3$)$_2$
      $\vert$
      CH$_3$
	88.0
	(1/20)
		29.5
		(1/12)
				15.0
				(1/50)
					792
					(1/2.3)
						9

Prochlorperazine R = CH$_2$CH$_2$CH$_2$N⟨piperazine⟩N—CH$_3$ X = Cl	6 (1/1.4)		6.2 (1.7/1)	0.35 (6/1)	2050 (1/6)	342

[a] Dose producing a 50% depression of motor activity.
[b] Chlorpromazine has been assigned an activity of 1. The ratios in parentheses refer to activity in that column relative to chlorpromazine.

The effect of chlorpromazine on the permeability of resting cells of *T. pyriformis* has been studied by Nathan and Friedman (1962). Incubation of cell suspensions of *T. pyriformis* with chlorpromazine increased permeability of cell membrane. The authors suggest that various cells and organ systems be screened for sensitivity of their cell membranes to permeability changes caused by chlorpromazine. They conclude that chlorpromazine may be used in combination therapy to increase intracellular absorption of the second drug; also, it may be used as a laboratory tool for increasing the range of compounds which can reach the interior of a cell without resorting to complete cell breakage. Guttman and Friedman (1963a,b) have studied the immobilization of *T. pyriformis* by various phenothiazines. The activity in this organism correlates with the clinical effectiveness of the various phenothiazines. Higher doses of chlorpromazine are reported to reduce phagocytosis *in vivo* (Greenberg and Ingalls, 1962; Guttman, 1962).

The action of reserpine, chlorpromazine, and serotonin on the metamorphosis of *Rana temporaria* tadpole were compared by Kehl *et al.* (1961). Chlorpromazine and reserpine, given 16 days before metamorphosis, accelerated this process in tadpoles. Serotonin at high doses was toxic; lower doses had no effect. Chlorpromazine has been found to potentiate the effects of pentylenetetrazole in the frog (Deshpande, 1963). It also causes a release of melanocyte stimulating hormone in the frog, *Rana pipiens*, and the flat fish, *Lophosetta maculata* (Scott, 1962). Antidiuretic-hormone-like effects in amphibians have also been reported (Khazan *et al.*, 1963). Effects on *Betta splendens* are described by Opitz (1962c).

It has been reported that there is considerable correlation between the psychotherapeutic and anthelmintic activities of the phenothiazines (Minchin and Holdaway, 1964).

The effect of hypnotics, tranquilizers, and neuroplegics on aggressive behavior of the praying mantis have been reported by Mercier and Dessaigne (1962). Mebubarbital, procalmadiol, chlorpromazine, and reserpine affected the praying mantis in a manner analogous to that of higher species. Chlorpromazine (5–10 μg/gm) suppressed aggressiveness, hunting instinct, and defense reactions; it had no effect on motor reactions. Higher doses (50 μg/gm) disturbed motor reactions. Inhibitory effects on the larvae of *Tribolium confusum* (brown beetles) with high concentrations of chlorpromazine are reported by Huot *et al.* (1963).

In Hydromedusae, a primitive invertebrate, chlorpromazine and perphenazine abolished the rhythmic movement of the mantle for a period of 15 to 25 minutes, and no response to electric stimulation was observed. The addition of perphenazine to the Hirudineae produced a complete inertia lasting 4 to 6 hours during which normal spontaneous movements, reactions to aversive stimuli, and feeding reactions disappeared. Holothuriae became inert after treatment with perphenazine and chlorpromazine. The addition of perphenazine to *Octopoda* produced an inert condition and movement could be invoked only on tactile stimulation. It is presumed that phenothiazine derivatives act on the highest nervous center of each animal since metabolism is maintained and no general toxicosis is observed. The lower the phylum to which the animals belong, the greater the amount of phenothiazine required to produce the necessary effect (Katona, 1962).

V. Structure-Activity Relationships in the Phenothiazines

Although a great deal of information in this area has been published, most of the studies involved only a few compounds and hence quantitative inter-comparisons can only be made for small groups of compounds.

Table III (p. 116) gives structure-activity relationships of a number of phenothiazines (Cook, 1956).

Comparing chlorpromazine with promazine, we see that the former is more active on a milligram basis in reducing motor activity in mice and in blocking the conditioned escape response and apomorphine-induced emesis, although the acute toxicity of the two phenothiazines is about the same. Oddly enough, introduction of a chloro-group into promethazine gives a decrease, rather than an increase in activity. Replacement of the dimethylaminopropyl chain of chlorpromazine by the N-methylpiperazinopropyl chain of prochlorperazine gives an increase in activity and a decrease in acute toxicity.

Table IV gives some additional structure-activity relationships (Burke *et al.*, 1956).

In this table it will be seen that substitution in 2-position of the phenothiazine seems optimal for activity. The substituents had about the following order of activity:

$$CF_3 > Cl > H \approx OCH_3 \approx CONHNH_2$$

Correlation between the rat and the monkey activity is only approximate and should be reserved for qualitative comparison. The pentobarbital data emphasize the specificity of the phenothiazine tranquilizers. The barbiturates produce little specific effect in the conditioned response test at low doses, and at higher doses physical incapacity or analgesia results.

The structure-activity relationships of some phenothiazine substituted nortropane derivatives have been published by Long *et al.* (1957). A summary of their data is shown in Table V (p. 122).

Here it is seen that the 2-chloro-10-propyl (trans) isomer is the most active, based on barbiturate potentiation and the production of hypothermia.

TABLE IV

Effect of Structural Variations on Conditioned Reflex and Tranquilization

[Phenothiazine structure with S at top, N at bottom bearing $(CH_2)_3N(CH_3)_2$ side chain, and X substituent at positions 2, 3, or 4 on one benzene ring]

Structural formula		Conditioned reflex in rats		Tranquilization in monkeys	
X	Position	CR_{50}[a] (mg/kg i.p.)	SR_{50}[b]/CR_{50}	Dose (mg/kg p.o.)	Rating score[c]
H	2	52.0	1.6	40	0.7
Cl	2	3.7	3.9	20	3.2
Cl	3	20.5	3.7	20	2.0
OCH_3	2	55.5	3.4	40	2.7
CO_2CH_3	2	7.5	3.8	60	0.0
$CONHNH_2$	2	54.0	1.8	56	2.0
CF_3	2	2.2	4.1	5	4.1
CF_3	3	8.5	3.0	30	1.0
CF_3	4	62.0	3.1	40	0.5
Pentobarbital	—	24.8	1.1	40	0
				80	Anesthesia

[a] CR_{50} = dose blocking conditioned reflex in 50% of rats.

[b] SR_{50} = dose blocking response to shock in 50% of rats.

[c] In monkey tranquilization, the following rating scores were used: 0 = normal; 1 = slightly reduced spontaneous motor activity; 2 = little or no spontaneous motor activity; 3 = approachable, but cannot be touched; 4 = can be touched and gently petted; 5 = is not antagonized by vigorous handling.

Wirth et al. (1958) have studied the pharmacology of a number of ring-acylated phenothiazine derivatives, in comparison with standards, using (1) the defense reaction in the golden hamster, where the propionyl and butyryl promazines showed the greatest activity; (2) the Siamese fighting fish assay, where the compounds with a 10-morpholinopropyl side chain showed the greatest activity; (3) the inclined plane test, where 2-acetyl > 2-propionyl > 2-butyryl > H; (4) potentiation of hexobarbital, where the 2-propionylpromazine was the most active compound; (5) the climbing test in rats, where the 2-acetyl and 3-acetylpromazines were equal to chlorpromazine in activity and the morpholinopropyl compounds were consistently less active; (6) catalepsy tests in rats, where the compounds having N-methylpiperazinopropyl side chains were the most active; (7) anticonvulsant activity (MES = maximal electroshock seizures), where results were equivocal; and (8) antagonism of apomorphine, where again the prochlorperazine side chain compounds were the most active.

Tiwari et al. (1960a,b) have studied structure-activity relationships of chlorpromazine and related compounds in their atropine-like activity on the rabbit intestine.

Nieschulz et al. (1956) have published pharmacological studies on N-alkylpiperidylphenothiazine derivatives, including blood pressure effects, antihistaminic activity, local anesthesia, and effects on nicotine tremor.

Structure-activity reviews on phenothiazines has been published by Viaud (1954), Martin et al. (1956), Takayanagi (1964), Hamacher and Hildebrandt (1964), and Wunderlich (1962). Janssen (1961b) has summarized the activity of a number of 4'-fluorobutyrophenone derivatives in comparison with chlorpromazine and perphenazine.

A paper by Gordon et al. (1963) reports that consideration of structure-activity relationships in the phenothiazines has resulted in a degree of predictability being possible in this area. Admittedly these correlations were not possible until after a large number of phenothiazines had been made and tested.

A. Side Chain Modifications

The hypothesis of Pfeiffer (1956) stated that the degree of structural specificity of any biologically active molecule is directly related to the ratio of activities of its optical isomers. This seemed reasonable since, if there is specificity among the enantiomorphs, the fit at receptor surfaces must be a critical factor.

The early work in the phenothiazine tranquilizers gave little clue to the structural specificity of the side chain, in the light of Pfeiffer's hypothesis, since normal propyl groups were involved in both chlorpromazine (**XXXIII**) and prochlorperazine (**XXXIV**).

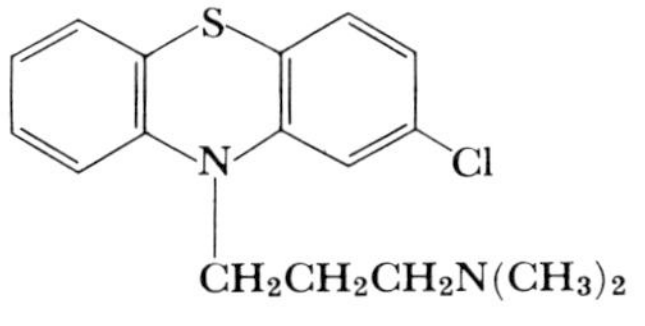

$CH_2CH_2CH_2N(CH_3)_2$

Chlorpromazine index (CI) = 1.0

(**XXXIII**)

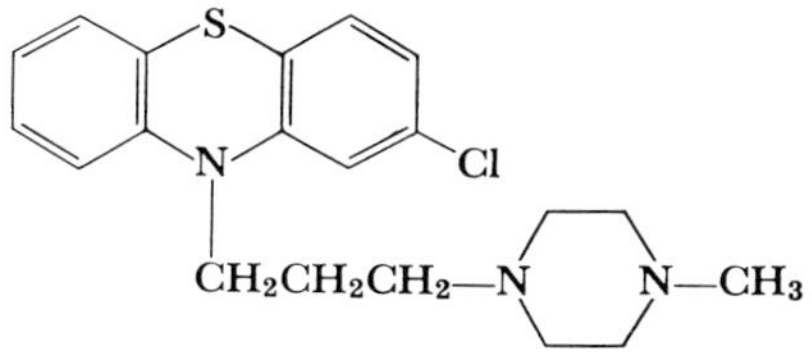

$CH_2CH_2CH_2$—N⟨ ⟩N—CH_3

CI = 3

(**XXXIV**)

Activity is shown as a fraction of chlorpromazine activity called the chlorpromazine index (CI) in this section. The principal index of activity used for purposes of this discussion is blockade of the conditioned escape response.

However, when the French workers prepared the isobutyl series [cf. trimeprazine (**XXXV**)], it was found that the levo isomer was many times

TABLE V
Relationship between Chemical Structure and Biological Activity of Phenothiazine-Substituted Nortropane Derivatives

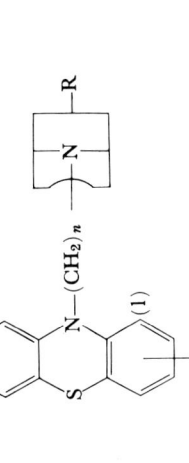

Compound number	X	n	R to N configuration	R	Central nervous system activity[a]		Adrenolytic activity[b] mg/kg for reversal	
					Barbiturate potentiation	Rectal temperature	Average	Range
1	H	3	trans	OH	14.0	8.5	0.27	0.1–0.5
2	H	3	cis[c]	OH	6.5	6.0	0.58	0.2–1.6
3	2—Cl	3	trans	OH	100.0[d]	100.0[e]	0.24	0.1–0.6
4	2—Cl	3	cis	OH	34.0	25.5	1.1	0.2–2.0
5	H	3	—	H	10.0	3.5	0.3	0.1–0.4
6	2—Cl	3	—	H	22.5	16.5	0.9	0.2–1.6

No.	R	n	isomer	Structure/X			
7	H	3	trans	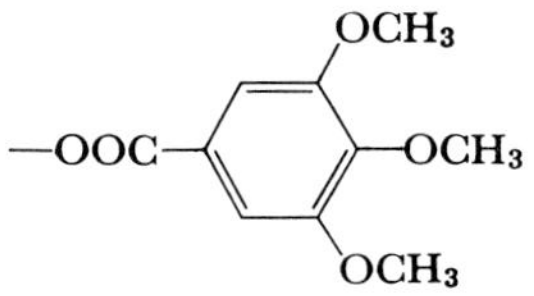 —OOC—C₆H₂(OCH₃)₃	<1.0	<1.0	0.13	0.05–0.2
8	H	3	cis	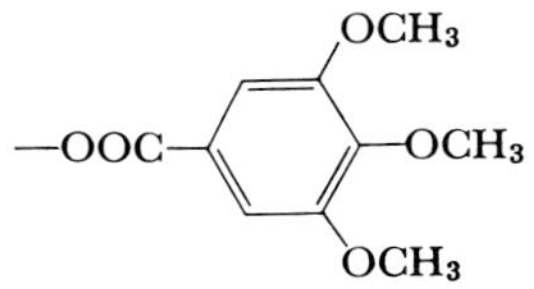 OH	<1.0	<1.0	8.0	6.0–10.0
9	H	2	trans	OH	<1.0	<1.0	>10.0	
10	H	4	trans	OH	<1.0	<1.0	4.5	2.0–8.0
11	H	5	trans	OH	<1.0	<1.0	>10.0	
12	3—Cl	3	trans	OH	8.0	3.0	0.4	0.2–0.8
13	2—Br	3	trans	OH	100.0	94.0	0.26	0.1–0.4

[a] Activity expressed as per cent of compound No. 3.
[b] Minimal dose (mg/kg) to produce reversal of control doses of epinephrine.
[c] In the cis isomers the parent structure refers to the form frequently designated as pseudo.
[d] A 100% increase in the sleeping time is equivalent to 1.7 mg/kg.
[e] A 5°F drop in the rectal temperature is equivalent to 1.3 mg/kg.

more active than the dextro. It could therefore be postulated that groups

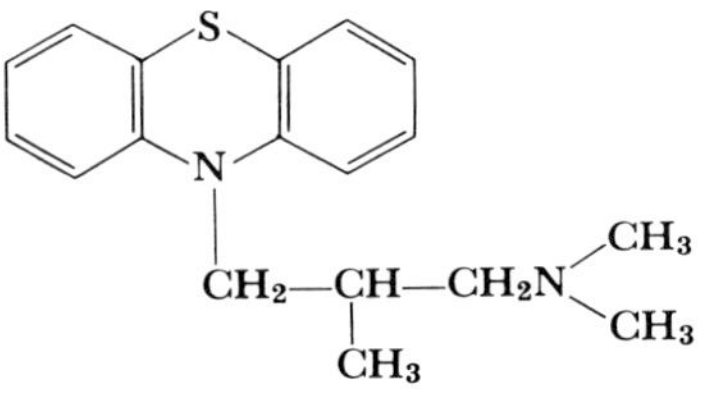

(XXXV)

larger than the methyl in the 2-position of the propyl chain should have reduced activity. It was indeed subsequently found that the following side chains led to less active compounds when compared with chlorpromazine.

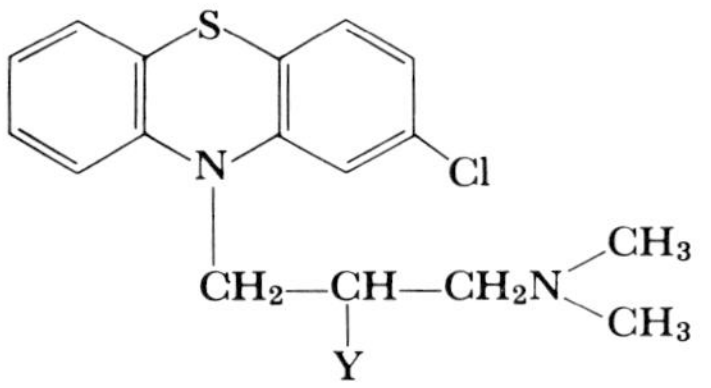

Y = phenyl   (CI = <0.1)
  = CH$_2$N(CH$_3$)$_2$ (CI = <0.1)
  = OH   (CI = <0.1)

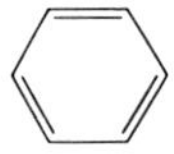

The 2-hydroxy group is not particularly large when compared with the methyl, but here it may be presumed that nonspecific binding elsewhere may be interfering with transport of the molecule to the specific receptor site.

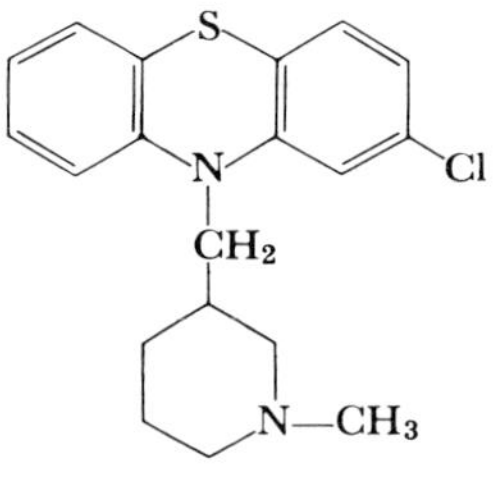

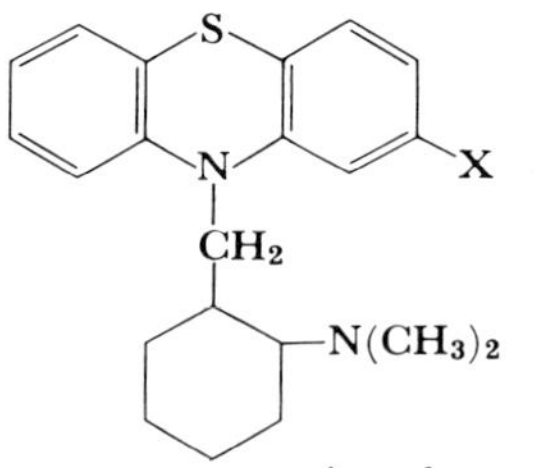

(CI = <0.1)   (CI = <0.1)   (CI = 0.2)
(XXXVI)   (XXXVII)   (XXXVIII)

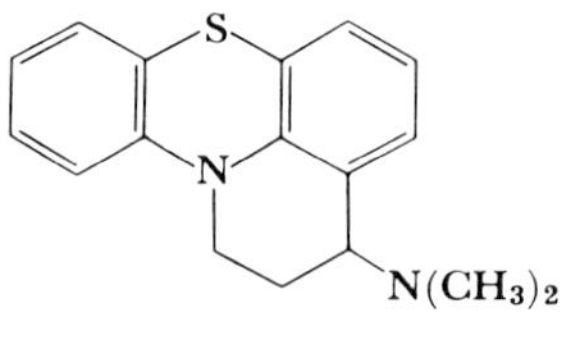

One may further speculate that the structural requirements of the 2-carbon include freedom of rotation, in addition to the limitation of the size of 2-substituents. Thus it was predicted that XXXVI, XXXVII, and XXXVIII would be less active since the 2-carbon is tied back in a ring, and test results have shown that these predictions were reliable.

It may be seen that in all of these instances (XXXVI–XXXVIII) there are 3 carbons between the ring and side-chain nitrogens. However, in every case, the critical 2-carbon of the side chain is tied back in a ring and the compounds are for this reason relatively devoid of chlorpromazine-like activity.

Other attributes of chlorpromazine such as antiemetic activity and depression of spontaneous motor activity are usually also reduced in these hindered congeners.

On the other hand, a compound like XXXIX, even though part of the side chain is in a ring, could be expected to have reasonable activity in the

(CI=0.6)

(XXXIX)

conditioned escape response test, since the 2-carbon of the side chain is unsubstituted. This expectation is supported by experimental evidence.

Some difficulty was found in explaining, initially, the activity of compounds like prochlorperazine, since increasing the size of the alkyl groups in the chlorpromazine side chain results in a loss of activity. It is now felt that the presently known facts may be accommodated in the approximation of the

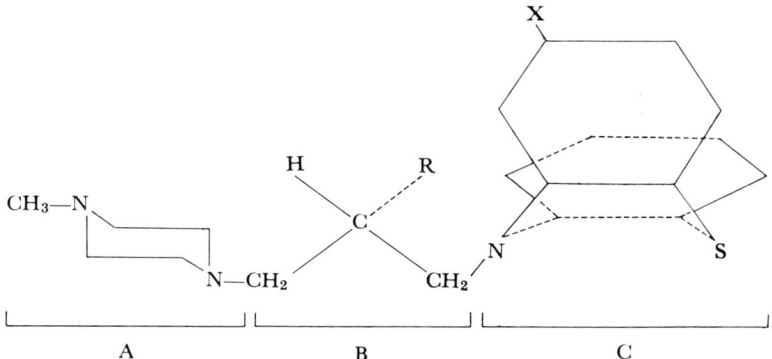

FIG. 1. Approximate configuration of prochlorperazine.

configuration of prochlorperazine (Fig. 1, XL) that may attach to the enzyme receptor.

In this model, the highest degree of structural specificity is believed to be in the B position of the molecule, where almost no leeway is permissible. The increased activity in some tests where $R = CH_3$ may reflect the fact that the presence of the methyl group tends to restrict rotation sufficiently to facilitate three-point attachment, without being large enough to get in the way. Alternatively, the methyl group might be said to improve the fit on the receptor. The structural requirements of the C portion of the molecule are very nearly as specific as those of the 3-carbon side chain, except that considerable variation in the nature of X is possible. The phenothiazine ring system has a fold along the nitrogen-sulfur axis. Hence the X-group may not be too close to the receptor surface and its only function might be to influence the resonance forms of the ring system and/or the electron density of the sulfur.

The A portion of the molecule has a low order of specificity in the longitudinal direction and a high order along the transverse axis. This may indicate that the molecule fits in a rather narrow slot. The terminal nitrogen of A must be somewhat removed from the receptor surface since rather bulky groups can be introduced here, as will be seen later. It is possible that the major influence of terminal groups is on the basicity of the nitrogen. The ease of removal of the residues on the terminal nitrogen may also play a role in the activity of these compounds.

The postulation of a long, rather narrow slot to accommodate the A part of the side chain is based on the activity of prochlorperazine and other ring compounds like XLI and XLII, whereas higher alkyl groups on the nitrogen reduce activity in the promazine series.

The pyrrolidino compound (XL) is about as active as chlorpromazine.

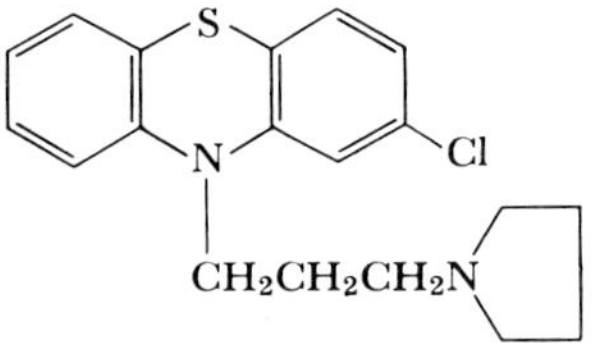

(CI = 0.7)
(XLI)

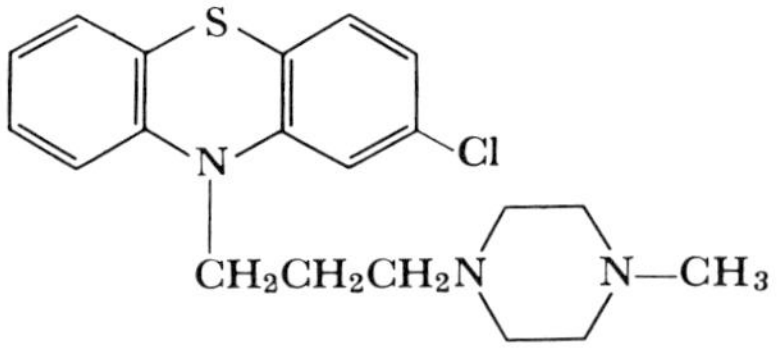

(CI = 3)
(XLII)

Free-rotating alkyl groups which are larger than methyl sweep a wider path than the piperazine, piperidino, or pyrrolidino group where the ends are tied back. The steric comparison is shown in Fig. 2.

The speculations above on the length of the area which accommodates the A portion of the side chain in Fig. 1 are based on the fact that bulky groups like *p*-aminophenethyl (XLIII) may be introduced with beneficial results. It is presumed that this part of the side chain is not hanging free in

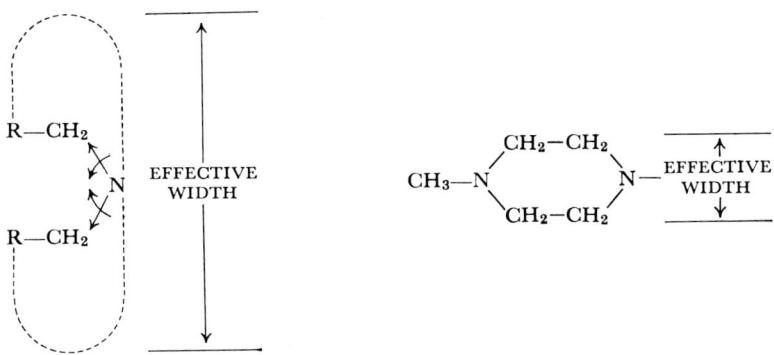

FIG. 2. Steric comparison of diethylamino and piperidino groups.

space since the *p*-aminophenethyl group is more active than the unsubstituted phenethyl (XLIIIa).

(CI = 9)
(XLIII)

(CI = 3)
(XLIIIa)

It was originally thought that further elaboration on the terminal nitrogen of prochlorperazine might not be productive since the *N*-ethyl compound was somewhat less active than the *N*-methyl and the *N*-propyl was even less. However, the development of the *N*-β-hydroxyethylpiperazinopropyl-phenothiazines (Cusic, 1956; Cusic and Hamilton, 1958) and the fact that phenethyl could be substituted for methyl on the nitrogen in meperidine (for review see Beckett and Casy, 1957) and morphine (Clark *et al.*, 1953) with resulting increases in activity, led to this substitution in the phenothiazine series.

The possible spatial limitation of the width of the piperazine ring, together with the interesting results found in substituting the *n*-propyl side chain by isobutyl (XXXV), led to the investigation of the effects of methyl substitution on the piperazine ring (XLIV).

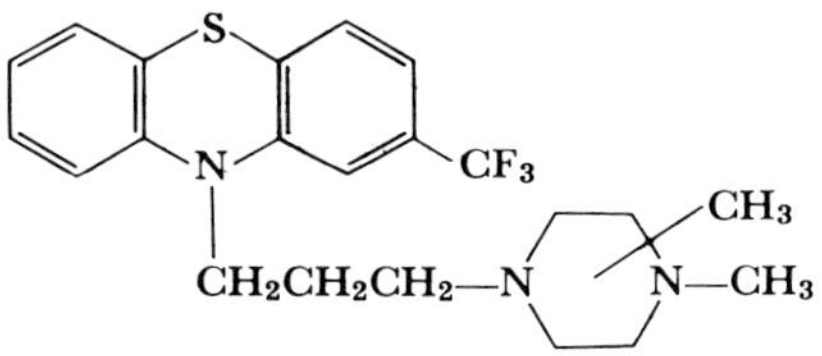

(XLIV)

There is some preliminary indication that the ring carbon-substituted piperazines may be less active than their unsubstituted analogs, thus providing additional confirmation for the effective width concept in Fig. 2.

B. Ring Substituents

The early French work showed that chlorine substitution at the 2-position of the phenothiazine nucleus led to optimal activity. Studies have therefore been concentrated on mono-substitution in this position.

The original work in the phenothiazine area showed that as far as substitution on the 2-position was concerned, $H < Cl \approx CH_3 \approx OCH_3$. Very little by way of conclusions could be reached from this information. However, the finding of a high order of activity in the 2-trifluoromethyl series (Craig *et al.*, 1957; Yale *et al.*, 1957) definitely indicated that electron-withdrawing groups at the 2-position had a favorable effect on activity. Shortly thereafter, the *N,N*-dimethyl-2-sulfonamido group (XLVa) was developed in France by Rhône-Poulenc, and it then seemed certain that this was a line worth following (Bhargava and Chandra, 1963). However, subsequently the methylsulfone (XLVb) and the hydroxy analog (XLVc) were synthesized, and the latter was found to be relatively inactive and the former active, but perhaps less active than expected based on the electron-withdrawing properties of the methylsulfonyl group.

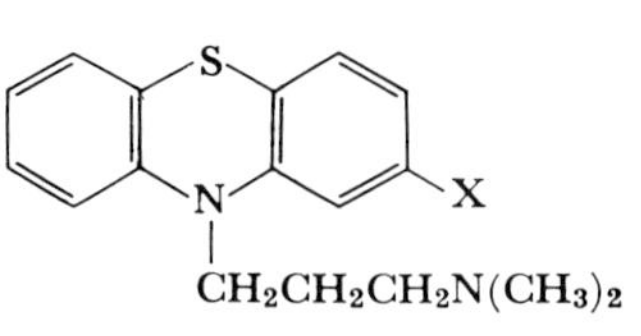

a, $X = SO_2N(CH_3)_2$
b, $X = SO_2CH_3$ (Cl = 0.6)
c, $X = OH$ (Cl = < 0.1)
d, $X = S-CF_3$ (Cl = 1)
e, $X = SO_2CH_3$ (Cl = 4)
f, $X = S-CH_3$ (Cl = 1)

(XLV)

At this point in the structure-activity correlations, a significant Russian paper came to the author's attention. Shemyakin *et al.* (1956), who had carried out extensive structure-activity correlations among chloramphenicol analogs, postulated that the activity of various *para*-substituted phenylacylaminopropanediols (XLVI) was proportional to the electron-withdrawing properties of the *para*-substituents. They made the further observation that these

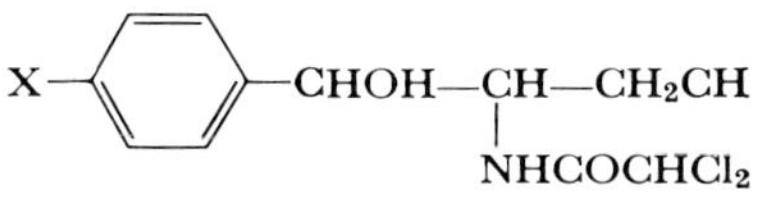

$$X-\langle\bigcirc\rangle-CHOH-\underset{NHCOCHCl_2}{CH}-CH_2CH$$

(XLVI)

relationships hold only if the substituent groups have a low order of what Shemyakin calls "ionogenicity." Shemyakin speculated that ionic (polar) groups, in this instance, permitted nonspecific binding of the molecule which prevented the drug from reaching specific receptor sites. Application of this speculation resolved most of the inconsistencies in the series of 2-substituted phenothiazines so that with a few exceptions like the OCH_3 and SCH_3 groups (which Shemyakin also observed in the choloramphenicols), the activity of a 2-substituted phenothiazine was proportional to the electron-withdrawing character of substituents—provided that the latter had no ionic character.

These theoretical considerations together with some of the recent Russian chemical literature, as well as the high activity of the 2-trifluoromethylphenothiazines, led certain investigators to two new series of phenothiazines. These were the trifluoromethylsulfide (XLVd) and the trifluoromethylsulfones (XLVe) (Nodiff *et al.*, 1960; Craig *et al.*, 1960).

Gordon *et al.* (1963) mentioned earlier the disappointing activity of the methyl sulfone group (XLVb). The ionogenicity concept suggested that the acidic hydrogens of this compound might be responsible for the relatively low activity. The replacement of these hydrogens by fluorines eliminated the acidic hydrogens and also increased the total electron-withdrawing effect of the 2-substituent. The effect of this change on biological activity was dramatic.

In the methylsulfide (XLVf) the hydrogens are not very acidic and hence the compound has good activity. Replacement of hydrogens by fluorine atoms to give SCF_3 analogs resulted in some increase in activity.

Thus, by examining a large number of phenothiazine compounds, the authors have arrived at certain structure-activity correlations, on an empirical basis, which have proved useful in predicting the activity of new ring substituents and side chains, as well as guiding the synthesis of new active compounds. Unfortunately these correlations have so far been found to have limited utility in areas outside the phenothiazines.

TABLE VI

ABSOLUTE POTENCIES OF PHENOTHIAZINES BY VARIOUS TEST PROCEDURES[a]

Drug	Conditioned response (ED$_{50}$ mg/kg)	Unconditioned response (ED$_{50}$ mg/kg)	Catalepsy (ED$_{50}$ mg/kg)	Locomotor depression (DD$_{50}$ mg/kg)	Serotonin antagonism (ED$_{50}$ mg/kg)	Tryptamine antagonism (ED$_{50}$ mg/kg)
Trifluoperazine	1.0 (0.7–2.2)	12.8 (7.2–22.5)	2.6 (1.5–4.7)	1.5 (0.9–5.7)	11.9 (6.3–22.6)	11.9 (10.0–13.4)
Perphenazine	1.0 (0.8–1.3)	14.0 (8.8–22.4)	2.1 (1.2–3.7)	1.7 (1.0–4.7)	2.8 (1.7–4.6)	5.6 (3.8–8.3)
Prochlorperazine	4.0 (3.2–4.3)	48.5 (33.2–71.0)	3.9 (2.6–5.8)	5.3 (3.5–8.8)	4.6 (2.4–8.7)	9.4 (7.1–12.6)
Triflupromazine	4.0 (2.6–6.3)	33.6 (22.3–50.7)	5.5 (2.8–11.0)	3.5 (2.0–6.7)	4.3 (3.0–6.3)	5.2 (3.8–7.2)
Chlorpromazine	11.9 (6.6–21.4)	166 (113–242)	21.0 (14.9–29.6)	8.5 (5.2–16.5)	9.7 (5.7–16.4)	8.0 (4.8–13.8)
Promazine	28.2 (19.1–41.6)	352 (248–520)	97.9 (70–134)	49.4 (44.6–195)	>400	522 (330–825)
Thioridazine	114.5 (54.6–238)	>400	39.8 (12.0–30.6)	103 (22.6–76.6)	103 (68–154)	182 (101–327.6)
Promethazine	312 (101–965)	>425	>400	>425	400 (292–551)	320 (247–415)
Mepazine	430 (333–556)	>600	>600	326 (131–820)	>600	>600

[a] Figures in parentheses are 95% fiducial limits. Potency of compounds expressed in terms of free bases.
All compounds tested orally at time of peak effect as determined for each procedure.

TABLE VII

RANK ORDER OF POTENCY OF PHENOTHIAZINES BY VARIOUS TEST PROCEDURES

Conditioned response	Unconditioned response	Catalepsy	Locomotor activity	Serotonin antagonism	Tryptamine antagonism
Trifluoperazine Perphenazine	Trifluoperazine Perphenazine	Perphenazine Trifluoperazine Prochlorperazine	Trifluoperazine Perphenazine	Perphenazine Trifluoperazine Prochlorperazine	Triflupromazine Perphenazine Chlorpromazine
Prochlorperazine Triflupromazine	Triflupromazine Prochlorperazine	Trifluoperazine Prochlorperazine Triflupromazine	Perphenazine Triflupromazine	Prochlorperazine Chlorpromazine	Chlorpromazine Prochlorperazine Trifluoperazine
Chlorpromazine	Chlorpromazine	Thioridazine Chlorpromazine	Triflupromazine Prochlorperazine Chlorpromazine	Chlorpromazine Trifluoperazine	Thioridazine
Promazine	Promazine	Promazine		Thioridazine	Promethazine Promazine
Thioridazine Promethazine Mepazine	Thioridazine Promethazine Mepazine	Promethazine Mepazine	Thioridazine Promazine	Promethazine	Mepazine
			Mepazine	Promazine Mepazine	
			Promethazine		

[a] Compounds grouped together in the table did not differ significantly from one another in potency ($P > 0.05$).

The comparative potencies of a series of phenothiazines were investigated by the conditioned response, unconditioned response, catalepsy, locomotor activity depression, serotonin antagonism, and tryptamine antagonism test procedures. In general, the rank order of potency of the compounds as conditioned response (CR) blockers (Table VI) agreed favorably (thioridazine is a notable exception) with their rank order of potency as tranquilizers in man (Table VII). In addition, rank orders of potencies of these compounds as unconditioned response blockers, motor activity depressants, and cataleptogenics were also generally similar to the CR rank order (Tedeschi et al., 1961a,b).

All of the compounds tested were found to be as effective (or as ineffective) in antagonizing tryptamine as they were in antagonizing serotonin, a finding which supports the hypothesis that tryptamine and serotonin share similar receptors in the central nervous system as well as in the periphery.

A fair degree of correlation was found between the activity of the compounds investigated as serotonin antagonists and their activity as tranquilizers. It was concluded, however, that tranquilizing activity is not always associated with serotonin antagonist activity and vice versa (Tedeschi et al., 1961a,b).

VI. *In Vivo* Distribution and Metabolism of Phenothiazines

The metabolic fate and tissue distribution of phenothiazines, especially chlorpromazine has been studied by many investigators in both animals and man. Unfortunately, the complex path of the metabolic fate of phenothiazines, coupled with the fact that many of the metabolites of phenothiazines are excreted as glucuronides (Posner, 1959) of hydroxylated (Kinbergen, 1959) derivatives which are difficult to isolate and characterize, means that relatively small definitive progress has been made toward the complete elucidation of the metabolic fate, tissue distribution, and especially mode of action of the phenothiazines.

Use of radioactively labeled phenothiazines (C^{14} or S^{35}) has been very useful in studying the tissue distribution and metabolic fate of these drugs. However, in some species, perhaps 80% of an administered dose of chlorpromazine was still unaccounted for by the end of 1963.

Bousquet (1962) has reviewed the general area of drug metabolism. The metabolism of the phenothiazine tranquilizers has been reviewed by Emmerson and Miya (1963) and by Carr (1962). Domino (1962) has published an excellent review of the pharmacology of the tranquilizers which includes material on their metabolic fate.

The scheme in Fig. 3 for the metabolism of chlorpromazine may be suggested.

Thus, by using only four reactions, namely demethylation, hydroxylation, glucuronide formation, and sulfoxide formation, it is possible to postulate at least sixteen metabolites. The major uncertainty is in the position of hydroxylation and whether multiple positions are susceptible to metabolic attack. Of

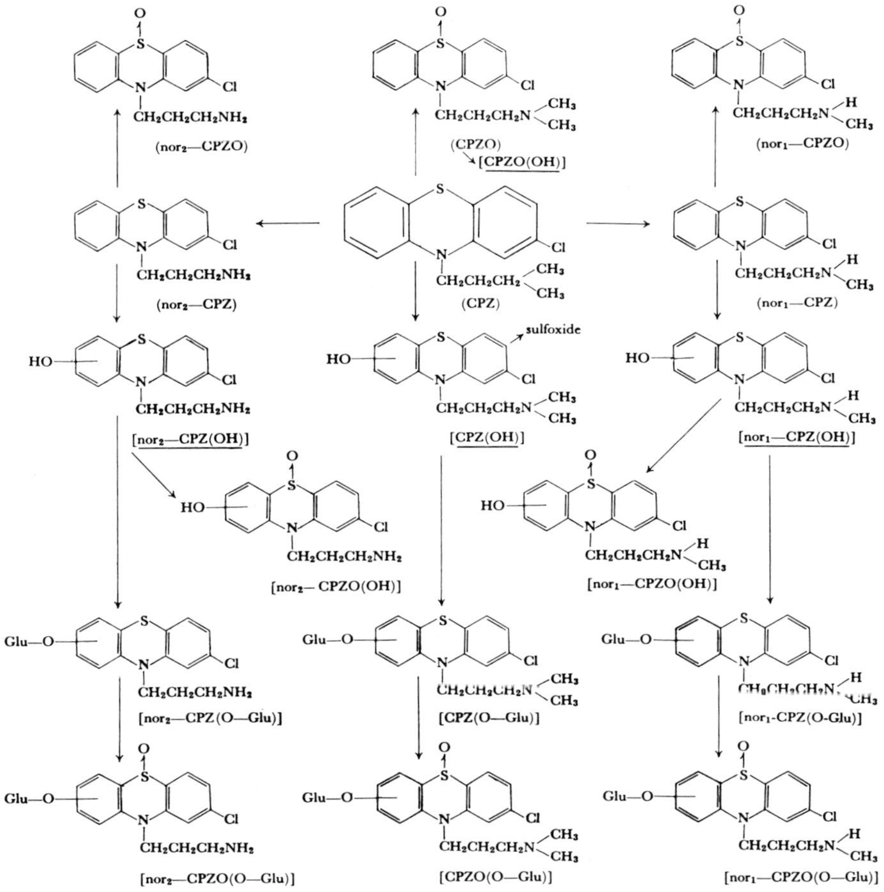

FIG. 3. Metabolic fate of chlorpromazine in animals.

the sixteen metabolites, several have not yet been identified and these are underlined in Fig. 3. Furthermore, some ethereal sulfates have been isolated, in addition to glucuronides.

If one takes into account all of the above metabolic pathways, and adds the possibility of sulfone formation, N-oxide formation, and side-chain removal, one finds more than one hundred metabolites of chlorpromazine theoretically possible.

Humans excrete 2–3 times as much phenolic as nonphenolic metabolites of chlorpromazine. The phenols are almost completely conjugated with glucuronic acid. At least five phenolic metabolites were found by Posner et al. (1962a,b, 1963), including a dioxygenated product. It was suggested that the monophenolic metabolite of chlorpromazine is hydroxylated in the 8-position, in contrast to promazine which is said to be hydroxylated in the 3-position. It was further suggested that the dioxygenated metabolite has a 7,8-dihydroxy structure. The urine of humans receiving single doses of chlorpromazine showed only small quantities of phenolic compounds and mainly the sulfoxides. Demethylation was observed in both nonphenolic and phenolic metabolites, with the mono and didemethylated compounds predominating over the intact forms (Posner et al., 1962a,b, 1963).

It has been shown, in an *in vitro* enzyme system, that liver homogenates from various species can oxidize chlorpromazine to the sulfoxide, sulfone, and other products (Kamm et al., 1958) (cf. Forrest and Forrest, 1963).

In view of the difficulty in isolating hydroxylated metabolites of the phenothiazines, and because of the unavailability of reference compounds, Craig et al. (1965) studied nuclear magnetic resonance spectra of phenothiazines and observed chemical shifts in NMR spectra with various substituents in the 1, 2, 3, 7, and 8-positions of phenothiazines.

A. Tissue Distribution

A number of phenothiazines were injected intraperitoneally into rats and their tissue distribution determined, with no significant differences being seen in tissue distribution of the various phenothiazines employed. It would appear that all tissues take up phenothiazines very rapidly after they have gotten into the blood stream. For example, in less than 2 minutes the brain was found to contain two to three times the concentration found in the blood. The highest concentrations of phenothiazines were found in the lungs and liver. As expected there was a large animal to animal variability, and most of the drugs were barely detectable after 24 hours in any of the tissues studied (Ragland, 1962).

Employing the dog as a test animal, the uptake of three different drugs by various areas of the brain was studied after intraperitoneal injection (DeJaramillo and Guth, 1963). The drugs employed were the phenothiazines chlorpromazine, prochlorperazine, and thiethylperazine. Chlorpromazine and prochlorperazine exhibit similar spectra of localization in the fourteen areas of the dog brain surveyed. Thiethylperazine, which is a weak anti-psychotic agent, but potent anti-nauseant, antiemetic and antivertige agent, concentrates differently from chlorpromazine and prochlorperazine, exhibiting highest concentrations in the cerebellar areas.

The distribution of thioridazine in rats after intraperitoneal injection was studied in the brain and liver. In both these organs more than half of the drug was found in the microsomal and supernatant fractions, and no more than

30% of the drug could be extracted from these tissues without drastic hydrolytic conditions—either acid or base.

Zehnder et al. (1962) have shown, using S^{35}-labeling and a reverse isotope-dilution technique, that thioridazine disulfone is found in rat bile and urine after administration of the drug. In addition, the ring (5) and 2-methyl-mercaptosulfoxides, and the disulfoxide, were identified.

Further investigation by Wollemann (1962) showed that the oxidized intermediate of the phenothiazines could be determined in brain tissue 30 to 60 minutes after administration. Giving the oxidized intermediate of chlorpromazine intravenously to rabbits produced characteristic phenothiazine-like changes in the EEG earlier than observed after the injection of chlorpromazine itself. The intermediate also potentiated the effects of narcotic drugs in rats and dogs, and the potentiating action was more pronounced than with chlorpromazine, but of shorter duration. During the same period (30 to 60 minutes after injection) it was also possible to demonstrate the presence of chlorpromazine sulfoxide, but it has been shown by Salzman and Brodie (1956; Salzman et al., 1955) and by Moran and Butler (1956) that the sulfoxide produces only slight pharmacological effects in comparison with chlorpromazine [cf. Davidson et al. (1957) for studies in man]. The oxidation of chlorpromazine to the sulfoxide has been observed in liver microsomes by Gillette and Kamm (1960) and in the urine of rodents by Forrest and Forrest (1957), as well as by Cavanaugh (1957) during the oxidation of chlorpromazine with catalase and hydrogen peroxide.

Wollemann (1962) has concluded that the intermediate compound, presumed to be a free radical, is responsible for the inhibitory biochemical and pharmacological effects produced *in vitro* as well as *in vivo*.

The metabolic fate of six different S^{35}-labeled phenothiazines, including chlorpromazine, methoxypromazine, levomepromazine, thioridazine, promethazine, and Secergan® (10-α-dimethylaminopropionylphenothiazine methobromide) was studied by Allgén et al. (1960; Allgén, 1962). The last named, an antispasmodic agent, was studied in mice and rats after subcutaneous and oral administration. There was a small accumulation of the antispasmodic in the liver, intestines, gastric mucosa, pancreas, and kidney. The accumulation in the gastrointestinal tract may be responsible for its pharmacological properties and its clinical application as an anti-ulcer drug.

The elimination and metabolism of these drugs was studied in man (patients receiving prolonged treatment) using mainly urine analyses. In some cases, however, blood serum and feces were analyzed as well. The aim of the studies was primarily to make possible the identification of the drug taken by a patient.

The analytical methods used include extractions, color reactions, ultraviolet spectrophotometry, spectrofluorometry, tracer techniques, and chromatography on paper, thin layer, and columns.

Ultraviolet absorption was measured on acid aqueous extracts obtained from heptane extracts of alkaline urine. The sulfoxide of the various drugs gave characteristic ultraviolet peaks. Surprisingly, elimination of metabolites in the urine was slow, being detectable after 1 week. Although large numbers of metabolites were found in the urine, none were detectable in the feces.

Berti and Cima (1954a,b,c, 1955, 1956, 1957, 1962) have studied the influence of species, sex, and environmental temperature on the metabolism of phenothiazines. Phenothiazines were detected by absorption on ion exchange resins, or preferably by paper chromatography or thin-layer chromatography. The CNS effects of phenothiazines in various species seems to correlate well with the quantity of unchanged drug in that species. For example, in guinea pigs, the very minor CNS depression observed correlates with the rapid biotransformation of the phenothiazine. In rabbits, there is also very little drug excreted unchanged (Berti and Cima, 1956). In mice and rats, on the other hand, which are very sensitive to chlorpromazine, higher unchanged drug levels are observed. It is further seen that in guinea pigs the hydroxylated metabolites predominate, while more autoxidation seems to take place in man. In rats, a greater amount of chlorpromazine was detected in the liver and brain in females than in males.

The pharmacological effects of chlorpromazine on mice and rats is quite dependent on the environmental temperature. At temperatures of 13° to 18°C, the CNS depression produced by chlorpromazine is marked. At room temperature, the CNS depression is less marked, and at 33° to 38°C, chlorpromazine produced excitation and death at normally depressant doses. It is thought that the biotransformation of chlorpromazine at various temperatures differs only in amount, and not qualitatively. Thus Berti and Cima (1962) conclude that the drug effects of chlorpromazine are due to unchanged drug, in contrast to the conclusions of Wollemann mentioned previously.

In a study of the pharmacological activity of some actual and model metabolites of chlorpromazine, the sulfoxide was the least active (Posner et al., 1962a,b, 1963). The N-oxide was somewhat active though less so than chlorpromazine or the norchlorpromazine. A delay in onset of activity of the N-oxide was noted in the conditioned response tests; this phenomenon was not seen with the other drugs and suggests that the N-oxide may be converted to a more active compound *in vivo*.

The norchlorpromazine derivative was only slightly less active than chlorpromazine alone. In the promazine series the 4-hydroxy derivative (cf. Fujimoto, 1959) was about equal to promazine in activity, whereas the 2-hydroxypromazine was less active than promazine except in the prolongation of sleeping time or by the intravenous route. 1-Hydroxypromazine was less active than promazine. As has been reported previously, promazine was less active than chlorpromazine in all the tests (cf. Goldenberg et al., 1964).

Chlorpromazine metabolism by mitochondria isolated from rat brain, liver, lung, and kidney was studied by Wechsler (1962). The drug was incubated with varying amounts of mitochondria in the presence of buffers and drug and metabolites determined as previously described by Wechsler and Forrest (1959). Shifts in ultraviolet absorption peaks have indicated that chlorpromazine was partially converted to its metabolites, and the identification of these was being attempted.

The metabolism of fluphenazine enanthate in the rat was studied by Hess et al. (1962). The interest in this compound derives from the fact that a single subcutaneous injection of fluphenazine enanthate in oil can cause pharmacodynamic effects for periods of 2 to 4 weeks depending on the species and test employed (Burke et al., 1962), whereas fluphenazine alone is much shorter acting. The fluphenazine was labeled with carbon-14 and injected into rats and feces and urine were collected daily.

The enzymatic formation of sulfoxides in the oxidation of chlorpromazine by guinea pig liver microsomes was described by Gillette and Kamm (1960). Chlorpromazine is oxidized to its sulfoxides by an enzyme system requiring reduced triphosphopyridine nucleotide and oxygen, in microsomes of guinea pig liver homogenates. The enzyme system is probably not a peroxidase. SK&F 525-A did not affect the sulfoxidation. An unidentified metabolite of chlorpromazine noticed in the incubation mixture may have been formed by either hydroxylation or dealkylation reactions (cf. Robinson, 1965).

Wechsler and Roizin (1960) have studied tissue levels of chlorpromazine in experimental animals. Chlorpromazine (10–25 mg/100 gm i.m.) as a single dose in rats or 15 mg/100 gm in monkeys, reached highest concentration in the lungs when animals were sacrificed within 16–18 hours. The concentration was less in liver, spleen, stomach, kidney, intestine, and brain. Chronic experiments (0.6 mg/100 gm/day for 2 weeks to 3 months in rats and for 20–30 months in monkeys) showed no chlorpromazine in any rat tissue or liver and brain samples of monkeys. The data suggest that there is no accumulation of chlorpromazine in tissues of patients treated for long periods.

The metabolism of drugs by microsomes from alloxan-diabetic rats was studied by Dixon et al. (1961). Alloxan diabetes decreased the ability of rat liver to metabolize hexobarbital, chlorpromazine, and codeine in vitro; it also prolonged hexobarbital-induced sleeping time in vivo. Insulin reversed these effects in vivo but not in vitro. The decreased enzyme activity cannot be explained by lack of TPNH (reduced TPN), presence of enzyme inhibitors, or direct action of alloxan. It may be due to increased destruction, decreased synthesis, or denaturation of the enzymes.

These results have been confirmed in in vitro studies where the drug was found to be bound by nuclei, mitochondria (Dingell et al., 1961) and by microsomes. It has been shown by Wollemann et al. (1961, 1962) that chlorpromazine and related compounds inhibit various dehydrogenases, while at the same time being chemically transformed. Similar alterations on the phenothiazines can be achieved by oxidation with ceric sulfate or by photo-oxidation. The intermediate product has an intensive wine red color and has absorption maxima at 530 millimicrons and 510 millimicrons, and at 256 and 275 millimicrons in the ultraviolet. This oxidized intermediate is readily separable from chlorpromazine sulfoxide by the method of Salzman and Brodie (1956). The two metabolites are also separable on paper chromatography. The intermediate is stable for weeks if precipitated with alkali and freeze dried. It is immediately decolorized by reduced diphosphopyridine nucleotide.

The metabolism of chlorpromazine (8 mg/kg p.o.) was compared in dogs and man by Goldenberg and Fishman (1961). Humans tended to favor excretion of polar derivatives, together with one or two major nonpolar metabolites, monodemethyl- or didemethylchlorpromazine sulfoxide. Human output of chlorpromazine and its sulfoxide was trivial. Dogs excreted less polar material, less didemethylchlorpromazine sulfoxide, more monodemethylchlorpromazine sulfoxide, and substantial amounts of both chlorpromazine and its sulfoxide. Human polar fractions contained persulfate-blue as well as persulfate-lavender staining metabolites; the blue series was absent from dog urine.

The metabolism of drugs by subfractions of hepatic microsomes was studied by Fouts (1961). Drug-metabolizing enzyme activities and the nitrogen content of rough- and smooth-surfaced microsomes of rat liver were studied. Chlorpromazine, codeine, hexobarbital, aminopyrine, TPNH, and nitrogen were used as substrates. Drug-metabolizing enzyme activity of smooth-surfaced microsomes was 3–5 times greater than that of rough-surfaced microsomes. The TPNH oxidase activity of smooth-surfaced microsomes was 5 times greater than that of rough-surfaced microsomes. The nitrogen content was roughly equivalent.

The concentration of phenothiazines in the eye has been reported by Potts (1962) and by Rutschmann et al. (1962). There seems to be no correlation between phenothiazine levels in the eye and the production of retinopathies by certain phenothiazines (cf. Whitten and Filmer, 1947). The uptake of phenothiazines in the brain receives indirect evidence from the finding of Gordon et al. (1962) that injection of chlorpromazine inhibits the uptake of d-aminoisobutyric acid by rat brain.

An interesting paper by Fouts and Adamson (1959) reports that the lesser degree of metabolism of drugs by livers of newborn rabbits may be due to the presence of enzyme inhibitors (cf. Fouts, 1961, 1963).

Chlorpromazine and its metabolites were found by Kohl et al. (1964) to concentrate in the guinea pig small intestine. The comparative accumulations were as follows: didemethylchlorpromazine > monodemethyl > chlorpromazine > chlorpromazine sulfoxide.

Studies by Van Loon et al. (1962) have showed that there is rapid absorption of S^{35}-labeled chlorpromazine, prochlorperazine, and trifluoperazine from the gastrointestinal tract. It was shown that 20% of administered labeled chlorpromazine appeared in the bowel in 10 hours, while greater than 60% of the prochlorperazine and 70% of the trifluoperazine were excreted by this route during this time (cf. Emmerson and Miya, 1962; Flanagan et al., 1962a,b; Ross et al., 1962; Phillips and Miya, 1962; Gold et al., 1962). The urinary excretion pattern differed in that the recovery of chlorpromazine was greatest (18%) followed by prochlorperazine (7%) and trifluoperazine (2%). The total biliary and urinary excretion for 10 hours was 78% for chlorpromazine, 77% for prochlorperazine, and 72% for trifluoperazine. The systemic and hepatic blood levels of the three phenothiazines did not exceed 10 µg/ml at any one time. During the early hours of the experiment, the portal blood contained 2–3 times as much drug as did the hepatic blood, thus demonstrating rapid removal by the liver. An additional study in dogs showed active hepatic recirculation of biliary-excreted phenothiazines.

Tissue distribution studies have also been done in animals by Besson and Leder, 1955; Christensen and Wase, 1956a,b; Henriksen et al., 1957; Wechsler and Roizin, 1960; Young et al., 1959; Ross et al., 1958, 1962; Berti and Cima, 1954a,b,c; Berti, 1954a,b; Gouzon et al., 1954; Kok, 1955; Wase et al., 1956; Block, 1961; Budinsky and Votava, 1960; Dubost and Pascal, 1953; Duhm et al., 1958; Eger and Poppe, 1960; Federov, 1957, 1958a,b; Grebennik, 1957; Hoffmann et al., 1959; Ogawa et al., 1958; Smith and Burke, 1960; Walkenstein and Seifter, 1958; Weikel et al., 1960; Whitten and Filmer, 1947; Emmerson and Miya, 1962; Flanagan et al., 1962a,b; Phillips and Miya, 1962; Gold et al., 1962; Kinross-Wright and Ragland, 1961.

B. Metabolic Fate

It has been demonstrated that the demethylation of chlorpromazine takes place *in vivo* in the rat, using labeled chlorpromazine (N-methyl-C^{14}), by the oral or intravenous route. In this experiment the methyl group of chlorpromazine was oxidized to carbon dioxide-C^{14} (Ross et al., 1958). Later Young et al. (1959) also demonstrated that this N-demethylation takes place *in vitro* in rat and rabbit liver homogenates. Walkenstein and Seifter (1959) have also demonstrated that promazine-S^{35} is demethylated in the dog to the corresponding monomethyl and monomethyl sulfoxide derivatives.

Ross et al. (1962) have studied the metabolism of C^{14}- or S^{35}-labeled chlorpromazine in rat and rabbit liver homogenates. Metabolic products identified were $C^{14}O_2$, C^{14}-labeled formaldehyde, and the N-demethyl derivative of chlorpromazine.

Of interest is the fact that it has been shown by Fouts (1961, 1963) that agents like chlordan can stimulate the chlorpromazine metabolizing activity of the hepatic microsomes of adult rats. On the other hand, ethylmorphine was found to inhibit the chlorpromazine metabolizing properties of hepatic microsomes (Rubin, 1964).

The isolation and characterization of chlorpromazine derivatives produced by ultraviolet irradiation was studied by Huang (1962). Some of these are thought to be similar to free radical containing products produced in the metabolism of chlorpromazine. The nature of the other products is not known. Some of the ultraviolet-transformation products have the same physical properties as those of the phenolic derivatives and the hydrolysis products of chlorpromazine glucuronides, and they may be possible precursors of the chlorpromazine metabolites. Wollemann and Keleti (1962) have shown that *in vitro* photooxidation of chlorpromazine yields, in addition to the sulfoxide, a "red chlorpromazine" which is a dehydrogenase inhibitor. Oxidation to a red product has also been accomplished by the use of peroxidase and catalase (Cavanaugh, 1957).

It has been shown by the techniques of electron spin resonance (E.S.R.) that free radicals can be formed from phenothiazine derivatives by a variety of procedures including the action of ultraviolet light (Lagercrantz, 1961; Piette *et al.*, 1961; Forrest *et al.*, 1958; Laborit *et al.*, 1960; Ravin *et al.*, 1958). Twelve different compounds were isolated after ultraviolet irradiation of a solution of chlorpromazine hydrochloride (Huang and Sands, 1964). On the other hand, Borg and Cotzias (1962b) could detect only a very weak E.S.R. signal in solutions of chlorpromazine irradiated with ultraviolet. Lagercrantz (1962) has reported that free radicals are obtained by ultraviolet irradiation of solutions of various phenothiazine derivatives in buffers near the neutral point. It is well known that free radicals can be induced by the action of light on a variety of substances in solution in the presence of such sensitizing agents as eosine (Schenck and Wohlgast, 1961; Lagercrantz and Yhland, 1962). It is speculated that a complex is formed of electron donors and electron acceptors, so that the radiant energy absorbed promotes a charge-transfer giving rise to the production of free radicals. It is further speculated that chlorpromazine is transformed by irradiation to a colored substance, not a radical, which may behave as a sensitizer to form the acceptor part of the complex with unreacted chlorpromazine. These mechanisms may be related to the photosensitivity sometimes seen with patients on large doses of chlorpromazine. Merkle (1964) has reported on the synthesis of a solid stable free radical of chlorpromazine.

Schieser and Tuck (1962) have reported that E.S.R. studies indicate the existence of stable free radical semiquinoid intermediates in the oxidation products of several phenothiazines.

Borg and Cotzias (1962a,b,c) have studied the interaction of phenothiazines with trace metals and have identified the chromophore produced by this interaction as being a semiquinone free radical ion. The latter is thought to be involved in the biological activity of this drug (cf. Piette and Forrest, 1962; Forrest *et al.*, 1958; Fels and Kaufman, 1959).

In related investigations Piette *et al.* (1962) and Piette and Forrest (1962) have studied the oxidation mechanisms of chlorpromazine using both nuclear magnetic resonance (N.M.R.) and electron paramagnetic resonance (E.P.R.), the latter being the only spectroscopic device for studying one electron intermediates (free radicals). Using ceric salts, chlorpromazine oxidizes in two univalent steps via competitive, consecutive second-order reaction. These mechanisms indicate that any simple enzymatic oxidation of chlorpromazine would always result only in the formation of sulfoxide. Inasmuch as this mechanism accounts for less than 20% of the drug in the urine, it is obvious that a simple oxidation of chlorpromazine cannot be the predominant metabolic mechanism. Fels and Kaufman (1959) have felt, from the stoichiometry involved, that the red oxidation product of chlorpromazine is a quinone rather than a free radical.

In attempts to establish the glucuronide structure for chlorpromazine metabolites, free radical spectra of the chlorpromazine-glucuronide type have been compared with selectively synthesized phenothiazine derivatives. It is believed that more than half of the metabolites of chlorpromazine appear as mono- or disubstituted glucuronide adducts, but the position of substitution on the phenothiazine ring had not been established until Price *et al.* (1964) recently reported isolation of 7-hydroxy chlorpromazine from the urine of schizophrenics receiving chlorpromazine. In an effort to use N.M.R. to identify the exact site of substitution, model compounds of known structures substituted in the 1-, 2-, 3-, 7-, and 8-positions as well as disubstituted phenothiazines, have been catalogued according to their N.M.R. spectra.

Metabolites from the urine of patients on chlorpromazine were separated by solvent extraction and purified by thin-layer chromatography. So far only the dimethyl, monomethyl, and demethylated sulfoxides in the organic soluble fractions have been characterized. Separation of at least six different glucuronides have been made from the aqueous fraction of the urine using thin-layer chromatography (cf. Huang and Ruskin, 1964).

Fedorov and Shnol' (1956) have studied the distribution of chlorpromazine using S^{35}-tagged material. In studies in the rat, maximal accumulation (identified by counting only) occurred in the lungs whereas the concentration in the blood was very low. Chlorpromazine was presumed to cross the blood-brain barrier easily, and the highest concentration of S^{35}-containing material was found in the cortex of the large hemispheres. After subcutaneous injection in the rat, metabolic products were found only in the urine, and after 4 days, 97.4% of the administered dose had been excreted. After oral administration of chlorpromazine, only about 16% is absorbed; the unabsorbed portion is excreted in the feces in the course of 8 to 9 days. The chlorpromazine in the feces was thought to be unmetabolized.

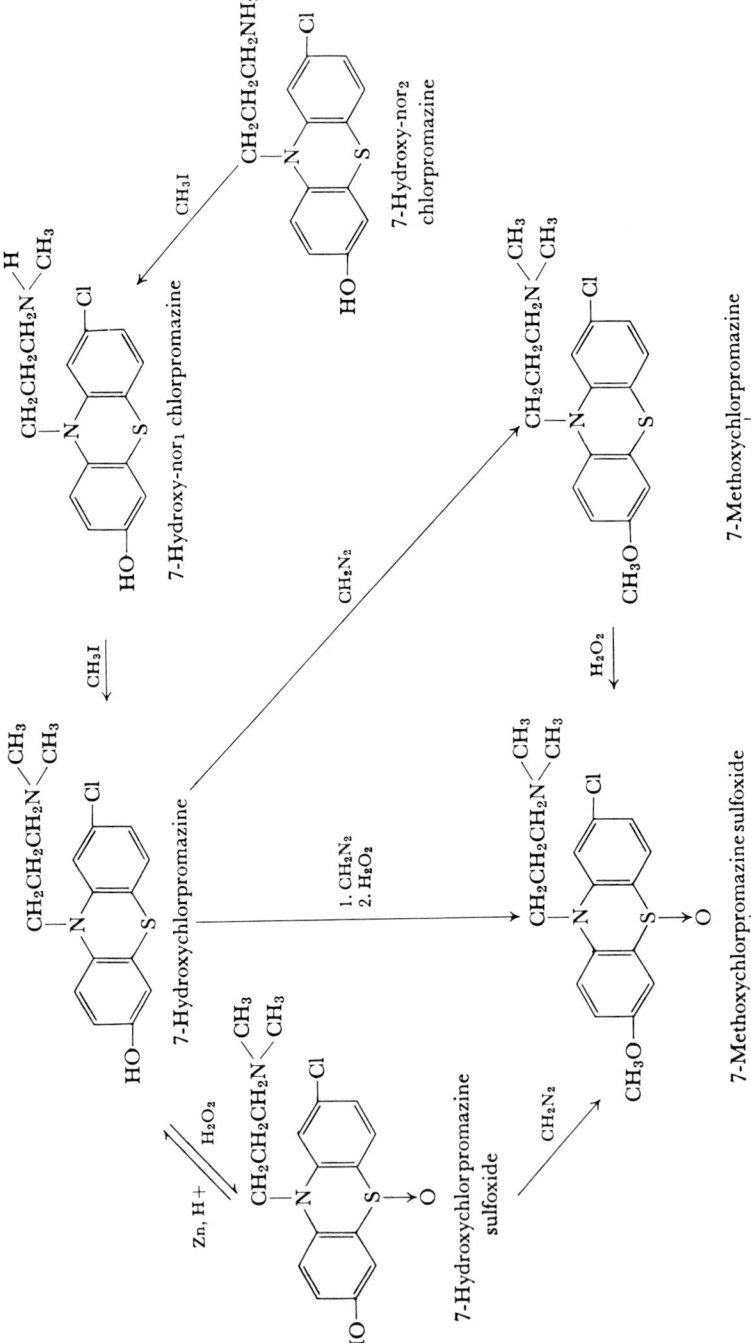

Fig. 4. New phenolic metabolites of chlorpromazine.

The metabolism of perphenazine has been studied by Symchowicz et al. (1962) and promethazine-S^{35} has been reported on by Hansson and Schmitleröw (1961), both groups found the sulfoxide of the respective drugs.

The metabolism of unsubstituted phenothiazine has been studied by a number of investigators (Craig, 1962; Clare, 1962; Collier et al., 1943; Harwood, 1953), but these experiments are not pertinent to the psychopharmacological area and hence will not be discussed here, except to say that 3-hydroxyphenothiazine is a metabolite which has been isolated and is excreted as the glucuronide or the ethereal sulfate (Esserman, 1952; Lazarus and Rogers, 1951; Harpur et al., 1950; Swales and Collier, 1940; Alexander et al., 1958). Finally Craig (1962) has reviewed the use of phenothiazines as anthelmintics.

In recent studies (Goldenberg and Fishman, 1964; Fishman and Goldenberg, 1963), the following metabolites of chlorpromazine were identified by comparison with reference compounds: 7-hydroxychlorpromazine, its sulfoxide, 7-hydroxy-N-demethylchlorpromazine, and 7-hydroxydidemethylchlorpromazine. These compounds were excreted both in the free form and as glucuronic acid conjugates. The interconversions used in the structure proof are shown in Fig. 4.

Huang et al. (1963) have speculated, on grounds of potential oxidizability, that hydroxylation *in vivo* takes place at the 3- or 7-positions. They have found in man that glucuronides are major metabolites. It is of interest that in a patient given 400 mg of chlorpromazine three times a day for 1 month, metabolites could be found in the urine for three weeks after discontinuance of the medication.

C. Distribution and Metabolism of Phenothiazines in Man

Beckett et al. (1962) have studied the metabolism of chlorpromazine in human urine. As a result of these studies, a tentative scheme for the metabolism of chlorpromazine in humans was suggested. One pathway postulates the conversion of chlorpromazine to a hydroxychlorpromazine (not yet detected free in human urine) and conjugation of this hydroxychlorpromazine with either glucuronic acid or sulfuric acid to give a glucuronide or an ethereal sulfate derivative. Another pathway shows the conversion of chlorpromazine to the sulfoxide followed by the hydroxylation of the sulfoxide (not yet demonstrated in human urine) and conjugation of the hydroxychlorpromazine sulfoxide with glucuronic acid. The chlorpromazine sulfoxide may also be N-demethylated to give monodemethylchlorpromazine sulfoxide which is in equilibrium with the monodemethylchlorpromazine. The monodemethylchlorpromazine may also arise from chlorpromazine directly and the demethylchlorpromazine can be hydroxylated (not yet demonstrated in human urine) and this hydroxydemethylchlorpromazine can also be conjugated with glucuronic acid or sulfuric acid as postulated above. Either the demethylchlorpromazine or its sulfoxide may be further demethylated to give the didemethylchlorpromazine sulfoxide or didemethylchlorpromazine, which in turn can be hydroxylated (the free hydroxydidemethylchlorpromazine has not yet been demonstrated in human urine) and this hydroxy compound can be converted to the corresponding glucuronide or ethereal sulfate, both of which have been demonstrated in human urine (cf. Beckett et al., 1963).

On the basis of very preliminary observations (Huang et al., 1961a,b; Kurland and Huang, 1962) it is suggested that the duration of the excretion of chlorpromazine glucuronides following the discontinuation of chlorpromazine therapy might serve to indicate the period in which a patient may remain in a state of remission without further drug therapy. This postulate was based on the fact that the chlorpromazine glucuronides seemed to disappear most rapidly in those patients who relapse more quickly, whereas patients in whom the excretion of glucuronides persisted were less likely to relapse (cf. Huang and Kurland, 1961a,b,c; Garetz and Leider, 1963). These suggestions were later withdrawn by Huang (1964) (cf. Kurland et al., 1965).

The use of thin film chromatography to separate phenothiazine metabolites from neuropsychiatric patients, and the metabolism of tritium, and sulfur-labeled thioridazine was studied by Eiduson and Geller (1962). The synthesis of tritium-labeled phenothiazines has been described by Kalberer and Rutschmann (1963).

Fishman et al. (1962) have reported the isolation and identification of chlorpromazine-N-oxide from human urine. This compound, although not a major human metabolite, is excreted in somewhat larger amounts than chlorpromazine sulfoxide. Dogs surpass humans in their output of the N-oxide. Recent behavioral and pharmacological tests indicate that norchlorpromazine and the N-oxide approach chlorpromazine in activity.

In a study on the isolation and characterization of glucuronic acid conjugates of chlorpromazine in human urine, Lin et al. (1959) isolated four polar, water-soluble metabolites of chlorpromazine by use of a cation exchange resin. These were shown to be glucuronides by release of free glucuronic acid, and less polar, ether-extractable phenothiazines as a result of beta-glucuronidase hydrolysis. The presence of phenolic functions in these liberated phenothiazines was shown by their extractability from an acetic medium. These results strongly suggest hydroxylation of chlorpromazine and subsequent conjugation with glucuronic acid as a route of chlorpromazine metabolism in man.

Fishman and Goldenberg (1960) have studied an organic extractable fraction from the urine of patients administered chlorpromazine. Chromatographic studies revealed the presence of ten compounds which produced a Dragendorff color reaction following organic extraction of alkalinized human urine. Six of these appear to be sulfoxides, including chlorpromazine sulfoxide which is a relatively minor product. Two major metabolites had chromatographic behavior indistinguishable from demethylchlorpromazine sulfoxide and didemethylchlorpromazine sulfoxide. A third major metabolite remained unidentified, but was not a sulfoxide derivative. It was found that the residual urine remaining after extraction contained numerous additional polar metabolites (see Fig. 4).

The isolation and characterization of phenothiazine and metabolites from body fluids by use of thin-layer chromatography, paper chromatography, and solvent extraction has been studied by Nadeau and Sobolewski (1959a,b,c). They have developed a rapid method for routine analysis using potassium iodoplatinate to give a blue color that can be estimated with a colorimeter at levels of 0–20 μg/ml. The free phenothiazine derivatives are readily extractable from urine with isobutanol under alkaline conditions. The conjugated portion of the drug in the remaining urine can be liberated by either chemical or enzymatic hydrolysis.

Other distribution studies in man have been carried out by Allgén et al. (1959), Behn et al. (1956), Berti and Cima (1957), Davidson et al. (1957), I. S. Forrest and F. M. Forrest (1960a–c, 1961); F. M. Forrest and I. S. Forrest (1960), Haynes (1960), Heyman and Merlis (1961), Hollister et al. (1960), Kinberger (1957), Kinberger and Lassenius (1956), Kleinsorge et al. (1959), Neve (1961), Zielinski and Eynetten (1960), Fedorov (1958a,b), Iwasa et al. (1957), Johnson and Masters (1962), Heimlich et al. (1961), Rosen and Swintosky (1960), Eiduson et al. (1960), Lubin et al. (1960), Hollester (1962), Beckett (1964), Beckett et al. (1963).

Three new metabolites of chlorpromazine have recently been isolated from the urine of mental patients by Johnson et al. (1965). These were identified as 2-chlorophenothiazine, 2-chlorophenothiazine sulfoxide, and 2-chlorophenothiazine-10-propionic acid. The first two metabolites, of interest because of the complete loss of the side chain, were isolated by extracting alkaline urine with dichloromethane, and the acidic compound was extracted from urine at pH 3 with chloroform. The compounds were identified by microcoulometric gas chromatography and thin-layer chromatography by comparison of the unknown with standards. Ion exchange chromatography was used to isolate larger quantities of the acidic metabolite and its infrared spectrum was identical with synthetic 2-chlorophenothiazine-10-propionic acid.

Extraction of urine at acid pH removed at least three other acidic phenothiazines in addition to the propionic acid metabolite. The identity of these is as yet unconfirmed. These metabolites were obtained in patients ranging in age from 18 to 81 years who received from 200 to 1000 mg of chlorpromazine per day.

A summary on metabolism of drugs has been published by Brodie et al. (1958). An interesting paper by Conney et al. (1960) reported that repeated administration of drugs resulted in an adaptive increase in drug-metabolizing enzymes. Thus pretreatment of rats with phenobarbital, aminopyrine, phenylbutazone, etc. caused a marked increase in the ability of enzymes in the liver microsomes to metabolize quite unrelated drugs.

VII. Analytical Methods for Phenothiazines

Fundamental to studies on the metabolic fate, and especially the study of *in vivo* distribution and excretion, of the phenothiazines has been the development of analytical procedures for their detection and estimation. Basic to much of this work is the use of isotopically labeled phenothiazines and many of the metabolism studies in Section VI have used isotopic techniques (C^{14}, S^{35}, or tritium labeling). However these procedures cannot be used broadly in human subjects, so analytical techniques were developed for the estimation of low levels of phenothiazines in urine and blood samples. Not the least of the objectives of this work is the determination of whether patients have in fact taken their intended medication. In this connection, Swintosky (1962) has reported an interesting method for ascertaining whether medication has been taken. The addition of 3 mg of riboflavin to, for example, 10 mg of chlorpromazine, 5 mg of prochlorperazine, 1 mg of trifluoperazine, or 10 mg of thioridazine followed by examination of the urine 3 hours after drug plus riboflavin marker, reveals a bright yellow fluorescence under ultraviolet light if drug has been taken (cf. Léider, 1964).

Forrest *et al.* (1961) have published a useful review of analytical procedures for the determination of phenothiazine in urine. It is of interest, for example, that chlorpromazine produces a pink color with ferric chloride in acid solution, whereas the sulfoxide metabolite does not. Various intermediate free radicals produce intense purple colors.

An extensive review of methods for the identification of tranquilizing drugs was published by Rajeswaran and Kirk (1961a,b, 1962). The methods employed include direct color tests and color tests with nitrated products (Rajeswaran and Kirk, 1961a). Also described are microscopic crystal tests Rajeswaran and Kirk, 1961b) and x-ray diffraction powder analysis (Rajeswaran and Kirk, 1962). The 1962 reference also reports on ultraviolet absorption characteristics of about fifty tranquilizing and related drugs. Other reviews have been published by Yung and Pernarowski (1963) and by Chuen and Riedel (1961), and by Kiger and Kiger (1965).

Inasmuch as phenothiazine metabolites are often bound to glucuronic acid, in urine, hydrolysis with beta-glucuronidases has been used to liberate the phenothiazine prior to extraction (Posner, 1959; F. M. Forrest and I. S. Forrest, 1960; I. S. Forrest and F. M. Forrest, 1960a–c, 1961). Obviously techniques for the detection of metabolites in urine and other body fluids often do little more than ascertain whether the phenothiazine has been taken. For identification purposes, techniques like counter-current distribution (Salzman el al., 1955; Smith and Burke, 1960), ion exchange chromatography using IRC-50 resin (Eiduson and Wallace, 1958a,b; Blazek et al., 1962) or Dowex 50 (H) (Lin et al., 1959), paper chromatography (Vačerková et al., 1962; Blazek et al., 1962; Huang and Kurland, 1961a,b; Allgén, 1959; Allgén et al., 1959, 1960; Behn et al., 1956; Berti and Cima, 1957; Walkenstein and Seifter, 1958, 1959; Cavanaugh, 1957; Eisdorfer and Ellenbogen, 1960; Fedorov, 1958a,b; Fedorov and Shnol', 1956; Fishman and Goldenberg, 1960; Frahm et al., 1956; Gillette and Kamm, 1960; Glowinski et al., 1960; Kleinsorge et al., 1959; Lin et al., 1959; Posner, 1959; Tabau and Vigne, 1958), electrophoresis on paper (Blazek et al., 1962; Mellinger and Keeler, 1962; Calo et al., 1956, 1958; Collier et al., 1943), thin-layer chromatography (Ragland, 1962; Cochin and Daly, 1962a,b, 1963; Eberhardt et al., 1963), gas chromatography (Ragland, 1962; Parker et al., 1963a,b; Vanden Heuvel et al., 1962; Craig et al., 1964), spectrophotometric techniques (Rieder, 1960; Ragland, 1962; I. S. Forrest and F. M. Forrest, 1960a–c, 1961; F. M. Forrest and I. S. Forrest, 1960; Allgén, 1959; Allgén et al., 1959, 1960; Berti and Cima, 1957; Calo et al., 1958; Cavanaugh, 1957; Cavanaugh and Ervin, 1957; Collier et al., 1943; Dubost and Pascal, 1953; Huang and Kurland, 1961a,b,c; Eiduson and Wallace, 1958a,b; Fels et al., 1958a,b; Flanagan et al., 1959; Haynes, 1960; Kinberger, 1957; Kinberger and Lassenius, 1956; Kok, 1955; Meyre, 1957; Neve, 1961; Pungor, 1960; Ryan, 1959; Salzman and Brodie, 1956; Smith and Burke, 1960; Wechsler and Forrest, 1959; Wechsler and Roizin, 1960; Weikel et al., 1960; Zielinski and Eynetten, 1960; Lucas and Fabierkiewicz, 1963; Beckett and Curry, 1963; Henricksen et al., 1960), column chromatography (Meyre, 1957), spectrofluometric methods (Davidson et al., 1957; Ragland and Kinross-Wright, 1961) and radioautographs for localization in tissues (Eger and Poppe, 1960) have been utilized.

A recent paper by Warren et al. reported detailed infrared, ultraviolet, and nuclear magnetic resonance spectra of seventeen clinically used phenothiazines, together with spectra for some intermediates. Spectra–structure correlations were made which should be useful in future analytical work.

Methods have been developed for the quantitative determination of phenothiazines in tablets and other dosage forms. Thus nonaqueous titrations have been used by Milne (1959), nonaqueous titrations with mercuric acetate and perchloric acid have been used by Milne and Chatten (1957) and by Fossoul (1950), potassium bromate titration by Cavicchi Sandri (1955) and by Dusinsky (1957, 1958), titration with silicotungstic acid by Thieme (1956) and by Blazek (1956), and polarographic methods by Blazek et al. (1962). Gravimetric procedures for phenothiazines have been developed by Milne and Chatten (1957), by Blazek and Stejskal (1955, 1956), and by Uyeo and Oishi (1952).

Colorimetric procedures have been the basis of both qualitative and quantitative procedures for the estimation of phenothiazines (Sobolewski and Nadeau, 1960; F. M. Forrest et al., 1961; Deviller, 1961; Gold et al., 1962; Brignon, 1955a,b; Allgén, 1959; Behn et al., 1956; I. S. Forrest and F. M. Forrest, 1960a–c, 1961; F. M. Forrest and I. S. Forrest, 1960; I. S. Forrest et al., 1960; Hetzel, 1961; Hollister et al., 1960; Kotionis, 1961).

Careful control of experimental conditions, especially pH, is required in the use of color reactions on biological materials. Thus the ferric chloride test of Vesell (1959) could not be confirmed by F. M. Forrest et al. (1959a,b,c). Other procedures for the use of ferric chloride in dilute sulfuric or nitric acid have been published by Brewer et al. (1959), Fellman (1956), Fels et al. (1958b), Fels and Kaufman (1959), Forrest and Forrest (1957), Cordier and Dupontreue (1962), I. S. Forrest et al. (1958), F. M. Forrest et al. (1960), Fossoul (1950, 1951), Lin and Reynolds (1960), Nellhaus (1959), and Vol'pe (1961). The combination of ferric nitrate and sulfuric acid has been used by Kleinsorge et al. (1959) and by Leach and Crimmin (1956). Ferric chloride and dilute perchloric acid and/or nitric acid has been used by I. S. Forrest and F. M. Forrest (1961), F. M. Forrest and I. S. Forrest (1959), and by F. M. Forrest et al. (1961).

Dubost and Pascal (1953) have found that sulfuric acid develops a red color with phenothiazines, and Dubost and Pascal (1955) have found that this color is stabilized by the addition of ethanol or formaldehyde. The use of 85% phosphoric acid has been reported to produce a more stable color than is obtained with sulfuric acid (Cavanaugh and Ervin, 1957; Eiduson and Wallace, 1958a,b). Other investigators who have used sulfuric acid as a color-developing reagent include Behn et al. (1956), Berti and Cima (1955), Eiduson and Wallace (1958a,b), Fedorov (1958a,b), Gouzon et al. (1954), Grebennik (1957), Haynes (1960), Henricksen et al. (1957), Kinberger and Lassenius (1956), Kok (1955), Neuhoff and Auterhoff (1955), Posner (1959), Omarova (1958), and Franchi and Gianni (1957). Heyman and Merlis (1961) have reported the development of false positives with mercuric nitrate and sulfuric acid, and Frahm et al. (1956) and Gillette and Kamm (1960) have used a sulfuric-acid–ethanol spray for detecting phenothiazines on paper chromatograms.

Other reagents that have been used to detect phenothiazines include nitrites (Berti and Cima, 1954a,b,c, 1955; Neve, 1958; Franchi and Gianni, 1957), iodic and phosphoric acids (Calo et al., 1958), nitric acid (Citterio, 1957; Citterio and Mattei, 1957; Fossoul, 1950, 1951; Hetzel, 1961; Grover, 1957), and uranyl nitrate (Deviller, 1961; Heyman et al., 1960; F. M. Forrest et al., 1959; Heyman et al., 1960). Uranyl nitrate in concentrated hydrochloric acid is said to be specific for triflupromazine (F. M. Forrest et al., 1959), and uranyl nitrate in trichloroacetic acid has also been used (F. M. Forrest et al., 1959a).

Among the other oxidative reagents used for the phenothiazines are ferric perchlorate (Deviller, 1961), sodium or ammonium persulfate (Deviller, 1961; Fossoul, 1951; Pungor, 1960; Waaler, 1960; Heyman et al., 1960), ceric sulfate (Blazek et al., 1962; Dusinsky, 1957), hydrogen peroxide (Heyman et al., 1960; Solsona and Mora, 1951; Wechsler and Forrest, 1959), bromine in sulfuric acid (Brignon, 1955a,b; Fossoul, 1950, 1951; Waddell, 1959), and potassium ferricyanide and ferric chloride (Kosir and Kosir, 1956).

Still other analytical techniques for phenothiazines have involved reineckates and silver acetate complexes (Blazek et al., 1962), a palladium lauryl sulfate complex salt (Ryan, 1959), vanadium sulfate in sulfuric acid (Neuhoff and Auterhoff, 1955), potassium iodoplatinate (Nadeau and Sobolewski, 1959a,b,c), bromthymol blue (Kotionis, 1961; Dubost and Pascal, 1956), diazotized sulfanilic acid (Fellman, 1956; Gillette and Kamm, 1960; Kinberger, 1957; Neuhoff and Auterhoff, 1955), mercuric nitrate and trichloroacetic acid (F. M. Forrest et al., 1959b), mercuric iodide (Grebennik, 1957), and palladium chloride (Cavatorta, 1959).

Various procedures for impregnation of filter papers have been used with varying success in the detection of phenothiazines in urine and other body fluids. Thus, Heyman et al. (1959) sprayed a sulfonic-acid-resin-impregnated paper treated with ferric chloride solution and sulfuric acid. He also used a mercuric nitrate sprayed paper (Heyman et al., 1960).

Indican (Levine et al., 1961) is said to interfere with the urine color tests for phenothiazines by giving false positives or poor dose-color correspondence. In particular, indican is reported to interfere with the triflupromazine test (F. M. Forrest et al., 1959a), the piperazine-linked phenothiazine test (F. M. Forrest et al., 1959b), the universal test (I. S. Forrest and F. M. Forrest, 1961), and the thioridazine test (F. M. Forrest et al., 1960) by producing a blue color. Indican does not interfere with the chlorpromazine (F. M. Forrest and I. S. Forrest, 1957), the promazine, or the mepazine tests (I. S. Forrest et al., 1958). According to F. M. Forrest et al. (1961) the indican interference is not critical since this color appears slowly, whereas the phenothiazine colors appear immediately and should be read within 10 seconds. Furthermore (I. S. Forrest et al., 1963), the addition of Dowex AG 3 × 4 anion exchange resin in the chloride form to urine will remove, by selective absorption, indican and other colored principles that might interfere with phenothiazine color tests. Posner and Levine (1963), on the other hand, did not find the use of Dowex AG 3 × 4 resin helpful.

Posner and Solomon (1960) found the chlorpromazine test satisfactory but obtained many false positives with the piperazine-linked phenothiazine test in volunteers who had not received drugs.

I. S. Forrest and F. M. Forrest (1960b) found false positives in the phenothiazine color reactions due to (a) phenylketonuria, (b) high doses of p-aminosalicylic acid, (c) impaired liver function, (d) high doses of estrogens, and (e) infrequently, unknown causes.

VIII. Miscellaneous Properties of Phenothiazines

Orloff and Fitts (1961) have done a molecular orbital treatment of phenothiazine and some related molecules (cf. Pullman and Pullman, 1959). Orloff and Fitts determined the electron energy levels of chlorpromazine, phenothiazine, and leuco-methylene blue and concluded that in the ground state delocalized electrons occupy only bonding orbitals if "d" orbitals on sulfur are taken into consideration. Paramagnetic resonance studies of certain phenothiazines have been made by Billon et al. (1961).

Gutmann and Netschey (1961) have studied the semiconductor properties of chlorpromazine. They found that it was an impurity semiconductor at low temperatures and an intrinsic semiconductor at temperatures above $32°C$.

Sorby and Plein (1961) found that considerable amounts of chlorpromazine and fourteen other phenothiazines were adsorbed by kaolin, talc, and activated carbon. A study is being made of the factors which influence this absorption process.

Chlorpromazine has been used as an analytical reagent for gold, iron, and other metals (Kum-Tatt, 1962; Kum-Tatt and Tong, 1962). The use of phenothiazine derivatives in analytical chemistry has been reviewed by Blazek (1963b).

Karreman et al. (1959) have studied the mechanism of action of chlorpromazine and have concluded that the therapeutic properties of chlorpromazine are related to the powerful electron donor properties of this drug.

IX. Summary of Clinical Applications

A. CNS Activity

As in the case of the pharmacology section, there are many thousands of papers on the clinical applications of the phenothiazines. Accordingly we have selected chlorpromazine as the prototype and will summarize its clinical applications citing some recent references (see Chapter 1, Volume I). Most of the other tranquilizing phenothiazines share qualitatively the properties of chlorpromazine, although there are important quantitative differences. Ten years of experience with chlorpromazine have been reviewed by Ayd (1963, 1964) and by Winkelman (1964).

The scope of the clinical applications of the phenothiazines is so broad that it may exceed even that of the corticosteroids. Reviews on the applications of phenothiazines in clinical medicine have been published by Altschule

(1960), DiPalma (1963), Goldman (1961), Hordern (1961), Saunders (1961), Schiele (1962), Smith et al. (1963), Voigt (1962), Rees (1962), Hemphill (1962), Cole (1962), Weatherall (1962), Wortis (1963, 1964), Bowes and Natarajan (1963), Kraines (1963), Haase (1963), Bortnik and Kalandarishvili (1963), Welsh (1964), Braceland (1964), Winkelman (1964), Witt (1961), Zakusov (1964), and Hippius (1965).

Altschule, for example, has speculated that various chemical and neural changes may explain tranquilizer action. Among these are depletion of epinephrine and its precursors, increased rate of oxidation of epinephrine, chelation of epinephrine, depression of ascending reticular activating system, inactivation of conditioned responses, combination with indoles, and competitive inhibition of indoles.

For the convenience of the researcher, we have provided, in Appendix A, a bibliography on prochlorperazine, trifluoperazine, trimeprazine, triflupromazine, promazine, methoxypromazine, propiamazine, acetophenazine, fluphenazine, perphenazine, thiopropazote, mepazine, pipamazine, thiethylperazine, thioridazine, and methdilazine.

An interesting discussion of the testing of tranquilizers has been published recently by Bain and Doughty (1963). It is of consequence to point out that medical education tends to emphasize the experimental aspects of pharmacology, with relative neglect of drug pharmacology, particularly with regard to the critical assessment of new therapeutic agents. Thus there is a severe shortage of qualified clinical pharmacologists who can evaluate new therapy (Wilson, 1963).

Chlorpromazine is the reference compound in the treatment of hospitalized psychiatric patients. It is used to control agitation, modify delusions and hallucinations, and to restore or increase the patient's response to psychotherapy.

The use of chlorpromazine in acute cases has been studied by Cutler et al. (1957), Hankoff et al. (1960), Kant and Abele (1961), Smelson and Foy (1962), Jenkins et al. (1962), Lovett Doust and Harrington (1962), Childers (1961a), Kurland et al. (1961a,b), Richards (1964), Rosati (1964), and Nishizono (1964). It has been reviewed by Cole (1964) and by Michaux et al. (1964) (cf. Pfeiffer and Bente, 1961).

Studies on the effects of chlorpromazine in chronic schizophrenic patients have been carried out by Zeleba (1961), Morozova (1961), Wilson et al. (1961), Ainslie (1961), Hackstein (1960), Engelhardt et al. (1960), Remvig and Sonne (1961), Schiele et al. (1961), Bennett and Kooi (1961), Ashcroft et al. (1961), Childers and Therrien (1961), Childers (1961b, 1962a,b), Waldrop et al. (1961), Tuteur et al. (1962), Tachezy (1962), Schweich et al. (1961), Rosati (1963), Walker et al. (1960), Rothstein et al. (1962), Judah et al. (1961), LeVay (1960), Glick and Margolis (1962), Kutin (1961), and Cameron et al. (1962), Haward (1964), Vaillant (1964), Engelhardt (1964), Frogel

(1964), Gittelman (1964), with generally favorable results. Results were particularly noteworthy in chronic delirium, mania, melancholia, conceptual types of disorders, hypermotor activity, impeded affect and verbal communication, catatonia, and paranoia.

Chlorpromazine has proved useful in many so-called "psychosomatic" conditions or diseases complicated by stress such as arthritis, tuberculosis, severe tension headaches, gastrointestinal disorders, dermatological conditions, and asthmatic states (Lester et al., 1962; Wolf, 1962; Endicott and Gralnick, 1961).

Chlorpromazine has been widely used as an antiemetic, with often dramatic results in severe and refractory cases (Kent et al., 1954a,b; Krais, 1955). This subject has been widely reviewed (see Section IV) and will not be treated further.

Chlorpromazine has been found to be useful in acute or chronic alcoholism to control agitation, delirium tremens, nausea and vomiting, and to prepare the way for psychotherapy and social rehabilitation (Hoover, 1960). It has been used in the treatment of mental defectives (Robb, 1960; Swain and Litteral, 1960; Abse and Dahlstrom, 1960; Freed and Frignito, 1961). Chlorpromazine has also been used successfully to facilitate withdrawal from narcotics and other drugs (Frankau and Stanwell, 1960; Litin, 1964).

Chlorpromazine and other phenothiazines have been used as adjuvants to control apprehension, pain, and nausea and vomiting. They allow a reduction in the amounts of drugs ordinarily used in obstetrical management, thus reducing the risk of respiratory depression in mother and infant (De Senarclens, 1961; Rodgers et al., 1961). The incidence of vomiting was only 2% in contrast to usual incidence of 12–20%. It is of interest here that chlorpromazine has apparently never been implicated in a case of neonatal jaundice.

There has been some controversy as to whether chlorpromazine dosage induces false positives in the male-frog pregnancy test. This literature has been reviewed by Wert and Greenhill (1961) and it is of interest that no true pregnancies have remained undetected due to the presence of chlorpromazine. Instances of abnormal lactation in female psychiatric patients have been reported (Hooper et al., 1961).

Marks and Shackcloth (1963) reported that the use of recently developed immunological pregnancy tests may eliminate many of the false-positive results obtained in women taking phenothiazines.

Chlorpromazine and other phenothiazines have been used in surgery, as both a pre- and post-anesthetic medication, to control anxiety and apprehension, pain, and nausea and vomiting, and to reduce, by potentiation (see also pages 60–63), the amounts of narcotics, sedatives, and anesthetics needed (Lear et al., 1961; Veghelyi, 1962; Gowen and Lindemuth, 1961; Hoagland and Bishop, 1961; Russell, 1961; Hoffenberg et al., 1961; Soehring, 1956; Vroom et al., 1962; Sainz, 1964).

It is significant that chlorpromazine (and other phenothiazine tranquilizers) will not suppress withdrawal signs in morphine-addicted monkeys (McCarthy et al., 1958), or humans (Fraser and Isbell, 1956). Challenge with nalorphine in patients given chlorpromazine chronically will not precipitate abstinence (cf. Haden, 1964; Gallant et al., 1964). Finally, after prolonged administration of chlorpromazine in monkeys (McCarthy et al., 1960) and prochlorperazine in humans (Fraser and Isbell, 1959), no withdrawal signs were seen following abrupt withdrawal. Similarly, methotrimeprazine showed no ability to suppress morphine abstinence in man, nor to produce habituation in chronic administration (Fraser and Rosenberg, 1963) (cf. Simpson, 1965). Hence the phenothiazines do not produce drug dependence of the opiate type. Other experiments have shown that the phenothiazines do not produce dependence of the barbiturate type.

B. Use of Rating Scales or Psychometric Techniques

Inasmuch as the estimation of improvement in psychiatric patients is highly subjective, a number of objective techniques have been devised to assist in estimating drug effects (Follin et al., 1961; Loftus et al., 1961; Blackburn and Allen, 1961; Nodine, 1963). Among the measuring procedures employed are:

1. Psychomotor (Kornetsky et al., 1958, 1959a,b; Kornetsky and Humphries, 1958; Mead et al., 1958; Idestrom, 1960; Wright and Kyne, 1960; Klugman, 1960; Wentzel and Rutledge, 1962; Pearl, 1960; Clark et al., 1961; Shatin, 1956; Kornetsky and Orzack, 1964)
    Tapping Rate
    Purdue Pegboard
    Reaction Time
    Tracking Test
    Hand Grip

2. Behavior rating scales (Gardner et al., 1955; Abrams, 1958; Ware, 1955; Gaitz et al., 1955; Whitehead, 1956; Mefferd et al., 1958; Moss et al., 1958; Good et al., 1958; Pearl et al., 1958; Heilizer, 1959; Roebuck et al., 1959; Casey et al., 1960; Lasky et al., 1962; Levin, 1959; Mendelsohn et al., 1959; May et al., 1959; Shawver et al., 1962; Kurland et al., 1962; Gwynne et al., 1962; Caffey, 1961; Adelson and Epstein, 1962; Gorham and Overall, 1960; Toms, 1961; Hawkins et al., 1961; Vestre, 1961; McCourt et al., 1961; Davidson and Ades, 1961; Kurland et al., 1961a,b)
    Multidimensional Scale for Rating Psychiatric Patients (Lorr)
    Inpatient Multidimensional Psychiatric Scale (IMPS)
    Psychotic Reaction Profile (PRP)
    Wittenborn Psychiatric Rating Scale

3. Intelligence factors (Sternberg et al., 1957; Kovitz et al., 1955; Thorpe and Baker, 1958a,b; Bair and Herold, 1955; Petrie, 1956; Porteus, 1957; Mason-Browne, 1958; Judson and MacCasland, 1960; Bennett and Hamilton, 1961; Bennett and Kooi, 1961; Childers and Therrien, 1961; Gilgash, 1961)
   Wechsler Bellevue Intelligence Scale
   Wechsler Adult Intelligence Scale
   Raven Progressive Matrix
   Stanford-Binet
   Columbia Mental Maturity Scale
   Porteus Maze

4. Personality tests (Gibbs et al., 1956; Winter and Frederickson, 1956; Simon et al., 1958; Toms, 1961; Freed, 1956; Castner et al., 1958; Motz, 1955)
   Minnesota Multiphasic Personality Inventory
   Rorschach
   Thematic Apperception Test

5. Sensory methods (Rosner et al., 1955; Bennett and Kooi, 1961; Hoehn-Saric, 1964)
   Flicker Fusion
   Archimedes Spiral After-Image
   Auditory Flutter Fusion

6. Other techniques (Tourlentes, 1958; Thorpe and Baker, 1958a,b; Barry and Degelman, 1961; Hawkins et al., 1961; Tuason and Guze, 1961; Mirsky, 1959; Dews and Morse, 1958)
   Operant Conditioning
   Sociometric Ratings
   Standardized Interview with Inter-action Chronograph
   Continuous Performance
   Time Perception
   Memory

In addition, the various statistical techniques like the t-test (Loftus et al., 1961), the chi-square method, and cluster analysis from correlation matrix (Gorham and Overall, 1960) have been employed.

C. Pediatric Applications

Much of the pediatric use of chlorpromazine is comparable to its application in adults. Moffitt et al. (1961) used chlorpromazine as a preanesthetic medication for pediatric cardiac catherization and angiocardiography. The inconclusive use of chlorpromazine in difficult pediatric dental patients has been described by Harrison and Sawusch (1961). Its use in schizophrenia has been described by Delage (1960). Chlorpromazine has been used to enhance reading in retarded children, and to treat children with behavioral disorders (Stell, 1964). In over 400 children no harmful personality effects were observed with long-term therapy (Freed and Frignito, 1961; Roux, 1959).

Denhoff and Holden (1961) have used chlorpromazine in cerebral palsy with beneficial results, primarily in behavior, in over half the cases.

D. Vascular and Respiratory Effects

The hypotensive effects of chlorpromazine (usually orthostatic) are variable and they are insufficient to be useful in treating hypertension (Witton, 1961; Blumberg, 1964). Chlorpromazine has also been reported to cause an increase in cerebral circulation (Lechner et al., 1961), changes in blood pressure of the central retinal artery (Shminke, 1961), and changes in vascular permeability in acute glomerulonephritis, leading to beneficial results in pediatric patients (Malossi, 1962). Coppolino and Wallace (1960) treated excessive peripheral vasoconstriction, in the immediate postanesthetic period, with chlorpromazine with dramatic results. Symptoms of cyanosis and shivering were relieved in 52 patients without affecting pulse rate or respiration. Chlorpromazine has been used successfully in the treatment of shock (see page 95).

Lambertsen et al. (1961) found that chlorpromazine did not consistently depress respiration, but it tended to improve tolerance to elevated pCO_2. Chlorpromazine at 25 mg/70 kg i.m. tended to potentiate the respiratory depressant effects of meperidine.

E. Miscellaneous Effects

Mirsky and Cardon (1962) and Traugott (1961a,b) have studied the effects of chlorpromazine and sleep deprivation on EEG (see Section IV,B,5).

The anticonvulsant effects of chlorpromazine are reviewed in Section IV,B,6.

Weight changes produced by chlorpromazine have been reviewed by Caffey (1961), Klett and Caffey (1961), Gordon and Groth (1964), and Crisp and Roberts (1962).

The effects of chlorpromazine in tetanus have been studied by Wilkinson (1961), Gerster and Moeschlin (1961), Sinha (1961), Kochhar (1961), and Fairley (1963).

Studies of the effects of chlorpromazine in man in nontherapeutic applications have been reported by Simpson and Kline (1961), Dundas et al. (1961), Kalinovskaya (1961), Kulikov (1961), McDonald and Weise (1962), Bennett and Hamilton (1961), Laxdal et al. (1961), Kornetsky and Humphries (1958) and by DiMascio et al. (1963).

There have been many reports of the successful use of chlorpromazine in combination with other drugs. Often these combinations will lower the side effect incidence of the individual drugs and permit the administration of lower doses of each. Thus chlorpromazine has been combined with d-amphetamine (Caffey and Klett, 1961; Casey et al., 1961), with nialamide (Pennington, 1962), with isocarboxazid (Caffey and Klett, 1961; Casey et al., 1961), with imipramine (Pennington, 1962; Casey et al., 1961; Caffey and Klett, 1961), with prochlorperazine (Noble and Castner, 1962), with trifluoperazine (Caffey and Klett, 1961; Casey et al., 1961; Terrell, 1962; McNichol and Seale, 1964), with meprobamate (Pennington, 1962), with butyrylperazine (Bryk and Moldenhauer, 1962), and with chlordiazepoxide (Dye, 1961). Rohde and Sargant (1961) report that combination of chlorpromazine with insulin therapy and electroshock is useful for treating early schizophrenia and reducing the length of hospital stay.

Tranylcypromine has been combined with chlorpromazine, trifluoperazine, and other phenothiazines (Barsa and Saunders, 1962; Bennett and Hamilton, 1963; Schiele et al., 1961; Antony et al., 1961; Clout, 1962; Milligan, 1962).

F. Side Effects

1. Jaundice

In the more than 14 million patients who have been treated with chlorpromazine in the United States, the incidence of jaundice—regardless of indication, dosage, or mode of administration—has been low (less than 0.5%—Ayd, 1963). Few cases have occurred in less than 1 week or after 6 weeks. Jaundice due to phenothiazines is of the so-called "obstructive" type, is without parenchymal damage, and is usually promptly reversible upon the withdrawal of the drug. Because detailed liver function tests of chlorpromazine-induced jaundice give a picture which mimics extrahepatic obstruction, exploratory laparotomy should be withheld if possible until determination of hepatic function after withdrawal of chlorpromazine.

Some recent reports on chlorpromazine-induced jaundice have been published by Klatskin (1961), Spellberg (1961), Eliakim (1960), Slocum (1961), Read et al. (1961), Kohn and Myerson (1961), Waitzkin and MacMahon (1962), Huete-Armijo and Exton-Smith (1962), Chatagnon et al. (1961a,b), Becker (1962), Ruttner et al. (1962), in an anonymous letter (Anonymous, 1962), and in a Symposium (1961), also cf. Michaux (1961).

A number of observers have remarked (Hollister, 1959; Pollack, 1957; Feldman, 1957a,b; Ayd, 1963; Sargant, 1964; West, 1964) that the number of cases of chlorpromazine jaundice seen today are far fewer than were reported during the introduction of the drug in 1953-1954. A recent United States Public Health Service Report (Morbidity and Mortality, 1963) (Fig. 5) showed a large outbreak of viral hepatitis in 1954. The low incidence of jaundice attributed to chlorpromazine in the viral hepatitis outbreak of 1961–1962 may have been due to better methods of differential diagnosis

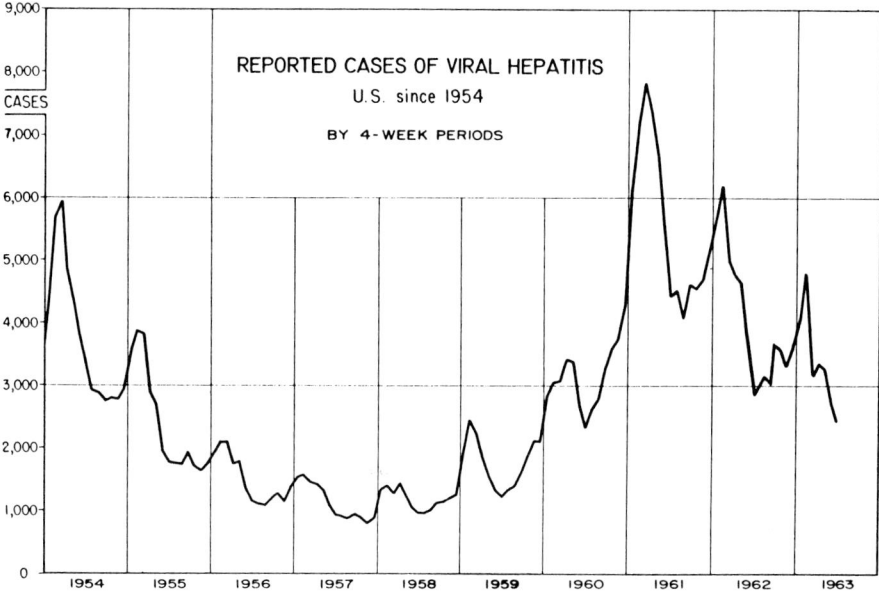

FIG. 5. Incidence of viral hepatitis in the United States 1953–1963.

(cf. Yakson, 1963; Wruble, 1966). By 1966 more than 25 million patients had been treated with chlorpromazine in the United States.

2. AGRANULOCYTOSIS

Agranulocytosis, although rare (one in 50,000–250,000 cases—Ayd, 1963), has been reported in patients on phenothiazine therapy (cf. Pisciotta et al., 1964; Pisciotta and Daly, 1960; Pisciotta and Kaldahl, 1962). Patients receiving chlorpromazine should be observed regularly and asked to report at once the sudden appearance of sore throat or other signs of infection. If white blood counts and differential smears give an indication of granulocytic depression, the drug should be discontinued, and antibiotic and other suitable therapy should be instituted. Because most reported cases have occurred between the fourth and tenth weeks of treatment, patients on prolonged therapy should be observed particularly during that period.

A moderate suppression of total white blood cells is sometimes observed in patients on chlorpromazine therapy. If not accompanied by other signs or symptoms, these occurrences do not necessarily require that chlorpromazine be discontinued, but the blood status of these patients should be followed carefully. Thus, it is advisable that routine blood counts be done on all patients receiving long-term chlorpromazine to detect the possible onset of agranulocytosis.

Some recent papers on chlorpromazine induced blood dyscrasias have been reported by Cuningham and Hannah (1960), Widmann and Eckle (1961), Carfagno and Magee (1961), Cares and Buckman (1961), Council on Drugs (1962), Erslev and Wintrobe (1962), Fau et al. (1962), Chatagnon and Chatagnon (1961), Karpovich (1962), Häfner and Kutscher (1964), Bacon (1964), Collins (1964), and Shelton et al. (1960).

3. Neuromuscular Reactions

With very large doses of chlorpromazine, as frequently used in psychiatric cases over long periods, there have been a few patients who have exhibited neuromuscular reactions (extrapyramidal symptoms) which closely resemble parkinsonism. Such symptoms are reversible and usually disappear within a short time after the dosage has been decreased or the drug withdrawn. These neuromuscular reactions can also be controlled by the concomitant administration of standard anti-parkinsonism agents (Burger, 1960).

Some reports on extrapyramidal symptoms have been published by Gowdey and Forster (1961), Hirsch and Hirsch (1961), Hollister (1961), Vates and Masucci (1960), Chicoine (1961), Cornman (1961), Blom and Ekbom (1961), Chatagnon et al. (1961a,b), Hunter et al. (1964a,b), and Mackiewicz and Gershon (1964). Anti-parkinson agents like triphenidyl have been used successfully to treat chlorpromazine-induced extrapyramidal symptoms (Mandel and Oliver, 1961). Ayd (1961) has pointed out that dystonic reactions are not a contraindication of phenothiazine therapy.

In rare instances some extrapyramidal symptoms have lasted months and even years, particularly in elderly patients with previous brain damage (Faurbye et al., 1964; Hunter et al., 1964a,b).

The possible role of heredity in drug-induced parkinsonism has been studied (Evans, 1963) and it has been suggested that further examination of the extrapyramidal side effects of phenothiazines, on a pharmacogenetic basis, be undertaken. In this connection, Fischer et al. (1965) have reported that a relation exists between the taste sensitivity of drugs in man and the appearance of phenothiazine-tranquilizer induced extrapyramidal symptoms.

4. Hypotensive Effect

Postural hypotension and simple tachycardia may be noted in some patients. In these patients, momentary fainting and some dizziness are characteristic and usually occur shortly after the first parenteral dose, occasionally after a subsequent parenteral dose—very rarely after the first oral dose. In most cases, prompt recovery is spontaneous and all symptoms disappear within ½ to 2 hours with no subsequent ill effects. Occasionally, however, this hypotensive effect may be more severe and prolonged, producing a shock-like condition. In consideration of possible hypotensive effects, the patient should be kept under observation (preferably lying down) for some time after the initial parenteral dose. If, on rare occasions, hypotension does occur, it can ordinarily be controlled by placing the patient in a recumbent position with head lowered and legs raised. If it is desirable to administer a vasoconstrictor, l-norepinephrine and phenylephrine are the most suitable. Other pressor agents, including epinephrine, are not recommended because phenothiazine derivatives may reverse the usual elevating action of these agents and cause a further lowering of blood pressure.

5. Dermatological Reactions

Dermatological reactions of a mild urticarial type (suggesting allergic origin) or photosensitivity may be seen. Patients should avoid undue exposure to sun. More severe reactions, including exfoliative dermatitis, have been reported occasionally from systemic use as well as from contact.

Drug sensitization and photosensitivity have been discussed by Hartman and Dickey (1964), Knox (1961), Somerville et al. (1960), Sams (1960), and Schreiber and Naylor (1962).

6. Miscellaneous Side Effects

Recently a few reports have been published on skin pigmentation and opacities of the cornea and lens in patients who had been treated with high doses of chlorpromazine for prolonged periods. The authors speculated that this skin pigmentation is due to melanin deposition (see Anonymous, 1964; Feldman and Frierson, 1964; Greiner and Berry, 1964; Greiner and Nicholson, 1964; Greiner et al., 1964; Hays et al., 1964; Perrot and Bourjala, 1962; Perry et al., 1964; Satanove, 1965; Sulman, 1964; Zelickson and Zeller, 1964; Ban, 1965; Ban and Lehman, 1965; Barsa et al., 1965a,b; Barsa and Saunders, 1965; Blois, 1965; Brill et al., 1965; Cairns et al., 1965; DeLong et al., 1965; Ellis, 1965; Greiner and Nicholson, 1965a,b; Hashimoto et al., 1965; Liljestrand, 1965; Margolis and Goble, 1965; Massey, 1965; Mathalone, 1965; Nicholson et al., 1966; Richards, 1965; Rives and Pellerat, 1965; Satanove, 1965; Saunders, 1959; Siddall, 1965; Tredici et al., 1965; Watt, 1966; Wetterholm et al., 1965; Zelickson, 1965; Reboton et al. (1962) found no retinopathy with chlorpromazine (cf. Ayd, 1966).

Moderate breast engorgement with lactation has been observed in some female patients receiving very large doses of chlorpromazine. However, this effect is transitory and disappears upon reduction of dosage or withdrawal of the drug. Amenorrhea may also be seen on chlorpromazine administration.

The phenothiazines are contraindicated in cases of organic phosphate poisoning, since they delay recovery of enzyme activity inhibited by organic phosphate.

In a few instances unexplained deaths have occurred with phenothiazine therapy and some evidence for intramyocardial lesions has been reported in the one or two cases a year seen in a 2000-bed neuropsychiatric hospital (Richardson et al., 1966).

G. Phenothiazine Overdosage

Hollister (1961) has stated that: "Successful suicide with phenothiazine derivatives is virtually unknown despite doses of 10–20 gm; among central nervous system depressants, these drugs are as suicide-proof as any might be." Summaries on this subject have been published by Algeri et al. (1959) and in an anonymous note (Anonymous, 1961). The last reference described 280 case of accidental poisoning with tranquilizers in the United States. The largest group consisted of 112 cases of overdosage with meprobamate or related compounds. The remaining cases were due almost equally to *Rauwolfia* alkaloids and phenothiazines, usually chlorpromazine. Nearly two-thirds of all cases were in children under 5 years, with toxic manifestations occurring in 45% of the 280 cases. Treatment consisted of removal of the offending substance, maintenance of pulmonary ventilation, and administration of CNS stimulants. Exchange transfusions may be useful in cases of chlorpromazine overdosage in children, following the other measures listed previously (Gordon and McCandless, 1959; McDonald, 1962; Chicoine, 1961; Epps and Scott, 1961; Cann and Verhulst, 1960; Goldsmith, 1959; Cain and Malcolm, 1960; Carter, 1959; Freed and Frignito, 1961; Waugh and Metts, 1960; De Gennes and Bricaire, 1957; Denham, 1958; Scime and Tallant, 1959; Bucher, 1959; Gailitis et al., 1960; Ayd, 1959, 1960, 1961; Broussolle et al., 1957; King and Weinberger, 1959; Wilcox, 1958; Wetterholm et al., 1959; Jacobziner and Raybin, 1958, 1960, 1962; Massonnat and Arroyo, 1958; Shaw et al., 1959; Mahrer et al., 1958; Nelson, 1959; Plummer et al., 1960; Sobel, 1960a,b; Smith and Denner, 1962; Griffin, 1962; Freyhan, 1958; Sherman et al., 1960; Bordeleau and Gratton, 1958; Fanning, 1961; Walker, 1959; Reznikoff, 1960; Robinson, 1960; Shafer et al., 1962; Childers, 1962a,b; Tedeschi et al., 1961a,b; Kline et al., 1956; Mauceri and Strauss, 1956; Denber, 1957; Sacks, 1957; Brill and Patton, 1959; Sainz, 1956; Hodge, 1959; Brooks, 1956; Rajapurkar and Panjwani, 1960; Paulson, 1960).

In spite of the fairly large number of cases of intentional and accidental overdosage of chlorpromazine in the literature, there are only one or two authenticated reports of death resulting from overdosage in each category (Hagerty, 1957; Algeri et al., 1959; Denber, 1957). Reports on chlorpromazine overdosage have been published by Algeri et al. (1959), Hagerty (1957),

Fontan (1955), Henne and Henne (1956), Beal (1955), Tofte (1957), Langeron et al. (1956), Aubertin et al. (1954a,b) Graux et al. (1956), Haarstad (1957), Hopkin (1955), Rainaut (1956), Ferguson (1957), Dotevall (1957), Spratt and Dean (1957), Winkelman (1954), Vallat (1954), Sinha and Mitra (1955), Kline et al. (1956), Mauceri and Strauss (1956), Samuels (1957), Douglas and Bates (1957), Denber (1957), Sacks (1957), Brill and Patton (1959), Ollendorff (1960), Master (1964), Anonymous (1964), and by Hollister (1961) (cf. Hollister, 1965).

The treatment of phenothiazine overdosage by dialysis has been reported recently by McGinn and Avram (1966).

Reports on suicidal attempts with trifluoperazine (Barker and Kerr, 1960; Vates and Masucci, 1960), prochlorperazine (McDonald, 1962), and thioridazine (Enticknap and Gordon, 1961; Guerin, 1960) have been published.

H. Veterinary Use

Chlorpromazine has found wide use as a tranquilizer and antiemetic in animals, especially dogs (Estrada, 1956). The use of chlorpromazine in the dog was reviewed by Macko et al. (1958). It has also been used for preanesthetic medication, as a treatment for heat stroke, in shock, tetanus, colic, and as a local anesthetic (Troughton et al., 1955; Schmiterlöw and Tufvesson, 1956). Studies in the horse have been published by Hall (1960) and by Alexander (1960).

References

Abernathy, R. S., and Halberg, F. (1955). *J. Lab. Clin. Med.* **46**, 790.
Abernathy, R. S., and Spink, W. W. (1957). *Proc. Soc. Exptl. Biol. Med.* **95**, 580.
Abernathy, R. S., Halberg, F., and Spink, W. W. (1957). *J. Lab. Clin. Med.* **49**, 708.
Abood, L. G. (1955). *Proc. Soc. Exptl. Biol. Med.* **88**, 688.
Abrams, J. (1958). *Diseases Nervous System* **19**, 20.
Abse, D. W., and Dahlstrom, W. G. (1960). *J. Am. Med. Assoc.* **174**, 2036.
Aceto, M. D., Lynch, V. D., and Thoms, R. K. (1961). *J. Pharm. Sci.* **50**, 823.
Adam, H. M., and Hye, H. K. A. (1964). *J. Physiol.* **171**, 37P.
Adelson, D., and Epstein, E. J. (1962). *J. Nervous Mental Disease* **134**, 543.
Ader, R., and Clink, D. W. (1957). *J. Pharmacol. Exptl. Therap.* **121**, 144.
Adriani, J., and Kerr, M. (1955). *Southern Med. J.* **48**, 858.
Aganyants, E. K. (1960). *Zh. Vyshei. Nervnoi Deyatel'nosti im J.P. Pavlova* **10**, 842.
Aghajanian, G. (1963). *Biochem. Pharmacol.* **12**, 7.
Ahrens, A., and Witzleb, E. (1955). *Arch. Intern. Pharmacodyn.* **104**, 42.
Ainslie, J. D. (1961). *J. Florida Med. Assoc.* **47**, 901.
Albaum, H. G., and Milch, L. J. (1962). *Ann. N.Y. Acad. Sci.* **96**, 190.
Alexander, F. (1960). *Res. Vet. Sci.* **1**, 355.
Alexander, F., Mackie, A., Ghatge, N., and Waddell, A. W. (1958). *Arch. Intern. Pharmacodyn.* **113**, 254.
Alexander, L., and Horner, S. R. (1961). *J. Neuropsychiat.* **2**, 246.
Algeri, E. J., Katsas, G. G., and McBay, A. J. (1959). *J. Forensic Sci.* **4**, 111.

Allgén, L. G. (1959). *Proc. 7th Scand. Congr. of Clin. Chem. & Clin. Physiol.*, 1959.
Allgén, L. G. (1962). *International Conference on Action Mechanism and Metabolism of Psychoactive Drugs Derived from Phenothiazine and Related Compounds, Paris, Sept.* 7–8; (1962). *Psychopharmacol. Serv. Center Bull.* **2**, 29.
Allgén, L. G., Jönsson, B., Rappe, A., and Dahlbom, R. (1959). *Experientia* **15**, 318.
Allgén, L. G., Ekman, L., Reio, L., and Ullberg, S. (1960). *Arch. Intern. Pharmacodyn.* **126**, 1.
Alloiteau, J. J. (1957). *Compt. Rend. Soc. Biol.* **151**, 207.
Altman, J., Wakim, K. G., and Winkelmann, R. K. (1962). *J. Invest. Dermatol.* **38**, 215.
Altschule, M. D. (1960). *J. Neuropsychiat.* **2**, 102.
Altschule, M. D., Bower, W., and Cook, L. (1955). *Am. Practitioner Dig. Treat.* **6**, 90.
Andén, N. E. (1964). *Life Sci.* **3**, 149.
Anderson, E. L., Bellinzona, G. B., Craig, P. N., Jaffe, G. E., Janeway, K. P., Kaiser, C., Lester, B. M., Nikawitz, E. J., Pavloff, A. M., Reiff, H. E., and Zirkle, C. L. (1962). *Arzneimittel-Forsch.* **12**, 397.
Andrejew, A., and Rosenberg, A. J. (1956). *Compt. Rend. Soc. Biol.* **150**, 639.
Andrejew, A., and Rosenberg, A. J. (1958). *Compt. Rend. Soc. Biol.* **152**, 1366.
Andrejew, A., Ducet, G., Louw, J., and Rosenberg, A. J. (1956a). *Compt. Rend. Soc. Biol.* **150**, 484.
Andrejew, A., Ducet, G., Louw, J., and Rosenberg, A. J. (1956b). *Compt. Rend. Soc. Biol.* **150**, 509.
Anokhina-Itskova, I. P. (1961). *Sechenov Physiol. J. USSR (English Transl.)* **47**, 170.
Anonymous (1961). *Lancet* **I**, 270.
Anonymous (1962). *Lancet* **I**, 1056.
Anonymous (1964). *Mind* **2**, 165.
Anonymous (1964). *Presse Med.* **72**, 2116.
Ansell, G. B., and Dohmen, H. (1957). *Biochem. J.* **65**, 1P.
Antony, G. S., *et al.* (1961). *Med. Observer* **2**, 255.
Archdeacon, J. W., and Giles, J. K. (1956). *Am. J. Physiol.* **186**, 60.
Archer, J. D. (1954). *Federation Proc.* **13**, 332.
Ariens, E. J., and Simonis, A. M. (1964). *J. Pharm. Pharmacol.* **16**, 137.
Arnold, E. T. (1955). *Med. Times* **83**, 707.
Arnold, O. H., Solms, W., and Hift, S. (1952). *Wien Med. Wochschr.* **48**, 964.
Aron, E. (1954). *Anesthesie Analgesie* **11**, 399.
Aron, E., Chambon, Y., and Voisin, A. (1953). *Bull. Acad. Natl. Med. (Paris)* **137**, 417.
Aron, E., Nezelof, C., and Guesle, J. (1954). *Arch. Maladies App. Digest Maladies Nutr.* **43**, 496.
Aronsen, K. F., Bergh, N. P., and Haeger, K. (1957). *Acta Pharmacol. Toxicol.* **13**, 30.
Arora, R. B., and Das, P. K. (1956). *Arch. Intern. Pharmacodyn.* **107**, 202.
Árvay, A., Lampé, L., Kertész, L., and Medveczky, L. (1960). *Acta Endocrinol.* **35**, 469.
Ashby, W., Bushrod, M. A., and Schuster, E. M. (1957). *Diseases Nervous System* **18**, 226.
Ashcroft, G. W., MacDougall, E. J., and Barker, P. A. (1961). *J. Mental Sci.* **107**, 287.
Aston, R., and Cullumbine, H. (1960). *Arch. Intern. Pharmacodyn.* **126**, 219.
Aston, R., Sekino, E., and Greifenstein, F. E. (1962). *Toxicol. Appl. Pharmacol.* **4**, 393.
Aubertin, E., Martin-Dupont, C., and Tavernier, J. (1954a). *Presse Med.* **62**, 752.
Aubertin, E., Martin-Dupont, C., and Tavernier, J. (1954b). *Semaine Hop. Paris* **30**, 2307.
Axelrod, J., Brady, R. O., Witkop, B., and Evarts, E. V. (1956). *Nature* **178**, 143.
Axelrod, J., Hertting, G., and Patrick, R. W. (1961a). *J. Pharmacol. Exptl. Therap.* **134**, 325.
Axelrod, J., Whitby, L. G., Hertting, G., and Kopin, I. L. (1961b). *Circulation Res.* **9**, 715.
Axelrod, J., Whitby, L. G., and Hertting, G. (1961c). *Science* **133**, 383.
Axelrod, J., Hertting, G., and Potter, L. (1962). *Nature* **194**, 297.
Ayd, F. J., Jr. (1959). *Clin. Med.* **6**, 387.
Ayd, F. J., Jr. (1960). *Psychosomatics* **1**, 143.
Ayd, F. J., Jr. (1961). *J. Am. Med. Assoc.* **175**, 1054.

Ayd, F. J., Jr. (1963) *J. Am. Med. Ascso.* **184**, 51.
Ayd, F. J., Jr. (1964). *J. Am. Med. Assoc.* **184**, 51.
Ayd, F. J., Jr. (1966). *International Drug Therapy Newsltr.* **1**, 1.
Azima, H., and Richman, A. (1956). *A.M.A. Arch. Neurol. Psychiat.* **75**, 163.
Bacon, H. M. (1964). *Am. J. Psychiat.* **120**, 915.
Bain, W. A., and Doughty, R. B. (1963). *Practitioner* **190**, 129.
Bair, H. V., and Herold, W. (1955). *A.M.A. Arch. Neurol. Psychiat.* **74**, 363.
Baker, W. W., Szeely, E. G., and Spiegel, E. A. (1956). *Federation Proc.* **15**, 397.
Balestrieri, A., and Fadiga, E. (1954). *Boll. Soc. Ital. Biol. Sper.* **30**, 1241.
Baltzly, R., Harfenist, M., and Webb, F. J. (1946). *J. Am. Chem. Soc.* **68**, 2673.
Ban, T. A. (1965). *Union Med. Canada* **94**, 305.
Ban, T. A. and Lehman, H. E. (1965). *Can. Psychiat. Assoc. J.* **10**, 112.
Bangham, A. D., Rees, K. R., and Shotlander, V. (1962). *Nature* **193**, 754.
Barker, J. C., and Kerr, E. M. (1960). *Lancet* **II**, 1304.
Barkov, N. K. (1961). *Byul. Eksperim. Biol. i Med.* **51**, 60.
Barraclough, C. A., and Sawyer, C. H. (1957). *Endocrinology* **61**, 341.
Barraclough, C. A., and Sawyer, C. H. (1959). *Endocrinology* **65**, 563.
Barry, H., and Miller, N. E. (1962). *J. Comp. Physiol. Psychol.* **55**, 201.
Barry, H., Wagner, S. A., and Miller, N. E. (1963). *Psychol. Rept.* **12**, 215.
Barry, J. J., Jr., and Degelman, J. (1961). *J. Exptl. Anal. Behavior* **4**, 85.
Barsa, J. A., and Saunders, J. C. (1962). *Am. J. Psychiat.* **118**, 933.
Barsa, J. A., Newton, J. C., and Saunders, J. C. (1965a). *Am. J. Psychiat.* **122**, 331.
Barsa, J. A., Newton, J. C., and Saunders, J. C. (1965b). *J. Am. Med. Assoc.* **193**, 10.
Barsa, J. A., and Saunders, J. C. (1965). *Psychopharmacologia*, **7**, 138.
Bartholini, G., Pletscher, A., and Gey, K. F. (1961). *Experientia* **17**, 541.
Bartlett, R. G., and Register, U. D. (1955). *Proc. Soc. Exptl. Biol. Med.* **90**, 500.
Baruk, H., Launay, J., and Berges, J. (1955a). *Ann. Med.-Psychol.* **113**, 439.
Baruk, H., Launay, J., and Berges, J. (1955b). *Ann. Med.-Psychol.* **113**, 705.
Basmajian, J. V., and Szatmari, A. (1955). *Neurology* **5**, 856.
Basu, S. N. (1956). *J. Indian Med. Assoc.* **26**, 269.
Beal, J. A. (1955). *Brit. Med. J.* **II**, 1620.
Bean, J. W. (1956). *Am. J. Physiol.* **187**, 389.
Bean, J. W., and Wagemaker, H. (1960). *Am. J. Physiol.* **198**, 341.
Beck, L. V., and Redick, T. F. (1956). *Proc. Soc. Exptl. Biol. Med.* **92**, 851.
Becker, K. L. (1962). *Am. J. Med. Sci.* **243**, 222.
Beckett, A. H. (1964). *J. Pharm. Pharmacol.* **16**, 500.
Beckett, A. H., and Casy, A. F. (1957). *Bull. Narcotics, U.N. Dept. Social Affairs* **9**, 37.
Beckett, A. H., and Curry, S. H. (1963). *J. Pharm. Pharmacol.* **15-S**, 246T.
Beckett, A. H., Beaven, M. A., and Robinson, A. E. (1962). *International Conference on Action Mechanism and Metabolism of Psychoactive Drugs Derived from Phenothiazine and Structurally Related Compounds, Paris, Sept.* 7–8.
Beckett, A. H., Beaven, M. A., and Robinson, A. E. (1963). *Biochem. Pharmacol.* **12**, 779.
Beeler, E. C. (1942). *Bull. Natl. Formulary Comm.* **10**, 84.
Behn, W., Frahm, M., and Fretwurst, E. (1956). *Klin. Wochschr.* **34**, 872.
Belkin, M., and Hardy, W. G. (1957). *Science* **125**, 233.
Benaron, H. B. W. (1955). *Am. J. Obstet. Gynecol.* **69**, 776.
Benditt, E. P., and Rowley, D. A. (1956). *Science* **123**, 24.
Benfey, B. G., and Greeff, K. (1961). *Brit. J. Pharmacol.* **17**, 232.
Bennett, G. M. (1953). *J. Chem. Soc.* 4192.
Bennett, J. L., and Hamilton, L. D. (1961). *J. Neuropsychiat.* **3**, 118.
Bennett, J. L., and Hamilton L. D. (1963). *Psychiat. Quart.* **37**, 53.
Bennett, J. L., and Kooi, K. A. (1961). *Arch. Gen. Psychiat.* **4**, 413.

Benson, G. K. (1960). *Proc. Soc. Exptl. Biol. Med.* **103**, 132.
Bensoussan, P. A., and Klein, F. (1953). *Ann. Med.-Psychol.* **111**, 529.
Bente, D., and Itil, T. (1954). *Arzneimittel-Forsch.* **4**, 418.
Berg, S. S., and Nicholson, J. (1952). U.S. Patent 2,606,773.
Berger, M. (1957). *J. Neurochem.* **2**, 30.
Berger, M., Strecker, H. J., and Waelsch, H. (1956). *Nature* **177**, 1234.
Bergmann, F., and Gutman, J. (1962). *International Conference on Action Mechanism and Metabolism of Psychoactive Drugs Derived from Phenothiazine and Structurally Related Compounds, Paris, Sept.* 7–8.
Bernheim, M. L. C. (1959). *Proc. Soc. Exptl. Biol. Med.* **102**, 660.
Bernsohn, J., Namajuska, I., and Cochrane, L. S. G. (1955). *Federation Proc.* **14**, 182.
Bernsohn, J., Namajuska, I., and Boshes, B. (1956a). *J. Neurochem.* **1**, 145.
Bernsohn, J., Namajuska, I., and Cochrane, L. S. G. (1956b). *Arch. Biochem. Biophys.* **62**, 274.
Bernsohn, J., Gylys, I., and Boshes, B. (1958). *J. Neurochem.* **2**, 312.
Bernthsen, A. (1883). *Ber. Deut. Chem. Ges.* **16**, 2896.
Berti, T. (1954a). *Arch. Ital. Sci. Farmacol.* **4**, 272.
Berti, T. (1954b). *Farmaco (Pavia) Ed. Sci.* **9**, 374.
Berti, T. (1961). *Gior. Mal. Infettive Parassit.* **13**, 326.
Berti, T., and Cima, L. (1954a). *Arch. Intern. Pharmacodyn.* **98**, 452.
Berti, T., and Cima, L. (1954b). *Arch. Ital. Sci. Farmacol.* **4**, 273.
Berti, T., and Cima, L. (1954c). *Boll. Soc. Ital. Biol. Sper.* **30**, 100.
Berti, T., and Cima, L. (1955). *Arch. Intern. Pharmacodyn.* **100**, 373.
Berti, T., and Cima, L. (1956). *Farmaco (Pavia) Ed. Sci.* **11**, 451.
Berti, T., and Cima, L. (1957). *Farmaco (Pavia) Ed. Sci.* **12**, 159.
Berti, T., and Cima, L. (1962). *International Conference on Action Mechanism and Metabolism of Psychoactive Drugs Derived from Phenothiazines and Structurally Related Compounds, Paris, Sept.* 7–8.
Bertrand, I., Quivy, D., and Gayet-Hallion, T. (1954). *Compt. Rend. Soc. Biol.* **148**, 1170.
Besse, J. H., and Patay, R. (1953). *Compt. Rend. Soc. Biol.* **147**, 1721.
Besson, S., and Leder, M. (1955). *Bull. Soc. Pharm. Nancy* No. 25.
Bhargava, K. P., and Chandra, O. (1963). *Brit. J. Pharmacol.* **21**, 436.
Bhargava, K. P., and Chandra, O. (1964). *Brit. J. Pharmacol.* **22**, 154.
Bhargava, K. P., and Jaitly, K. D. (1964). *Brit. J. Pharmacol.* **22**, 162.
Bhose, L. (1964). *Am. J. Obstet. Gynecol.* **89**, 898.
Bianchi, R. G., and Craig, R. L. (1960). *Am. J. Digest. Diseases* **5**, 419.
Bianco, M., Belloni, F., and Verga, G. (1955). *Minerva Anestesiol.* **21**, 91.
Billon, J. P., Cauquis, G., and Combrisson, J. (1961). *Compt. Rend.* **253**, 1593.
Binet, P., and Decaud, J. (1954). *Compt. Rend. Soc. Biol.* **148**, 1557.
Blackburn, H. L., and Allen, J. L. (1961). *J. Nervous Mental Disease* **133**, 303.
Blacker, K. H., Weinstein, B. J., and Ellman, G. L. (1962). *Am. J. Psychiat.* **119**, 178.
Blazek, J. (1956). *Cesk. Farm.* **5**, 210.
Blazek, J. (1963a). *Pharmazie* **18**, 85.
Blazek, J. (1963b). *Pharmazie* **18**, 391.
Blazek, J., and Stejskal, Z. (1955). *Cesk. Farm.* No. 5. cf. Negwer, 1961.
Blazek, J., and Stejskal, Z. (1956). *Pharmazie* **11**, 27.
Blazek, J., Spinkova, V., and Stejskal, Z. (1962). *Pharmazie* **17**, 497.
Bloch, M., Bloom, H. J., Penman, J., and Walsh, L. (1961). *Lancet* **II**, 906.
Block, W. (1961). *Arzneimittel-Forsch.* **11**, 266.
Blois, M. S. (1965). *J. Invest. Dermatol.* **45**, 475.
Blom, S., and Ekbom, K. A. (1961). *Acta Med. Scand.* **170**, 689.
Bloomfield, S. (1964). *Can. Med. Assoc. J.* **90**, 1156.
Blough, D. S. (1958). *Science* **127**, 586.

Blumberg, A. G. (1964). *J. Psychiat. Res.* **2**, 51.
Blumberg, H., and Dayton, H. B. (1959). *Proc. Soc. Exptl. Biol. Med.* **101**, 594.
Boeles, J. T. F., and Blok, J. (1956). *Arch. Intern. Pharmacodyn.* **106**, 381.
Boer, G. E. (1955). *Acta Paediat. Latina* **89**, 37.
Bogdansky, D. F., Sulser, F., and Brodie, B. B. (1961). *J. Pharmacol. Exptl. Therap.* **132**, 176.
Boissier, J. R., Tardy, J., and Diverres, J. C. (1960). *Med. Exptl.* **3**, 81.
Bonafede, V. I. (1955). *A.M.A. Arch Neurol. Psychiat.* **72**, 158.
Bonomolo, A., and Mariani, E. (1955). *Riv. Neurol.* **25**, 824.
Bonvicino, G. E., Yogodzinski, L. H., and Hardy, R. A., Jr. (1962). *J. Org. Chem.* **27**, 4272.
Bordeleau, J. M., and Gratton, L. (1958). *Union Med. Canada* **87**, 1552.
Borg, D. C., and Cotzias, G. C. (1962a). *Proc. Natl. Acad. Sci. U.S.* **48**, 617.
Borg, D. C., and Cotzias, G. C. (1962b). *Proc. Natl. Acad. Sci. U.S.* **48**, 623.
Borg, D. C., and Cotzias, G. C. (1962c). *Proc. Natl. Acad. Sci. U.S.* **48**, 643.
Boriani, A. (1955). *Riv. Neurol.* **25**, 67.
Borison, H. L., Bayer, K. F., and Clawson, J. (1955). *J. Pharmacol. Exptl. Therap.* **113**, 6a.
Bornmann, G. (1961). *Arzneimittel-Forsch.* **11**, 89.
Bortnick, T. L., and Kalandarishvili, A. S. (1963). *Zh. Nevropatol. i Psikhiatr.* **63**, 263.
Bose, B. C., Vijayvargiya, R., and Saifi, A. Q. (1959). *Indian J. Med. Res.* **47**, 1.
Boulton, T. B. (1955). *Anaesthesia* **10**, 233.
Bourgeois-Gavardin, M., Nowill, W. K., Margolis, G., and Stephen, C. R. (1955). *Anesthesiology* **16**, 829.
Bourgeois-Gavardin, M., Fabian, L. W., and Stephen, C. R. (1957). *Anesthesia Analgesia, Current Res.* **36**, No. 1, 50.
Bousquet, W. F. (1962). *J. Pharm. Sci.* **51**, 297.
Bowes, H. A., and Natarajan, R. (1963). *Psychosomatics* **4**, 22.
Boyd, E. M., Boyd, C. E., and Cassell, W. A. (1954). *Can. Med. Assoc. J.* **70**, 276.
Boyd, E. M., and Miller, J. K. (1954). *Federation Proc.* **13**, 338.
Boyd, E. M., Cassell, W. A., Boyd, C. E., and Miller, J. K. (1955). *J. Pharmacol. Exptl. Therap.* **113**, 299.
Boyd, E. S., Hutchinson, E. D., Gardner, L. C., and Meritt, D. A. (1963). *Arch. Intern. Pharmacodyn* **144**, 533.
Braceland, F. J. (1964). *Postgrad. Med.* **35**, 237.
Bradley, P. B., and Hance, A. J. (1955). *J. Physiol. (London)* **129**, 50P.
Bradley, P. B., and Hance, A. J. (1956). *Electroencephalog. Clin. Neurophysiol.* **8**, 700.
Bradley, P. B., and Hance, A. J. (1957). *Electroencephalog. Clin. Neurophysiol.* **9**, 191.
Bradley, P. B., and Key, B. J. (1958). *Electroencephalog. Clin. Neurophysiol.* **10**, 97.
Bradshaw, A. K., Fraser, R. S., and McIntyre, J. W. R. (1958). *Can. Anaesthesiol. Soc. J.* **5**, 337.
Brand, E. D., Harris, T. D., Borison, H. L., and Goodman, L. S. (1954). *J. Pharmacol. Exptl. Therap.* **110**, 860.
Brena, S., and Marocco, F. (1953). *Minerva Anestesiol.* **19**, 334.
Brendel, W., and L'Allemand, H. (1955). *Arch. Exptl. Pathol. Pharmakol.* **225**, 87.
Breuninger, H., and Schmid, W. (1955). *Arch. Exptl. Pathol. Pharmakol.* **225**, 251.
Brewer, W. R., Picchioni, A. L., and Chin, L. (1959). *Ariz. Med.* **16**, 646.
Brignon, J. J. (1955a). *Bull. Soc. Pharm. Nancy* **24**, 13.
Brignon, J. J. (1955b). *Bull. Soc. Pharm. Nancy* **25**, 17.
Brill, H. and Patton, R. E. (1959). *Am. J. Psychiat.* **116**, 495.
Brill, H., Scheie, H. G., and DeLong, S. L. (1965). *Am. J. Psychiat.* **122**, 326.
Brillhart, J. R. (1959). *Obstet. Gynecol.* **14**, 581.
Brodie, B. B. (1955). *J. Am. Med. Assoc.* **159**, 1146.
Brodie, B. B., Shore, P. A., and Silver, S. L. (1955). *Nature* **175**, 1133.
Brodie, B. B., Gillette, J. R., and La Du, N. (1958). *Ann. Rev. Biochem.* **27**, 427.

Brooks, G. W. (1956). *New Engl. J. Med.* **254**, 1119.
Broussolle, P., Perrin, J., Maurel, H., Lambert, P., and Berthier, C. (1957). *Presse Med.* **65**, 1628.
Brown, B. B. (1960). *Arch. Intern. Pharmacodyn.* **128**, 391.
Brown, W. L., Elam, C. B., and Wortz, E. C. (1957). *J. Psychol.* **43**, 101.
Browne, A. D. H., and Mannion, P. L. (1955). *Irish J. Med. Sci.* **6**, 117.
Bruecke, F. T. (1956). *Proc. Intern. Physiol. Congr. Brussels*, 1956 p. 20.
Brunaud, M., Brunaud, S., and Lecourt, P. (1953). *Compt. Rend. Soc. Biol.* **147**. 1764.
Bruscha, W. (1954). *Klin. Wochschr.* **32**, 805.
Bryk, B., and Moldenhauer, B. (1962). *Med. Welt* No. 25, 1426.
Bubnoff, M. V., Hoffman, D., and Schmid, E. (1955). *Arch. Exptl. Pathol. Pharmakol.* **224**, 443.
Bucher, W. H. (1959). *Bull. Los Angeles Children's Hosp.* **6**, 77.
Budde, H., and Witzleb, E. (1955). *Arch. Intern. Pharmacodyn.* **102**, 126.
Budinsky, J., and Votava, Z. (1960). *Acta Biol. Med. Ger.* **4**, 35.
Buisson, P. J. C., Gailliot, P., and Gaudechon, J. (1956). U.S. Patent 2,769,002.
Bulle, P. H. (1957a). *Proc. Soc. Exptl. Biol. Med.* **94**, 553.
Bulle, P. H. (1957b). *Science* **126**, 24.
Burbridge, T. N., Tipton, D., Sutherland, V. C., and Simon, A. (1958). *Federation Proc.* **17**, 355.
Burger, A. (1960). "Medicinal Chemistry," 2nd Ed. p. 505, Wiley (Interscience), New York.
Burke, J. C., Piala, J., and Yale, H. (1956). *Meeting Soc. Pharmacol. Exptl. Therap.* 1956, French Lick, Indiana.
Burke, J. C., High, J., Laffan, R., and Ravaris, C. L. (1962). *Federation Proc.* **21**, 339.
Burkman, A. M. (1961a). *J. Pharm. Sci.* **50**, 156.
Burkman, A. M. (1961b). *J. Pharm. Sci.* **50**, 771.
Burkman, A. M. (1962a). *Arch. Intern. Pharmacodyn.* **37**, 396.
Burkman, A. M. (1962b). *Arch. Intern. Pharmacodyn.* **37**, 404.
Burns, J. H. (1954). *Proc. Roy. Soc. Med.* **47**, 617.
Burton, R. M., and Salvador, R. (1962). *Ann. N.Y. Acad. Sci.* **96**, 353.
Burton, R. M., Kaplan, N. O., Goldin, A., Leitenberg, M., and Humphreys, S. R. (1960a). *Arch. Intern. Pharmacodyn.* **128**, 260.
Burton, R. M., Salvador, R. A., Goldin, A., and Humphreys, S. R. (1960b). *Arch. Intern. Pharmacodyn.* **128**, 253.
Burton, R. M., Salvador, R., Smith K., and Howard, R. E. (1962). *Ann. N.Y. Acad. Sci.* **96**, 185.
Busse, W., and Loennecken, S. J. (1953). *Arch. Exptl. Pathol. Pharmakol.* **22C**, 232.
Buzard, J. A. (1960). *Experientia* **16**, 153.
Caffey, E. M., Jr. (1961). *Am. J. Psychiat.* **117**, 713.
Caffey, E. M., Jr., and Klett, C. J. (1961). *Diseases Nervous System* **22**, 370.
Cahen, R. L. (1964). *Proc. Soc. Exptl. Biol. Med.* **116**, 402.
Cain, H. D., and Malcolm, M. (1960). *Calif. Med.* **93**, 24.
Cairns, R. J., Capoore, H. S., and Gregory, I. D. R. (1965). *Lancet* **1**, 239.
Calo, A., Mariani, A., and Mariani Marelli, O. (1956). *Svensk Farm. Tidskr.* **35**, 842.
Calo, A., Mariani, A., and Mariani Marelli, O. (1958). *Pharm. Acta Helv.* **33**, 126.
Camanni, F., Molinatti, G. M., and Olivetti, M. (1959). *Nature* **184**, 65.
Camba, R. (1955). *Rass. Med. Sarda* **9**, 1.
Cameron, D. E., Lohrenz, J. G., and Handcock, K. A. (1962). *Comprehensive Psychiat.* **3**, 65.
Campbell, F. L., Sullivan, W. N., Smith, L. E., and Haller, H. L. (1934). *J. Econ. Entomol.* **27**, 1176.
Cann, H. M., and Verhulst, H. L. (1960). *New Engl. J. Med.* **263**, 719.
Cares, R. M., and Buckman, C. (1961). *Diseases Nervous System* **22**, 97.
Carfagno, S. C., and Magee, J. T. (1961). *Am. J. Med. Sci.* **241**, 44.
Carneiro, J., and Cardoso, A. C. S. Q. (1962). *Experientia* **18**, 220.
Carr, C. J. (1962). *Ann. N.Y. Acad. Sci.* **96**, 170.

Carr, C. J. (1963). *J. New Drugs* **3**, 135.
Carreras, M., and Angeleri, F. (1957). *Intern. Record Med.* **170**, 67.
Carruthers, G. F., and Gowdey, C. W. (1956). *Can. J. Biochem. Physiol.* **34**, 217.
Carson, R. P., and Domino, E. F. (1962). *Anesthesiology* **23**, 187.
Carter, C. B., and David, N. A. (1960). *Toxicol. Appl. Pharmacol.* **2**, 564.
Carter, C. H. (1959). *Southern Med. J.* **52**, 174.
Carver, M. J. (1963). *Biochem. Pharmacol.* **12**, 19.
Casey, J. F., Bennett, I. F., Lindley, C. L., Hollister, L. E., Gordon, M. H., and Springer, N. N. (1960). *A.M.A. Arch. Gen. Psychiat.* **2**, 210.
Casey, J. F., Hollister, L. E., Klett, C. J., Lasky, J. J. and Caffey, E. M., Jr. (1961). *Am. J. Psychiat.* **117**, 997.
Castaigne, A. (1954). *Semaine Hop. Paris* **30**, 321.
Castner, C. W., Covington, C. M., and Nichols, J. E. (1958). *Texas Rept. Biol. Med.* **16**, 21.
Cathala, H. P., and Pocidalo, J. J. (1952). *Compt. Rend. Soc. Biol.* **146**, 1709.
Caussade, L., Neimann, N., Stehlin, S., and Pierson, M. (1954). *Rev. Med. Nancy* No. 2, 1.
Cavanaugh, D. J. (1957). *Science* **125**, 1040.
Cavanaugh, D. J., and Ervin, F. R. (1957). *Am. J. Psychiat.* **114**, 171.
Cavatorta, L. (1959). *J. Pharm. Pharmacol.* **11**, 49.
Cavicchi Sandri, G. (1955). *Farmaco (Pavia) Ed. Sci.* **10**, 444.
Celice, J., Forcher, P., and Plas, F. (1955). *Therapie* **10**, 30.
Century, B., and Horwitt, M. K. (1956). *Proc. Soc. Exptl. Biol. Med.* **91**, 493.
Chamberlain, T. J., Rothschild, G. H., and Gerrard, R. W. (1963). *Proc. Natl. Acad. Sci. U.S.* **49**, 918.
Chambon, Y. (1955). *Ann. Endocrinol. (Paris)* **16**, 912.
Chambon, Y. (1957). *Ann. Endocrinol. (Paris)* **18**, 80.
Chardon, G. (1955). *Compt. Rend. Soc. Biol.* **149**, 1539.
Charpentier, P. (1950a). U.S. Patent 2,519,886.
Charpentier, P. (1950b). U.S. Patent 2,530,451.
Charpentier, P. (1953). U.S. Patent 2,645, 640.
Chartan, F. B. E., and Bartlett, N. G. (1955). *J. Mental Sci.* **101**, 351.
Chatagnon, C., and Chatagnon, P. (1961). *Ann. Med.-Psychol.* **119** (2/3), 509.
Chatagnon, C., Chatagnon, P., and Mortier, D. (1961a). *Ann. Med.-Psychol.* **119**, No. 2, 753.
Chatagnon, P., Chatagnon, C., Wilkin, M. O., Fournier, M., and Lorcy, P. (1961b). *Ann. Med.-Psychol.* **119**, No. 1, 310.
Chatonnet, J., and Tanche, M. (1955). *Compt. Rend. Soc. Biol.* **149**, 950.
Chauchard, B., and Chauchard, P. (1952a). *Compt. Rend. Soc. Biol.* **146**, 528.
Chauchard, B., and Chauchard, P. (1952b). *Compt. Rend. Soc. Biol.* **146**, 681.
Chauchard, B., and Chauchard, P. (1952c). *Compt. Rend. Soc. Biol.* **146**, 1721.
Chaudhury, R. R., Chaudhury, M. R., and Lu, F. C. (1961). *Brit. J. Pharmacol.* **17**, 305.
Chedid, L. (1954). *Compt. Rend. Soc. Biol.* **148**, 1039.
Chen, G. (1963). *Arch. Intern. Pharmacodyn.* **142**, 30.
Chessin, M., Kramer, E. R., and Scott, C. C. (1957). *J. Pharmacol. Exptl. Therap.* **119**, 453.
Cheymol, J., and Levassort, C. (1955). *Compt. Rend. Soc. Biol.* **149**, 475.
Cheymol, J., deLeeuw, J., and Oger, J. (1954). *Compt. Rend. Soc. Biol.* **148**, 1213.
Chicoine, L. (1961). *Union Med. Canada* **90**, 469.
Child, K. J., Sutherland, P., and Tomich, E. G. (1960). *Biochem. Pharmacol.* **5**, 87.
Childers, R. T., Jr. (1962a). *Am. J. Psychiat.* **119**, 462.
Childers, R. T., Jr. (1962b). *Diseases Nervous System* **23**, 156.
Childers, R. T., Jr., and Therrien, R. (1961). *Am. J. Psychiat.* **118**, 552.
Chin, J. H. (1964). *Federation Proc.* **23**, 248.
Chin, J. H., and Smith, C. M. (1962). *J. Pharmacol. Exptl. Therap.* **136**, 276.
Chinn, H. I., and Sheldon, G. L. (1954). *Proc. Soc. Exptl. Biol. Med.* **86**, 293.

Chinn, H. I., Mitchell, R. B., Bieberdorf, F. W., and Arnold, A. C. (1954). *Antibiot. Chemotherapy* **4**, 982.
Cho, M. H. (1961). *J. Appl. Physiol.* **16**, 390.
Chorazy, M. (1959). *Nature* **184**, 200.
Christensen, J., and Wase, A. W. (1956a). *Acta Pharmacol. Toxicol.* **12**, 81.
Christensen, J., and Wase, A. W. (1956b). *Federation Proc.* **15**, 410.
Christensen, J. A., and Wase, A. W. (1960). *Federation Proc.* **19**, 228.
Chuen, N., and Riedel, B. E. (1961). *Can. Pharm. J.* **94**, 51.
Citterio, C. (1957). *Lavoro Neuorpsichiat.* **20**, 201.
Citterio, C., and Mattei, F. (1957). *Lavoro Neuropsichiat.* **20**, 189.
Clare, N. T. (1962). *International Conference on Action Mechanism and Metabolism of Psychoactive Drugs Derived from Phenothiazine and Structurally Related Compounds*, Paris, Sept. 7–8.
Clark, L. C., Jr., Fox, R. P., Morin, R., and Benington, F. (1956). *J. Nervous Mental Disease* **124**, 466.
Clark, M. L., Ray, T. S., Paredes, A., Costiloe, J. P., Chappell, J. S., Hagans, J. A., and Wolf, S. (1961). *Psychopharmacologia* **2**, 107.
Clark, R., Jackson, J. A., and Brady, J. V. (1962). *Science* **135**, 1132.
Clark, R. L., Pessolano, A. A., Weijlard, J., and Pfister, K., III (1953). *J. Am. Chem. Soc.* **75**, 4963.
Clement, A. J., and Benazon, D. (1962). *Lancet* **II**, 197.
Clerc, N. A., Turner, M., and Berard, E. (1955). *Anesthesie Analgesie* **12**, 466.
Cliche, F., and Fortin, R. (1953). *Union Med. Canada* **84**, 945.
Clodi, P., and Schnack, H. (1960). *Wien. Klin. Wochschr.* **77**, 801.
Clodi, P., and Schnack, H. (1961). *Gastroenterologia* **95**, 176.
Clout, I. R. (1962). *Med. World* **96**, 383.
Cochin, J., and Daly, J. W. (1962a). *Experientia* **18**, 294.
Cochin, J., and Daly, J. W. (1962b). *Pharmacologist* **4**, 171.
Cochin, J., and Daly, J. W. (1963). *J. Pharmacol. Exptl. Therap.* **139**, 160.
Cohen, I. M. (1955). *Am. J. Med. Sci.* **229**, 355.
Cohen, I. M., and Archer, J. D. (1955). *J. Am. Med. Assoc.* **159**, 99.
Cohen, I. M., and Nelson, J. W. (1964). *J. Pharm. Sci.* **53**, 863.
Cole, A. C. E., and Robertson, D. H. (1955). *Lancet* **II**, 1063.
Cole, J. O. (1962). *J. New Drugs* **2**, 264.
Cole, J. O. (1964). *Arch. Gen. Psychiat.* **10**, 246.
Collier, H. B., Allen, D. E., and Swales, W. E. (1943). *Can. J. Res.* **21**, 151.
Collins, I. S. (1964). *Med. J. Australia* **1**, 222.
Collins, V. J. (1962). *Illinois Med. J.* **122**, 350.
Collins, V. J. (1964). *Surg. Clin. North Am.* **44**, 173.
Conner, P. K., and Moyer, J. H. (1957). *Antibiot. Med. Clin. Therapy* **4**, 508.
Conney, A. G., Clarke, D., Gastel, R., and Burns, J. J. (1960). *J. Pharmacol. Exptl. Therap.* **130**, 1.
Conqvist, S., Rayner, S., and Wretmark, G. (1955). *Nord. Med.* **53**, 730.
Constant, M. A., and Becker, B. (1956). *Am. J. Ophthalmol.* **41**, 1071.
Cook, L. (1956). *Meeting American Psychiatric Association*, Philadelphia, Pennsylvania, 1956.
Cook, L., and Kelleher, R. T. (1962). *Ann. N.Y. Acad. Sci.* **96**, 315.
Cook, L., and Kelleher, R. T. (1963). *Ann. Rev. Pharmacol.* **3**, 205.
Cook, L., and Toner, J. J. (1954). *J. Pharmacol. Exptl. Therap.* **110**, 12.
Cook, L., Weidley, E. F., and Morris, R. W. (1955). *J. Pharmacol. Exptl. Therap.* **113**, 11a.
Coppolino, C. A., and Wallace, G. (1960). *Anesthesia Analgesia, Current Res.* **39**, 548.
Coraboeuf, E., Lavigne, S., Distel, R., and Boistel, J. (1955). *Compt. Rend.* **149**, 58.
Cordier, P., and Dupontreue, J. (1962). *Boll. Chim. Farm.* **101**, 462.
Corne, S. J., Pickering, R. W., and Warner, B. T. (1963). *Brit. J. Pharmacol.* **20**, 106.

Cornman, H. D., III (1961). In "Extrapyramidal System and Neuroleptics," p. 479. Editions Psychiatriques, Montreal.
Cosnier, J., and Drouin, M. (1954). *Bull. Soc. Med. Mil. Franc.* **48**, 185.
Costa, E. (1956). *Proc. Soc. Exptl. Biol. Med.* **91**, 39.
Costa, E., and Rinaldi, F. (1958). *Am. J. Physiol.* **194**, 214.
Costa, E., Garattini, S., and Valzelli, L. (1960). *Experientia* **16**, 461.
Council on Drugs (1962). *J. Am. Med. Assoc.* **179**, 888.
Courvoisier, S., and Cosar, C. (1955). *Compt. Rend.* **240**, 2026.
Courvoisier, S., and Ducrot, R. (1954). *Compt. Rend. Soc. Biol.* **148**, 462.
Courvoisier, S., Fournel, J., Ducrot, R., Kolsky, M., and Koetschet, P. (1953). *Arch. Intern. Pharmacodyn.* **92**, 305.
Craig, J. C. (1962). *International Conference on Action Mechanism and Metabolism of Psychoactive Drugs Derived from Phenothiazine and Structurally Related Compounds, Paris, Sept. 7–8.*
Craig, J. C., Green, D. E., Roy, S. K., Piette, L. H., and Loeffler, K. O. (1965). *J. Med. Chem.* **8**, 392.
Craig, J. C., and Tate, M. R. (1961). *Progr. Drug Res.* **3**, 75.
Craig, J. C., Mary, N. Y., and Roy, S. V. (1964). *Anal. Chem.* **36**, 1142.
Craig, P. N., Nodiff, E. A., Lafferty, J. J., and Ullyot, G. E. (1957). *J. Org. Chem.* **22**, 709.
Craig, P. N., Gordon, M., Lafferty, J. J., Lester, B. M., Pavloff, A. M., and Zirkle, C. L. (1960). *J. Org. Chem.* **25**, 944.
Craig, P. N., Gordon, M., Lafferty, J. J., Lester, B. M., Saggiomo, A. J., and Zirkle, C. L. (1961). *J. Org. Chem.* **26**, 1138.
Cranston, E. M. (1958a). *Cancer Res.* **18**, 897.
Cranston, E. M. (1958b). *Proc. Soc. Exptl. Biol. Med.* **98**, 320.
Cranston, E. M. (1961). *Proc. Soc. Exptl. Biol. Med.* **108**, 514.
Cremer, J. E. (1961). *Biochem. Pharmacol.* **6**, 153.
Creze, J. (1955). *Gynecol. Obstet.* **54**, 622.
Crisp, A. H., and Roberts, F. J. (1962). *Postgrad. Med. J.* **38**, 350.
Cuningham, J. A., and Hannah, E. E. (1960). *New Zealand Med. J.* **59**, 528.
Cusic, J. W. (1956). U.S. Patent 2,766,235.
Cusic, J. W., and Hamilton, R. W. (1956). U.S. Patent 2,766,235.
Cusic, J. W., and Hamilton, R. W. (1958). U.S. Patent 2,838,507.
Cutler, R. P., Munroe, J., and Anderson, T. E. (1957). *A.M.A. Arch. Neurol. Psychiat.* **77**, 616.
daCruz, A. (1955). *Compt. Rend. Soc. Biol.* **149**, 1829.
Dahlbom, R. (1951). Swedish Patent 129,843.
Dandiya, P. C. (1963). *Arch. Intern. Pharmacodyn.* **141**, 216.
Dandiya, P. C., Johnson, G., and Sellers, E. A. (1960). *Can. J. Biochem. Physiol.* **38**, 591.
Danese, C., and Cesare, E. D. (1955). *Policlin. (Rome) Sez. Chir.* **62**, 116.
Danhof, I. E. (1958). *Texas Rept. Biol. Med.* **16**, 443.
Das, N. N., Dasgupta, S. R., and Werner, G. (1954). *Bull. Calcutta School Trop. Med.* **1**, 5.
Das, N. N., Dasgupta, S. R., and Werner, G. (1955). *Arch. Exptl. Pathol. Pharmakol.* **224**, 248.
Dasgupta, S. R. (1955). *Bull. Calcutta School Trop. Med.* **3**, 17.
Dasgupta, S. R. (1957). *Arch. Intern. Pharmacodyn.* **112**, 264.
Dasgupta, S. R., Mukherjee, K. L., and Werner, G. (1954). *Arch. Intern. Pharmacodyn.* **97**, 149.
Dasgupta, S. R., and Hausler, H. F. (1955a). *Bull. Calcutta School Trop. Med.* **3**, 69.
Dasgupta, S. R., and Hausler, H. F. (1955b). *Bull. Calcutta School Trop. Med.* **3**, 112.
Dasgupta, S. R., and Hausler, H. F. (1955c). *Bull. Calcutta School Trop. Med.* **3**, 113.
Dasgupta, S. R., and Mukherjee, K. L. (1956). *Bull. Calcutta School Trop. Med.* **4**, 123.
Dasgupta, S. R., and Werner, G. (1954). *Brit. J. Pharmacol.* **9**, 389.
Dasgupta, S. R., and Werner, G. (1955). *Arch. Intern. Pharmacodyn.* **100**, 409.

Dasgupta, S. R., Chatterjee, A., and Ray, H. N. (1956). *Bull. Calcutta School Trop. Med.* **4**, 124.
David, M., Benda, P., and Klein, F. (1953). *Bull. Mem. Soc. Med. Hop. Paris* **69**, 691.
Davidson, G. M., and Ades, F. (1961). *Diseases Nervous System* **22**, 273.
Davidson, J. D., Terry, L., and Sjoerdsma, A. (1957). *J. Pharmacol. Exptl. Therap.* **121**, 8.
Davies, J. I. (1955). *Can. Anesthesiol. Soc. J.* **2**, 327.
Davis, W. M., Capehart, J., and Llewellin, W. L. (1961). *Psychopharmacologia* **2**, 268.
Dawkins, M. J. R., Judah, J. D., and Rees, K. R. (1958). *Nature* **182**, 875.
Dawkins, M. J. R., Judah, J. D., and Rees, K. R. (1959a). *Biochem. J.* **72**, 204.
Dawkins, M. J. R., Judah, J. D., and Rees, K. R. (1959b). *Biochem. J.* **73**, 16.
Dawkins, M. J. R., Judah, J. D., and Rees, K. R. (1959c). *Biochem. Pharmacol.* **2**, 112.
Dawkins, M. J. R., Judah, J. D., and Rees, K. R. (1960). *Biochem. J.* **76**, 200.
Dawson, J. F., Jr., and Hiestand, W. A. (1955). *Federation Proc.* **14**, 36.
DeBias, D. A., Paschkis, K. E., and Cantarow, A. (1958). *Am. J. Physiol.* **193**, 553.
Decortis, A., and Lecomte, J. (1953). *Compt. Rend. Soc. Biol.* **147**, 1640.
Decourt, P. (1953). *Therapie* **8**, 846.
Decourt, P. (1955). *Anaesthesia* **10**, 221.
Decourt, P., and Anguera, G. (1953). *Compt. Rend.* **236**, 1445.
Decourt, P., Anguera, G., and Grenat, R. (1953b). *Compt. Rend.* **236**, 2268.
Decourt, P., Brunaud, M., and Brunaud, S. (1953a). *Compt. Rend. Soc. Biol.* **147**, 1602.
Décsi, L. (1961). *Psychopharmacologia* **2**, 224.
Décsi, L., and Méhes, J. (1957). *Arch. Exptl. Pathol. Pharmakol.* **230**, 462.
Décsi, L., and Méhes, J. (1958). *Experientia* **14**, 145.
De Eds, F., and Thomas, J. O. (1942). *J. Parasitol.* **24**, 363.
De Gennes, L., and Bricaire, H. (1957). *Presse Med.* **65**, 499.
De Jaramillo, G. A. V., and Guth, P. S. (1963). *Biochem. Pharmacol.* **12**, 525.
Delage, J. (1960). *Laval Med.* **30**, 652.
Delay, J., and Deniker, P. (1952a). *Compt. Rend. Congr. Med. Alienistes Neurologistes, Luxembourg* p. 19.
Delay, J., and Deniker, P. (1952b). *Compt. Rend. Congr. Med. Alienistes Neurologistes, Luxembourg* p. 497.
Delay, J., Deniker, P., and Harl, J. M. (1952a). *Ann. Med.-Psychol.* **110**, No. 2, 112.
Delay, J., Deniker, P., Harl, J. M., and Grasset, A. (1952b). *Ann. Med.-Psychol.* **110**, No. 2, 398.
Delay, J., Deniker, P., Ropert, M., and Thuillier, J. (1956). *Compt. Rend. Soc. Biol.* **150**, 512.
DeLong, S. L., Poley, B. S., and McFarlane, J. R. (1965). *Arch. Ophthalmol.* **73**, 611.
Delphaut, J. (1963). *Compt. Rend. Soc. Biol.* **157**, 2229.
DeMaar, E. W. J., Martin, W. R., and Unna, K. R. (1958). *J. Pharmacol. Exptl. Therap.* **124**, 77.
Denber, H. C. B. (1957). *Diseases Nervous System* **18**, 76.
Denber, H. C. B. (1961). *Psychiat. Quart.* **35**, 18.
Denenberg, V. H., Ross, S., and Ellsworth, J. (1959). *Psychopharmacologia* **1**, 59.
Denham, J. (1958). *J. Mental Sci.* **104**, 1190.
Denhoff, E., and Holden, R. H. (1961). *New Engl. J. Med.* **264**, 475.
De Risio, C., and Manghi, E. (1954). *Boll. Soc. Ital. Biol. Sper.* **30**, 1352.
De Ropp, R. S., and Snedeker, E. H. (1961). *Proc. Soc. Exptl. Biol. Med.* **106**, 696.
De Senarclens, F. (1961). *Intern. Abstr. Surg.* **113**, 375; (1961). *Gynaecologia* **151** 165.
Deshpande, V. R. (1963). *Arch. Intern. Pharmacodyn.* **141**, 525.
Deshpande, V. R., and Tiwaskar, H. V. (1960). *Indian J. Med. Res.* **48**, 478.
Deviller, M. (1961). *Ann. Pharm. Franc.* **19**, 131.
De Vleeschhouwer, G. R., King, T. O., Poulsen, E., and Rovati, A. L. (1957). *Arch. Intern. Pharmacodyn.* **112**, 485.
de Wied, D., and Jinks, R. (1958). *Proc. Soc. Exptl. Biol. Med.* **99**, 44.

Dews, P. B. (1956). *J. Pharmacol. Exptl. Therap.* **116**, 16.
Dews, P. B. (1958). *J. Exptl. Anal. Behavior* **1**, 73.
Dews, P. B., and Morse, W. H. (1958). *J. Exptl. Anal. Behaviour* **1**, 359.
Dhawan, B. N., Saxena, P. N., and Gupta, G. P. (1961). *Brit. J. Pharmacol.* **16**, 137.
Di Mascio, A., Havens, L. L., and Klerman, G. L. (1963). *J. Nerv. Ment. Dis.* **136**, 15, 168.
Dimmling, T., and Staib, F. (1955). *Arzneimittel-Forsch.* **5**, 393.
Dingell, J. V., Duncan, W. A. M., and Gillette, J. R. (1961). *Federation Proc.* **20**, 173.
Di Palma, J. R. (1963). *Clin. Pediat.* **2**, 225.
Di Palma, J. R., and Catenacci, A. J. (1955). *Federation Proc.* **14**, 333.
Dixon, R. L., Hart, L. G., and Fouts, J. R. (1961). *J. Pharmacol. Exptl. Therap.* **133**, 7.
Dobkin, A. B., and Gilbert, R. G. B. (1956). *Anesthesiology* **17**, 135.
Dobkin, A. B., Gilbert, R. G. B., and Lamoureux, L. (1954a). *Anaesthesia* **9**, 157.
Dobkin, A. B., Lamoureux, L., and Gilbert, R. G. B. (1954b). *Treatment Serv. Bull.* **9**, 324.
Dobkin, A. B., Lamoureux, L., Letienne, R., and Gilbert, R. G. B. (1954c). *Can. Med. Assoc. J.* **70**, 626.
Domer, F. R., and Feldberg, W. (1960). *Brit. J. Pharmacol.* **15**, 578.
Domino, E. F. (1962). *Clin. Pharmacol. Therap.* **3**, 599.
Donnadieu, A., Florentin, M., and Florentin, M. M. (1955). *Ann. Med.-Psychol.* **113**, 205.
Donnet, V., Zwirn, P., and Ardisson, J. L. (1954). *Compt. Rend. Soc. Biol.* **148**, 1617.
Dotevall, G. (1957). *Nord. Med.* **57**, 687.
Doty, B. A., and Doty, L. A. (1963). *Can. J. Psychol.* **17**, 45.
Douglas, A. D. M., and Bates, T. J. N. (1957). *Brit. Med. J.* **I**, 1514.
Dripps, R. D., Vandam, L. D., and Pierce, E. C. (1955). *Ann. Surg.* **142**, 774.
Dubost, P., and Pascal, S. (1953). *Ann. Pharm. Franc.* **11**, 615.
Dubost, P. and Pascal, S. (1955). *Ann. Pharm. Franc.* **13**, 56.
Dubost, M., and Pascal, S. (1956). Private communication.
Ducommun, P. (1952). *Praxis (Bern)* **30**, 641.
Duff, R. S., McIntyre, J. W. R., and Butler, N. G. P. (1956). *Brit. Med. J.* **I**, 264.
Duhm, B., Koester, L., Maul, W., and Medenwald, H. (1958). *Z. Naturforsch.* **13**b, 756.
Dundas, E., Toogood, J. H., and Wanklin, J. (1961). *J. Allergy* **32**, 1.
Dundee, J. W., Mesham, P. R., and Scott, W. E. B. (1954). *Anesthesia* **9**, 296.
Dusinsky, G. (1957). *Cesk. Farm.* **6**, 302.
Dusinsky, G. (1958). *Pharmazie* **13**, 478.
Dye, E. N. (1961). *Am. J. Psychiat.* **118**, 548.
Eberhard, F., Wilke, G., and Ansorg, W. (1961). *Psychopharmacologia* **2**, 160.
Eberhardt, H., Lerbs, O. W., and Freundt, K. J. (1963). *Arzneimittel-Forsch.* **9**, 804.
Eckhardt, E. T., and Govier, W. M. (1958). *Proc. Soc. Exptl. Biol. Med.* **97**, 124.
Eddy, N. B. (1963). Private communication (ED_{50} 3.1 mg/kg s.c.).
Edgerton, W. H., Gordon, M., and Wilson, J. W. (1961). U.S. Patent 3,000,886.
Edgren, R. A. (1956). *Anat. Record* **125**, 602.
Egdahl, R. H., and Richards, J. B. (1956). *Am. J. Physiol.* **185**, 235.
Eger, W., and Poppe, H. (1960). *Arzneimittel-Forsch.* **14**, 262.
Eggers, G. W. N., Jr., Corssen, G., and Allen, C. R. (1959). *Anesthesiology* **20**, 261.
Ehringer, H., Hornykiewicz, O., and Lechner, K. (1960). *Arch. Exptl. Pathol. Pharmakol.* **239**, 507.
Eiduson, S., and Geller, E. (1962). *International Conference on Action Mechanism and Metabolism of Psychoactive Drugs Derived from Phenothiazine and Structurally Related Compounds, Paris, Sept.* 7–8.
Eiduson, S., and Wallace, R. D. (1958a). *Trans. 2nd Res. Conf. Chemotherapy Psychiat., VA, Washington, D.C.* **2**, 88.
Eiduson, S., and Wallace, R. D. (1958b). *Federation Proc.* **17**, 365.

Eiduson, S., Crockett, J. T., and Cohen, S. (1960). *Trans. 4th Res. Conf. Chemotherapy Psychiat.*, *VA, Washington, D.C.* **4**, 248.
Eisdorfer, I. B., and Ellenbogen, W. C. (1960). *J. Chromatog.* **4**, 329.
Elder, J. T., Jr., and Dille, J. M. (1962). *J. Pharmacol. Exptl. Therap.* **136**, 162.
Eliakim, M. (1960). *Harefuah* **58**, 119.
Eliakim, M., and Feldman, S. (1958). *Exptl. Med. Surg.* **16**, 240.
Ellis, P. P. (1965). *Arch. Ophthalmol.* **74**, 96.
Elo, R., and Turunen, M. (1955). *Ann. Chir. Gynaecol. Fenniae* **44**, 10.
Emmelin, N. (1955). *Acta Physiol. Scand.* **34**, 29.
Emmerson, J. L., and Miya, T. S. (1962). *J. Pharmacol. Exptl. Therap.* **137**, 148.
Emmerson, J. L., and Miya, T. S. (1963). *J. Pharma. Sci.* **52**, 411.
Endicott, N. A., and Gralnick, A. (1961). *Diseases Nervous System* **22**, 680.
Engelhardt, D. M. (1964). *Arch. Gen. Psychiat.* **11**, 162.
Engelhardt, D. M., Freedman, N., Hankoff, L. D., Mann, D., and Margolis, R. (1960). *Comprehensive Psychiat.* **1**, 313.
Enticknap, J. B., and Gordon, B. (1961). *Brit. Med. J.* **II**, 522.
Epps, R. P., and Scott, R. B. (1961). *Med. Ann. District Columbia* **30**, 317.
Erdos, E. G., Baart, N., Shanor, S. P., and Foldes, F. F. (1958). *Arch. Intern. Pharmacodyn.* **117**, 163.
Ernsting, M. J. E., Kafoe, W. F., Nauta, W. T., Oosterhuis, H. K., and de Waart, C. (1960). *J. Neurochem.* **5**, 121.
Erslev, A. J., and Wintrobe, M. M. (1962). *J. Am. Med. Assoc.* **181**, 114.
Esserman, H. B. (1952). *Can. J. Res.* **30E**, 485.
Essig, C. F., and Carter, W. W. (1957). *Proc. Soc. Exptl. Biol. Med.* **95**, 726.
Estler, C. J. (1961). *Med. Exptl.* **4**, 209.
Estrada, E. (1956). *J. Am. Vet. Med. Assoc.* **128**, 292.
Evans, D. A. P. (1963). *Am. J. Med.* **34**, 639.
Evans, W. J., and Smiles, S. (1935a). *J. Chem. Soc.* p. 1263.
Evans, W. J., and Smiles, S. (1935b). *J. Chem. Soc.* p. 181.
Evans, W. O. and Jewett, A. (1962). *Psychopharmacologia* **3**, 134.
Fabisch, W. (1955). *Lancet* **I**, 1277.
Faguet, M. M., Goudet, A., and Tréfouel, M. J. (1963). *Presse Med.* **71**, 579.
Fairley, H. B. (1963), *Appl. Therap.* **5**, 322.
Fanning, W. J. (1961). *Can. Med. J.* **85**, 1459.
Fau, R., Flandrin, P., and Hollard, D. (1962). *Ann. Med.-Psychol.* **120**, No. 1, 571.
Faurbye, A. Rasch, P. J., Petersen, P. B., Brandborg, G., and Pakkenberg, H. (1964). *Acta Physiol. Scand.* **40**, 10.
Fazekas, J. F., Albert, S. N., and Alman, R. W. (1955). *Am. J. Med. Sci.* **230**, 128.
Fedorov, N. A. (1957). *Zh. Nevropatol. i Psikhiatr.* **57**, 761.
Fedorov, N. A. (1958a). *Zh. Nevropatol. i Psikhiatr.* **58**, 137.
Fedorov, N. A. (1958b). *Proc. Intern. Conf. Peaceful Uses At. Energy, 2nd, Geneva, 1958.* Vol. **24**, p. 205. I. D.S., Columbia Univ. Press, New York.
Fedorov, N. A., and Shnol', S. E. (1956). *Zh. Nevropatol. i Psikhiatr.* **56**, 137.
Feldman, P. E. (1957a). *J. Clin. Exptl. Psychopathol.* **18**, 1.
Feldman, P. E. (1957b). *Am. J. Psychiat.* **13**, 59.
Feldman, P. E., and Frierson, B. D. (1964). *Am. J. Psychiat.* **121**, 187.
Feldman, R. G., and Brown, B. B. (1955). *J. Pharmacol. Exptl. Therap.* **113**, 20.
Feldman, R. S. (1962). *J. Neuropsychiat.* **3**, 254.
Feldman, S., and Eliakim, M. (1958). *Arch. Intern. Pharmacodyn.* **116**, 340.
Feldman, S., and Kidron, D. P. (1957). *Arch. Intern. Pharmacodyn.* **151**, 70.
Feller, K. (1955a). *Arch. Exptl. Pathol. Pharmakol.* **225**, 90.
Feller, K. (1955b). *Arch. Exptl. Pathol. Pharmakol.* **226**, 269.

Feller, K., and Staib, A. H. (1964). *Arch. Intern. Pharmacodyn.* **148**, 255.
Fellman, J. H. (1956). *J. Nervous Mental Diseases* **123**, 575.
Fels, I. G., and Kaufman, M. (1959). *Nature* **183**, 1392.
Fels, I. G., Kaufman, M., and Karczmar, A. G. (1958a). American Society for Pharmacology and Experimental Therapeutics, August 25–28.
Fels, I. G., Kaufman, M., and Karczmar, A. G. (1958b). *Nature* **181**, 1266.
Fenters, J. D., and Jeter, W. S. (1961). *J. Bacteriol.* **82**, 156.
Ferguson, J. T. (1957). *J. Am. Med. Assoc.* **165**, 1677.
Ferster, C. B., Appel, J. B., and Hiss, R. A. (1962). *J. Exptl. Anal. Behavior* **5**, 73.
Filk, H., and Loeser, A. (1954). *Klin. Wochschr.* **32**, 661.
Filk, H., Ritter, K., Sturmer, E., and Loeser, A. (1954). *Klin. Wochschr.* **32**, 265.
Findlay, G. M. (1950). "Recent Advances in Chemotherapy," 3rd ed., Vol. I, p. 124. McGraw-Hill (Blakiston), New York.
Fink, G. B., and Swinyard, E. A. (1960). *J. Am. Pharm. Assoc. Sci. Ed.* **49**, 510.
Fink, G. B., and Swinyard, E. A. (1962). *J. Pharm. Sci.* **51**, 548.
Fink, M. (1961). *Med. Exptl.* **5**, 364.
Finkelstein, M., Spencer, W. A., Hammen, C. S., and Albert, S. N. (1954a). *Federation Proc.* **13**, 354.
Finkelstein, M., Spencer, W. A., and Ridgeway, E. R. (1954b). *Proc. Soc. Exptl. Biol. Med.* **87**, 343.
Fischer, R., Knopp, W., and Griffin, F. (1965). *Arzneimittel-Forsch.* **12**, 1369.
Fishman, V., and Goldenberg, H. (1960). *Proc. Soc. Exptl. Biol. Med.* **104**, 99.
Fishman, V., and Goldenberg, H. (1963). *Proc. Soc. Exptl. Biol. Med.* **112**, 501.
Fishman, V., Heaton, A., and Goldenberg, H. (1962). *Proc. Soc. Exptl. Biol. Med.* **109**, 548.
Flacke, W., Mulke, G., and Schulz, R. (1953). *Arch. Exptl. Pathol. Pharmakol.* **220**, 469.
Flanagan, T. L., Lin, T. H., Novick, W. J., Rondish, I. M., Bocher, C. A., and Van Loon, E. J. (1959). *J. Med. Pharm. Chem.* **1**, 263.
Flanagan, T. L., Reynolds, L. W., Novick, W. J., Lin, T. H., Rondish, I. M., and Van Loon, E. J. (1962a). *J. Pharm. Sci.* **51**, 833.
Flanagan, T. L., Newman, J. H., Maass, A. R., and Van Loon, E. J. (1962b). *J. Pharm. Sci.* **51**, 996.
Follin, S., Chanoit, P., and Pilon, L. (1961). *Ann. Med.-Psychol.* **119**, No. 1, 976.
Fontan, V., (1955). *Semaine Hop. Paris* **31**, 2255.
Foote, R. H., and Gray, L. C. (1960). *J. Dairy Sci.* **43**, 1499.
Forrest, F. M., and Forrest, I. S. (1957). *Am. J. Psychiat.* **113**, 931.
Forrest, F. M., and Forrest, I. S. (1960). *Trans. 4th Res. Conf. Chemotherapy Psychiat., VA, Washington, D.C.* **4**, 245.
Forrest, F. M., Forrest, I. S., and Mason, A. S. (1959a). *New Engl. J. Med.* **261**, 254.
Forrest, F. M., Forrest, I. S., and Mason, A. S. (1959b). *Am. J. Psychiat.* **115**, 1114.
Forrest, F. M., Forrest, I. S., and Mason, A. S. (1959c). *Am. J. Psychiat.* **116**, 549.
Forrest, F. M., Forrest, I. S., and Mason, A. S. (1960a). *Am. J. Psychiat.* **117**, 561.
Forrest, F. M., Forrest, I. S., and Mason, A. S. (1961). *Am. J. Psychiat.* **118**, 300.
Forrest, I. S., and Forrest, F. M. (1963). *Exptl. Med. Surg.* **21**, 231.
Forrest, I. S., and Forrest, F. M. (1960a). *Trans. 5th Res. Conf. Chemotherapy Psychiat., VA, Washington, D.C.* **5**, 128.
Forrest, I. S., and Forrest, F. M. (1960b). *Clin. Chem.* **6**, 11.
Forrest, I. S., and Forrest, F. M. (1960c). *Clin. Chem.* **6**, 362.
Forrest, I. S., and Forrest, F. M. (1961). *Proc. 4th Intern. Congr. Clin. Chem., Edinburgh*, 1960 p. 160. Williams & Wilkins, Baltimore, Maryland.
Forrest, I. S., Forrest, F. M., and Berger, M. (1958). *Biochim. Biophys. Acta* **29**, 441.
Forrest, I. S., Forrest, F. M., and Mason, A. S. (1960). *Am. J. Psychiat.* **116**, 928.
Forrest, I. S., Wechsler, M. B., and Sperco, J. E. (1963). *Am. J. Psychiat.* **120**, 44.

Fossoul, C. (1950). *J. Pharm. Belg.* **5**, 202.
Fossoul, C. (1951). *J. Pharm. Belg.* **6**, 383.
Foster, C. A., and O'Mullane, E. J. (1954). *Lancet* **II**, 614.
Fotherby, K. (1959). *Acta Endocrinol.* **32**, 425.
Fournel, J. (1952). *Compt. Rend. Soc. Biol.* **146**, 561.
Fouts, J. R. (1961). *Biochem. Biophys. Res. Commun.* **6**, 373.
Fouts, J. R. (1963). *Ann. N.Y. Acad. Sci.* **104**, 875.
Fouts, J. R., and Adamson, R. H. (1959). *Science*, **129**, 897.
Fowler, P. J., Tedeschi, O. H., Cromley, W. H., Pauls, J. F., Eby, R. Z., and Fellows, E. J. (1964). *Federation Proc.* **23**, 198.
Frahm, M., Fretwurst, E., and Soehring, K. (1956). *Klin. Wochschr.* **34**, 1259.
Franchi, G., and Gianni, A. M. (1957). *Acta Anaesthesiol.* **8**, 197.
Franco-Browder, S., Masson, G. M. C., and Corcoran, A. C. (1958). *Proc. Soc. Exptl. Biol. Med.* **97**, 778.
Frankau, I. M., and Stanwell, P. M. (1960). *Lancet* **II**, 1377.
Fraser, H. F., and Isbell, H. (1956). *A.M.A. Arch. Neurol. Psychiat.* **76**, 257.
Fraser, H. F., and Isbell, H. (1959). *Bull. Drug. Addict. Narcotics* Add. 2, p. 1.
Fraser, H. F., and Rosenberg, D. E. (1963). *Bull. Drug. Addict. Narcotics* Add. 8, p. 1.
Freed, H. (1956). *Am. J. Psychiat.* **113**, 22.
Freed, H., and Frignito, N. (1961). *Pennsa. Psychiat. Quart.* **1**, 39.
Freedman, D. X., and Giarman, N. J. (1956). *Science* **124**, 264.
Freeman, A. R., and Spirtes, M. A. (1962). *Biochem. Pharmacol.* **11**, 161.
Freeman, A. R., and Spirtes, M. A. (1963). *Biochem. Pharmacol.* **12**, 47.
Freund, R. B., and Levine, N. M. (1958). *Psychiat. Quart.* **32**, 758.
Freyhan, F. A. (1958). "Trifluoperazine," p. 195. Lea & Febiger, Philadelphia, Pennsylvania.
Friebel, H., and Kastner, H. (1955). *Arch. Exptl. Pathol. Pharmakol.* **225**, 210.
Friebel, H., and Reichle, C. (1955). *Arch. Expt. Pathol. Pharmakol.* **226**, 551.
Friend, D. G., and Cummins, J. F. (1953). *J. Am. Med. Assoc.* **153**, 481.
Frogel, M. (1964). *Psychiat. Neurol.* **147**, 267.
Frommel, E., and Fleury, C. (1959a). *Med. Exptl.* **1**, 223.
Frommel, E., and Fleury, C. (1959b). *Med. Exptl.* **1**, 264.
Frommel, E., von Ledebur, I., and Béguin, M. (1963). *Arch. Intern. Pharmacodyn.* **143**, 52.
Fry, W., Kelleher, R. T., and Cook, L. (1960). *J. Exptl. Anal. Behavior* **3**, 193.
Fujii, K. (1956a). *J. Pharm. Soc. Japan* **76**, 637.
Fujii, K. (1956b). *J. Pharm. Soc. Japan* **76**, 640.
Fujii, K. (1956c). *J. Pharm. Soc. Japan* **76**, 644.
Fujimoto, M. (1959). *Bull. Chem. Soc. Japan* **32**, 371.
Fujita, K., Iwase, S., Ito, T., and Matsuyama, M. (1958). *Nature* **181**, 54.
Fuller, J. L., Clark, L. D., and Waller, M. B. (1960). *Psychopharmacologia* **1**, 393.
Furgiuele, A. R., Kinnard, W. J., and Buckley, J. P. (1961). *J. Pharm. Sci.* **50**, 252.
Gadermann, E., and Donat, K. (1955). *Arch. Intern. Pharmacodyn.* **102**, 85.
Gailitis, J., Knowles, R. R., and Longobardi, A. (1960). *Ann. Internal Med.* **52**, 538.
Gaitz, C. M., Roy, H., Thompson, W., Kimbell, I., Mullen, A. J., and Pokorny, A. D. (1955). *Psychiat. Res. Rept.* **1**, 84.
Gallant, D. M., Edwards, C. G., Bishop, M. P., and Galbraith, G. C. (1964). *Am. J. Psychiat.* **121**, 491.
Gangloff, H., and Monnier, M. (1957). *Helv. Physiol. Pharmacol. Acta* **15**, 83.
Ganshirt, H., and Brilmayer, H. (1954). *Arch. Intern. Pharmacodyn.* **90**, 467.
Gardner, M. J., Hawkins, H. M., Judah, L. N., and Murphree, O. D. (1955). *Psychiat. Res. Rept.* **1**, 77.
Garetz, F. K., and Léider, L. L. (1963). *Minn. Med.* **46**, 973.
Garner, R. J., and Skude, I. M. (1956). *Nature* **178**, 1348.

Gati, T., Harmos, G., and Ludany, G. (1958). *Arch. Intern. Pharmacodyn.* **114**, 251.
Geiger, H., and Finkelstein, B. A. (1954). *Schweiz. Med. Wochschr.* **84**, 1063.
Gelfand, M. (1955). *Central African J. Med.* **1**, 5.
Gerster, P., and Moeschlin, S. (1961). *Deut. Med. Wochschr.* **86**, 890.
Gey, K. F., and Pletscher, A. (1961). *J. Pharmacol. Exptl. Therap.* **133**, 18.
Gey, K. F., and Pletscher, A. (1962). *Nature* **194**, 387.
Gey, K. F., and Pletscher, A. (1964). *J. Pharmacol. Exptl. Therap.* **145**, 337.
Giaja, J., and Markovic-Giaja, L. (1954). *Compt. Rend. Soc. Biol.* **148**, 842.
Giao, T., and Rico, J. M. (1961). *Compt. Rend. Soc. Biol.* **155**, 1744.
Gibbons, T. B., Reeves, R. L., and Hill, L. D. (1955). *Bull. Mason Clin.* **9**, 125.
Gibbs, J. J., Wilkens, B., and Laüterback, C. G. (1956). *Am. J. Psychiat.* **113**, 254.
Gilgash, C. A. (1961). *J. Clin. Psychol.* **17**, 95.
Gillett, E. (1960). *Proc. Soc. Exptl. Biol. Med.* **103**, 392.
Gillette, J. R., and Kamm, J. J. (1960). *J. Pharmacol. Exptl. Therap.* **130**, 262.
Gilman, H., and Shirley, D. A. (1944a). *J. Am. Chem. Soc.* **66**, 626.
Gilman, H., and Shirley, D. A. (1944b). *J. Am. Chem. Soc.* **66**, 888.
Giro, C. (1960). *Boll. Soc. Ital. Biol. Sper.* **36**, 1348.
Gittelman, R. K. (1964). *Psychopharmacologia* **5**, 317.
Glasky, A. (1963). *Federation Proc.* **22**, 272.
Glaviano, V. V., and Wang, S. C. (1954). *Federation Proc.* **13**, 358.
Glende, E. A., and Cornatzer, W. E. (1963). *J. Pharmacol. Exptl. Therap.* **139**, 377.
Glick, B. S., and Margolis, R. (1962). *Am. J. Psychiat.* **118**, 1087.
Gliedman, L. H., and Gantt, W. H. (1956). *Southern Med. J.* **49**, 880.
Glowinski, M., Limanski, M., and Sieron, G. (1960). *Polski Tygod. Lekar.* **15**, 497.
Göschke, H. (1963). *Med. Exptl.* **8**, 256.
Gold, S., Griffiths, P. D., and Huntsman, R. G. (1962). *J. Mental Sci.* **108**, 88.
Goldberg, M. E., and Johnson, H. E. (1964). *J. Pharm. Pharmacol.* **16**, 60.
Goldenberg, H., and Fishman, V. (1961). *Proc. Soc. Exptl. Biol. Med.* **108**, 178.
Goldenberg, H., and Fishman, V. (1964). *Biochem. Biophys. Res. Commun.* **14**, 404.
Goldenberg, H., Fishman, V., and Burnett, R. (1964). *Proc. Soc. Exptl. Biol. Med.* **115**, 1044.
Goldman, D. (1955). *J. Am. Med. Assoc.* **157**, 1274.
Goldman, D. (1961). *Psychosomatics* **11**, 379.
Goldring, S., Metcalf, J. S., Huang, S. H., Shields, J., and O'Leary, J. L. (1959). *J. Nervous Mental Disease* **128**, 1.
Goldsmith, R. W. (1959). *J. Am. Med. Assoc.* **170**, 361.
Gonzalez, R. C., and Ross, S. (1961). *J. Comp. Physiol. Psychol.* **54**, 645.
Gonzalez, R. C., and Shepp, B. (1962). *Can. J. Psychol.* **16**, 64.
Good, W. W., Sterling, M., and Holzman, W. H. (1958). *Am. J. Psychiat.* **115**, 443.
Gordon, H. L., and Groth, C. (1964). *Arch. Gen. Psychiat.* **10**, 187.
Gordon, M. (1960a). U.S. Patent 2,945,030.
Gordon, M. (1960b). U.S. Patent 2,945,031.
Gordon, M. (1960c). U.S. Patent 2,944,054.
Gordon, M. (1960d). "Medicinal Chemistry" (A. Burger, ed.) 2nd Ed. p. 397, Wiley (Interscience), New York.
Gordon, M. (1961). French Patent 1,261,186.
Gordon, M. (1962a). *New Engl. J. Med.* **267**, 730.
Gordon, M. (1962b). U.S. Patent 3,063,996.
Gordon, M. (1962c). *Penna. Med. J.* **65**, 191.
Gordon, M. (1962d). *Pharma. Ind.* **24**, 461.
Gordon, M. (1962e). British Patent 894,913.
Gordon, M., and Ullyot, G. E. (1957). *In* "Encyclopedia of Chemical Technology" (R. E. Kirk and D. F. Othmer, eds.), 1st Suppl. Vol., pp. 720–743. Wiley (Interscience), New York.

Gordon, M., and McCandless, R. F. J. (1959). Tranquilizers. *In* "Handbook of Toxicology," Vol. IV, Saunders, Philadelphia, Pennsylvania.
Gordon, M., Craig, P. N., and Saggiomo, A. J. (1958). *J. Org. Chem.* **23**, 1906.
Gordon, M., Cook, L., Tedeschi, D. H., and Tedeschi, R. E. (1963). *Arzneimittel-Forsch.* **13**, 318.
Gordon, M. W., Sims, J. A., Hanson, R. K., and Kuttner, R. E. (1962). *J. Neurochem.* **9**, 477.
Gorham, D. R., and Overall, J. E. (1960). *J. Nervous Mental Disease* **131**, 528.
Gottlieb, L. S., Hazel, M., Broitman, S., and Zamcheck, N. (1960). *Federation Proc.* **19**, 181.
Gouzon, B., Pruneyre, A., and Donnet, V. (1954). *Compt. Rend. Soc. Biol.* **148**, 2039 and 2040.
Gowdey, C. W., and Forster, K. S. (1961). *Can. Psychiat. Assoc. J.* **6**, 79.
Gowdey, C. W., McKay, A. R., and Torney, D. (1960). *Arch Intern. Pharmacodyn.* **123**, 352.
Gowen, G. F., and Lindenmuth, W. W. (1961). *J. Am. Med. Assoc.* **175**, 29.
Gözsy, B., and Kátó, L. (1960). *Arch. Intern. Pharmacodyn.* **128**, 75.
Grandjean, E., and Bättig, K. (1962). *Helv. Physiol. Pharmacol. Acta* **20**, 373.
Graux, P., Rabache, R., Milbled, G., Galibert, P., and Druart, R. (1956). *Presse Med.* **64**, 1675.
Grebennik, L. I. (1957). *Zh. Nevropatol. i Psikhiatr.* **57**, 208.
Greenberg, L., and Ingalls, J. W. (1962). *J. Pharm. Sci.* **51**, 71.
Greenberg, R., and Sabelli, H. C. (1964). *Proc. Soc. Exptl. Biol. Med.* **116**, 705.
Greenberg, S. M., Masurat, T., Rice, E. G., Herndon, J. F., and Van Loon, E. J. (1959). *Biochem. Pharmacol.* **2**, 308.
Greengard, P., and Quinn, G. P. (1962). *Ann. N.Y. Acad. Sci.* **96**, 179.
Greig, M. E., and Gibbons, A. J. (1955). *Am. J. Physiol.* **181**, 313.
Greiner, A. C., and Berry, K. (1964). *Can. Med. Assoc. J.* **90**, 663.
Greiner, A. C., and Nicolson, G. A. (1964). *Can. Med. Assoc. J.* **91**, 627.
Greiner, A. C., Nicolson, G. A., and Baker, R. A. (1964). *Can. Med. Assoc. J.* **91**, 638.
Greiner, A. C., and Nicolson, G. A. (1965a). *Can. Psychiat. Assoc. J.* **10**, 109.
Greiner, A. C., and Nicolson, G. A. (1965b). *Lancet* **II**, 1165.
Grenell, R. G., Mendelson, J., and McElroy, W. D. (1955). *A.M.A. Arch. Neurol. Psychiat.* **73**, 347.
Griffin, P. J. (1962). *Gen. Practice* **26**, 110.
Grönroos, M., Kalliomäki, J. L., Keyriläinen, T. O., and Marjanen, P. (1959). *Acta Endocrinol.* **31**, 154.
Gromova, E. A., Tkachenko, K. N., and Romanova, G. A. (1962). *Bull. Exptl. Biol. Med. USSR (English Transl.)* **52**, 1378.
Grossi, E., Paoletti, P., and Paoletti, R. (1960). *J. Neurochem.* **6**, 73
Grossman, S. P. (1961). *J. Comp. Physiol. Psychol.* **54**, 517.
Grossman, S. P., and Miller, N. E. (1961). *Psychopharmacologia* **2**, 342.
Grosz, H. J., and Norton, J. (1959). *Science* **129**, 784.
Grover, J. (1957). *Tidsskr. Norske Laegeforen.* **77**, 638.
Guerin, A. (1960). *J. Med. Bordeaux Sud-Ouest* **137**, 748.
Guha, G., Dasgupta, S. R., and Werner, G. (1954). *Bull. Calcutta School Trop. Med.* **2**, 46.
Gujral, M. L., and Dhawan, B. N. (1957). *J. Sci. Ind. Res. (India)* **16C**, 161.
Gujral, M. L., Saxena, P. N., and Khanna, B. K. (1956). *J. Indian Med. Profess.* **3**, 1098.
Gunn, C. G., Jr., Jouvet, M., and King, E. E. (1955). *Circulation* **12**, 717.
Gupta, S. K., Patel, M. A., and Joseph, A. D. (1960). *Arch. Intern. Pharmacodyn.* **128**, 82.
Guth, P. S., and Spirtes, M. A. (1961). *Biochem. Pharmacol.* **8**, 170.
Gutmann, F., and Netschey, A. (1961). *Nature* **191**, 1390.
Guttman, H. N. (1962). *International Conference on Action Mechanism and Metabolism of Psychoactive Drugs Derived from Phenothiazine and Structurally Related Compounds, Paris, Sept. 7–8.*
Guttman, H. N., and Friedman, W. (1963a). *Federation Proc.* **22**, 569.
Guttman, H. N., and Friedman, W. (1963b). *Trans. N.Y. Acad. Sci.* **26**, 75.

Gwynne, P. H., Hundziak, M., Kautschitsch, J., Lefton, M., and Pasananick, B. (1962). *J. Nervous Mental Disease* **134**, 451.
Gyermek, L. (1955). *Lancet* **II**, 724.
Gyermek, L., Lázár, I., and Csák, A. Z. (1956). *Arch. Intern. Pharmacodyn.* **107**, 62.
Haarstad, J. (1957). *Tidsskr. Norske Laegeforen.* **77**, 385.
Haase, H. J. (1963). *Deut. Med. Wochenschr.* **88**, 505.
Hackstein, F. G. (1960). *Nervenarzt* **31**, 541.
Haden, P. (1964). *Can. Med. Assoc. J.* **91**, 974.
Hadnagy, C., Eperjessy, Á., Kiss, A., Csegedy, J., Dézsi, Z., Huntz, A., and Erdei, P. (1958). *Arch. Intern. Pharmacodyn.* **117**, 395.
Häfner, H., and Kutscher, I. (1964). *Arzneimittel-Forsch.* **18**, 18.
Hafs, H. D., and Williams, J. A. (1964). *Am. J. Vet. Res.* **25**, 523.
Hagerty, R. J. (1957). *New Engl. J. Med.* **256**, 527.
Halasz, M. F., and Marrazzi, A. S. (1964). *Federation Proc.* **23**, 103.
Haley, T. J. (1957). *Acta Pharmacol. Toxicol.* **13**, 107.
Haley, T. J., McCormick, W. G., and McCulloh, E. F. (1955). *Proc. Soc. Exptl. Biol. Med.* **88**, 475.
Hall, G. H., and Ryman, B. E. (1958). *Arch. Intern. Pharmacodyn.* **117**, 81.
Hall, L. W. (1960). *Vet. Record* **72**, 85.
Hall, L. W., and Stevenson, D. E. (1960). *Nature* **187**, 696.
Halpern, B. N. (1946). *Compt. Rend. Soc. Biol.* **140**, 363.
Halpern, B. N., and Ducrot, R. (1946). *Compt. Rend. Soc. Biol.* **140**, 361.
Hamburger, C. (1955). *Acta Endocrinol.* **20**, 383.
Hamacher, J., and Hildebrandt, G. (1964). *Arzneimittel-Forsch.* **14**, 977.
Handford, S. W., Cone, T. E., Jr., Chinn, H. I., and Smith, P. K. (1954). *J. Pharmacol. Exptl. Therap.* **111**, 447.
Hankoff, L. D., Engelhardt, D. M., Freedman, N., Mann, D., and Margolis, R. (1960). *Arch. Gen. Psychiat.* **3**, 657.
Hankoff, L. D., Rudorfer, L., and Paley, H. M. (1962). *J. New Drugs* **2**, 173.
Hanson, H. M. (1964). *Federation Proc.* **23**, 104.
Hansson, E., and Schmitlerōw, C. G. (1961). *Arch. Intern. Pharmacodyn.* **131**, 309.
Hapke, II. J. (1964). *Arch Exptl. Pathol.* **247**, 307.
Hardinge, M. G. (1964). *Federation Proc.* **23**, 405.
Harper, J., and Tait, A. (1964). *Practitioner* **192**, 5.
Harpur, R. P., Swales, W. E., and Denstedt, O. R. (1950). *Can. J. Res.* **D28**, 143.
Harris, A. F., and Teodoru, C. V. (1961). *Proc. Soc. Exptl. Biol. Med.* **107**, 953.
Harris, A. F., Saifer, A., and Volk, B. W. (1960). *Proc. Soc. Exptl. Biol. Med.* **104**, 542.
Harrison, S. I., and Sawusch, R. H. (1961). *Diseases Nervous System* **22**, 282.
Hartman, D. L., and Dickey, R. F. (1964). *Skin* **3**, 198.
Harwood, C. T. (1956). *J. Clin. Endocrinol. Metab.* **16**, 938.
Harwood, C. T., and Mason, J. W. (1957). *Endocrinology* **60**, 239.
Harwood, P. D. (1953). *Exptl. Parasitol.* **2**, 428.
Hashimoto, K., Wiener, W., and Albert, J. (1965). *Clin. Res.* **13**, 530.
Haverback, B. J., Stevenson, T. D., Sjoerdsma, A., and Terry, L. L. (1955). *Am. J. Med. Sci.* **230**, 601.
Haward, L. R. C. (1964). *Brit. J. Psychiat.* **110**, 514.
Hawkins, D. R., Pace, R., Pasternack, B., and Sandifer, M. G., Jr. (1961). *Psychosomat. Med.* **23**, 1.
Haynes, E. E. (1960). *J. Lab. Clin. Med.* **56**, 570.
Hays, G. B., Lyle, C. B., and Wheeler, C. E. (1964). *Arch. Dermatol.* **90**, 471.
Hazard, R., Fanchamps, A., and Renier-Cornec, A. (1961). *Compt. Rend. Soc. Biol.* **155**, 1223.
Heilizer, F. (1959). *J. Nervous Mental Disease* **128**, 358.

Heimlich, K. R., MacDonnell, D. R., Polk, A., and Flanagan, T. L. (1961). *J. Pharm. Sci.* **50**, 213.
Heistad, G. T. (1958). *J. Comp. Physiol. Psychol.* **51**, 209.
Hemphill, R. E. (1962). *Med. J. South Wales* **77**, 18.
Henne, M., and Henne, S. (1956). *Ann. Med.-Psychol.* **114**, 309.
Henricksen, R. I., Odell, G. V., Costello, W. J., and Reuber, H. W. (1960). *J. Animal Sci.* **19**, 26.
Henriksen, U., Huus, I., and Kopf, R. (1957). *Arch. Intern. Pharmacodyn.* **109**, 39.
Herman, E. H., and Barnes, C. D. (1964). *Federation Proc.* **23**, 456.
Herr, F., Stewart, J., and Charest, M. P. (1961). *Arch. Intern. Pharmacodyn.* **134**, 328.
Hershey, S. G., Guccione, I., and Zweifach, B. W. (1955). *Surg., Gynecol. Obstet.* **101**, 431.
Herxheimer, H. (1956). *Arch. Intern. Pharmacodyn.* **106**, 371.
Hess, S. M., Yale, H., and Ebert, A. G. (1962). *International Conference on Action Mechanism and Metabolism of Psychoactive Drugs Derived from Phenothiazine and Structurally Related Compounds, Paris, Sept. 7–8.*
Hetzel, C. A. (1961). *Clin. Chem.* **7**, 130.
Heyck, H. (1962). *Nervenarzt* **33**, 66.
Heyman, J. J., and Merlis, S. (1961). *Am. J. Psychiat.* **117**, 924.
Heyman, J. J., Almudejar, M., and Merlis, S. (1959). *Am. J. Psychiat.* **116**, 259.
Heyman, J. J., Bayne, B., and Merlis, S. (1960). *Am. J. Psychiat.* **116**, 1108.
Hiebel, G., Bonvallet, M., and Dell, P. (1954). *Semaine Hop. Paris* **30**, 2346.
Hippius, H. (1965). *Anglo-German Med. Rev.* **2**, 634.
Hirsch, S., and Hirsch, D. L. (1961). *Am. J. Psychiat.* **117**, 1037.
Hoagland, R. J., and Bishop, R. H., Jr. (1961). *Am. J. Med. Sci.* **241**, 415.
Hodge, J. R. (1959). *Am. J. Psychiat.* **116**, 337.
Hoehn-Saric, R. (1964). *J. Nervous Mental Disease* **138**, 287.
Hoffenberg, R., Louw, J. H., and Voss, T. J. (1961). *Lancet* **II**, 687.
Hoffman, R. A. (1959). *Am. J. Physiol.* **196**, 876.
Hoffman, R. A., and Zarrow, M. X. (1958). *Am. J. Physiol.* **193**, 547.
Hoffmann, I., Nieschulz, O., Popendiker, K., and Tauchert, E. (1959). *Arzneimittel-Forsch.* **9**, 133.
Holliday, A. R., and Dille, J. M. (1958). *J. Comp. Physiol. Psychol.* **51**, 811.
Hollister, L. E. (1959). *J. Am. Med. Assoc.* **169**, 1235.
Hollister, L. E. (1961). *New Engl. J. Med.* **264**, 291.
Hollister, L. E. (1962). *Current Therap. Res.* **4**, 471.
Hollister, L. E. (1962). *J. Am. Med. Assoc.* **192**, 1035.
Hollister, L. E., and Kanter, S. L. (1955). *Gastroenterology* **29**, 1069.
Hollister, L. E., Traub, L. and Prusmack, J. J. (1960). *J. Neuropsychiat.* **1**, 200.
Holmstedt, B. (1964). *Acta Physiol. Scand.* **61**, 177.
Holzbauer, M., and Vogt, M. (1954). *Brit. J. Pharmacol.* **9**, 402.
Holzmann, C. (1888). *Ber. Deut. Chem. Ges.* **21**, 2069.
Hooper, J. H., Jr., Welch, V. C., and Shackelford, R. T. (1961). *J. Am. Med. Assoc.* **178**, 506.
Hoover, M. P. (1960). *Can. Med. Assoc. J.* **83**, 1352.
Hopkin, D. A. B. (1955). *Brit. Med. J.* **I**, 166.
Horclois, R. J. (1959). U.S. Patent 2,902,484.
Hordern, A. (1961). *New Engl. J. Med.* **265**, 584.
Hormia, A. (1959). *Acta Psychiat. Neurol. Scand.* **34**, 62.
Horn, L., and Converse, J. M. (1963). *Proc. Soc. Exptl. Biol. Med.* **113**, 194.
Hornykiewicz, O., Ehringer, H., and Lechner, K. (1961). *Arch. Exptl. Pathol. Pharmakol.* **241**, 198.
Horovitz, Z. P., and Chow, M. I. (1962). *J. Pharmacol. Exptl. Therap.* **137**, 127.
Horvath, S. M., Spurr, G. B., and Blatteis, C. (1956). *Am. J. Physiol.* **185**, 505.

Hoskin, F. C. G. (1960). *Biochim. Biophys. Acta* **40**, 309.
Houde, R. W., and Wallenstein, S. L. (1955). *Federation Proc.* **14**, 353.
Hougs, W., and Andersen, E. W. (1954). *Acta Pharmacol. Toxicol.* **10**, 227.
Hrdek, J. (1964). *Activatis Nervosa Super.* **6**, 73.
Hsi-Jui, W. (1961). *Bull. Exptl. Biol. Med. USSR (English Transl.)* **51**, 461.
Huang, C. L. (1962). *International Conference on Action Mechanism and Metabolism of Psychoactive Drugs Derived from Phenothiazines and Structurally Related Compounds, Paris, Sept.* 7–8.
Huang, C. L. (1964). *Am. Psychiat. Assoc. Sci. Proc.* p. 213. Los Angeles, May 4–8.
Huang, C. L., and Kurland, A. A. (1961a). *Am. J. Psychiat.* **118**, 428.
Huang, C. L., and Kurland, A. A. (1961b). *Arch. Gen. Psychiat.* **5**, 509.
Huang, C. L. and Kurland, A. A. (1961c). *Clin. Chem.* **7**, 574.
Huang, C. L., and Ruskin, . (1964). *J. Nervous Mental Disease* **139**, 381.
Huang, C. L., and Sands, F. L. (1964). *J. Chromatography* **13**, 246.
Huang, C. L., Sands, F. L., and Kurland, A. A. (1961a). *Clin. Chem.* **7**, 573.
Huang, C. L., Vyner, R. H., and Kurland, A. A. (1961b). *Clin. Chem.* **7**, 574.
Huang, C. L., Sands, F. L., and Kurland, A. A. (1963). *Arch. Gen. Psychiat.* **8**, 301.
Hudson, R. D., and Domino, E. F. (1964). *Arch. Intern. Pharmocodyn.* **147**, 36.
Huete-Armijo, A., and Exton-Smith, A. N. (1962). *Brit. Med. J.* **I**, 1113.
Hughes, F. W., and Kopmann, E. (1960). *Arch. Intern. Pharmacodyn,* **126**, 158.
Hughes, F. W., and Rountree, C. B. (1961). *Arch. Intern. Pharmacodyn.* **133**, 418.
Huidobro, F. (1954). *Arch. Intern. Pharmacodyn.* **98**, 308.
Hunder, G., and Spink, W. W. (1957). *Proc. Soc. Exptl. Biol. Med.* **95**, 55.
Hunter, R., Earl, C. J., and Thornicroft, S. (1964a). *Proc. Roy. Soc. Med.* **57**, 75.
Hunter, R., Earl, C. J., and Janz, D. (1964b). *J. Neurol. Neurosurg. Psychiat.* **27**, 219.
Huntzinger, J. A., Witoslawski, J. J., and Hanson, H. M. (1959). *J. Am. Pharm. Assoc., Sci. Ed.* **48**, 605.
Huot, L., Corrivault, G. W., and LeBlanc, J. A. (1963). *Arch. Intern. Physiol.* **71**, 215.
Hussey, L. M. (1963). *Gen. Practice* **26**, 6.
Ideström, C. M. (1960). *Acta Psychiat. Neurol. Scand.* **35**, 302.
Inglis, F. G., Hampson, L. G., and Gurd, F. R. N. (1959). *Ann. Surg.* **149**, 43.
Ingram, C. G. (1962). *Clin. Pharmacol. Therap.* **3**, 345.
Ingvar, D. H., and Söderberg, U. (1957). *A.M.A. Arch. Neurol. Psychiat.* **78**, 254.
Irwin, S. (1961). *Arch. Intern. Pharmacodyn.* **132**, 279.
Irwin, S. (1963). *Arch. Intern. Pharmacodyn.* **142**, 152.
Irwin, S. (1964). *Psychosomatics* **5**, 174.
Irwin, S., Slabok, M., and Thomas, G. (1958). *J. Pharmacol. Exptl. Therap.* **123**, 206.
Isaacs, B., and MacArthur, J. G. (1954). *Lancet* **II**, 570.
Iwasa, K., Hara, T., Hayashi, K., and Tokui, T. (1957). *Keio J. Med.* **6**, 93.
Izquierdo, I. (1962). *J. Pharm. Pharmacol.* **14**, 316.
Jackson, D., White, L., and Moyer, J. H. (1959). *Proc. Soc. Exptl. Biol. Med.* **100**, 332.
Jackson, J. (1964). *Federation Proc.* **23**, 103.
Jacob, R. M., and Jacques, G. R. (1958). U.S. Patent 2,837,518.
Jacobziner, H., and Raybin, H. W. (1958). *N.Y. State J. Med.* **58**, 1535.
Jacobziner, H., and Raybin, H. W. (1960). *N.Y. State J. Med.* **60**, 894.
Jacobziner, H., and Raybin, H. W. (1962). *N.Y. State J. Med.* **62**, 3804.
Jamieson, D., and Van Den Brenck, H. A. (1961). *Biochem. Pharmacol.* **7**, 35.
Janssen, P. A. J. (1961a). *Arzneimittel-Forsch.* **11**, 932.
Janssen, P. A. J. (1961b). *Psychopharmacologia* **2**, 141.
Janssen, P. A. J., Niemegeers, C. J. E., and Jageneau, A. H. M. (1960a). *Arzneimittel-Forsch.* **10**, 1003.
Janssen, P. A. J., Jageneau, A. H. M., and Niemegeers, C. J. E. (1960b). *J. Pharmacol. Exptl. Therap.* **129**, 471.

Janssens, J. (1954). *Nouveautes Med.* **3**, 467.
Jarrett, R. J. (1963). *Brit. J. Pharmacol.* **20**, 497.
Jasmin. G., and Bois, P. (1960). *Lab. Invest.* **9**, 503.
Jaulmes, C., Laborit, H., and Benitte, A. (1952). *Compt. Rend.* **234**, 372.
Jenkins, S. B., and Samborski, A. H. (1964). *J. Michigan State Med. Soc.* **63**, 187.
Jenkins, S. B., Revita, D. M., and Tousignant, A. (1962). *Am. J. Psychiat.* **118**, 1048.
Jindal, M. N., and Deshpande, V. R. (1961). *Arch. Intern. Pharmacodyn.* **132**, 322.
Jindal, M. N., Tiwari, N. M., and Kherdikar, P. R. (1960). *Arch. Intern. Pharmacodyn.* **129**, 166.
Jóhannesson, T., and Lausen, H. H. (1961). *Acta Pharmacol. Toxicol.* **18**, 398.
Johansson, M., Lindell, S. E., Roos, B. E., and Westling, H. (1961). *Med. Exptl.* **4**, 239.
Johnson, D. E., Rodriguez, C. F., and Burchfield, H. P. (1965). 149th Mtg. American Chemical Society, April 5, 1965, Detroit, Michigan.
Johnson, P. C., and Masters, Y. F. (1962). *J. Lab. Clin. Med.* **59**, 993.
Johnson, G. E. (1964). *Acta Physiol. Scand.* **60**, 181.
Jones, C. J., and Ripstein, C. B. (1957). *Surgery* **41**, 589.
Jongkees, L. B. W., and Philipszoon, A. J. (1960). *Acta Physiol. Pharmacol. Neerl.* **9**, 240.
Jourdan, F., Duchene-Marullaz, P., and Boissier, P. (1955). *Arch. Intern. Pharmacodyn.* **101**, 253.
Judah, J. D. (1961). *Biochim. Biophys. Acta* **53**, 375.
Judah, L. N., Josephs, Z. M., and Murphree, O. D. (1961). *Am. J. Psychiat.* **118**, 156.
Judson, A. J., and MacCasland, B. W. (1960). *J. Consulting Psychol.* **24**, 192.
Juszkiewicz, T. (1961). *Am. J. Vet. Res.* **22**, 537.
Juszkiewicz, T., and Jones, L. M. (1961a). *Am. J. Vet. Res.* **22**, 544.
Juszkiewicz, T., and Jones, L. M. (1961b). *Am. J. Vet. Res.* **22**, 553.
Kaelber, W. W., and Correll, R. E. (1958). *A.M.A. Arch. Neurol. Psychiat.* **80**, 544.
Kaelber, W. W., and Joynt, R. J. (1956). *Proc. Soc. Exptl. Biol. Med.* **92**, 399.
Kajikuri, H., Shumacker, H. B., and Riberi, A. (1957). *Ann. Surg.* **146**, 799.
Kalberer, F., and Rutschmann, J. (1963). *Helv. Chim. Acta* **46**, 586.
Kalinovskaya, R. Y. (1961). *Zh. Nevropatol. i Psikhiatr.* **61**, 1143.
Kalkoff, W. (1955). *Arch. Exptl. Pathol. Pharmakol.* **225**, 92.
Kamm, J. J., Gillette, J. R., and Brodie, B. B. (1958). *Federation Proc.* **17**, 382.
Kant, F., and Abele, H. B. (1961). *Diseases Nervous System* **22**, 45.
Karoly, A. J. (1964). *Arch. Intern. Pharmacodyn.* **148**, 40.
Karp, M., Lamb, V. E., and Benaron, H. B. W. (1955). *Am. J. Obstet. Gynecol.* **69**, 780.
Karpovich, J. A. (1962). *Zh. Nevropatol. i Psikhiatr.* **62**, 758.
Karreman, G., Isenberg, I., and Szent-Györgyi, A. (1959). *Science* **130**, 1191.
Kátó, L., and Gözsy, B. (1960). *J. Pharmacol. Exptl. Therap.* **129**, 231.
Kátó, L., and Gözsy, B. (1961a). *Indian J. Med. Res.* **49**, 788.
Kátó, L., and Gözsy, B. (1961b). *Toxicol. Appl. Pharmacol.* **3**, 145.
Kátó, L., Gözsy, B., Lehmann, H. E., and Ban, T. A. (1962). *J. Clin. Exptl. Psychopathtl.* **23**, 75.
Kátó, R. (1960). *Experientia* **16**, 427.
Kátó, R., and Chiesara, E. (1962). *Brit. J. Pharmacol.* **18**, 29.
Katona, F. (1962). *International Conference on Action Mechanism and Metabolism of Psychoactive Drugs Derived from Phenothiazine and Structurally Related Compounds, Paris, Sept.* 7–8.
Kaufmann, M. J. (1955). *Arch. Intern. Pharmacodyn.* **102**, 167.
Keating, V. (1954). *Brit. Med. J.* **II**, 470.
Kehl, R., Dumont, L., and Czyba, J. C. (1961). *Compt. Rend. Soc. Biol.* **155**, 1667.
Kelemen, K., and Bovet, D. (1961). *Acta Physiol. Acad. Sci. Hung.* **19**, 142.
Kelleher, R. T., and Cook, L. (1959). *J. Exptl. Anal. Behavior* **2**, 267.
Kelleher, R. T., Fry, W., Deegan, J., and Cook, L. (1961). *J. Pharmacol. Exptl. Therap.* **133**, 271.
Kelleher, R. T., Riddle, W. C., and Cook, L. (1962). *J. Exptl. Anal. Behavior* **5**, 3.

Kelly, R. E., and Laurence, D. R. (1956). *Lancet* **I**, 118.
Kelsey, J. R., Jr., Moyer, J. H., Brown, W. G., and Bennett, H. D. (1955). *Gastroenterology* **29**, 865.
Kent, B., Knight, R., Morris, G., Dizon, M., and Moyer, J. H. (1954a). *Med. Record. Ann.* **48**, 758.
Kent, B., Morris, G., Rogers, S., and Knight, R. (1954b). *J. Pharmacol. Exptl. Therap.* **110**, 29.
Keranen, G. M., Zaratzian, V. L., and Coleman, R. (1961). *Toxicol. Appl. Pharmacol.* **3**, 481.
Key, B. J. (1961a). *Psychopharmacologia* **2**, 352.
Key, B. J. (1961b). *Nature* **190**, 275.
Key, B. J. (1965). *Electroenceph. Clin. Neurophysiol.* **18**, 670.
Key, B. J., and Bradley, P. B. (1958). *Nature* **182**, 1517.
Key, B. J., and Bradley, P. B. (1960). *Psychopharmacologia* **1**, 450.
Khazan, N., Primo, C., Danon, A., Assael, M., Sulman, F. G., and Winnik, H. Z. (1962). *Arch. Intern. Pharmacodyn.* **136**, 291.
Khazan, N., Ben-David, M., and Sulman, F. G. (1963). *Proc. Soc. Exptl. Biol. Med.* **112**, 490.
Khouw, L. B., Burbridge, T. N., and Simon, A. (1960) *Federation Proc.* **19**, 280.
Khrabrova, O. P. (1961). *Bull. Exptl. Biol. Med. USSR (English Transl.)* **51**, 23.
Kiger, J. L., and Kiger, J. G. (1965). *Ann. Pharm. Franc.* **23**, 489.
Killam, E. K., and Killam, K. F. (1956). *J. Pharmacol. Exptl. Therap.* **116**, 35.
Kimura, T. (1957). *Japan. J. Pharmacol.* **6**, 162.
Kinbergen, B. A. (1959). "Psychopharmacology Frontiers," p. 373. Little, Brown, Boston, Massachusetts.
Kinberger, B. (1957). *Proc. Intern. Congr. Psychiat.* 1957.
Kinberger, B., and Lassenius, B. (1956). *Svenska Lakartidn.* **53**, 501.
King, P. D., and Weinberger, W. (1959). *Am. J. Psychiat.* **115**, 1026.
Kinnard, W. J., Jr., and Carr, C. J. (1957). *J. Pharmacol. Exptl. Therap.* **121**, 354.
Kinross-Wright, J. V. (1954). *Diseases Nervous System* **16**, 114.
Kinross-Wright, J. V., and Ragland, J. B. (1961). *Biochem. Pharmacol.* **8**, 46.
Kirpekar, S. M., and Lewis, J. J. (1960). *Brit. J. Pharmacol.* **15**, 175.
Kistner, R. W., and Duncan, C. J. (1956). *N. Engl. J. Med.* **254**, 507.
Kistner, S. (1960). *Acta Chem. Scand.* **14**, 1389.
Kivalo, E., Rinne, U. K., and Mäkelä, S. (1958). *Experientia* **14**, 293.
Klatskin, G. (1961). *Bull. N.Y. Acad. Med.* **37**, 767.
Kleinsorge, H., Thalmann, K., and Rosner, K. (1959). *Arzneimittel-Forsch.* **9**, 121.
Klett, C. J., and Caffey, E. M., Jr. (1960). *J. Neuropsychiat.* **2**, 102.
Kline, N. S., Barsa, J., and Gosline, E. (1956). *Diseases Nervous System* **17**, 352.
Klugman, S. (1960). *Chemotherapy Psychiat.* **4**, 111.
Knox, J. M. (1961). *Ann. Allergy* **19**, 749.
Kochhar, K. S. (1961). *Brit. Med. J.* **II**, 789.
Koeze, T. H., and Telford, I. R. (1958). *Proc. Soc. Exptl. Biol. Med.* **98**, 775.
Kohl, H. H., Kamano, A., and Haber, B. (1964). *Federation Proc.* **23**, 489.
Kohn, N. N., and Myerson, R. M. (1961). *Am. J. Med.* **31**, 665.
Kok, K. (1955). *Acta Physiol. Pharmacol. Neerl.* **4**, 388.
Kok, K. (1956). *Acta Physiol. Pharmacol. Neerl.* **5**, 1.
Kollias, J. and Bullard, R. W. (1964). *J. Pharmacol. Exptl. Therap.* **45**, 373.
Kopeloff, L. M., Chusid, J. G., and Kopeloff, N. (1955). *Proc. Soc. Exptl. Biol. Med.* **90**, 282.
Kopera, J., and Armitage, A. K. (1954). *Brit. J. Pharmacol.* **9**, 392.
Kopmann, E., and Hughes, F. W. (1958). *Experientia* **14**, 301.
Kornetsky, C., and Humphries, O. (1958). *J. Mental Sci.* **104**, 1093.
Kornetsky, C., and Orzack, M. H. (1964). *Psychopharmacologia* **6**, 79.
Kornetsky, C., Pettit, M., Wynne, R., and Evarts, E. (1958). *Federation Proc.* **17**, 385.
Kornetsky, C., Pettit, M., Wynne, R., and Evarts, E. (1959a). *J. Mental Sci.* **105**, 190.

Kornetsky, C., Vates, T. S., and Kessler, E. K. (1959b). *J. Pharmacol. Exptl. Therap.* **127**, 51.
Korneva, E. A., and Yakovleva, M. I. (1962). *Bull. Exptl. Biol. Med. USSR (English Transl.)* **53**, 78.
Kosir, B., and Kosir, J. (1956). *Acta Pharm. Jugoslav.* **6**, 671.
Kotionis, A. Z. (1961). *Arzneimittel.-Forsch.* **11**, 108.
Kotkin, S., Lear, E., Chiron, A. E., Pallin, I. M., and Dickler, D. (1956). *Anesthesiology* **17**, 494.
Kovács, B. M., Kovács, G. S., and Petri, G. (1956). *Experientia* **12**, 376.
Kovács, K., Horváth, E., Kovács, B. M., Kovács, G. S., and Petri, G. (1956). *Arch. Intern. Pharmacodyn.* **108**, 170.
Kovács, K., Kovács, G. S., Kovács, B. M., and Petri, G. (1957). *Arch. Intern. Pharmacodyn.* **109**, 1.
Kovitz, B., Carter, J. T., and Addison, W. P. (1955). *A.M.A. Arch. Neurol. Psychiat.* **74**, 467.
Kozák, J., Lang, N., and Zelený, A. (1958). *Experientia* **15**, 454.
Kozák, J., Zelený, A., and Lang, N. (1960). *Nature* **185**, 107.
Kraines, S. H. (1963). *Diseases Nervous System* **24**, 181.
Krais, W. (1955). *Medizinische* **51**, 1779.
Krais, W., Lehr, H., and Riess, W. (1954). *Arch. Gynaekol.* **185**, 40.
Krais, W., Lehr, H., and Riess, W. (1954b). *Arch. Gynaekol.* **185**, 248.
Krause, D., and Schmidtke-Ruhnau, D. (1955). *Arch. Exptl. Pathol. Pharmakol.* **226**, 243.
Kreindler, A., Zuckerman, E., Steriade, M., and Chimion, D. (1959). *Arch. Intern. Pharmacodyn.* **120**, 263.
Kris, E. B. (1962). *Recent. Advan. Biol. Psychiat.*, Plenum Press., **4**, 180.
Kris, E. B., and Carmichael, D. M. (1957). *Psychiat. Quart.* **31**, 690.
Krishna, S., and Jain, M. S. (1931). *Proc. 15th Indian Sci. Congr.*, 1928, p. 153.
Krivoy, W. A. (1957). *Proc. Soc. Exptl. Biol. Med.* **96**, 18.
Krivoy, W. A., and Guillemin, R. (1962). *Experientia* **18**, 20.
Krivoy, W. A., and Kroeger, D. C. (1962). *Proc. Soc. Exptl. Biol. Med.* **109**, 30.
Kruger, S., Robison, G. A., and Schueler, F. W. (1960). *Arch. Intern. Pharmacodyn.* **129**, 125.
Kuchler, A., and Koch, R. (1954). *Klin. Wochschr.* **32**, 1098.
Kuchler, A., and Koch, R. (1955). *Klin. Wochschr.* **33**, 426.
Kulikov, L. S. (1961). *Zh. Nevropatol. i Psikhiatr.* **61**, 201.
Kum-Tatt, L. (1962). *Anal. Chim. Acta* **26**, 285.
Kum-Tatt, L., and Tong, H. K. (1962). *Anal. Chim. Acta* **26**, 583.
Kurland, A. A., Hanlon, T. E., Tatom, M. H., Ota, K. Y., and Simopoulos, A. M. (1961a). *J. Nervous Mental Disease* **133**, 1.
Kurland, A. A., Hanlon, T. E., Tatom, M. H., and Simopoulos, A. M. (1961b). *J. Nervous Mental Disease* **132**, 61.
Kurland, A. A., and Huang, C. L. (1962). *International Conference on Action Mechanism and Metabolism of Psychoactive Drugs Derived from Phenothiazine and Structurally Related Compounds*, Paris, Sept. 7–8; *Psychopharmacol. Serv. Center Bull.*, **2** (1962).
Kurland, A. A., Huang, C. L., Hallam, K. J., and Hanlon, T. E. (1965). *J. Psych. Res.* **3**, 27.
Kurland, A. A., Michaux, M. H., Hanlon, T. E., Ota, K. Y., and Simopoulos, A. M. (1962). *J. Nervous Mental Disease* **134**, 48.
Kutin, V. P. (1961). *Zh. Nevropatol. i Psikhiatr.* **61**, 228.
Laborit, H. (1964). *Presse Med.* **72**, 1.
Laborit, H., and Huguenard, P. (1951). *Presse Med.* **59**, 1329.
Laborit, H., Huguenard, P., and Alluaume, R. (1952a). *Presse Med.* **60**, 206–347.
Laborit, H., Jaulmes, C., and Benitte, A. (1952b). *Anesthesie Analgesie* **9**, 232.
Laborit, H., Drouet, J., Gerard, J., Jouany, J. M., Nervacs, C., Niaussat, P., and Weber, B. (1960). *Intern. Record Med.* **173**, 351.

Laborit, H., Leterrier, F., and Brue, F. (1962). *International Conference on Action Mechanisms and Metabolism of Psychoactive Drugs Derived from Phenothiazine and Structurally Related Compounds, Paris, Sept.* 7-8.
Lacomme, M., and LeLorier, G. (1955). *Bull. Federation Soc. Gynecol. Obstet. Langue Franc.* **7**, 119.
Lacassagne, A. (1959). *Compt. Rend.* **249**, 903.
Ladinskaya, M. Y. (1958). *Bull. Exptl. Biol. Med. USSR (English Transl.)* **44**, 1491.
Lagercrantz, C. (1961). *Acta Chem. Scand.* **15**, 1545.
Lagercrantz, C. (1962). *International Conference on Action Mechanism and Metabolism of Psychoactive Drugs Derived from Phenothiazine and Structurally Related Compounds, Paris, Sept.* 7-8.
Lagercrantz, C., and Yhland, M. (1962). *Acta Chem. Scand.* **16**, 508.
Lamarche, M., and Arnould, P. (1954). *Compt. Rend. Soc. Biol.* **148**, 565.
Lambertsen, C. J., Wendel, H., and Longenhagen, J. B. (1961). *J. Pharmacol. Exptl. Therap.* **131**, 381.
Lancaster, N. P., and Jones, D. H. (1954). *Brit. Med. J.* **II**, 565.
Langeron, L., Noif, N., Fruchart, G., Destombes, N., and Lemaire, E. (1956). *J. Sci. Med. Lille* **74**, 16.
Laporte, J. (1964). *J. Med. Exp.* (Basel) **10**, 369.
Larsson, S. (1961). *Acta Physiol. Scand.* **53**, 68.
Lasagna, L., and McCann, W. P. (1957). *Science* **125**, 1241.
Lasagna, L., De Kornfeld, J. J., and Pearson, J. W. (1963). Private communication.
Lasky, J. J., Klett, C. J., Caffey, E. M., Bennett, J. L., Rosenblum, M. P., and Hollister, L. E. (1962). *Diseases Nervous System* **23**, 698.
Laties, V. G., and Weiss, B. (1964). *Federation Proc.* **23**, 104.
Laurence, D. R., and Webster, R. A. (1958). *Brit. J. Pharmacol.* **13**, 334.
Laurence, D. R., and Webster, R. A. (1961). *Brit. J. Pharmacol.* **16**, 296.
Laxdal, O. E., Khera, S., and Haworth, D. H. (1961). *Can. Med. Assoc. J.* **84**, 828.
Lazarus, M., and Rogers, W. P. (1951). *Can. J. Res.* **29E**, 163.
Leach, H., and Crimmin, W. R. C. (1956). *J. Clin. Pathol.* **9**, 164.
Lear, E., Chiron, A. E., and Pallin, I. M. (1955). *N.Y. State J. Med.* **55**, 1853.
Lear, E., Suntay, R., Fisch, H. J., Chiron, A. E., and Pallin, I. M. (1961). *Anesthesiology* **22**, 529.
Leary, R. W., and Stynes, A. J (1959). *A.M.A. Arch. Gen. Psychiat.* **1**, 67.
LeBlanc, J. A. (1958a). *J. Appl. Physiol.* **13**, 237.
LeBlanc, J. A. (1958b). *Proc. Soc. Exptl. Biol. Med.* **97**, 238.
LeBlanc, J. A. (1958c). *Proc. Soc. Exptl. Biol. Med.* **98**, 406.
LeBlanc, J. A. (1958d). *Proc. Soc. Exptl. Biol. Med.* **98**, 648.
LeBlanc, J. A. (1959). *Proc. Soc. Exptl. Biol. Med.* **100**, 635.
LeBlanc, J. A. (1960a). *Proc. Soc. Exptl. Biol. Med.* **103**, 621.
LeBlanc, J. A. (1960b). *Proc. Soc. Exptl. Biol. Med.* **105**, 109.
LeBlanc, J. A., and Rosenberg, F. (1958). *Proc. Soc. Exptl. Biol. Med.* **97**, 95.
Le Breton, R., Rondepierre, J. J., Ropert, R., and Nizard, I. (1962). *Ann. Med. Psychol.* **120**, No. 1, 755.
Lechner, H., Mayr, F., Geyer, N., and Rodler, H. (1961). *Med. Exptl.* **5**, 291.
Lehman, H. E. (1964). *Comprehensive Psychiat.* **5**, 36.
Lehmann, H. E., and Hanrahan, G. E. (1954). *A.M.A. Arch. Neurol. Psychiat.* **71**, 227.
Léider, L. L. (1964). *Postgrad. Med.* **35**, A-22.
Leme, J. G., and Rocha e Silva, M. (1961). *J. Pharm. Pharmacol.* **13**, 734.
Lenke, D. (1961). *Arzneimittel-Forsch.* **11**, 874.
Lesinski, J., and Podlewska, A. (1957). *Ginekol. Polska* **28**, 669.
Lessin, A. W. (1959). *Brit. J. Pharmacol.* **14**, 251.
Lessin, A. W., and Parkes, M. W. (1957). *Brit. J. Pharmacol.* **12**, 245.
Lester, E. P., Wittkower, E. D., Kalz, F., and Azima, H. (1962). *Am. J. Psychiat.* **119**, 136.

Le Vay, M. K. (1960). *Lancet* **II**, 1403.
Levin, M. L. (1959). *J. Consulting Psychol.* **23**, 167.
Levine, J., Levine, D., and Small, S. M. (1961). *Am. J. Psychiat.* **117**, 747.
Levine, S., and Klein, M. (1959). *Proc. Soc. Exptl. Biol. Med.* **102**, 192.
Lewis, J. J. (1964). *Practitioner* **192**, 12.
Lewis, W. H., Jr., Richardson, D. J., and Gahagan, L. H. (1955). *New Engl. J. Med.* **252**, 1016.
Liberson, W. T. (1964). *J. Nervous Mental Disease* **138**, 131.
Liberson, W. T., Karczmar, A., Schwartz, E., Ellen, P., and Thomas, L. (1962). *International Conference on Action Mechanism and Metabolism of Psychoactive Drugs Derived from Phenothiazine and Related Compounds*, Paris, Sept. 7–8; (1963), *Psychopharmacol. Serv. Center Bull.* **2**, 79.
Liljestrand, A. (1965). *Svenska a Kartidn.* **62**, (Suppl. II), 63.
Lillehei, R. C. (1963). *Am. J. Cardiol.* **12**, 599.
Lin, T. H., and Reynolds, L. W. (1960). *Am. J. Psychiat.* **116**, 752.
Lin, T. H., Reynolds, L. W., Rondish, I. M., and Van Loon, E. J. (1959). *Proc. Soc. Exptl. Biol. Med.* **102**, 602.
Lindan, O., Quastel, J. H., and Sved, S. (1957). *Can. J. Biochem. Physiol.* **35**, 1145.
Lipton, B., and Hershey, S. G. (1955). *N.Y. State J. Med.* **55**, 2463.
Litin, E. H. (1964). *Minnesota Med.* **47**, 547.
Litteral, E. B. (1955). *Psychiat. Res. Rept.* **1**, 63.
Loewe, S. (1956). *Arch. Intern. Pharmacodyn.* **158**, 453.
Loftus, T. A., Clark, D. L., Crouse, F. R., Dillon, T. E., Jones, D. J., III, and Lefever, H. E., Jr. (1961). *Psychiat. Quart.* **35**, 121.
Long, J. P., Lands, A. M., and Zenitz, B. L. (1957). *J. Pharmacol. Exptl. Therap.* **119**, 479.
Long, R. F., and Lessin, A. W. (1962). *Biochem. J.* **82**, 4P.
Longo, V. G., Von Berger, G. P., and Bovet, D. (1954). *J. Pharmacol. Exptl. Therap.* **111**, 349.
Lorr, M., McNair, D. M., Weinstein, G. J., Michaux, W. W., and Raskin, A. (1961). *Arch. Gen. Psychiat.* **4**, 381.
Lovett Doust, J. W., and Harrington, R. W. (1962). *Can. Psychiat. Assoc. J.* **7**, 76.
Løvtrup, S. (1964). *J. Neurochem.* **11**, 377.
Low, H. (1959). *Biochim. Biophys. Acta* **32**, 11.
Lubin, G. T., Crockett, J. T., Eiduson, S., and Cohen, S. (1960). *Trans. 4th Res. Conf. Chemotherapy Psychiat.*, VA, Washington, D.C. **4**, 251.
Lucas, G. H., and Fabierkiewicz, C. (1963). *J. Forensic Sci.* **8**, 462.
Lutzenkirchen, A., and Schoog, M. (1954). *Arzneimittel-Forsch.* **4**, 560.
Mackiewicz, J., and Gershon, S. (1964). *J. Neuropsychiat.* **5**, 159.
McCarthy, D. A., Burns, R. H., Deneau, G. A., and Seevers, M. H. (1958). *Bull. Drug Addict. Narcotics* Add. 2, p. 15.
McCarthy, D. A., Deneau, G. A., and Seevers, M. H. (1960). *Bull. Drug Addict. Narcotics* Add. 7, p. 2225.
McCourt, W. F., Sidley, N. T., Browne, I., and Solomon, P. (1961). *New Engl. J. Med.* **265**, 201.
McDonald, J. K. (1962). *Am. J. Psychiat.* **118**, 746.
McDonald, R. K., and Weise, V. K. (1962). *J. Pharmacol. Exptl. Therap.* **136**, 26.
McGinn, J. T., and Avram, M. M. (1966). *J. Am. Med. Assoc.* **197**, 142.
McGrath, W. R., and Jenkins, H. J. (1958). *J. Am. Pharm. Assoc. Sci. Ed.* **47**, 827.
McIlwain, H., and Greengard, O. (1957). *J. Neurochem.* **1**, 348.
Macko, E., Scheidy, S. F., and Tucker, R. G. (1958). *Vet. Med.* **53**, 378.
McLaughlan, J. M., Shenoy, K. G., and Campbell, J. A. (1961). *J. Pharm. Sci.* **50**, 59.
McNichol, R. W., and Seale, A. L. (1964). *Diseases Nervous System* **25**, 240.
Madjerek, Z., and Stern, P. (1956). *Arch. Intern. Pharmacodyn.* **104**, 404.
Maffii, G. (1959). *J. Pharm. Pharmacol.* **11**, 129.

Magee, W. L., and Rossiter. R. J. (1963). *Can. J. Biochem, Physiol.* **41**, 1155.
Magee, W. L., Berry, J. F., and Rossiter, R. J. (1956). *Biochim. Biophys. Acta* **21**, 408.
Mahfouz, M., and Ezz, E. A. (1958). *J. Pharmacol. Exptl. Therap.* **123**, 39.
Mahrer, P. R., Bergman, P. S., and Estren, S. (1958). *Am. J. Psychiat.* **115**, 337.
Maickel, R. P., Stern, D. N., and Takabataki, T. (1964). *Federation Proc.* **23**, 567.
Maier, A., Forster, E., and Kayser, C. (1955). *Compt. Rend. Soc. Biol.* **149**, 398.
Maier, A., Forster, E., Schaff, G., and Kayser, C. (1955b). *Compt. Rend. Soc. Biol.* **149**, 568.
Malhotra, C. L., and Prasad, K. (1962). *Brit. J. Pharmacol.* **18**, 595.
Mallov, S., and Witt, P. N. (1961). *J. Pharmacol. Exptl. Therap.* **132**, 126.
Malmejac, J., Chardon, G., and Neverre, G. (1954). *Compt. Rend. Soc. Biol.* **148**, 1397.
Malossi, M. (1962). *Boll. Soc. Ital. Biol. Sper.* **38**, 102.
Mandel, W., and Oliver, W. A. (1961). *Am. J. Psychiat.* **118**, 350.
Mandell, A. J. (1963). *Am. Heart J.* **65**, 572.
Manghi, E. (1954). *Giorn. Psichiat. Neuropatol.* **82**, 959.
Marconi, M. (1961). *Clin. Terap.* **20**, 274.
Marcus, S., and Sperling. H. H. (1960). *Calif. Med.* **92**, 226.
Margolis, L. H., and Goble, S. L. (1965). *J. Am. Med. Assoc.* **193**, 7.
Marks, V., and Shackcloth, P. (1963). *Brit. Med. J.* **II**, 52.
Marocco, F., and Brena, S. (1953). *Minerva Anestesiol.* **19**, 332.
Marquardt, P. (1953). *Therapie* **8**, 787.
Marquardt, P., Puppel, H., and Schumacher, H. (1955). *Klin. Wochschr.* **33**, 211.
Marrazzi, A. S., and Hart, E. R. (1956). *J. Nervous Mental Disease* **124**, 388.
Mars, G., and Morpurgo, M. (1955). *J. Am. Med. Assoc.* **159**, 816.
Martin, G. J., Brendel, R., and Beiler, J. M. (1956). *Arzneimittel-Forsch* **6**, 408.
Martin, W. R., and Eades, C. G. (1960). *Psychopharmacologia* **1**, 303.
Martin, W. R., DeMaar, E. W. J., and Unna, K. R. (1958). *J. Pharmacol. Exptl. Therap.* **122**, 343.
Martin, W. R., Riehl, J. L., and Unna, K. R. (1960). *J. Pharmacol. Exptl. Therap.* **130**, 37.
Mashkovsky, M. D. (1956). *Zh. Nevropatol. i Psikhiatr.* **56**, 81.
Mashkovsky, M. D., and Medvedev, B. A. (1956). *Bull. Exptl. Biol. Med. (USSR) (English Transl.)* **41**, 335.
Mason-Browne, N. L. (1958). *Can. Med. Assoc. J.* **79**, 985.
Masse, G., and Chollot, M.-L. (1962). *Compt. Rend. Soc. Biol.* **156**, 145.
Massey, L. W. C. (1965). *Can. Med. Assoc. J.* **92**, 186.
Massie, S. (1954). *Chem. Rev.* **54**, 797.
Masson, G. M. C., Corcoran, A. C., and Franco-Browder, S. (1958). *Am. J. Physiol.* **195**, 407.
Masson, G. M. C., Nairn, R. C., and Corcoran, A. C. (1955). *Endocrinology* **57**, 670.
Massonnat, J., and Arroyo, H. (1958). *Presse Med.* **66**, 963.
Master, R. S. (1964). *Am. J. Psychiat.* **120**, 1126.
Masurat, T., Greenberg, S. M., Rice, E. G., Herndon, J. F., and Van Loon, E. J. (1960). *Biochem. Pharmacol.* **5**, 20.
Mathalone, M. B. R. (1965). *Lancet* **II**, 240.
Máthé, V., Kassay, G., and Hunkar, K. (1961). *Psychopharmacologia* **2**, 334.
Mathues, J. K., Greenberg, S. M., Herndon, J. F., Parmelee, E. T., and Van Loon, E. J. (1959). *Proc. Soc. Exptl. Biol. Med.* **102**, 594.
Mauceri, J., and Strauss, H. (1956). *Electroencephalog. Clin. Neurophysiol.* **8**, 671.
May, A. R., Whiteley, J. S., and Gradwell, B. G. (1959). *J. Mental Sci.* **105**, 1059.
Mayer, S. W., Kelly, F. H., Morton, M. E. (1956). *J. Pharmacol. Exptl. Therap.* **117**, 197.
Mazurkiewicz, I. M., and Lu, F. C. (1960). *J. Pharm. Pharmacol.* **12**, 103.
Mead, B. T., Ellsworth, R. B., and Grimmett, J. D. (1958). *J. Nervous Mental Disease* **127**, 351.
Mefferd, R. B., Labrosse, E. H., Gawienowski, A. M., and Williams, R. J. (1958). *J. Nervous Mental Disease* **127**, 167.

Meidinger, F. (1955). *Compt. Rend. Soc. Biol.* **149**, 1426.
Meidinger, F. (1956). *Compt. Rend. Soc. Biol.* **150**, 1340.
Meier, R., Bruni, C., and Tripod, J. (1955). *Arch. Intern. Pharmacodyn.* **104**, 137.
Mellinger, T. J., and Keeler, C. E. (1962). *J. Pharm. Sci.* **51**, 1169.
Melville, K. I. (1954). *Federation Proc.* **13**, 386.
Melville, K. I. (1958). *Arch. Intern. Pharmacodyn.* **115**, 278.
Mendelsohn, R. M., Penman, A. S., and Schiele, B. C. (1959). *Psychiat. Quart.* **33**, 55.
Menguy, R. B., Grindlay, J. H., and Cain, J. B. (1955). *Proc. Staff Meetings Mayo Clinic* **30**, 601.
Mennear, J. H., Miya, T. S., and Yim, G. K. W. (1962). *J. Pharm. Sci.* **51**, 420.
Mercier, J. (1955). *Compt. Rend. Soc. Biol.* **149**, 379.
Mercier, J., and Dessaigne, S. (1962). *Compt. Rend. Soc. Biol.* **156**, 110.
Mercier, J., Dessaigne, S., and Etzensperger, P. (1962). *Ann. Pharm. Franc.* **20**, 131.
Merck Index (1960). 7th Ed., Rahway, New Jersey.
Merkle, F. H. (1964). *J. Pharm. Sci.* **53**, 965.
Messer, M. (1958). *Australian J. Exptl. Biol. Med. Sci.* **36**, 65.
Metcalf, R. L. (1948). *Chemistry Biology Coordination Center, National Research Council*, Review No. 1, Washington, D.C.
Meyer, H. J. and Meyer-Burg, J. (1964). *Arch. Intern. Pharmacodyn.* **148**, 97.
Meyer, V., and Jacobsen, P. (1920). "Lehrbuch der Organischen Chemie," Vol 2, p. 1490. Veit, Leipzig.
Meyre, F. (1957). *Arzneimittel-Forsch.* **7**, 296.
Michaux, M. H., Hanlon, T. E., Ota, K. Y., and Kurland, A. A. (1964). *Current Therap. Res.* **6**, 331.
Michaux, W. W. (1961). *J. Nervous Mental Disease* **133**, 203.
Milcou, S. M., Negoesco, I., Lupulesco, A., and Cocou, F. (1957). *Ann. Endocrinol. (Paris)* **18**, 902.
Miletzky, O., Rieunau, J., and Espagno, G. (1955). *Anesthesie Analgesie* **12**, 495.
Millar, R. A., and Benfey, B. G. (1959). *Brit. J. Anaesthesia* **31**, 258.
Miller, R. E., Murphy, J. V., and Mirsky, I. A. (1957a). *J. Pharmacol. Exptl. Therap.* **120**, 379.
Miller, R. E., Murphy, J. V., and Mirsky, I. A. (1957b). *A.M.A. Arch. Neurol. Psychiat.* **78**, 526.
Millican, R. C., and Rhodes, C. J. (1958a). *J. Pharmacol Exptl. Therap.* **122**, 255.
Millican, R. C., and Rhodes, C. J. (1958b). *J. Pharmacol. Exptl. Therap.* **122**, 262.
Milligan, W. L. (1962). *Med. Proc. (Johannesburg)*, **8**, 237.
Milne, J. J. (1959). *J. Am. Pharm. Assoc., Sci. Ed.* **48**, 117.
Milne, J. B., and Chatten, L. G. (1957). *J. Pharm. Pharmacol.* **9**, 686.
Minard, F. N., and Davis, R. V. (1962). *Nature* **193**, 277.
Minchin, R. L. H., and Holdaway, I. (1964). *Brit. J. Psychiat.* **110**, 411.
Mirsky, A. F. (1959). *J. Nervous Mental Disease* **128**, 12.
Mirsky, A. F., and Cardon, P. V., Jr. (1962). *Electroencephalog. Clin. Neurophysiol.* **14**, 1.
Mitchell, J. C., and King, F. A. (1960). *Psychopharmacologia* **1**, 463.
Moe, R., Bagdon, R., and Zbinden, G. (1962). *Angiology* **13**, 4.
Moffitt, E. A., Dawson, B., and O'Neill, N. C. (1961). *Anesthesia Analgesia, Current Res.* **40**, 483.
Monnier, M., and Krupp, P. (1959). *Schweiz. Med. Wochschr.* **89**, 430.
Monroe, R. R., Heath, R. G., and Mickle, W. A. (1955). *Ann. N.Y. Acad. Sci.* **61**, 56.
Moraczewski, A. S., and DuBois, K. P. (1959). *Arch. Intern. Pharmacodyn.* **120**, 201.
Moran, N. C., and Butler, W. M. (1956). *J. Pharmacol. Exptl. Therap.* **118**, 328.
Moran, N. C., and Perkins, M. E. (1961). *J. Pharmacol. Therap.* **133**, 192.
Morand, P., and Gay, J. L. (1953). *Compt. Rend. Soc. Biol.* **147**, 1447.
Morbidity and Mortality (1963). Weekly Report. U.S. Public Health Service, Aug. 9.
Moriarity, A. J. (1963). *Can. Med. Assoc. J.* **88**, 97.
Moriarity, A. J., and Nance, M. R. (1963). *Can. Med. Assoc. J.* **88**, 375.
Morocutti, C. (1957). *Riv. Neurobiol.* **3**, 523.

Morozova, T. N. (1961). *Zh. Nevropatol. i Psikhiatr.* **61**, 589.
Morpurgo, C. (1962). *Biochem. Pharmacol.* **11**, 967.
Morrell, F., and Baker, L. (1961). *Neurology* **11**, 651.
Morris, G., Pontius, R., Herschberger, R., and Moyer, J. H. (1955). *Federation Proc.* **14**, 371.
Moses, A. H. (1964). *Endocrinology* **74**, 889.
Moss, C. S., Jenson, R. E., Morrow, W., and Freund, H. G. (1958). *Am. J. Psychiat.* **115**, 449.
Motz, G. (1955). *Dissertation Abstr.* **15**, 1903.
Moyer, J. H. (1955). *Intern. Record Med.* **168**, 301.
Moyer, J. H., Kent, B., Knight, R. W., Morris, G., Dizon, M., Rogers, S., and Spurr, C. (1954a). *Am. J. Med. Sci.* **228**, 174.
Moyer, J. H., Kent, B., Knight, R., Morris, G., Huggins, R., and Handley, C. A. (1954b). *Am. J. Med. Sci.* **227**, 283.
Moyer, J. H., Greenfield, L., Heider, C., and Handley, C. (1957). *Ann. Surg.* **146**, 12.
Mráz, M. (1963). *Arch. Intern. Pharmacodyn.* **141**, 423.
Murphree, H. B. (1962). *Clin. Pharmacol. Therap.* **3**, 314.
Murphree, O. D., Monroe, B. L., and Seager, L. D. (1962). *J. Neuropsychiat.* **3**, 295.
Murphree, O. D., and Peters, J. E. (1956). *J. Nervous Mental Disease* **124**, 78.
Murphy, C. M., Rainer, H., and Smith, N. L. (1950). *Anal. Chem.* **42**, 2479.
Nadeau, G., and Sobolewski, G. (1959a). *J. Chromatog.* **2**, 544.
Nadeau, G., and Sobolewski, G. (1959b). *Can. Med. Assoc. J.* **80**, 826.
Nadeau, G., and Sobolewski, G. (1959c). *Can. Med. Assoc. J.* **81**, 658.
Nasmyth, P. A. (1955). *Brit. J. Pharmacol.* **10**, 336.
Nathan, H. A., and Friedman, W. (1962). *Science* **135**, 793.
Negwer, M. (1961). "Organisch-Chemische Arzneimittel," Akademie Verlag, Berlin.
Nellhaus, G. (1959). *Pediatrics* **23**, 1018.
Nelson, N. M. (1959). *New Engl. J. Med.* **260**, 1296.
Nelson, R. D. (1951). Ph.D. Thesis, Iowa State College, Ames, Iowa.
Neuhoff, E. W., and Auterhoff, H. (1955). *Arch. Pharm.* **288**, 400.
Neuman, M. (1960). *Nouveautes Med.* **9**, 181.
Neve, H. K. (1958). *J. Mental Sci.* **104**, 488.
Neve, H. K. (1961). *Acta Pharmacol. Toxicol.* **17**, 404.
Ngai, S. H., Wang, S. C. (1955). *J. Pharmacol. Exptl. Therap.* **113**, 41a.
Nicholson, G. A., Greiner, A. C., McFarlane, W. J. G., and Baker, R. A. (1966). *Lancet* **I**, 344.
Nieschulz, O., Hoffmann, I., and Popendiker, K. (1956). *Arzneimittel-Forsch.* **6**, 651.
Nikitina, G. M. (1961). *Pavlov J. Higher Nervous Activity (English Transl.)* **11**, 341.
Nishizono, M. (1964). *Psychosomatics* **5**, 34.
Noack, H. (1963). *Zentr. Gynaekol.* **85**, 938.
Noble, R. C., and Castner, C. W. (1962). *Diseases Nervous System* **19**, 531.
Nodiff, E. A., and Hausman, M. (1964). *J. Org. Chem.* **29**, 2453.
Nodiff, E. A., Lipschutz, S., Craig, P. N., and Gordon, M. (1960). *J. Org. Chem.* **25**, 60.
Nodine, J. H. (1963). *Psychosomatics* **3**, 351.
Norman, D., and Hiestand, W. A. (1955a). *Anat. Record* **122**, 461.
Norman, D., and Hiestand, W. A. (1955b). *Proc. Soc. Exptl. Biol. Med.* **90**, 89.
Noyes, H. E., Sanford, J. P., and Nelson, R. M. (1956). *Proc. Soc. Exptl. Biol. Med.* **92**, 617.
Ogasawara, J., and Nakayama, M. (1958). *Virology* **6**, 288.
Ogasawara, K., and Yasue, T. (1959). *Virology* **8**, 268.
Ogawa, Y., Kawasaki, A., and Yamamoto, K. (1958). *Ann. Rept. Shiongi Res. Lab.* 229.
Ohler, E. A., Sevy, R. W., and Weiner, A. (1956). *J. Clin. Endocrinol. Metab.* **16**, 915.
Olds, J. (1958). *Science* **127**, 315.
Olds, J., Killam, K. F., and Bach-Y-Rita, P. (1956). *Science* **124**, 265.
Olds, M. E. (1964). *Am. J. Physiol.* **206**, 515.
Ollendorff, H. V. (1960). *Am. J. Psychiat.* **116**, 729.

Olling, C. C. J., and de Wied, D. (1956a). *Acta Endocrinol.* **22**, 283.
Olling, C. C. J., and de Wied, D. (1956b). *Acta Physiol. Pharmacol. Neerl.* **5**, 240.
Olmstead, M. P., Craig, P. N., Lafferty, J. J., Pavloff, A. M., and Zirkle, C. L. (1961). *J. Org. Chem.* **26**, 1901.
Omarova, V. A. (1958). *Farmakol. i Toksikol.* **21**, No. 6, 14.
Opitz, K. (1962a). *Arzneimittel-Forsch.* **12**, 333.
Opitz, K. (1962b). *Arzneimittel-Forsch.* **12**, 525.
Opitz, K. (1962c). *Arzneimittel-Forsch.* **12**, 618.
Opitz, K., and Loeser, A. (1962). *Deut. Med. Wochschr.* **87**, 105.
Orgel, S. Z. (1962). *N.Y. State J. Med.* **62**, 2378.
Orloff, M. K., and Fitts, D. D. (1961). *Biochim. Biophys. Acta* **47**, 529.
Otis, L. S. (1964). *Science* **143**, 1347.
Overton, R. C., and DeBakey, M. E. (1956). *Ann. Surg.* **143**, 439.
Paasonen, M. K. (1964). *Arch. Exptl. Pathol. Pharmakol.* **248**, 223.
Palazzetti, P., and Torsello, R. (1955). *Minerva Ginecol.* **7**, 819.
Parker, K. D., Fontan, C. R., and Kirk, P. L. (1963a). *Anal. Chem.* **35**, 356.
Parker, K. D., Fontan, C. R., and Kirk, P. L. (1963b). *Anal. Chem.* **34**, 757.
Parrish, A. E., and Levine, E. H. (1956). *Clin. Res. Proc.* **4**, No. 1, 42.
Paul, S. D., and Leopold, I. H. (1956a). *Am. J. Ophthalmol.* **42**, 107.
Paul, S. D., and Leopold, I. H. (1956b). *Am. J. Opthalmol.* **42**, 752.
Paulson, G. (1960). *Diseases Nervous System* **21**, 447.
Pearl, D. (1960). *Chemotherapy Psychiat.* **4**, 99.
Pearl, D., Herman, L., Vander Kamp, H., Olson, A., and Armitage, S. G. (1958). *Psychiat. Quart.* **32**, 565.
Pennington, V. M. (1962). *Am. J. Psychiat.* **118**, 935.
Perrot, and Bourjala (1962). *Bull. Soc. Franc. Dermatol. Syph.* **69**, 631.
Perry, T. L., Culling, C. F. A., Berry, K., and Hansen, S. (1964). *Science* **146**, 81.
Peruzzo, L., and Forni, R. B. (1953a). *J. Am. Med. Assoc.* **154**, 722.
Peruzzo, L., and Forni, R. B. (1953b). *Minerva Anestesiol.* **19**, 278.
Peters, K. (1955). *Arch. Exptl. Pathol. Pharmakol.* **226**, 570.
Peters, K. (1956). *Arch. Exptl. Pathol. Pharmakol.* **229**, 182.
Peters, K., Gartner, H., and Krais, W. (1955). *Strahlentherapie* **97**, 579.
Peters, R. A. (1959). *Biochem. Pharmacol.* **3**, 77.
Peterson, R. D., Beatty, C. H., Dixon, H. H., and West, E. S. (1960). *Federation Proc.* **19**, 259.
Petrie, A. (1956). *J. Clin. Exptl. Psychopathol.* **17**, 170.
Pfeiffer, A. K., Satory, E., and Pataky, I. (1961). *Acta Physiol. Acad. Sci. Hung.* **19**, 225.
Pfeiffer, C. J., Gass, G. H., and Schwartz, C. S. (1963). *Nature* **197**, 1014.
Pfeiffer, E. (1956). *Science* **124**, 29.
Pfeiffer, W. M., and Bente, D. (1961). *Med. Exptl.* **5**, 280.
Phillips, B. M., and Miya, T. S. (1962). *Pharmacologist* **4**, 170.
Piala, J. J., High, J. P., Hassert, G. L., Jr., Burke, J. C., and Craver, B. N. (1959). *J. Pharmacol. Exptl. Therap.* **127**, 55.
Pidevich, I. N. (1961). *Bull. Exptl. Biol. Med. (USSR) (English Transl.)* **51**, 51.
Piette, L. H., and Forrest, I. S. (1962). *Biochim. Biophys. Acta* **57**, 419.
Piette, L. H., Ludwig, P., and Adams, R. N. (1961). *J. Am. Chem. Soc.* **83**, 3909.
Piette, L. H., Bulow, G., and Forrest, I. S. (1962). *International Conference on Action Mechanism and Metabolism of Psychoactive Drugs Derived from Phenothiazines and Structurally Related Compounds, Paris, Sept. 7–8.*
Piette, Y. (1961). *Arch. Intern. Pharmacodyn.* **130**, 220.
Pisciotta, A. V., and Daly, M. (1960). *Blood* **16**, 1572.
Pisciotta, A. V., and Hinz, J. E. (1964). *Federation Proc.* **23**, 281.
Pisciotta, A. V., and Kaldahl, T. (1962). *Blood* **20**, 364.

Pisciotta, A. V., Santos, A. S., and Keller, C. (1964). *J. Lab. Clin. Med.* **63**, 445.
Plaa, G. L., McGough, E. C., Blacker, G. J., and Fujimoto, J. M. (1960). *Am. J. Physiol.* **199**, 793.
Pletscher, A., and Gey, K. F. (1960). *Med. Exptl.* **2**, 259.
Pletscher, A., and Gey, K. F. (1962). *Med. Exptl.* **6**, 165.
Plotnikoff, N. N. (1961). *Science* **134**, 1881.
Plotnikoff, N. P. (1958). *Arch. Intern. Pharmacodyn.* **116**, 130.
Plotnikoff, N. P. (1960). *Psychopharmacologia* **1**, 429.
Plotnikoff, N. P., and Green, D. M. (1957). *J. Pharmacol. Exptl. Therap.* **119**, 294.
Plummer, H. B., Harrison, T., and Trever, R. W. (1960). *J. Am. Med. Assoc.* **172**, 600.
Pocidalo, J. J., and Tardieu, C. (1954). *Compt. Rend. Soc. Biol.* **148**, 452.
Pocidalo, J. J., Cathala, H. P., Himbert, J., and Tardieu, C. (1953). *Anesthesie Analgesie* **10**, 111.
Polishuk, W. Z., and Kulcsar, S. (1956). *J. Clin. Endocrinol. Metab.* **16**, 292.
Pollack, B. (1957). *Am. J. Psychiat.* **113**, 1115.
Pomerat, C. M., Finerty, M., and Perry, C. (1955). *Neurology* **5**, 787.
Popovic, V. (1954). *Compt. Rend. Soc. Biol.* **148**, 845.
Popper, H., Dubin, A., Bruce, C., Kent, G., and Kushner, D. (1957). *J. Lab. Clin. Med.* **49**, 767.
Popper, M., and Lorian, V. (1959). *Presse Med.* **67**, 212.
Porteus, S. D. (1957). *J. Consulting Psychol.* **21**, 15.
Posner, H. S. (1959). *Abstr. Am. Chem. Soc. 136th Meeting, Atlantic City, New Jersey, Sept. 1959*, p. 81C.
Posner, H. S., and Levine, J. (1963). *J. Nervous Mental Disease* **136**, 591.
Posner, H. S., and Solomon, J. D. (1960). *Am. J. Psychiat.* **117**, 561.
Posner, H. S., Hearst, E., Taylor, W. L., and Cosmides, G. J. (1962a). *Federation Proc.* **21**, 418.
Posner, H. S., Hearst, E., Taylor, W. L., and Cosmides, G. J. (1962b). *J. Pharmacol. Exptl. Therap.* **137**, 84.
Posner, H. S., Culpan, R., and Levine, J. (1963). *Federation Proc.* **22**, 540.
Potts, A. M. (1962). *Invest. Ophthalmol.* **1**, 522.
Pozdnyakov, V. S. (1963). *Zh. Nevropatol. i Psikhiat.* **63**, 276.
Preston, J. B. (1956). *J. Pharmacol. Exptl. Therap.* **118**, 100.
Price, S., Martin, H. F., and Gudzinowicz, B. J. (1964). *Biochem. Pharmacol.* **13**, 659.
Protiva, M. (1955). *Chem. Antihistaminovych Latek Histaminove Skupiny*, Prague.
Prueter, G. W. (1959). *Can. Med. Assoc. J.* **81**, 21.
Pullman, B., and Pullman, A. (1959). *Biochim. Biophys. Acta* **35**, 535.
Pungor, E. (1960). *Pharm. Acta Helv.* **35**, 173.
Purshottam, N. (1962). *Am. J. Obstet. Gynecol.* **83**, 1405.
Purshottam, N., Mason, M. M., and Pincus, G. (1961). *Fertility Sterility* **12**, 346.
Quadbeck, G. (1962). *International Conference on Action Mechanism and Metabolism of Psychoactive Drugs Derived from Phenothiazines and Structurally Related Compounds*, Paris, Sept. 7–8.
Quastel, J. H. (1962). *International Conference on Action Mechanism and Metabolism of Psychoactive Drugs Derived from Phenothiazine and Structurally Related Compounds*, Paris, Sept. 7–8.
Quinn, G., and Brodie, B. B. (1961). *Med. Exptl.* **4**, 349.
Raab, W., Stark, E., MacMillan, W. H., and Gigee, W. R. (1961). *Am. J. Cardiol.* **8**, 203.
Raevsky, K. S. (1957). *Bull. Exptl. Biol. Med. (USSR) (English Transl.)* **43**, 675.
Raevsky, K. S. (1961). *Bull. Exptl. Biol. Med. (USSR) (English Transl.)* **51**, 189.
Rafaelsen, O. J. (1959). *Acta Psychiat. Neurol. Scand.* **34**, 62.
Rafaelsen, O. J. (1961). *Psychopharmacologia* **2**, 185.
Raffel, S., Kochan, I., Poland, N., and Hollister, L. E. (1960). *Am. Rev. Respirat. Diseases* **81**, 555.

Ragland, J. B. (1962). *International Conference on Action Mechanism and Metabolism of Psychoactive Drugs Derived from Phenothiazines and Structurally Related Compounds, Paris, Sept. 7–8.*
Ragland, J. B., and Kinross-Wright, J. (1961). *Federation Proc.* **20**, 397.
Rahmann, H., and Engels, W. (1964). *Psychopharmacologia* **6**, 71.
Rainaut, J. (1956). *Presse Med.* **64**, 246.
Raitt, J. R., Nelson, J. W., and Tye, A. (1961). *Brit. J. Pharmacol.* **17**, 473.
Rajapurkar, M. V., and Panjwani, M. H. (1960). *Arch. Intern. Pharmacodyn.* **128**, 89.
Rajeswaran, P., and Kirk, P. L. (1961a). *Bull. Narcotics, U.N. Dept. Social Affairs* **13**, No. 3, 15.
Rajeswaran, P., and Kirk, P. L. (1961b). *Bull. Narcotics, U.N. Dept. Social Affairs* **13**, No. 4, 21.
Rajeswaran, P., and Kirk, P. L. (1962). *Bull. Narcotics, U.N. Dept. Social Affairs* **14**, No. 1, 19.
Ravin, L. J., Kennon, L., and Swintosky, J. (1958). *J. Pharm. Sci.* **47**, 460.
Ray, O. S., and Marrazzi, A. S. (1961). *Science* **133**, 1705.
Rea, E. L., Shea, J., and Fazekas, J. F. (1954). *J. Am. Med. Assoc.* **156**, 1249.
Read, A. E., Harrison, C. V., and Sherlock, S. (1961). *Am. J. Med.* **31**, 249.
Read, G. W., Cutting, W., and Furst, A. (1960). *Psychopharmacologia* **1**, 346.
Reboton, J., Jr., Weekly, R. D., Bylenga, N. D., and May, R. H. (1962). *J. Neuropsychiat.* **3**, 311.
Reckless, D., and Hopkin, D. A. B. (1954). *Brit. Med. J.* **I**, 1035.
Rees, L. (1962). *Anglo-Ger. Med. Rev.* **1**, 448.
Reid, A. A. (1964). *Med. J. Australia* **1**, 187.
Reid, W. B., Wright, J. B., Kolloff, H. G., and Hunter, J. H. (1948). *J. Am. Chem. Soc.* **70**, 3100.
Reilly, J., and Tournier, P. (1953). *Bull. Acad. Natl. Med. (Paris)* **137**, 385.
Remvig, J., and Sonne, L. M. (1961). *Psychopharmacologia* **2**, 203.
Reynolds, G. S., and Catania, A. C. (1962). *Science* **135**, 314.
Reynolds, R. W., and Carlisle, H. J. (1961). *J. Comp. Physiol. Psychol.* **54**, 354.
Reznikoff, L. (1960). *Am. J. Psychiat.* **116**, 1024.
Richards, A. D. (1964). *Brit. J. Psychiat.* **110**, 46.
Richards, F. (1965). *Lancet*, **II**, 437.
Richardson, H. L., Graupner, K. I., and Richardson, M. E. (1966). *J. Am. Med. Assoc.* **195**, 254.
Rieder, H. P. (1960). *Med. Exptl.* **3**, 353.
Riley, P. A., Jr., Mixon, B. M., Jr., and Barila, T. G. (1957). *Surgery* **42**, 936.
Ripstein, C. B., Friedgood, C. E., and Solomon, N. (1954). *Surgery* **35**, 90.
Ritchie, J. M., and Greengard, P. (1961). *J. Pharmacol. Exptl. Therap.* **133**, 241.
Ritschel, W. (1959). *Pharm. Acta Helv.* **34**, 189.
Rives, H., and Pellerat, J. (1965). *Presse Med.* **73**, 1597.
Rizzo, E. M., and Russo, S. (1953). *Rass. Studi Psichiat.* **42**, 677 and 709.
Robb, H. P. (1955). *Brit. Med. J.* **II**, 1086.
Robb, H. P. (1960). *J. Mental Sci.* **106**, 1413.
Robinson, A. E. (1965). *J. Pharm. Pharmacol.* **18**, 19.
Robinson, A. S. (1960). *J. Am. Med. Assoc.* **173**, 504.
Rocha e Silva, M., and Antonio, A. (1960). *Med. Exptl.* **3**, 371.
Rodgers, C. D., Wickard, C. P., McCaskill, M. R. (1961). *Obstet. Gynecol.* **17**, 92.
Rodig, O. R., Culliér, R. E., and Schlatzer, R. K. (1964). *J. Org. Chem.* **29**, 2652.
Roebuck, B. E., Chambers, J. L., and Williams, E. (1959). *J. Nervous Mental Disease* **129**, 184.
Rohde, P., and Sargant, W. (1961). *Brit. Med. J.* **II**, 67.
Roizin, L. (1959). *Res. Publ. Assoc. Res. Nervous Mental Disease* **37**, 285.
Roizin, L., Kaufman, M. A., and Miles, B. (1960). *Federation Proc.* **19**, 391.
Roizin, L., True, C., and Knight, M. (1959). *Res. Publ. Assoc. Res. Nervous Mental Disease* **37**, 285.
Rosati, D. (1963). *Am. J. Psychiat.* **119**, 360.
Rosati, D. (1964). *Brit. J. Psychiat.* **110**, 61.
Rosen, E., and Swintosky, J. V. (1960). *J. Pharm. Pharmacol.* **12**, 237T.

Rosenberg, F. J., and Savarie, P. J. (1963). *Federation Proc.* **22**, 568.
Rosner, H., Levine, S., Hess, H., and Kaye, H. (1955). *J. Nervous Mental Disease* **122**, 505.
Ross, J. J., Young, R. L., and Maass, A. R. (1958). *Science* **128**, 1279.
Ross, J. J., Flanagan, T. L., and Maass, A. R. (1962). *J. Med. Pharm. Chem.* **5**, 1035.
Ross, S., and Rhoades, M. V. (1961). *Psychol. Rept.* **9**, 639.
Roth, F. E., McKenna, J. M., and Govier, W. M. (1958). *Proc. Soc. Exptl. Biol. Med.* **99**, 157.
Rothstein, C., Zeltzerman, I., and White, H. R. (1962). *J. Nervous Mental Disease* **134**, 555.
Roux, C. (1959). *Arch. Franc. Pediat.* **16**, 969.
Rubin, A. (1964). *Biochem. Pharmacol.* **13**, 1007.
Rupp, J. J., and Paschkis, K. E. (1957). *Proc. Soc. Exptl. Biol. Med.* **95**, 477.
Russell, E. S. (1961). *Can. Med. Assoc. J.* **85**, 846.
Rutledge, L. T., and Doty, R. W. (1955). *Federation Proc.* **14**, 126.
Rutledge, L. T., and Doty, R. W. (1957). *Am. J. Physiol.* **191**, 189.
Rutschmann, J., Kalberer, F., Schalch, W., and Stahelin, H. (1962). *International Conference on Action Mechanism and Metabolism of Psychoactive Drugs Derived from Phenothiazine and Structurally Related Compounds, Paris, Sept.* 7–8.
Ruttner, J. R., Rondez, R., and Maier, C. (1962). *Deut. Med. Wochschr.* **87**, 1107.
Ryall, R. W. (1956). *Brit. J. Pharmacol.* **11**, 339.
Ryan, J. A. (1959). *J. Am. Pharm. Assoc. Sci. Ed.* **48**, 240.
Saarima, H. S. (1963). *Acta Psychiat. Scand.* **39**, Suppl. 169, 362.
Sackler, A. M., Weltman, A. S., and Sackler, R. R. (1959). *Nature* **183**, 896.
Sacks, N. Z. (1957). *Lancet* **II**, 983.
Sadove, M. S., Balagot, R. C. (1955). *Intern. Record Med.* **168**, 346.
Sadove, M. S., Levin, M. J., Rose, R. F., Schwartz, L., and Witt, F. W. (1954). *J. Am. Med. Assoc.* **155**, 626.
Sadove, M. S., Balagot, R. C., and Reyes, R. M. (1956). *Current Res. Anesthesia Analgesia* **35**, 165.
Saggiomo, A. J., Craig, P. N., and Gordon, M. (1958). *J. Org. Chem.* **23**, 1906.
Sainz, A. A. (1956). *Psychiat. Quart.* **30**, 647.
Sainz, A. A. (1964). *Psychosomatics* **5**, 167.
Salzman, N. P., and Brodie, B. B. (1956). *J. Pharmacol. Exptl. Therap.* **118**, 46.
Salzman, N. P., Moran, N. C., and Brodie, B. B. (1955). *Nature* **176**, 1122.
Sámel, M. (1958). *Arch. Intern. Pharmacodyn.* **117**, 151.
Sams, W. M. (1960). *J. Am. Med. Assoc.* **174**, 2043.
Samuels, A. S. (1957). *Am. J. Psychiat.* **113**, 746.
Sankar, D. V. S., Phipps, E., Gold, E., and Sankar, D. B. (1962). *Ann. N.Y. Acad. Sci.* **96**, 93.
Sapeika, N. (1959). *Arch. Intern. Pharmacodyn.* **122**, 196.
Sargant, W. (1964). *Brit. Med. J.* **I**, 694.
Satanove, A. (1965). *J. Am. Med. Assoc.* **191**, 263.
Saunders, J. C. (1961). *J. Mental Sci.* **107**, 31.
Saunders, J. C. (1959). "Pharmacological Frontiers," pp. 407–412. Little, Brown, Boston.
Sautet, J., Jullien, G., Leandri, M., and Rampal, C. (1960). *Compt. Rend. Soc. Biol.* **154**, 1852.
Sautet, J., Jullien, G., Leandri, M., and Rampal, C. (1961). *Presse Med.* **69**, 335.
Savlov, E. D. (1959). *Surgery* **45**, 229.
Saxena, P. N. (1960). *Arch. Intern. Pharmacodyn.* **126**, 228.
Schallek, W. (1962). *Ann. N.Y. Acad. Sci.* **96**, 303.
Schanberg, S. M., and Giarman, N. J. (1962). *Biochem. Pharmacol.* **11**, 187.
Schanker, L. S., Fuks, Z., and Lanman, R. C. (1963). *Pharmacologist* **5**, 247.
Schaumkell, K. W. (1955a). *Acta Endocrinol.* **20**, 371.
Schaumkell, K. W. (1955b). *Arch. Exptl. Pathol. Pharmakol.* **225**, 381.
Schaumkell, K. W. (1955c). *Klin. Wochschr.* **33**, 282.
Scheckel, C. L., and Dahlen, P. (1964). *Physiologist* **7**, 245.

Schellenberg, H. (1961b). *Med. Exptl.* **5**, 459.
Schellenberg, H. (1961a). *Med. Exptl.* **5**, 467.
Schenck, G. O., and Wohlgast, R. (1961). *Naturwissenschaften* **48**, 737.
Schenker, E., and Herbst, H. (1963). *Progr. Drug Res.* **5**, 269.
Schiele, B. C. (1962). *J. Am. Med. Assoc.* **181**, 126.
Schiele, B. C., Vestre, N. D., and Stein, K. E. (1961). *J. Clin. Exptl. Psychopathol.* **22**, 151.
Schieser, D. W., and Tuck, L. D. (1962). *J. Pharm. Sci.* **51**, 694.
Schmidt, H., Jr. (1958). *J. Comp. Physiol. Psychol.* **51**, 26.
Schmidt, H., Jr., and Van Meter, W. G. (1958). *J. Comp. Physiol. Psychol.* **51**, 29.
Schmiterlöw, C. G., and Tufvesson, G. (1956). *Nord. Veterinarmed.* **8**, 1.
Schmitt, H., and Schmitt, H. (1961). *Arch. Intern. Pharmacodyn.* **132**, 74.
Schmitt, J., Hallot, A., Comoy, P., Suquet, M., Fallard, R., and Boitard, J. (1957). *Bull. Soc. Chim. France* p. 1474.
Schneider, J. A. (1954). *Proc. Soc. Exptl. Biol. Med.* **87**, 614.
Schneider, R. A. (1955). *Psychiat. Res. Rept.* **1**, 1.
Schneider, R. A., and Costiloe, J. P. (1956). *Clin. Res. Proc.* **4**, 45.
Scholz, O., and Kretzschmar, E. (1956). *Arch. Klin. Chir.* **283**, 515.
Scholz, O., and Kretzschmar, E. (1958). *Klin. Wochschr.* **36**, 38.
Schreiber, M. M., and Naylor, L. Z. (1962). *Arch. Dermatol.* **86**, 58.
Schrire, I. (1963). *Lancet* **I**, 174.
Schültz, E. (1960). *Arzneimittel-Forsch.* **10**, 958.
Schuette, D. V., and Gulick, W. L. (1961). *Ann. Otol. Rhinol. Laryngol.* **70**, 143.
Schuler, W. A. (1959). U.S. Patent 2,901,478.
Schuler, W. A., Klebe, H., and Schlictegroll, A. V. (1964). *Ann. Chem.* **673**, 102.
Schwarz, B. E., Bickford, R. G., and Rome, H. P. (1955). *Proc. Staff Meetings Mayo Clinic* **30**, 407.
Schweich, M. J., Martel, J., and Rondepierre, A. (1961). *Ann. Med.-Psychol.* **119**, No. 1, 755.
Scime, I. A., and Tallant, E. J. (1959). *J. Am. Med. Assoc.* **171**, 1813.
Scott, G. T. (1962). *International Conference on Action Mechanism and Metabolism of Psychoactive Drugs Derived from Phenothiazine and Structurally Related Compounds*, Paris, Sept. 7–8.
Scott, G. T., and Nading, L. K. (1961). *Proc. Soc. Exptl. Biol. Med.* **106**, 88.
Sedivec, V. (1964). *Activatis Nervosa Super.* **6**, 204.
Selbach, H. (1956). *Encephale* **45**, 1124.
Serbinenko, M. V. (1960a). *Fiziol. Zh. SSSR* **46**, 1111.
Serbinenko, M. V. (1960b). *Fiziol. Zh. SSSR* **46**, 1105.
Sergio, C., and Alemà, G. (1957). *Boll. Soc. Ital. Biol. Sper.* **33**, 290.
Setekleiv, J., Andersen, P., Bruland, H., and Kaada, B. R. (1960). *Acta Pharmacol. Toxicol.* **16**, 357.
Sevy, R. W., Ohler, E. A., and Weiner, A. (1957). *Endocrinology* **61**, 45.
Shafer, S., Joseph, L., and Anderson, J. P. (1962). *Lancet* **I**, 221.
Shaklee, A. B. (1958). *J. Genet. Psychol.* **93**, 59.
Sharma, P. L., and Arora, R. B. (1961). *Indian J. Med. Res.* **49**, 1099.
Shatin, L. (1956). *Psychiat. Quart.* **30**, 402.
Shaw, E. B., Dermott, R. V., Lee, R., and Burbridge, T. N. (1959). *Pediatrics* **23**, 485.
Shawver, J. R., Scarborough, J. S., and Frank, T. V. (1962). *Diseases Nervous System* **23**, 392.
Shay, H., Sun, D. C. H., and Gruenstein, M. (1959). *In* "Proceedings of the World Congress of Gastroenterology," p. 108. Williams & Wilkins, Baltimore, Maryland.
Sheatz, G. C., and Fazekas, J. F. (1955). *J. Pharmacol. Exptl. Therap.* **113**, 47a.
Shelton, J. G., Kingston, W. R., and McRae, C. (1960). *Med. J. Australia* **47**, 130.
Shemano, I., and Nickerson, M. (1958). *Can. J. Biochem. Physiol.* **36**, 1243.
Shemyakin, M. M., Kolosov, M. N., Levitov, M. M., Germanova, K. I., Karapetyan, M. G., Shvetsov, Y. B., and Bamdas, E. M. (1956). *J. Gen. Chem. USSR (English Transl.)* **26**, 885.

Sherif, M. A. F., Chata, M. K., and Madkour, M. K. (1958). *Arch. Intern. Pharmacodyn.* **115**, 269.
Sherman, S., Dussik, K. T., and Lever, P. G. (1960). *Diseases Nervous System* **21**, 333.
Shibusawa, K., Saito, S., and Fukuda, M. (1955). *Endocrinol. Japon.* **2**, 189.
Shibusawa, K., Saito, S., Nishi, K., Yamamoto, T., Abe, C., and Tomizawa, K. (1956). *Endocrinol. Japon.* **3**, 138.
Shirley, D. A. (1943). Ph.D. Thesis, Iowa State College, Ames, Iowa.
Shlyafer, T. P. (1961). *Pavlov J. Higher Nervous Activity (English Transl.)* **11**, 783.
Shminke, G. A. (1961). *Pavlov J. Higher Nervous Activity (English Transl.)* **11**, 237.
Siddall, J. R. (1965). *Arch. Ophthalmol.* **74**, 460.
Sidley, N. A., and Schoenfeld, W. N. (1963). *J. Exptl. Anal. Behavior* **6**, 293.
Silvestrini, B., and Maffii, G. (1959). *J. Pharm. Pharmacol.* **11**, 224.
Simoes, M. S., and Osswald, W. (1955). *Metab., Clin. Exptl.* **4**, 333.
Simon, W., Wirt, R. D., Wirt, A. L., Halloran, A. V., and Hopkins, G. W. (1958). *Am. J. Psychiat.* **114**, 1077.
Simpson, G. M. (1965). *Comp. Psychiat.* **6**, 347.
Simpson, G. M., and Kline, N. S. (1961). *J. Nervous Mental Disease* **133**, 19.
Sines, J. O., and Sines, L. K. (1958). *Psychol. Rept.* **4**, 519.
Singleton, A. R., and Witt, R. W. (1956). *Obstet. Gynecol.* **7**, 540.
Sinha, B. N. (1961). *J. Indian Med. Assoc.* **36**, 288; *J. Am. Med. Assoc.* **176**, 822.
Sinha, G. B., and Mitra, S. K. (1955). *J. Indian Med. Assoc.* **24**, 557.
Sinigaglia, M. G. (1955). *Boll. Soc. Ital. Biol. Sper.* **31**, 1628.
Siva Sankar, D. V. (1961). *J. Neuropsychiat.* **3**, 123.
Skinner, B. F. (1955). *Trans. N.Y. Acad. Sci.* **17**, 547.
Slocum, Y. K. (1961). *Am. J. Psychiat.* **118**, 75.
Smelson, H., and Foy, J. L. (1962). *Diseases Nervous System* **23**, 36.
Smilevich, A. B. (1961). *Zh. Nevropatol. i Psikhiatr.* **61**, 236.
Smith Kline and French Laboratories (1956). Unpublished data.
Smith, E. E. (1964). *Biochem. Pharmacol.* **13**, 643.
Smith, C. I., and Burke, J. C. (1960). *Toxicol. Appl. Pharmacol.* **2**, 553.
Smith, J. A., Willrich, K., and Rudy, L. H., (1963). *Diseases Nervous System* **24**, 310.
Smith, M. J., and Denner, J. L. (1962). *Diseases Nervous System* **23**, 466.
Smith, N. L. (1950). *J. Org. Chem.* **15**, 1125.
Smith, N. L. (1951). *J. Org. Chem.* **16**, 415.
Smith, R. P., Wagman, A. I., Wagman, W., Pfeiffer, C. C., and Riopelle, A. J. (1957). *J. Pharmacol. Exptl. Therap.* **119**, 317.
Sobel, A. M. (1960a). *U.S. Armed Forces Med. J.* **11**, 1446.
Sobel, D. E. (1960b). *Arch. Gen. Psychiat.* **2**, 606.
Sobolewski, G., and Nadeau, G. (1960). *Clin. Chem.* **6**, 153.
Söderberg, U. (1956). *Experientia* **12**, 299.
Soehring, K. (1956). *Arzneimittel-Forsch.* **6**, 773.
Solsona, M., and Mora, A. (1951). *Rev. Espan. Fisiol.* **7**, 221.
Somerville, D. M., Cohen, P. H., and Graves, G. D. (1960). *J. Mental Sci.* **106**, 1417.
Sorby, D. L., and Plein, E. M. (1961). *J. Pharm. Sci.* **50**, 355.
Spellberg, M. A. (1961). *Postgrad. Med.* **29**, 622.
Spirtes, M. A., and Guth, P. S. (1961). *Nature* **190**, 274.
Spirtes, M. A., and Guth, P. S. (1963). *Biochem. Pharmacol.* **12**, 37.
Spratt, R. J., and Dean, E. F. (1957). *Rocky Mt. Med. J.* **54**, 153.
Spurr, G. B., Farrand, E. A., and Horvath, S. M. (1956a). *Am. J. Physiol.* **185**, 499.
Spurr, G. B., Horvath, S. M., and Farrand, E. A. (1956b). *Am. J. Physiol.* **186**, 525.
Stacey, C. H., Azima, H., Huestis, D. W., Howlett, J. G., and Hoffman, M. M. (1955). *Can. Med. Assoc. J.* **73**, 386.

Staniszewski, K. (1960). *Arch. Intern. Pharmacodyn.* **124**, 263.
Starbuck, W. C., and Heim, H. C. (1959). *J. Am. Pharm. Assoc., Sci. Ed.* **48**, 251.
Stefko, P. L., and Zbinden, G. (1963). *Am. J. Gastroenterol.* **39**, 410.
Stein, L., and Seifter, J. (1961). *Science* **134**, 286.
Steiner, W. G., and Himwich, H. E. (1962). *Science* **136**, 873.
Stell, B. S. (1964). *Am. J. Psychiat.* **121**, 75.
Stephen, C. R., Bourgeois-Gavardin, M., and Martin, R. C. (1955). *Ann. N.Y. Acad. Sci.* **61**, 236.
Sternberg, U., Spitz, H., and Goyne, J. B. (1957). *J. Clin. Exptl. Psychopathol.* **18**, 258.
Stevenson, T. D., and Sjoerdsma, A. (1954). *Proc. Soc. Exptl. Biol. Med.* **86**, 726.
Stewart, J. (1962). *Psychopharmacologia* **3**, 132.
Stewart, L., and Redeker, A. G. (1954). *Calif. Med.* **81**, 203.
Stone, G. C., Calhoun, D. W., and Kloppenstein, M. H. (1958). *J. Comp. Physiol. Psychol.* **51**, 315.
Streicher, E., and Garbus, J. (1955). *J. Gerontol.* **10**, 441.
Stucki, J. C., and Thompson, C. R. (1958). *Am. J. Physiol.* **193**, 275.
Sturtevant, F. M., and Drill, V. A. (1956). *Proc. Soc. Exptl. Biol. Med.* **92**, 383.
Sturtevant, F. M., and Drill, V. A. (1957). *Nature* **179**, 1253.
Su, C., and Lee, C. Y. (1960). *Brit. J. Pharmacol.* **15**, 88.
Sullivan, C. L. (1957). *Postgrad. Med.* **22**, 429.
Sullivan, C. L. (1958). *New Engl. J. Med.* **258**, 232.
Sulman, F. G. (1964). *Lancet* **II**, 592.
Sulman, F. G., and Winnik, H. Z. (1956a). *Lancet* **I**, 161.
Sulman, F. G., and Winnik, H. Z. (1956b). *Nature* **178**, 365.
Summerfield, A. (1964). *Brit. Med. J.* **20**, 70.
Sun, D. C. H., and Shay, H. (1956). *Am. J. Physiol.* **187**, 635.
Sun, D. C. H., and Shay, H. (1959). *J. Pharmacol. Exptl. Therap.* **126**, 155.
Supek, Z., Uroić, B., Gjuriš, V., and Kečkeš, S. (1959). *J. Pharm. Pharmacol.* **11**, 448.
Supek, Z., Kečkeš, S., and Vojvodić, S. (1960a). *Arch. Intern. Pharmacodyn.* **123**, 260.
Supek, Z., Kečkeš, S., and Vojvodić, S. (1960b). *Arch. Intern. Pharmacodyn.* **123**, 253.
Supek, Z., Uroic, B., Gjuris, V., and Marijan, N. (1962). *J. Pharm. Pharmacol.* **14**, 284.
Suva, J. (1964). *Activatis Nervose Super.* **6**, 29.
Suzuki, M., Kamio, K., Yasuda, M., and Yamashita, T. (1956). *Endocrinol. Japon.* **3**, 67.
Swain, J. M., and Litteral, E. B. (1960). *J. Nervous Mental Disease* **131**, 550.
Swales, W. E., and Collier, H. B. (1940). *Can. J. Res.* **D18**, 279.
Swinehart, L. A. (1955). *Henry Ford Hosp. Med. Bull.* **3**, 136.
Swintosky, J. V. (1962). *J. Pharm. Sci.* **51**, 1015.
Symchowicz, S., Peckham, W. D., Korduba, C. A., and Perlman, P. L. (1962). *Biochem. Pharmacol.* **11**, 499.
Symposium. (1961). *Brit. Med. J.* **I**, 268.
Szilágyi, T., Csaba, B., and Szabó, E. (1961). *Acta Physiol. Acad. Sci. Hung.* **20**, 145.
Tabau, R., and Vigne, J. (1958). *Bull. Soc. Chim. France* p. 458.
Tachezy, R. (1962). *Casopis Lekaru Ceskych* **101**, 467.
Taeschler, M., and Cerletti, A. (1959). *Nature* **184**, 823.
Takayanagi, I. (1964). *Arzneimittel-Forsch.* **14**, 694.
Talwalker, P. K., Meites, J., Nicoll, C. S., and Hopkins, T. H. (1960). *Am. J. Physiol.* **199**, 1073.
Tanaka, K. (1955). *J. Pharmacol. Exptl. Therap.* **113**, 89.
Tanche, M., and Klepping, J. (1955). *Compt. Rend. Soc. Biol.* **149**, 1564.
Taterka-Seiler, W. (1958). *Arzneimittel-Forsch.* **8**, 304.
Taylor, D. B., and Winters, W. D. (1964). *Federation Proc.* **23**, 455.
Tedeschi, D. H., Tedeschi, R. E., and Fellows, E. J. (1961a). *Arch. Intern. Pharmacodyn.* **132**, 172.

Tedeschi, D. H., Tedeschi, R. E., and Fellows, E. J. (1961b). *In* "Extrapyramidal System and Neuroleptics," p. 113. Editions Psychiatrigues, Montreal.
Telkka, A. (1964). *Experientia* **20**, 27.
Terrace, H. S. (1963). *Science* **140**, 318.
Terrell, M. S. (1962). *Diseases Nervous System* **23**, 41.
Terzian, H. (1952). *Rass. Neurol. Vegetativa* **9**, 211.
Terzioğlu, M., and Özer, F. (1956). *Arch. Intern. Physiol. Biochim.* **64**, 1.
Theret, C. (1962a). *Compt. Rend.* **254**, 4100.
Theret, C. (1962b). *Compt. Rend.* **254**, 4233.
Theret, C. (1962c). *Compt. Rend. Soc. Biol.* **156**, 31.
Thieme, H. (1956). *Pharmazie* **11**, 460.
Thomas, L. (1956). *J. Exptl. Med.* **104**, 865.
Thompson, T. (1961). *J. Comp. Physiol. Psychol.* **54**, 398.
Thorpe, J. G., and Baker, A. A. (1958a). *J. Mental Sci.* **104**, 801.
Thorpe, J. G., and Baker, A. A. (1958b). *J. Mental Sci.* **104**, 865.
Tipton, D. L., Jr., Sutherland, V. C., Burbridge, T. N., and Simon, A. (1961). *Am. J. Physiol.* **200**, 1007.
Tiwari, N. M., Sharma, M. L., Gupta, S. K., and Dashputra, P. G. (1960a). *Arch. Intern. Pharmacodyn.* **125**, 456.
Tiwari, N. M., Jindal, M. N., and Jaiswal, C. L. (1960b). *Arch. Intern. Pharmacodyn.* **128**, 383.
Tofte, F. (1957). *Ugeskrift Laeger* **119**, 388.
Tokizane, T., Kawakami, M., and Gellhorn, E. (1957). *Arch. Intern. Pharmacodyn.* **113**, 217.
Toms, E. C. (1961). *J. Nervous Mental Disease* **132**, 425.
Torres, A. A. (1964). *Psychol. Rept.* **14**, 359.
Torres-Acero Fernandez, J. M., and De La Pena Regidor, P. (1955). *Rev. Espan. Obstet. Ginecol.* **12**, 213.
Torsello, R., and Palazzetti, P. (1955). *Minerva Ginecol.* **7**, 824.
Tourlentes, T. T. (1958). *A.M.A. Arch. Neurol. Psychiat.* **79**, 468.
Traugott, N. N. (1961a). *Pavlov J. Higher Nervous Activity (English Transl.)* **11**, 599.
Traugott, N. N. (1961b). *Pavlov J. Higher Nervous Activity (English Transl.)* **11**, 850.
Tredici, L. M., Schiele, B. C., and McClanahan, W. S. (1965). *Minn. Med.* **48**, 569.
Trigos, G., and McCullough, W. (1955). *Diseases Nervous System* **16**, 309.
Triner, L., and Mráz, M. (1962). *Physiol. Bohemoslov.* **11**, 24.
Troughton, S. E., Gould, G. N., and Anderson, J. A. (1955). *Vet. Record* **67**, 903.
Truitt, E. B., Jr., and Ebersberger, E. M. (1960). *Arch. Intern. Pharmacodyn*, **129**, 223.
Tuason, V. B., and Guze, S. B. (1961). *Clin. Pharmacol. Therap.* **2**, 152.
Turner, A. W., and Hodgetts, V. E. (1960). *Nature* **185**, 43.
Turner, M., Berard, E., Turner, N., and Franco, N. (1955). *Anesthesie Analgesie* **12**, 453.
Tuteur, W., Stiller, R., and Glotzer, J. (1962). *Current Therap. Res.* **4**, 206.
Ullyot, G. E. (1962). U.S. Patent 3,058,979.
Usdin, V. R., Su, S.-C., and Usdin, E. (1961). *Proc. Soc. Exptl. Biol. Med.* **108**, 457.
Uyeo, S., and Oishi, H. (1952). *J. Pharm. Soc. Japan* **72**, 443.
Vácerková, J., Sulcová, M., and Kácl, K. (1962). *Pharmazie* **17**, 22.
Vaillant, G. E. (1964). *New Engl. J. Med.* **271**, 280.
Vallat, J. N. (1954). *Presse Med.* **62**, 752.
Vanden Heuval, W. J. A., Haahti, E. O. A., and Horning, E. C. (1962). *Clin. Chem.* **8**, 351.
Vanderbrook, M. J., Olson, K. J., Richmond, M. R., and Kuizenea, M. H. (1948). *J. Pharmacol. Exptl. Therap.* **94**, 197.
Vandewater, S. L., and Gordon, R. A. (1955). *Can. Anaesthesiol. Soc. J.* **2**, 23.
Van Ess, P. R. (1936). Ph.D. Thesis, Iowa State College, Ames, Iowa.
Vanlerenverghe, J., Robelet, A., and Milbled, G. (1954). *Arch. Intern. Pharmacodyn.* **98**, 421.
Vanlerenverghe, J., Robelet, A., and Guerrin, F. (1960). *Compt. Rend. Soc. Biol.* **154**, 1243.

Van Loon, E. J., Flanagan, T. L., Novick, W. J., and Maass, A. R. (1962). *International Conference on Action Mechanism and Metabolism of Psychoactive Drugs Derived from Phenothiazine and Structurally Related Compounds, Paris, Sept.* 7–8.
van Proosdij-Hartzema, E. G. (1955). *Acta Physiol. Pharmacol. Neerl.* **4**, 378.
Vates, T. S., and Masucci, E. F. (1960). *Med. Ann. District Columbia* **29**, 670.
Veghelyi, P. V. (1962). *J. Pediat.* **60**, 122.
Venkataraman, K. (1952). "The Chemistry of Synthetic Dyes." Vol. 2, p. 791. Academic Press, New York.
Verhave, T., Owen, J. E., and Robbins, E. B. (1958). *Arch. Intern. Pharmacodyn.* **116**, 45.
Vesell, E. S. (1959). *New Engl. J. Med.* **260**, 1078.
Vestre, N. D. (1961). *J. Abnormal Social Psychol.* **63**, 432.
Viaud, P. (1954). *J. Pharm. Pharmacol.* **6**, 361.
Vinař, O., Hausner, M., Sčudlik, M., Horanská, D., and Tautermann, P. (1965). *Activitatio Nervosa Super.* **7**, 300.
Vinegar, R., and Berger, F. M. (1959). *Proc. Soc. Exptl. Biol. Med.* **102**, 88.
Virtue, R. W., and Jones, B. E. (1956). *Anesthesiology* **17**, 601.
Visentini, P. (1954). *Arch. Ital. Sci. Farmacol.* **4**, 78.
Vivoli, G. (1960). *Bull. Soc. Med. Chir. Modena*, **60**, 105.
Vogel, G. (1961). *Arzneimittel-Forsch.* **11**, 978.
Vogel, G., and Tervooren, U. (1961). *Med. Exptl.* **4**, 59.
Voigt, R. (1962). *Pharmazie* **17**, 269.
Vol'pe, M. M. (1961). *Zh. Nevropatol. i Psikhiatr.* **61**, 232.
von Ledebur, I., Frommel, E., and Béguin, M. (1962). *Med. Exptl.* **7**, 177.
Vroom, F. Q., Brown, R. E., Dempsey, H., and Hill, S. R., Jr. (1962). *Ann. Internal Med.* **56**, 941.
Waaler, T. (1960). *Pharm. Acta Helv.* **35**, 168.
Wada, J. A. (1963). *Arch. Neurol.* **9**, 69.
Waddell, A. W. (1959). *Arch. Intern. Pharmacodyn.* **121**, 368.
Waitzkin, L., and MacMahon, H. E. (1962). *Ann. Internal Med.* **56**, 220.
Waldrop, F. N., Robertson, R. H., and Vourlekis, A. (1961). *Comprehensive Psychiat.* **2**, 96.
Walkenstein, S. S., and Seifter, J. (1958). *Federation Proc.* **17**, 417.
Walkenstein, S. S., and Seifter, J. (1959). *J. Pharmacol. Exptl. Therap.* **125**, 293.
Walker, M. F. (1959). *Can. Med. Assoc. J.* **81**, 109.
Walker, R. G., Williams, R. A., and Kelly, F. E. (1959). *J. Clin. Exptl. Psychopathol.* **21**, 304.
Waller, M. B. (1961). *J. Exptl. Anal. Behavior* **4**, 351.
Waller, M. B., and Waller, P. F. (1962). *J. Exptl. Anal. Behavior* **5**, 259.
Ware, K. (1955). *Dissertation Abstr.* **15**, 2580.
Warecka, K. (1960). *Acta Physiol. Pharmacol. Neerl.* **9**, 452.
Warren, R. J., Eisdorfer, I. B., Thompson, W. E., and Zarembo, J. E. (1966). *Pharm. Sciences*, **55**, 144.
Wase, A. W., Christensen, J., and Polley, E. (1956). *A.M.A. Arch. Neurol. Psychiat.* **75**, 54.
Watt, J. (1966). *Lancet* **I**, 366.
Waugh, W. H., and Metts, J. C. (1960). *New Engl. J. Med.* **262**, 353.
Weatherall, M. (1962). *Brit. Med. J.* **I**, 1219.
Weaver, J. E., and Miya, T. S. (1961). *J. Pharm. Sci.* **50**, 910.
Webster, R. A. (1961). *Brit. J. Pharmacol.* **17**, 507.
Webster, R. A. (1962). *Brit. J. Pharmacol.* **18**, 150.
Wechsler, M. B. (1962). *International Conference on Action Mechanism and Metabolism of Psychoactive Drugs Derived from Phenothiazine and Structurally Related Compounds, Paris, Sept.* 7–8.
Wechsler, M. B., and Forrest, I. S., (1959). *J. Neurochem* **4**, 366.
Wechsler, M. B., and Roizin, L. (1960). *J. Mental Sci.* **106**, 1501.
Weikel, J. H., Jr., Wheeler, A. G., and Joiner, P. D. (1960). *Toxicol. Appl. Pharmacol.* **2**, 68.

Weinberg, S. J., and Haley, T. J. (1956). *Arch. Intern. Pharmacodyn.* **105**, 209.
Weiss, B., and Laties, V. G. (1964). *J. Pharmacol. Exptl. Therap.* **144**, 17.
Weitzman, E. D., and Ross, G. S. (1962). *Neurology* **12**, 264.
Wellhöner, H. H., Hartmann, H., and Hauschild, F. (1960). *Arch. Exptl. Pathol. Pharmakol.* **240**, 224.
Welsh, A. L. (1964). *Med. Clin. N. Am.* **48**, 459.
Wendel, O. W., and Charkey, L. W. (1958). *Proc. Soc. Exptl. Biol. Med.* **98**, 463.
Wentzel, D. G., and Rutledge, C. O. (1962). *J. Pharm. Sci.* **51**, 631.
Werboff, J., and Dembicki, E. L. (1962). *J. Neuropsychiat.* **4**, 87.
Werboff, J., and Kesner, R. (1963). *Nature* **197**, 102.
Wert, E. B., and Greenhill, J. P. (1961). *J. Am. Med. Assoc.* **177**, 279.
West, E. D. (1964). *Brit. Med. J.* **2**, 445.
Wetterholm, B., Aborg, S., and Olin, K. (1959). *Svenska Lakartidn.* **56**, 2512.
Wetterholm, D. H., Snow, H. L., and Winter, F. C. (1965). *Arch. Ophthalmol.* **74**, 55.
White, R. P., and Boyajy, L. D. (1959). *Proc. Soc. Exptl. Biol. Med.* **102**, 479.
White, T. (1961). *J. Physiol. (London)* **159**, 191.
Whitehead, W. A. (1956). Doctoral Thesis, Vanderbilt University, Nashville, Tennessee.
Whitten, L. K., and Filmer, D. B. (1947). *Australian Vet. J.* **23**, 336.
Widmann, H., and Eckle, U. (1961). *Med. Welt* **15**, 797.
Wight, C. F., and Smiles, S. (1935). *J. Chem. Soc.* p. 2774.
Wilcox, F. (1958). *Diseases Nervous System* **19**, 118.
Wilens, S. L., and Gallo, G. (1957). *A.M.A. Arch. Pathol.* **64**, 570.
Wilens, S. L., McCluskey, R. T., and Somoza, C. (1956). *Proc. Soc. Exptl. Biol. Med.* **93**, 121.
Wilhelmi, G. (1961). *Chemotherapia* **2**, 210.
Wilke, G., and Iizuka, R. (1960). *Nervenarzt* **31**, 515.
Wilkinson, J. L. (1961). *Brit. Med. J.* **I**, 1721.
Wilson, G. M. (1963). *Clin. Pharmacol. Therap.* **4**, 255.
Wilson, I. C., McKay, J., and Sandifer, M. G., Jr. (1961). *J. Mental Sci.* **107**, 90.
Winbury, M. M., Hausler, L. M., Wolf, J. K., Klein, M. J., and Govier, W. M. (1958). *Anesthesiology* **19**, 743.
Winkelbauer, R. G., and Kimsey, L. R. (1956). *Am. J. Obstet. Gynecol.* **71**, 1353.
Winkelman, N. W. (1954). *J. Am. Med. Assoc.* **155**, 18.
Winkelman, N. W. (1964). *Am. J. Psychiat.* **120**, 861.
Winter, W. D., and Frederickson, W. K. (1956). *J. Consulting Psychol.* **20**, 431.
Winters, E. P., and Husa, W. J. (1960). *J. Am. Pharm. Assoc.* **49**, 709.
Wirth, W. (1954). *Arch. Exptl. Pathol. Pharmakol.* **222**, 75.
Wirth, W., Groesswald, R., Hoerlein, U., Risse, K. H., and Kreiskott, H. (1958). *Arch. Intern. Pharmacodyn.* **115**, 1.
Wislicki, L. (1958). *Arch. Intern. Pharmacodyn.* **115**, 52.
Witherspoon, J. D., Short, H. W., and Hiestand, W. A. (1957). *Proc. Soc. Exptl. Biol. Med.* **95**, 560.
Witkin, L. B., Spitaletta, P., and Plummer, A. J. (1959). *J. Pharmacol. Exptl. Therap.* **126**, 330.
Witt, P. N. (1955). *Monatsschr. Psychiat. Neurol.* **129**, 123.
Witt, P. N. (1961). *Trans. Studies Coll. Physicians Phila.* **29**, 9.
Witton, K. J. (1961). *Diseases Nervous System* **22**, 189.
Witzleb, E., and Budde, H. (1955). *Arch. Intern. Pharmacodyn.* **104**, 33.
Wolf, J. W. (1962). *Missouri Med.* **59**, 495.
Wollemann, M. (1962). *International Conference on Action Mechanism and Metabolism of Psychoactive Drugs Derived from Phenothiazine and Structurally Related Compounds*, Paris, Sept. 7–8.
Wollemann, M., and Elödi, P. (1961). *Biochem. Pharmacol.* **6**, 228.
Wollemann, M., and Keleti, T. (1962). *Arzneimittel-Forsch.* **12**, 360.
Wortis, J. (1963). *Am. J. Psychiat.* **119**, 621.

Wortis, J. (1964). *Am. J. Psychiat.* **120**, 643.
Wright, R. L. D. and Kyne, W. P. (1960). *Psychopharmacologia* **1**, 437.
Wruble, L. D. (1966). *J. Am. Med. Assoc.* **195**, 184.
Wunderlich, H. (1962). *Pharmazie* **17**, 269.
Yagi, K., Nagatsu, T., and Ozawa, T. (1956). *Nature* **177**, 891.
Yagi, K., Ozawa, T., and Nagatsu, T. (1959). *Nature* **184**, 982.
Yagi, K., Ozawa, T., Ando, M., and Nagatsu, T. (1960a). *J. Neurochem.* **5**, 304.
Yagi, K., Ozawa, T., and Nagatsu, T. (1960b). *Biochim. Biophys. Acta* **43**, 310.
Yakson, Z. P. (1963). *Zh. Nevropatol. i Psikhiatr.* **63**, 280.
Yakubovskaya, V. I., and Kiseleva, N. A. (1961). *Vopr. Med. Khim.* **7**, 93.
Yale, H., Sowinski, F., and Bernstein, J. (1957). *J. Am. Chem. Soc.* **79**, 4375.
Yamamoto, I., Tsujimoto, A., Tsujimura, Y., Minami, M., and Kurogochi, Y. (1957). *Japan. J. Pharmacol.* **6**, 138.
Yamamoto, I., Adachi, N., Kurogochi, Y., and Tsujimoto, A. (1960). *Japan. J. Pharmacol.* **10**, 38.
Yoshitani, H. (1963). *Japan. Circulation J. (Full Ed.)* **27**, 487.
Young, R. L., Ross, J. J., and Maass, A. R. (1959). *Nature* **183**, 1396.
Yung, D. K., and Pernarowski, M. (1963). *J. Pharm. Sci.* **52**, 365.
Zakusov, V. V. (1964). *Farmakol. Toksikol.* **27**, 107.
Zapata-Ortiz, V., and Stastny, P. (1956). *Arch. Intern. Pharmacodyn.* **107**, 431.
Zehnder, K., Kalberer, F., Kreis, W., and Rutschmann, J. (1962). *Biochem. Pharmacol.* **11**, 535.
Zeleba, M. S. (1961). *Zh. Nevropatol. i Psikhiatr.* **61**, 581.
Zelickson, A. S. (1965). *J. Am. Med. Assoc.* **194**, 670.
Zelickson, A. S., and Zeller, H. C. (1964). *J. Am. Med. Assoc.* **188**, 394.
Zetler, G., and Moog, E. (1958). *Arch. Exptl. Pathol. Pharmakol.* **232**, 442.
Zielinski, J., and Eynetten, A. (1960). *Polski Tygod. Lekar.* **15**, 626.
Zimbardo, P. G., and Barry, H., III (1958). *Science* **127**, 84.
Zimmerman, G. R. (1962). *Arch. Pathol.* **74**, 47.
Zipf, H. F., and Alstaedter, R. (1954). *Arzneimittel-Forsch.* **4**, 14.
Zografi, G. (1964). *J. Pharm. Sci.* **53**, 573.
Zoller, E., Schreiner, K., and Yang, P. R. (1958). *Arzneimittel-Forsch.* **8**, 238.

~2~
Haloperidol and Related Butyrophenones

∽

Paul A. J. Janssen

Janssen Pharmaceutica, Research Laboratories, Beerse, Belgium

I. Origin	199
II. Structure-Activity Relationships	206
III. Pharmacological Activity of the Butyrophenones	209
IV. Clinical Uses	217
A. Haloperidol (R1625)	217
B. Trifluperidol (R2498)	221
C. Methylperidol or Moperone (R1658)	225
D. Fluanisone or Haloanisone (R2028)	226
E. Floropipamide or Dipiperon (R3345)	227
F. Benperidol (R4584)	228
G. Droperidol (R4749)	229
H. Other Butyrophenones	230
References	231

I. Origin

The butyrophenone series of neuroleptic drugs originated in this laboratory from a systematic investigation of the relationship between the chemical

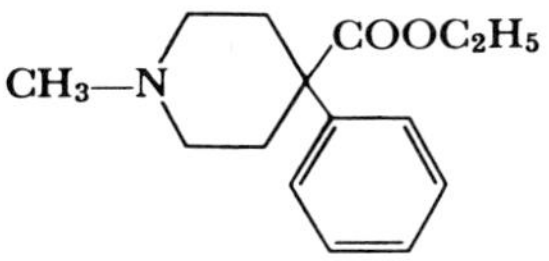

(I)

structure of 4-phenyl-piperidines related to meperidine (I) and their pharmacological properties (Haase and Janssen, 1965; Janssen, 1962d, 1964b,d,

TABLE I

COMMERCIALLY AVAILABLE NEUROLEPTICS (MAJOR TRANQUILLIZERS) OF THE BUTYROPHENONE SERIES

Chemical structure and serial number	Generic name, formula, and melting point	Trade names	Pharmaceutical forms for human use		
			tablets mg	drops mg/ml	ampules mg/ml
R 1625 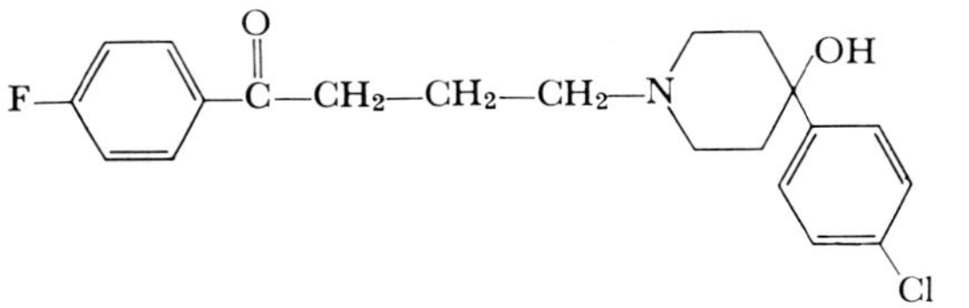	Haloperidol, $C_{21}H_{23}ClFNO_2$ · base 151–152	Haloperidol, Halopidol, Haldol, Aloperidin, Serenase, Serenace, Serenelfi, Vesalium,[a] Ulcolind,[a] Pernox,[b] Lealgin compositum,[a] Halopal[a]	0.5 1 1.5 2 5	0.5 2	2 2.5 5
R 1658 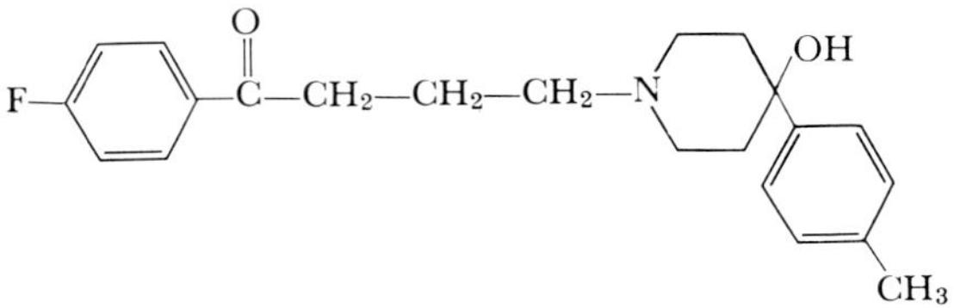	Methylperidol, Moperone, $C_{22}H_{26}NNO_2$ · HCl 216–217	Luvatrena, Luvatren, Luvatrene	5	5	5
R 2028, 2028 MD 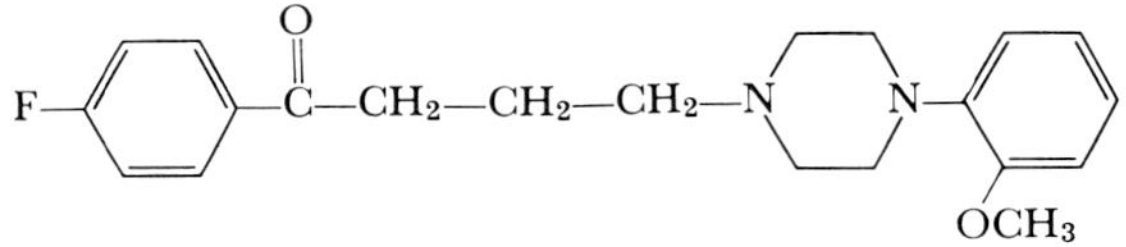	Fluanisone, Haloanisone, $C_{21}H_{25}FN_2O_2$ · base 74–75	Haloanisone, Sedalande, Anti-pica,[b] Hypnorm,[b] Haloanisone compositum,[b] Solusediv,[b] Sedavic[b]	5 10 20	5 25	5

Compound	Structure	Name, formula, m.p. (°C)	Other names	col1	col2	col3	col4
R 2498	(structure: 4-[3-(trifluoromethyl)phenyl]-4-hydroxypiperidine with 4'-fluorobutyrophenone)	Trifluperidol, triperidol, $C_{22}H_{23}F_4NO_2 \cdot HCl$, 207–209	Triperidol, Psicoperidol	1	1	1	2.5, 5
R 3345 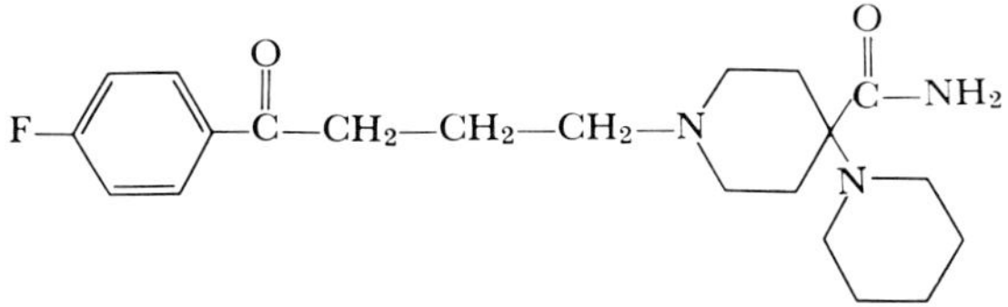	(structure: 4-piperidino-piperidine-4-carboxamide with 4'-fluorobutyrophenone)	Floropipamide, $C_{21}H_{30}FN_3O_2 \cdot 2HCl$, 259–261	Dipiperon, Propitan, Piperonyl	25, 40, 100	—	—	—
R 4584, 8089 CB 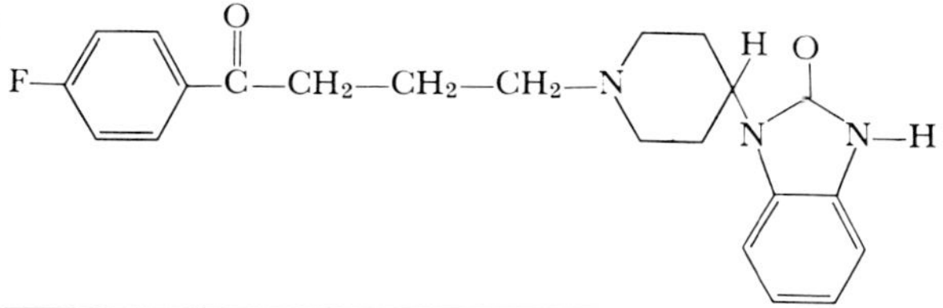	(structure: 2,3-dihydro-1H-benzimidazol-2-ol piperidine with 4'-fluorobutyrophenone)	Benperidol, Benzperidol, $C_{22}H_{24}FN_3O_2 \cdot$ base, 173–174	Frenactyl	2	2	2	0.5
R 4749 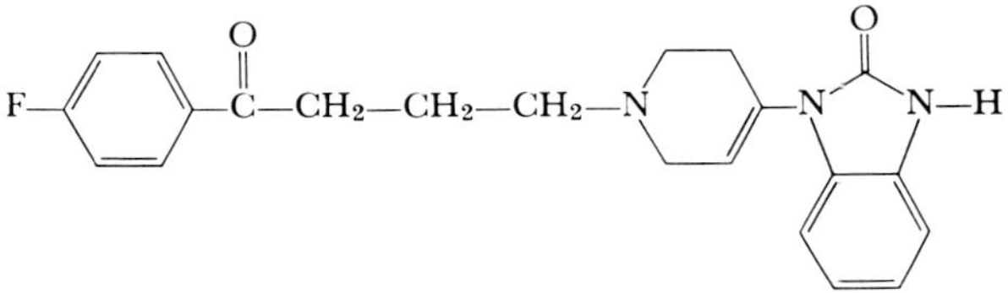	(structure: 1,3-dihydro-2H-benzimidazol-2-one tetrahydropyridine with 4'-fluorobutyrophenone)	Droperidol, dehydrobenzperidol, $C_{22}H_{22}FN_3O_2 \cdot$ base, 145–147	Dehydrobenzperidol, Deidrobenzperidolo, Inapsin, Droperidol, Thalamonal,[a] Innovar.[a] Leptofen[a], Vetkalm,[b] Innovar-vet,[b] R 4749,[b] Innovan, Inoval[a]	—	—	2.5	5

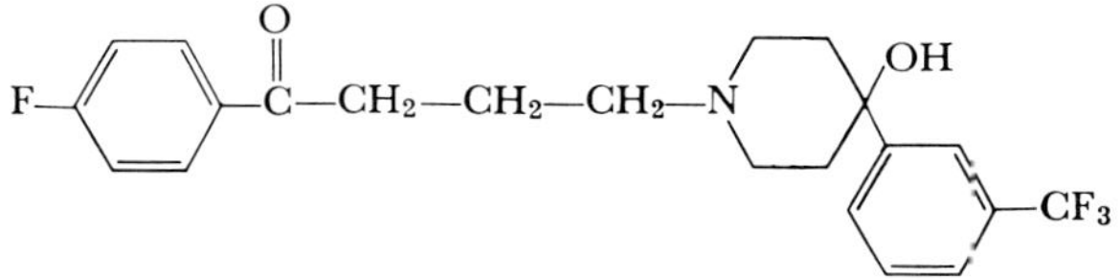

[a] combination product.
[b] veterinary product.

TABLE II

OTHER NEUROLEPTICS OF THE BUTYROPHENONE SERIES (CLINICALLY TESTED, BUT NOT AVAILABLE COMMERCIALLY)

Chemical structure and serial number	Generic name, formula, and melting point	Pharmaceutical forms for human use			References
		tablets mg	drops mg/ml	ampules mg/ml	
R 1647 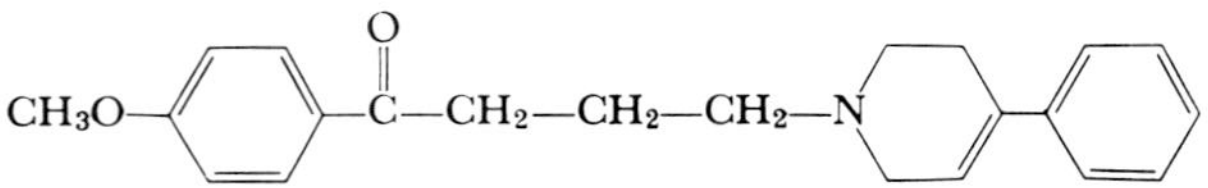	Anisoperidone, $C_{22}H_{25}NO_2 \cdot HCl$ 202–204	10 20 50	—	—	Collard (1961); Divry et al. (1959b); Janssen et al. (1965a, b, 1966).
R 1892 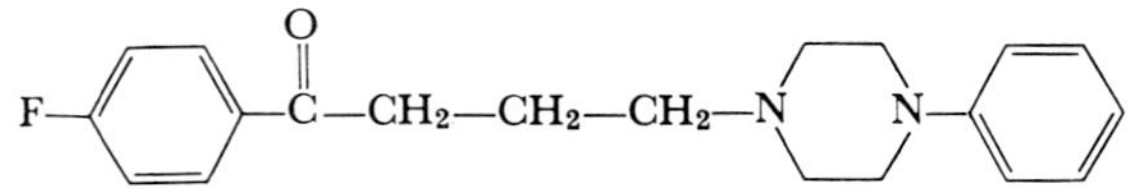	Butropipazone, $C_{20}H_{23}FN_2O \cdot$ base 105–107	50 100 200	—	15	Janssen et al. (1965a,b, 1966).
R 2962 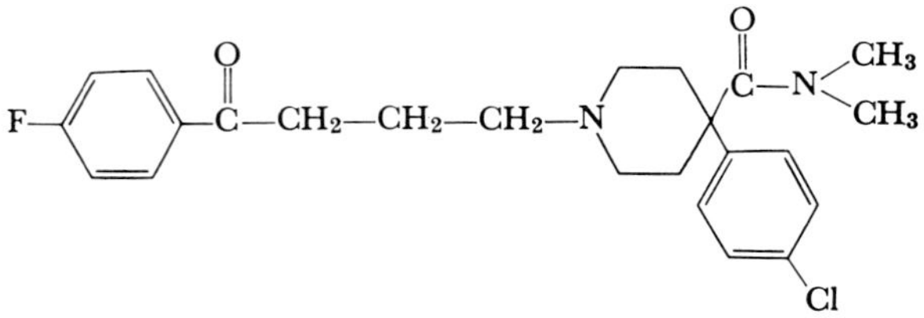	Paraperidide, Amiperone $C_{24}H_{28}ClFN_2O_2 \cdot$ base 135–137	5	—	2.5	Janssen et al. (1965a,b, 1966).
R 2963 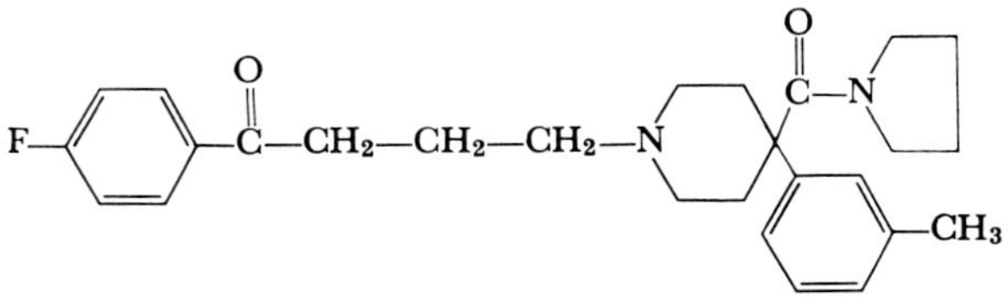	Methylperidide, $C_{27}H_{33}FN_2O_2$ 112–113	5 20	—	1 2 5	Collard (1961); Divry et al. (1960c); Janssen (1961c,d); Janssen et al. (1965a, b, 1966).

Code	Structure	Name, Formula, M.p. (°C)	Col3	Col4	Col5	Col6	Reference
R 3201 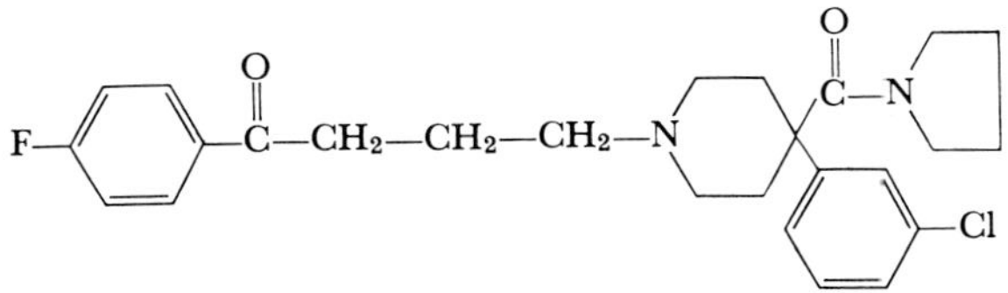		Haloperidide, $C_{26}H_{30}ClFN_2O_2 \cdot C_2H_2O_4$ 218–220	—	2.5	—	2.5	Janssen (1961c,d); Janssen and Niemegeers (1961a); Janssen et al. (1965a, b, 1966).
R 3248 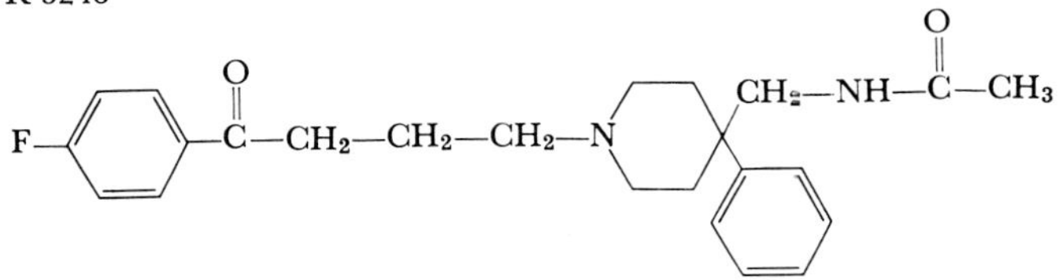		Acetabuton, aceperone $C_{24}H_{29}FN_2O_2$ 110–111	10	—	—	2 10 20	Janssen et al. (1965a,b, 1966); Schaper et al. 1962.
R 3264 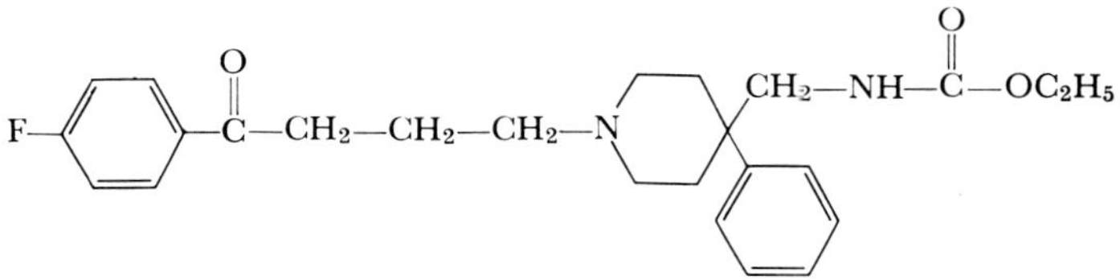		$C_{25}H_{31}FN_2O_3 \cdot HCl$ 146–148	—	—	—	10	—
R 4082 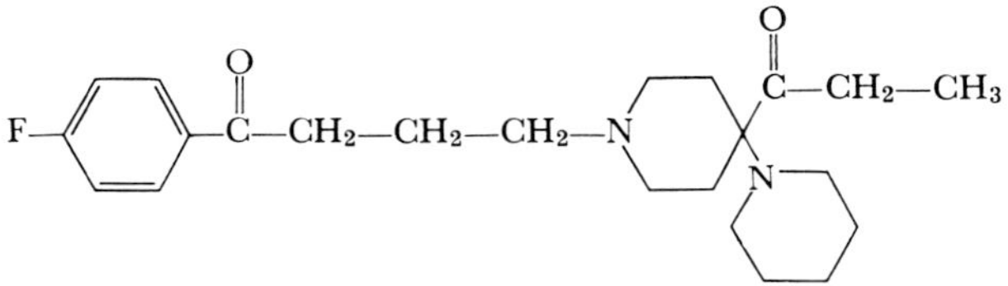		Floropipeton, $C_{23}F_{33}FN_2O_2 \cdot 2HCl$ 206–208	—	40	—	—	Janssen et al. (1966).

TABLE II—continued

Chemical structure and serial number	Generic name, formula, and melting point	Pharmaceutical forms for human use			References
		tablets mg	drops mg/ml	ampules mg/ml	
R 5147 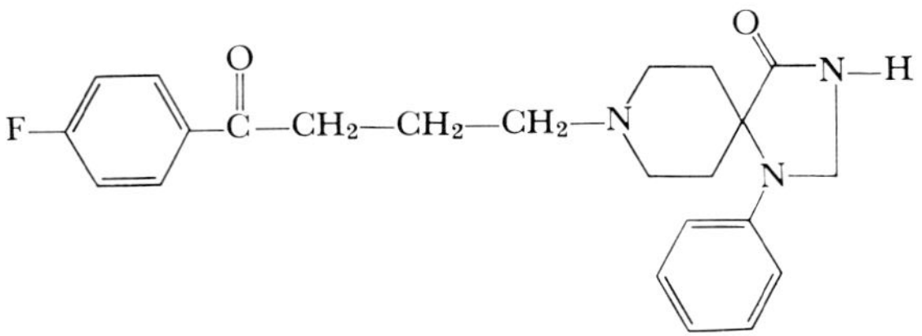	Spiroperidol, $C_{23}H_{26}FN_3O_2$ 207–208	—	1 2	0.1	Bobon et al. (1963b); Janssen et al. (1965a, b, 1966).
F 33, R 7158 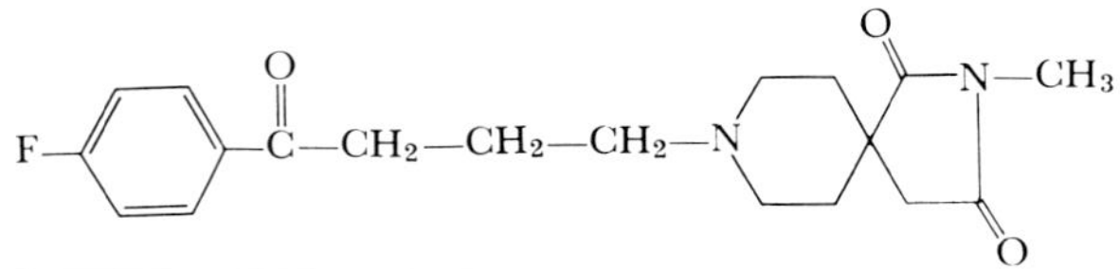	$C_{19}H_{23}FN_2O_3 \cdot HCl$ 285–287	—	—	—	Jucker (1963).
WY 3457, R 4006 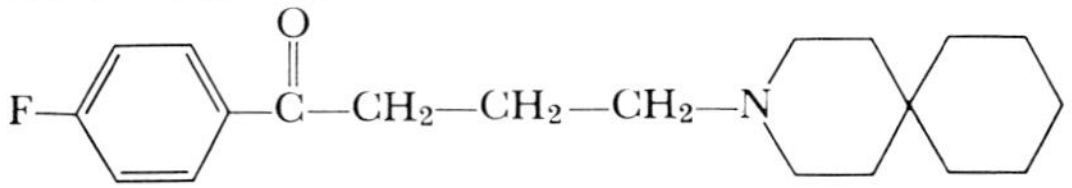	$C_{20}H_{28}FNO \cdot HCl$ 254–256	25	—	—	Simpson et al. (1964a,b).
WY 6123, R 4457 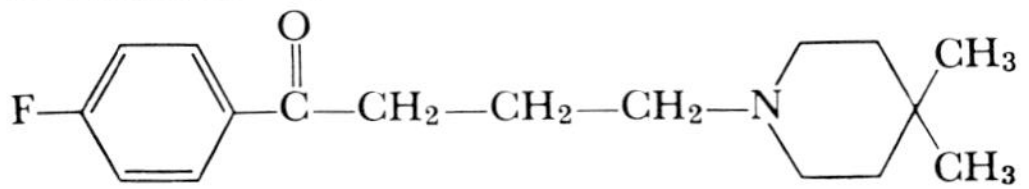	$C_{17}H_{24}FNO \cdot HCl$ 233–234	50	—	—	Simpson et al. (1965).

(1966); Janssen et al., 1959). The surprising finding that the propiophenone derived from normeperidine (II) was about 200 times more potent than

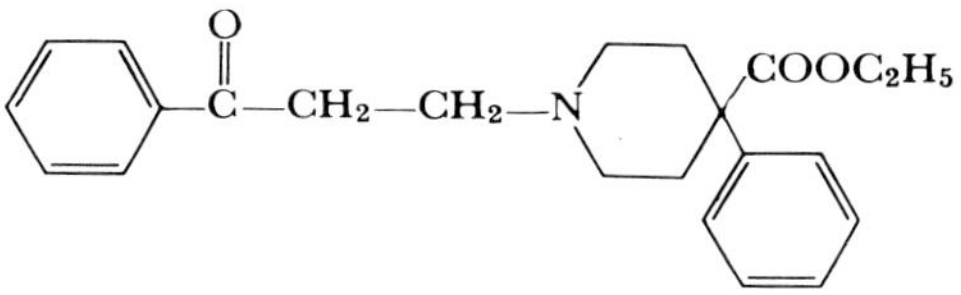

(II)

meperidine (I) itself lead to the synthesis of a series of related compounds, i.e. the butyrophenone derivative of normeperidine (III), which was found to

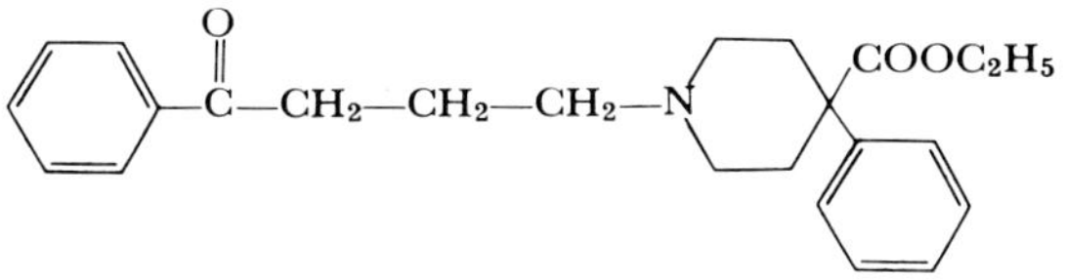

(III)

possess mixed morphine-like and chlorpromazine-like properties. The corresponding butyrophenone derived from 4-phenylpiperidin-4-ol (IV) however

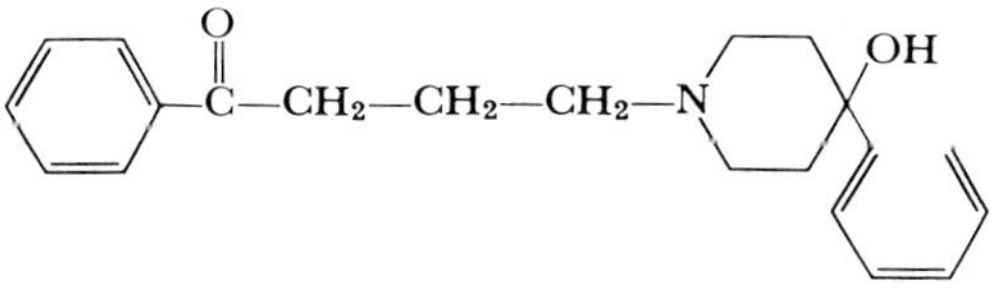

(IV)

was clearly a typical chlorpromazine-like drug, completely devoid of morphinomimetic effects.

Further systematic studies showed that it is possible to increase neuroleptic potency considerably by introducing selected aromatic substituents in both benzene rings, preferably a fluorine atom in the para position of the ketonic ring and chlorine, trifluoromethyl or lower alkyl in the meta or para position of the other ring (V).

Serial number R 1625, haloperidol (V:X=4-Cl), was finally selected for clinical investigation in psychiatry as a potential antipsychotic neuroleptic agent (Janssen, 1961c,d, 1964c; Janssen et al., 1959, 1965a,b, 1966).

More than 5000 tertiary amines related to haloperidol have since been prepared and pharmacologically investigated.

At least nineteen of these compounds underwent clinical trial (Tables I and II). Seven butyrophenone derivatives are now commercially available (Table I) and extensively used in psychiatry, neurology, and anesthesiology

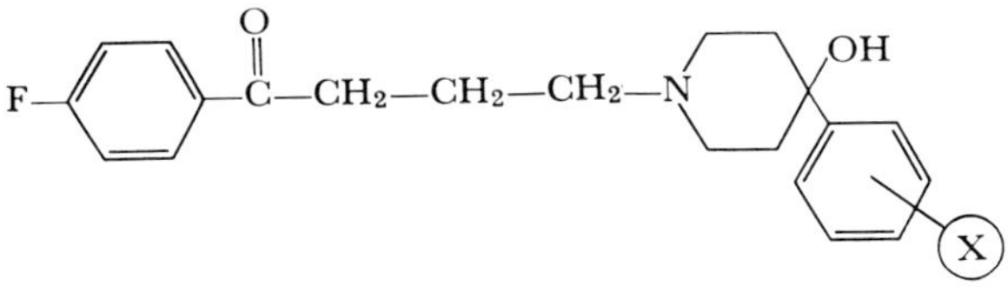

(V)

(as antiemetic drugs) as well as in veterinary medicine, i.e., haloperidol (R 1625), methylperidol (R 1658), fluanisone (R 2028), trifluperidol (R 2498), floropipamide (R 3345), benperidol (R 4584), and droperidol (R 4749).

II. Structure–Activity Relationships

All known potent neuroleptics derived from butyrophenone are tertiary amines of general structure (VI), i.e., derivatives of a 4-substituted piperidine

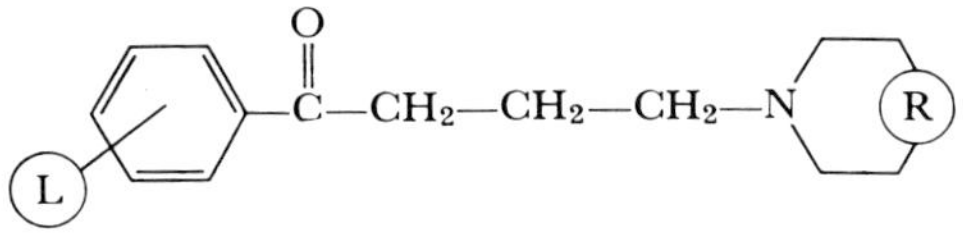

(VI)

(VII), a 4-substituted tetrahydropyridine (VIII), or a 4-substituted piperazine (IX).

In each series, the highest neuroleptic potency is associated with the presence of a fluorine substituent in para position of the ketonic benzene ring (VI:L=4–F).

The following chemical modifications of structure (VI) have as a rule a large potency-lowering effect: (a) shortening, lengthening or branching of the propylene side-chain, (b) replacement of the ketonic moiety, (c) replacement of the ketonic benzene ring by a non-isosteric moiety, (d) substitution of positions 2 or 3 of the six-membered heterocyclic amine, and (e) replacement of the six-membered basic ring by smaller or larger heterocyclic rings or by uncyclized amines.

A number of isosteric butyrothienones however are potent neuroleptic agents, only a few times less active than the corresponding butyrophenones.

All butyrophenones of type (VI) are conveniently prepared by condensation of a selected secondary amine (piperidine, tetrahydropyridine, or piperazine) with a suitably substituted ω-halogenobutyrophenone.

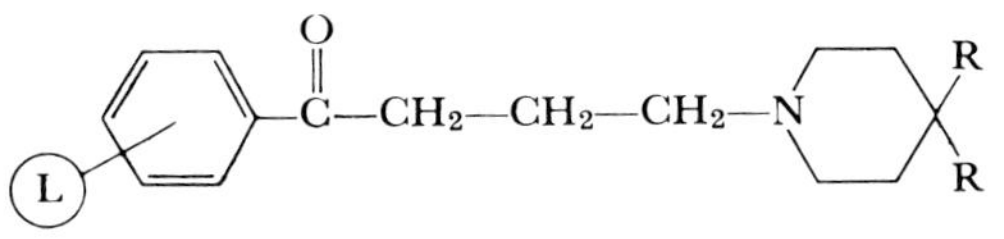

(VII)

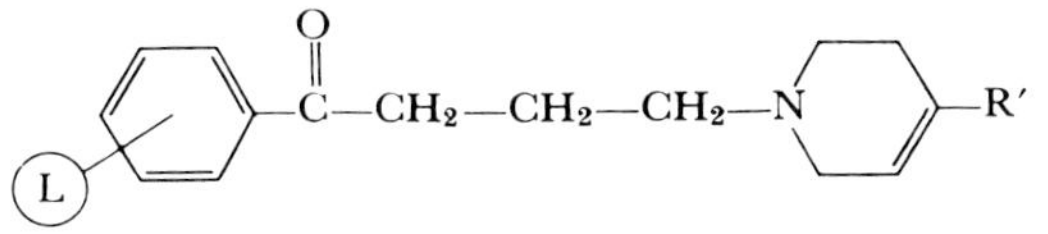

(VIII)

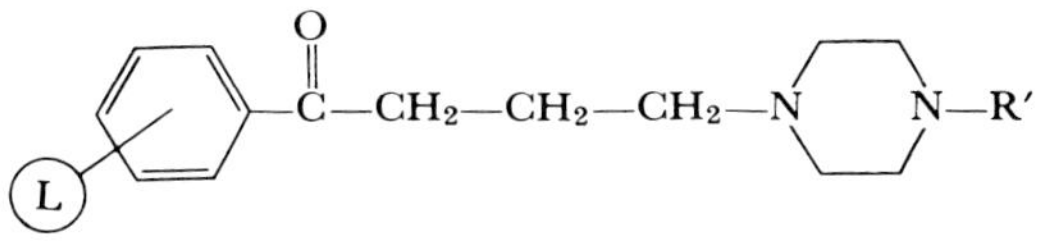

(IX)

The most interesting butyrophenones derived from piperidine (VII) are derivatives of either 4-phenylpiperidine (X) or of 4-anilinopiperidine (XI).

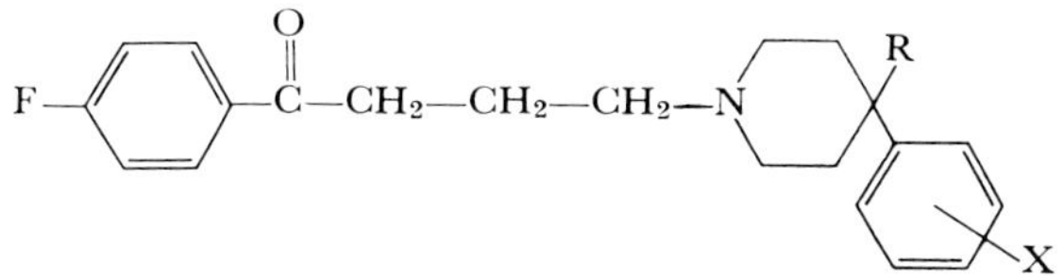

(X)

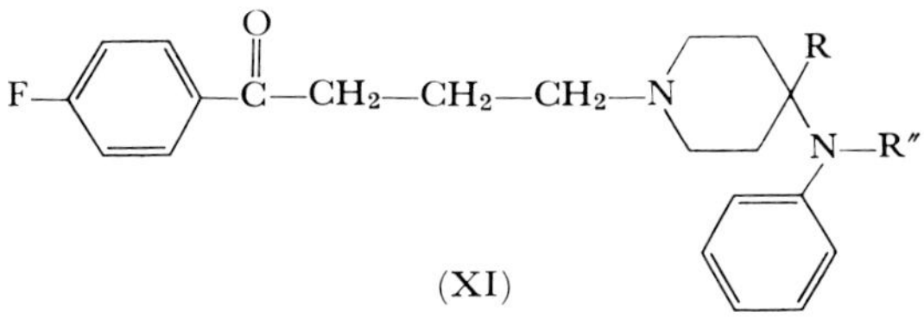

(XI)

Among the phenylpiperidines of type X, highest neuroleptic potency is found among structures (a) with a small substituent R in position 4 of the piperidine ring, e.g., OH (haloperidol, trifluperidol, methylperidol, Table I) or a tertiary amide (haloperidide, methylperidide, paraperidide, Table II), and (b) with one or two suitable aromatic substituents (X), e.g., 4-Cl (haloperidol, paraperidide), 3-CF$_3$ (trifluperidol), 3-Cl (haloperidide), 4-CH$_3$ (methylperidol), or 3-CH$_3$ (methylperidide).

The most interesting butyrophenones derived from 4-anilinopiperidine (XI) are compounds related to the benzimidazolone derivative, benperidol (XIII, Table I) or to the spiropiperidine, spiroperidol (XV, Table II).

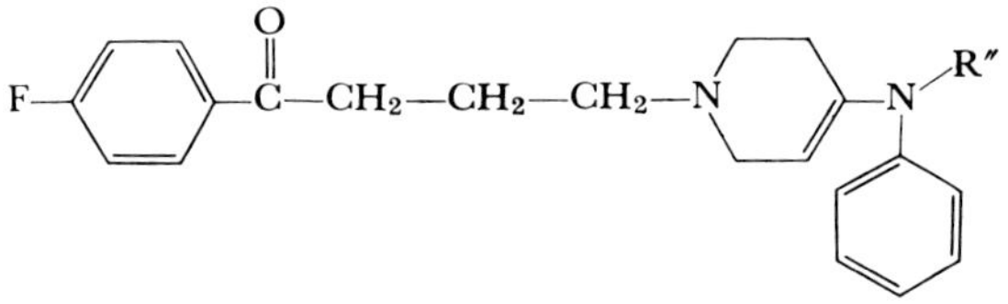

(XII)

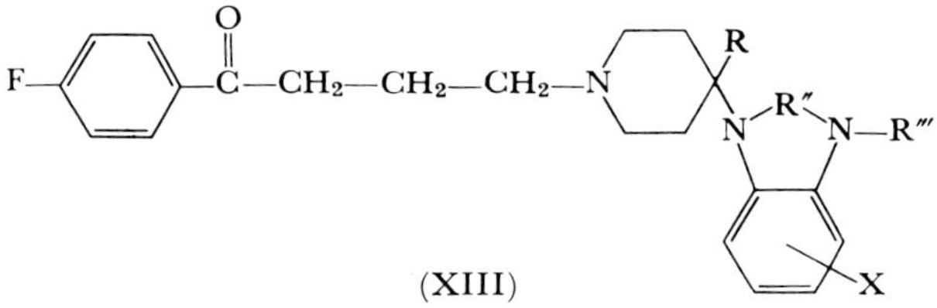

(XIII)

Droperidol (Table I) is the prototype of a series of potent neuroleptics of general structure (XIV) which are 4-anilinotetrahydropyridine derivatives of

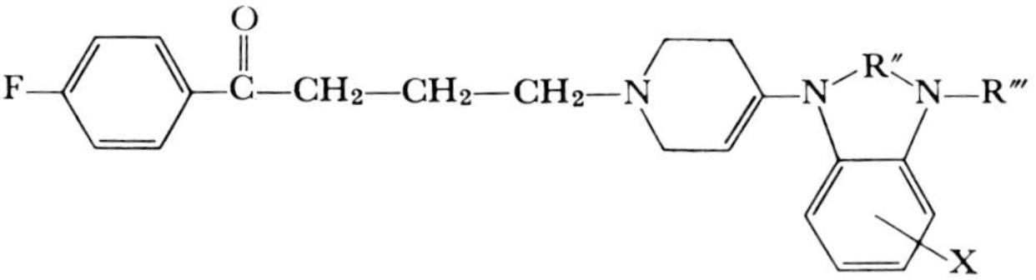

(XIV)

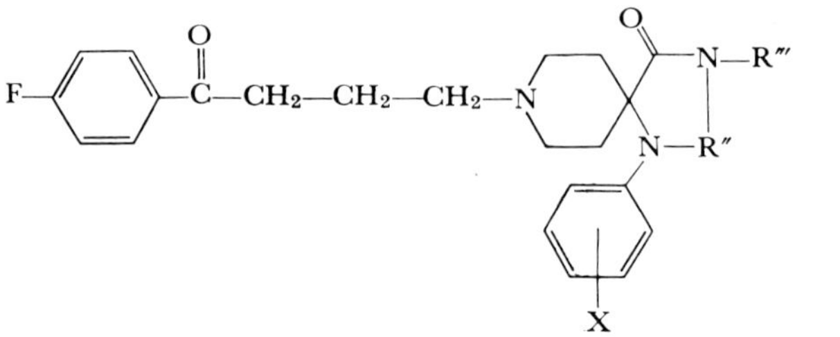

(XV)

butyrophenone (XII) closely related to the compounds of the benperidol series (XIII).

Floropipamide (Table I) is an α-aminoamide derived from 4-piperidinopiperidine (XVI: R = CONH$_2$) and floropipeton (Table II) is the corresponding ethylketone (XVI: R = COC$_2$H$_5$).

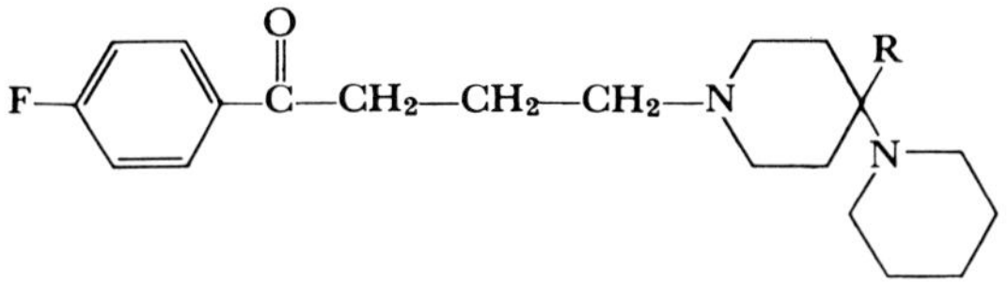

(XVI)

Among the derivatives of 4-piperazinobutyrophenone (IX), high neuroleptic potency requires the presence of an aromatic moiety R', e.g., a benzene ring (XVII) such as in fluanisone (Table I) or in butropipazone (Table II).

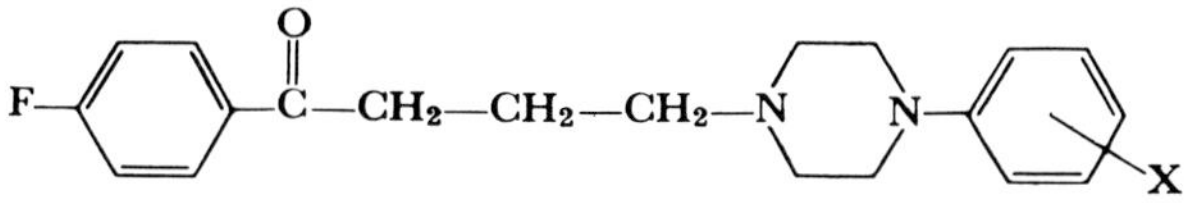

(XVII)

III. Pharmacological Activity of the Butyrophenones

Haloperidol and the other neuroleptics of the butyrophenone series are pharmacologically closely related to chlorpromazine and similar major tranquilizers derived from phenothiazine, e.g., fluphenazine, trifluperazine, prochlorperazine, thioridazine, and promazine.

An essentially comparative method of pharmacological classification of these various neuroleptic drugs, based on experimental data from use with dogs and rats, is illustrated in Table III.

The following tests were used for constructing Table III.
1. The jumping box test in dogs (Niemegeers and Janssen, 1960).

A trained dog is required to cross a hurdle when presented with an auditory warning signal in order to avoid electric shock. One, five, and twenty-five hours after subcutaneous injection or after oral administration of the experimental drug, the dog is subjected to ten consecutive 1-minute trials per session. A typical neuroleptic drug induces prolongation of the reaction time and hence leads to avoidance loss at low dose levels. There is no overt behavioral deficit at the ED$_{50}$ level.

The ratio "oral ED$_{50}$:s.c. ED$_{50}$", defined as the oral effectiveness ratio (OER), is a useful expression of the degree of gastrointestinal absorption of the drug.

TABLE III

Pharmacological Classification of a Series of Neuroleptic Drugs Based on Experimental Data in Dogs and in Rats[a]

Drugs	Dog: Jumping box test, ED_{50} (mg/kg), p.o.	Dog: Jumping box test, ED_{50} (mg/kg), s.c.	Dog: Jumping box test, OER[b]	Dog: Anti-apomorphine test, Lowest ED_{50}g (mg/k) s.c.	Dog: Anti-apomorphine test, Time-effect parameters, Peak effect (hours), onset	Dog: Anti-apomorphine test, Time-effect parameters, Peak effect (hours), duration	Dog: Anti-apomorphine test, Time-effect parameters, RRC[c]	Dog: ASR[d]	Rat: ED_{50}(mg/kg) s.c., Jumping box test	Rat: ED_{50}(mg/kg) s.c., Anti-amphetamine test	Rat: ED_{50}(mg/kg) s.c., Anti-norepinephrine test	Rat: Relative peripheral adrenolytic potency	Rat: Relative tendency to produce palpebral ptosis	Rat: Acute toxicity LD_{50} mg/kg subc	Prototype of category
	a	b	a/b	c				b/c	d	e	f	e/f	g	h	
1. Spiroperidol	0.01	0.005	2	0.00025	4	8	10	20	0.01	0.03	1	1/33	+	>320	Haloperidol
2. Benperidol	0.01	0.005	2	0.0005	¾	4	4	10	0.03	0.03	0.3	1/10	+	220	
3. Droperidol	0.02	0.01	2	0.001	<½	2	3.5	10	0.03	0.03	0.1	1/3	+	>640	
4. Trifluperidol	0.1	0.05	2	0.005	¾	3	3	10	0.03	0.03	0.3	1/10	+	70	
5. Haloperidol	0.1	0.05	2	0.015	<½	6	3	3.5	0.06	0.03	2	1/70	+	65	
6. Paraperidide	0.1	0.1	1	0.010	<½	6	6	10	0.2	0.1	7	1/70	+	320	
7. Methylperidol	0.3	0.1	3	0.015	¾	4	6	7	0.1	0.03	1	1/33	+	65	
8. Fluphenazine	0.6	0.06	10	0.006	3	6	5	10	0.03	0.01	1	1/10	+	640	
9. Haloperidide	0.6	0.06	10	0.002	<½	12	10	30	0.2	0.1	10	1/100	+	>160	
10. Methylperidide	1	0.02	50	0.002	<½	6	5	10	0.1	0.1	5	1/50	+	280	
11. Trifluperazine	1	0.5	2	0.03	¾	6	4	17	0.1	0.3	7	1/23	+	>320	
12. Prochlorperazine	3	3	1	0.7	<½	6	3	4	1	0.5	7	1/14	+	>320	
13. Fluanisone	1	0.2	5	0.15	<½	2	2.5	1.3	0.3	0.3	0.06	5	++	420	Chlorpromazine
14. Floropipamide	2	2	1	1.5	<½	4	3	1.3	10	5	2.5	2	+++	>265	
15. Butropipazone	3	4	¾	1.5	¾	1.5	2	2.6	2	1	0.15	6	++	550	
16. Chlorpromazine	5	2.5	2	0.7	¾	1.5	2	3.6	1	1	0.5	2	++	140	
17. Anisoperidone	40	>80	<½	1.5	<½	¾	1.5	>50	2	1	0.35	3	+++	>320	
18. Thioridazine	15	20	¾	3.5	3	16	2	5.7	20	100	0.7	143	+++	≥640	Promazine
19. Promazine	20	30	⅔	12	<½	6	1.5	2.5	10	30	0.7	43	++	300	
20. Aceperone	10	20	½	0.7	<½	3	3	30	10	>160	0.4	>400	++	>640	Aceperone

[a] Fourteen butyrophenone and six phenothiazine derivatives.
[b] Oral effectiveness ratio.
[c] Recovery rate constant.
[d] Antiemetic specificity ratio.

As seen in Table III, the twenty neuroleptics listed vary greatly in neuroleptic potency, the most active ones (spiroperidol and benperidol) being more than 1000 times more potent than the weakest neuroleptics of the series (anisoperidone, thioridazine, promazine, and aceperone). Chlorpromazine is a neuroleptic of moderate potency in dogs; doses of 1 to 10 mg/kg are required to produce significant avoidance failure. Fluphenazine is the most potent of the six phenothiazines listed, but it is poorly effective orally. Prochlorperazine is slightly more active than chlorpromazine but less active than trifluperazine. Thioridazine and promazine are roughly equiactive and well absorbed orally.

The most potent neuroleptics of the butyrophenone series (spiroperidol, benperidol, droperidol) are several times more active than fluphenazine, particularly when given orally. Fluphenazine is also a few times less active orally than trifluperidol, haloperidol, methylperidol and paraperidide, but about equally potent by the subcutaneous route.

By both routes of administration in dogs, fluphenazine and haloperidide are equipotent neuroleptics. The very poor oral effectiveness of methylperidide, an extremely potent parenteral drug, is particularly striking (OER = 50).

Fluanisone is comparable with trifluperazine in potency, whereas floropipamide and butropipazone are in the same activity class as prochlorperazine. Aceperone and anisoperidone, the two remaining butyrophenones of the series, are only effective at high dose levels, anisoperidone being surprisingly more active orally than subcutaneously. It should be noted that the relative oral effectiveness of weakly active neuroleptics is generally high (OER = $\frac{1}{2}$ to 2).

2. The anti-apomorphine test in dogs (Janssen et al., 1965b; Niemegeers, 1960).

A dog is given a subcutaneous dose of the experimental drug and challenged, $\frac{1}{2}$, 1, 2, 4, 8, 16, 32, or 64 hours thereafter, with an emetic dose of 0.31 mg/kg of apomorphine hydrochloride subcutaneously. By probit analysis independent ED_{50}'s (no emesis in half of the pretreated dogs) are thus obtained for each time interval. These ED_{50}'s are plotted on log–log paper to estimate the following parameters: (a) the lowest ED_{50}-value (mg/kg s.c.); (b) onset and duration of the period of peak activity (lowest ED_{50}); (c) the recovery rate constant (RRC), calculated as illustrated in Fig. 1, an expression of the rate at which the effect of the drug disappears following the period of peak activity. A compound with a low RRC will tend to accumulate in the body when repeatedly administered.

The ratio "s.c. ED_{50}, jumping box: lowest ED_{50}, anti-apomorphine test" is defined as the antiemetic specificity ratio of the experimental drug.

It is seen in Table III that all twenty compounds listed as powerful antagonists of apomorphine-induced emesis at dose levels that are slightly lower to more than 50 times lower than ED_{50} levels of the jumping box test. In this sense, all these neuroleptics are "specific" apomorphine-antagonists.

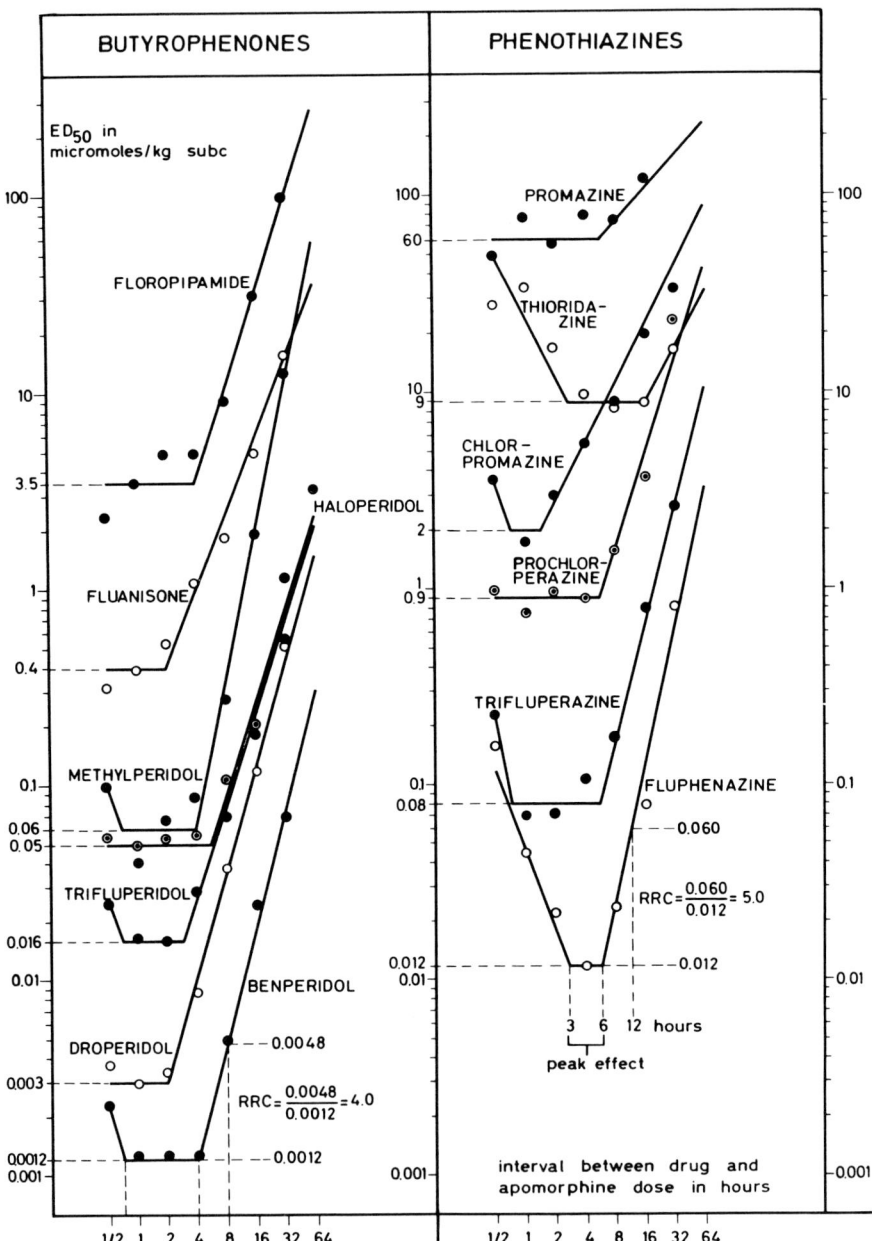

FIG. 1. Time-effect parameters of seven derivatives of butyrophenone and of six derivatives of phenothiazine in the anti-apomorphine test in dogs.

The antiemetic specificity of fluanisone and floropipamide is of a lower order than that of the other eighteen drugs of Table III (ASR = 1.3). Haloperidol, methylperidol, prochlorperazine, butropipazone, chlorpromazine, thioridazine and promazine have a somewhat higher ASR (2.6 to 4). Haloperidide (ASR = 30), aceperone (ASR = 30) and particularly anisoperidone (ASR > 50) are extremely specific antiemetic agents within the framework of the definition as previously outlined. The eight remaining drugs have specificity ratios of 10 to 20.

As compared with most other central nervous system (CNS) drugs, neuroleptics in general have a rather slow onset and a prolonged duration of action. With the slowest acting compounds of Table III (spiroperidol, fluphenazine, and thioridazine) the period of maximal antiemetic effectiveness in dogs has an onset of 3 to 4 hours after subcutaneous injection, all other compounds listed reach peak activity within 0.75 hour. Among the potent neuroleptics, droperidol and haloperidol are the fastest acting ones.

Half of the twenty drugs listed in Table III are long acting, with a peak effect period of 6 to 16 hours; spiroperidol, haloperidide, and thioridazine have the longest duration of action. Spiroperidol and haloperidide however have the highest recovery rate constants (RRC = 10) of the series. Among the other long acting neuroleptics, haloperidol has the lowest RRC (3), and may therefore be expected to accumulate in the body more easily when given on a chronic administration schedule. Droperidol, on the other hand, is the shortest acting potent neuroleptic known.

It should be noted that the least potent antiemetics of the series (lowest $ED_{50} = 0.15$ to 3.5 mg/kg s.c.) tend to recover more slowly (RRC = 1.5 to 3) than the more potent ones ($ED_{50} - 0.00025$ to 0.03; RRC = 3 to 10) (Janssen et al., 1965b).

3. The jumping box test in rats (Table III), (Janssen 1961c, d); (Janssen et al. 1963b, 1965a, 1966).

The experimental details of this test are identical to those described previously for the jumping box experiment in dogs. In both species a typical neuroleptic drug induces a similar abnormal behavioral state in which the trained animal, without showing overt signs of neurological deficit, will fail to avoid shock by crossing a hurdle when presented with the auditory warning signal. The ED_{50}'s are similarly computed for both species by probit analysis.

The ratio "ED_{50} rat: ED_{50} dog" (jumping box test, s.c.) is therefore an expression of species differences in sensitivity to a given drug (ratio d/b in Table III).

Except for anisoperidone, which is almost inactive by subcutaneous route in the dog's jumping box test, but clearly active in rats (d/b < 1/40), the d/b ratios for the nineteen other neuroleptics of Table III scatter around unity.

For some reasons, possibly metabolic ones, the Wistar rat seems to be more sensitive than the dog (on a mg/kg basis) for phenothiazine derivatives, for compounds having an aromatic trifluoromethyl group, and generally for neuroleptics of low potency.

On the same basis, the dog appears to be more sensitive than the rat to butyrophenones derived from 4-anilinopiperidine, for the basic amides of the peridide group and, in general, for neuroleptics of high potency.

For slightly more than half of the neuroleptics tested, however, we found no significant quantitative difference in the jumping box test (s.c.) between ED_{50} (dog) and ED_{50} (rat).

4. The anti-amphetamine test (Table III), (Janssen, 1961c,d; Janssen et al., 1965a).

All rats react with compulsory gnawing or chewing movements to an intravenous dose of 10 mg/kg of amphetamine and pretreatment with a low dose of a typical neuroleptic drug will prevent this reaction.

All twenty neuroleptics listed in Table III, except aceperone ($ED_{50} > 160$ mg/kg) are potent antagonists of amphetamine, as measured 1 hour after subcutaneous injection, at dose levels that are about the same as the doses needed for inhibiting learned behavioral habits in the jumping box test. When $d = ED_{50}$ (jumping box test, s.c., rat) and $e = ED_{50}$ (anti-amphetamine test, s.c., rat), then eighteen of the twenty d/e ratios for the twenty neuroleptics of Table III scatter around unity ($d/e = \frac{1}{3}$ to 3); thirteen of them are not significantly different from unity (P 0.05). The low ratios of thioridazine ($d/e = \frac{1}{5}$) and of aceperone ($d/e < \frac{1}{16}$) are the only noteworthy exceptions to the general rule.

A typical neuroleptic drug may therefore be said to be a specific antagonist of amphetamine-induced gnawing in the rat.

5. The anti-norepinephrine test in rats (Table III) (Janssen 1961c,d; Janssen et al., 1965a).

The twenty neuroleptic drugs listed in Table III are all peripheral adrenolytic agents in the sense that they antagonize a number of epinephrine- or norepinephrine-induced peripheral effects, particularly those that are said to be caused by alpha-receptor stimulation. Reversal of epinephrine-induced pressor effects or inhibition of epinephrine-induced contractions of the isolated rabbit spleen are classical procedures for evaluating this type of peripheral alpha-adrenolytic activity. We have found however that the results of these classical tests correlate very well with the results obtained by measuring the ability of neuroleptic drugs in preventing the toxic effects of a lethal intravenous dose of epinephrine or norepinephrine. For the purpose of classifying neuroleptic agents as in Table III, we prefer to use the antinorepinephrine test, which shows excellent correlation with a similar antiepinephrine test, but is more sensitive (lower ED_{50}'s) and somewhat more reproducible.

The ED_{50} in this test is the estimated subcutaneous dose (probit analysis) which protects half of the treated rats against the lethal effect of an intravenous dose of 1.25 mg/kg of norepinephrine, given 1 hour after the experimental drug.

The e/f ratio (e = ED_{50}, anti-amphetamine test; f = ED_{50}, anti-norepinephrine test) is used as a measurement of the relative peripheral adrenolytic potency of the experimental drug, i.e., the extent to which it tends to induce alpha-receptor blockade at "therapeutic," i.e., neuroleptic dose levels.

As seen in Table III, the twenty compounds listed vary greatly in terms of both absolute and relative adrenolytic potency. The most potent alpha-blocker of the series, fluanisone (ED_{50} = 0.06 mg/kg s.c.), is about 170 times more potent that haloperidide, the weakest one (ED_{50} = 10 mg/kg), aceperone (e/f > 400), is relatively more than 40,000 times more potent than haloperidide (e/f = $\frac{1}{100}$).

On the basis of relative peripheral adrenolytic potency, the twenty neuroleptics of Table III can be classified as follows in four distinct categories:

(a) The haloperidol category (e/f = $\frac{1}{3}$ to $\frac{1}{100}$). These drugs are practically devoid of peripheral adrenolytic effects at neuroleptic dose levels.

(b) The chlorpromazine category (e/f = 2 to 6). These drugs are moderately active as peripheral adrenolytics at neuroleptic dose levels.

(c) The promazine category (e/f = 43 to 143). These drugs exert potent peripheral adrenolytic effects at neuroleptic dose levels.

(d) The aceperone category (e/f > 400). Aceperone is almost a specific adrenolytic agent, being devoid of significant anti-amphetamine activity within the framework of the definitions as previously outlined.

Among the twelve compounds of the haloperidol category, droperidol (e/f = $\frac{1}{3}$) is relatively more active as an adrenolytic agent than the other drugs. It is followed, in order of decreasing relative adrenolytic potency, by benperidol, trifluperidol and fluphenazine (e/f = $\frac{1}{10}$), prochlorperazine ($\frac{1}{14}$), trifluperazine ($\frac{1}{23}$), spiroperidol and methylperidol ($\frac{1}{33}$), methylperidide ($\frac{1}{50}$), haloperidol and parapcrididc ($\frac{1}{70}$), and finally haloperidide ($\frac{1}{100}$).

Fluanisone is the most potent representative of the chlorpromazine category, followed by butropipazone, anisoperidone, chlorpromazine, and floropipamide. Fluanisone and butropipazone are relatively somewhat more potent than the three other drugs of this category, but relatively much less potent than promazine, thioridazine, and particularly aceperone.

6. The catalepsy-ptosis observation test in rats (Janssen 1961a, c, d; Janssen et al., 1965b).

This test consists of determining the subcutaneous ED_{50} of the experimental drug that induces a state of typical cataleptic immobility in 50% of treated rats. The tendency of rats, treated with this dose, to keep their eyes closed during handling is simultaneously evaluated.

As shown in Table III, there is a striking correlation between relative tendency to produce palpebral ptosis and relative peripheral adrenolytic potency. The twelve "specific" neuroleptics of the haloperidol category are relatively weakly active in both respects, the eight other compounds are not only relatively more active as adrenolytics, but also as ptosis-inducing drugs.

Floropipamide, anisoperidone, and thioridazine are relatively more active in the ptosis test in rats than fluanisone, butropipazone, chlorpromazine, and promazine.

Table III also shows all twenty listed drugs to be relatively atoxic in rats, the LD_{50} exceeding the lowest ED_{50} by a factor of 250 or more; the most potent neuroleptics tend to show the highest safety ratio. Droperidol, for example, is atoxic at 20,000 times its neuroleptic ED_{50}.

Taking the jumping box data in dogs (Table III) as a parameter for predicting equiactive "neuroleptic" dose levels in man, the time-effect parameters of the anti-apomorphine test in dogs for predicting clinical duration of action and tendency to produce cumulative effects, the relative adrenolytic potency data in rats for predicting the expected intensity of orthostatic hypotension and tachycardia at neuroleptic dose levels in man, and relative tendency to produce palpebral ptosis in rats as a parameter for predicting the clinical tendency of the drug to produce symptoms of oversedation or drowsiness at neuroleptic dose levels, one would arrive at the following predictive conclusions:

(a) The drugs of the haloperidol category are "selective" neuroleptic agents, inducing a typical neuroleptic syndrome at minimal active dose levels, orthostatic hypotension and oversedation are observed with significantly higher doses only. Droperidol, the shortest acting drug of this category, is however more likely to induce adrenolytic effects at therapeutic dose levels than the eleven other members of the group. Fluphenazine, haloperidide, and methylperidide are relatively less active orally than the other drugs of Table III. The first symptoms of overdosage are side effects of the extrapyramidal type.

(b) The five members of the chlorpromazine category are expected to produce orthostatic hypotension and tachycardia regularly at neuroleptic dose levels, floropipamide and anisoperidone are more active as sedatives than fluanisone, butropipazone, and chlorpromazine.

Neurological side effects are uncommon at minimal active dose levels at which autonomic effects and sedation are expected to dominate the clinical picture.

(c) Thioridazine and promazine are expected to induce sedation and orthostatic hypotension at dose levels that are much lower than the neuroleptic dose levels. With these relatively weak and aspecific neuroleptic drugs, it should be practically difficult to induce a typical neurological neuroleptic syndrome in man.

(d) With the almost specific adrenolytic drug aceperone, blood pressure effects should predominate clinically, with CNS effects occurring at extremely high doses only.

Detailed studies on the pharmacology, chemistry, toxicology, use in animals, metabolism, and biochemical mechanism of action of haloperidol, trifluperidol, droperidol, and other butyrophenones have been published by several authors, i.e. Andén *et al*. (1964); Bhargava (1965); Boissier and Pagny (1960); Boissier and Simon (1963, 1964a,b); Boissier *et al*. (1960, 1961, 1964a,b, 1965); Bruno and Allegranza (1965); Buchel and Lévy (1962a,b); Buchel *et al*. (1962); Carlsson and Lindqvist (1963); Carlsson and Waldeck (1965); Carlsson *et al*. (1962); Cession-Fossion *et al*. (1961); Chen (1965); Chen and Ensor (1962); Chodoff and Domino (1965); Demoen (1961); Dobkin and Criswick (1961); Dresse and Cession-Fossion (1962); Dresse and De Meyer (1964, 1965); Dresse *et al*. (1962); Frommel and Chmouliovsky (1964); Frommel and Joye (1963); Frommel *et al*. (1960); Gardocki *et al*. (1964); Goldwurm and Vanni (1961); Groh and Lemieux (1964); Ingvar and Nilsson (1961); Janssen (1961a,b,c,d, 1962a,b,c,d, 1964a, b,c,d); Janssen and Niemegeers (1959, 1961a,b); Janssen *et al*. (1959, 1960a,b,c,d, 1962, 1963a,b, 1965a,b, 1966); Kakolewski (1964); Kandaurova (1964); Kato *et al*. (1964); Kreuscher (1965a); La Barre (1962, 1963); Lechat and Deleau (1965); Lechner *et al*. (1961); Lecomte and Dresse (1962); Marriott and Spencer (1965) Marsboom (1963); Marsboom and Allewijn (1964); Marsboom and Mortelmans (1964); Marsboom and Sierens (1962a,b); Marsboom *et al*. (1962, 1963a,b, 1964b); McIlwain (1964); Morpurgo (1965); Mortelmans *et al*. (1962); Munkvad (1962); Niemegeers (1960); Niemegeers and Janssen (1960); Niemegeers *et al*. (1964); Nilsson and Janssen (1961); Nordström and Kugelberg (1964); Oskam (1965); Randrup *et al*. (1963); Revol (1961); Revol and Miachon (1963); Roos (1965); Schaper and Jageneau (1961); Schaper *et al*. (1960, 1962, 1963); Schmitt and Schmitt (1962); Sodoyez *et al*. (1962); Soep (1961a,b); Soep and Janssen (1961); Soyka (1964); Spencer (1965); Stille *et al*. (1965); Thomas and Dryon (1964); Usdin and Usdin (1961); Van de Westeringh *et al*. (1964); Van Nueten (1962); Van Rossum (1965); Venning (1963); Verstraete *et al*. (1962); Yelnosky and Field (1964); Yelnosky and Gardocki (1964); Yelnosky *et al*. (1964). A detailed discussion of the available data is not within the scope of this review.

IV. Clinical Uses

A. Haloperidol (R 1625)

Haloperidol is a powerful neuroleptic drug in man. Its clinical properties are documented in over 400 published studies and an estimated 200 million daily doses of haloperidol were used therapeutically between 1958 and 1965. The original pilot studies were conducted at Liège University by Divry *et al*. (1958, 1959a). In the first 400 clinical papers on haloperidol published between 1959 and October 1965, a total of 35,364 haloperidol-treated patients are described in more or less detail, i.e., 11,948 adult psychiatric cases, 238 children with mental disease, 1885 patients in which the drug was used for preventing or treating nausea and vomiting, 18,611 patients undergoing surgery in which haloperidol was used as an adjunct to anesthesia, generally neuroleptanalgesia (NLA), and 2682 obstetrical cases.

The results of a total of twenty-eight controlled trials are available, i.e., nineteen in psychiatry, two in psychology, five in anesthesiology, and two in obstetrics.

Haloperidol is about equally active orally as parenterally. In adults the recommended parenteral dose is 2.5 to 5 mg. The optimal oral maintenance dose, usually between 0.5 mg and 30 mg daily (average, 3 mg), depends on many factors such as the severity of the symptoms and the individual susceptibility of the patient to neuroleptic drugs in general, and should be determined by individual titration.

In severely ill acute psychotic episodes, the recommended practice is to initiate haloperidol therapy with relatively high parenteral doses and to continue, as soon as the situation is brought under control, with oral maintenance doses, i.e., drops or tablets, once or twice daily.

In psychiatry, haloperidol is particularly useful as an antipsychotic drug and for patients with psychomotor agitation of various etiology, for example, manic reactions, alcoholic delirium, aggressive and destructive behavior, tic nerveux, and chorea, both in adults (Aleksandrovskii, 1964; Alema and Gianniotti, 1962; Alemà et al., 1961, 1962a,b; Alleva, 1962b; Amati and Procaccini, 1962; Baccaglini and Caprini, 1960; Baciocchi, 1961; Balducci and Frascella, 1962; Balducci and Loguloso, 1962; Ban, 1962, 1964; Ban and Stonehill, 1964; Bandettini Di Poggio and Levi, 1960; Bianchi and Ronchi, 1963; Bishop et al., 1965; Bister, 1961; Blandin et al., 1961; Bobon and Collard, 1962; Bobon et al., 1963a; Bohacek, 1961, 1964; Bonhoure, 1962; Borenstein and Blès, 1963; Borenstein et al., 1962a,b,c,d,e; Borghesi, 1964; Bouchard, 1965; Bozzi et al., 1962; Brandrup and Kristjansen, 1961; Buffardi, 1962; Buis, 1962; Buis and Flohil, 1964; Burgermeister, 1965; Caldonazzo, 1960; Cameron, 1965; Caprini and Melotti, 1961; Capron, 1962; Carbonell Cadenas De Llano and Herrero Aldama, 1960; Cardani and Goldwurm, 1960; Cardo et al., 1965; Caron et al., 1961; Cenacchi, 1962; Challas and Brauer, 1963; Chapel et al., 1964; Collard, 1962; Cook, 1966; Corneli and Rotondi, 1961; Cossa and Paoli, 1961; Court and Cameron, 1963; Craft, 1965; Cwynar and Bukowczyk, 1962; Dagan et al., 1963; Danik and Goverdhan, 1962; Davies, 1962; Davoli et al., 1960; De Haene, 1960; Delay and Deniker, 1961a,b; Delay et al., (1960a,c,d, 1962b, 1964; De Lerma Penasco, 1961; Della Beffa, 1962; Della Pietra, 1962; Della Pietra and Fina, 1960; Della Rovere, 1960; De Maio et al., 1960; De Mondragon, 1964; Denber and Collard, 1962; Denber et al., 1959, 1962; Deniker, 1963, 1964; Deprez, 1961; Dick, 1962; Di

Cristo, 1960; Divry *et al.*, 1958, 1959a, 1960a; Dolley, 1962; Durost *et al.*, 1964; Enoch and Robin, 1960; Entwistle *et al.*, 1962; Evrard *et al.*, 1960; Failla *et al.*, 1962; Fajardo, 1965; Favier *et al.*, 1963; Ferrero, 1962; Ferro-Milone and Lorizio, 1964; Flegel, 1961, 1962, 1964a; Flegel and Neller, 1963; Flegel *et al.*, 1960; Fiume and Argenta, 1962; Fourny *et al.*, 1961, 1962; Fox *et al.*, 1964; Franchini *et al.*, 1962; Galindez *et al.*, 1963; Garry and Leonard, 1962; Gatti and Bertini, 1960; Gattuso and Lanteri, 1962; Gavaudan *et al.*, 1962; Géraud *et al.*, 1963; Gerle, 1960, 1962, 1963, 1964a,b; Gerle *et al.*, 1961; Geyer and Mayr, 1962; Giacobini and Lassenius, 1961; Giannelli and Invernizzi, 1960; Gillet, 1965; Giordano and Cipriani, 1964; Gjerris, 1965; Goldman, 1961; Goldwurm and Torrigiani, 1962; Gonçalves and Newton Lacerda, 1964; Guilbert *et al.*, 1961; Harder, 1961; Haward, 1964, 1965; Hekimian and Friedhoff, 1964; Hollister and Motzenbecker, 1963; Hollister *et al.*, 1962; Holstein and Chen, 1965; Houillon *et al.*, 1961; Hulak, 1964; Humbeeck, 1960; Jacob and Marie, 1961; Jacobs, 1959, 1960; Jensen, 1962; Kabat, 1961; Kaczynski *et al.*, 1965; Kakolewski, 1964; Kamenskaia and Aleksandrovskij, 1964; Kamphausen, 1962; Kent, 1965; Kivalo and Amneli, 1961; Kristjansen, 1960, 1962; Kristjansen and Hansen, 1961; Kurland *et al.*, 1964; Labhardt, 1964; Lacourt, 1963; Lambert, 1964; Lassner, 1964; Lavitola and Santorelli, 1962; Lecoeur, 1965; Ledesma Jimeno, 1963; Lehmann *et al.*, 1964; Lehoczki and Halasy, 1961; Leone, 1962; Leyritz *et al.*, 1961; Lindqvist, 1961; Linford Rees, 1965; Linford Rees and Davies, 1965; Lods *et al.*, 1964; Loret, 1960; Luna, 1964; Luria and Rizzuto, 1964; Maccagnani and Albonetti, 1960; Maccagnani *et al.*, 1962; Madalena *et al.*, 1963; Madeddu and Leone, 1960a,b; Manganaro and De Casi, 1961; Marquez *et al.*, 1964; Martin and Carranza Sanchez, 1960; Masciocchi and Marino, 1962; Masciocchi *et al.*, 1961, 1962; Mendigutia *et al.*, 1960; Meurice, 1960a,b; Milani, 1962; Milne, 1965; Monceaux, 1961; Monnerot *et al.*, 1961; Montigneaux, 1962; Morosini, 1962; Mueller and Warnes, 1964; Nayrac *et al.*, 1964; Neumann, 1960; Nick and Nicolle, 1964, 1965; Nistri and Mori, 1962; Okasha and Tewfik, 1964; Oles, 1960a,b, 1962; Olsson, 1961; Oosterbaan and Van Wijk, 1962; Pagliano *et al.*, 1962; Paleologue *et al.*, 1962; Paley *et al.*, 1962; Pancer, 1964; Paquay *et al.*, 1959a,b, 1960a,c, 1962a,b; Pavlou-Karageorgiadou *et al.*, 1962; Pelaz, 1960a,b, 1962; Périer, 1961; Pigem *et al.*, 1960; Piret, 1965; Piret-Pilachon, 1962; Pratt *et al.*, 1964; Puca and Cascella, 1960; Renald *et al.*, 1965; Riggi and Vanni, 1962; Ronchi, 1962; Rosa *et al.*, 1964; Rouleau and Jean, 1964; Rovetta, 1962; Royer, 1962; Ruggerini and Zecca, 1964; Ruiz, 1962; Ruiz and Leyla, 1963; Santiago Barrios, 1961; Sarwer-Foner, 1964; Schneider *et al.*, 1963; Schwarz *et al.*, 1961, 1962; Schweigh *et al.*, 1961; Seabra-Dinis and da Silva, 1960; Seignot, 1961; Songar, 1959; Soulairac *et al.*, 1962a; Steenfeldt-Foss, 1962, 1963; St. Jean *et al.*, 1964; Stucke, 1963; Subra *et al.*, 1962; Sugerman *et al.*, 1964; Svendsen and Willadsen, 1963; Szobor, 1962; Temkov and Daskalov, 1962; Tewfik, 1965; Van der Spek, 1962; Varela, 1961; Warnes *et al.*, 1964; Zerbe,

1964; Zerbini et al., 1962) and in children (Aldeghi and Maderna, 1961; Blackford Rogers, 1965; Brauner, 1964; Dongier et al., 1961; Duché, 1961; Dykyj and Nodine, 1964; Feldmann, 1963; Gastaut et al., 1962; Gayral et al., 1965; Haberlandt, 1963; Jancar, 1965; Jaeggi et al., 1960; Merland and Aubin, 1961; Schmitz et al., 1961).

As an antipsychotic drug, haloperidol is particularly effective against hallucinations and somewhat less effective against delirious symptoms. Withdrawn schizophrenics tend to be less responsive than active schizophrenics.

Haloperidol treatment gave excellent results in 86.3% of 572 manic patients, reported on by forty-nine different investigators, in 83.9% of 1371 adults with severe psychomotor agitation of various etiology (twenty investigators), in 75.4% of 541 acute schizophrenic episodes, and in 53.0% of 2930 chronic schizophrenics (sixty-two investigators). In many of these patients, haloperidol was not given at optimal dose levels, as determined by careful titration. The calculated percentages are therefore on the low side.

Haloperidol is useful as a tranquillizer in certain types of neurosis (Azima et al., 1960; Böcher et al., 1964; Domanowsky, 1963; Fierlafyn, 1963b; Friedrich, 1963; Hilgers, 1964; Lehoczki and Halasy, 1961; Mahoudeau and Elissalde, 1963; Nodine et al., 1962; Pelaz and Sanz, 1964; Perini, 1964; Perini and Lampo, 1964; Pöldinger, 1964; Prumm, 1963; Samuels, 1961; von Eiff and Jesdinski, 1960; Waelkens, 1960a; Wambsganss, 1965a,b), in anesthesiology (Bergmann, 1962, 1964; Brown, 1962, 1963, 1964, 1965; Brown et al., 1963; Citro and Calligari, 1964; Civai and Chesi, 1964; Deligné, 1961a,b; Gianasi and Nanni Costa, 1964; Gürtner et al., 1964; Helrich and Atwood, 1964; Hofmann, 1965; Kapferer, 1961, 1962; Kapferer et al., 1962; Laffargue-Leguerinel, 1963; Le Goaziou, 1962; Mainardi and Ardillo, 1965; Marsico, 1964; Mostert and Milner, 1961; Mundeleer and De Castro, 1962; Nilsson, 1962a,b,c, 1963; Nilsson and Janssen, 1961; Nordström and Kugelberg, 1964; Rossi, 1964; Saarne, 1963; Sabathié, 1962; Schweder, 1964; Soergel, 1963; Vanzelli and Andreoli, 1964) and in obstetrics (Ardillo et al., 1965; Beck, 1962; Lawson and McGowan, 1962; Pomarede-Ravoir, 1963).

Haloperidol is also a powerful antiemetic drug (Appiani, 1960; Casaglia, 1960; Cipriani and Giordano, 1961; Cuocolo and Messina, 1961; Dyrberg, 1962; Kandaperredy-Tellier, 1964; Magnier, 1964; Mainardi, 1964; Nanni Costa and Cianasi, 1960; Riding, 1963; Saarne, 1963; Stoll, 1962).

The most important undesirable features associated with intensive haloperidol therapy are the typical signs and symptoms of the so-called extrapyramidal type, which are common to all neuroleptic drugs, i.e., akinesia, akathisia, dyskinesia, and Parkinson-like rigidity and tremor (Ayd, 1961).

The incidence of these side effects in adults is negligible below 1.5 mg of haloperidol daily, low below 3 mg daily, significant between 3 and 6 mg daily, common between 6 and 12 mg daily, and very common above 12 mg daily. Women are more apt to have unpleasant neurological reactions to neuroleptic drugs in general than men, although dyskinesia happens more often in men. Parkinsonism develops more easily in elderly patients, akathisia in middle-aged patients, and dyskinesia in young patients. Dyskinesia occurs as a rule during the few first days of treatment, akathisia several days later, and parkinsonism is usually the last side effect to appear.

Severely agitated patients are much less likely to develop these side effects than others, whereas hysterical patients are quite sensitive. Environmental factors and suggestion can have striking positive or negative effects on reactions of the neurodysleptic type.

Autonomic side reactions, such as orthostatic hypotension and tachycardia as well as oversedation and somnolence, are relatively rare in haloperidol-treated patients. In general, therefore, the side-effect liability of haloperidol is predictable from animal data and quite comparable with the side effect liability of fluphenazine, trifluperazine, prochlorperazine, perphenazine, and other potent neuroleptic drugs.

The incidence of chronic toxic reactions associated with long-term therapy is extremely low. In a series of 12,500 analyzed patients (Gerle, 1964a), there was no significant hematological, hepatological, gastrointestinal, endocrine, dermatological, or ophthalmological pathology. Haloperidol-induced neurological symptoms disappear spontaneously. Furthermore, they can be counteracted with an effective anti-Parkinson agent.

Insomnia has been reported in patients treated with fairly large maintenance doses. Therefore, most psychiatrists prefer to give haloperidol in the morning and eventually a second dose at noon, but not in the evening.

Depressive reactions have been observed in haloperidol-treated patients, particularly in manic depressive states after the manic episode was brought under control. This is also a common finding with all potent and specific neuroleptic drugs.

As with most other drugs, the extent of the therapeutic benefit derived from haloperidol therapy, more predictable in certain types of patients than in others, not only depends on the selection of the patient but also on the environmental setting and on the ability of the treating physician to prescribe and administer adequate dose levels.

B. Trifluperidol (R 2498)

The clinical results obtained with trifluperidol in the treatment of 1347 patients with severe mental disease are reported upon in fifty-four publications; nine of which describe controlled trials. Between 1961 and 1965, an estimated 15 million doses of trifluperidol have been used clinically.

In the original publication by Divry *et al.* (1960b), trifluperidol is described as a potent neuroleptic drug, about twice as active as haloperidol. Optimal activity was obtained with 2.5 mg (1 to 5 mg) daily in acute cases and 1 mg (0.3 to 1.8 mg) daily in oral maintenance therapy. As an antipsychotic agent, trifluperidol possesses powerful hallucinolytic properties. Withdrawn, autistic schizophrenics generally derive more therapeutic benefit from trifluperidol than from haloperidol, whereas the latter drug is superior in the treatment of severe psychomotor agitation. The side-effect liability of both drugs is qualitatively similar; excitomotor symptoms, such as akathisia and neurodysleptic reactions, occurring relatively more frequently in trifluperidol-treated patients. Subsequent investigators essentially confirmed these original conclusions.

A group of fifty-seven newly admitted 20- to 52-year-old schizophrenic men with slightly above average symptomatology were treated by Hollister et al. (1965) for six weeks with trifluperidol tablets. Following a 2-week period of initial build-up (1, 2, 4 mg daily), daily doses ranged between 1.5 and 12 mg (average 5.5 mg). Significant improvement was noted in thirteen of the sixteen syndromes scored on the BPRS, on all ten factors of the IMPS, and on each of four syndrome factors derived from the BPRS, i.e., somatic concern, anxiety, emotional withdrawal, conceptual disorganization, tension, mannerism-posturing, grandiosity, hostility, suspiciousness, hallucinatory behavior, uncooperativeness, unusual thought content and blunted affect (BPRS), excitement, hostile belligerence, paranoid projection, grandiose expansiveness, perceptual distortion, anxious intropunitiveness, retardation-apathy, disorientation, motor disturbance and conceptual disorganization (IMPS), thinking disturbance, withdrawal-retardation, paranoid interpersonal and depressive disturbance BPRS syndrome factors. The results of this study place trifluperidol among the most effective antipsychotic drugs known. Computer analysis of pretreatment-rating profiles was used for classifying the fifty-seven patients: eleven "paranoids," forty "schizophrenics," and six "depressives," i.e., three diagnostic categories.

The results indicate that trifluperidol is not only quite effective across the total patient sample, but also superior to any other drug for the treatment of patients of the "paranoid" type, i.e., those with maximal elevations in grandiosity, hostility, and suspiciousness, and with minimum guilt feelings, depressive mood, and motor retardation. The most frequent side effects were muscular rigidity, observed in half of the patients. Akathisia occurred in about $\frac{1}{3}$ and dystonia in $\frac{1}{5}$ of the cases.

Three different rigorous double-blind studies of trifluperidol versus "prototype drug" in a total of fifty-seven acute and ninety-six chronic schizophrenics were conducted in New Orleans by Bishop and Gallant (1965), Bishop et al. (1965), Gallant et al. (1963a,b, 1965) and Pratt et al. (1964). In the first 10-week test, oral trifluperidol had a significantly greater therapeutic effect in chronic schizophrenia than oral chlorpromazine, not only in the global ratings of improvement but in the majority of the objective psychological tests as well. Trifluperidol (6 mg daily) produced much less hypotension and sedation, but more extrapyramidal side effects than 1200 mg of chlorpromazine. Benztropine was quite effective in counteracting these neurological symptoms.

In a similar 10-week double-blind test, both trifluperidol and trifluoperazine were clearly superior to phenobarbital in a group of sixty hospitalized chronic schizophrenics. Trifluperidol had a greater and more rapid effect than trifluoperazine as measured in the global ratings of improvement, suggesting that trifluperidol may well be the drug of choice for schizophrenic patients. The side-effect liability of both drugs was similar (Gallant et al., 1965).

In a third double-blind test conducted at Tulane University (Pratt et al., 1964), trifluperidol was compared with haloperidol and with chlorpromazine in fifty-eight hospitalized schizophrenic patients. Capsules were given for a period of 30 days. Dosage was gradually increased and maximal doses were 4 mg of trifluperidol, 16 mg of haloperidol, and 800 mg of chlorpromazine. The psychiatric and psychological evaluation techniques included the Beckomberga rating scale for the schizophrenia factor, the MACC behavioral adjustment scale for evaluation of ward behavior, subjective global ratings of improvement by the responsible psychiatrist, and the Tulane test battery, comprised of measures of perceptual response speed, memory, comprehension or judgment, psychomotor speed, and aspects of general test behavior.

Both butyrophenones were clearly superior to chlorpromazine as indicated by analysis of the combined measures ($P < 0.05$). Somnolence was more notable in the chlorpromazine group, whereas the incidence of extrapyramidal reactions was higher with the butyrophenones. It is concluded that haloperidol and trifluperidol are both highly and about equally effective in the treatment of acute schizophrenic disorders.

Reviewing the data of these three double-blind studies, Bishop and Gallant (1965) failed to find evidence for selective efficacy of trifluperidol on the paranoid schizophrenic patient. The findings rather suggested the superior efficacy of the drug in both paranoid and non-paranoid schizophrenics, as ordinarily defined.

In another double-blind study involving forty-five chronic schizophrenic women, Fox et al. (1964) found oral trifluperidol (2 to 4 mg daily) somewhat more effective than haloperidol (8 to 16 mg daily) and significantly more effective than chlorpromazine (200 to 800 mg daily) at the end of 1 month of treatment. There were very few extrapyramidal side effects in this study, probably because of the administration of benztropine to patients treated with high doses of the three neuroleptic drugs.

A series of twenty hospitalized acutely agitated trifluperidol-treated female schizophrenics were carefully studied by Keitel (1963, 1964). A significant decrease in the amplitude of handwriting was noted within the first 4 days of treatment in all cases and with 0.5 mg to 1.5 mg of trifluperidol intramuscularly i.e., about $\frac{1}{300}$ of the corresponding chlorpromazine dose (Haase and Janssen, 1965).

A simultaneous decrease of the intensity of the psychotic symptoms was observed in eighteen patients. Hallucinations, psychomotor agitation, and affective tension were fully and rapidly controllable. Overdosage was regularly associated with typical extrapyramidal symptomatology.

Optimal oral maintenance therapy was achieved with 0.4 mg to 2.0 mg daily. Trifluperidol is therefore about equally active orally and parenterally.

After having treated a series of fifty chronic, previously treated schizophrenic women over a period of 1 year, Flegel (1964a,b) concluded that striking therapeutic benefit can be expected from oral trifluperidol even in patients who failed to respond to a variety of other antipsychotic drugs.

Dick (Dubois et al., 1963; Dick, 1963) treated forty hospitalized schizophrenics with an average of 2 to 3 mg of trifluperidol daily; thirty-four of these patients improved. Clear-cut and rapid antipsychotic effects were observed in acute schizophrenia, significant effects in chronic hallucinatory psychoses, hebephrenia, and chronic paranoid schizophrenia. Side effects remained within tolerable limits. As compared with other neuroleptic drugs, trifluperidol produced more akathisia, restlessness, and clinical improvement in autistic patients with psychomotor inhibition.

Comparing haloperidol and trifluperidol by statistical analysis of global clinical ratings and Wittenborn profiles before and after treatment Delay (Delay and Deniker, 1961a; Delay et al. 1962a) arrived at the following conclusions: (a) both butyrophenones are about equally effective in paranoid schizophrenia; chlorpromazine and perchlorperazine are less effective; (b) trifluperidol gives better results than haloperidol in withdrawn hebephrenic schizophrenia, where autism, lack of social contact, and apragmatism are predominant symptoms; (c) haloperidol is the drug of choice in manic states; (d) depression is unlikely to occur during maintenance therapy with trifluperidol.

Essentially similar results with trifluperidol in psychotic patients have been described by Alema and Gianniotti (1962); Alemà et al. (1962a); Alleva (1962a); Benayoun (1965); Bobon et al. (1962, 1964a); Cenacchi (1962); Clos et al. (1964); Collard (1961); Delay et al. (1962c); Della Beffa (1962); Della Beffa et al. (1962); Della Pietra and Semprevivo (1962); Della Rovere and Varraso (1962); Di Piazza et al. (1963); Doussinet et al. (1964); Flegel (1964a,b); Fiume and Argenta (1962); German (1962); Goldwurm and Torrigiani (1962); Haase (1962); Kristjansen (1962); Laurans (1964); Le Guen (1965); Lehembre (1962); Levi (1962), Lods (1962); Lods et al. (1964); Maccagnani and Albonetti (1961); Madalena (1964, 1965); Masciocchi (1962); Megre Velloso and Paprocki (1963, 1965) O'Reilly et al. (1964); Pariante et al. (1963); Pelaz (1962, 1963); Pigem et al. (1962); Romildo Bueno (1965); Rosadini et al. (1961); Rovetta (1962); Samulak (1964); Santaella (1965); Sivadjian et al. (1963); Trethowan (1965a,b); Warnes et al. (1964).

The chronic toxicity of trifluperidol seems to be negligible, no significant complications during long-term therapy having been described.

C. Methylperidol or Moperone (R 1658)

In the first seventeen clinical publications and reports on methylperidol, results obtained in a total of 925 mostly psychotic patients are discussed. An excellent controlled experimental psychological study on the effect of methylperidol in normal volunteers was published by Janke.

A single 5-mg tablet induced the following significant behavioral changes: inhibition of the speed of verbal expression and of handwriting without effecting accuracy; tendency to induce emotional stability. There was no effect on vigilance or on various reaction times in several motor task tests. No side effects were reported.

Quite different psychological effects were obtained with 10 mg of diazepoxide, 400 mg of meprobamate, or 25 mg of promazine.

In their pilot study on twenty chronic patients Bobon et al. (1963a) found oral methylperidol generally somewhat less active as an antipsychotic drug than oral haloperidol. At the dose levels used (20 ± 15 mg daily), methylperidol also produced less neurological side effects than haloperidol (7.5 ± 4 mg daily).

In a series of 122 hospitalized psychotics (Angst and Pöldinger, 1963), oral treatment with 20 ± 10 mg of methylperidol daily induced relatively few neurological side effects. They could be largely avoided by introducing the drug gradually. Dyskinesia, occurring in twelve patients during the first days of treatment, was very sensitive to antiparkinson drugs. The drug was more effective against hallucinations than against psychomotor agitation in schizophrenic patients. The incidence of somnolence, hypotension, or other autonomic symptoms was negligible.

Low side-effect liability improved social contact in withdrawn patients, and striking anti hallucinatory effects were also noted in methylperidol-treated schizophrenics (Angst and Pöldinger, 1963; Bobon et al., 1963a; Eckmann, 1963; Eckmann and Immich, 1963; Gastager and Gruber, 1965; Hackstein, 1963; Stelter and Bielinski, 1964; Uyterschaut and Jacobs, 1962; Vitger, 1965).

In a recent well-controlled double-blind study, Cook (1966) found considerable improvement in twenty-two out of thirty-three senile, confused, and disoriented patients after three weeks on methylperidol. Only two developed extrapyramidal side effects. Placebo administration was significantly less effective than methylperidol. All patients received 5 mg t.i.d. during the first week of treatment. Adjustments to the dosage were subsequently made so that by the end of the third week an optimum dosage level had been found for each patient. Senile dementia is therefore an excellent indication for methylperidol.

The surprisingly low incidence of extrapyramidal reactions in patients on methylperidol is most likely related to its relatively short duration of action. For Parkinsonian symptoms to develop, it appears necessary to maintain the patient under the continuous influence of a neuroleptic drug for several days.

The psychopharmacological effects of methylperidol in volunteers have been carefully studied by Janke (1961/1962; 1964).

Between 1960 and 1965 an estimated 1,000,000 daily doses of methylperidol have been used clinically. No serious toxic reactions during maintenance therapy have been reported.

D. Fluanisone or Haloanisone (R 2028)

In the first 58 clinical publications on the use of haloanisone, a total of 2892 patients are reported upon, i.e., 2152 psychiatric cases, including 97 children, and 740 cases in which haloanisone was used as an anesthesiological adjunct. Between 1960 and 1965 an estimated 2.5 million daily doses of fluanisone have been used clinically.

The most important clinical properties of haloanisone or fluanisone are predictable from animal data: (*a*) As a neuroleptic drug, haloanisone is active at higher dose levels than haloperidol and lower than chlorpromazine. (*b*) It is one of the fastest acting neuroleptics known but its duration of action is relatively short. (*c*) Its side-effect liability, more similar to chlorpromazine than to haloperidol is characterized by a relatively high incidence of autonomic effects, particularly orthostatic hypotension and tachycardia during the first days of treatment, a pronounced tendency to produce somnolence or oversedation, and a relatively low incidence of neurological symptoms of the extrapyramidal type. The incidence of these side effects is much less in agitated patients than in others.

Good results are obtained with intramuscular doses of 5 mg to 20 mg of fluanisone in psychiatric emergency situation, for example, in patients with severe psychomotor agitation where the drug has a strikingly short onset of action (Avroutzki and Gourovitch, 1963; Bertolotti and Solime, 1963; Bissière, 1961; Blanck *et al.*, 1964; Brousolle *et al.*, 1961; Camplo and Torrubia, 1962; Caustier, 1962; Coirault *et al.*, 1961; Crémiaux *et al.*, 1963; Daumézon *et al.*, 1960; Deberdt, 1960; Delay and Deniker, 1961a; Delay *et al.*, 1960b; De Ryck, 1962; Ey *et al.*, 1963; Favre-Tissot and Robert, 1963; Fouks *et al.*, 1961a,b; Geissmann *et al.*, 1962; Gutbub, 1963; Hekimian and Friedhoff, 1964; Hekimian *et al.*, 1963; Israel *et al.*, 1964; Kammerer *et al.*, 1962a,b; Katila and Pihkanen, 1963; Kurland *et al.*, 1962, 1964; Le Gaudu, 1964; Maer and Kohler, 1963; Maitron *et al.*, 1965; Masquin and Dermenghem, 1960, 1961; Monnerot and Barre, 1963; Monteverdi, 1963; Morin *et al.*, 1960a,b, 1961; Naviau *et al.*, 1963; Nodine *et al.*, 1962; Paquay *et al.*, 1960b; Pariente, 1961; Pariente *et al.*, 1960; Perrin and Siffermann, 1961; Roux *et al.*, 1963; Scherrer and Dermenghem, 1962; Singer *et al.*, 1961; Soulairac *et al.*, 1962a,b; 1964; Vauterin and Robert, 1961; Villa 1964).

In oral maintenance therapy of psychotic patients, at daily dose levels of 40 to 400 mg daily, fluanisone possesses undesirable antipsychotic properties. Its sedative properties are sometimes beneficial, e.g., in oligophrenia.

As compared with other neuroleptics, the usefulness of fluanisone as an antipsychotic agent is rated somewhat differently by different groups of investigators.

According to Paquay et al. (1960b) fluanisone, inferior to haloperidol in combatting hallucinations and delirious episodes, may be a useful adjunct to haloperidol therapy in oligophrenics. Mental retardation associated with impulsive, turbulent, and aggressive behavior is generally said to be an excellent indication for fluanisone therapy both in adults and in children (Brousolle et al., 1961; Maer and Kohler, 1963; Paquay et al., 1960b; Roux et al., 1963; Scherrer and Dermenghem, 1962).

In two double-blind tests, Deberdt (1960) found oral fluanisone (40 mg daily) and oral chlorpromazine (200 mg daily) equally effective in chronic schizophrenics.

In a similar double-blind test by De Ryck (1962), fluanisone was somewhat more effective than chlorpromazine and possessed similar side-effect liability.

Fluanisone has been used in anesthesiology as the neuroleptic component of neuroleptanalgesia (Deligné, 1961a,b; Deligné et al., 1960; Marchais and Jason, 1962; Racinet, 1963; Thuries and Miech, 1964; Touraine, 1961).

In veterinary medicine, fluanisone is a useful tranquillizer for dogs, poultry, monkeys, pigs, and horses.

In dogs, the drug is used in combination with the powerful narcotic fentanyl to produce a state of surgical analgesia in a quiet animal.

In chickens, the administration of fluanisone in the drinking water is quite effective in the treatment of cannibalism and agitation (Kiel, 1963; Marsboom and Allewijn, 1964; Marsboom and Sierens, 1962a,b; Marsboom et al., 1964b; Oskam, 1965; Verstraete et al., 1962).

E. Floropipamide or Dipiperon (R 3345)

In the first twenty-four clinical studies on floropipamide (dipiperon, R 3345), a total of 1233 treated patients are reported on. Between 1961 and 1965 an estimated 8,000,000 daily doses of floropipamide were used clinically.

In the original paper by Bobon, Collard, and Demaret (1961) the following effects were observed in fifty-four patients: (a) good hallucinolytic activity and remarkable resocializing effects in chronic delusions at oral dose levels of 300 to 600 mg daily; (b) delayed hypnogenic activity, i.e., normalization of disturbed diurnal sleep pattern; potentiation of the hypnogenic effects of barbiturates on 80 to 160 mg daily; (c) inactive against mania and melancholia, unpredictable anti-anxiety effects in neurotic patients; (d) extrapyramidal side effects were rare and of very low intensity; the most common side effect was orthostatic hypotension.

The results of similar clinical studies on the effect of floropipamide on psychotic patients have been reported by Andersen and Søvsø (1965); Bente and Pfeiffer (1964); Bente et al. (1962, 1963); Flegel and Neller (1963);

Fierlafyn (1963a); Gross and Langner (1964); Hartung *et al.* (1964); Heinrich (1961); Heinrich and Rumpf (1964); Ideström and Cadenius (1963); Katscher (1962); Nuyts (1963); Schwarz *et al.* (1962, 1964); Sugerman (1964); Toledo and Zimerman (1965); Warnes *et al.* (1964).

There is common agreement on the fact that floropipamide is a well-tolerated antipsychotic agent. It appears to be unusually effective in the treatment of chronic schizophrenic patients (Sugerman, 1964) including those who have proven refractory to treatment with currently available psychotropic drugs. Primary antipsychotic effects are observed in the areas of emotional withdrawal, blunted affect, and hallucinations, and reduction of tension, increased cooperation, and lessened retardation follows. Treated patients also tend to sleep longer. Dosage must be adjusted individually for each patient according to tolerance.

F. Benperidol (R 4584)

In the first twenty-four clinical papers and twenty-nine unpublished reports on benperidol a total of 2464 patients were reported on. Between 1962 and 1965 an estimated 1,000,000 daily doses of benperidol were used clinically, mostly in the treatment of various psychotic symptoms.

Benperidol is described in the original paper by Bobon, Collard, and Pinchard (1962) as a well-tolerated neuroleptic drug, effective at low dose levels in chronic psychotic patients. In contrast with most other potent neuroleptic drugs, benperidol tends to improve sleep.

According to Haase *et al.* (1964), who investigated the action of benperidol in thirty agitated female acute schizophrenics by the Haase method, the compound produces reduction of the amplitude of handwriting at daily doses of 0.1 to 1.5 mg. It is equally active orally and parenterally. The average antipsychotically active dose is 0.5 mg, i.e., about 8.3 times lower than the equiactive haloperidol dose. Haloperidol, however, is longer acting than benperidol. Typical neuroleptic side effects are observed at dose levels exceeding 1 mg daily. Somnolence was a regular feature in patients treated with high intravenous doses. Autonomic side effects were absent at useful dose levels.

Pronounced antipsychotic effects in adults and children were also observed in benperidol-treated patients by Achaintre *et al.* (1965); Bardenat and Corman (1964); Bobon *et al.* (1963c); Brousolle and Grunthaler (1965); Chatagnon and Chatagnon (1964); Collard and Lecoq (1964); Cossa *et al.* (1965); Guyotat and Miraillet (1965); Iwamoto (1964); Juillet *et al.* (1964); Kaneko *et al.* (1964a,b); Lambert *et al.* (1965); Milette and Sacco (1963); Miura (1964); Nomura *et al.* (1964); Poire *et al.* (1965); Riser and Déro (1965); Sato *et al.* (1965); Schönbeck (1964); Tsuchimoto and Nishigori (1964); Vallade *et al.* (1963).

Control of psychomotor agitation of different etiology, hallucinolytic activity, and improved social behavior have been regularly observed by all investigators. The side effects are essentially of the extrapyramidal type and easily controllable with effective anti-Parkinson agents. The most commonly employed doses are 0.5 to 5 mg daily, depending on the type and the severity of the psychotic symptoms.

G. Droperidol (R 4749)

Droperidol was selected as the neuroleptic of choice in anesthesiology because of its high potency, the short onset and the relatively short duration of its peak effect, its high anti-shock activity, its pronounced antiemetic properties, its extremely low acute toxicity, and its specificity of action (Janssen *et al.*, 1963a, 1965a,b, 1966).

Between 1962 and 1965, an estimated 1.2 million patients were treated with droperidol, 21,521 of whom are mentioned in the first eighty-five publications and reports on its clinical use.

The majority of these patients were given droperidol in combination with the powerful, fast and short acting analgesic drug fentanyl when undergoing major surgery using a technique which is known as neuroleptanalgesia (N.L.A.).

Droperidol alone or in combination with fentanyl or another potent morphine-like drug is also being used in premedication, minor surgery, bronchoscopy, arteriography, obstetrics, and psychiatry, both in adults and in children (Appiani and Pedronetto, 1963a,b,c, 1964; Arnozis and Miyahara, 1964; Arosio and Pedrazzini, 1964; Aubry *et al.*, 1965; Audet *et al.*, 1964; Berti *et al.*, 1965; Brambilla, 1964; Calligari *et al.*, 1964; Carignan *et al.*, 1964; Carpino Boeri, 1964; Ceraso, 1965; Ceraso *et al.*, 1963, 1965; Cetrullo and Zattoni, 1963; Colombo *et al.*, 1964; Corssen *et al.*, 1964, 1965a,b; Couadau *et al.*, 1964; Cremonesi, 1964; Cuocolo *et al.*, 1964; De Blasi *et al.*, 1964; Dobkin, 1964; Dobkin and Lee, 1965; Dobkin *et al.*, 1963, 1964, 1965a,b; Doenicke, 1965; Doenicke *et al.*, 1965; Du Cailar and Jaquenoud, 1963; Elder *et al.*, 1964; Ferrari and Ceraso, 1963; Ferrari and Fuentes, 1964; Foldes *et al.*, 1964; Fratello *et al.*, 1964; Frey and Kreuscher, 1965; Frey *et al.*, 1962; Fuentes, 1964; Gemperle, 1964; Gemperle and Grüninger, 1964; Gianfranchi and Carpino Boeri, 1964; Gonçalves and Cols, 1965; Grabow and Allemand, 1964; Gruvel *et al.*, 1963a,b; Gürtner *et al.*, 1964; Henschel, 1962, 1963, 1964; Henschel *et al.*, 1963, 1964; Hoffmann, 1965; Hofmann, 1965; Holderness *et al.*, 1963; Horton, 1962; Israel *et al.*, 1965; Jaquenoud *et al.*, 1963; Just *et al.*, 1965; Keéri-Szànto *et al.*, 1963; Kern, 1965; Kreuscher, 1965a,b; Kreuscher *et al.*, 1965; Langer and Zierach, 1964; Larson, 1963; Lavallée, 1964; Lawin, 1965; Madjidi, 1965; Manni and Trifogli, 1964; Manni *et al.*, 1963, 1965; Mazzarella and Memoli, 1964; Moran *et al.*, 1964; Nalda Felipe, 1963; Nicoletti and Cols, 1965; Nicoletti *et al.*, 1964a,b; Nigro *et al.*, 1965; Pereira, 1965; Pérez Sanfelix *et al.*, 1962; Polaczek-Kornecki, 1963; Pöntinen and

Miettinen, 1964; Pöntinen *et al.*, 1964; Prinzhorn, 1964; Rajagopalan and Ramamurthi, 1964; Ruggerini, 1962; Schneider and Zeller, 1964; Sforza and Siciliano, 1964; Sironi and Varesi, 1964; Soma and Shields, 1964; Tasker and Marshall, 1965; Terrassier, 1965; Timmermans *et al.*, 1965; Torelli and Schiavi, 1965; Tornetta and Boger, 1964; Trifogli and Manni, 1964; Trop and Brindle, 1964; Vourc'h *et al.*, 1964; Walker and McIntyre, 1965; Winckler, 1963; Zauder *et al.*, 1965; Zecca and Molinaroli, 1965; Zegveld, 1963; Zindler *et al.*, 1964; Zugliani, 1964).

In man, a single parenteral dose of 5 to 20 mg of droperidol rapidly produces a state of tranquillity without loss of consciousness. Environment-induced anxiety disappears, voluntary movements are rare and are absent while the subject remains cooperative. The cardiovascular system remains surprisingly stable with no detectable depressant action on the myocardium (Kreuscher, 1965a). Droperidol possesses adrenolytic properties at these dose levels; the pressor effects of epinephrine are reserved. Orthostatic hypotension can occur in the upright position. The emetic effects of morphine-like narcotics are prevented, droperidol acting as a potent blocker of the chemoreceptor trigger zone. Droperidol is also strikingly effective in the treatment of traumatic shock. The administration of doses in excess of 20 mg, particularly in normal volunteers not undergoing surgery, is sometimes associated with neurological Parkinson-like effects, which are effectively treated with an active anti-Parkinson agent such as benztropine or trihexyphenidyl.

In psychiatry, the droperidol-fentanyl combination is extremely effective in controlling psychomotor agitation (Bobon *et al.*, 1964b).

In veterinary medicine, droperidol is used as an effective tranquillizer in monkeys and in dogs (Marsboom, 1963c; Marsboom and Mortelmans, 1964; Marsboom *et al.*, 1962, 1963a; Mortelmans *et al.*, 1962).

H. Other Butyrophenones

The other butyrophenones that underwent clinical trial, but are not available commercially are listed in Table II.

Spiroperidol (R 5147) is an extremely potent and specific neuroleptic drug in man (Bobon *et al.*, 1963b; Haase and Janssen, 1965; Mattke, 1964; Paquay *et al.*, 1964). At dose levels of 0.1 to 5 mg daily, antipsychotic activity and Parkinson-like side effects are regularly observed.

Methylperidide (R 2963) and haloperidide (R 3201) are potent and specific neuroleptic drugs in man. They are however relatively inactive when given orally (Collard, 1961; Divry *et al.*, 1960c). The related compound paraperidide (R 2962) appears to be greatly absorbed by the gastrointestinal tract (unpublished observations, 1961).

Butropipazone (R 1892) produces clinical effects that are very similar to those of chlorpromazine at about the same dose levels (unpublished results).

Anisoperidone (R 1647) is a sedative in man without obvious antipsychotic or neuroleptic properties (Collard, 1961; Divry et al., 1959b; Nodine et al., 1962; Waelkens, 1960b).

Acetabuton (R 3248) is currently being studied in hypertensive disease. At oral daily dose levels of 2.5 to 50 mg, the drug is an effective hypotensive agent and devoid of obvious sedative properties (unpublished results).

The butyrophenones WY 3457 (Simpson et al., 1964a,b), WY 6123 (Simpson et al., 1965), and F 33 (Jucker, 1963) are of no practical interest in the treatment of psychosis (Table II).

References

Achaintre, A., Burgat, R., Desmettre, G., and Petrod, S. (1965). *J. Med. Lyon* **46**, 403.
Aldeghi, E., and Maderna, A. (1961). *Freniatria* **85**, 216.
Aleksandrovskii, I. A. (1964). *Zh. Nevropatol. Psikhiatr.* **64**, 131.
Alemà, G., and Gianniotti, G. (1962). In "International Symposium on Haloperidol and Triperidol" p. 79. Istituto Luso Farmaco d'Italia, Milan.
Alemà, G., Gianniotti, G., and Rosadini, G. (1961). *Riv. Sper. Freniat.* **85**, fasc. II.
Alemà, G., Gianniotti, G., and Fiorito, L. (1962a). In "International Symposium on Haloperidol and Triperidol" p. 99. Istituto Luso Farmaco d'Italia, Milan.
Alemà, G., Gianniotti, G., Rosadini, G., Giberti Rosadini, I., and Fiorito, L. (1962b). In "International Symposium on Haloperidol and Triperidol" p. 113. Istituto Luso Farmaco d'Italia, Milan.
Alleva, P. M. (1962a). In "International Symposium on Haloperidol and Triperidol" p. 121. Istituto Luso Farmaco d'Italia, Milan.
Alleva, P. M. (1962b). In "International Symposium on Haloperidol and Triperidol" p. 131. Istituto Luso Farmaco d'Italia, Milan.
Amati, G., and Procaccini, S. (1962). In "International Symposium on Haloperidol and Triperidol" p. 147. Istituto Luso Farmaco d'Italia, Milan.
Andén, N. E., Roos, B. E., and Werdinius, B. (1964). *Life Sci.* **3**, 149.
Andersen, P., and Søvsø, H. (1965). *Saertryk Ugeskrift Laeger* **127**, 70.
Angst, J., and Pöldinger, W. (1963). *Praxis (Bern)* **52**, 1348.
Appiani, L. (1960). *Minerva Anestesiol.* **26**.
Appiani, L., and Pedronetto, S. (1963a). *Anestesia Rianimazione* **4**, 413.
Appiani, L., and Pedronetto, S. (1963b). *Anestesia Rianimazione* **4**, 423.
Appiani, L., and Pedronetto, S. (1963c). *Anestesia Rianimazione* **4**, 429.
Appiani, L., and Pedronetto, S. (1964). *Anestesia Rianimazione* **5**, 299.
Ardillo, L., et al. (1965). *Minerva Ginecol.* **17**, 133.
Arnozis, J. H. R., and Miyahara, R. C. (1964). *Proc. 3rd World Congress of Anesthesiology, Sao Paulo, 1964.*
Arosio, G., and Pedrazzini, A. (1964). *Minerva Anestesiol.* **30**, 522.
Aubry, U., Denis, R., Keéri-Szanto, M., and Parent, M. (1965). *Can. Anaesthiol. Soc. J.* **12**, 510.
Audet, J., Beaudoin, G., Keéri-Szanto, N., and Trop, D. (1964). *Proc. 3rd World Congress of Anesthesiology, Sao Paulo, 1964.*
Avroutzki, G. Y., and Gourovitch, I. Y. (1963). *J. Neuropathol. Psychiat.* **63**, 87.
Ayd, F. (1961). In "Extrapyramidal System and Neuroleptics" (J. M. Bordeleau, ed.), p. 355. Editions psychiatriques, Montreal, Canada.
Azima, H., Durost, H., and Arthurs, D. (1960). *Am. J. Psychiat.* **117**, 546.
Baccaglini, B., and Caprini, G. (1960). *Girn. Psichiat. Neurol.* III.
Baciocchi, M. (1961). *Ann. Medico-Psychol.* **119**, 781.

Balducci, M., and Frascella, G. (1962). *In* "International Symposium on Haloperidol and Triperidol", p. 177. Istituto Luso Farmaco d'Italia, Milan.
Balducci, M., and Loguloso, R. (1962). *In* "International Symposium on Haloperidol and Triperidol", p. 181. Istituto Luso Farmaco d'Italia, Milan.
Ban, T. A. (1962). *In* "International Symposium on Haloperidol and Triperidol", p. 187. Istituto Luso Farmaco d'Italia, Milan.
Ban, T. A. (1964). *In* "The Butyrophenones in Psychiatry," p. 120. (First North American Symposium held at "Hospitaldes Laurentides", L'Annonciation, Quebec, January 10, 1964.)
Ban, T. A., and Stonehill, E. (1964). *In* "The Butyrophenones in Psychiatry," p. 113.
Bandettini Di Poggio, U., and Levi, P. G. (1960). *Riv. Neuropsichiat. Sci. Affini* **6**, 27.
Bardenat, C., and Corman, M. (1964). *Rev. Neuro-Psychiat Ouest.* No. 6.
Beck, L. (1962). *Geburtsh. Frauenheilk.* **22**, 1519.
Benayoun, C. (1965). M. D. Thesis, Univ. Toulouse.
Bente, D., and Pfeiffer, W. M. (1964). *Arzneimittel-Forsch.* **14**, 523.
Bente, D., Pfeiffer, W. M., and Müller, M. L. (1962). *Proc. 60th Session Congr. Psychiat. Neurol. Langue Française, Anvers, 1962.*
Bente, D., Engelmeier, M. P., Heinrich, H., Hippius, H., and Schmitt, W. (1963). *Nervenarzt* **34**, 426.
Bergmann, H. (1962). *Anaesthesist* **11**, 109.
Bergmann, H. (1964). *Wien Klin. Wochschr.* **76**, 969.
Berti, F., Bisiani, M., Laveneziana, D., and Zocche, G. P. (1965). *Minerva Anestesiol.* **31**, 80.
Bertolotti, P., and Solime, F. (1963). *Riv. Freniat.* **87**, fasc. 2.
Bhargava, K. P. (1965). *Brit. J. Pharmacol.* **25**, 74.
Bianchi, G., and Ronchi, E. (1963). *Proc. 61st Session Congrès Psychiatrie Neurologie Langue Française, Nancy, 1963.*
Bishop, M. P., and Gallant, D. M. (1965). *Current Therap. Res*, **7**, 96.
Bishop, M. P., Gallant, D. M., and Sykes, T. F. (1965). *Arch. Gen Psychiat.* **13**, 155.
Bissière, H. (1961). M.D. Thesis, Univ. Lyon.
Bister, W. (1961). *Med. Exptl.* **5**, 255.
Blackford Rogers, W. J. (1965). *Clin. Trials J.* **2**, 162.
Blanc, M., Bourgeois, M., and Vincent, J. D. (1964). *J. Med. Bordeaux Sud-Ouest* **141**, 575.
Blandin, J., Bonhoure, J., and Soucachet, P. (1961). *Ann. Medico-Psychol.* **119**, 988.
Bobon, J., and Collard, J. (1962). *In* "International Symposium on Haloperidol and Triperidol", p. 193. Istituto Luso Farmaco d'Italia, Milan.
Bobon, J., Collard, J., and Demaret, A. (1961). *Acta Neurol. Psychiat. Belg.* **61**, 611.
Bobon, J., Collard, J., and Pinchard, A. (1962). *Acta Neurol. Psychiat. Belg.* **62**, 566.
Bobon, J., Collard, J., and Daigneux-Delhez, R. (1963a). *Acta Neurol. Psychiat. Belg.* **63**, 67.
Bobon, J., Collard, J., Delrée, C., and Gernay, J. M. (1963b). *Acta Neurol. Psychiat. Belg.* **63**, 991.
Bobon, J., Collard, J., and Lecoq, R. (1963c). *Acta Neurol. Psychiat. Belg.* **63**, 839.
Bobon, J., Gernay, J. M., Goffioul, F., and Maccagnani, C. (1964a). *Soc. Med. Mentale Belg.* séance du 25 avril.
Bobon, J., Collard, J., Pinchard, A., Bury, J., and Colinet, M. (1964b). *Acta Neurol. Psychiat. Belg.* **64**, 1165.
Böcher, W., Nieschke, W., Schmidt, D., Schubert, G., and Senf, E. (1964). *Med. Exptl.* **11**, 308.
Bohacek, N. (1961). *Neuropsihijatria* **9**, 177.
Bohacek, N. (1964). *Wien Med. Wochschr.* **114**, 76.
Boissier, J. R., and Pagny, J. (1960). *Therapie* **15**, 479.
Boissier, J. R., and Simon, P. (1963). *Therapie* **18**, 1257.
Boissier, J. R., and Simon, P. (1964a). *Encephale* **53**, 109.
Boissier, J. R., and Simon, P. (1964b). *Arch. Intern. Pharmacodyn.* **147**, 372.
Boissier, J. R., Pagny, J., Mouille, P., and Forrest, J. (1960). *Acta Neurol. Psychiat. Belg.* **60**, 39.
Boissier, J. R., Pagny, J., and Font du Picard, Y. (1961). *Therapie* **16**, 279.

Boissier, J. R., Simon, P., and Lwoff, J. M. (1964a). *Therapie* **19**, 571.
Boissier, J. R., Pagny, J., and Font du Picard, Y. A. (1964b). *Neuropsychopharmacol.* **3**, 59.
Boissier, J. R., Simon, P., Lwoff, J. M., and Giudicelli, J. F. (1965). *Therapie* **20**, 895.
Bonhoure J. (1962). M.D. Thesis, Univ. Clermont-Ferrand.
Borenstein, P., and Blès, G. (1963). *Ann. Med. Psychol.* **121**, 440.
Borenstein, P., Dabbah, M., and Blès, G. (1962a). *Ann. Med. Psychol.* **120**, 133.
Borenstein, P., Dabbah, M., and Blès, G. (1962b). *Ann. Med. Psychol.* **120**, 279.
Borenstein, P., Dabbah, M., Blès, G., Roussel, A., and Rosemberger (1962c). *Ann. Med. Psychol.* **120**, 281.
Borenstein, P., Dabbah, M., and Blès, G. (1962d). *Ann. Med. Psychol.* **120**, 396.
Borenstein, P., Dabbah, M., and Blès, G. (1962e). *Ann. Med. Psychol.* **120**, 506.
Borghesi, R. (1964). *Rass. Stud. Psichiat.* **53**, 627.
Bouchard, J. M. (1965). *In* "Bilan actuel de l'apport thérapeutique des neuroleptiques dans le traitement des psychoses hallucinatoires chroniques." R. Foulon & Cie, Paris.
Bozzi, R., Allegranza, A., and Bruni, A. (1962). *In* "International Symposium on Haloperidol and Triperidol," p. 199. Istituto Luso Farmaco d'Italia, Milan.
Brambilla, G. (1964). *Rass. Intern. Clin. Terap.* **44**, 810.
Brandrup, E., and Kristjansen, P. (1961). *J. Mental Sci.* **107**, 778.
Brauner, F. (1964). *Encephale* **53**, 215.
Brousolle, P., and Grunthaler, C. (1965). *J. Med. Lyon* **46**, 407.
Brousolle, P., Bouvard, R. J. M., and Reynaud, R. (1961). *Ann. Med. Psychol.* **119**, 586.
Brown, A. S. (1962). *Anaesthesist* **11**, 22.
Brown, A. S. (1963). *Irish J. Med. Sci.* p. 535.
Brown, A. S. (1964). *Anaesthesia* **19**, 70.
Brown, A. S. (1965). *Med. News* p. 11.
Brown, A. S., Horton, J. M., and MacRae, W. R. (1963). *Anaesthesia* **18**, 143.
Bruno, A., and Allegranza, A. (1965). *Psychopharmacologia* **8**, 60.
Buchel, L., and Lévy, J. (1962a). *J. Physiol. (Paris)* **54**, 304.
Buchel, L., and Lévy, J. (1962b). *In* "International Symposium on Haloperidol and Triperidol," p. 205. Istituto Luso Farmaco d'Italia, Milan.
Buchel, L., Lévy, J., and Tissier, M. (1962). *Therapie* **17**, 1053.
Buffardi, R. (1962). *Riv. Sper. Freniat.* **86**, fasc. II.
Buis, C. (1962). *Geneesk. Gids* **40**, 205.
Buis, C., and Flohil, J. M. (1964). *Ned. Tijdschr. Geneesk.* **108**, 796.
Burgermeister, J. J., Dick, P., Miche, F., and Tissot, R. (1965). *Schweiz. Arch. Neurol. Neurochir. Psychiat.* **95**, 345.
Caldonazzo, C. (1960). *Riv. Neuropsichiat. Sci Affini* **6**, 227.
Calligari, G., Citro, A., and Ferraris, E. (1964). *Rass. Intern. Clin. Terap.* **44**, 761.
Cameron, I. A. (1965). *Clin. Trials J.* **2**, 143.
Camplo, J., and Torrubia, H. (1962). *Ann. Med. Psychol.* **120**, 146.
Caprini, G., and Melotti, V. (1961). *Riv. Sper. Freniat.* **85**, fasc. 4.
Capron, H. (1962). M.D. Thesis, Univ. Paris.
Carbonell Cadenas De Llano, J., and Herrero Aldama, P. (1960). *Medicamenta* **18**, 264.
Cardani, A. J., and Goldwurm, G. F. (1960). *Freniatria* **84**, fasc. III.
Cardo, W. N., de Carvalho, H. M., de Albuquerque Fortes, J. R., and Gonçalves, J. (1965). *Arquiv. Neuro-Psiquiat.* **23**, 37.
Carignan, G., Keéri-Szanto, M., Lavallée, J. P., and Lepage, C. (1964). *Anesthesia Analgesia, Current Res.* **43**, 560.
Carlsson, A., and Lindqvist, M. (1963). *Acta Pharmacol. Toxicol.* **20**, 140.
Carlsson, A., and Waldeck, B. (1965). *J. Pharm. Pharmacol.* **17**, 243.
Carlsson, A., Hilarp, N. A., and Waldeck, B. (1962). *Med. Exptl.* **6**, 47.
Caron, M., Dussartre, J., and Gerandal, C. (1961). *Ann. Med. Psychol.* **119**, 966.

Carpino Boeri, A. (1964). *Rass. Intern. Clin. Terap.* **44**, 800.
Casaglia, G. (1960). *Clin. Ginecol.* **2**, 98.
Caustier, M. (1962). M.D. Thesis, Univ. Paris.
Cenacchi, G. (1962). *In* "International Symposium on Haloperidol and Triperidol," p. 221. Istituto Luso Farmaco d'Italia, Milan.
Ceraso, O. L. (1965). *Proc. 3rd World Congr. Anesthiol., Sao Paulo, 1964. Med. Panamericana* **23**, 107.
Ceraso, O. L., Elder, R., and Ferrari, H. (1963). *Proc. 34th Argentine Congr. Surg.*
Ceraso, O. L., Elder, R., and Ferrari, H. (1965). *Prensa Med. Argent.* **52**, 1292.
Cession-Fossion, A., Monard, Y., and Dresse, A. (1961). *Compt. Rend. Soc. Biol.* **155**, 2452.
Cetrullo, C., and Zattoni, J. (1963). *Minerva Anestesiol.* **29**.
Challas, G., and Brauer, W. (1963). *Am. J. Psychiat.* **120**, 283.
Chapel, J. I., Brown, N., and Jenkins, R. L. (1964). *Am. J. Psychiat.* **121**, 608.
Chatagnon, P. A., and Chatagnon, C. (1964). *Ann. med. Psychol.* **122**, 809; *Presse Med.* **72**, 2151.
Chen, G. (1965). *Arch. Intern. Pharmacodyn.* **157**, 193.
Chen, G., and Ensor, Ch. R. (1962). *Pharmacologist* **4**, 155.
Chodoff, P., and Domino, E. F. (1965). *Anaesthesia Analgesia, Current Res.* **44**, 558.
Cipriani, G., and Giordano, G. B. (1961). *Giorn. Psichiat. Neuropatol.* fasc. II.
Citro, A., and Calligari, G. (1964). *Rass. Intern. Clin. Terap.* **44**, 816.
Civai, O., and Chesi, R. (1964). *Acta Anaesthesiol. (Padova)* **15**, 331.
Clos, M., Gobble, I., Balling, J., and Fox, W. (1964). *Current Therap. Res.* **6**, 703.
Coirault, R., Herschberg, A. D., Damasio, R., Rigal, J., Alliot, B., and Bissière, H. (1961). *Presse Med.* **69**, 2373.
Collard, J. (1961). *In* "Psychopharmacologie comparée du halopéridol et de ses dérivés (tripéridol, méthylpéridide, R1647). Extrapyramidal System and Neuroleptics" (J. M. Bordelau, ed.), p. 369. Editions Psychiatriques, Montreal, Canada.
Collard, J. (1962). *Symp. Newest Psychotic Drugs and Human Behavior. San Francisco, California, 1962.*
Collard, J., and Lecoq, R. (1964). *Acta Neurol. Psychiat. Belg.* **64**, 353.
Colombo, P. A., Ferrero, A., and Diego, M. (1964). *Rass. Intern. Clin. Terap.* **44**, 824.
Cook, W. A. (1966). *Med. J. Australia.*
Corneli, R., and Rotondi, A. (1961). *Ann. Med. Psychol.* **119**, 619.
Corssen, G., Domino, E. F., and Sweet, R. B. (1964). *Anesthesia Analgesia, Current Res.* **43**, 748.
Corssen, G., Chodoff, P., Domino, E. F., and Kahn, D. R. (1965a). *J. Thoracic Cardiovascular Surg.* **49**, 901.
Corssen, G., Chodoff, P., and Domino, E. F. (1965b). *Med. Tribune* p. 10.
Cossa, P., and Paoli, F. (1961). *Gaz. Med. France* **68**, 901.
Cossa, P., Valéry, B., Darcourt, G., and Lavagna, J. (1965). *Ann. Med. Psychol.* **123**, 484.
Couadau, A., Couadau, H., and Campan, L. (1964). *Arch. Ophthalmol. (Paris)* **24**, 333.
Court, J. H., and Cameron, I. A. (1963). *Perceptual Motor Skills* **17**, 168.
Craft, M. (1965). *Clin Trials J.* **2**, 140.
Crémiaux, A., Pache, R., Tollinchi, G., and Danjard, J. (1963). *Ann. Med. Psychol.* **121**, 263.
Cremonesi, E. (1964). M.D. Thesis, Univ. Sao Paulo. (1964). *Rev. Brasil. Anestesiol.* **14** (Suppl.) pp. 1–76.
Cuocolo, R., and Messina, N. (1961). *Rass. Intern. Clin. Terap.* **41**, 435.
Cuocolo, R., Pica, M., Spampinato, N., and De Santis, S. (1964). *Rass. Intern. Clin. Terap.* **44**, 742.
Cwynar, S., and Bukowczyk, A. (1962). *Neurol. Neurochir. Psychiat. (Polska)* **12**, 421.
Dagan, Hachon, Dauch, Nondedeu, and Louars, (1963). *Ann. Med. Psychol.*, **121**, 261.
Danik, J. J., and Goverdhan, M. (1962). *In* "International Symposium on Haloperidol and Triperidol," p. 287. Istituto Luso Farmaco d'Italia, Milan.

Daumézon, G., Audisio, M., Conte, C., and Huguet, P. (1960). *Ann. Med. Psychol.* **118**, 539.
Davies, B. M. (1962). In "International Symposium on Haloperidol and Triperidol," p. 299. Istituto Luso Farmaco d'Italia, Milan.
Davoli, P., Coppola, F., and Grisanti, M. (1960). *Riv. Neuropsichiat. Sci. Affini* **6**, 219.
Deberdt, R. (1960). *Acta Neurol. Psychiat. Belg.* **60**, 663.
De Blasi, S., Brienta, A., De Bellis, V., and Trizio, W. (1964). *Rass. Intern. Clin. Terap.* **44**, 768.
De Haene, A. (1960). *Acta Neurol. Psychiat. Belg.* **60**, 58.
Delay, J., and Deniker, P. (1961a). In "Méthodes chimiothérapeutiques en psychiatrie. Les nouveaux médicaments psychotropes," p. 150. Masson et Cie, Paris.
Delay, J., and Deniker, P. (1961b). In "Apport de la clinique à la connaissance de l'action des neuroleptiques. Extrapyramidal System and Neuroleptics," p. 369. Editions Psychiatriques, Montreal, Canada.
Delay, J., Pichot, P., Lempérière, T., Elissalde, B., and Peigne, F. (1960a). *Ann. Med. Psychol.* **118**, 145.
Delay, J., Deniker, P., Levrie, J., and Donnet, J. L. (1960b). *Ann. Med. Psychol.* **118**, 749.
Delay, J., Pichot, P., Lempérière, T., and Elissalde, B. (1960c). *Acta Neurol. Psychiat. Belg.* **60**, 21.
Delay, J., Pichot, P., Lempérière, T., and Elissalde, B. (1960d). *Presse Med.* **68**, 1353.
Delay, J., Pichot, P., Lempérière, T., Bailly, R., Cattan, F., and Basquin, R. (1962a). *Presse Med.* **70**, 2147.
Delay, J., Pichot, P. Lempérière, T., and Piret, J. (1962b). *C.I.N.P. 3rd Congr. Intern. Munich, 1962.* Fränkischer Tag GmbH & Co., Bamberg, Germany.
Delay, J., Pichot, P., Lempérière, T. and Bailly, R. (1962c). In "International Symposium on Haloperidol and Triperidol," p. 305. Istituto Luso Farmaco d'Italia, Milan.
Delay, J., Pichot, P., Lempérière, T., and Piret, J. (1964). In "Neuropsychopharmacology," (P. Bradley, F. Flügel, and P. Hoch, eds.), vol. 3, p. 89. Elsevier, Amsterdam.
De Lerma Penasco, J. L. (1961). *Medicamenta* **19**, 348.
Deligné, P. (1961a). *Agressologie* **2**, 363.
Deligné, P. (1961b). *Agressologie* **2**, 493.
Deligné, P., Talairach, J., and David, M. (1960). *Neuro-Chirurg.* **6**, 356.
Della Beffa, A. (1962). In "International Symposium on Haloperidol and Triperidol," p. 31. Istituto Luso Farmaco d'Italia, Milan.
Della Beffa, A., Ronchi, E., and Barberini, E. (1962). In "International Symposium on Haloperidol and Triperidol," p. 229. Istituto Luso Farmaco d'Italia, Milan.
Della Pietra, V. (1962). In "International Symposium on Haloperidol and Triperidol," p. 255. Istituto Luso Farmaco d'Italia, Milan.
Della Pietra, V., and Fina, G. (1960). *Ospedale Psichiat.* **1**, 39.
Della Pietra, V., and Semprevivo, A. (1962). In "International Symposium on Haloperidol and Triperidol," p. 271. Istituto Luso Farmaco d'Italia, Milan.
Della Rovere, M. (1960). *Giorn. Psichiat. Neuropatol.* **88**, 431.
Della Rovere, M., and Varraso, A. (1962). *Freniatria* **86**, 252.
De Maio, D., Faggioli, L., and Carini, A. (1960). *Gazz. Med. Ital.* **119**, 511.
Demoen, P. J. A. W. (1961). *J. Pharm. Sci.* **50**, 350.
De Mondragon, C. (1964). *Rev. Neuro-Psychiat. Ouest* **2**, 25.
Denber, H. C. B., and Collard, J. (1962). *Acta Neurol. Psychiat. Belg.* **62**, 577.
Denber, H. C. B., Rajotte, P., and Kauffman, D. (1959). *Am. J. Psychiat.* **116**, 356.
Denber, H. C. B., Florio, D., and Rajotte, P. (1962). *Am. J. Psychiat.* **119**, 172.
Deniker, P. (1963). *Therapie* **18**, 1079.
Deniker, P. (1964). In "Neuropsychopharmacology" (P. Bradley, F. Flügel, and P. Hoch, eds.) Vol. 3, p. 126. Elsevier, Amsterdam.
Deprez, M. (1961). *Med Libre* **35**, 45.
De Ryck, A. (1962). *Acta Neurol. Psychiat. Belg.* **62**, 598.

Dick, P. (1962). In "International Symposium on Haloperidol and Triperidol," p. 321, Istituto Luso Farmaco d'Italia, Milan.
Di Cristo, G. (1960). Riv. Patol. Nerv. Ment. **81**, 363.
Di Piazza, P., Gori, E. C., and Levi-Minzi, S. (1963). Rass Stud. Psichiat. **52**, 595.
Divry, P., Bobon, J., and Collard, J. (1958). Acta Neurol. Psychiat. Belg. **58**, 878.
Divry, P., Bobon, J., Collard, J., Pinchard, A., and Nols, E. (1959a). Acta Neurol. Psychiat. Belg. **59**, 337.
Divry, P., Bobon, J., Collard, J., Pinchard, A., and Nols, E. (1959b). Acta Neurol. Psychiat. Belg. **59**, 1033.
Divry, P., Bobon, J., and Collard, J. (1960a). Acta Neurol. Psychiat. Belg. **60**, 7.
Divry, P., Bobon, J., Collard, J., and Demaret, A. (1960b). Acta Neurol. Psychiat. Belg. **60**, 465.
Divry, P., Bobon, J., Collard, J., and Demaret, A. (1960c). Acta Neurol. Psychiat. Belg. **60**, 1073.
Dobkin, A. B. (1964). Can. Anaesthesiol. Soc. J. **11**, 252.
Dobkin, A. B., and Criswick, V. G. (1961). Can. Anaesthesiol. Soc. J. **8**, 387.
Dobkin, A. B., and Lee, P. K. Y. (1965). Can. Anaesthesiol. Soc. J. **12**, 34.
Dobkin, A. B., Kwang Yi Lee, P., Byles, P., and Israel, J. S. (1963). Brit. J. Anaesthesiol. **35**, 694.
Dobkin, A. B., Israel, J. S., and Byles, P. H. (1964). Can. Anaesthesiol. Soc. J. **11**, 41.
Dobkin, A. B., Lee, P. K. Y., and Byles, P. H. (1965a). Can. Anaesthesiol. Soc. J. **12**, 39.
Dobkin, A. B., Byles, P. H., and Cho, M. H. (1965b). Can. Anaesthesiol. Soc. J. **12**, 349.
Doenicke, A. (1965). Acta Obstet. Gynecol. Scand. **43**, 269.
Doenicke, A., Kugler, J., Schellenberger, A., Gürtner, Th., and Spiess, W. (1965). Arzneimittel-Forsch. **15**, 269.
Dolley, M. (1962). M.D. Thesis, Univ. Paris.
Domanowsky, K. (1963). Med. Welt p. 2508.
Dongier, S., Dongier, M., Faidherbe, J., and Gastaut, H. (1961). Ann. Med. Psychol. **119**, 993.
Doussinet, P., Peyronnaud, G., and Bonhour, J. (1964). Ann. Med. Psychol. **122**, 435.
Dresse, A., and Cession-Fossion, A. (1962). Arch. Intern. Pharmacodyn. **135**, 485.
Dresse, A., and De Meyer, R. (1964). Life Sci. **3**, 759.
Dresse, A., and De Meyer, R. (1965). Biochem. Pharmacol. **14**, 1129.
Dresse, A., Otto-Servais, M., and Lecomte, J. (1962). Compt. Rend. Soc. Biol. **156**, 386.
Dubois, C., Dick, P., and Rey-Bellet, J. (1963). Schweiz. Med. Wochschr. **93**, 1600.
Du Cailar, J., and Jaquenoud, P. (1963). Proc. 3rd Congr. Français d'Anesthésiologie, Bordeaux, 1963.
Duché, D. J. (1961). Rev. Neuropsychiat. Infant. **9**, Nos. 7–8.
Durost, H., Lee, H., and Arthurs, D. (1964). In "The Butyrophenones in Psychiatry," p. 53.
Dykyj, R., and Nodine, J. H. (1964). Clin. Med. **71**, 491.
Dyrberg, V. (1962). Acta Anaesthesiol. Scand. **6**, 37.
Eckmann, F. (1963). Therapiewoche **13**, 350.
Eckmann, F., and Immich, H. (1963). Nervenarzt **34**, 374.
Elder, O., Ferrari, F., Ceraso, O., de Leonardis, M., Fuentes, O., Ferro, J., and Cambareri, P. Proc. 3rd World Congr. Anesthesiol., Sao Paulo, 1964.
Enoch, M. D., and Robin, A. A. (1960). J. Mental Sci. **106**, 1459.
Entwistle, C., Taylor, R. M., and MacDonald, I. A. (1962). J. Mental Sci. **108**, 373.
Evrard, E., Molders, V., and de Bruyne-Mottard (1960). Acta Neurol. Psychiat. Belg. **60**, 811.
Ey, H., Cor, M., and Yvonneau, M. (1963). Ouest Medical **16**, 657.
Failla, E., Stefanachi, L., and Stancati, G. (1962). In "International Symposium on Haloperidol and Triperidol," p. 337. Istituto Luso Farmaco d'Italia, Milan.
Fajardo, S. G. (1965). M.D. Thesis, Univ. Mexico D.F.
Favier, M., Savelli, A., Romani, B., and Jenny, B. (1963). Soc. Med. Militaire Franç. **57**, 339.
Favre-Tissot, M., and Robert, J. (1963). Société de neuro-psychiatrie médico-sociale de la région lyonnaise. (1963). Ann. Med. Psychol. **121**, 798.
Feldmann, H. (1963). Schweiz. Med. Wochschr. **93**, 81.

Ferrari, H., and Ceraso, O. (1963). *Actas del IX Congr. Argentino Anestesiol.*, *Buenos Aires, 1963.* p. 291.
Ferrari, H. A., and Fuentes, O. A. (1964). *Proc. 3rd World Congr. Anesthesiol.*, *Sao Paulo, 1964.*
Ferrero, M. (1962). *In* "International Symposium on Haloperidol and Triperidol," p. 357. Istituto Luso Farmaco d'Italia, Milan.
Ferro-Milone, F., and Lorizio, A.(1964). *Rev. Neurobiol.* **10**, 17.
Fierlafyn, E. (1963a). *Nouveautes Med.* **12**, 7.
Fierlafyn, E. (1963b). *Brux. Med.* **43**, 985.
Fiume, S., and Argenta, G. (1962). *In* "International Symposium on Haloperidol and Triperidol," p. 363. Istituto Luso Farmaco d'Italia, Milan.
Flegel, H. (1961). *Med. Exptl.* **5**, 311.
Flegel, H. (1962). *In* "International Symposium on Haloperidol and Triperidol," p. 367. Istituto Luso Farmaco d'Italia, Milan.
Flegel, H. (1963). *Proc. Compt. Rend. Congr. Psychiat. Neurol.*, *Nancy, 1963.* p. 364.
Flegel, H. (1964a). *Ann. Med. Psychol.* **122**, 176.
Flegel, H. (1964b). *Therap. Gegenw.* **103**, 115.
Flegel, H., and Neller, K. (1963). *Nervenarzt* **34**, 85.
Flegel, H., Rasper, A., and Lauber, H. (1960). *Nervenarzt* **31**, 133.
Foldes, F. F., Kepes, E. R., Torda, T.A. G., Bailey, R., and Wulfsohn, N. L. (1964). *Proc. 3rd World Congr. Anesthesiol.*, *Sao Paulo, 1964.*
Fouks, Laine, Mathis, Pagot, Ferrant, Delavalade, and Riou (1961a). *Ann. Med. Psychol.* **119**, 135.
Fouks, Laine, Mathis, Pagot, Ferrant, Delavalade, and Riou (1961b). *Ann. Med. Psychol.* **119**, 589.
Fourny, L., Ségal, J., Combette, H., and Stéphanopoli, M. J. (1961). *Ann. Med. Psychol.* **119**, 991.
Fourny, L., Combette, H., Stéphanopoli, M. J., and Ségal, J. (1962). *Ann. Med. Psychol.* **120**, 146.
Fox, W., Gobble, I. F., and Clos, M. (1964). *Current Therap. Res.* **6**, 409.
Franchini, C., Zaccala, M., and Ferutta, A. M. (1962). *In* "International Symposium on Haloperidol and Triperidol," p. 377. Istituto Luso Farmaco d'Italia, Milan.
Fratello, U., D'Auria, C., and Palmentieri, P. (1964). *Rass. Intern. Clin. Terap.* **44**, 755.
Frey, R., and Kreuscher, H. (1965). *Proc. 6th Intern. Congr. European Assoc. Anaesthesiol.*, *Athens, 1965.*
Frey, R., Kreuscher, H., and Madjidi, A. (1962). *Proc. Symp. Neuroleptanalgesia in relation to the 1st European Congr. Anesthesiol.*, *Vienna, 1962.*
Friedrich, R. (1963). *Arztl. Praxis* **15**, 333.
Frommel, E., and Chmouliovsky, M. (1964). *Compt. Rend. Soc. Biol.* **158**, 48.
Frommel, E., and Joye, E. (1963). *Med. Hyg.* **21**, 675.
Frommel, E., Fleury, C., Schmidt-Ginzkey, J., and Béguin, M. (1960). *Therapie* **15**, 1175.
Fuentes, O. A. (1964). *Semana Medica* **125**, 2356.
Galindez, L., Santos, M. R., and Borel, R. O. (1963). *Dia Medico* **35**, 1435.
Gallant, D. M., Bishop, M. P., Timmons, E., and Steele, C. A. (1963a). *Current Therap. Res.* **5**, 463.
Gallant, D. M., Bishop, M. P., Timmons, E., and Steele, C. A. (1963b). *Am. J. Psychiat.* **120**, 485.
Gallant, D. M., Bishop, M. P., Nesselhof, W. M., and Sprehe, D. J. (1965). *Psychopharmacologia* **7**, 37.
Gardocki, J. F., Yelnosky, J., Kuehn, W. F., and Gunster, J. C. (1964). *Toxicol. Appl. Pharmacol.* **6**, 593.
Garry, J. W., and Leonard, T. J. (1962). *J. Mental Sci.* **108**, 105.
Gastager, H., and Gruber, H. (1965). *Wien. Med. Wochschr.* **115**, 14.

Gastaut, H., Dongier, S., Dongier, M., and Faidherbe, J. (1962). *Rev. Med. Liege* **17**, 288.
Gatti, G., and Bertini, F. (1960). *Gazz. Med. Ital.* **119**, 398.
Gattuso, R., and Lanteri, G. (1962). *In* "International Symposium on Haloperidol and Triperidol," p. 385. Istituto Luso Farmaco d'Italia, Milan.
Gavaudan L., *et al.* (1962). *Gaz. Med. France* **69**, 3765.
Gayral, L., Turnin, J., Roux, G., and Puyuelo, R. (1965). *Therapie* **20**, 817.
Geissmann, P., Rohmer, F., Israel, L., and Singer, L. (1962). *Rev. Neurol.* **106**, 166.
Gemperle, M. (1964). *Anaesthesist* **13**, 181.
Gemperle, M., and Grüninger, B. (1964). *Anaesthesist* **13**, 6.
Géraud, J., Rascol, A., Bès, A., Benazet, J., and Arbus (1963). *Proc. Soc. Med. Chir. Pharmacie Toulouse, 1963. Presse Med.* **71**, 1818.
Gerle, B. (1960). *Acta Neurol. Psychiat. Belg.* **60**, 70.
Gerle, B. (1962). *In* "International Symposium on Haloperidol and Triperidol," p. 397. Istituto Luso Farmaco d'Italia, Milan.
Gerle, B. (1963). *Acta Psychiat. Scand.* **39**, 348.
Gerle, B. (1964a). *Acta Psychiat. Scand.* **40**, 65.
Gerle, B. (1964b). *Nord. Psykiat. Tidsskr.* **18**, 68.
Gerle, B., Petersson, B., and Widmark, M. (1961). *Svenska Lakartidn.* **58**, 1415.
German, E. (1962). M.D. Thesis, Univ. Paris.
Geyer, N., and Mayr, F. (1962). *Wien. Med. Wochschr.* **112**, 603.
Giacobini, E., and Lassenius, B. (1961). *Svenska Lakartidn.* **58**, 1429.
Gianasi, G. C., and Nanni Costa, P. (1964). *Acta Anaesthesiol.* **15**, 65.
Gianfranchi, M., and Carpino Boeri, A. (1964). *Rass. Intern. Clin. Terap.* **44**, 805.
Giannelli, A., and Invernizzi, G. (1960). *Riv. Patol. Nerv. Ment.* **81**, 543.
Gillet, G. (1965). M.D. Thesis, Univ. Paris.
Giordano, G. B., and Cipriani, G. (1964). *Acta Anaesthesiol.* **15**, 91.
Gjerris, F. (1965). *Ugeskrift Laeger* **127**, 229.
Goldman, D. (1961). *Rev. Can. Biol.* **20**, 549.
Goldwurm, G. F., and Torrigiani, G. (1962). *In* "International Symposium on Haloperidol and Triperidol," p. 425. Istituto Luso Farmaco d'Italia, Milan.
Goldwurm, G. F., and Vanni, F. (1961). *Diseases Nervous System* **22**, nr 11.
Gonçalves, B., and Cols, B. (1965). *Rev. Brasil. Anestesiol.* **15**, 332.
Gonçalves, J. A. and Lacerda, N. (1964). *Vida Cultura* **28–29**, 25.
Grabow, L., and Allemand, H. L. (1964). *Anaesthesist* **13**, 220.
Groh, G., and Lemieux, M. (1964). *In* "The Butyrophenones in Psychiatry," p. 53.
Gross, H., and Langner, E. (1964). *Wien. Med. Wochschr.* **114**, 686.
Gruvel, G., Bloch, A., Piéchaud, C., and Sabathié, M. (1963a). *Proc. 3rd Congr. Français d'Anesthésiol., Bordeaux, 1963.*
Gruvel, M., Sabathié, M., Piéchaud, C., and Bloch, A. (1963b). *Proc. 3rd Congr. Français d'Anesthésiol., Bordeaux, 1963.*
Guilbert, P., Féron, A., and Monceaux, J. P. (1961). *Ann. Med. Psychol.* **119**, 543.
Gürtner, Th., Doenicke, A., and Spiess, W. (1964). *Anaesthesist* **13**, 183.
Gutbub, T. (1963). M.D. Thesis, Univ. Strasbourg.
Guyotat, J., and Miraillet, P. (1965). *J. Med. Lyon* **46**, 411.
Haase, H. J. (1962). *In* "International Symposium on Haloperidol and Triperidol," p. 467. Istituto Luso Farmaco d'Italia, Milan.
Haase, H. J., and Janssen, P. A. J. (1965). *In* "The Action of Neuroleptic Drugs. A Psychiatric Neurologic and Pharmacologic Investigation." North-Holland Publishing Company, Amsterdam.
Haase, H. J., Mattke, D., and Schönbeck, M. (1964). *Psychopharmacologia* **6**, 435.
Haberlandt, W. F. (1963). *Med. Welt* p. 210.
Hackstein, F. G. (1963). *Therapiewoche* **13**, 485.

Harder, A. (1961). *Praxis* **50**, 868.
Hartung, M. L., Bente, D., and Schneewind, K. A. (1964). *Arzneimittel-Forsch.* **14**, 584.
Haward, L. R. C. (1964). *Brit. J. Psychiat.* **110**, 514.
Haward, L. R. C. (1965). *Clin. Trials J. (London)* **2**, 135.
Heinrich, K. (1961). *Med. Welt* **7**, 335.
Heinrich, K., and Rumpf, K. (1964). *Arzneimittel-Forsch.* **14**, 587.
Hekimian, L. J., and Friedhoff, A. J. (1964). *J. New Drugs* **4**, 264.
Hekimian, L., Friedhoff, A., Arnold, J., and Handley, P. (1963). *Current Therap. Res.* **5**, 437.
Helrich, M., and Atwood, J. M. (1964). *Anesthesia Analgesia, Current Res.* **43**, 471.
Henschel, W. F. (1962). *Proc. Symp. Neuroleptanalgesia in relation to 1st European Congr. Anaesthesiol.*, Vienna, 1962.
Henschel, W. F. (1963). *Proc. 3rd Congr. Français d'Anesthésiol.*, Bordeaux, 1963.
Henschel, W. F. (1964). *Bremer Arzteblatt* **17**, 10.
Henschel, W. F., Hammer, H., and Buhr, G. (1963). Bericht über die gemeinsame Tagung der Oesterreichischen, Schweizerischen und Deutschen Anaesthesiologen, Freiburg.
Henschel, W. F., Wilken, G., and Buhr, G. (1964). *Proc. 8th Congr. Scand. Soc. Anaesthesiol., Turku, 1964. Acta Anaesthesiol. Scand.* (Suppl. 15) 124.
Hilgers, H. (1964). *Med. Monatschr.* **18**, 83.
Hoffmann, M. (1965). M.D. Thesis, Univ. Paris.
Hofmann, S. (1965). *Z. Kinderchir. Grenzgeb.* **2**, 249.
Holderness, M. C., Chase, P. E., and Dripps, R. D. (1963). *J. Anaesthesiol.* **24**, 336.
Hollister, F. P., and Motzenbecker, F. P. (1963). *J. Neuropsychiat.* **4**, 386.
Hollister, L. E., Overall, J. E., Caffey, E., Bennett, J. L., Meyer, F., Kimbell, I., and Honigfeld, G. (1962). *J. Nervous Mental Disease* **135**, 544.
Hollister, L. E., Overall, J. E., Bennett, J. L., Kimbell, I., and Shelton, J. (1965). *J. New Drugs* **5**, 34.
Holstein, A. P., and Chen, C. H. (1965). *Am. J. Psychiat.* **122**, 462.
Horton, J. M. (1962). *Proc. Symp. Neuroleptanalgesia in relation to 1st European Congr. Anaesthesiol.*, Vienna, 1962.
Houillon, Salles, Féron, A., and Monceaux, J. P. (1961). *Ann. Med. Psychol.* **119**, 337.
Hulak, S. (1964). *Neurobiologia* **27**, 170.
Humbeeck, L. (1960). *Acta Neurol. Psychiat. Belg.* **60**, 75.
Ideström, C. M., and Cadenius, B. (1963). *Psychopharmacologia*, **4**, 235.
Ingvar, D., and Nilsson, E. (1961). *Acta Anaesthesiol. Scand.* **5**, 85.
Israel, L., Croufer, F., and Wartel, R. (1964). *Proc. Réunion Psychiat. de l'Est 1964. Ann. Med. Psychol.* **122**, 769.
Israel, J. S., Janssen, G. T., and Dobkin, A. B. (1965). *Anesthesiology* **26**, 253.
Iwamoto, S. (1964). *Japan. Clin. Exptl. Med.* **41**, 2398.
Jancar, J. (1965). *Clin. Trials* **2**, 153.
Jacob, E., and Marie, C. (1961). *Ann. Med. Psychol.* **119**, 948.
Jacobs, R. (1959). *Psychiat. Verpleging.* 8, 20; (1960), 16.
Jacobs, R. (1960). *Acta Neurol. Psychiat. Belg.* **60**, 560.
Jaeggi, F., Amati-Sas, S., and da Silva, A. M. (1960). *Med. Hyg.* **18**, 818.
Janke, W. (1961-1962). Sitzungsberichte der Gesellschaft zur Beförderung der gesamten Naturwissenschaften, Marburg **83–85**, 277.
Janke, W. (1964). *Arzneimittel-Forsch.* **14**, 582.
Janssen, P. A. J. (1961a). *Psychopharmacologia* **2**, 141.
Janssen, P. A. J. (1961b). *Lancet* p. 111.
Janssen, P. A. J. (1961c). *Arzneimittel-Forsch.* **11**, 819.
Janssen, P. A. J. (1961d). *Arzneimittel-Forsch.* **11**, 932.
Janssen, P. A. J. (1962a). *Proc. Symp. Neuroleptanalgesia in relation to 1st European Congr. Anaesthesiol.*, Vienna, 1962.

Janssen, P. A. J. (1962b). *In* "International Symposium on Haloperidol and Triperidol," p. 9. Istituto Luso Farmaco d'Italia, Milan.
Janssen, P. A. J. (1962c). *Compt. Rend. Séances Soc. Psychopharmacol. Langue Française* **51**, 582.
Janssen, P. A. J. (1962d). *Intern. J. Neuropharmacol.* **1**, 145.
Janssen, P. A. J. (1964a). *Proc. 2nd Bremer Neuroleptanalgesie Symp.* Springer-Verlag, 1966.
Janssen, P. A. J. (1964b). *In* "Neuropsychopharmacology," (P. Bradley, F. Flügel, P. Hoch, eds.), Vol. 3, p. 33. Elsevier, Amsterdam.
Janssen, P. A. J. (1964c). *In* "Ciba Foundation Symposium, Session 4," p. 264. Churchill, London.
Janssen, P. A. J. (1964d). *Proc. 4th Intern. C.I.N.P. Meeting, Birmingham, 1964*.
Janssen, P. A. J. (1966). *Intern. Rev. Neurobiol.* (in press).
Janssen, P. A. J., and Niemegeers, C. J. E. (1959). *Arzneimittel-Forsch.* **9**, 765.
Janssen, P. A. J., and Niemegeers, C. J. E. (1961a). *Nature*, **190**, 911.
Janssen, P. A. J., and Niemegeers, C. J. E. (1961b). *Arzneimittel-Forsch.* **11**, 1037.
Janssen, P. A. J., Van de Westeringh, C., Jageneau, A. H. M., Demoen, P., Hermans, B., Van Daele, P., Schellekens, K. H. L., Van der Eycken, C., and Niemegeers, C. J. E. (1959). *J. Med. Pharm. Chem.* **1**, 281.
Janssen, P. A. J., Niemegeers, C. J. E., Schellekens, K. H. L. (1960a). *Arzneimittel-Forsch.* **10**, 955.
Janssen, P. A. J., Jageneau, A. H. M., and Schellekens, K. H. L. (1960b). *Psychopharmacologia* **1**, 389.
Janssen, P. A. J., Jageneau, A. H. M., and Niemegeers, C. J. E. (1960c). *J. Pharmacol. Exptl. Therap.* **129**, 411.
Janssen, P. A. J., Niemegeers, C. J. E., and Jageneau, A. H. M. (1960d). *Arzneimittel-Forsch.* **10**, 1003.
Janssen, P. A. J., Niemegeers, C. J. E., and Verbruggen, F. J. (1962). *Psychopharmacologia* **3**, 114.
Janssen, P. A. J., Niemegeers, C. J. E., Schellekens, K. H. L., Verbruggen, F. J., and Van Nueten, J. M. (1963a). *Arzneimittel-Forsch.* **13**, 205.
Janssen, P. A. J., Niemegeers, C. J. E., and Dony, J. G. H. (1963b). *Arzneimittel-Forsch.* **13**, 401.
Janssen, P. A. J., Niemegeers, C. J. E., and Schellekens, K. H. L. (1965a). *Arzneimittel-Forsch.* **15**, 104.
Janssen, P. A. J., Niemegeers, C. J. E., and Schellekens, K. H. L. (1965b). *Arzneimittel-Forsch.* **15**, 1196.
Janssen, P. A. J., Niemegeers, C. J. E. and Schellekens, K. H. L. (1966). *Arzneimittel-Forsch.* **16**, 339.
Jaquenoud, P., Grolleau, D., and du Cailar, J. (1963). *Agressologie* **4**, 533.
Jensen, O. (1962). *Ugeskrift Laeger* **124**, 1138.
Jucker, E. (1963). *Angew. Chem.* **75**, 524.
Juillet, P., Savelli, A., Bouvier, S., and Trystram, D. (1964). *Ann. Med. Psychol.* **122**, 81.
Just, O. H., Lutz, H., and Müller, C. (1965). *Anaesthesist* **14**, 280.
Kabat, H. (1961). *Rev. Can. Biol.* **20**, 475.
Kaczynski, M., Bernaskiewicz, E., Wypych, M., and Wojnicka, H. (1965). *Neurol. Neurochir. Psychiat. Polska* **15**, 281.
Kakolewski, J. (1964). *Neurol. Neurochir. Psychiat. Polska* **14**, 93.
Kamenskaia, V. M. and Aleksandrovskij, Yu, A. (1964). *Zh. Nevropatol. Psikhiat.* **64**, 896.
Kammerer, T., Singer, L., Geissmann, P., Depoutot, J.-C., and Gutbub, Th. (1962a). *Ann. Med. Psychol.* **120**, 402.
Kammerer, T., Singer, L., Geissmann, P., Gutbub, Th., Sichel, C., and Wagner, M. (1962b). *Ann. Med. Psychol.* **120**, 535.
Kamphausen, H. (1962). *Arztl. Praxis* **14**, 1869.
Kandaperredy-Tellier, C. (1964). M.D. Thesis, Univ. Paris.
Kandaurova, Yu. N. (1964). *Vopr. Klin. Patog. Lecheniya Schizofr.* (*Moscow*) p. 50.

Kaneko, J., Ichimary, S., and Takesada, H. (1964a). *Proc. Meeting Japan. Assoc. Neuropsychiat. Osaka, 1964.*
Kaneko, J., et al. (1964b). *Clin. Psychiat.* **6**, 690.
Kapferer, J. M. (1961). *Anaesthesist* **10**, 101.
Kapferer, J. M. (1962). *Anaesthesist* **11**, 25.
Kapferer, J. M., Kraus, B., Bergmann, H., and Purtscheller, W. (1962). *Agressologie* **3**, 49.
Katila, O., and Pihkanen, T. (1963). *Acta Neurol. Psychiat. Belg.* **63**, 291.
Kátó, L., Gözsy, B., Lemieux, M., and St. Jean, A. (1964). *In* "The Butyrophenones in Psychiatry," p. 12.
Katscher, J. (1962). *Proc. Congr. Psychiat. Neurol. de Langue Française, Anvers, 1962.*
Keéri-Szànto, M., Telmosse, F., and Trop, D. (1963). *Can. Anaes. Soc. J.* **10**, 484.
Keitel, P. (1963). *Med. Welt* 1380.
Keitel, P. (1964). M.D. Thesis, Univ. Düsseldorf.
Kent, D. A. (1965). *Clin. Trials J.* **2**, 166.
Kern, R. (1965). *Anaesthesist* **14**, 54.
Kiel, H. (1963). *Deut. Geflugelwirtsch.* **14**, 699. (1963). *Tierärtl. Umschau* **18**, 636.
Kivalo, E., and Amneli, G. (1961). *Ann. Paediat. Fenniae* **7**, 320.
Kreuscher, H. (1965a). *Acta Anaesthesiol. Scand.* **9**, 155.
Kreuscher, H. (1965b). *Anaesthesist* **14**, 21.
Kreuscher, H., Frey, R., and Madjidi, A. (1965). *Deut. Med. Wochschr.* **90**, 721.
Kristjansen, P. (1960). *Acta Neurol. Psychiat. Belg.* **60**, 82.
Kristjansen, P. (1962). *In* "International Symposium of Haloperidol and Triperidol," p. 471. Istituto Luso Farmaco d'Italia, Milan.
Kristjansen, P., and Hansen, G. (1961). *Nord. Med.* **65**, 812.
Kurland, A. A., MacCusker, K., and Michaux, W. W. (1962). *J. New Drugs* **2**, 352.
Kurland, A. A., Ferro-Diaz, P., and MacCusker, K. (1964). *Comprehensive Psychiat.* **5**, 179.
La Barre, J. (1962). *Agressologie* **3**, 23.
La Barre, J. (1963). *Ann. Soc. Roy. Sci. Med. Nat. Bruxelles* **16**, 5.
Labhardt, F. (1964). *Praxis (Bern)* **53**, 1553.
Lacourt, J. (1963). *In* " Le champ thérapeutique de l'Halopéridol." Imprimerie E. Drouillard, Bordeaux.
Laffargue-Leguerinel, B. (1963). Thesis, Paris.
Lambert, P. A. (1964). *Encephale* **53**, 262.
Lambert, P. A., Marcou, G., Midenet, J., and Bouchardy, M. (1965). *J. Med. Lyon* **46**, 419.
Langer, R., and Zierach, H. J. (1964). *Wehrmed. Mitteil.* **9**, 129.
Larson, A. G. (1963). *Lancet* **1**, 128.
Lassner, J. (1964). *Cahiers Anesthesiol.* **12**, 122.
Laurans, J. (1964). M.D. Thesis, Univ. Clermont.
Lavallée, J. P. (1964). *Union Med. Canada* **93**, 567.
Lavitola, G., and Santorelli, G. (1962). *In* "International Symposium on Haloperidol and Triperidol," p. 475. Istituto Luso Farmaco d'Italia, Milan.
Lawin, P. (1965). *Anaesthesist* **14**, 103.
Lawson, J. I. M., and McGowan, St. W. (1962). *Lancet* **1**, 1205.
Lechat, P., and Deleau, D. (1965). *Therapie* **20**, 565.
Lechner, H., Mayr, F., Geyer, N., and Rodler, H. (1961). *Med. Exptl.* **5**, 291.
Lecoeur, J. L. J. (1965). M.D. Thesis, Univ. Paris.
Lecomte, J., and Dresse, A. (1962). *Arch. Intern. Pharmacodyn.* **139**, 604.
Ledesma Jimeno, A. (1963). *Medicamenta* **21**, 98.
Le Gaudu, J. Fr. (1964). M.D. Thesis, Univ. Paris.
Le Goaziou, F. (1962). *Presse Med.* **70**, 578.
Le Guen, C. (1965). M.D. Thesis, Univ. Paris.
Lehembre, J. (1962). *Acta Neurol. Psychiat. Belg.* **62**, 611.

Lehmann, H. E., Ban, T. A., Matthews, V., and Garcia-Rill, T. (1964). *First N. Am. Symp. "Hospital des Laurentides," L'Annonciation, Quebec. In* "The Butyrophenones in Psychiatry," p. 77.
Lehoczki, T., and Halasy, M. (1961). *Chemotherap. Rev.* **2**, 138.
Leone, B. N. (1962). *In* "International Symposium on Haloperidol and Triperidol," p. 493. Istituto Luso Farmaco d'Italia, Milan.
Levi, P. G. (1962). *Freniatria* **86**, fasc. 1.
Leyritz, M., Capron, H., and Timsit, M. (1961). *Ann. Med. Psychol.* **119**, 529.
Lindqvist, R. (1961). *Svenska Lakartidn.* **58**, 1422.
Linford Rees, W. L. (1965). *Clin. Trials J.* **2**, 149.
Linford Rees, W. L., and Davies, B. (1965). *Intern. J. Neuropsychiat.* **1**, 263.
Lods, J. C. (1962). *In* "International Symposium on Haloperidol and Triperidol," p. 499. Istituto Luso Farmaco d'Italia, Milan.
Lods, J. C., Vallin, J., and Dupuy, R. (1964). *Arch. Maladies Appl. Digest.* **53**, 93.
Loret, L. (1960). *Acta Neurol. Psychiat. Belg.* **60**, 86.
Luna, N. E. (1964). *Semana Medica (Buenos Aires)* **124**, 973.
Luria, E., and Rizzuto, N. (1964). *Rass. Studi Psichiat.* **53**, 168.
Maccagnani, G., and Albonetti, G. (1960). *Riv. Neuropsichiat. Sci. Affini* **6**, 43.
Maccagnani, G., and Albonetti, G. (1961). *Riv. Neuropsichiat. Sci. Affini* **7**, 33.
Maccagnani, G., Albonetti, G., and Ferri, G. (1962). *In* "International Symposium on Haloperidol and Triperidol," p. 507. Istituto Luso Farmaco d'Italia, Milan.
McIlwain, H. (1964). *Biochem. Pharmacol.* **13**, 523.
Madalena, J. C. (1964). *Hospital* **66**, 69.
Madalena, J. C. (1965). *Hospital* **68**, 279.
Madalena, J. C., Ferreira, L. F., and Bello, H. (1963). *Riv. Assoc. Med. Brasil* **9**, 375.
Madeddu, A., and Leone, B. (1960a). *Minerva Med.*
Madeddu, A., and Leone, B. (1960b). *Minerva Med.*
Madjidi, A., (1965). *Geburtsh. Frauenheilk.* **25**, 827.
Maer, M., and Kohler, C. (1963). *Ann. Med. Psychol.* **121**, 798.
Magnier, P. (1964). *Gynec. Prat.* **1**, 17.
Mahoudeau, D., and Elissalde, B. (1963). *Presse Med.* **71**, 401.
Mainardi, C. (1964). *Acta Anaesthesiol.* **15**, 323.
Mainardi, C., and Ardillo, L. (1965). *Minerva Chir.* **20**, 65.
Maitron, Luxembourger, C., and Wagner, J. (1965). *Proc. Reunion Psychiat. de l'Est, Strasbourg, 1964. Ann. Med. Psychol.* **123**, 649.
Manganaro, D., and De Casi, A. (1961). *Policlinico* **68**, 546.
Manni, C., and Trifogli, L. (1964). *Rev. Brasil. Anestesiol.* **14**, 247.
Manni, C., Trifogli, R., and Mazzoni, P. (1963). *Policlinico* **70**, 961.
Manni, C., Sarcinelli, L., and Reale, A. (1965). *Rev. Brasil. Anestesiol.* **15**, 161.
Marchais, P., and Jason, M. (1962). *Ann. Med. Psychol.* **120**, 734.
Marquez, C., Gago, M. I., Lagocki, A. M., Luciano, M., Pasqualini, G., Quinci, A., Saradjieff, P., and Shyster, M. (1964). *Dia Medico* **36**, 247.
Marriott, A. S., and Spencer, P. S. J. (1965). *Brit. J. Pharmacol.* **25**, 432.
Marsboom, R. (1963). *Vlaams Diergeneesk. Tijdschr.* **88**, 482.
Marsboom, R., and Allewijn, A. (1964). *Poultry Sci.* **43**, 1225.
Marsboom, R., and Mortelmans, J. (1964). "Symposium on Small Animal Anaesthesia," p. 31. Macmillan (Pergamon), New York.
Marsboom, R., and Sierens, G. (1962a). *Poultry Sci.* **41**, 776.
Marsboom, R., and Sierens, G. (1962b). *Poultry Sci.* **41**, 1346.
Marsboom, R., Mortelmans, J., Vercruysse, J., and Thienpont, D. (1962). *Nord. Veterinarmed.* **14**, 95.
Marsboom, R., Mortelmans, J., and Vercruysse, J. (1963a). *Vet. Record* **75**, 132.

Marsboom, R., Mortelmans, J., and Vercruysse, J. (1963b). *Kleintierpraxis* **3**, 61.
Marsboom, R., Verstraete, A., Thienpont, D., and Mattheeuws, D. (1964b). *Brit. Vet. J.* **120**, 466.
Marsico, V. (1964). *Riv. Patol. Clin.* **19**, 763.
Martin, Gabriel Narros, and Carranza Sanchez, L. J. (1960). *Medicamenta* **18**, 271.
Masciocchi, A. (1962). *In* "International Symposium on Haloperidol and Triperidol," p. 541. Istituto Luso Farmaco d'Italia, Milan.
Masciocchi, A., and Marino, A. (1962). *In* "International Symposium on Haloperidol and Triperidol," p. 547. Istituto Luso Farmaco d'Italia, Milan.
Masciocchi, A., Marino, A., and Sfondrini, E. (1961). *Rass. Studi Psichiat.* **50**, 781.
Masciocchi, A., Marino, A., and Monteverdi, T. (1962). *In* "International Symposium on Haloperidol and Triperidol," p. 557. Istituto Luso Farmaco d'Italia, Milan.
Masquin, P., and Dermenghem, J. F. (1960). *Ann. Med. Psychol.* **118**, 943.
Masquin, P., and Dermenghem, J. F. (1961). *Compt. Rend. Congr. Med. Alienistes Neurol., Montpellier, 1961*.
Mattke, D. (1964). M.D. Thesis, Univ. Düsseldorf.
Mazzarella, B., and Memoli, G. (1964). *Rass. Intern. Clin. Terap.* **44**, 794.
Megre, Velloso, F., and Paprocki, J. (1963). *Hospital* **63**, 1427.
Megre Velloso, F., and Paprocki, J. (1965). *Hospital* **68**, 47.
Mendigutia, C., Perèz, R., and Hospigliosi, L. (1960). *Medicamenta* **18**.
Merland, A., and Aubin, B. (1961). *Proc. Soc. Psychiat. Marseille Sud-Est Mediteraneen, 1961. Ann. Med. Psychol.* **119**, 373.
Meurice, E. (1960a). *Acta Neurol. Psychiat. Belg.* **60**, 91.
Meurice, E. (1960b). *Acta Neurol. Psychiat. Belg.* **60**, 96.
Milani, B. (1962). *In* "International Symposium on Haloperidol and Triperidol," p. 573. Istituto Luso Farmaco d'Italia, Milan.
Milette, G., and Sacco, J. J. (1963). *Ann. Med. Psychol.* **121**, 228.
Milne, H. B. (1965). *Clin. Trials J.* **2**, 167.
Miura, T. (1964). *Japan. J. Clin. Exp. Med.* **41**, 2389.
Monceaux, J. P. (1961). *In* "Psychoses et halopéridol." Maloine, Paris.
Monnerot, E., and Barre, R. (1962). *Proc. Soc. Psychiat. Marseille Sud-Est Mediterraneen., 1963. Presse Med.* **71**, 370.
Monnerot, E., Chancel, M., and Danjard, J. (1961). *Ann. Med. Psychol.* **119**, 669.
Monteverdi, T. (1963). *Rass. Neuropsichiat.* **17**, 283.
Montigneaux, P. (1962). M.D. Thesis, Univ. Strasbourg.
Moran, J., Marshall, B. M., and Gordon, R. A. (1964). *Can. Anaesthetists Soc. Ann. Meeting, Montebello, Quebec, 1964*.
Morin, G., Vignot, P., and Bouchacourt, A. (1960a). *Rev. Neurol.* **103**, 272.
Morin, G., Vignot, P., and Bouchacourt, A. (1960b). *Congr. d'E.E.G., Paris*, 1960.
Morin, G., Bouchacourt, A., Vignot, P., and Coulonjou, R. (1961). *Presse Med.* **69**, 915.
Morosini, C. (1962). *In* "International Symposium on Haloperidol and Triperidol," p. 581. Istituto Luso Farmaco d'Italia, Milan.
Morpurgo, C. (1965). *Psychopharmacologia (Berlin)* **8**, 91.
Mortelmans, J., Marsboom, R., and Vercruysse, J. (1962). *Bull. Soc. Roy. Zool. Anvers* no. 23.
Mostert, J. W., and Milner, L. (1961). *Med. Proc.* **7**, 468.
Mueller, H. F., and Warnes, H. (1964). *First N. Am. Symp. "Hospital des Laurentides," L'Annonciation, Quebec. In* "The Butyrophenones in Psychiatry," p. 29.
Mundeleer, P., and De Castro, G. (1962). *Cahiers Anesthesiol.* **10**, 23.
Munkvad, I. (1962). *In* "International Symposium on Haloperidol and Triperidol," p. 599. Istituto Luso Farmaco d'Italia, Milan.
Nalda Felipe, M. A. (1963). *Proc. 3rd Congr. Francais Anesthesiol. Bordeaux, France, 1963*.
Nanni Costa, P., and Cianasi, G. C. (1960). *Acta Anaesthesiol.* **11**, 349.

Naviau, J., Baré, Cl., and Duquesne, J. P. (1963). *Ann. Med. Psychol.* **121**, 118.
Nayrac, P., Arnott, G., and Milbled, G. (1964). *Encephale* **53**, 221; *Lille Med.* p. 765.
Neumann, H. (1960). *Med. Exptl.* **2**, 174.
Nick, J., and Nicolle, M. (1964). *Soc. Med. Hop. Paris* **115**, 275.
Nick, J., and Nicolle, M. H. (1965). *Exp. Sci. Franç.* p. 51.
Nicoletti, R. L., and Cols, B. (1965). *Rev. Brasil. Anestesiol.* **15**, 341.
Nicoletti, R. L., Sato, M., Soares, P. M., Lourenço, C. F. S., and Elias, L. (1964a). *Rev. Brasil. Anestesiol.* **14**, 239.
Nicoletti, R. L., Sato, M., Soares, P. M., Lourenço, C. F. S., and Elias, L. (1964b). *Rev. Brasil. Anestesiol.* **14**, 247.
Niemegeers, C. (1960). Ph.D. Thesis, Univ. Paris.
Niemegeers, C. J. E., and Janssen, P. A. J. (1960). *J. Pharm. Pharmacol.* **12**, 744.
Niemegeers, C. J. E., Verbruggen, F. J., and Janssen, P. A. J. (1964). *J. Pharm. Pharmacol.* **16**, 810.
Nigro, R., Bayerlein, L., Zolnerkiek, P., Pernet, A., and Taques, L. C. (1965). *Proc. 1st Congr. Intern. Cirurgia da Mao, Rio de Janeiro, Brazil, 1965*.
Nilsson, E. (1962a). *Surv. Anesthesiol.* **6**, 610.
Nilsson, E. (1962b). *Anaesthesist* **11**, 17.
Nilsson, E. (1962c). *Proc. Symp. Neuroleptanalgesia in relation to 1st European Congr. Anaesthesiol., Vienna, 1962*.
Nilsson, E. (1963). *Anesthesiology* **24**, 267.
Nilsson, E., and Janssen, P. A. J. (1961). *Acta Anaesthesiol. Scand.* **5**, 73.
Nistri, M., and Mori, F. (1962). *In* "International Symposium on Haloperidol and Triperidol," p. 601. Istituto Luso Farmaco d'Italia, Milan.
Nodine, J. H., Bodi, T., Levy, H. A., Siegler, P. E., Slap, J. W., Mapp, Y., and Khorsandian, R. (1962). *Clin. Pharmacol. Therap.* **3**, 432.
Nomura, A., *et al.* (1964). *Japan. J. Clin. Exptl. Med.* **41**, 2203.
Nordström, L., and Kugelberg, J. (1964). *Acta Anaesthesiol. Scand. Suppl.* **15**, 122.
Nuyts, A. (1963). *Acta Neurol. Psychiat. Belg.* **63**, 326.
Okasha, A., and Tewfik, G. I. (1964). *Brit. J. Psychiat.* **110**, 56.
Oles, M. (1960a). *Acta Neurol. Psychiat. Belg.* **60**, 100.
Oles, M. (1960b). *Med. Monatsschr.* **7**, 452.
Oles, M. (1962). *In* "International Symposium on Haloperidol and Triperidol," p. 609. Istituto Luso Farmaco d'Italia, Milan.
Olsson, O. (1961). *Svenska Lakartidn.* **58**, 1433.
Oosterbaan, W. M., and Van Wijk, L. (1962). *Ned. Tijdschr. Geneesk.* **106**, 1978.
O'Reilly, P. O., O'Regan, J. B., and Lioanag, E. M. (1964). *Diseases Nervous System* **25**, 221.
Oskam, A. C. W. (1965). *Tijdschr. Diergeneesk.* **90**, 940.
Pagliano, S., Somazzi, D., and Susini, R. (1962). *In* "International Symposium on Haloperidol and Triperidol," p. 611. Istituto Luso Farmaco d'Italia, Milan.
Paleologue, A., Sigalos, J., Spatharas, G., and Terentios, E. (1962). *In* "International Symposium on Haloperidol and Triperidol," p. 619. Istituto Luso Farmaco d'Italia, Milan.
Paley, H., Hankoff, L., Kawi, D., Ali, A., and Mendelsohn, F. (1962). *J. Neuropsychiat.* **4**, 39.
Pancer, E. (1964). *Acta Psiquiat. Psicol. Am. Lat.* **10**, 50.
Paquay, J., Arnould, F., and Burton, P. (1959a). *Ann. Med. Psychol.* **117**, 344.
Paquay, J., Arnould, F., and Burton, P. (1959b). *Acta Neurol. Psychiat. Belg.* **59**, 882.
Paquay, J., Arnould, F., and Burton, P. (1960a). *Acta Neurol. Psychiat. Belg.* **60**, 108.
Paquay, J., Arnould, F., and Burton, P. (1960b). *Acta Neurol. Psychiat. Belg.* **60**, 677.
Paquay, J., Arnould, F., and Burton, P. (1960c). *Proc. 58th Congr. Psychiat. Neurol. Langue Française, Lille, France, 1960*.
Paquay, J., Arnould, F., Burton, P., and Tinant, M. (1962a). *Acta Neurol. Psychiat. Belg.* **62**, 539.

Paquay, J., Arnould, F., Burton, P., and Tinant, M. (1962b). *In* "International Symposium on Haloperidol and Triperidol," p. 637. Istituto Luso Farmaco d'Italia, Milan.
Paquay, J., Arnould, F., Burton, P., and Tinant, M. (1964). *Proc. 62nd Congr. Psychiat. Neurol. Langue Française, Marseille, France, 1964.*
Pariante, F., Stefanachi, L., and Grassi, F. (1963). *Lavoro Neuropsichiat.* **33**, fasc. III.
Pariente, M. (1961). *Ann. Med. Psychol.* **119**, 589.
Pariente, M., Madre, J. C., and Kipman, S. D. (1960). *Ann. Med. Psychol.* **118**, 938.
Pavlou-Karageorgiadou, A., Yanniris, M., and Papachristou, C. (1962). *Iatrika Chronica* **1**, 706.
Pelaz, E. (1960a). *Arch. Neurobiol.* **23**, 207.
Pelaz, E. (1960b). *Medicamenta* **18**, 89.
Pelaz, E. (1962). *In* "International Symposium on Haloperidol and Triperidol," p. 643. Istituto Luso Farmaco d'Italia, Milan.
Pelaz, E. (1963). *Medicamenta* **21**, 237.
Pelaz, E. M., and Sanz, J. J. (1964). *Medicamenta* **22**, 31.
Pereira, F. B. L. (1965). M.D. Thesis, Univ. Sao Paulo.
Pérez Sanfelix, J., Clérigo Delgado, J., and Pigem, J. M. (1962). *In* "International Symposium on Haliperidol and Triperidol," p. 647. Istituto Luso Farmaco d'Italia, Milan.
Périer, M. (1961). M.D. Thesis, Univ. Paris.
Perini, U. (1964). *Minerva Med.* **55**, 4387.
Perini, U., and Lampo, B. (1964). *Minerva Med.* **55**, 3387.
Perrin, J., and Siffermann, A. (1961). *Proc. Soc. Psychiat. de l'Est (France)*.
Pigem, J. M., Pérez Sanfelix, J., and Sanchez-Ruis, L. (1960). *Medicamenta* **18**, 284.
Pigem, J. M., Pérez Sanfelix, J., Delgado, J. C., and Clerigo, J. (1962). *Congr. National de Psychiatrie*, Gerona.
Piret, J. M. (1965). M.D. Thesis, Univ. Paris.
Piret-Pilachon, J. (1962). M.D. Thesis, Univ. Paris.
Poire, R., Stoianoffnenoff, S., and Steiner, M. (1965). *Ann. Med. Psychol.* **123**, 648.
Polaczek-Kornecki, T. (1963). *Polski Tygod. Lekar.* **18**, 1683.
Pöldinger, W. (1964). *Praxis* **53**, 926.
Pomarede-Ravoir, A. (1963). M.D. Thesis, Univ. Toulouse.
Pöntinen, P. J., and Miettinen, P. (1964). *Acta Ophthalmol.* Suppl. 179.
Pöntinen, P. J., Söderholm, R., and Leslie, N. H. (1964). *Duodecim* **80**, 1015.
Pratt, J. P., Bishop, M. P., and Gallant, D. M. (1964). *Current Therap. Res.* **6**, 562.
Prinzhorn, G. (1964). *Wehrmed. Mitt.* nr 6, 81.
Prumm, E. (1963). *Landarzt* **39**, 1186.
Puca, A., and Cascella, G. (1960). *Riv. Neuropsychiat. Sci. Affini* **6**, 60.
Racinet, P. (1963). M.D. Thesis, Univ. Lyon.
Rajagopalan, V., and Ramamurthi, B. (1964). *Indian J. Anaesth.* **12**, 291.
Randrup, A. Munkvad, I., and Udsen, P. (1963). *Acta Pharmacol. Toxicol.* **20**, 145.
Renald, P., Larrostis-Bicheron, C., and Morin, Y. (1965). *Gaz. Med. France (Paris)* **72**, 1746.
Revol, M. L., and Miachon, S. (1963). *Bull. Trav. Soc. Pharm. Lyon* **7**, 70.
Revol, M. L. (1961). *Bull. Trav. Soc. Pharm. Lyon* **5**, 69.
Riding, J. E. (1963). *Brit. J. Anaesthesia* **35**, 180.
Riggi, F., and Vanni, F. (1962). *In* "International Symposium on Haloperidol and Triperidol," Istituto Luso Farmaco d'Italia, Milan.
Riser, M., and Déro, M. (1965). *Ann. Med. Psychol.* **123**, 256.
Romildo Bueno, J. (1965). *Hospital (Rio de Janeiro)* **67**, 1035.
Ronchi, E. (1962). *In* "International Symposium on Haloperidol and Triperidol," p. 667. Istituto Luso Farmaco d'Italia, Milan.
Roos, B. E. (1965). *Acta Psychiat. Scand.* **40**, Suppl. 180, 421.
Rosa, J. J., Schroeder, E., and Barros Hurtado, A. (1964). *Rev. Arg. Neurol. Psiquiat.* **1**, 262.
Rosadini, G., Gianniotti, G., and Rosadini, L. (1961). *Riv. Neuropsichiat. Scienze Affini* **7**, 76.

Rossi, G. (1964). *Osped. Ital. Chir.* **10**, 349.
Rouleau, Y., and Jean, B. (1964). *In* "The Butyrophenones in Psychiatry," p. 89.
Roux, G., Mouton, P., Bardis, Cl., and Gayral, L. (1963). *Ann. Med. Psychol.* **121**, 84.
Rovetta, P. (1962). *In* "International Symposium on Haloperidol and Triperidol," p. 673. Istituto Luso Farmaco d'Italia, Milan.
Royer, R. (1962). *In* "International Symposium on Haloperidol and Triperidol," p. 677. Istituto Luso Farmaco d'Italia, Milan.
Ruggerini, R. (1962). *Ateneo Parmense* **33**, Suppl. 1.
Ruggerini, R., and Zecca, C. (1964). *Acta Anesthesiol. Belg.* **15**, 85.
Ruiz, A. B. (1962). *Medicamenta* **20**, 85.
Ruiz, D. C. A., and Leyla, M. (1963). *Prensa Med. Arg.* **50**, 2348.
Saarne, A. (1963). *Acta Anesthesiol. Scand.* **7**, 21.
Sabathié, M. (1962). *Proc. Symp. Neuroleptanalgesia in relation to 1st European Congr. Anaesthesiol. Vienna, 1962.*
Samuels, A. S. (1961). *Am. J. Psychiat.* **118**, 253.
Samulak, G. (1964). M.D. Thesis, Univ. Lille.
Santaella, A. (1965). *Folha Med.* **50**, 313.
Santiago Barrios, F. (1961). *Medicamenta* **19**, 154.
Sarwer-Foner, G. J. (1964). *In* "The Butyrophenones in Psychiatry," p. 74.
Sato, R., et al. (1965). *J. New Remed. Clin.* **14**, 53.
Schaper, W. K. A., and Jageneau, A. H. M. (1961). *Arzneimittel-Forsch.* **11**, 1102.
Schaper, W. K. A., Jageneau, A. H. M., Huygens, J., and Janssen, P. A. J. (1960). *Med. Exptl.* **3**, 169.
Schaper, W. K. A., Jageneau, A. H. M., and Xhonneux, R. (1962). *Arzneimittel-Forsch.* **12**, 1015.
Schaper, W. K. A., Jageneau, A. H. M., and Bogaard, J. M. (1963). *Arzneimittel-Forsch.* **13**, 316.
Scherrer, P., and Dermenghem, J. F. (1962). *Ann. Med. Psychol.* **120**, 623.
Schmitt, H., and Schmitt, H. (1962). *Arch. Intern. Pharmacodyn.* **137**, 91.
Schmitz, B., Hoyon, A., Tarkian, M., and Weck, G. (1961). *Ann. Med. Psychol.* **119**, 949.
Schneider, J., Thomalske, G., Perrin, J., and Siffermann, A. (1963). *Nervenarzt* **34**, 521.
Schneider, P., and Zeller, K. (1964). *Therap. Umschau* **21**, 166.
Schönbeck, M. (1964). M.D. Thesis, Univ. Düsseldorf.
Schwarz, H., Jünemann, H. J., and Krüger, H. J. (1961). *Med. Welt* p. 1438.
Schwarz, H., Krüger, H. J., and Jünemann, H. J. (1962). *Arztl. Praxis* **14**, 1449.
Schwarz, H., Krüger, H. J., and Jünemann, H. J. (1964). *Acta Neurol. Psychiat. Belg.* **64**, 401.
Schweder, N. (1964). *Anaesthesist* **13**, 108.
Schweigh, M., Capron, C., and Sanchez, F. (1961). *Ann. Med. Psychol.* **119**, 348.
Seabra-Dinis, J., and da Silva, A. M. (1960). *Acta Neurol. Psychiat. Belg.* **60**, 123.
Seignot, J.-N. (1961). *Ann. Med. Psychol.* **119**, 578.
Sforza, I., and Siciliano, C. (1964). *Minerva Anestesiol.* **30**, 552.
Simpson, G. M., Farkas, T., and Saunders, J. C. (1964a). *Psychopharmacologia* **5**, 306.
Simpson, G. M., Blair, J. H., and Cranswick, E. H. (1964b). *Clin. Pharmacol. Therap.* **5**, 310.
Simpson, G. M., Kunz, E., and Watts, T. P. S. (1965). *Psychopharmacologia* **8**, 223.
Singer, L., Geissmann, P., and Gutbub, T. (1961). Reunion Psychiatrique de l'Est, Centre Psychothérapique de Nancy-Laxou. *Agressologie* **3**, 31 (1962).
Sironi, P. G., and Varesi, E. M. (1964). *Anestesiol. Rianim.* **5**, 315.
Sivadjian, J., Vautrin, M., and Matge, H. (1963). *Therapie* **18**, 1279.
Sodoyez, J. C., Dresse, A., and Lecomte, J. (1962). *Compt. Rend Soc. Biol.* **156**, 384.
Soep, H. (1961a). *Nature*, **192**, 67.
Soep, H. (1961b). *J. Chromatog.* **6**, 122.
Soep, H., and Janssen, P. A. J. (1961). *Biochem. Pharmacol.* **7**, 81.
Soergel, W. (1963). *Geburtsh. Frauenheilk.* **33**, 453.

Soma, L. R., and Shields, D. R. (1964). *J. Am. Vet. Med. Assoc.* **145**, 897.
Songar, A. (1959). *Turk Hekimler Dergisi* **1**, 3.
Soulairac, A., Halpern, B., Grisoni, F., Brunhes, M., Frélot, Cl., Geier, S., and Ochonisky, J. (1962a). *Ann. Med. Psychol.* **120**, 384.
Soulairac, A., Schaub, Cl., and Morel, P. (1962b). *Presse Med.* **70**, 805.
Soulairac, A., Geier, S., Ochonisky, J., and Poyart (1964). *Ann. Med. Psychol.* **122**, 271.
Soyka, D. (1964). *Arzneimittel-Forsch.* **14**, 1182.
Spencer, P. S. J. (1965). *Brit. J. Pharmacol.* **25**, 442.
Steenfeldt-Foss, O. W. (1962). In "International Symposium on Haloperidol and Triperidol," p. 699. Istituto Luso Farmaco d'Italia, Milan.
Steenfeldt-Foss, O. W. (1963). *Tidskr. Norske Laegeforen.* **83**, 1038.
Stelter, E., and Bielinski, C. (1964). *Therap. Umschau* **21**, 63.
Stille, G., Lauener, H., Eichenberger, E., Hunziker, F., and Schmutz, J. (1965). *Arzneimittel-Forsch.* **15**, 841.
St. Jean, A., Lidsky, A., Ban, T. A., and Lehmann, H. E. (1964). In "The Butyrophenones in Psychiatry," p. 38.
Stoll, B.A. (1962). *Brit. Med. J.* **II**, 507.
Stucke, W. (1963). *Landarzt* **13**, 540.
Subra, Dagand, Auge, and Dauch (1962). *Gaz. Hop.* **134**, 645.
Sugerman, A. A. (1964). *Diseases Nervous System* **25**, 355.
Sugerman, A. A., Williams, B. H., and Adlerstein, A. M. (1964). *Am. J. Psychiat.* **120**, 1190.
Svendsen, B. B., and Willadsen, J. (1963). *Acta Psychiat. Scand.* **39**, 351.
Szobor, A. (1962) *Acta Neurol. Psychiat Belg.* **62**, 662.
Tasker, R. R., and Marshall, B. M. (1965). *Can. Anaesthesiol. Soc. J.* **12**, 29.
Temkov, I., and Daskalov, Z. (1962). *Suvremenna Meditsina (Sofia)* **13**, 31.
Terrassier, J. (1965). M.D. Thesis, Univ. Bordeaux.
Tewfik, G. I. (1965). *Clin. Trials J.* **2**, 150.
Thomas, J. J., and Dryon, L. (1964). *J. Pharm. Belg.* p. 481.
Thuries, J., and Miech, G. (1964). *Strasbourg Med.* **15**, 239.
Timmermans, F. J. M., Bush, H. J., and Crul, J. F. (1965). *Ned. Tijdschr. Geneesk.* **109**, 955.
Toledo, J. B., and Zimerman, C. (1965). *Ann. Argent. Med.* **10**, 35.
Torelli, L., and Schiavi, F. (1965). *Agressologie* **6**, 327.
Tornetta, F. J., and Boger, W. P. (1964). *Anesthesia Analgesia Current Res.* **43**, 544.
Touraine, J. (1961). *Agressologie* **2**, 357.
Trethowan, W. H. (1965a). *Brit. Med. J.* **i**, 647.
Trethowan, W. H. (1965b). "Proceedings of a symposium at St. Bartholomew's Hospital, London, 1964." Macmillan (Pergamon), New York.
Trifogli, L., and Manni, C. (1964). *Proc. 3rd World Congr. Anesthesiol.*, Sao Paulo, 1964.
Trop, D., and Brindle, G. F. (1964). *Can. Anaesthetists Soc. Ann. Meeting, Montebello, Quebec, 1964.*
Tsuchimoto, T., and Nishigori, T. (1964). Meeting of the Japanese Association of Neuropsychiatry, Osaka.
Usdin, E., and Usdin, V. R. (1961). *Proc. Soc. Exptl. Biol Med.* **108**, 461.
Uyterschaut, P., and Jacobs, R. (1962). *Acta Neurol. Psychiat. Belg.* **62**, 677.
Vallade, B., Boutillier, Corsetti, Raybaud, and Ducamin (1963). *Ann. Med. Psychol.* **121**, 233.
Van der Spek, P. A. F. (1962). In "International Symposium on Haloperidol and Triperidol," p. 685. Istituto Luso Farmaco d'Italia, Milan.
Van de Westeringh, C., Van Daele, P., Hermans, B., Van der Eycken, C., Boey, J., and Janssen, P. A. J. (1964). *J. Med. Chem.* **7**, 619.
Van Nueten, J. (1962). Ph.D. Thesis, Univ. Paris.
Van Rossum, J. M. (1965). *J. Pharm. Pharmacol.* **17**, 202.
Vanzelli, U. and Andreoli, F. A. (1964). *Acta Anaesthesiol.* **15**, 31.

Varela, L. B. (1961). *Medicamenta* **35**, 210.
Vauterin, C., and Robert, J. (1961). *Journees de Bichat, Paris*.
Venning, G. R. (1963). *J. New Drugs* **3**, 351.
Verstraete, A., Marsboom, R., and Mattheeuws, D. (1962). *Vlaams Diergeneesk. Tijdschr.* **31**, 81.
Villa, J. L. (1964). *Praxis* **53**, 1725.
Vitger, J. (1965). *Praxis* **54**, 162.
von Eiff, A. W., and Jesdinski, H. J. (1960). *Acta Neurol. Psychiat. Belg.* **60**, 63.
Vourc'h, G., Arfel, G., Denavit, M., Millan, E., Besson, J. M., and Brown, H. (1964). *Actualites Pharmacol.* **17**, 213.
Waelkens, J. (1960a). *Acta Neurol. Psychiat. Belg.* **60**, 128.
Waelkens, J. (1960b). *Acta Neurol. Psychiat. Belg.* **60**, 576.
Walker, R., and McIntyre, J. W. (1965). *Can. Anaes. Soc. J.* **12**, 361.
Wambsganss, E. (1965a). *Psychopharmacologia* **7**, 61.
Wambsganss, E. (1965b). *Arzneimittel-Forsch.* **15**, 1063.
Warnes, H., Lee, H., and Ban, T. (1964). *In* "The Butyrophenones in Psychiatry," p. 100.
Winckler, C. (1963). *Acta Inst. Anesthesiol.* **12**.
Yelnosky, J., and Field, W. E. (1964). *Am. Vet. Res.* **25**, 1751.
Yelnosky, J., and Gardocki, J. F. (1964). *Toxicol. Appl. Pharmacol.* **6**, 63.
Yelnosky, J., Katz, R., and Dietrich, E. V. (1964). *Toxicol. Appl. Pharmacol.* **6**, 37.
Zauder, H. L., Del Guerciom, L. R. M., Feins, N., Barton, N., and Wollman, S. (1965). *Anesthesiology* **26**, 266.
Zecca, C., and Molinaroli, P. (1965). *Minerva Anestesiol.* **33**, 138.
Zegveld, C. (1963). *Nerderl. Tijdschr. Geneesk.* **107**, 2209.
Zerbe, H. (1964). M.D. Thesis, Univ. Paris.
Zerbini, E., Petromilli, M., and Tiberi, F. (1962). *In* "International Symposium on Haloperidol and Triperidol," p. 733. Istituto Luso Farmaco d'Italia, Milan.
Zindler, M., Eunike, S., and Satter, P. (1964). Third World Congress of Anesthesiology, Sao Paulo.
Zugliani, J. A. (1964). *Riv. Brasileira Anestesiol.* **14**, 255.

~3~
Biochemical Basis of Mental Disease

Louise H. Greenberg, R. F. J. McCandless, and Maxwell Gordon

Smith Kline & French Laboratories, Philadelphia, Pennsylvania

I.	Introduction	249
II.	Theories of Mental Disease	251
	A. Abnormal Protein Factors	251
	B. Endogenous Amines and Related Substances	255
	C. Faulty Energy Metabolism	273
	D. Genetically Linked Defects	274
	E. Nutritional Disorders	275
	F. Conclusion	276
	References	277

I. Introduction

The possibility of a biochemical basis for mental disease has been attractive to medicinal chemists and pharmacologists because they are always trying to find fundamental biochemical characteristics of diseases which can be modified through the antimetabolite, or other, approach. Unfortunately in mental disease, as in most other diseases, medicinal agents are usually discovered by screening techniques or by accident. Thus, the medicinal chemist's goal of designing new chemical agents, based on theoretical considerations, continues to elude him.

Although the main thrust of investigations as to possible biochemical bases underlying mental disease has been in schizophrenia and related disorders, it is in this area that our knowledge is imprecise and fragmentary, and our therapy, where there is any, is empirical. On the other hand, the mental aberrations associated with vitamin deficiencies are better understood and their therapy is more rational. This chapter will emphasize the biochemical aspects of schizophrenia and depressions, and a brief discussion of nutritionally and genetically based disorders will be given at the end of the chapter.

There are many "schools" of thought regarding the etiology of mental illness. Of the many points of view which have been expressed, two of the most extreme views are represented by those who would attribute diseases such as schizophrenia to constitutional causes (e.g., physiological or biochemical derangements), and those who feel that mental disease is primarily an environmental, behavioral aberration (psychoanalytical school), ignoring completely biochemical concepts. The majority of members of both "schools," however, probably assume an interaction between many factors, some constitutional and some environmental.

Irrespective of these arguments, it is known that drugs can modify behavior. Certain of these, e.g., the phenothiazine derivatives, can provide, by some as yet unknown biochemical action, relief of certain of the symptoms of schizophrenia. Others, e.g., LSD or psilocybin, can mimic some of the symptoms of this same disease. This would lend support to the thesis that some biochemical abnormality is of etiologic significance in mental illness. The evidence that genetic factors may be important in certain of these disorders (at least the predisposition to them) would also be suggestive of a specific biochemical lesion. However, the problem of identifying a biochemical difference between normal individuals and psychotic patients, and then establishing that this difference is, in fact, the cause of the psychotic symptoms, is vast and complicated. Certainly one must consider that all behavior, whether normal or abnormal, has a biochemical basis, since all neuronal processes are dependent upon biochemical events within the neuron and at neuronal synapses. Thus, the aberrant brain function apparent in various mental illnesses can be assumed to be mediated in some manner (if not wholly caused) by alterations in local biochemical phenomena.

But these alterations may be only quantitative rather than qualitative. That is, there may simply be alterations in the rates at which critical neurochemical reactions proceed (e.g., the synthesis or metabolism of a neurotransmitter substance or the transport of ions) leading to a change in the functional levels of normally occurring substances. Such changes could lead to altered neuronal function and transmission of nerve impulses in one small area of the brain, or to an imbalance in the normal interrelationships between various brain structures or levels of integration. Needless to say, local quantitive changes in biochemical processes would be very difficult to detect. It is not surprising, therefore, that most researchers have directed their efforts toward finding qualitatively different chemical substances in psychotic patients which are absent in normal persons or present to only a limited extent. Furthermore, most of the search has been directed to the blood and urine of psychotic patients, since, obviously, such samples are readily available.

But it is conceivable that even if there is an abnormal substance formed or concentrated in the brain of a schizophrenic patient, for example, this could be such a highly localized phenomenon that one could not detect its presence when diluted out in blood and urine along with substances from all parts of the body. Thus, it is not hard to understand why research to date has not led to a single incontrovertible biochemical defect in psychotic individuals, despite the plethora of interesting leads, provocative hypotheses, and extensive investigative effort.

The question, therefore, as to whether there is a characteristic biochemical lesion in mental disease and, if so, what the nature of that lesion may be, has been the source of much controversy which we cannot resolve at this time. We can merely briefly summarize the various speculations and lines of research that have been pursued. In this connection, the reader's attention is directed to excellent reviews by Kety (1959, 1965a,b) of the biochemical theories of schizophrenia and the possible sources of errors and difficulty inherent in research in this area (cf. Eiduson et al., 1964). However inconclusive the results of this effort may be at this time, the effort has not been without value, if only in providing impetus for further research and improved methodology which may lead to a greater understanding of normal as well as abnormal brain function and, hopefully, to the eventual prevention or cure of mental illness.

II. Theories of Mental Disease

A. Abnormal Protein Factors

Many of the protein factors described here are probably related to each other, and some may be identical, but they are described separately for historical perspective and because of the absence of objective structural comparative data.

1. Akerfeldt's Ceruloplasmin

In investigations carried out in Sweden in 1955, Akerfeldt (1957) reported that serum obtained from patients with mental disease, including schizophrenic, manic depressive, and senile psychoses, had the capacity to oxidize N,N-dimethyl-p-phenylene diamine (DPP) more rapidly than serum from control subjects. It was postulated that elevated ceruloplasmin (a copper-containing protein) levels in schizophrenic serum, as indicated by high serum copper, was responsible for the rapid oxidizability of DPP. It was speculated that this DPP color development might be used as a diagnostic tool for mental disease.

However, Wurtman et al. (1958) reported that measurement of serum oxidative activity by means of a modification of the Akerfeldt test revealed no abnormalities in the sera of patients with various psychoses. Furthermore, these authors stated that the Akerfeldt test does not measure serum ceruloplasmin content. They found that even though the test can be made to measure oxidative activity, the latter is so subject to variations in plasma ascorbic acid level [ceruloplasmin is an ascorbate oxidase, hence, the sensitivity of the test to ascorbic acid levels (Osaki *et al.*, 1962)], due to both dietary factors and disease, as to make it impossible to use the test to diagnose any specific condition. Similarly, Frank and Wurtman (1958) stated that the Akerfeldt test results depend on the temperature and the pH at which the reaction is carried out, in addition to the great potential for variability caused by diet and the physical condition of the patient.

More importantly, however, the ceruloplasmin test was found to be very nonspecific, since other conditions such as tuberculosis, arthritis, liver disease, or pregnancy could also produce positive reactions in the test. Since then literally hundreds of papers on ceruloplasmin have been published, and in general, later workers have found that the ceruloplasmin test was too nonspecific to be of value diagnostically.

2. Heath's Taraxein

Heath *et al.* (1957, 1958; Heath and Leach, 1958) have reported on the isolation of a factor called taraxein from the blood of schizophrenic patients. The readministration of this factor to monkeys, to nonpsychotic human volunteers, and to schizophrenic patients in remission is said to produce schizophrenic-like symptoms.

Taraxein is thought to be a coenzyme or a co-factor dialyzable from a protein fraction which has been called taraxinogen. Taraxein itself is a small, chemically unidentified molecule, possibly an indole. Heath has suggested that taraxinogen is qualitatively different from ceruloplasmin, but to date it must be stated that the relationship between the two proteins is not clear.

In 1961, Heath published data suggesting that his taraxein fraction isolated from schizophrenic serum not only produced changes in the behavior of monkeys and nonpsychotic human volunteers which resembled certain aspects of schizophrenia, but also produced at the same time alterations in EEG recordings (taken from implanted depth electrodes) which correlated well with the behavioral changes. Heath has suggested (1960) that the taraxein fraction may be a biochemical manifestation of a genetic defect present in the schizophrenic patient. Attempts to confirm Heath's taraxein work have been successful in a few laboratories, but unsuccessful in many others. Work in this area is continuing (Redick, 1963).

3. The α-Globulin Factor of Frohman and Gottlieb

Frohman *et al.* (1960a) found that chicken erythrocytes incubated with plasma from schizophrenic patients had higher lactate/pyruvate ratios than those incubated with plasma from normal subjects. It was suggested that this difference was due to a substance, perhaps a protein, present in altered or excessive amounts in the plasma of schizophrenic patients. Results with rat diaphragms were in the same direction, with both carbohydrate metabolism and protein synthesis being inhibited (Walaas et al., 1964, 1965).

Further work by Frohman et al. (1960b,c) suggested that this factor from schizophrenic patients stimulated energy production by forcing glucose through the Emden-Meyerhof metabolic path rather than through the hexose-monophosphate shunt. Strains of Hela cells in culture were also reported to be inhibited when schizophrenic rather than normal serum was used to supplement the growth medium (Stone et al., 1965).

This factor was readily affected by pH and temperature, remaining relatively stable between pH 6 and 9 at 4°C. It appeared to be an α-globulin or a prosthetic group attached to an α-globulin. It was suggested by these authors that the taraxein protein might be related to this active principle and that inconsistency in reports regarding the activity of sera might be related to the lability of the substance to changes in pH and temperature.

Further experiments by Frohman et al. (1961) carried out on a blind basis demonstrated that schizophrenic patients could be differentiated from non-schizophrenic subjects biochemically in a significant number of cases as mentioned above.

However, it should be noted that the same investigators (Frohman et al., 1963) found that the amount of motor activity or exercise in which subjects engaged had a pronounced effect on the lactate/pyruvate ratio, so that only when normal subjects were moderately exercised before the test could a difference between schizophrenics and normal subjects be demonstrated. Subsequently it was found that injection of norepinephrine into the chickens prior to studying the effect of schizophrenic plasma on chicken erythrocytes blocked the elevation of the lactate/pyruvate ratio produced by the serum factor (Latham et al., 1964, 1965). This blocking was not by a direct inhibitory effect on the factor, but perhaps by a mobilization of some inhibitor substance which alters the reactivity of the chicken erythrocytes to the schizophrenic plasma. Following the norepinephrine injection, the protein fraction from chickens that was most active in depressing the normal lactate/pyruvate ratios had the electrophoretic mobility of a gamma globulin (Frohman et al., 1964).

Frohman et al. (1966) also reported that the schizophrenic plasma factor significantly increased transport of glutamic acid and histamine across membranes of chicken erythrocytes. No significant differences were found in lysine or methionine transport.

Along similar lines, Lees et al. (1965) found, using rat liver homogenates, that succinic oxidase activity was significantly lower in the presence of dialyzed serum from 27 schizophrenics, when compared with normal controls.

4. Other Protein Factors

Other work on the isolation and identification of protein factors from schizophrenic plasma was stimulated by the report of Winter and Flataker

(1958) that the intraperitoneal injection of plasma from the majority of schizophrenic and other severely psychotic patients into rats produced a deficit in rope climbing resembling, but not identical with, that produced by injection of LSD. In a rat trained to climb a rope, injection of 1 ml of plasma produced a deficiency in performance which could be measured quantitatively. Comparison of the effects of plasma from 80 psychotic patients and 82 non-psychotic subjects, including both general hospital patients and normal subjects, showed a highly significant difference between the two groups. Cerebrospinal fluid had much less effect than plasma. Winter et al. (1961) further reported that serum or plasma from humans injected intraperitoneally retards the performance of rats trained to climb a rope. On the average, the effect of serum from schizophrenic donors was much greater than that from normal donors when individual sera were examined. When the serum from schizophrenics was pooled, however, most of the pooled sera did not affect the rats in the rope climbing test. On this basis it was suggested by the authors that inhibitors may be present in some sera.

When the pooled serum cited above was fractionated by the method of Lever et al. (1951), the principle producing the decrement in rope climbing performance of rats was in fraction III.[1] The fraction III from normal and schizophrenic sera still showed the same differences as the whole sera.

Plasma "rope climbing factors" were further studied by Sanders et al., (1965) who could find no chemical differences by a variety of procedures (including cellulose acetate electrophoresis and immunoelectrophoresis) in either whole plasma or fraction III between schizophrenics and control subjects. Neither could he demonstrate any differences in the rope climbing procedure.

Bergen (1965) summarized the work on the plasma globulin fractions and suggested that the active principle in producing the decrement in rope climbing performance may be a small molecule bound to a globulin. He also suggested that the small molecule may be an amine since it appeared to have been protected by monoamine oxidase inhibitors, and by ascorbic acid and storage under nitrogen gas. Furthermore, on the basis of several behavioral tests in animals, he hypothesized that this amine may be 3,4-dimethoxyphenethylamine (or be closely related to it). Friedhoff and Van Winkle (1962, 1963a,b) had isolated 3,4-dimethoxyphenethylamine (DMPEA) from the urine of schizophrenics. Work on DMPEA will be discussed in greater detail in Section II,B,1).

A number of other groups have also obtained evidence which suggests that an abnormal protein may exist in the blood of schizophrenics which is not present (or is present in lesser amounts) in normal individuals. One of the most

[1] A heterogeneous fraction, the major components of which include α_2-macroglobulins and β_{2A}-globulins. Some of the minor components include haptoglobulin, β-lipoprotein, prothrombin, ceruloplasmin, albumin, and several others (Sanders et al., 1965).

provocative findings was that of Haddad and Rabe (1963). These investigators, in well-controlled experiments, sensitized rabbits with serum pooled from chronically ill schizophrenic patients, desensitized the animals with serum from nonschizophrenic individuals, and then challenged with schizophrenic serum. In this manner they found an abnormal antigen in the pooled schizophrenic serum which may be of some significance in the disease.

Other reports include that of Kemali (1960) who found that extracts made from the urine of schizophrenic patients, when applied to the cerebral cortex of the unanesthetized rabbit, produced an epileptic type of activity on the electroencephalographic records. This EEG activity was not seen when equivalent amounts of extracts from the urine of healthy subjects were used. The above urine principle was further fractionated by German and Kemali (1963) and the fraction evoked similar responses when applied to the cerebral cortex of the rat. Extracts from sera of schizophrenic patients showed similar effects (German, 1963), although the relationship between the urine and serum principles is not known.

Clarification of the confusion in this area, however, must await the current attempts by many laboratories to fractionate the plasma proteins of schizophrenics and to isolate and characterize the abnormal substance or substances responsible for the various biological effects which have been attributed specifically to schizophrenic blood.

B. Endogenous Amines and Related Substances

A number of well-known substances, such as acetylcholine, noradrenalin, dopamine, serotonin, γ-aminobutyric acid, and histamine, have been implicated as neurohumoral transmitter agents, both in the central nervous system and in the periphery. Some of the most interesting hypotheses regarding biochemical lesions in mental disease have involved a variety of derivatives or suspected abnormal metabolites of these substances, leading to the so-called "neurotoxin" theories. Such theories have been attractive, not only because it might be imagined that such abnormal derivatives might function much the same as antimetabolites, interfering with nerve transmission by antagonizing the action of the "neurotransmitter" at nerve synapses, but also because several psychotomimetic agents (e.g., mescaline, bufotenine, dimethyltryptamine, etc.) are close chemical relatives of the proposed neurotransmitters, particularly serotonin and noradrenalin.

1. Catecholamine Derivatives

a. *Metabolism*. Before reviewing some of the neurotoxin theories proposing various abnormal metabolites of catecholamines such as dopamine, norepinephrine, and epinephrine, it might be well to review first what has now been fairly well established regarding the biosynthesis and degradation of these agents. The major pathway for the biosynthesis of norepinephrine and epinephrine (Axelrod, 1959) via phenylalanine, tyrosine, and dihydroxyphenylalanine (dopamine) is shown in Fig. 1. The conversion of p-tyrosine

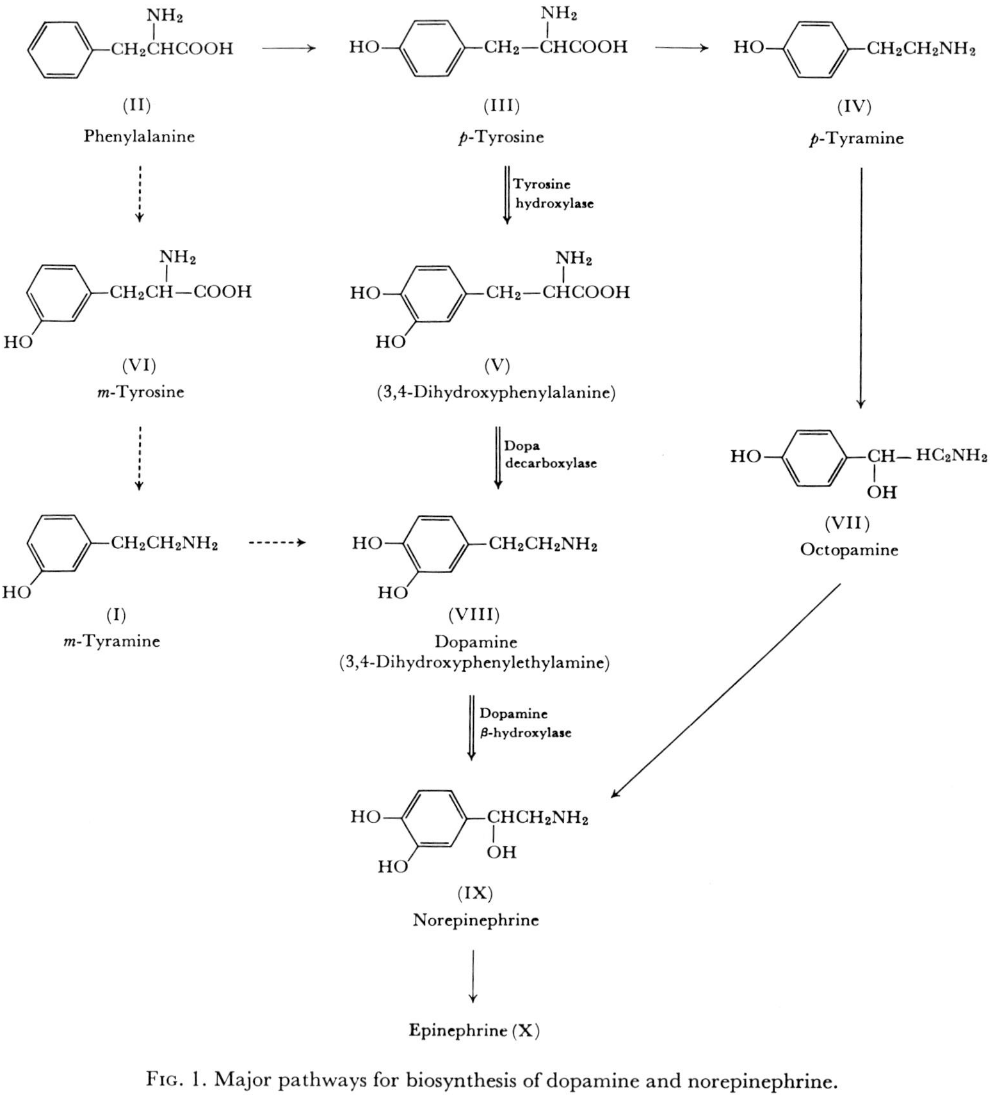

FIG. 1. Major pathways for biosynthesis of dopamine and norepinephrine.

(III) to dopa (V) is slow and may be the rate-limiting step (Levitt et al., 1965; see also Bunney and Davis, 1965). Additional alternate pathways for epinephrine biosynthesis have been cited by Kirshner (1966).

Fig. 2 illustrates the degradation of these catecholamines. Major

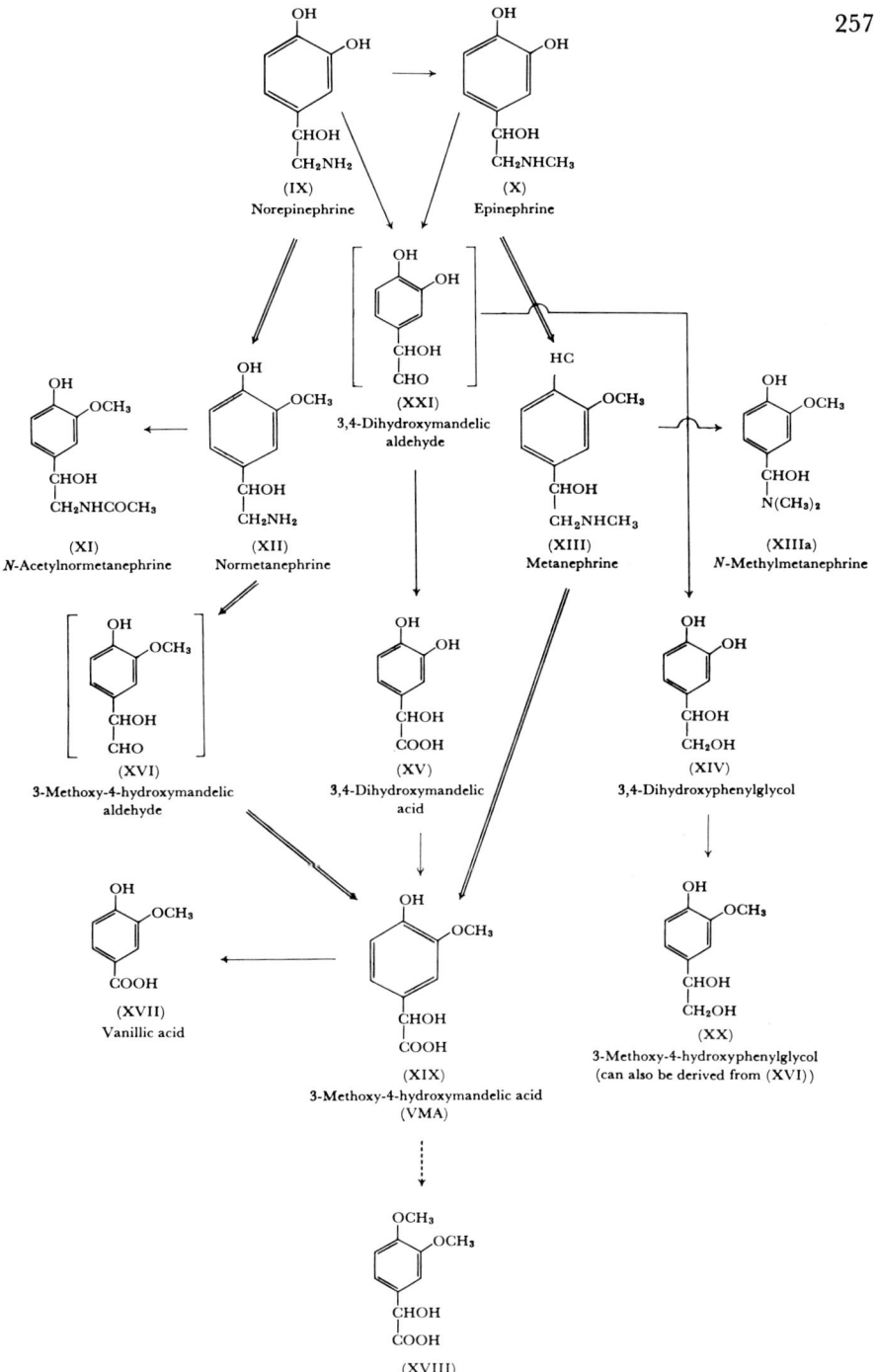

Fig. 2. Metabolic products of catecholamines.

pathways are indicated by bold arrows, speculations are indicated by dotted lines. This subject has been well reviewed by Daly and Witkop (1963). Hartung et al. (1964) have described the synthesis and Hess (1960) has studied the action of potential antimetabolites of catecholamines.

In Fig. 2, major excretion products of norepinephrine (IX) in man are 3-methoxy-4-hydroxymandelic acid (XIX) (cf. Daly et al., 1965), normetanephrine (XII), 3,4-dihydroxymandelic acid (XV) (Goodall et al., 1959), and 3,4-dihydroxyphenylglycol (XIV) in rats (Axelrod et al., 1959). Suspected intermediates are 3,4-dihydroxymandelic aldehyde (XXI), and 3-methoxy-4-hydroxymandelic aldehyde (XVI).

Other probable metabolites include vanillic acid (XVII) in man (Rosen and Goodall, 1962), N-acetylnormetanephrine (XI) (Weissbach et al., 1961), and N-methylmetanephrine (XX) (Perry, 1963) and their conjugates.

The major excretion products of epinephrine in man are formed via O-methylation or deamination. The glycols (XIV) and (XVI) are minor products in man, but are major metabolites in the rodent (Axelrod et al., 1959; Kopin and Axelrod, 1960).

Some of the enzymes involved in Fig. 2 are: IX→X, XIII→XIIIa, N-methyl transferase; IX→XXI, X→XXI, XII→XVI and XIII→XVI monoamine oxidase; IX→XII, X→XIII, and XIV→XX, catechol O-methyl transferase; and XXI→XV and XVI→XIX, aldehyde oxidase (Hayaishi, 1962) (cf. Daly and Witkop, 1963).

The biosynthesis of dopamine (cf. Anton and Sayre, 1964) can be seen in Fig. 1, and its metabolism is traced in Fig. 3 (not including its conversion to norepinephrine, which is in Fig. 1). The close resemblance between these amines and the hallucinogen, mescaline (XXII) is apparent from Fig. 3. In rats, dopamine is metabolized mainly via 3,4-dihydroxyphenylacetic acid (XXIV) with about a 20% conversion to 3-methoxytyramine (XXVI) (Goldstein et al., 1959), and with ultimate urinary excretion as 3-methoxy-4-hydroxyphenylacetic acid (XXVII) and its conjugates (cf. Furchgott, 1966).

b. *Neurotoxin Theories*. One of the first neurotoxin theories suggested that norepinephrine or epinephrine might be abnormally metabolized in schizophrenics to form hallucinogenic derivatives such as mescaline (see Fig. 3), adrenochrome, or adrenolutin. The adrenochrome and adrenolutin theories

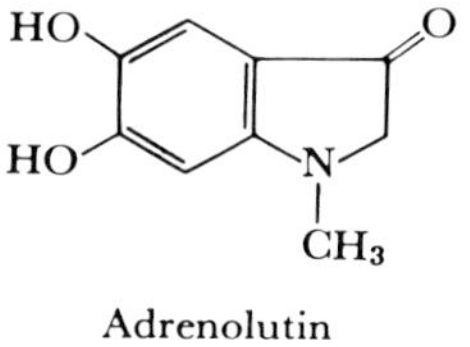

Adrenolutin

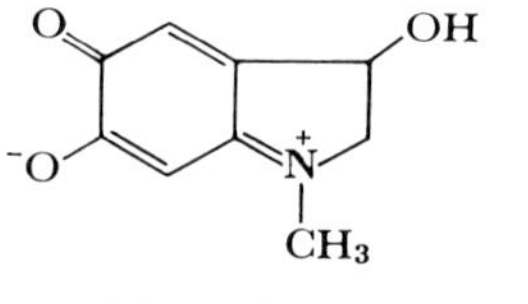

Adrenochrome

were discussed in Volume I on p. 578. On the basis of recent research and improved analytical procedures, however, it is unlikely that mescaline, adrenochrome, and adrenolutin are present in the urine or serum of normal or schizophrenic patients.

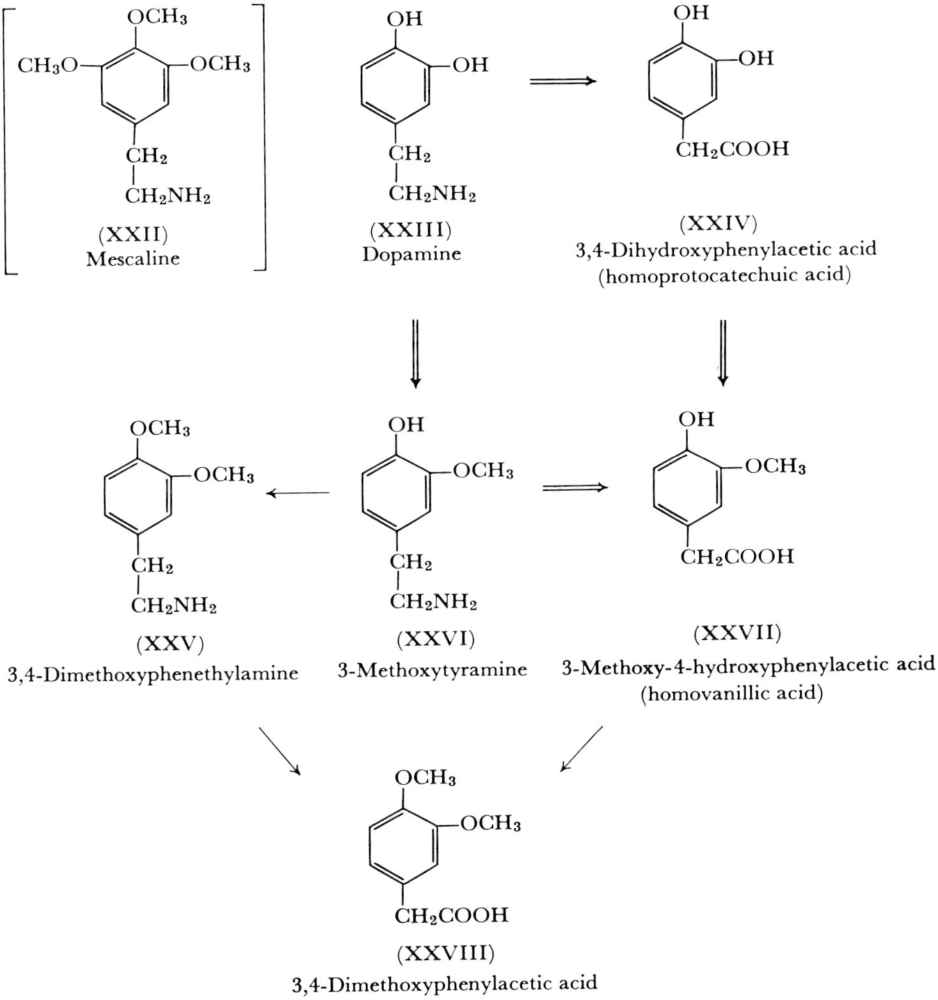

FIG. 3. Metabolism of dopamine.

Szara et al. (1958), utilizing a specific and sensitive method for the estimation of adrenochrome in plasma, could not detect this substance in the plasma of normal or schizophrenic subjects. Similarly, Feldstein (1959) did not detect any abnormal adrenaline metabolites in the blood of schizophrenics, and other workers have not noted any qualitative difference between the way schizophrenics and normal individuals react to injected adrenalin (Pollin and Goldin, 1961; Cardon et al., 1961), although differences in sensitivity to adrenalin at receptor sites has not been ruled out.

In addition, studies with labeled epinephrine and norepinephrine have shown that at least 95 to 98% of the radioactivity can be accounted for by the metabolites in Fig. 2 (to be discussed later). Also, a paper by LaBrosse et al. (1961) reported studies of the metabolism and excretion of epinephrine, labeled with tritium, in both schizophrenic and normal males and found no difference in the metabolism of circulating epinephrine between normal and schizophrenic patients (cf. Kety, 1962).

Furthermore, except for the reports of the original proponents, there has been only one report that adrenochrome or adrenolutin are psychotogenic in their activity. This was a report of a double-blind study by Grof et al. (1961) which indicated that certain individuals did get psychotic reactions and EEG changes from certain batches of sublingually administered adrenochrome. They claimed that the lability of this substance has contributed to the confusion regarding its activity. In view of all of the negative evidence, however, the adrenochrome-adrenolutin hypothesis does not appear to be tenable.

Along similar lines, perhaps, Veech et al. (1961) carried out chromatographic studies on material precipitated from schizophrenic urine with lead acetate. They reported that this precipitate consisted, at least in part, of aminochromes whose properties resembled those of adrenolutin and adrenochrome. These investigators further reported that aminochromes were found in the urine of 14 of 19 patients diagnosed as having schizophrenia. Of 20 control subjects, two had aminochromes present. Diet was ruled out as a factor, although it has been shown by many investigators that dietary factors can be critical when examining urine for the presence or absence of specific substances, particularly indoles, catecholamines, and their metabolites. For example, foods such as bananas and coffee contain large amounts of serotonin, norepinephrine, etc., which may confound analytical procedures (Waalkes et al., 1958; Mann and LaBrosse, 1959). This work remains unsubstantiated.

A more recent addition to the neurotoxin theories is the isolation of 3,4-dimethoxyphenethylamine (DMPEA, see Fig. 3 and p. 254, Section A,4) from the urine of schizophrenics by Friedhoff and Van Winkle (1962a,b, 1963a,b). This substance could be formed from dopamine (Fig. 3) by two successive O-methylations. The most prominent pathway for the degradation of dopamine involves one O-methylation to 3-methoxytyramine and then oxidation to homovanillic acid.

The work of Friedhoff and Van Winkle has been confirmed by Sen and McGeer (1964) (who also reported the isolation of 4-methoxyphenethylamine —a substance not yet found in normal urine) and by Kuehl et al. (1964), and Horwitt (1965), as cited and confirmed by Bourdillon et al. (1965). Friedhoff and Van Winkle did not find 3,4-dimethoxyphenethylamine in normal urine, but Takesada *et al.* (1963) found this amine in 92% of a group of schizophrenics and in about 40% of a normal control group. Perry *et al.* (1964) could not find DMPEA in either normal or schizophrenic urine and Nishimura and Gjessing (1965) and Faurbye and Pind (1964) also could not confirm the findings of Friedhoff and Van Winkle. Bourdillon *et al.* (1965), in an extensive, well-controlled study, found DMPEA ("pink spot") in the urine of a high percentage of schizophrenics of the Schneider-positive type (Schneider, 1957), but this factor was extremely rare in nonpsychotic controls, unless they were close relatives of psychotic patients (cf. Clarke, 1964). Howorth (1966) cautioned that phenothiazine administration may lead to erroneous identification of the "pink spot."

Friedhoff (1963b) subsequently provided additional evidence for the *in vivo* methylation of both hydroxyl groups of dopamine in schizophrenics by his finding that upon administering tritium-labeled dopamine to these patients, incorporation of the tritium label into their urinary 3,4-dimethoxyphenylacetic acid (oxidative degradation product of DMPEA) was observed. Furthermore, he found that liver tissue from schizophrenic, but to date not from normal, subjects has an enzyme system capable of methylating both hydroxyl groups of dopamine (Friedhoff and Van Winkle, 1964, 1965). It has been found that S-adenosylmethionine is the methyl donor for the O-methylation discussed above and incubation of C^{14}-labeled S-adenosylmethionine with liver biopsy material and tritium-labeled dopamine gave mono- and di-O-methylated phenethylamines.

Of particular interest with regard to this theory are the findings of Pollin *et al.* (1961), Brune and Himwich (1962a,b, 1963), and Park *et al.* (1965) that two precursors of methyl donors, methionine and betaine, administered to schizophrenic patients produced acute exacerbation of their illness, particularly when these patients had been pretreated with a monoamine oxidase inhibitor (Giarman and Freedman, 1965). These findings suggest the possibility that schizophrenics may have defective transmethylations, a theory thought to be further supported by the fact that methylated derivatives of two other amines, serotonin and tryptamine, are potent hallucinogens (see p. 269). Furthermore, it has been reported that methyl acceptors, niacin diphosphopyridine nucleotide (DPN), and nicotinamide, may be beneficial in treating acute schizophrenics (Hoffer, 1957; Osmund and Hoffer, 1962). However, a recent double-blind study (Kline *et al.*, 1966) showed no difference in improvement rates between DPN and placebo in the treatment of chronic schizophrenics.

Little has been reported as yet about the pharmacological effects of DMPEA in man, although it (and 4-methoxyphenethylamine) have been reported to produce catatonic effects in animals resembling those of mescaline (Ernst, 1962; Michaux and Verly, 1963; cf. Noteboom, 1934). The general pharmacology of DMPEA has been reviewed by Brown *et al.* (1965). A further similarity in the effects of 3,4-dimethoxyphenethylamine and mescaline is found in the work of Takeo and Himwich (1965) who found that EEG arousal in transected rabbit brain took place at the medullary level with these two substances, while adrenalin arousal took place at the midbrain level.

Although preliminary evidence suggests that DMPEA is formed endogenously rather than originating from dietary sources, this must be further explored, particularly since Nishimura and Gjessing (1965) and Perry et al. (1964) were unable to find the compound in the urine of patients on plant-free diets. Even if DMPEA is enzymatically formed in schizophrenics, it will remain to be shown that sufficient amounts of it could be synthesized to have a causal relationship to the disease, unless its synthesis and action are highly localized phenomena in the brain. Another abnormal catecholamine metabolite was reported by Perry (1963) who found that three of eighteen psychotic children excreted N-methylmetanephrine (**XIIIa**) (Fig. 2).

c. *Faulty Adrenergic Nerve Transmission.* Norepinephrine has been found to be the neurotransmitter agent released from adrenergic nerve terminals in the peripheral sympathetic nervous system, while norepinephrine as well as dopamine have been purported to play a similar role in the central nervous system. Interfering with the function of released norepinephrine by abnormal derivatives, as proposed in the various neurotoxin theories, is, therefore, an attractive hypothesis (Costa *et al.*, 1961; Decsi, 1965; Monnier, 1960; Rothballer, 1956).

However, one must consider the adrenergic nerve, particularly the nerve ending, as a very complex, highly integrated biophysical unit, the function of which can be impaired in many ways. But first, let us consider how this unit is believed to function. (For a review of this subject the reader's attention is directed to the Proceedings of the Second Symposium on Catecholamines, published in the first 1966 issue of Pharmacological Reviews.)

Costa and Brodie (1964) have described the sympathetic nerve ending as a "neurochemical transducer" where the input into the nerve ending (electrical energy of the nerve impulse) is changed to an output in the form of a quantity of free neurohumoral transmitter. The latter crosses the synaptic junction and acts as the input of another transducer system (i.e., a target organ in the peripheral nervous system or another neuron in the brain).

Recent research has suggested that norepinephrine is stored in the brain, as well as in peripheral tissue in granules or vesicles concentrated at the nerve endings (Grillo, 1966; Stjärne, 1966; Maynert, 1966; von Euler, 1966; Kopin, 1966; and Chang *et al.*, 1964) in which is contained the enzyme for converting dopamine to norepinephrine (dopa-β-oxidase; see Fig. 1). This norepinephrine appears to exist in essentially two functionally different metabolic pools which are in dynamic equilibrium (reviewed by Schildkraut, 1965; Bunney and Davis, 1965; Wurtman, 1965; and Kopin, 1964).

The smaller of these pools contains norepinephrine which is loosely bound and readily released by nerve stimulation and by indirectly acting sympathomimetic amines like tyramine or amphetamine (see Daly *et al.*, 1966

Creveling *et al.*, 1966). This norepinephrine, released from the storage granules to receptor sites, is inactivated by reuptake into the axon or granules in the nerve ending, or by the action of the enzyme catechol-*O*-methyl transferase, forming normetanephrine (Fig. 2, XII).

The larger of these pools contains norepinephrine in a more firmly bound form, from which it can be released by reserpine, guanethidine, and α-methyl dopa. This pool is thought to act much like a storage reservoir. Norepinephrine released from this reservoir spontaneously or by reserpine-like drugs is inactivated mainly by mitochondrial monoamine oxidase, intraneuronally, to give primarily 3,4-dihydroxymandelic acid (XV) which may undergo *O*-methylation in the circulation to give 3-methoxy-4-hydroxymandelic acid (VMA) (XIX).

Thus, since all of the processes of synthesis, storage, release, and metabolism of catecholamines operate as an integrated unit, adrenergic nerve transmission conceivably could be impaired by a defect in any one of the following mechanisms (which may result in too much or too little functionally active norepinephrine at the receptor site): (1) formation of the catecholamine synthesis enzymes and storage granules and their transport down the nerve axon to the nerve terminal where they are concentrated, (2) synthesis of norepinephrine (or dopamine), (3) binding and storage of the catecholamine in the granules, (4) control of the size of the catecholamine store by monoamine oxidase, (5) release of the catecholamine at the synapse in response to the nerve impulse, (6) response of the receptor site to the released norepinephrine, (7) recapture or reuptake (pump mechanism) to get the released norepinephrine back into the granules, (8) action of catechol-*O*-methyl transferase in inactivating that norepinephrine not recaptured into the nerve ending.

As a matter of act, most drugs which have been found to affect the function of the sympathetic nervous system, many of which also influence mood and behavior, have been found to interfere with at least one of these processes (based primarily on what is known about peripheral sympathetic nerve endings). A few of these may be cited as follows (Costa and Brodie, 1964):

(1) By mimicking norepinephrine directly (i.e., phenylephrine)
(2) By mimicking norepinephrine indirectly by releasing it (i.e., amphetamine)
(3) By blocking its action (i.e., phenoxybenzamine)
(4) By blocking its metabolism (i.e., monoamine oxidase inhibitors)
(5) By blocking its synthesis or uptake of its precursors (inhibitors of dopa decarboxylase, tyrosine-hydroxylase, or dopamine-β-oxidase)
(6) By blocking its binding or storage mechanism (i.e., reserpine)
(7) By blocking its release by nerve impulses (i.e., bretylium)
(8) By persistent stimulation of the processes through which nerve impulses release it (i.e., guanethidine)

(9) By acting as a "false transmitter"—a substance which appears to displace norepinephrine from its binding sites but is not an effective neurotransmitter agent [i.e., octopamine (VII, Fig. 1) (Gillespie, 1966; Kirschner, 1966; Gitlow, 1966)].

The role of catecholamines in the periphery, including their release into the circulation (from the adrenals and other peripheral catecholamine-containing tissues) in various conditions of stress is now fairly well defined and has been thoroughly reviewed by Kety (1966). Their role in the central nervous system in mediating mood and behavior is still uncertain. However, a better understanding of adrenergic nerve function and of the mechanisms of action of many classes of drugs which interfere with this function has led to some interesting speculation regarding the role of catecholamines, particularly norepinephrine, in various affective states. Thus, Rosenblatt (1960), Pare and Sandler (1959) and Schildkraut (1965) have suggested that some, if not all depressive illnesses might be associated with an absolute or relative decrease in norepinephrine available at central adrenergic receptor sites. [Conversely, Nickerson (1966) has suggested that elation may be associated with an excess of these amines.] The evidence for involvement of norepinephrine in the etiology of depressive illnesses has been the subject of three excellent reviews (Schildkraut, 1965; Bunney and Davis, 1965; and Kety, 1966). Some of the primary evidence cited in these reviews is listed briefly as follows:

(1) Drugs which elevate brain levels of norepinephrine (presumably by increasing the level of free amine at receptor sites), e.g., monoamine oxidase inhibitors such as iproniazid, are effective in the treatment of certain depressive illnesses.

(2) Drugs which deplete brain levels of norepinephrine by interfering with the binding mechanism, e.g., reserpine, tetrabenazine, and α-methyl dopa, have been found to produce a severe depression of mood, not unlike the symptoms of endogenous depression, in patients treated with these agents. Furthermore, dopa (precursor to norepinephrine) has been found to reverse reserpine-induced sedation in man. In animals, antidepressant drugs such as monoamine oxidase inhibitors and imipramine prevent reserpine-induced sedation.

(3) A drug which inhibits the synthesis of norepinephrine by inhibiting tyrosine hydroxylase, α-methyl tyrosine, produces sedation.

4. Amphetamine, which is a psychic stimulant and mood elevator, does not increase brain levels of norepinephrine but is believed to act by releasing this amine from nerve endings and at the same time blocking its inactivation by reuptake.

5. Imipramine, demethylimipramine, and other clinically effective antidepressant drugs in man do not appear to alter absolute levels of norepinephrine or to inhibit either monamine oxidase or catechol-O-methyl transferase. However these agents have been found to: (a) potentiate many of the peri-

pheral effects of norepinephrine and amphetamine in animals and man, (b) potentiate the effects of adrenergic nerve stimulation, and (c) prevent the effects of reserpine in animals (unless the stores of norepinephrine have been previously depleted by a specific norepinephrine releaser, α-methyl m-tyrosine), perhaps by blocking the inactivation of norepinephrine by reuptake, thus increasing the level of free neurotransmitter at the adrenergic receptor site peripherally and centrally.

6. VMA (XIX, Fig. 2) excretion appears to be decreased and normetanephrine excretion increased in depressed patients during treatment with MAO inhibitors and with imipramine. This suggests that both of these types of drugs (by different mechanisms) may increase the functional level of norepinephrine at the receptor sites, since increased urinary normetanephrine appears to be a reflection of increased adrenergic nerve function and decreased urinary VMA suggests less intracellular deamination of norepinephrine, thus allowing more to be available at the receptor site.

While all of this evidence is merely suggestive and not conclusive, it does illustrate that interference with adrenergic nerve function by any one of a variety of mechanisms may play some role in the etiology of at least one type of mental disease, namely depressive illness (see also p. 268). It is conceivable, therefore, that altered nerve transmission may have etiologic significance in other mental diseases as well, and that this impaired transmission may not necessarily result from an abnormal catecholamine metabolite, although of course this possibility has not been completely ruled out.

2. Serotonin, Tryptamine, and Related Indoles

The serotonin hypothesis as related to normal brain function and mental illness was introduced on p. 600 of Volume I and will not be discussed in detail here. There has been a great deal of speculation that serotonin (5-hydroxytryptamine), a proposed neurotransmitter, might be involved in mental disease. These speculations have been in three directions. The first suggests that serotonin levels in the brain may be excessive in schizophrenia, and that certain tranquilizers, such as the phenothiazines, antagonize serotonin, or others, such as reserpine, decrease its level in the brain. Conversely, it has been suggested that in depressive illnesses serotonin may be present in inadequate amounts, since antidepressants of the monoamine oxidase inhibitor class increase the absolute brain levels of this amine.

A second theory, suggested by Woolley and Shaw (1954), proposes that too little brain serotonin may be involved in schizophrenic psychoses, since LSD, a potent serotonin antagonist on peripheral smooth muscle tissue, has psychotomimetic effects (although there has been no correlation between the activity of agents as peripheral serotonin antagonists and as psychotomimetic agents).

A third serotonin hypothesis suggests that an abnormal metabolite of serotonin may play a role in mental illness.

Experimental evidence in animals supporting both an excess and a deficiency of brain serotonin in various behavioral conditions has accumulated through the years without any clear cut solution or definition of the role of this amine in the brain. Nevertheless, as Page (1958) has pointed out, there is no proof of serotonin control of normal mental processes, but there is a body of evidence which indicates that tampering with the brain levels or the action of serotonin can result in behavioral changes in man and laboratory animals. Unfortunately, the drugs used as tools in studying brain serotonin (e.g., reserpine which depletes brain levels and monoamine oxidase inhibitors which increase the levels) also influence the levels of brain catecholamines (norepinephrine and dopamine) and perhaps other amines as well. No drug has yet been found which will selectively deplete brain serotonin; however, Brodie (1960) has suggested that reserpine sedation may be due to the release of brain serotonin from its binding sites, resulting in the persistence of small amounts of "free" serotonin acting at receptor sites. [For discussions of some of the experimental interrelationships of LSD and serotonin and other aspects of the serotonin theories see Cerletti and Rothlin (1955), Schneckloth et al. (1956), Giarman and Freedman (1965), Gaddum (1957), Gallant et al. (1963), Freedman (1963), Woolley et al. (1957), Woolley and Van Der Hoeven (1963), Inouye et al. (1962), and Potter and Axelrod (1962).]

Since the role of serotonin as a neurotransmitter in the peripheral nervous system, as well as in the brain, is still unclear, speculation on the consequences of interfering with its normal function is necessarily more limited than in the case of norepinephrine. Thus, aside from such vague suggestions as excessive or inadequate amounts of this amine in the brains of psychotic patients, most of the theories have been directed to the possibility of abnormal metabolites. Before reviewing these, however, it might be well to review what is known regarding serotonin (and tryptophan) metabolism and the attempts which have been made to measure the excretion of normal metabolites of these agents in psychotic patients.

a. *Tryptophan, Serotonin, and Tryptamine Metabolism.* The metabolism of tryptophan, showing the biosynthesis and degradation of serotonin and tryptamine, are shown in Fig. 4 (major pathways are along double lines).

The transformation of tryptophan (XXIX) to 5-hydroxytryptophan is accomplished by tryptophan hydroxylase. The transformations of tryptophan (XXIX) to tryptamine (XXX) and 5-hydroxytryptophan (XXXI) to 5-hydroxytryptamine (XXXII) are carried out by decarboxylases. The transformation of serotonin (XXXII) to melatonin (XXXIII), 5-hydroxyindoleacetic acid (XXXIV) to 5-methoxyindole acetic acid (XXXVI), and 5-hydroxy-N-acetyltryptamine (XXXV) to 5-methoxy-N-acetyltryptamine (XXXVII) are carried out by O-methyl transferase. The conversion of

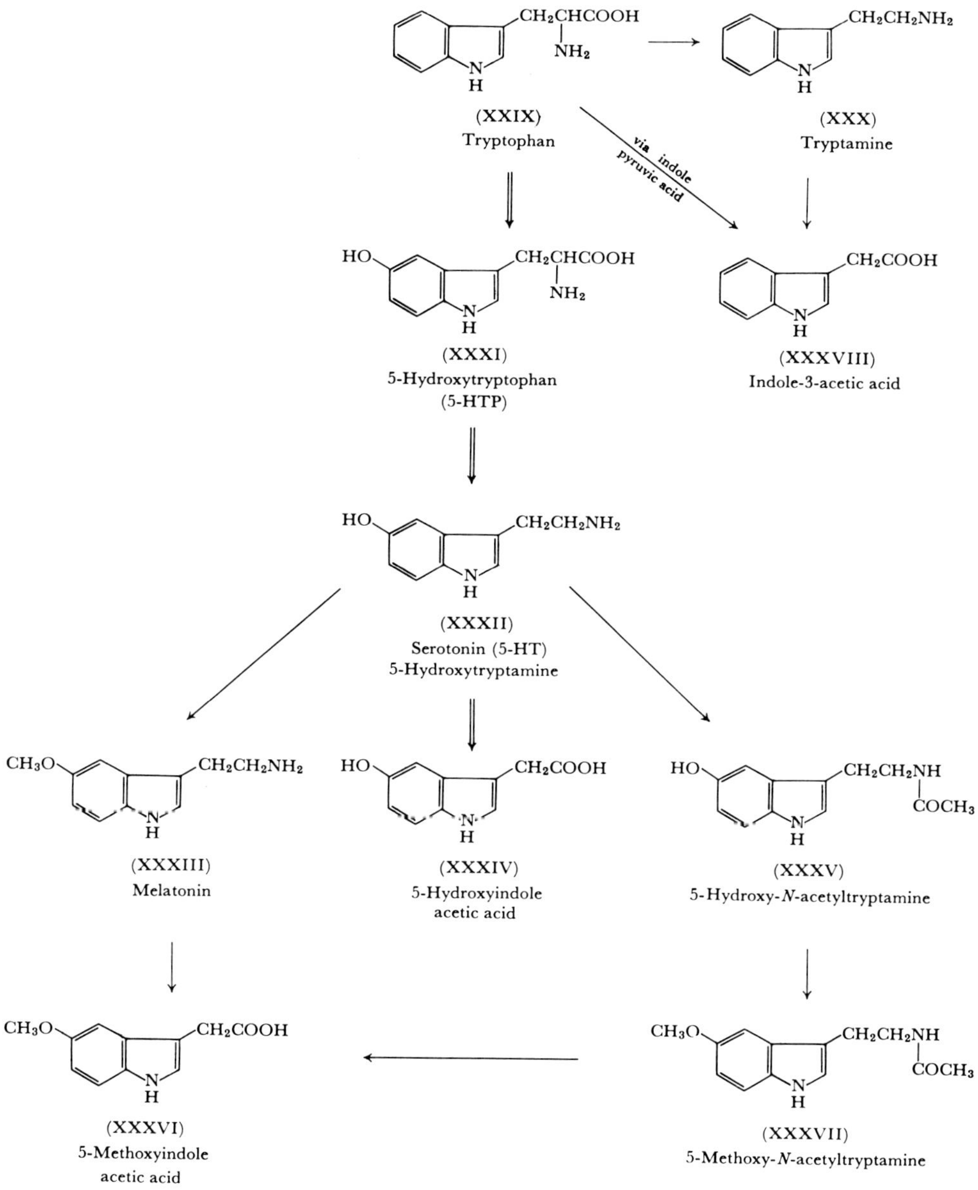

FIG. 4. Metabolism of tryptophan, serotonin, and tryptamine.

serotonin (XXXII) to 5-hydroxyindoleacetic acid (XXXIV), tryptamine (XXX) to indole-3-acetic acid (XXXVIII), and melatonin (XXXIII) to 5-methoxyindole acetic acid (XXXVI) is accomplished by monoamine oxidase.

With regard to the excretion of normal serotonin or tryptophan metabolites in psychotic patients, numerous investigators have studied the major metabolite of serotonin, 5-hydroxyindole acetic acid (5-HIAA, Fig. 4, XXXIV), in schizophrenics in comparison with normal individuals. However, contradictory results have been reported ranging from abnormally low values to abnormally high levels in schizophrenics, most workers having reported values in the normal range with perhaps greater variability (see Buscaino and Stefanachi 1958; Feldstein *et al.*, 1958). Kopin (1959) found no significant differences in the rate of 5-HIAA excretion in schizophrenics versus normal subjects before or after administration of tryptophan, in contrast to the work of Zeller (1957) (cf. Schanberg, 1963). Recently Yuwiler (1965) added further confirmation to the reports that schizophrenics and nonschizophrenics do not differ in 5-HIAA excretion. In this study they did not differ in variability of excretion either.

Brune and Himwich (1960, 1963) determined the urinary excretion of tryptamine (see Fig. 4) and its major metabolite, indole-3-acetic acid, in three groups of patients: mental defectives, schizophrenics, and two boys with phenylpyruvic oligophrenia. When the patients did not show any overt psychotic symptoms, all values for tryptamine and indole-3-acetic acid were in the normal range. In those patients who experienced activation of agitated psychotic behavior, an elevation in the excretion of both substances was found before and during the behavioral aberrations. The same group (Bertlet *et al.*, 1965) suggested, on the basis of their work on indole and catecholamine excretion, that symptoms such as increased motor activity or restlessness, anxiety and tension appear to be associated with increased urinary levels of catecholamines, while psychotic symptoms such as intensification of hallucinatory and delusional experiences and hostile, aggressive, and combative behavior appear to be associated with increased urinary indole (primarily tryptamine and indole-3-acetic acid) excretion. The working hypothesis suggested by this group relating indoles to psychotic symptomatology will be presented below under abnormal tryptophan metabolites (p. 269).

Coppen *et al.* (1965) also investigated tryptamine excretion in depressed patients and found that urinary excretion of this amine was abnormally low during the period when they were severely depressed (compared with that of normal subjects and with themselves after recovery). After recovery the values rose by an average of 70% to approximately normal levels. This change apparently did not result from dietary factors (which were carefully controlled) nor from differences in concentration of plasma tryptophan, or urinary pH, or volume. Indole-3-acetic acid excretion, on the other hand, showed no significant alterations from normal values throughout. The investigators were unable to demonstrate any CNS effects, however, after intravenous administration of tryptamine to depressed patients receiving a monoamine oxidase inhibitor. Confirmation and further investigation of these findings would appear to be warranted.

(b) *Abnormal Metabolites of Tryptophan, Serotonin and Tryptamine.* It has been found that N-methylation of serotonin and tryptamine can take place in the presence of the methyl donor, S-adenosylmethionine. This methylating enzyme may be responsible for the methylation of these indoles to produce psychotomimetic substances like N,N-dimethylserotonin (bufotenine) and N,N-dimethyltryptamine. Axelrod's demonstration (1961) that mammalian

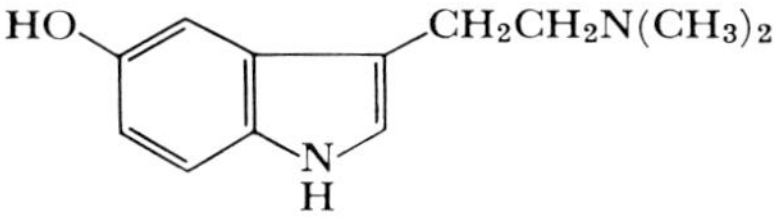

N,N-Dimethylserotonin (bufotenine) 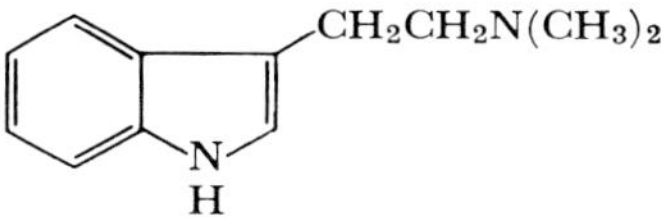 N,N-Dimethyltryptamine

tissue is capable of N-methylating tryptamine and derivatives to such potent hallucinogens (Szara, 1961) is of added interest in view of the previously discussed (p. 261) effect of methionine (precursor to S-adenosylmethionine) when given to schizophrenics. It is perhaps additional suggestive evidence for a defect in transmethylating enzymes in schizophrenics. Of course, in evaluating the possibility of whether these methylated metabolites may have any etiologic significance in diseases like schizophrenia, it is essential to consider the rates of formation of these metabolites, their concentration in tissues, and whether they are formed in brain and in liver, or in liver only.

There has been much controversy as to whether or not bufotenine is excreted in normal individuals or in the urine of schizophrenics (see Bumpus and Page, 1955; Fischer *et al.*, 1961; Perry, 1963; Brune and Himwich, 1963). Recently, however, Siegel (1965) reported development of an improved, sensitive (< 1 μgm per l. of urine) method for detection of bufotenine. Using this method he could not find any bufotenine in the urine of five normal individuals or of twenty-one schizophrenics. [Additional early work in the area has been reported by Rodnight (1956), McIsaac (1961a,b), and Märki and Witkop (1963).]

Bertlet *et al.* (1964) presented a hypothesis involving abnormal tryptophan metabolites which may be presented briefly as follows: An initiating cause of unknown origin precipitates psychotic behavior which is accompanied by a loss of appetite. As a consequence of the latter, methionine and tryptophan (among other amino acids) are released (perhaps from muscle protein since creatinine excretion is increased concomitantly) to compensate for the decreased food intake and may act together to intensify the behavioral disturbance—the methionine acting as a source of methyl groups in the formation of methylated indole derivatives of tryptophan with psychotogenic properties (e.g., N,N-dimethyltryptamine). In this connection, however, it should be noted that Sprince *et al.* (1963) were unable to detect any methylated derivatives of tryptamine or serotonin in the urine of four schizophrenic and two psychoneurotic patients treated with placebo, an MAO inhibitor, and/or methionine or tryptophan. The combination of the monamine oxidase inhibitor and methionine, however, consistently resulted in increased tryptamine and indoleacetamide excretion (greater than with either agent alone) in both groups. These findings were related to the onset of mental aberrations and confirmation of these findings would appear warranted.

Other miscellaneous reports of abnormal indoles in schizophrenic patients include that of Sprince *et al.* (1960) who published a procedure for the differential extraction of indolic compounds from the urine of schizophrenics. On chromatography a substance tentatively identified as 6-hydroxyskatole was reported. This substance occurred more frequently and with greater intensity in overnight urine pools of male schizophrenics than in normal subjects. Krall *et al.* (1963) also made a chromatographic study of the urinary levels of 6-hydroxyskatole and indole-3-acetamide from a group of 72 schizophrenics, 101 manic depressives, and 55 other psychotic subjects, and a comparison was made with a group of 76 normal controls. In contrast with earlier findings, neither compound was significantly different in level in the urine from psychotics compared with the urine from normal subjects.

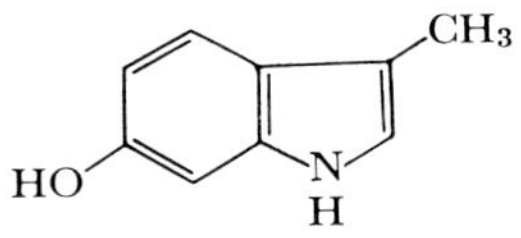

6-Hydroxyskatole

Also, McIsaac (1961a,b) reported that presumed carboline metabolites of melatonin (Fig. 4, XXXIII) produced behavioral and serotonin antagonist effects in animals. Other possible psychotomimetic metabolites of tryptamine that have been reported include 6-methoxytryptamines (Szara, 1964) and 10-methoxyharmalan (McIsaac, 1961a,b).

It may be concluded that while there has been an abundance of indole theories of mental illness (and many suggested abnormal indole metabolites), some of these have been refuted and the remainder may be considered no more than working hypotheses at the present time.

3. Other Agents

Cerebral levels of γ-aminobutyric acid (GABA) (Elliott and Jasper, 1959; Roberts *et al.*, 1960), glutamine, glutamic acid, etc. are importantly related to metabolic activity (energy metabolism) in the brain. It is thought that the GABA-glutamic acid pathway provides a shunt to the Krebs cycle (reviewed by Tower, 1959; Elliott, 1959). The metabolism of glutamic acid and the relationship between GABA and the Krebs cycle is shown in Fig. 5 (Elliott, 1959; Fishbein and Bessman, 1963). GABA also has been found

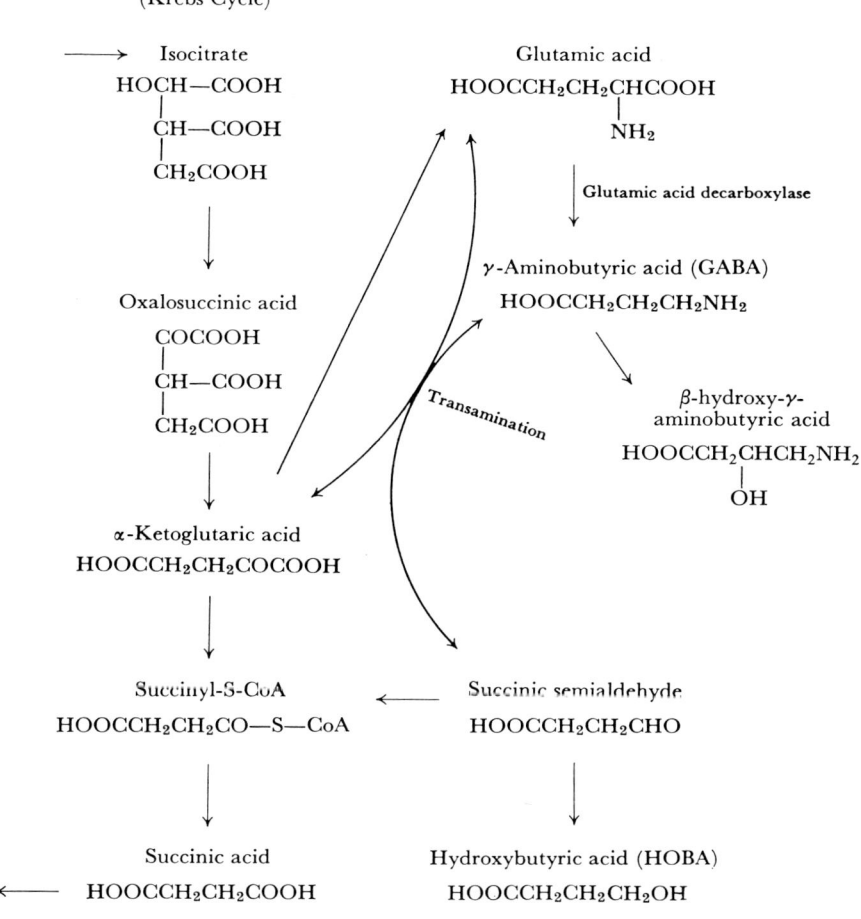

FIG. 5. Metabolism of glutamic acid.
(HOBA has been employed as a local anesthetic, and this application may be relevant to the role played by GABA in brain metabolism.)

to exert a depressant effect on mammalian neurons, which has led to the suggestion that this substance may be a neurotransmitter agent of inhibitory neuronal pathways. The question of whether or not GABA is a synaptic neurotransmitter agent or simply influences nerve function by playing a role in energy metabolism can not be answered at present (see review by Curtis and Watkins, 1965).

The psychotomimetic effects of some atropine-like compounds has been reported (see Volume I, p. 579), and this has led to the suggestion (reviewed by Giarman and Freedman, 1965) that acetylcholine plays a role in central nervous system transmission, as it does in the peripheral nervous system.

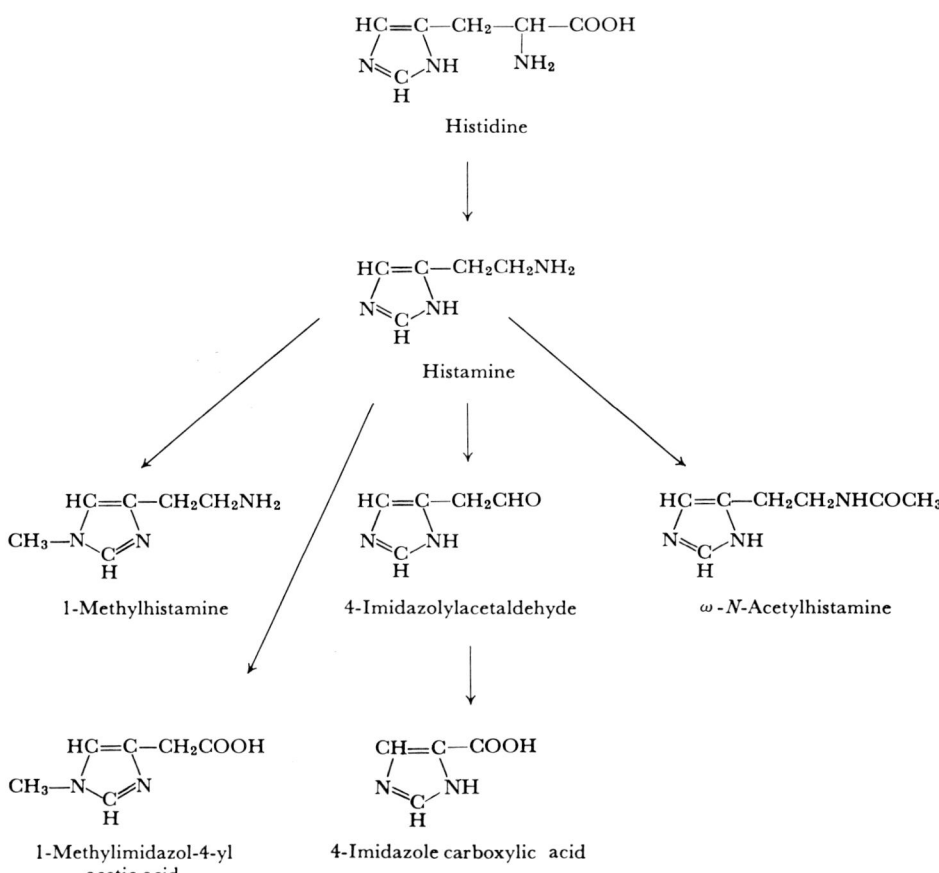

FIG. 6. Metabolism of histamine.

However, with the recent interest and emphasis in amines such as catecholamines and serotonin in the brain, research on acetylcholine has been somewhat neglected and its role in the central nervous system has remained largely undefined.

The discovery of large amounts of histamine in the brain has led to the suggestion that it too may function as a neurotransmitter agent, particularly since it appears to be bound in particles which sediment with synaptic vesicles

(Carlini and Green, 1963) as is true of norepinephrine. However, as in the case of many other proposed neurotransmitter agents, the role of histamine in the brain remains obscure despite many studies (Green, 1964; White, 1964; see review by Kahlson and Rosengren, 1965). The metabolism of histamine is shown in Fig. 6.

C. Faulty Energy Metabolism

Considerable evidence has been reported which suggests that some psychotic patients have abnormalities in their energy metabolism (see Ahlquist, 1966, and Lundholm *et al.*, 1966, for reviews). Obviously, hormonal effects must play some role in these abnormalities. Victor *et al.* (1957) reported that patients with Wernicke's encephalopathy, associated with alcoholism, showed a marked disturbance of carbohydrate intermediary metabolism. The pyruvic and alpha-ketoglutaric acids were most regularly affected. Altschule *et al.* (1957a,b) reported that patients with chronic Korsakoff's psychosis, and patients with paranoid hallucinatory syndrome due to chronic alcoholism, show abnormalities in carbohydrate metabolism after ingestion of glucose. These abnormalities were indistinguishable from those seen in patients with schizophrenic, manic depressive, and involutional psychoses, and in nonpsychotic patients with multiple sclerosis.

On the other hand, several workers have not found any abnormal rate of cerebral circulation, oxygen consumption, or cerebral glucose consumption in schizophrenia (Kety *et al.*, 1948; Wilson *et al.*, 1952; Sokoloff *et al.*, 1957). Richter (1957) has also failed to confirm a decrease in basal metabolism in schizophrenics (cf. Altschule, 1957, 1961; Altschule *et al.*, 1952a,b,c,d, 1953).

Kety (1965a) has reviewed the suggestion of greater than normal antiinsulin or hyperglycemic activity in the blood or urine of schizophrenics, of aberrant phosphate metabolism, and of the reported beneficial effects of glutathione in schizophrenia (Altschule *et al.*, 1951, 1954; Frohman *et al.*, 1960a; Altschule and Giancola, 1960; Eldred *et al.*, 1960). Kety aptly concluded, "It is difficult for some to believe that a generalized defect in energy metabolism—a process so fundamental to every cell in the body—could be responsible for the highly specialized features of schizophrenia. On the other hand, a moderate lack of oxygen, an essential requirement of practically every tissue, produces highly selective manifestations involving especially the higher mental functions and as suggestive of schizophrenia as manifestations produced by many of the more popular hallucinogens. It may not, therefore, be completely appropriate that, in a search for biochemical factors etiologically related to schizophrenic psychoses, the center of interest today appears to have shifted to other, more specialized aspects of metabolism."

D. Genetically Linked Defects

Genetic studies in recent years have provided provocative evidence suggesting that certain mental illnesses (e.g., schizophrenia, manic depressive psychoses), or at least the predisposition to these illnesses, may be inherited. Such studies have given added impetus to the search for specific, inherited biochemical lesions. The most compelling data have come from the study of twins, both monozygotic and dizygotic. In a few cases twins have been separated at birth and thus presumably subjected to different environments. Kety (1965a) and Essen-Möller (1965) have recently reviewed and evaluated the techniques which have been utilized in twin studies and the resulting data. To date it would appear that genetic influences may have important etiologic significance, but one cannot completely rule out the operation of environmental factors.

It should also be pointed out that mental retardation may result from any one of a number of genetically linked biochemical defects. Although these defects usually bear little or no relationship to the mental disorders discussed in this chapter, they will be listed briefly below. This subject has been reviewed by Stanbury *et al.* (1960), by Sourkes (1962), by Penrose (1963) and by Quastel and Scholefield (1958).

1. Phenylketonuria

It has been suggested that the mental retardation seen in children with phenylketonuria results from intoxication by unmetabolized phenylalanine, and thus this condition could be avoided by feeding a diet low in this amino acid (Pare *et al.*, 1957; Spencer, 1963; Lyman, 1963).

2. Cretinism

This condition is usually due to a congenital absence of thyroid hormone. Supplementation with the hormone, if started early enough, usually leads to normal development.

3. Leucinosis or Maple Syrup Urine Disease

Leucine, isoleucine, and valine are normally metabolized first to the corresponding alpha-keto acid and then, by oxidative decarboxylation, to the fatty acid with one less carbon. In the above disease, the decarboxylating enzyme is absent and hence alpha-keto acids accumulate. These are partially reconverted to amino acids which can result in cerebral degeneration and early death. Treatment with a diet low in leucine, isoleucine, and valine is effective.

4. Galactosemia

The enzyme responsible for metabolizing galactose is absent in some infants and the accumulation of this sugar can lead to mental and physical degeneration. Treatment with a galactose-free diet from birth is usually effective in preventing mental or physical damage (Harris, 1962).

5. Hartnup's Disease (Congenital Pellagra)

In this disease there is thought to be a defect in the jejunal and renal transport of tryptophan, resulting in a mental deficiency.

6. Cystathionuria

Mental defects can also result from deficiencies in cystathione metabolism.

7. Neurolipoidosis

This disease manifests itself in a variety of forms. Thus, in Gaucher's disease there is a degeneration of nerve cells with an accumulation of lipids thought to be galacto and glucocerebrosides (Klenk, 1940, 1955; Ottenstein et al., 1948). In the Niemann-Pick disease the lipids stored in nerve and other cells are sphingomyelins, but the acid components of the sphingomyelins differ in the different tissues. This disease generally occurs in infancy with survival rarely going beyond 2 years.

8. Infantile Aumorotic Familial Idiocy

In this disease, controlled by a single recessive gene, only the brain is involved. There is an excess of gangliosides related to sphingomyelins and cerebrosides (Slone, 1933; Klenk, 1940, 1955). Pfaundler–Hurler's disease (gargoylism) may be regarded as a special form of aumorotic idiocy in which skeletal development is also impaired.

9. Wilson's Disease (Hepatolenticular Degeneration)

This disease, which involves a disturbance in copper metabolism, is a cause of certain mental defects (Ravin, 1956).

10. Idiopathic Hypercalcemia of Infancy with Mental Defect

This disease is thought to be due to disturbances of cholesterol metabolism which lead to excess calcification (Forfar et al., 1956).

E. Nutritional Disorders

1. Pellagra

In the 1930's it was discovered that the mental disorders that accompanied pellagra were due to a nicotinic acid deficiency, and that this disorder was alleviated by the administration of the missing vitamin (Lehman, 1952).

The loss of memory, lassitude, mental retardation, and depression or delusions that are characteristic of pellagra may easily be confused with mental disease, particularly since these symptoms may precede the appearance of other signs such as dermatitis and diarrhea by many weeks (cf. Sourkes, 1962).

It is of interest that nicotinic acid has been claimed, in some cases, to cause improvement in mental states not definitely related to pellagra.

2. Beri-Beri

Prolonged deprivation of thiamine can lead to central and peripheral neuropathy as a result of interruption of the Krebs cycle in the central nervous system (Himwich, 1951). Alcoholic polyneuritis is a deficiency disease, as is the polyneuritis of pregnancy and of certain gastrointestinal disorders in which vitamins and other nutrients are poorly absorbed.

3. Lathyrism

This is a crippling neurological disturbance which occurs in various Asian countries, presumably because of dietary peculiarities.

4. Methionine Sulfoximine

Epileptiform symptoms can be invoked by feeding flour treated with nitrogen trichloride. The offending agent is thought to be methionine sulfoximine, which interferes with glutamine synthesis (Braganca *et al.*, 1953).

5. Riboflavin

Deficiencies of this vitamin have led to depression, apathy and lethargy, but acute behavioral disturbances usually are not observed.

F. Conclusion

We are reminded by Kety (1965a) of the concept so well expressed by Thudicum in 1884.

> Many forms of insanity are unquestionably the external manifestations of the effects upon the brain substance of poisons fermented within the body, just as mental abberations accompanying chronic alcoholic intoxication are the accumulated effects of a relatively simple poison fermented out of the body. These poisons we shall, I have no doubt, be able to isolate after we know the normal chemistry to its uttermost detail. And then will come in their turn the crowning discoveries to which our efforts must ultimately be directed, namely, the discoveries of the antidotes to the poisons and to the fermenting causes and processes which produce them.

Perhaps by 1984 the nature of these brain "poisons," if such exist, will have been elucidated and a more positive chapter will have been written.

REFERENCES

Acheson, G. H. (1966). *Pharmacol. Rev.* **16**, 179.
Ahlquist, R. P. (1966). *J. Pharm. Sci.* **55**, 359.
Akerfeldt, S. (1957). *Science* **125**, 117.
Altschule, M. D. (1957). *New Engl. J. Med.* **257**, 919.
Altschule, M. D. (1961). "Chemical Pathology of the Nervous System," p. 497. Macmillan (Pergamon), New York.
Altschule, M. D., and Giancola, J. N. (1960). *Comprehensive Psychiat.* **1**, 250.
Altschule, M. D., Siegel, E. P., and Mora-Castaneda, F. (1951). *A.M.A. Arch. Neurol. Psychiat.* **65**, 589.
Altschule, M. D., Siegel, E. P., and Henneman, D. H. (1952a). *A.M.A. Arch. Neurol. Psychiat.* **67**, 64.
Altschule, M. D., Parkhurst, B. H., and Siegel, E. P. (1952b). *A.M.A. Arch. Neurol. Psychiat.* **67**, 754.
Altschule, M. D., Restaino, R. M., and Siegel, E. P. (1952c). *A.M.A. Arch. Neurol. Psychiat.* **68**, 561.
Altschule, M. D., Siegel, E. P., Restaino, R. M., and Parkhurst, B. H. (1952d). *A.M.A. Arch. Neurol. Psychiat.* **67**, 228.
Altschule, M. D., Grunebaum, H. U., Parkhurst, B. H., and Siegel, E. P. (1953). *A.M.A. Arch. Neurol. Psychiat.* **70**, 235.
Altschule, M. D., Siegel, E. P., Goncz, R. M., and Murnane, J. P. (1954). *A.M.A. Arch. Neurol. Psychiat.* **71**, 615.
Altschule, M. D., Victor, M., and Holliday, P. D. (1957a). *A.M.A. Arch. Intern. Med.* **99**, 40.
Altschule, M. D., Goncz, R. M., and Holliday, P. D. (1957b). *A.M.A. Arch. Intern. Med.* **99**, 892.
Altschule, M. D., Goncz, R. M., and Holliday, P. D. (1959). *A.M.A. Arch. Intern. Med.* **103**, 726.
Anton, A. H., and Sayre, D. F. (1964). *J. pharmacol. exptl. therap.* **145**, 326.
Axelrod, J. (1959). *Physiol. Rev.* **39**, 751.
Axelrod, J. (1961). *Science* **134**, 343.
Axelrod, J., Kopin, I. J., and Mann, J. S. (1959). *Biochim. Biophys. Acta* **36**, 576.
Barbeau, A., Jasmin, G., and Duchastel, Y. (1963). *Neurology* **13**, 56.
Bergen, J. R. (1965). *Trans. N.Y. Acad. Sci.* **28**, 40.
Bergen, J. R., Pennell, R. B., Freeman, H., and Hoagland, H. (1960). *A.M.A. Arch. Neurol.* **2**, 146.
Bertlet, H. H., Bull, C., Himwich, H. E., Kohl, H., Matsumoto, K., Pscheidt, G. R., Spude, J., Tourlentes, T. T., and Ualverde, J. M. (1964). *Science* **144**, 311.
Bertlet, H. H., Matsumoto, K., Pscheidt, G. R., Spude, J., Bull, C., and Himwich, H. E. (1965). *Arch. Gen. Psychiat.* **13**, 521.
Bickel, M. H., Sulser, F., and Brodie, B. B. (1963). *Life Sci.* **4**, 247.
Bourdillon, R. E., Clarke, C. A., Ridges, A. P., Sheppard, P. M., Harper, P., and Leslie, S. A. (1965). *Nature*, **208**, 453.
Braganca, B. M., Faulkner, P., and Quastel, J. H. (1953). *Biochim. Biophys. Acta* **10**, 83.
Brodie, B. B. (1960). *Diseases Nervous System* **21**, (March Suppl.), 1.
Brodie, B. B., Finger, K. F., Orlans, F. B., Quinn, G. P., and Sulser, F. (1960). *J. Pharmacol. Exptl. Therap.* **129**, 250.
Brown, M. L., Lang, W. J., and Gershon, S. (1965). *Arch. Intern. Pharmacodyn.* **158**, 439.
Brune, G. G., and Himwich, H. E., (1960). Acta Intern. Mtg. "Techniques for Study of Psychotropic Drugs," Bologna, June 26, 27; p. 1.
Brune, G. G., Himwich, H. E. (1962a). *Arch. Gen. Psychiat.* **6**, 324.
Brune, G. G., and Himwich, H. E. (1962b). *J. Nervous Mental Disease* **134**, 447.
Brune, G. G., and Himwich, H. E. (1963). *Recent Advan. Biol. Psychiat.* **5**, 144.

Brune, G. G., Hohl, H. H., and Himwich, H. E. (1963). *J. Neuropsychiat.* **5**, 14.
Bumpus, F. M., and Page, I. H. (1955), *J. Biol. Chem.* **212**, 111.
Buniatian, H. D. (1963). *J. Neurochem.* **10**, 461.
Bunney, W. E., and Davis, J. M. (1965). *Arch. Gen. Psychiat.* **13**, 495.
Buscaino, G. A., and Stefanachi, L. (1958). *A.M.A. Arch. Neurol. Psychiat.* **80**, 78.
Cameron, D. E. (1963). *Am. J. Psychiat.* **120**, 320.
Cardon, P. V., Sokoloff, L., Vates, T., and Kety, S. S. (1961). *Psychiat. Res.* **1**, 37.
Carlini, E. A., and Green, J. P. (1963). *Brit. J. Pharmacol.* **20**, 264.
Cerletti, A., and Rothlin, E. (1955). *Nature,* **176**, 785.
Chamberlain, T. J., Rothschild, G. H., and Gerard, R. W. (1963). *Proc. Natl. Acad. Sci. U.S.* **49**, 918.
Chang, C. C., Costa, E., and Brodie, B. B. (1964). *Life Sciences* **3**, 839.
Clarke, C. A. (1964). *Brit. Med. J.* II, 373.
Coppen, A., Shaw, D. M., Malleson, A., Eccleston, E., and Gundy, G. (1965). *Brit. J. Psychiat.* **111**, 993.
Costa, E., and Brodie, B. B. (1964). *In* "Biogenic Amines" (H. E. Himwich and W. A. Himwich, eds.), p. 168. Elsevier, New York.
Costa, E., Revzin, A. M., Kuntzman, R., Spector, S., and Brodie, B. B. (1961). *Science* **133**, 1822.
Creveling, C. R., Daly, J. W., and Witkop, B. (1966). *J. Med. Chem.* **9**, 284.
Curtis, D. R., and Watkins, J. C. (1965). *Pharmacol. Rev.* **17**, 347.
Daly, J., and Witkop, B. (1963). *Angew. Chem. Intern. Ed. Engl.* **2**, 421.
Daly, J., Inscoe, J. K., and Axelrod, J. (1965). *J. Med. Chem.* **8**, 153.
Daly, J. W., Creveling, C. R., and Witkop, B. (1966). *J. Med. Chem.* **9**, 273, 280.
Decsi, L. (1965). *Progr. Drug Res.* **8**, 54.
Ehringer, H., and Hornykiewicz, O. (1960). *Klin. Wochschr.* **38**, 1236.
Eiduson, S., Geller, E., Yuwiler, A., and Eiduson, B. T. (1964). "Biochemistry and Behavior." Van Nostrand, New York.
Eldred, S. H., Bell, N. W., and Sherman, L. J. (1960). *New Engl. J. Med.* **263**, 1330.
Elliott, K. A. C. (1959). *Proc. Intern. Congr. Biochem.*, 4th Vienna, 1958, **3**, 251.
Elliott, K. A. C., and Jasper, H. H. (1959). *Physiol. Rev.* **9**, 383.
Ernst, A. M. (1962). *Nature* **193**, 178.
Essen-Möller, C. (1965). *Intern. J. Psychiat.* **1**, 466.
Faurbye, A., and Pind, K. (1964). *Acta Psychiat. Scand.* **40**, 240.
Feldstein, A. M. (1959). *J. Psychiat.* **116**, 454.
Feldstein, A., Hoagland, H., and Freeman, H. (1958). *Science* **128**, 358.
Fischer, E., Fernandez Lagravere, T. A., Vazquez, A. J., and DiStefano, A. O. (1961). *J. Nervous Mental Disease* **133**, 441.
Fishbein, W. N., and Bessman, S. P. (1963). *J. Pediat.* **63**, 754.
Forfar, J. O., Balf, C. L., Maxwell, G. M., and Tompsett, S. L. (1956). *Lancet* **1**, 981.
Frank, M. M., and Wurtman, R. J. (1958). *Proc. Soc. Exptl. Biol. Med.* **97**, 478.
Freedman, D. X. (1963). *Am. J. Psychiat.* **119**, 843.
Friedhoff, A. J., and Van Winkle, E. (1962a). *Nature* **194**, 897.
Friedhoff, A. J., and Van Winkle, E. (1962b). *J. Nervous Mental Disease* **135**, 550.
Friedhoff, A. J., and Van Winkle, E. (1963a). *J. Chromatog.* **11**, 272.
Friedhoff, A. J., and Van Winkle, E. (1963b). *Nature* **199**, 1271.
Friedhoff, A. J., and Van Winkle, E. (1964a). *Meeting Am. Psychiat. Assoc., Los Angeles, Calif. 1964.*
Friedhoff, A. J., and Van Winkle, E. (1964). *Psychiat. Res. Rept. Am. Psychiat. Assoc.* **19**, 149.
Friedhoff, A. J., and Van Winkle, E. (1965). *Am. J. Psychiat.* **121**, 1054.
Frohman, C. E., Latham, L. K., Beckett, P. G. S., and Gottlieb, J. S. (1960a). *Arch Gen. Psychiat.* **2**, 255.

Frohman, C. E., Czajkowski, N. P., Luby, E. D., Gottlieb, J. S., and Senf, R. (1960b). *Arch. Gen. Psychiat.* **2**, 263.
Frohman, C. E., Luby, E. D., Tourney, G., Beckett, P. G. S., and Gottlieb, J. S. (1960c). *Am. J. Psychiat.* **117**, 401.
Frohman, C. E., Tourney, G., Beckett, P. G. S., Lees, H., Latham, L. K., and Gottlieb, J. S. (1961). *Arch. Gen. Psychiat.* **4**, 404.
Frohman, C. E., Latham, L. K., Warner, K. A., Brosius, C. O., Beckett, P. G. S., and Gottlieb, J. S. (1963). *Arch. Gen Psychiat.* **9**, 83.
Frohman, C. E., Beckett, P. G. S., and Gottlieb, J. S. (1964). *In* "Recent Advances in Biological Psychiatry" (J. Wortis, ed.), Vol. VII, p. 45. Plenum Press, New York.
Frohman, C. E., Latham, L. K., Warner, K., Beckett, P. G. S., and Gottlieb, J. S. (1966). *Federation Proc.* **25**, 800.
Furchgott, R. F. (1966). *Pharmacol. Rev.* **18**, 641.
Gaddum, J. E. (1957). *Ann. N.Y. Acad. Sci.* **66**, 643.
Gallant, D. M., Bishop, M. P., Steele, C. A., and Noblin, C. D. (1963). *Am. J. Psychiat.* **119**, 882.
German, G. A. (1963). *Brit. J. Psychiat.* **109**, 616.
German, G. A., and Kemali, D. (1963). *Nature* **198**, 791.
Giarman, N. J., and Freedman, D. X. (1965). *Pharmacol. Rev.* **17**, 1.
Gillespie, J. S. (1966). *Pharmacol. Rev.* **18**, 587.
Gitlow, S. E. (1966). *Pharmacol. Rev.* **18**, 707.
Goodall, M., Kirschner, M., and Rosen, L. (1959). *J. Clin. Invest.* **38**, 707.
Goldstein, L., Murphree, H. B., Sugerman, A. A., and Pfeiffer, C. C. (1963). *Clin. Pharmacol. Therap.* **4**, 10.
Goldstein, M., Friedhoff, A. J., and Simmons, C. (1959). *Biochem. Biophys. Acta* **33**, 572.
Green, J. P. (1964). *Federation Proc.* **23**, 1095.
Grillo, M. A. (1966). *Pharmacol. Rev.* **18**, 387.
Grof, S., Vojtechovsky, M., Vitek, V., and Frankova, S. (1961). *Abstr. 3rd World Congr. Psychiat. Montreal, Quebec, 1961*, p. 310. Univ. of Toronto Press, McGill Univ. Press, Canada.
Gross, H., and Frenken, F. (1964). *Biochem. Z.* **340**, 403.
Haddad, R. K., and Rabe, A. (1963). *In* "Serological Fractions in Schizophrenia" (R. G. Heath, ed.), pp. 151–157. Harper and Row, New York.
Haefely, W., and Hürlimann, A. (1962). *Experientia* **18**, 297.
Häkkinen, H. M., and Kulonen, E. (1963). *J. Neurochem.* **10**, 489.
Harris, H. (1962). *In* "Aspects of Psychiatric Research" (D. Richter, J. M. Tanner, L. Taylor, and O. L. Zangwill, eds.), p. 194. Oxford Univ. Press, New York.
Hartung, W. H., Mattocks, A. N., and Ellin, R. I. (1964). *J. Pharm. Sci.* **53**, 550.
Hayaishi, O. (1962). *Ann. Rev. Biochem.* **31**, 25.
Heath, R. G. (1960). "The Etiology of Schizophrenia" (D. D. Jackson, ed.), pp. 146–156. Basic Books, New York.
Heath, R. G. (1961). *J. Neuropsychiat.* **3**, 1.
Heath, R. G., and Leach, B. E. (1958). *Progr. Psychotherapy* **3**, 219.
Heath, R. G., Martens, S., Leach, B. E., Cohen, M., and Angel, C. (1957). *Am. J. Psychiat.* **114**, 1.
Heath, R. G., Martens, S., Leach, B. E., Cohen, M., and Feigley, C. A. (1958). *Am. J. Psychiat.* **114**, 917.
Hess, S. (1960). *Pharmacologist* **2**, 81.
Himwich, H. (1951). "Brain Metabolism and Cerebral Disorders." Williams & Wilkins, Baltimore.
Hoagland, H., Pennell, R. B., Bergen, J. R., Saravis, C. A., Freeman, H., and Koella, W. (1962). *Recent. Advan. Biol. Psychiat.* **4**, 329.

Hoffer, A. (1957). *In* "Hormones, Brain Function, and Behavior" (H. Hoagland, ed.), p. 181. Academic Press, New York.
Hoffer, A., Osmond, H., Calbeck, M. J., and Kahen, I. (1965). *Arch. Neurol. Psychiat.* **77**, 437.
Howorth, P. J. N. (1966). *Lancet* **1**, 202.
Inouye, A., Katoaka, K., and Shinagawa, J. (1962). *Nature* **194**, 286.
Kahlson, G., and Rosengren, E. (1965). *Ann. Rev. Pharmacol.* **5**, 305.
Kemali, D. (1960). *Nature* **185**, 540.
Kety, S. S. (1959). *Science* **129**, 528, 1590.
Kety, S. S. (1962). *Trans. Studies Coll. Physicians Phila.* **29**, 101.
Kety, S. S. (1965a). *Intern. J. Psychiat.* **1**, 409.
Kety, S. S. (1965b). *McGill Med. J.* **34**, 39.
Kety, S. S. (1966). *Pharmacol. Rev.* **18**, 787.
Kety, S. S., Woodford, R. B., Harnell, H., Freyhan, F. A., Appel, K. E., and Schmidt, C. F. (1948). *Am. J. Psychiat.* **104**, 165.
Kirshner, N. (1966). *Pharmacol. Rev.* **18**, 83.
Kitay, J. I., and Altschule, M. D. (1952). *A.M.A. Arch. Neurol. Psychiat.* **68**, 506.
Klenk, E. (1940). *Z. Physiol. Chem.* **272**, 280.
Klenk, E. (1955). *In* "Biochemistry of the Developing Nervous System" (H. Waelsch, ed.), p. 397. Academic Press, New York.
Kline, N. S., Cole, I., Lehmann, H., Wittenborn, I. P., Himwich, H. E., Esser, A. H., and Barclay, G. (1966). *J. Am. Med. Assoc.* **197**, 30.
Kopin, I. J. (1959). *Science* **29**, 835.
Kopin, I. J. (1964). *Pharmacol. Rev.* **16**, 179.
Kopin, I. J. (1966). *Pharmacol. Rev.* **18**, 513.
Kopin, I. J., and Axelrod, J. (1960). *Arch. Biochem. Biophys.* **89**, 148.
Krall, A. R., Lever, P. G., Villaverde, R. and Bilett, B. (1963). *J. Am. Med. Assoc.* **184**, 280.
Kuehl, F. A., Hickens, M., Ormond, R. E., Meisinger, M. A. P., Gale, P. H., Cuello, V. J., and Brink, N. G. (1964). *Nature* **203**, 154.
LaBrosse, E. H., Mann, J. D., and Kety, S. S. (1961). *J. Psychiat. Res.* **1**, 68.
Latham, L. K., Frohman, C. E., Warner, K., Beckett, P. G. S., and Gottlieb, J. S. (1964). *Federation Proc.* **23**, 177.
Latham, L. K., Warner, K., Beckett, P. G. S., Gottlieb, J. S., and Frohman, C. E. (1965). *Federation Proc.* **24**, 326.
Lees, H., Greenwood, D. J., Frohman, C. E., Beckett, P. G. S., and Gottlieb, J. S. (1965). *J. Neuropsychiat.* **5**, 534.
Lehman, H. (1952). "Biology of Mental Health and Disease". Harper and Row (Hoeber), New York.
Lever, W. F., Gurd, F. R. N., Uroma, E., Brown, R. K., Barnes, B. A., Schmid, K., and Schultz, E. L. (1951). *J. Clin. Invest.* **30**, 99.
Levitt, M., Spector, S., Sjoerdsma, A., and Udenfriend, S. (1965). *J. Pharmacol. Exptl. Therap.* **148**, 1.
Lundholm, L., Mohme-Lundholm, E., and Svedmyr, N. (1966). *Pharmacol. Rev.* **18**, 255.
Lyman, F. L. (1963). "Phenylketonuria". Thomas, Springfield, Illinois.
McGeer, P. L., Boulding, J. E., Gibson, W. C., and Foulks, R. G. (1961). *J. Am. Med. Assoc.* **177**, 665.
McGeer, P. L., and Williams, C. M. (1963). *Neurology* **23**, 73.
McIsaac, W. M. (1961a). *Biochim. Biophys. Acta* **52**, 607.
McIsaac, W. M. (1961b). *Postgrad. Med.* **30**, 111.
McLennan, H. (1957). *J. Physiol.* **139**, 79.
Mann, J. D., and LaBrosse, E. H. (1959). *Arch. Gen. Psychiat.* **1**, 547.
Märki, F., and Witkop, B. (1963). Unpublished results, cited in Daly and Witkop (1963).

Maynert, E. W. (1966). *Pharmacol. Rev.* **18**, 457.
Michaux, R., and Verly, W. G. (1963). *Life Sciences* **3**, 175.
Monnier, M. (1960). *Arch. Intern. Pharmacodyn.* **124**, 281.
Nickerson, M. (1966). *Pharmacol. Rev.* **18**, 801.
Nishimura, T., and Gjessing, L. R. (1965). *Nature* **206**, 963.
Noteboom, L. (1934). *Proc. Acad. Sci. (Amsterdam)* **37**, 562.
Osaki, S., Walter, C., and Frieden, E. (1962). *J. Biol. Chem.* **237**, 3455.
Osmund, H., and Hoffer, A. (1962) *Lancet* **1**, 316.
Ottenstein, B., Schmidt, G., and Thannhauser, S. J. (1948). *Blood* **3**, 1250.
Page, I. H. (1958). *Physiological Rev.* **38**, 277.
Pare, C. M. B., and Sandler, M. M. (1959). *J. Neurol. Neurosurg. Psychiat.* **22**, 247.
Pare, C. M. B., Sandler, M. M., and Stacey, R. S. (1957). *Lancet* **1**, 551.
Park, L. C., Baldessarini, R. J., and Kety, S. S. (1965). *Arch. Gen. Psychiat.* **12**, 346.
Penrose, L. S. (1963). "The Biology of Mental Defect," 3rd Ed. Sidgwick & Jackson, Ltd. London.
Perrin, G. M., Altschule, M. D., and Holliday, P. D. (1960). *A.M.A. Arch. Internal. Med.* **105**, 752.
Perrin, G. M., Altschule, M. D., Holliday, P. D., and Goncz, R. M. (1959). *A.M.A. Arch. Internal. Med.* **103**, 730.
Perry, T. L. (1963). *Science* **139**, 587.
Perry, T. L., Hansen, S. and MacIntyre, L. (1964). *Nature* **202**, 519.
Pisano, J. J., Abraham, D. and Udenfriend, S. (1963). *Arch. Biochem. Biophys.* **100**, 323.
Pisano, J. J., Wilson, J. D., Cohen, L., Abraham, D., and Udenfriend, S. (1961). *J. Bio. Chem.* **236**, 499.
Pollin, W., Cardon, P. V., Jr., and Kety, S. S. (1961). *Science* **133**, 104.
Pollin, W., and Goldin, S. (1961). *J. Psychiat. Res.* **1**, 50.
Potter, L. T., and Axelrod, J. (1962). *Nature* **194**, 581.
Quastel, J. H., and Scholefield, P. G. (1958). *Am. J. Med.* **25**, 420.
Ravin, H. A. (1956). *Lancet* **1**, 726.
Redick, T. F. (1963). *Science* **141**, 646.
Richter, D. (1957). *In* "Schizophrenia: Somatic Aspects" (D. Richter, ed.), pp. 53–75. Pergamon Press, London.
Roberts, E., Baxter, C. F., Harreveld, A. V., Wiersma, C. A. G., Adey, W. R., and Killam, K. F. (1960). "Inhibition in the Nervous System and Gamma-Aminobutyric Acid." Pergamon Press, London.
Rodnight, R. (1956). *Biochem. J.* **64**, 621.
Rosen, L., and Goodall, M. (1962). *Proc. Soc. Exptl. Biol. Med.* **110**, 767.
Rosenblatt, S. (1960). *J. Neurochem.* **5**, 172.
Rothballer, A. B. (1956). *EEG Clin. Neurophysiol.* **8**, 603.
Sanders, B. E., Smith, E. V. C., Flataker, L., and Winter, C. A. (1962). *Ann N.Y. Acad. Sci.* **96**, 448.
Sanders, B. E., Small, S. M., Ayers, W. J., Oh, Y. H., and Axelrod, S. (1965). *Trans. N.Y. Acad. Sci.* **28**, 22.
Schanberg, S. M. (1963). *J. Pharmacol. Exptl. Therap.* **139**, 191.
Schildkraut, J. J. (1965). *Am. J. Psychiat.* **122**, 509.
Schneckloth, R. E., Corcoran, A. C., Dustan, H. P., and Page, I. H. (1956). *J. Am. Med. Assoc.* **162**, 868.
Schneider, K. (1957). *Fortschr. Neurol. Psychol.* **25**, 487.
Sen, N. P., and McGeer, P. L. (1964). *Biochem. Biophys. Res. Comm.* **14**, 227.
Siegel, M. (1965). *J. Psychiat. Res.* **3**, 205.
Slone, D. (1933). *J. Genetics* **27**, 363.

Sokoloff, L., Perlin, S., Kornetsky, C., and Kety, S. S. (1957). *Ann N. Y. Acad. Sci.* **66**, 468.
Sourkes, T. L. (1962). "Biochemistry of Mental Disease." Harper and Row, New York.
Spencer, G. (1963). *Chem. Ind. (London)* p. 311.
Sprince, H., Houser, E., Jameson, D., and Dohan F. C. (1960). *Arch. Gen. Psychiat.* **2**, 268.
Sprince, H., Parker, C. A., Jameson, D., and Alexander, P. (1963). *J. Nervous Mental Disease* **137**, 246.
Stanbury, J. B., Wyngarden, J. B. and Frederickson, D. S., (1960). "The Metabolic Basis of Inherited Disease." McGraw-Hill, New York.
Stjärne, L. (1966). *Pharmacol. Rev.* **18**, 425.
Stone, D., Bridge, C. J., and Bernard, A. (1965). *Intern. J. Neuropsychiat.* **1**, 80.
Szara, S. (1961). *Federation Proc.* **20**, 855.
Szara, S. (1964). In "Comparative Neurochemistry" (D. Richter, ed.), p. 425. Pergamon Press, Oxford.
Szara, S., Axelrod, J., and Perlin, S. (1958). *Am. J. Psychiat.* **115**, 162.
Takeo, Y., and Himwich, H. E. (1965). *Science* **150**, 1309.
Takesada, M., KaKimoto, Y., and Sane, I. (1963). *Nature* **199**, 203.
Tower, D. B. (1959). *Proc. Intern. Congr. Biochem.*, 4th Vienna, 1958, **3**, 213.
Veech, R. L., Bigelow, L. B., Denckla, W. D., and Altschule, M. D. (1961). *Arch. Gen. Psychiat.* **5**, 127.
Victor, M., Altschule, M. D., Holliday, P. D., and Goncz, R. M. (1957). *A.M.A. Arch. Intern. Med.* **99**, 28.
von Euler, U.S. (1966). *Pharmacol. Rev.* **18**, 365.
Waalkes, T. P., Sjoerdsma, A., Creveling, C. R., Weissbach, H., and Udenfriend, S. (1958). *Science* **127**, 648.
Walaas, E., Lingjaerde, O., Sövik, O., Alertsen, A. R., and Walaas, O. (1964). *Acta Psychiat. Scand.* **40**, 423.
Walaas, O., Walaas, E., Sövik, O., Alertsen, A. R., and Lingjaerde, O. (1965). *Confin. Neurol.* **25**, 175.
Weissbach, H., Redfield, B. G., and Axelrod, J. (1961). *Biochim. Biophysica Acta* **54**, 190.
White, T. (1964). *Federation Proc.* **23**, 1105.
Wilson, W. P., Schieve, J. F., and Scheinberg, P. (1952). *A.M.A. Arch. Neurol. Psychiat.* **68**, 651.
Winter, C. A., and Flataker, L. (1958). *A.M.A. Arch. Neurol. Psychiat.* **80**, 441.
Winter, C. A., Flataker, L., Boger, W. P., Smith, E. V. C., and Sanders, B. E. (1961). "Chemical Pathology of the Nervous System," p. 641. MacMillan (Pergamon), New York.
Woolley, D. W., and Shaw, E. (1954). *Science* **119**, 587.
Woolley, D. W., and Van Der Hoeven, T. (1963). *Sicnce* **139**, 610.
Woolley, D. W., Van Winkle, E., and Shaw, E. (1957). *Proc. Natl. Acad. Sci.* **43**, 128.
Wurtman, R. J. (1965). *New Engl. J. Med.* **273**, 637, 693, 746.
Wurtman, R. J., Frank, M. M., and Altschule, M. D. (1958). *A.M.A. Arch. Intern. Med.* **102**, 790.
Yuwiler, A. (1965). *J. Psychiat. Res.* **3**, 125.
Zeller, E. A. (1957). *Naturwissenschaften* **15**, 427.

Note added in proof: Prada and Pletscher, 1966 (*J. Pharm. Pharmacol.*, *18*, 628) have recently reported on the mechanism of chlorpromazine-induced changes in cerebral homovanillic acid (XXVII, see pps. 258, 259) levels.

~4~
Miscellaneous Psychotherapeutic Agents

Maxwell Gordon
Smith Kline & French Laboratories, Philadelphia, Pennsylvania

A variety of miscellaneous agents are listed in Table I. Some of these may never be marketed. Others are covered in other chapters, but are listed here for purposes of indexing. The majority of agents in this chapter are of borderline pertinence to this book.

Thus, methylparafynol, ethchlorvynol, ethinamate, methyprylon, glutethimide, and petrichloral are primarily hypnotics, but their use in daytime sedation qualifies them for inclusion here. The barbiturates have been adequately reviewed elsewhere, and hence they are not included in this chapter.

The classical stimulants and anorexigenic agents like amphetamine, methamphetamine, pentylenetetrazole, bemegride, methylphenidate, phenmetrazine, and nikethamide are included even though they are only effective in neurotic depressions—rarely in the psychotic type.

In most instances only a single recent reference is given to each agent.

A useful review of newer developments in the chemistry of psychopharmacological agents has been published by Jucker (1963).

A comprehensive review on nonbarbiturate hypnotics has been published by Wheeler (1963), and spinal cord depressant drugs derived from polyhydroxy alcohols have been reviewed by Pribyl (1963).

A compilation of psychotropic and related compounds has been published by Usdin and Amai (1963).

TABLE I
Miscellaneous Psychopharmacological Agents

Structure	Molecular formula	Nonproprietary name	Proprietary name (Company)	Medical use	Reference
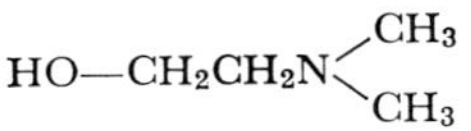 HO—CH$_2$CH$_2$N(CH$_3$)$_2$	C$_4$H$_{11}$NO	Deanol	Deaner (Riker) Elevol Elevan	Stimulant	Murphree et al. (1959)
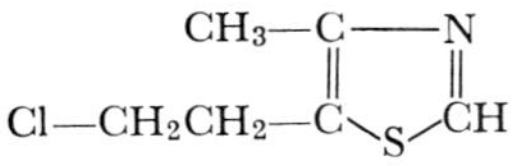 CH$_3$—C=N / Cl—CH$_2$CH$_2$—C—S—CH	C$_6$H$_8$ClNS	SCTZ	Hemineurin	Sedative-hypnotic	Osterman et al. (1959)
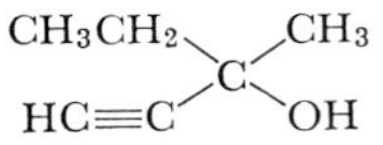 CH$_3$CH$_2$—C(CH$_3$)(OH)—C≡CH	C$_6$H$_{10}$O	Methylparafynol	Dormison	Hypnotic	Swinyard et al. (1954)
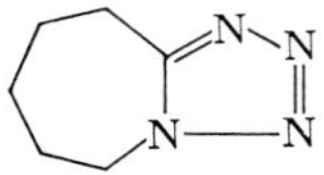 (triazepine structure)	C$_6$H$_{10}$N$_4$	Pentazol Pentylenetetrazole	Cardiazol Metrazol	Stimulant	Bennett (1962)
C$_2$H$_5$—C(OH)(C≡CH)—CH=CHCl	C$_7$H$_9$ClO	Ethchlorvynol	Placidyl (Abbott)	Hypnotic	Kuensberg (1962)
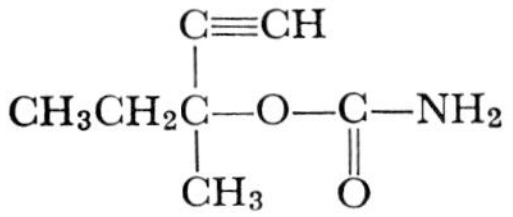 CH$_3$CH$_2$C(C≡CH)(CH$_3$)—O—C(=O)—NH$_2$	C$_7$H$_{10}$NO$_2$	—	Oblivon-C	Tranquilizer	Lewis (1964)

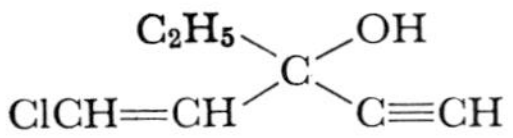

Structure	Formula	Generic name	Trade name (Company)	Action	Reference
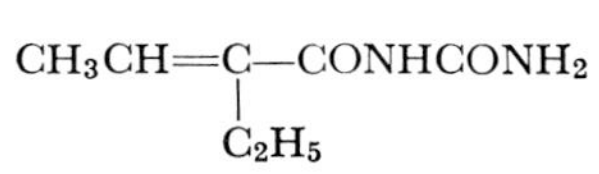 CH₃CH=C(C₂H₅)—CONHCONH₂	$C_7H_{12}N_2O_2$	Ectylurea	Ektyl Nostyn (Ames) Sedarex Nastyn Levanil (Upjohn)	Tranquilizer	Hukuhara (1962)
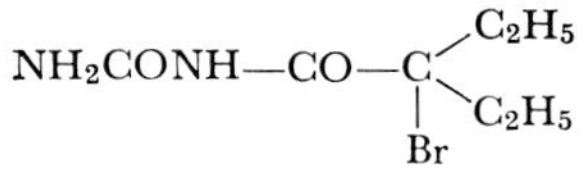 NH₂CONH—CO—C(C₂H₅)(C₂H₅)Br	$C_7H_{13}BrN_2O_2$	Carbromal	—	Sedative	Buck and Mitchell (1963)
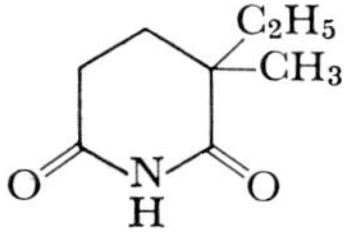 (piperidine-2,6-dione with C₂H₅ and CH₃)	$C_8H_{13}NO_2$	Bemegride	Megimide (Abbott)	Stimulant	Bennett (1962)
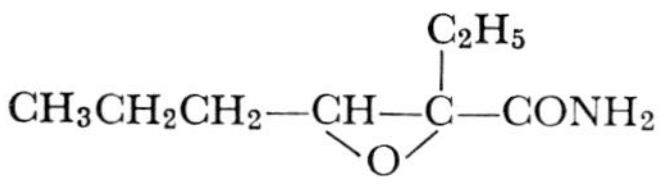 CH₃CH₂CH₂—CH(C₂H₅)—C(O)—CONH₂ (epoxide)	$C_8H_{15}NO_2$	Oxanamide	Quiactin (Merrell)	Tranquilizer	Warren et al. (1949) Proctor (1957)
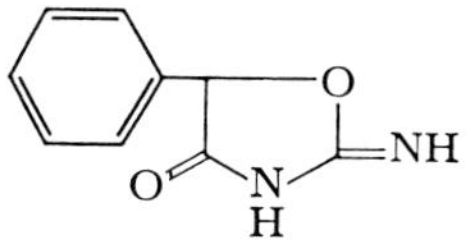 (2-imino-5-phenyl-oxazolidinone)	$C_9H_8N_2O_2$	Azoxodon	Tradon (Beiersdorf)	Stimulant	Bugard (1960) Polezhaieva (1962)
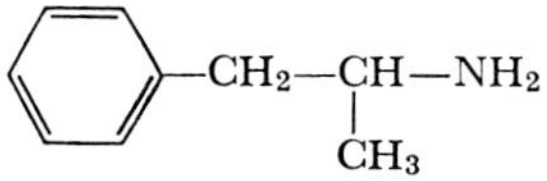 C₆H₅—CH₂—CH(NH₂)—CH₃	$C_9H_{13}N$	d-Amphetamine	Dexedrine (SK & F) and many others	Stimulant Anorexic	Livingston et al. (1948) Trendelenburg et al. (1962)

TABLE I—continued

Structure	Molecular formula	Nonproprietary name	Proprietary name (Company)	Medical use	Reference
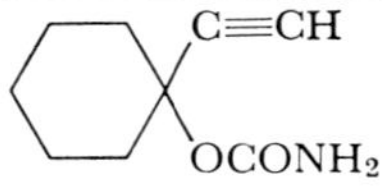 (cyclohexane with C≡CH and OCONH$_2$)	$C_9H_{13}NO_2$	Ethinamate	Valmid	Hypnotic	Finke and Schwab (1962)
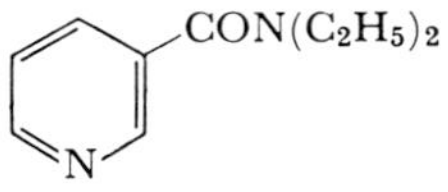 (pyridine with CON(C$_2$H$_5$)$_2$)	$C_{10}H_{14}N_2O$	Nikethamide	Coramine (Ciba)	Stimulant	Schulte et al. (1939)
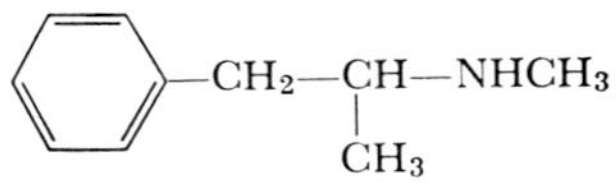 (phenyl-CH$_2$-CH(CH$_3$)-NHCH$_3$)	$C_{10}H_{15}N$	Methamphetamine	Amphedroxyn (Lilly) Desoxyn (Abbott) Desyphed (Winthrop) Dexoval (Vale) Doxyfed (Raymer) Drinalfa (Squibb) Efroxine (Maltbie) Gerobit Isophen Methedrinal Methedrine (Burroughs Wellcome) Norodin (Endo) Pervitin Psykoton	Stimulant	Ivy and Goetzl (1943) Haley (1947)

Formula	Structure	Generic name	Trade name (manufacturer)	Use	References
$C_{10}H_{17}NO_2$		Methyprylon	Semoxydrine (Massengill) Syndrox (McNeil) Noludar (Roche)	Hypnotic	Reiser et al. (1963) Hagenbucher and Kleh (1962)
$C_{11}H_{12}ClNO_3S$		Chlormethazanone	Trancopal (Winthrop)	Muscle relaxant	Surrey et al. (1958)
$C_{11}H_{12}O_2$		Kö 339	Centalun (Boehringer)	Sedative	Koch (1963)
$C_{11}H_{13}N$		Pargyline	Eutonyl (Abbott)	MAO inhibitor Hypotensive	See Chapter XII (Vol. I)
$C_{11}H_{14}N_2O$		Amphenidone	Dornwal (Maltbie)[a]	Tranquilizer	Pittman (1962) Rickels et al. (1963)

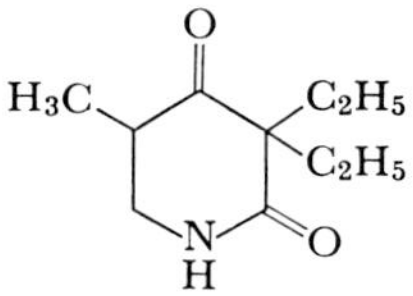

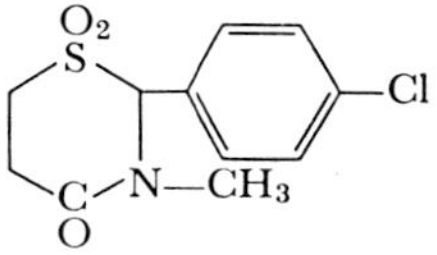

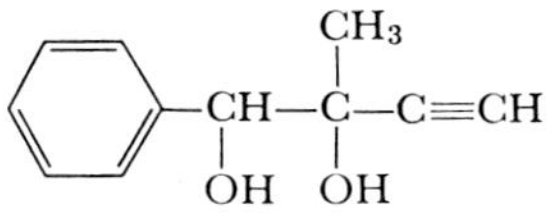

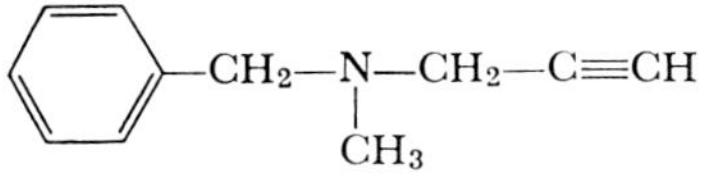

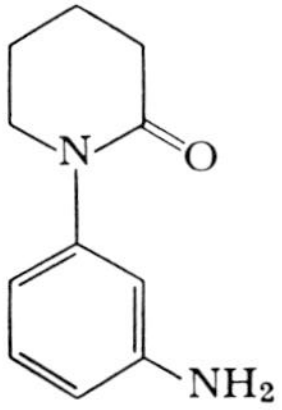

[a] Withdrawn from market.

TABLE I—continued

Structure	Molecular formula	Nonproprietary name	Proprietary name (Company)	Medical use	Reference
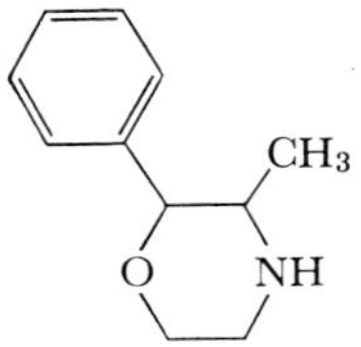 [phenmetrazine structure]	$C_{11}H_{15}NO$	Phenmetrazine	Preludin (Geigy)	Stimulant Anorexic	Rudolph and MacLachlan (1962)
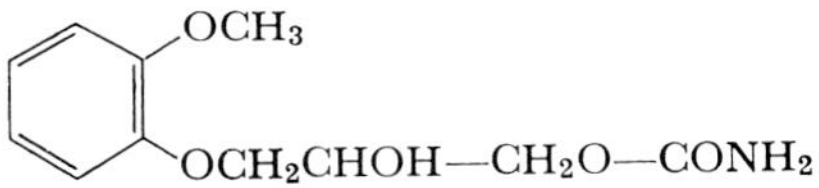 [methocarbamol structure]	$C_{11}H_{15}NO_5$	Methocarbamol	Robaxin (Robins) Tresortil	Muscle relaxant	Griffin (1962)
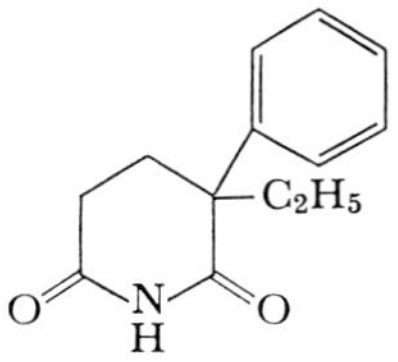 [glutethimide structure]	$C_{13}H_{15}NO_2$	Glutethimide	Doriden (Ciba)	Hypnotic	Rickels and Bass (1963)
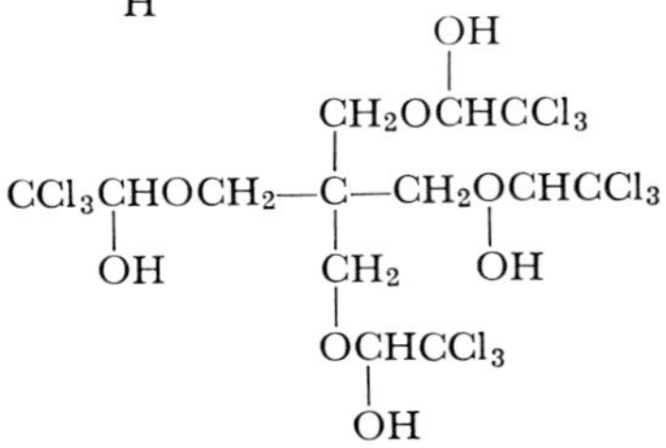 [petrichloral structure]	$C_{13}H_{16}Cl_{12}O_8$	Petrichloral	Periclor (Ives)	Hypnotic	Negwer (1961)

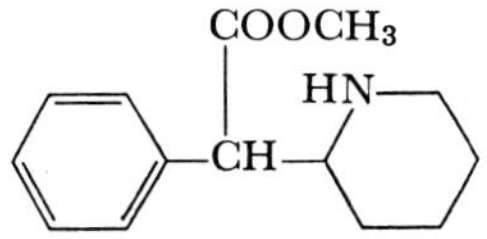 $C_{14}H_{19}NO_2$	Methylphenidate	Ritalin (Ciba) Rilatin Ritalina	Stimulant	See Chapter VI (Vol. I)
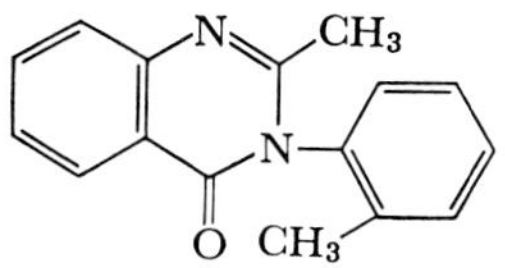 $C_{16}H_{13}N_2O$	Methaqualone	Tuazole (Strasenburgh) Hyminal (Eisai)	Depressant	Akagi et al. (1963)
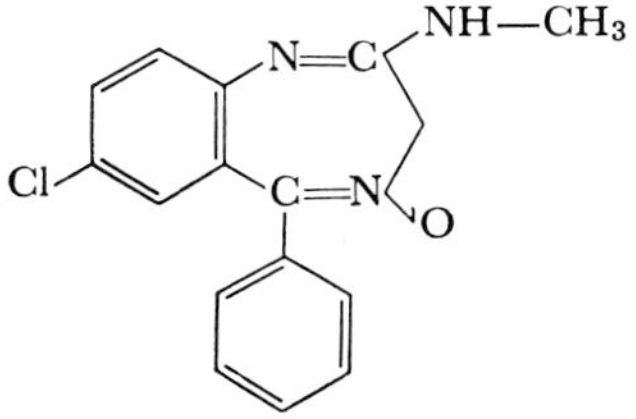 $C_{16}H_{14}ClN_3O$	Chlordiazepoxide	Librium (Roche)	Tranquilizer	See Chapter V (Vol. I)
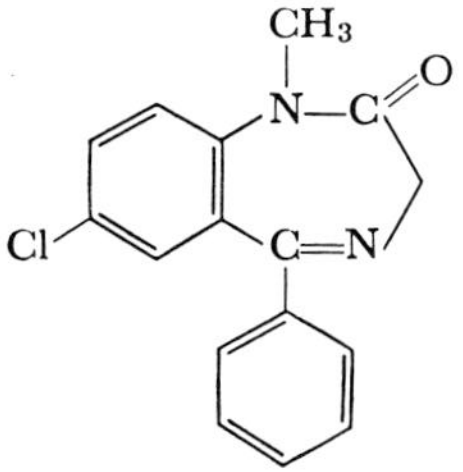 $C_{16}H_{13}ClN_2O$	Diazepam	Valium (Roche)	Tranquilizer	See Chapter V (Vol. I)

TABLE I—*continued*

Structure	Molecular formula	Nonproprietary name	Proprietary name (Company)	Medical use	Reference
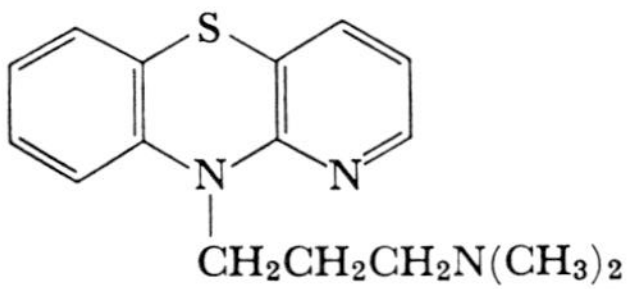 (phenothiazine with CH₂CH₂CH₂N(CH₃)₂ side chain, aza)	$C_{16}H_{19}N_3S$	Prothipendyl	Dominal (Homburg) Dominil Azacon Timovan (Ayerst)	Tranquilizer	Quandt et al. (1958) von Schlictergroll (1957, 1958)
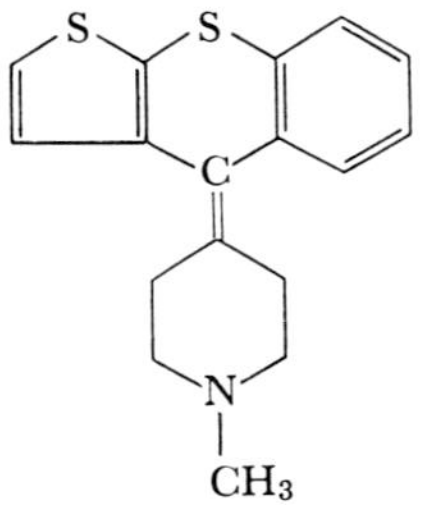 (thiophene-fused tricyclic with =C-piperidine-N-CH₃)	$C_{17}H_{17}NS_2$	—	BP401 (Sandoz)	—	Sandoz (1962b)
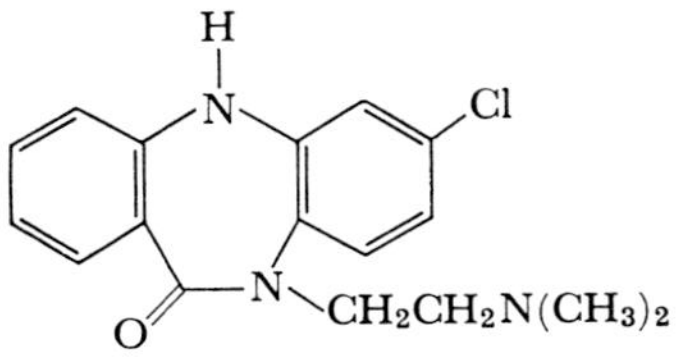 (chloro benzodiazepinone with CH₂CH₂N(CH₃)₂)	$C_{17}H_{18}ClN_3O$	—	Tarpan (Wander)	—	Hunziker et al. (1963)

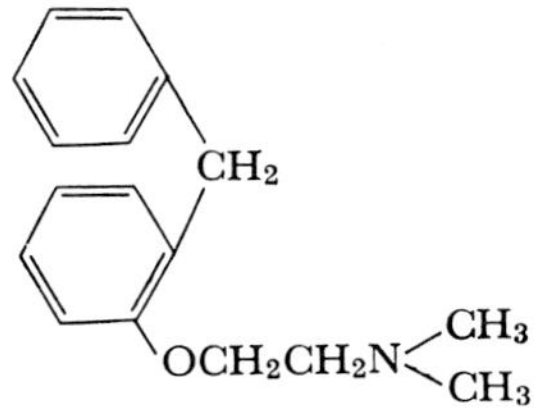 $C_{17}H_{21}NO$	Phenyltoloxamine[b]	P.R.N. (Bristol)	Tranquilizer	Gordon and McCandless (1959)
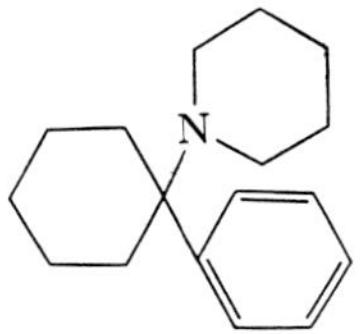 $C_{17}H_{25}N$	Phencyclidine	Sernyl (Parke-Davis)	Research compound	Wilkins and Barnes (1962) Van Meter et al. (1960)
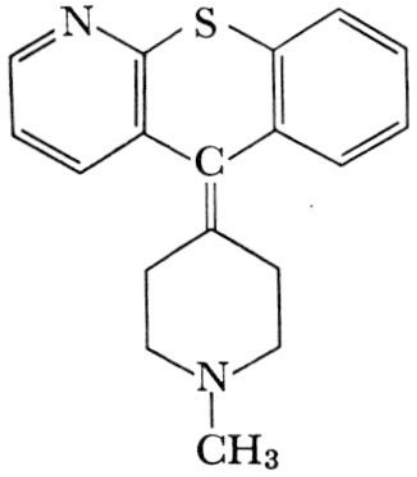 $C_{18}H_{18}N_2S$	—	AP800	—	
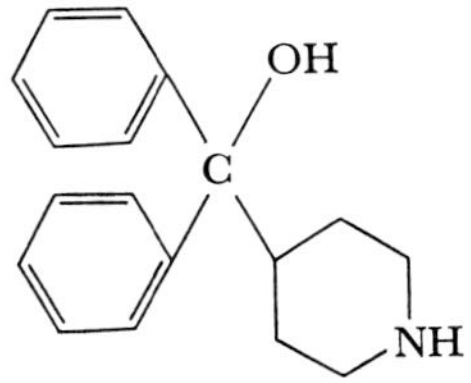 $C_{18}H_{21}NO$	Azacyclonol	10,906 (Sandoz) Frenquel (Merrell) Frenoton Calmeran Psychosan	Tranquilizer	Sandoz (1961, 1962a) See Chapter VI (Vol. I)

[b] Withdrawn from market as tranquilizer.

TABLE I—*continued*

Structure	Molecular formula	Nonproprietary name	Proprietary name (Company)	Medical use	Reference
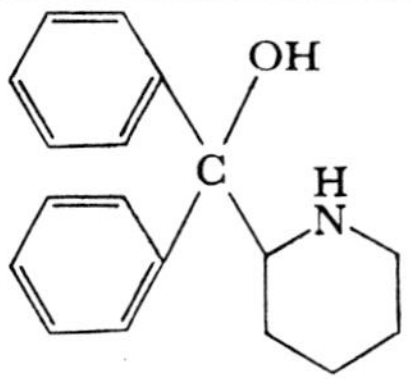	$C_{18}H_{21}NO$	Pipradrol	Meratran (Merrell) Gerodyl Pipradol	Stimulant	See Chapter VI (Vol. I)
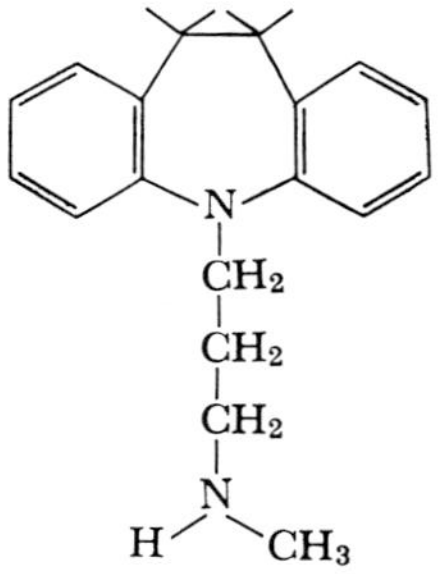	$C_{18}H_{22}N_2$	Desmethyl-imipramine Desipramine	Pertofrane (Geigy) Norpramine (Lakeside)	Antidepressant	Brodie *et al.* (1961) See Chapter XIII (Vol. I)
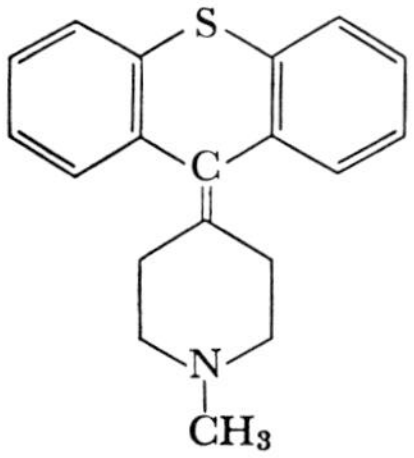	$C_{19}H_{19}NS$	—	BP 400/Sandoz	—	Sandoz (1961)

Structure	Formula	Name	Trade name (Company)	Use	References
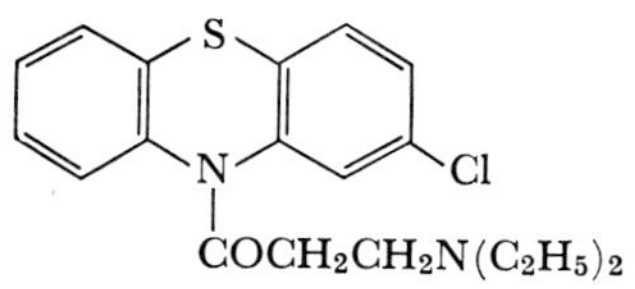 (chlorpromazine-thiazine with COCH₂CH₂N(C₂H₅)₂ and Cl)	$C_{19}H_{21}ClN_2OS$	Chloracizine	—	Antidepressant	Shchelkumov (1963)
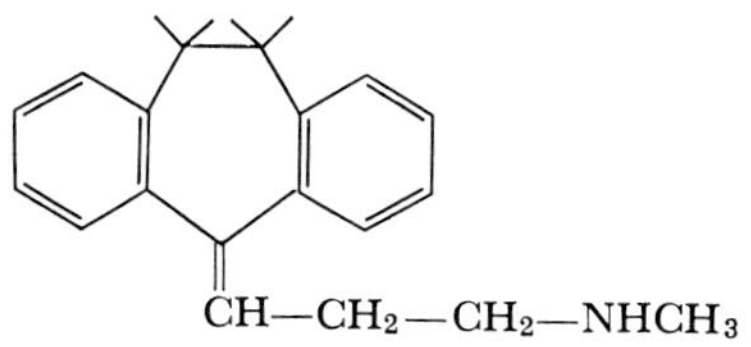 (dibenzosuberene with CH–CH₂–CH₂–NHCH₃)	$C_{19}H_{21}N$	Desmethylamitriptyline Nortriptyline	Aventyl (Lilly)	Antidepressant	See Chapter XIII (Vol. I) Chesrow (1964) Leahy and Rose (1964)
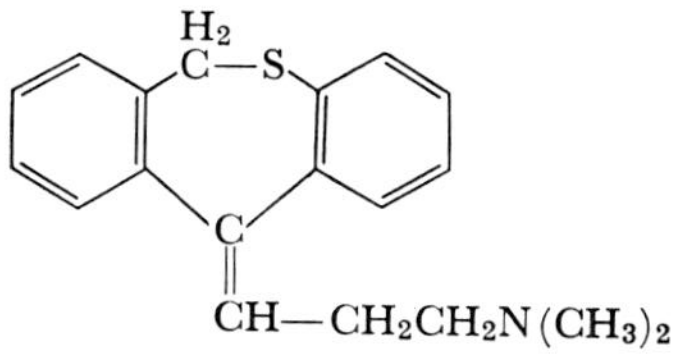 (dibenzothiepine with CH–CH₂CH₂N(CH₃)₂)	$C_{19}H_{21}NS$	—	10,914 (Sandoz) Prothiaden (Spofa) 1596 (Boehringer)	—	Gadient et al. (1962) Protiva et al. (1962) Stach and Bickelhaupt (1962)
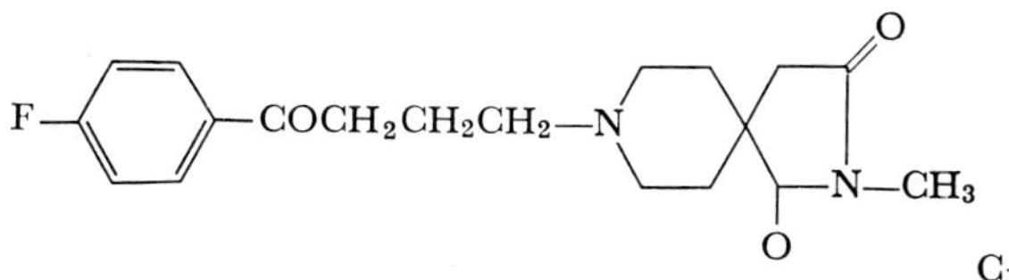 (4-fluorophenyl-COCH₂CH₂CH₂–N spiro piperidine-pyrrolidinedione with N–CH₃)	$C_{19}H_{23}FN_2O_3$	—	FR 33 (Sandoz)	—	Sandoz (1962c) Jucker (1962)

293

TABLE I—*continued*

Structure	Molecular formula	Nonproprietary name	Proprietary name (Company)	Medical use	Reference
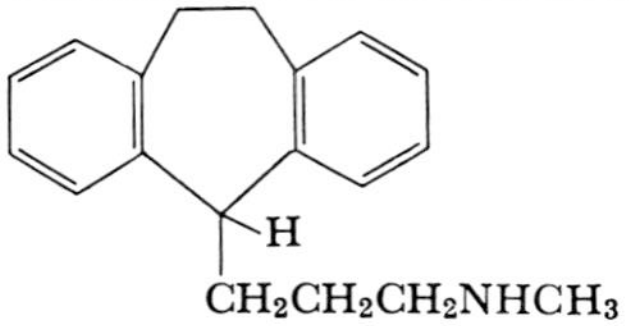 (dibenzosuberyl) CH₂CH₂NHCH₃	$C_{19}H_{23}N$	Protriptylene MK 240	Amimethylene (MSD)	Antidepressant	Stone (1963)
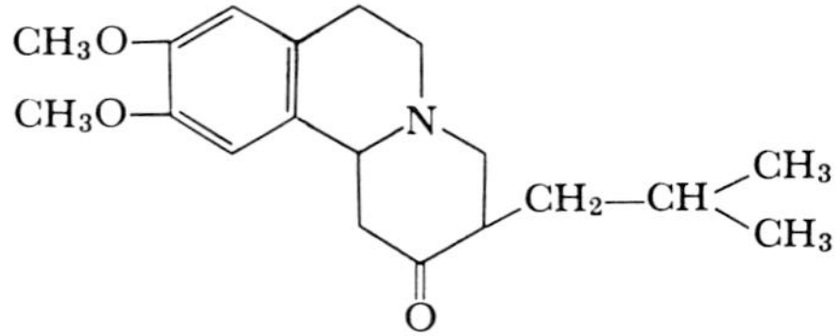 (benzoquinolizine with CH₂CH(CH₃)₂ and =O, CH₃O, CH₃O)	$C_{19}H_{27}NO_3$	Tetrabenazine	Nitoman (Roche)	Tranquilizer	Brossi *et al.* (1958) Eechaute *et al.* (1962) Quinn *et al.* (1959)
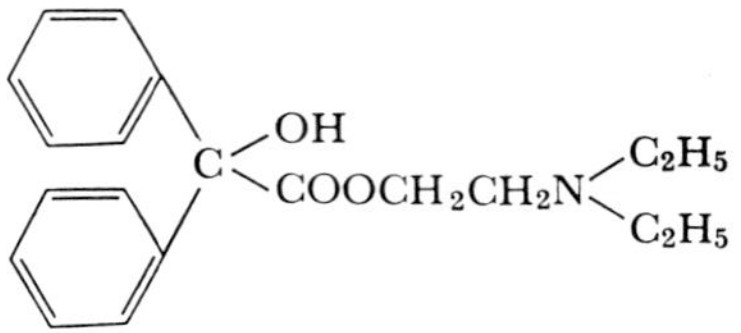 (diphenyl C(OH)COOCH₂CH₂N(C₂H₅)₂)	$C_{20}H_{25}NO_3$	Benactyzine	Phobex Parasan Suavitil (MSD) Stoikon Cevanol Lucidil Nutinal	Tranquilizer	See Chapter VIII (Vol. I)
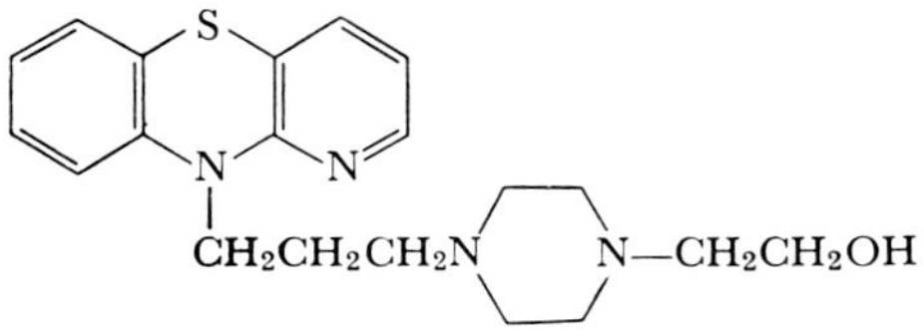 (phenothiazine-pyridine with CH₂CH₂CH₂–N(piperazine)–CH₂CH₂OH)	$C_{20}H_{26}N_4OS$	—	Pervetral	Tranquilizer	Goethe (1962)

Structure	Formula	Generic name	Trade name (manufacturer)	Activity	Reference
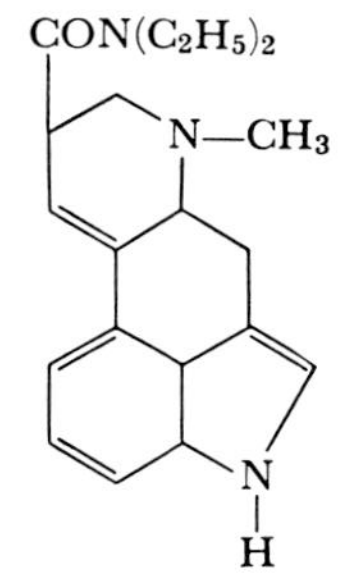 (lysergic acid diethylamide structure) CON(C₂H₅)₂, N—CH₃, N—H	$C_{20}H_{25}N_3O$	Lysergide LSD-25	Delysid (Sandoz)	Psychotomimetic	See Chapter XV (Vol. I)
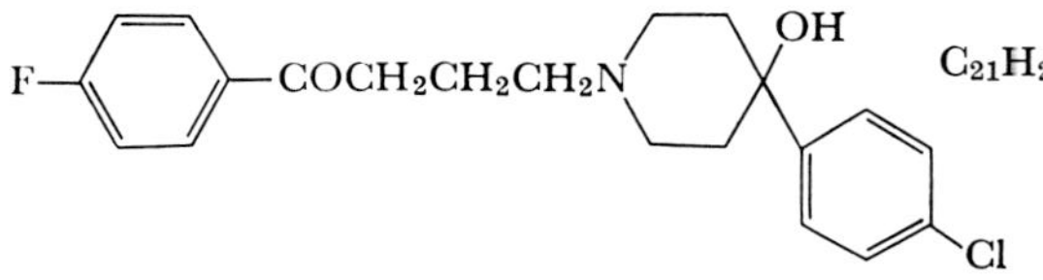 (haloperidol structure) F—C₆H₄—COCH₂CH₂CH₂N—(piperidine)—OH, —C₆H₄—Cl	$C_{21}H_{23}ClFNO_2$	Haloperidol	Haloperidol (Janssen) Serenase Aldol (Leo)	Tranquilizer	See Chapter VII (Vol. I) Janssen (1959)
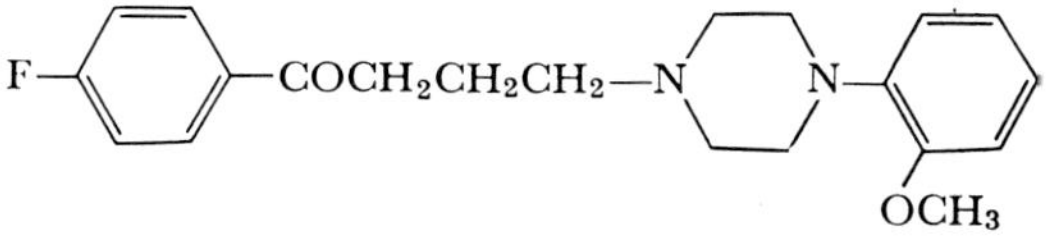 (haloanisone structure) F—C₆H₄—COCH₂CH₂CH₂—N(piperazine)N—C₆H₄—OCH₃	$C_{21}H_{25}FN_2O_2$	—	Haloanisone (Janssen)	Tranquilizer	Daumézon et al. (1960)
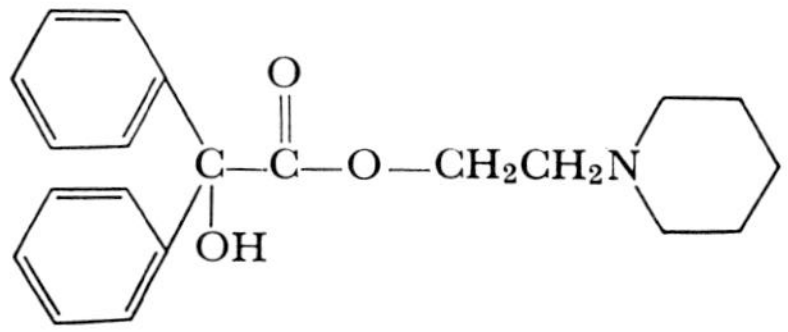 (pipethanate structure) (C₆H₅)₂C(OH)—C(=O)—O—CH₂CH₂N(piperidine)	$C_{21}H_{25}NO_3$	Pipethanate	Sycotrol (Reed-Carnick)	Tranquilizer	Welsh (1964)

295

TABLE I—*continued*

Structure	Molecular formula	Nonproprietary name	Proprietary name (Company)	Medical use	Reference
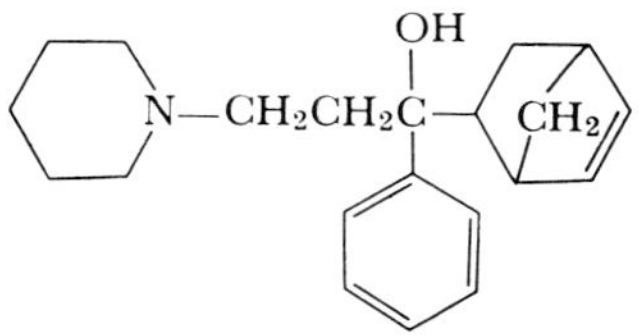	$C_{21}H_{29}NO$	Biperiden	Akineton	Tranquilizer	Lewis (1964)
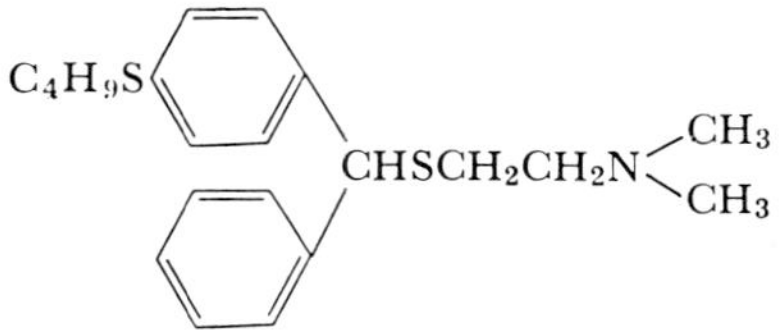	$C_{21}H_{29}NS_2$	Captodiamine	Covatin (Lundbeck) Covatix Suvren (Ayerst)	Tranquilizer	Gordon and McCandless (1959)
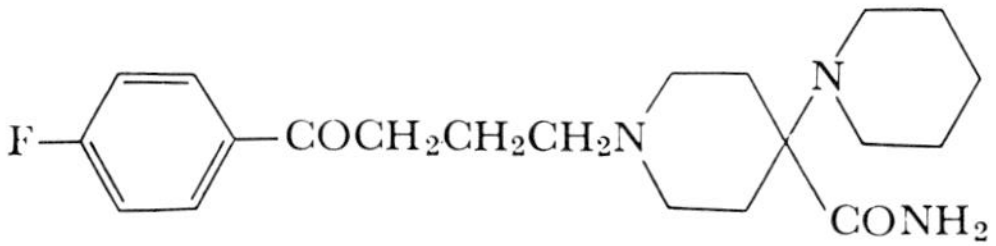	$C_{21}H_{30}FN_3O_2$	—	Dipiperon	—	Janssen (1961)

Structure	Formula	Name	Other name	Use	Reference
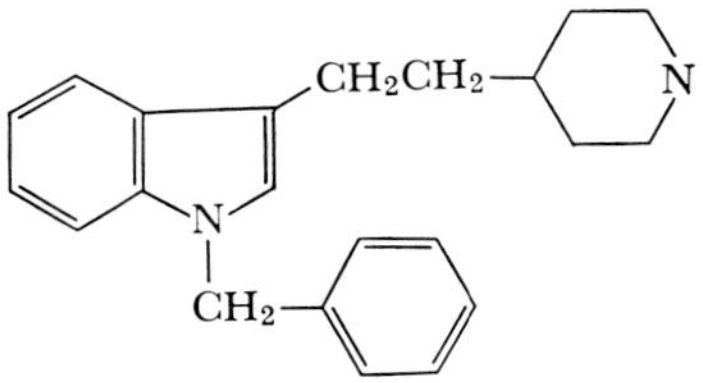 (indole with CH₂CH₂-piperidine and N-CH₂-phenyl)	$C_{22}H_{20}N_2$	Benzindopyrin Pyrbenzindol	—	—	—
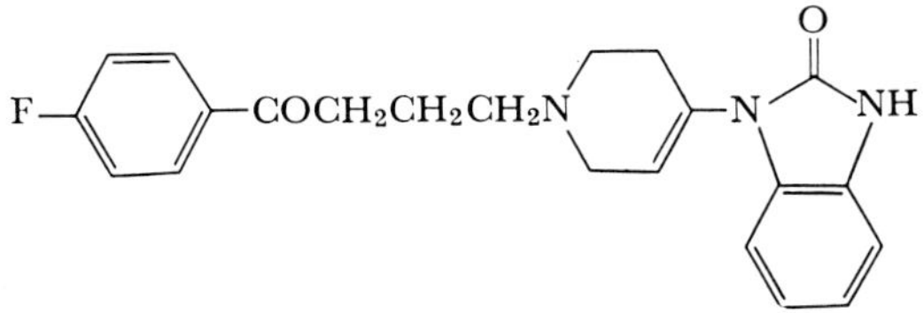 (fluorophenyl-COCH₂CH₂CH₂N-tetrahydropyridine-benzimidazolone)	$C_{22}H_{22}FN_3O_2$	Dehydrobenzperidol	(Janssen)	Tranquilizer	Janssen et al. (1963)
(chloro-dibenzosuberylidene-methylpiperidine)	$C_{22}F_{24}ClN$	PF 97 (Sandoz)	—	—	Swiss Patent application (Sandoz, A.G.)
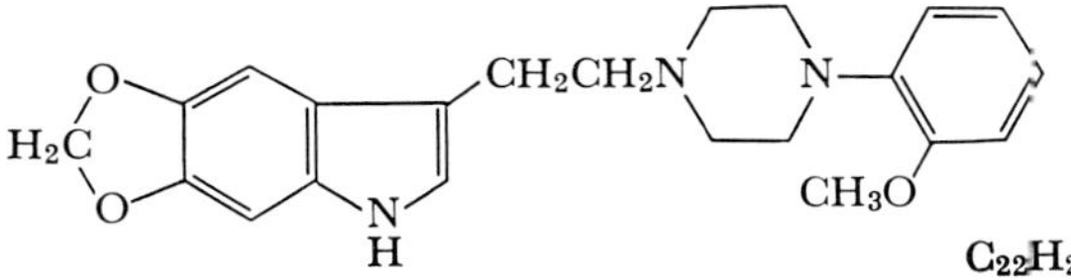 (methylenedioxy-indole with CH₂CH₂N-piperazine-methoxyphenyl)	$C_{22}H_{25}N_3O_3$	Solypertine (Sterling-Winthrop)	—	—	Archer et al. (1962) Wylie and Archer (1962)

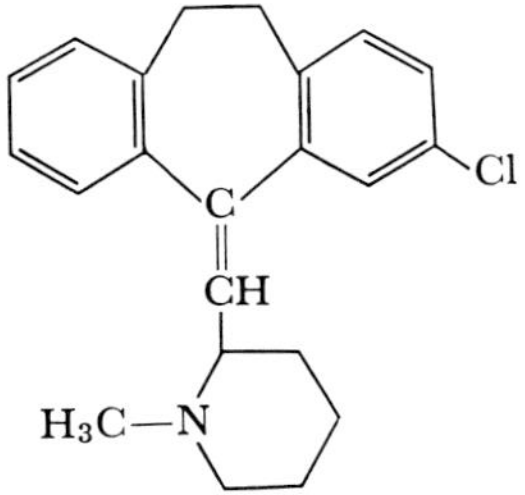

TABLE I—continued

Structure	Molecular formula	Nonproprietary name	Proprietary name (Company)	Medical use	Reference
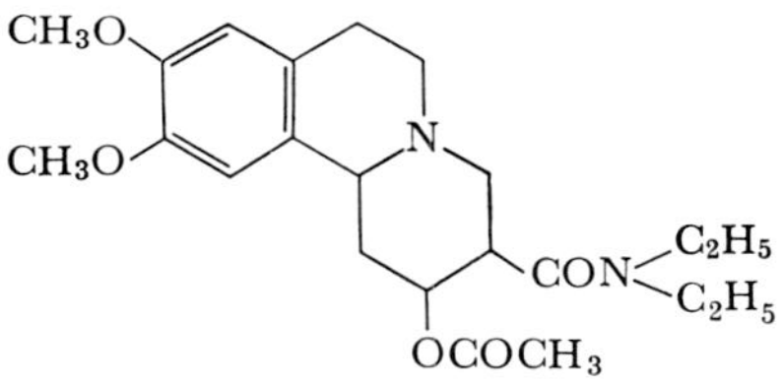 [structure with CH$_3$O, CH$_3$O, N, CON(C$_2$H$_5$)$_2$, OCOCH$_3$]	C$_{22}$H$_{32}$N$_2$O$_5$	Benzquinamide P-2647	Quantril (Pfizer)	Tranquilizer	Scriabine et al. (1963) Settel (1963) Smith (1962)
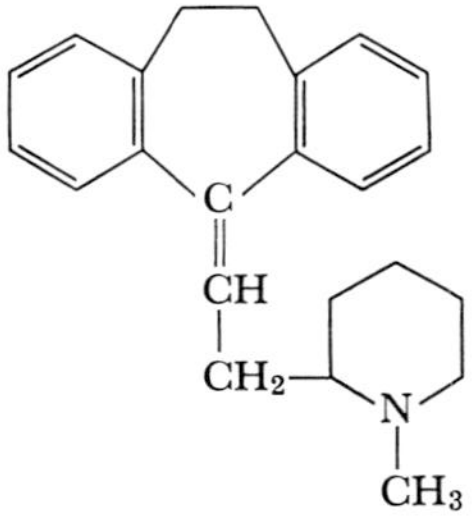 [dibenzo structure with =CH-CH$_2$-N(CH$_3$) piperidine]	C$_{23}$H$_{27}$N	—	ID 22 (Sandoz)	—	Sandoz (1962d)
			Compound 20B		Winthrop et al. (1962)
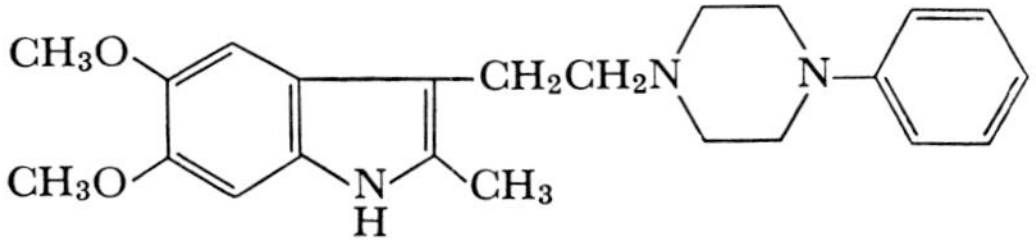 [indole structure with CH$_3$O, CH$_3$O, CH$_3$, CH$_2$CH$_2$N-piperazine-phenyl]	C$_{23}$H$_{29}$N$_3$O$_2$	Oxypertine	— (Sterling-Winthrop)	Tranquilizer	Edwards et al. (1962) Friedhoff and Hekimian (1963) Hollister et al. (1963)

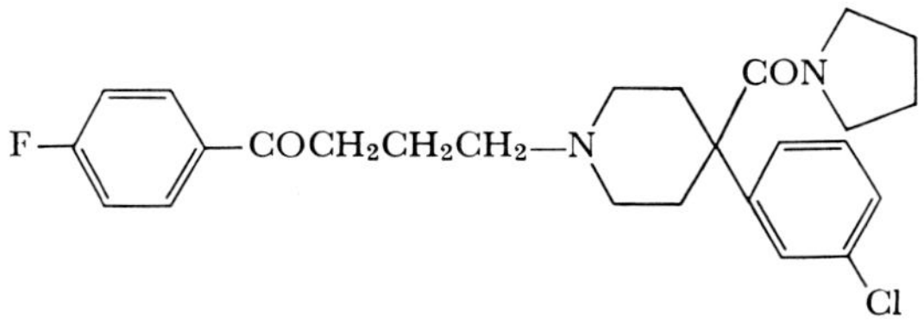

(structure: F-C6H4-COCH2CH2CH2-N(piperidine with 3-chlorophenyl and CON-pyrrolidine))	$C_{26}H_{30}ClFN_2O_2$	—	Haloperidid (Janssen)	—	Schaper et al. (1960)

ADDED IN PROOF

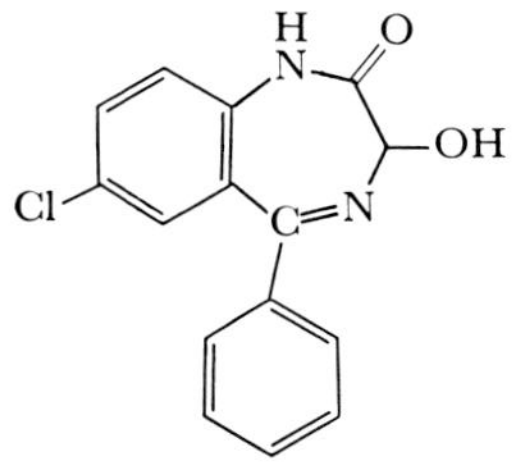

(structure: 7-chloro-3-hydroxy-5-phenyl-1,4-benzodiazepin-2-one)	$C_{15}H_{11}ClN_2O_8$	Oxazepam	Serax (Wyeth)	Anti-neurotic

REFERENCES

Akagi, M., Oketani, Y., Takada, M., and Suga, T. (1963). *Chem. Pharm. Bull.* (*Tokyo*) **11**, 321.
Archer, S., Wylie, D. W., Harris, L. S., Lewis, T. R., Schulenberg, J. W., Bell, M. R., Kulling, R. K., and Arnold, A. (1962). *J. Am. Chem. Soc.* **84**, 1306; Belgian Patent 595,341 (1961).
Bennett, P. B. (1962). *Life Sci.* **1**, 721.
Brodie, B. B., Bickel, M. H., and Sulser, F. (1961). *Med. Exptl.* **5**, 454.
Brossi, A., Lindlar, H., Walter, M., and Schnider, O. (1958). *Helv. Chim. Acta* **41**, 119.
Buck, H. W., and Mitchell, J. C. (1963). *Can. Med. Assoc. J.* **88**, 1116.
Bugard, P. (1960). *Presse Med.* **68**, 1785.
Chesrow, E. J. (1964). *J. Amer. Geriat. Soc.*, **12**, 271.
Condousis, G. A. (1961). *Am. J. Med. Sci.*, **242**, 574.
Daumézon, G. Audisio, M., Conte, C. and Huguet, P. (1960). *Ann. Med. Psychol.* **118**, 539.
Edwards, R. E., Moon, L. E., Jr., and Pearl, J. (1962). *Pharmacologist* **4**, 167.
Eechaute, W., Lacroix, E., and Leusen, I. (1962). *Experientia* **18**, 233.
Finke, J., and Schwab, G. (1962). *Deut. Med. Wochschr.* **87**, 2325.
Friedhoff, A. J., and Hekimian, L. (1963). *Diseases Nervous System* **24**, 241.
Gadient, F., Jucker, E., and Lindenmann, A. (1962). *Helv. Chim. Acta* **45**, 1860; Belgian Patent 607,503.
Gallant, D. M. (1965). *Curr. Ther. Res.*, **7**, 102.
Goethe, H. (1962). *Arzneimittel-Forsch.* **12**, 321.
Gordon, M., and McCandless, R. F. J. (1959). "Handbook of Toxicology," Vol. IV. Saunders, Philadelphia, Pennsylvania.
Griffin, P. J. (1962). *Gen. Practitioner* (*U.S.A.*) **26**, 110.
Hach, V. (1963). *Die Pharmazie*, **18**, 1.
Hagenbucher, J. T., and Kleh, J. (1962). *J. Am. Geriat. Soc.* **10**, 1038.
Haley, T. J. (1947). *J. Am. Pharm. Assoc. Sci. Ed.* **36**, 161.
Hollister, L. E., Overall, J. E., Kimbell, I., Bennett, J. L., Meyer, F., and Caffey, E., Jr. (1963) *J. New Drugs* **3**, 26.
Hukuhara, T. (1962). *Arzneimittel-Forsch.* **12**, 1134.
Hunziker, F., Lauener, H., and Schmutz, J. (1963). *Arzneimittel-Forsch.* **13**, 324; Belgian Patent 611,926 (Parke-Davis) (1962).
Ivy, A. C., and Goetzl, F. R. (1943). *War Med.* **3**, 60.
Jannsen, P. A. J. (1959). *J. Med. Pharm. Chem.* **1**, 281.
Jannsen, P. A. J. (1961). *Arzneimittel.-Forsch.* **11**, 819; U.S. Patent 3,041,344 (1964).
Janssen, P. A. J., Niemegeers, C. J. E., Schellekens, K. H. L., Verbruggen, F. J., and Van-Nueten, J. M. (1963). *Arzneimittel-Forsch.* **13**, 205.
Jucker, E. (1963). *Angew. Chem.* **75**, 524.
Jucker, E. (1962). *J. Sci. Ind. Res.*, Sect. A., **21**, 415.
Koch, L. (1963). *Med. Wochenschr.* **105**, 1273.
Kuenssberg, E. V. (1962). *Brit. Med. J.* **II**, 1610.
Leahy, M. R. and Rose, J. T. (1964). *Am. J. Psychiatry*, **121**, 72.
Lewis, J. J. (1964). *Practitioner*, **192**, 12.
Livingston, S., Kajdi, L., and Bridge, E. M. (1948). *J. Pediat.* **32**, 490.
Murphree, H. B., Jenney, E. H., and Pfeiffer, C. C. (1959). "The Effect of Pharmacologic Agents on the Nervous System." Williams and Wilkins, Baltimore.
Negwer, M. (1961). "Organisch-chemische Arzneimittel." Akademie Verlag, Berlin.
Osterman, E., Bellander-Löfvenberg, S., and Lassenius, B. (1959). *Rept. 12th Congr. Scand. Psychiat.* **34**, 344.
Pittman, J. A. (1962). *New Engl. J. Med.* **267**, 861.
Polezhaieva, A. I. (1962). *Farmakol. i Toksikol.* **25**, 515.

Pribyl, E. J. (1963). *In* "Medicinal Chemistry" (E. E. Campaigne and W. H. Hartung, eds.), Vol. VI, p. 246. Wiley, New York.
Proctor, R. C. (1957). *Diseases Nervous System* **18**, 223.
Protiva, M., Rajsner, M., Seidlová, V., Adlerová, E., and Vejdélek, Z. J. (1962). *Experientia* **18**, 326; Belgian Patent 618,591 (1962).
Quandt, J., von Horn, L., and Schliep, H. (1958). *Psychiat. Neurol.* **135**, 197.
Quinn, G. P., Shore, P. A., and Brodie, B. B. (1959). *J. Pharmacol. Exptl. Therap.* **127**, 103.
Reiser, P., Kay, L. L., Printz, S., Cherico, P., and Harris, S. B. (1963). *Clin. Med.* **70**, 395.
Rickels, K., and Bass, H. (1963). *Am. J. Med. Sci.* **245**, 142.
Rickels, K., Snow, L., Baumm, C., and Mock, J. (1963). *Am. J. Psychiat.* **119**, 1093.
Rudolph, L. A., and MacLachlan, I. (1962). *Current Therap. Res.* **4**, 629.
Sandoz, S. A. (1961). Belgian Pat. 601,668, Oct. 2.
Sandoz, S. A. (1961a). Belgian Pat. 603,154.
Sandoz, S. A. (1962a). Belgian Pat. 611,216.
Sandoz, S. A. (1962b). Belgian Pat. 616,813.
Sandoz, S. A. (1962c). Belgian Pat. 609,766.
Sandoz, S. A. (1962d). Belgian Pat. 610,038.
Schaper, W. K. A., Jageneau, A. H. M., Huggens, J., and Jannsen, P. A. J. (1960). *Med. Exptl.* **3**, 169.
Schulte, J. W., Tainter, M. L., and Dille, J. M. (1939). *Proc. Soc. Exptl. Biol. Med.* **42**, 242.
Scriabine, A., Weissman, A., Finger, K. F., Delahunt, C. S., Constantine, J. W., and Schneider, J. A. (1963). *J. Am. Med. Assoc.* **184**, 276.
Settel, E. (1963). *Clin. Med.* **70**, 957.
Shchelkumov, E. L. (1963). *Zh. Nevropat. Psikhiat. Korsakov*, **63**, 1415.
Smith, M. E. (1962). *Am. J. Psychiat.* **118**, 937.
Stach, K., and Bickelhaupt, F. (1962). *Monatsh. Chem.* **93**, 896.
Stone, C. A. (1963). *Federation Proc.* **22**, 627.
Surrey, A. R., Webb, W. G., and Gesler, R. M. (1958). *J. Am. Chem. Soc.* **80**, 3469.
Swinyard, E. A., Madsen, J. A., and Goodman, L. S. (1954). *J. Pharmacol. Exptl. Therap.* **111**, 54.
Trendelenburg, U., Muskus, A., Fleming, W. W., and Gomez Alonso de la Sierra, B. (1962). *J. Pharmacol. Exptl. Therap.* **138**, 170.
Usdin, E., and Amai, R. L. S. (1963). *Psychopharmacol. Serv. Center Bull.* **2**, 17.
Van Meter, W. G., Owens, H. F., and Himwich, H. E. (1960). *J. Neuropsychiat.* **1**, 129.
von Schlichtegroll, A. (1957). *Arzneimittel-Forsch.* **7**, 237.
von Schlichtegroll, A. (1958). *Arzneimittel-Forsch.* **8**, 489.
Warren, M. R., Thompson, C. R., and Werner, H. W. (1949). *J. Pharmacol. Exptl. Therap.* **96**, 209.
Welsh, A. L. (1964). *Med. Clin. N. Amer.*, **48**, 459.
Wheeler, K. W. (1963). *In* "Medicinal Chemistry" (E. E. Campaigne and W. H. Hartung, eds.), Vol. VI, p. 1. Wiley, New York.
Wilkins, J. H., and Barnes, J. H. (1962). *Nature* **195**, 1172.
Winthrop, S. O., Davis, M. A., Meyers, G. S., Gavin, J. G., Thomas, R., and Barber, R. (1962). *J. Org. Chem.* **27**, 230.
Wylie, D. W., and Archer, S. (1962). *J. Med. Pharm. Chem.* **5**, 932; *Federation Proc.* **21**, 322 (1962).

Appendix A
Phenothiazine Bibliographies

Compiled by MAXWELL GORDON

A.1	Acetophenazine	305
A.2	Carphenazine	308
A.3	Fluphenazine	311
A.4	Mepazine	323
A.5	Methdilazine	330
A.6	Methoxypromazine	332
A.7	Perphenazine	335
A.8	Pipamazine	363
A.9	Prochlorperazine	365
A.10	Promazine	389
A.11	Propiomazine	406
A.12	Prothipendyl	408
A.13	Thiethylperazine	414
A.14	Thiopropazate	416
A.15	Thioridazine	421
A.16	Trifluoperazine	435
A.17	Triflupromazine	460
A.18	Trimeprazine	469

~ A.1 ~
Acetophenazine

Chemistry

Forrest, F. M., et al. (1961). Review of rapid urine tests for phenothiazine and related drugs. *Am. J. Psychiat.* **118**, 300–307.

Mellinger, T. J., et al. (1962). Chromatography and electrophoresis of phenothiazine drugs. *J. Pharm. Sci.* **51**, 1169–1173.

Biology and Pharmacology

Guttman, H. N., et al. (1963). Evaluation of phenothiazines as membrane permeability alterants. Paper presented at 47th Annual Meeting, Atlantic City, New Jersey, April 16–20, 1963; (1963). *Federation Proc.* **22**, 569 (abstr.).

Hirshleifer, I. (1963). Cardiovascular disorders. Adjunctive treatment with psychopharmacologicals. *Gen. Practitioner* **26**, 6–8 (Kansas City, Missouri).

Knight, W. R., et al. (1963). Acetophenazine and fighting behavior in mice. *Science* **141**, 830–831.

Mapp, Y., et al. (1962). Psychopharmacology II: Tranquilizers and antipsychotic drugs. *Psychosomatics* **3**, 458–463.

Myers, H. M., et al. (1963). Pharmacology of the sedative-hypnotic and tranquilizing drugs. *Dental Clin. N. Am.* pp. 489–502.

Steiner, W. G., et al. (1963). An electroencephalographic study of some structural aspects of D-amphetamine antagonism in phenothiazine and related compounds. *Intern. J. Neuropharmacol.* **2**, 327–335.

Steiner, W. G., et al. (1963). Effects of antidepressant drugs on limbic structures of rabbit. *J. Nervous Mental Disease* **137**, 277–284.

Side Effects

Ayd, F. J., Jr. (1963). Uses and side effects of phenothiazines. *Mind* **1**, 326–348. *Appl. Therap.* **6**, 301 and 303 (abstr.) (1964).

Cares, R. M., et al. (1963). Comparative review of the structure and side-effects of newer psychotropic agents. *Diseases Nervous System* **24**, 92–105.

Goldman, D. (1961). Parkinsonism and related phenomena from administration of drugs: Their production and control under clinical conditions and possible relation to therapeutic effect. *Proc. Intern. Symp. Extrapyramidal System and Neuroleptics, Montreal,* Nov. 1960 pp. 453–464. Editions Psychiatriques.

Hollister, L. E. (1964). Adverse reactions to phenothiazines. *J. Am. Med. Assoc.* **189**, 311–313.

Simonson, M. (1964). Phenothiazine depressive reaction. *J. Neuropsychiat.* **5**, 259–265.

A.1. ACETOPHENAZINE

Clinical Use

Alexander, D. D. (1962). Observations in the use of Tindal. *Diseases Nervous System* **23**, 351.

Ayd, F. J., Jr. (1960). Tranquilizers and the ambulatory geriatric patient. *J. Am. Geriat. Soc.* **8**, 909–914.

Black, J. (1960). Phenothiazines as antiemetics and tranquilizers. *J. Med. Assoc. Alabama* **29**, 492–500.

Bowes, H. A. (1961). The Aberdeen experiment: A pioneering venture in community psychiatry. Presented at the 3rd World Congress of Psychiatry, Montreal, Canada, June 8, 1961.

Carter, C. H. (1962). Antiemetic specificity of carphenazine in brain damage; a blind crossover study with acetophenazine. *Am. J. Gastroenterol.* **38**, 587–591.

Chesrow, E. J., Kaplitz, S. E., Breme, J. T., and Sabatini, R. (1963). Acetophenazine (Tindal) in the treatment of 80 chronically ill patients with anxiety and tension: Double blind study. *J. Am. Geriat. Soc.* **11**, 445–448.

Cooper, I. S. (1964). Cryogenic surgery in the geriatric patient. *J. Am. Geriat. Soc.* **12**, 884–888.

Darling, H. F. (1961). Acetophenazine (Tindal) and thiopropazate (Dartal) in ambulatory psychoneurotic patients. *Am. J. Psychiat.* **118**, 358–359.

Darling, H. F. (1962). Acetophenazine in ambulatory schizophrenic adults. *Am. J. Psychiat.* **119**, 260–261.

Darling, H. F. (1963). The treatment of ambulatory adolescent schizophrenia with acetophenazine. *Am. J. Psychiat.* **120**, 68–69.

Freyhan, F. (1959). Therapeutic implications of differential effects of new phenothiazine compounds. *Am. J. Psychiat.* **115**, 577.

Frohman, I. P. (1961). The alleviation of stress in the elderly cardiac patient. Presented at the Conference on Aging, March 16, 1961, Hartford, Connecticut.

Gouldman, C., and Rutherford, A. (1960). Effects of a drug on the body odor of the chronically mentally ill. *Am. J. Psychiat.* **117**, 354–355.

Greenfield, A. R. (1961). Use of phenothiazines in alcoholic agitation. *Med. Ann. District Columbia* **30**, 726–728.

Hamilton, L. D., and Bennett, J. L. (1962). Acetophenazine for hyperactive geriatric patients. *Geriatrics* **17**, 596–601.

Himwich, H. E. (1959). Some drugs used in the treatment of mental disorders. *Am. J. Psychiat.* **115**, 756.

Hollister, L. E. (1958). The present status of tranquilizing drugs. *Calif. Med.* **89**.

Lapolla, A. (1963). Clinical study of a piperazine tranquilizer. *Clin. Med.* **70**, 347–348, and 351.

McLaughlin, B. E., Duffy, R. E., and Ryan, F. R. (1962). Chemotherapy as adjunctive treatment for emotionally disturbed children. *Diseases Nervous System* **23**, 95–98.

Moravec, C. L. (1961). Pathogenesis and therapy of stress in the menopause. Presented at Symposium on Office Practice and Problems of Women, Key West, Florida, Nov. 11, 1961.

Overall, J. E., et al. (1963). Comparison of acetophenazine with perphenazine in schizophrenics: Demonstration of differential effects based on computer-derived diagnostic models. *Clin. Pharmacol. Therap.* **4**, 200–208.

Riccitelli, M. L. (1964). Modern concepts in the management of anxiety and depression in the aged and infirm. *J. Am. Geriat. Soc.* **12**, 652–657.

Robin, B. A. (1961). Acetophenazine in the treatment of anxiety reactions. *Psychosomatics* **2**, 270–274.

Rodman, M. J. (1962). Drugs for treating high blood pressure. *R.N.* **25**, 75–79, 82, 84, and 86.

Rossi, G. V. (1964). The psychotherapeutic agents. *Am. J. Pharm.* **136**, 6–24.

Sainz, A., Ozerengin, F., Sanchez, N., and Ferreri, V. J. (1962). The phrenopraxic spectrum of acetophenazine. *Diseases Nervous System* **23**, 714–717.
Schiele, B. C. (1962). New drugs for mental illness. *J. Am. Med. Assoc.* **181**, 126–133.
Sheppard, C., et al. (1964). Effects of acetophenazine dimaleate on paranoid symptomatology in female geriatric patients: Double-blind study. *J. Am. Geriat. Soc.* **12**, 884–888.
Sines, L. K., and Hamlon, J. S. (1960). Clinical evaluation of a new phenothiazine in chronic psychiatric patients. *Diseases Nervous System* **21**, 86–90.
Smith, K., and Moody, A. C. (1961). The effect of meprobamate (Miltown (R)), RO 1-9569/12 (Nitoman (R)), and SCH-6673 (Tindal (R)) on the odor of schizophrenic sweat. *Am. J. Psychiat.* **117**, 1034–1035.
Smith, M. E. (1961). Clinical investigation of acetophenazine (Tindal), a new phenothiazine. *Psychosomatics* **2**, 112–116.
Taub, S. J. (1961). The management of anxiety in allergic disorders—a new approach. *Psychosomatics* **2**, 349–350.
Tortora, A. R. (1962). Influence of acetophenazine (Tindal) upon the attitude of cardiac patients. *J. Am. Geriat. Soc.* **10**, 270–273.
Welborn, W. S. (1961). A trial of a new tranquilizing agent in geriatric patients. *Psychosomatics* **2**, 450–452.
Welsh, A. L. (1964). The newer tranquilizing drugs. *Med. Clin. N. Am.* **48**, 459–481.
Witton, K., and Hermann, H. T. (1963). Clinical experiences with acetophenazine in the elderly psychotic. *Diseases Nervous System* **24**, 314–318.

~ A.2 ~
Carphenazine

Chemical Papers

Anonymous (1964). Qualitative and quantitative tests for carphenazine maleate. *J. Pharm. Sci.* **53**, 101–103.

Cares, R. M., and Buckman, C. (1963). Comparative review of the structure and side-effects of newer psychotropic agents. *Diseases Nervous System* **24**, Suppl., 91–105.

Heyman, J. J., Bayne, B., and Merlis, S. (1960). The estimation of phenothiazines using chemically impregnated paper strips. *Am. J. Psychiat.* **116**, 1108–1109.

Russell, P. B. (1961). Chemistry of carphenazine. *Diseases Nervous System* **22**, 5–6.

Seeman, P. M., and Bialy, H. S. (1963). The surface activity of tranquilizers. *Biochem. Pharmacol.* **12**, 1181–1191.

Sherlock, M. H., and Sperber, N. (1961). Piperazino derivatives and methods for their manufacture. U.S. Patent 2,985,654 Schering Corp.

Biology and Pharmacology

Collins, K., and Brunson, J. G. (1960). Further studies on the phenothiazine derivatives in experimental shock. *Circulation* **22**, 734 (abstr.).

Geller, I. (1961). Behavioral procedures used in evaluation of the psychopharmacological effects of carphenazine. *Diseases Nervous System* **22**, 19–22.

Hosko, M. J. (1961). EEG effects of carphenazine. *Diseases Nervous System* **22**, 14–18.

Kothari, N. J., Saunders, J. C., and Kline, N. S. (1961). Effect of phenothiazines and hydrazines on pituitary adrenal cortical response. *Psychopharmacologia* **2**, 22–26.

Stein, L. (1961). Inhibitory effects of phenothiazine compounds on self-stimulation of the brain. *Diseases Nervous System* **22**, 23–27.

Steiner, W. G., and Himwich, H. E. (1963). Effects of antidepressant drugs on limbic structures of rabbit. *J. Nervous Mental Disease* **137**, 277–284.

Tiangco, E., (1962). Intensive hepatological studies using carphenazine. *Am. J. Psychiat.* **118**, 845–846.

Tislow, R. (1961). Pharmacology and toxicity of carphenazine. *Diseases Nervous System* **22**, 7–13.

Tislow, R., Hosko, M. J., Wilson, S. P., Eckfeld, D. K., Gore, E. M., Hadley, F. V., and Begany, A. J. (1961). Pharmacological approach to neuroleptics. *Rev. Can. Biol.* **20**, 233–238; (1961). *Psychopharm. Abstr.* **1**, No. 12, 3139.

Side Effects

Freedman, D. X., and De Tong, J. (1961). Factors that determine drug-induced akathisia. *Diseases Nervous System* **22**, 69–76.

Goldman, D. (1961). Parkinsonism and related phenomena from administration of drugs: Their production and control under clinical conditions and possible relation to therapeutic effect. *Rev. Can. Biol.* **20**, 549–560.

Mendels, J. (1964). Transient toxicity with carphenazine hydrochloride. *Am. J. Psychiat.* **121**, 185–187.
Niver, E. O. (1962). Carphenazine and the extrapyramidal regulation of kinesthetic function. *Diseases Nervous System* **23**, 340–348.

Clinical Papers

Barron, A., Beckering, B., Rudy, L. H., and Smith, J. A. (1962). A comparison of a recently introduced phenothiazine derivative (MDS 92) and a placebo in chronically ill mental patients. *Am. J. Psychiat.* **119**, 68–69.
Barron, A., Rudy, L. H., and Smith, J. A. (1963). Comparison of a psychoactive drug and an anabolic steroid in chronically ill mental patients. *Am. J. Psychiat.* **119**, 1172–1173.
Barsa, J. A., and Saunders, J. C. (1962). Carphenazine in the treatment of chronic schizophrenics. *Am. J. Psychiat.* **119**, 169.
Bellville, T. P., Heistad, G. T., and Schiele, B. C. (1963). A comparative study of thioridazine and carphenazine using sequential analysis. *Psychopharmacologia* **4**, 53–65.
Cacioppo, J., Babikian, H., and Merlis, S. (1961). A comparison between trifluoperazine and carphenazine in chronically ill schizophrenic in-patients. *Diseases Nervous System* **22**, 46–50.
Carter, C. H. (1961). Carphenazine in mental defectives. A specific antiemetic. *Arch. Pediat.* **78**, 349–356.
Carter, C. H. (1962). Antiemetic specificity of carphenazine in brain damage. A blind crossover study with acetophenazine. *Am. J. Gastroenterol.* **38**, 587–591.
Chen, C. H., and Poim, S. (1963). Carphenazine in the treatment of schizophrenia. *Current Therap. Res.* **5**, 195–197.
Claffey, B., Margolis, L. H., and Mandel, W. (1962). Clinical evaluation of carphenazine and piperacetazine in previously placebo-treated chronic schizophrenics. *Am. J. Psychiat.* **119**, 75–76.
Goldman, D. (1961). Treatment of chronic schizophrenia with parenteral and oral carphenazine. *Diseases Nervous System* **22**, 51–57.
Kothari, N. J., Saunders, J. C., Kline, N. S., and Griffen, J. A. (1960). A comparison of perphenazine, Proketazine, nialamide and MO-482 in chronic schizophrenics. *Am. J. Psychiat.* **117**, 358–360.
Kothari, N. J., Park, I. H., Kline, N. S., and Saunders, J. C. (1961). Carphenazine therapy in hospitalized patients. *Diseases Nervous System* **22**, 58–59.
McCreight, D. W. (1961). Clinical evaluation of carphenazine. *Diseases Nervous System* **22**, 60–68.
Merlis, S. (1961). Use of carphenazine in severely ill psychiatric out-patients. *Diseases Nervous System* **22**, 42–45.
Oltman, J. E., and Friedman, S. (1961). Carphenazine in the treatment of schizophrenia. *Diseases Nervous System* **22**, 37–41.
Oltman, J. E., and Friedman, S. (1961). Treatment of schizophrenia with Proketazine. *Am. J. Psychiat.* **117**, 745–746.
Page, J. A. (1961). Discussion of paper on Proketazine. *Diseases Nervous System* **22**, 588–589.
Payne, R. W., Friedlander, D., Laverty, S. G., and Haden, P. (1963). Overinclusive thought disorder in chronic schizophrenics and its response to Proketazine. *Brit. J. Psychiat.* **109**, 523–530.
Peppel, H. H., and Joynes, T. (1963). Study design for clinical evaluation of phenothiazine derivatives. *Am. J. Psychiat.* **120**, 497–499.

Sainz, A. (1961). Comparison of the clinical effects of carphenazine and fluphenazine in chronic schizophrenics. *Diseases Nervous System* **22**, 77–79; pp. 585–587; Antipsychotic spectrum of Proketazine, Physiological reactivity of carphenazine in parenteral and oral use, pp. 28–29.

Solomon, S. (1963). Clinical trial of an antipsychotic agent with a low toxic index—carphenazine. *J. Neuropsychiat.* **5**, 80–85.

Stratas, N. E. (1964). Carphenazine in chronic schizophrenics. *Am. J. Psychiat.* **120**, 902–903.

Tobin, J. M. (1961). Summary of the findings in pharmacological and clinical studies of carphenazine. *Diseases Nervous System* **22**, 80–84.

Tyce, F. (1964). The chronic regressed schizophrenic. Prolonged oral treatment with carphenazine. *Minn. Med.* **47**, 795–798.

~ A.3 ~
Fluphenazine

Chemical Papers

Anders, M. W., and Mannering, G. J. (1962). Gas chromatography of some pharmacologically active phenothiazines. *J. Chromatog.* **7**, 258–260.

Berger, F. M. (1960). Classification and psychoactive drugs according to their chemical structures and sites of action. *In* "Drugs and Behavior" (L. Uhr and J. G. Miller, eds.), pp. 86–105. Wiley, New York.

Cares, R. M., *et al.* (1963). Comparative review of the structure and side-effects of newer psychotropic agents. *Diseases Nervous System* **24**, Pt. 2, 92–105. (Permitil).

Forrest, F. M., Forrest, I. S., and Mason A. S. (1959). A rapid, semi-quantitative urine color test for piperazine-linked phenothiazine drugs ('Compazine,' 'Trilafon' and analoguous compounds). *Am. J. Psychiat.* **116**, 549–551.

Forrest, F. M., Forrest, I. S., and Mason, A. S. (1961). Review of rapid urine tests for phenothiazine and related drugs. *Am. J. Psychiat.* **118**, 300–307.

Forrest, I. S., and Forrest, F. M. (1960). Urine color test for the detection of phenothiazine compounds. *Clin. Chem.* **6**, 11–15.

Forrest, I. S., *et al.* (1964). Comment on Posner's and Levine's "inability to validate the urinary FPN test for phenothiazine drugs." *J. Nervous Mental Disease* **138**, 90–91.

Gothelf, B., *et al.* (1963). Quantitative colorimetric method and extraction procedure for determination of chlorpromazine in animal tissues. *Intern. J. Neuropharmacol.* **2**, 95–99.

Parker, K. D., Rontan, C. R., and Kirk, P. L. (1962). Separation and identification of tranquilizers by gas chromatography. *Anal. Chem.* **34**, 757–760.

Rajeswaran, P., and Kirk, P. L. (1961). Tranquilizing and related drugs: Properties for their identification (Part I). *Bull. Narcotics, U.N., Dept. Social Affairs* **13**, 15–37. (Permitil cited as Trancin also.)

Rajeswaren, P., and Kirk, P. L. (1961). Tranquilizing and related drugs: Properties for their identification (Part II). *Bull. Narcotics, U.N., Dept. Social Affairs* **13**, 21–32.

Rajeswaren, P., and Kirk, P. L. (1962). Tranquilizing and related drugs: Properties for their identication (Part III). *Bull. Narcotics, U.N., Dept. Social Affairs* **14**, 19–33.

Sunshine, I. (1963). Use of thin layer chromatography in the diagnosis of poisoning. *Am. J. Clin. Pathol.* **40**, 576–582.

Yung, D. K., *et al.* (1963). Identification and differentiation of some phenothiazine-type tranquilizers. *J. Pharm. Sci.* **52**, 365–370.

Biology and Pharmacology

Bruns, W., *et al.* (1963). Tierexperimentelle Untersuchungen zur Beeinflussung des Radiojodtestes durch Hypnotica aund Sedativa. *Arzneimittel-Forsch.* **13**, 796–798.

Burke, J. C., *et al.* (1962). Depot action of fluphenazine (Prolixin) enanthate in oil. *Federation Proc.* **21**, 339. (Prolixin.)

Burkman, A. M. (1962). Potent anti-apomorphine action of fluphenazine in pigeons. *Arch. Intern. Pharmacodyn.* **137**, 396–403.

Denhoff, E. (1964). Cerebral palsy—a pharmacologic approach. *Clin. Pharmacol. Therap.* **5**, Pt. 2, 947–954.

Dobkin, A. B., and Purkin, N. (1960). The antisialogogue effect of phenothiazine derivatives. *Brit. J. Anaesthesia* **32**, 57–59. (Trancin.)

Dobkin, A. B., Keil, A. McL., and Wong, G. (1961). Circulatory response to tilt with phenothiazines. *Anaesthesia* **16**, 160–171, No. 2; *Psychopharmacol. Abstr.* **1**, 144–145.

Dobkin, A. B., Woodworth, H., and Israel, J. S. (1962). The antisialogogue effect of hydroxyzine, thiethylperazine, and N'-p-chloro-benzylhydryl-N'-methyl homopiperazine (SA 97). *Can. Anaesthesial. Soc. J.* **9**, 234–238.

Emmerson, J. L., *et al.* (1963). Metabolism of phenothiazine drugs. *J. Pharm. Sci.* **52**, 411–419.

Friend, D. G. (1964). Pharmacology of muscle relaxants. *Clin. Pharmacol. Therap.* **5**, 871–878.

Gozsy, G., and Kato, L. (1962). Prevention de la reaction anaphylactique chez le rat. *Compt. Rend. Soc. Biol.* **156**, 556–559.

Guttman, H. N., *et al.* (1963). Evaluation of phenothiazines as membrane permeability alterants. Paper presented at 47th Annual Meeting, Atlantic City, New Jersey, April 16–20, 1963; *Federation Proc.* **22**, 569 (abstr.).

Guttman, H. N., *et al.* (1963). Protozoa as pharmacological tools: The phenothiazine tranquilizers. *Trans. N.Y. Acad. Sci.* [2] **26**, 75–89.

Hendley, C. D., Chow, M.-I., and Mechner, F. (1959). A method for measuring effects of drugs on visual discrimination in the cat. *Pharmacologist* **1**, No. 2.

High, J. P., Hassert, G. L., Jr., Rubin, B., Piala, J. J., Burke, J. C., and Craver, B. N. (1960). Pharmacology of fluphenazine (Prolixin). *Toxicol. Appl. Pharmacol.* **2**, 540–552.

Irwin, S. (1959). Comparative potency of phenothiazine tranquilizers in suppressing avoidance and locomotor behavior: its implications. Paper presented at the Miami meeting of the American Society for Pharmacology and Experimental Therapeutics, Inc., Aug. 31–Sept. 3, 1959; *Pharmacologist* **1**, 51.

Kato, L., and Gozsy, B. (1961). Effect of psychopharmacological agents on the capillary endothelium. *Rev. Can. Biol.* **20**, No. 2, 261–270; *Psychopharmacol. Abstr.* **1**, 656.

Lieberman, W. (1964). Objective measurement of external anal. sphincter tension. *Am. J. Proctol.* **15**, 375–381. (Orpitil.)

Mercier, J., *et al.* (1964). Contribution a l'etude pharmacologique de la fluphenazine (3 trifluoromethyl) 10-phenothiazinyl-propyl-piperazine ethanol) II.–Actions exercees sur l'appareil respiratoire, l'appareil cardiovasculaire, l'appareil digestif. *Arch. Intern. Pharmacodyn.* **152**, 416–432.

Myers, H. M., *et al.* (1963). Pharmacology of the sedative-hypnotic and tranquilizing drugs. *Dental Clin. N. Am.* pp. 489–502. (Permitil.)

Rao, M. N., *et al.* (1963). The antiemetic efficacy of Fluphenazine with comparative results of the inventory and biometrical evaluation. *Anesthesia and Analgesia, Current Res.* **42**, 253–261. (Prolixin.)

Scott, G. T., and Nading, L. K. (1961). Relative effectiveness of phenothiazine tranquilizing drugs causing release of MSH. *Proc. Soc. Exptl. Biol. Med.* **106**, 88–90.

Smith, C. I., and Burke, J. C. (1960). Enzymatic hydrolysis of acetylfluphenazine to fluphenazine by certain mammalian tissues in vitro. *Toxicol. Appl. Pharmacol.* **2**, 553–557.

Steiner, W. G., *et al.* (1963). Effects of antidepressant drugs on limbic structures of rabbit. *J. Nervous Mental Disease* **137**, 277–284. (Permitil.)

Steiner, W. G., *et al.* (1963). An electroencephalographic study of some structural aspects of D-amphetamine antagonism in phenothiazine and related compounds. *Intern. J. Neuropharmacol.* **2**, 327–335.

Stevens, J. D. (1964). Psychopharmacology. *J. Neuropsychiat.* **5**, 566–576. (Permitil.)

Taber, R. I., Irwin, S., and Fox, J. E. (1964). Comparison of the enanthates of perphenazine and fluphenazine. Presented at the Fall Meeting of the American Society for Pharmacology and Experimental Therapy, Inc. Aug. 24–27, 1964; *Pharmacologist* **6**, 179. (Permitil.)

Usdin, E., and Usdin, V. R. (1961). Effects of psychotropic compounds on enzyme systems II. In vitro inhibition of monoamine oxidase. *Proc. Soc. Exptl. Biol. Med.* **108**, 461–463.

Side Effects

Anderson, J. H., and Sanchex-Longe, L. P. (1961). The complications and side effects of the phenothiazine ataraxics. A review of 173 clinical series of 10 phenothiazine derivates. *Bol. Asoc. Med. Puerto Rico* **53**, 123–151.
Anstreicher, K. (1960). Fatalities during or following fluphenazine therapy. *Delaware State Med. J.* **32**, 430–434.
Arneson, G. A. (1961). The risk of the new psychotropic drugs. *J. Louisiana State Med. Soc.* **113**, 372–376.
Ayd, F. J., Jr. (1960). Drug-induced extrapyramidal reactions: their clinical manifestations and treatment with Akineton. *Psychosomatics* **1**, 143–150.
Ayd, F. J., Jr. (1961). Neuroleptics and extrapyramidal reactions in psychiatric patients. *Proc. Intern. Symp. Extrapyramidal System and Neuroleptics, Montreal, 1960* (J. M. Bordeleau, ed.), pp. 355–363. Editions Psychiatriques, Montreal.
Ayd, F. J., Jr. (1961). A survey of drug-induced extra-pyramidal reactions. *J. Am. Med. Assoc.* **175**, 1054–1060.
Ayd, F. J., Jr. (1963). Uses and side effects of phenothiazines. *Mind* **1**, 326–348; (1964). *Appl. Therap.* **6**, 301 and 303 (abstr.).
Ben-David, M., et al. (1965). Production of lactation by non-sedative phenothiazine derivatives. *Proc. Soc. Exptl. Biol. Med.* **118**, 265–270. (Prolixin.)
Brooks, G., et al. (1963). The effect of potassium on phenothiazine-induced extrapyramidal system dysfunction. *Am. J. Psychiat.* **119**, 1096–1097. (Prolixin.)
Burns, R. P. (1961). Ocular side effects of systemic medication. *Northwest. Med.* **2**, 1083–1092.
Cares, R. M., and Buckman, C. (1961). A survey of side-effects and or toxicity of newer psychopharmacologic agents. *Diseases Nervous System* **22**, Pt. 2, 97–105.
Childers, R. T., Jr. (1962). Procyclidine and benztropine methansulfonate compared in drug induced extrapyramidal reactions. *Am. J. Psychiat.* **119**, 462–463.
Cole, J. O., and Clyde, D. J. (1961). Extrapyramidal side effects and clinical response to the phenothiazines. *Proc. Intern. Symp. Extrapyramidal System and Neuroleptics, Montreal, 1960* (J. M. Bordeleau, ed.), pp. 469–478. Editions Psychiatriques, Montreal.
Dubois, J. R., Jr. (1963). Neurologic complications of phenothiazine therapy. *Henry Ford Hosp. Med. Bull.* **11**, 59–63. (Permitil.)
Goldman, D. (1961). Parkinsonism and related phenomena from administration of drugs: Their production and control under clinical conditions and possible relation to therapeutic effect. *Proc. Intern. Symp. Extrapyramidal System and Neuroleptics, Montreal, 1960* (J. M. Bordeleau, ed.), pp. 453–464. Editions Psychiatriques, Montreal.
Goldman, D. (1961). Parkinsonism and related phenomena from administration of drugs: Their production and control under clinical conditions and possible relation to therapeutic effect. *Rev. Can. Biol.* **20**, No. 2, 549–560; *Psychopharmacol. Abstr.* **1**, 631.
Haase, H. J. (1961). Extrapyramidal modification of fine movements—a "conditio sine qua non" of the fundamental therapeutic action of neuroleptic drugs. *Proc. Intern. Symp. Extrapyramidal System and Neuroleptics, Montreal, 1960* (J. M. Bordeleau. ed.), pp. 329–353. Editions Psychiatriques, Montreal.
Hollister, L. E. (1964). Adverse reactions to phenothiazines. *J. Am. Med. Assoc.* **189**, 311–313. (Permitil.)
Hollister, L. E. (1961). Current concepts in therapy. Complications from psychotherapeutic drugs. I. *New Engl. J. Med.* **264**, 291–293.

Hollister, L. E. (1964). Complications from psychotherapeutic drugs—1964. *Clin. Pharmacol. Therap.* **5**, 322–333.

Hooper, J. H., Jr., Welch, V. C., and Shackelford, R. T. (1961). Abnormal lactation associated with tranquilizing drug therapy. *J. Am. Med. Assoc.* **178**, 506–507.

Kennedy, B., *et al.* (1961). Phototoxic and photoallergic skin reactions resulting from modern drug therapy. *J. Louisiana State Med. Soc.* **113**, 365–371.

Kothari, U. C. (1961). A case of accidental overdosage with Permitil. Clinical report. *Current Therap. Res.* **3**, 329–332.

Kruse, W. (1960). Treatment of drug-induced extrapyramidal symptoms. A comparative study of three antiparkinson agents. *Diseases Nervous System* **21**, 79–81.

Kruse, W. (1960). The relationship between the anti-hallucinatory effect and extrapyramidal symptoms induced by fluphenazine. (A study in 40 chronic schizophrenics.) *Current Therap. Res.* **3**, 19–22.

Kruse, W. (1963). Development of Parkinsonism after gradual reduction of fluphenazine dosage. *Am. J. Psychiat.* **119**, 995–996.

Lehmann, H. E. (1963). Use and abuse of phenothiazines. *Appl. Therap.* **5**, 1057–1060, 1062, 1067, and 1069. (Permitil.)

Mandel, W., and Oliver, W. A. (1961). Withdrawal of maintenance antiparkinson drug in the phenothiazine-induced extrapyramidal reaction. *Am. J. Psychiat.* **118**, 350–351.

Proctor, R. C. (1960). The use and abuse of tranquilizing drugs. *J. Tenn. State Med. Assoc.* **53**, 295–299.

Rodman, M. J. (1964). Management in drug abuse and addiction. *RN* **27**, 59–64 and 77–79.

Shideman, F. E. (1961). Toxicity of the phenothiazines. *Wisconsin Med. J.* **60**, 487–488.

Simonson, M. (1964). Phenothiazine depressive reaction. *J. Neuropsychiat.* **5**, 259–265. (Permitil.)

Wachsmuth, R. (1962). Problems der psychiatrischen Pharmakotherapie und die Stellung des Flugphenazine in der Behandlung der Psychosen. *Arzneimittel-Forsch.* **16**, 87–95.

Walters, G. M., *et al.* (1963). Jaundice following administration of fluphenazine dihydrochloride. *Am. J. Psychiat.* **120**, 81–82. (Prolixin.)

Clinical Papers

Aceves Ortega, R. (1961). Flufenazine en dormatologia. *Semana Med. Mex.* **28**, 289–290. (Teviral (Permitil).)

Adriani, J., Summers, F. W., and Antony, S. O. (1961). Is the prophylactic use of antiemetics in surgical patients justified. *J. Am. Med. Assoc.* **175**, 666–671.

Adriani, J., Arens, J., and Antony, S. O. (1962). Postanesthetic vomiting. *Am. J. Surg.* **103**, 2–5.

Ahumada, M. (1964). La utilidad del clorhidrato de flufenzina en dermatologia. *Medico, Mexico* **13**, 51–53.

Alexander, H. G. (1962). Combined fluphenazine and ECT in acute schizophrenia. *Diseases Nervous System* **23**, 526–532.

Alexander, J., *et al.* (1964). Anti-emetic effects of a phenothiazine compared with an antihistamine. *Practitioner* **193**, 358–360. (Moditen.)

Ancona, A. (1961). Fluphenazine (Anatensol): Characteristics and properties. *Boll. Chim. Farm.* **100**, 623–625. (In Italian.)

Archer, J. S., Smessaert, A. A., and Hicks, R. G. (1962). Phenothiazine tranquilizers in anesthesia. Review, with report on fluphenazine. *N. Y. State J. Med.* **62**, 828–833.

Archer, J. S. (1961). The amazing phenothiazines. *N. Y. Med.* **17**, 221–224.

Archer, J. S., and Hicks, R. G. (1962). Phenothiazine subgroups. *N. Y. State J. Med.* **62**, 3769–3772.

Arnedo Gutierrez, J. A. (1963). Indicaciones y eficacia de la flufenazina en preanestesia. *Dia. Med.* **35**, 1382–1383. (Siqualine.)
Auch, W. (1962). Neuroleptische Therapie bei antriebsbehemmten Patieten. *Med. Klin.* (*Munich*) **57**, 1266–1267.
Ayd, F. J., Jr. (1959). Fluphenazine: its spectrum of therapeutic application and clinical results in psychiatric patients. *Current Therap. Res.* **1**, 41–48.
Ayd, F. J., Jr. (1960). Current status of major tranquilizers. *J. Med. Soc. New Jersey* **57**, 4–14.
Ayd, F. J., Jr. (1960). Tranquilizers and the ambulatory geriatric patient. *J. Am. Geriat. Soc.* **8**, 909–914.
Ayd, F. J., Jr. (1961). Phenothiazine tranquilizers: Eight years of development. *Med. Clin. N. Am.* **45**, 1027–1040.
Ayd, F. J., Jr. (1962). Nialamide therapy for the depressed geriatric patient. *J. Am. Geriat. Soc.* **10**, 432–435.
Bailey, H. R., Blow, J. S., and Sandes, S. G. (1960). "Siqualine" (fluphenazine) in psychiatric practice: a preliminary report. *Med. J. Australia* **1**, 885–887.
Barsa, J. A. (1960). Combination drug therapy in psychiatry. *Am. J. Psychiat.* **117**, 448–449.
Barsa, J. A., and Saunders, J. C. (1961). Fluphenazine use with chronic psychotic patients. *Diseases Nervous System* **22**, 211–212.
Barsa, J. A., and Saunders, J. C. (1962). Carphenazine in the treatment of chronic schizophrenics. *Am. J. Psychiat.* **119**, 169.
Batterman, R. C., et al. (1963). Comparative treatment of the psychoneurotic reactive-type anxiety state with fluphenazine and chloriazepoxide. *J. New Drugs* **3**, 297–301. (Permiti Chronotab.)
Beavers, W. R. (1963). Evaluating drugs used in emotional illness. *Texas State J. Med.* **59**, 844–847. (Permitil.)
Bellville, J. W. (1961). Postanesthetic nausea and vomiting. *Anesthesiology* **22**, 773–780.
Bellville, J. W., Bross, I. D. J., and Howland, W. S. (1960). Postoperative nausea and vomiting IV: Factors related to postoperative nausea and vomiting. *Anesthesiology* **21**, 186–193.
Bellville, J. W., Howland, W. S., Bross, I. D. J. (1960) Postoperative nausea and vomiting. *J. Am. Med. Assoc.* **172**, 1488–1493.
Benson, W. M., and Schiele, B. C. (1960). Current status of tranquilizing and antidepressive drugs. *J. Lancet* **80**, 579–592.
Benzecry, E., et al. (1963). La flufenazina en la practica clinica y oftalmologica. *Dia Med.* **35**, 1527–1530. (Elinol Cronotabs.)
Berzewski, H. (1964). Die medikamentose Dauertherapie der Schizophrenein. *Pharmakotherapia* **2**, 181–189.
Black, J. (1960). Phenothiazines as antiemetics and tranquilizers. *J. Med. Assoc. Alabama* **29**, 492–500.
Bodi, T., et al. (1961). Clinical evaluation of fluphenazine in cases of anxiety and other psychoneuroses. *Postgrad. Med.* **29**, 408–414.
Bonica, J. J., et al. (1962). Clinical evaluation of fluphenazine dihydrochloride as antiemetic agent. *Anesthesia Analgesia Current Res.* **41**, 732–739. (Proxlixin.)
Braceland, F. J. (1964). Drugs effective in emotional disorders. *Postgrad. Med.* **35**, 237–242. (Permitil.)
Brett, R. J. (1961). A note on the tranquilizers. *Rocky Mt. Med. J.* **58**, 34–35 and 59–60.
Brougher, J. C. (1960). Use of an antiemetic agent in nausea and vomiting associated with pregnancy. *Western Med.* **1**, 9–11.
Buitragò, D. (1961). Flufenazina, un nuevo tranquilizante. Experiencia terapeutica. *Med. Panam.* **17**, 256–261.
Burke, J. C., High, J. P., Laffan, R. J., and Ravaris, C. L. (1962). Depot action of fluphenazine (Prolixin) enanthate in oil. *Federation Proc.* **21**, 339.

Burkman, A. M. (1962). Potent anti-apomorphine action of fluphenazine in pigeons. *Arch. Intern. Pharmacodyn.* **137**, 396–403.

Caffey, E. M., Jr. (1962). The use of drugs in outpatient and inpatient psychiatric practice. *Virginia Med. Monthly* **89**, 55–59. (Prolixin.)

Camba, M. E., et al. (1964). Diclohidrato de flufenazina. *Dia Med.* **36**, 116–117.

Cardenas, A., et al. (1963). La terapia farmacologica y los factores psicologicos en la emesis del embarazo. *Tribuna Med.* **3**, 1 and 12–13. (Emesil.)

Cardenas Torre, R. (1960). Fluphenazine in apprehension and anxiety neuroses. *Semana Med., Mex.* **27**, 173–176.

Carsley, S.H., and Olson, J. A. (1962). Use of fluphenazine dihydrochloride for relief of anxiety. *Clin. Med.* **69**, 717–720.

Cattell, J. P., and Malitz, S. (1960). Revised survey of selected psychopharmacological agents. *Am. J. Psychiat.* **117**, 449–453.

Chesrow, E. J. (1963). Fluphenazine in the treatment of the disturbed chronically ill and aged patient. *Illinois Med. J.* **124**, 238–241. (Permitil.)

Childers, R. T., Jr. (1961). Controlling the chronically disturbed patient with massive phenothiazine therapy. *Am. J. Psychiat.* **118**, 246–247.

Childers, R. T. (1962). Use of fluphenazine in acute and chronic schizophrenics. *Current Therap. Res.* **4**, Suppl., 224–227.

Childers, R. T., Jr. (1964). Comparison of four regimens in newly admitted female schizophrenics. *Am. J. Psychiat.* **120**, 1010–1011.

Collignon, C. (1963). Emesis gravidica. Su tratamiento con flufenazina-piridoxina. *Semana Med. Mex.* **36**, 478–480. (Pregnidox.)

Coodley, E. L. (1963). Clinical evaluation of combined orphenadrine-fluphenazine in acute and chornic musculoskeletal disorders. *Clin. Med.* **70**, 1843–1850. (Orpitil.)

Corum, L. T. (1962). Fluphenazine (Prolixin) as an antiemetic agent in children. *J. Florida Med. Assoc.* **68**, 890–891.

Cremieux, A., et al. (1963). Effects de la fluphenazine (Moditen) en therapeutique psychiatrique. A propos de 40 observations. Paper given at Soc. psychiat. Marseille, May 8, 1963. *Ann. Med.-Psychol.* **121**, 106 (abstr.). (Moditen.)

Cure, W. (1960–1961). Flufenazina en el tratamiento de los estados angustiosos de la practica medica general. *Med. Cir.* **24**, 232.

Dale, P. W. (1961). Current concepts in therapy. Medical management of mental problems in the aged. *New Engl. J. Med.* **265**, 84–86.

Darling, H. F. (1959). Prolixin in hospitalized female psychiatric patients. *Squibb Clin. Res. Notes* II 9–10.

Darling, H. F. (1959). Fluphenazine: A preliminary study. *Diseases Nervous System* **20**, 167–170.

Darling, H. F., Hess, G. H., Capistrano, A. C., and Hoermann, M. G. (1960). Fluphenazine: Comparative studies. *Disease Nervous System* **21**, 409–413.

Denber, H. C. B., et al. (1962). Peinture et effects secondaires des neuroleptiques majeurs. *Ann. Med.-Psychol.* **1**, 11–30; *Psychopharmacol. Abstr.* **2**, 172–173.

Denhoff, E. (1964). Cerebral palsy. *In* "Current Therapy" (H. F. Conn, ed.), pp. 504–508. Saunders, Philadelphia, Pennsylvania. (Permitil.)

Denzel, H. A. (1961). Fluphenazine in the treatment of psychotic patients. *J. Clin. Exptl. Psychopathol.* **22**, 34–37.

Deom, P., Buxbaum, H., and Gatski, R. L. (1962). Experience with fluphenazine in a psychiatric hospital. *Diseases Nervous System* **23**, 231–235.

Detre, T., and Jarecki, H. (1961). A practical guide to the use of psychopharmacological agents in general practice. *Conn. State Med. J.* **25**, 553–565.

DiPalma, J. R. (1963). The basic pharmacologic principles underlying the use of sedatives and tranquilizers. *Clin. Pediat.* **2**, 225–232. (Permitil.)

Dobkin, A. B., and Purkin, N. (1960). The antisialogogue effect of phenothiazine derivatives. *Brit. J. Anaesthesia* **32**, 57–59.

Dobkin, A. B. (1960). Potentiation of thiopentone anaesthesia. Comparisone of promethazine, chlorpromazine, perphenazine, fluphenazine, thiopropazate, pipamazine and triflupromazine. *Brit. J. Anaesthesia* **32**, 424–426.

Dube, A. H. (1960). A workable program for senile mental changes. *Virginia Med. Monthly* **87**, 614–618.

Dundee, J. W., et al. (1963). Alterations in response to somatic pain associated with anaesthesia. XV: Further studies with phenothiazine derivatives and similar drugs. *Brit. J. Anaesthesia* **35**, 597–610. (Prolixin.)

Dunlop, E. (1962). Fluphenazine dihydrochloride—an anti-anxiety agent. *J. Neuropsychiat.* **3**, 251–253.

Dundee, J. W., et al. (1964). Clinical studies of induction agents. X. The effect of phenothiazine premedication on thiopentone anaesthesia. *Brit. J. Anaesthesia* **36**, 106–109.

Dussik, K. T. (1960). The awakening from psychosis. *J. Neuropsychiat.* **2**, 41–48.

Ebert, A. G., et al. (1963). The metabolism of C^{14}-fluphenazine (Prolixin) enanthate. Paper presented at 47th Annual Meeting, Atlantic City, New Jersey, April 16–20, 1963; *Federation Proc.* **22**, 539 (abstr.). (Prolixin.)

Ebert, A. G. (1964). Studies on the mechanism of the prolonged action of fluphenazine (Prolixin) enanthate. *Federation Proc.* **23**, Pt. 1, 489 (2325).

Enelow, A. J. (1964). A brief review of clinical psychopharmacology. *Ariz. Med.* **21**, 161–163.

Ernst, E. M. (1960). Clinical study of fluphenazine in general practice. *Clin. Med.* **7**, No. 5, 1349–1353.

Flaherty, J. A. (1961). Permitil: An evaluation of its use in psychiatric outpatients. *Delaware State Med. J.* **33**, 217–224.

Fogel, E. J., and Matheu, H. (1962). Results with fluphenazine in chronic schizophrenia. *Current Therap. Res.* **4**, Suppl. 213–217.

Foltz, L. M. (1962). Critical evaluation of tranquilizers. *J. Kentucky Med. Assoc.* **60**, 733–738. (Permitil.)

Fouks, L. (1962). Pharmacopsychotherapy and geriatrics. *Geriatrie* pp. 209–215.

Fouks, L., et al. (1961). Rappors sur l'essai clinique de la fluphenazine en therapeutique psychiatrique. Paper presented at Groupe d'etutde de Psycho-Pharmacologie Biochimique Society Moreau-de-Tours, April 30, 1961; (1962). *Presse Med.* **69**, 2399 (abstr.).

Fouks, M. (1961). La fluphenazine. Indications cliniques. *Scalpel* **46**, 1061.

Fouks, M., et al. (1961). La fluphenazine, ses indications therapeutiques. *Ann. Med.-Psychol.* **119**, No. 3, 572–578; *Psychopharmacol. Abstr.* **1**, 231.

Fouks, M., et al. (1961). Rapport sur l'essai clinique de la fluphenazine en therapeutique, psychiatrique. *Semaine Hop. Paris* **37**, No. 59, 2858; *Psychopharmacol. Abstr.* **1**, 642.

Fox, V. (1960). The management of alcoholism. *J. Med. Assoc. Alabama* **29**, 501–505.

Freyhan, F. A. The relationship of drug-induced neurological phenomena on therapeutic outcome. *Proc. Intern. Symp. Extrapyramidal System and Neuroleptics*, Montreal, 1960 pp. 483–486. Editions Psychiatriques, J. M. Bordeleau, Ed., Montreal.

Frieberg, M. (1961). Clinical report on fluphenazine. *Svenska Lakartidn.* **58**, No. 12, 932–937; *Psychopharmacol. Abstr.* **1**, 437.

Funcia, R. A. J. (1961). Experiencias medicas psiquiatricas con un nuevo derivado fenotiazinico. *Prensa Med. Arg.* **48**, 896–897.

Garcia De La Villa, A., et al. (1964). Terapeutica con flufenazina en altas dosis en enfermos cronicos. *Med. Panam.* **22**, 199–200.

Gayral, L., Herve, Y., Stern, H., and Bardis, C. (1962). Notes sur la fluphenazine. *Presse Med.* **70**, 1415.
Goldman, D. (1959). Prolixin in the treatment of psychotic symptoms. *Squibb Clin. Res. Notes* II 3.
Gould, A. H. (1962). Combined dexbrompheniramine-fluphenazine (Diperm Chronotab) in the oral treatment of pruritus. *J. New Drugs* **2**, 179–182. (Diperm Chronotabs.)
Gray, W. D. (1960). A clinical evaluation of fluphenazine. *Intern. Record Med.* **173**, 375–379.
Grimaldi, R. (1960). The clinical use of fluphenazine in pregnancy. *J. N. Y. Med. Coll., Flower Fifth Ave. Hosp.* **2**, 42–49.
Gross, H., *et al.* (1963). La fluphenazine (Lyogen), nouvel antipsychotique phenothiazinique. *Wien. Med. Wochschr.* **113**, 112; *Nouveautes Med.* **12**, 495–497. (Lyogen.)
Haase, H. J. (1961). Das therapeutische Achsensyndrom neuroleptische Medikaments und seine Beziehungen zu extrapyramidaler Symptomatik. *Fortschr. Neurol. Psychiat.* **29**, 245–268; *Abstr. World Med.* **30**, 326–327.
Haase, H. J. (1963). Möglichkeiten und Grenzen der Psychopharmakotherapie mit Tranquilizern und Neuroleptika. *Deut. Med. Wochschr.* **88**, 505–514. (Permitil.)
Hankoff, L. D., Mendelsohn, F. S., and Paley, H. M. (1960). Fluphenazine treatment in a receiving hospital setting. *Diseases Nervous System* **21**, 467–472.
Heather, A. J. (1963). An evaluation of an orphenadrine-fluphenazine combination as an antispastic and muscle relaxant. *Current Therap. Res.* **5**, 37–81. (Orpitil.)
Heseltine, W. W. (ed.) (1961). "Fluphenazine in Anxiety and Tension", 92 pp. Birchall, Liverpool.
Hewitt, M. I. (1960). Which tranquilizer? *J. Indiana State Med. Assoc.* **53**, 1475–1483.
Himwich, H. W. (1959). The management of alcoholism. *Mod. Med. Minneapolis* **27**, 23–32.
Himwich, H. E. (1960). Some drugs useful in the treatment of emotional disorders-physiology, indications, and contraindications. *Am. Practitioner Dig. Treat.* **11**, 687–698.
Himwich, H. E. (1965). Psychoactive drugs. *Postgrad. Med.* **37**, 35–44.
Hoerner, E. F., *et al.* (1963). The effect of skeletal muscle relaxant on muscle extensibility. *Ind. Med. Surg.* **32**, 516–520.
Holt, J. P., and Wright, E. R. (1960). Preliminary results with fluphenazine in chronic psychotic patients. *Am. J. Psychiat.* **117**, 157–159.
Holt, J. P., and Wright, E. R. (1961). Clinical evaluation of fluphenazine in the treatment of psychotic patients. *Diseases Nervous System* **22**, 513–519.
Hordern, A. (1961). Psychiatry and the tranquilizers. *New Engl. J. Med.* **265**, 584–588.
Howell, R. J., Brown, H. M., Jr., and Beaghler, H. E. (1960). Fairway project: A comparison to two phenothiazine tranquilizers and a placebo. *Provo Papers* **4**, 1–49.
Howell, R. J., Brown, H. M., and Beaghler, H. E. (1961). A comparison of fluphenazine, trifluoperazine and a placebo in the context of an active treatment unit. *J. Nervous Mental Disease* **132**, 522–530.
Hurst, L. (1960). Phenothiazine derivatives in the treatment of schizophrenia. *J. Mental Sci.* **106**, 755–770.
Hyman, Y. K., and Orkin, L. R. (1962). Triflupromazine and fluphenazine as adjuncts in anesthetic management. *N. Y. State J. Med.* **62**, 480–485.
Iliopoulos, C., and Gatski, R. L. (1961). Fluphenazine treatment of behavioral disorders. *Comprehensive Psychiat.* **2**, 364–367.
Irwin, S. (1961). Correlation in rats between the locomotor and avoidance suppressant potencies of eight phenothiazine tranquilizers. *Arch. Intern. Pharmacodyn.* **132**, 279–286.
Irwin, S. (1959). Comparative potency of phenothiazine tranquilizers in suppressing avoidance and locomotor behaviour: its implications. *Pharmacologist* **1**, No. 2.
Jassin, A., and Jose Juliaa, J. (1962). La flufenazina en el tratamiento de la tension premenstrual. *Orient. Med.* **9**, 20–21.
Johnson, A. G., *et al.* (1964). Allergic pericarditis. *Brit. Med. J.* I, 481–482. (Diperm Chronotabs.)

Jordan, D. M. (1961). Some practical aspects of the antidepressant drugs. *Illinois Med. J.* **120**, 219–221.
Kalinowsky, L. B., and Hoch, P. H. (1961). Pharmacotherapy. *In* "Somatic treatments in psychiatry"(L. B. Kalinowsky, ed.), pp. 65–66. Grune & Stratton, New York.
King, J. T., et al. (1963). Perinatal findings in women treated during pregnancy with oral fluphenazine. *J. New Drugs* **3**, 21–25. (Permitil Chronotabs.)
Kinross-Wright, J., Rowell, R. C., and Otero, M. J. (1962). Fluphenazine in treatment of chronic schizophrenia. *Diseases Nervous System* **23**, 152–155.
Kinross-Wright, J., et al. (1963). A new method of drug therapy. *Am. J. Psychiat.* **119**, 779–780.
Klerman, G. L. (1961). NIMH collaborative study of phenothiazine treatment of acute schizophrenic psychoses. *Trans. 6th Res. Conf. Coop. Chemotherapy Studies Psychiat. Broad Res. Approaches to Mental Illness*, 1961 pp. 30–38, Psychopharmacology Service Center, Bethesda, Md.
Kline, N. S. (1961). The use of psychopharmaceuticals in office practice. *Med. Clin. N. Am.* **45**, 1677–1684.
Kline, N. S., et al. (1964). A long-acting phenothiazine in office practice. *Am. J. Psychiat.* **120**, 1012–1014. (Prolixin enanthate.)
Knoble, M., et al. (1963). Experiencia clinica con el dichlorhidrato de flufenazina, ansiolitico de amplio espectro. *Dia Med.* **35**, 1181–1182. (Elinol Chronotabs.)
Kossover, M. F., and Goldman, A. M. (1961). Clinical experience with fluphenazine (Prolixin) a new phenothiazine drug. *J. Louisiana State Med. Soc.* **113**, 516–520.
Kraines, S. H. (1964). Psychotropic drugs in general practice. *Memphis Mid-South Med. J.* **39**, 9–27.
Kris, E. B. (1962). Post-hospital care of patients in their community. *Current Therap. Res.* **4**, Suppl., 200–205.
Kruse, W. (1960). Persistent muscular restlessness after phenothiazine treatment: report of 3 cases. *Am. J. Psychiat.* **117**, 152–153.
Kudo, Y. (1961). Effect of fluphenazine in psychoneurosis. *J. New Drugs & Clin.* **10**, No. 5, 428–430; *Psychopharmacol. Abstr.* **1**, 642.
Kugele, L. (1961). Vegetative Fehlsteuerung an den Ableitenden Harnwegen und ihre Behandlung mit Fluphenazin. *Med. Welt* **43**, 2244–2245; *Psychopharmacol. Abstr.* **1**, 618.
Kurland, A. A., Hanlon, T. E., Tatom, M. H., and Simopoulos, A. M. (1961). Comparative studies of the phenothiazine tranquilizers: methodological and logistical considerations. *J. Nervous Mental Diseases* **132**, 61–74.
Kurland, A. A., Hanlon, T. E., and Ota, K. Y. (1961). Fluphenazine in the treatment of the hospitalized psychiatric patient. *Diseases Nervous System* **22**, 339–343.
Kurland, A. A., et al. (1964). Fluphenazine (Prolixin) enanthate a phenothiazine preparation of prolonged activity. *Current Therap. Res.* **6**, 137–147.
Laffan, R. J., Papandrianos, D. P., Burke, J. C., and Craver, B. N. (1961). Antiemetic action of fluphenazine (Prolixin) a comparison with other phenothiazines. *J. Pharmacol. Exptl. Therap.* **131**, 130–134.
Lapolla, A. (1961). Fluphenazine in the treatment of hospitalized psychotic females. *Western Med.* **11**, 110, 113–116, and 132. (Prolixin.)
LaSalle, M. W. (1964). Carphenazine in chronic schizophrenia. *Am. J. Psychiat.* **121**, 494–495.
Lavalle, A., et al. (1962). Vomiting of pregnancy: Its treatment with a combination of fluphenazine and pyridoxine. *Semana Med., Mex.* **29**, 373–374. (Pregnidox.)
La Veck, G. D., de la Cruz, F., and Simundson, E. (1960). Fluphenazine in the treatment of mentally retarded children with behavior disorders. *Diseases Nervous System* **21**, Pt. 1, 82–85.
LaVeck, G. D., and Buckley, P. (1961). The use of psychopharmacologic agents in retarded children with behavior disorders. *J. Chronic Diseases* **13**, 174–183.
Lear, E., Suntay, R., Fisch, H. J., Chiron, A. E., and Pallin, I. M. (1961). Ataraxic drugs in preanesthetic medication blind studies in 1,852 patients. *Anesthesiology* **22**, 529–536.

Lehmann, H. E. (1963). Psychopharmacology; a discussion of current problems. *Ohio Med. J.* **59**, 1091–1097. (Permitil.)

Lehmann, H. E., et al. (1964). Notes from the log-book of a psychopharmacological research unit. I. *Can. Psychiat. Assoc. J.* **9**, 28–32. (Permitil.)

Levinsky, W. J. (1961). Current therapy of common medical problems; the psychotherapeutic agent. *Delaware State Med. J.* **33**, 72–76.

Levy, L., and Ban, T. (1962). Phenothiazine drugs and the general practitioner. *Can. Med. Assoc. J.* **86**, 415–417.

Linn, E., et al. (1963). Itching dermatoses, treated with combined dexbrompheniramine-fluphenazine. A double-blind comparison with trimeprazine. *Skin* **2**, 374–376. (Diperm.)

Loianno, R. (1963). Experiencias clinicas con flufenazina, grageas de accion repetida. *Dia Med.* **35**, 1690–1692. (Elinol Cronotabs.)

Lopez de Nava, A. (1963). Tension y ansiedad en ginecologia. Consideraciones sobre su tratamiento con flufenazina. *Prensa Med., Mex.* **28**, 54–56; (1964). *Psychopharmacol. Abstr.* **3**, No. 3, 154.

Mockle, J. A. (1960). Aspects pharmacologique et therapeutique des derives de le phenothiazine. *Can. Pharm. J.* **93**, 25, 54–56, and 58.

Mapp, Y., et al. (1962). Psychopharmacology II: Tranquilizers and antipsychotic drugs. *Psychosomatics* **3**, 458–463.

Markey, H. (1961). Lazarus, come forth. A program to help the patient with chronic psychosis return to living. *New Engl. J. Med.* **265**, 580–584.

Matheu, H., and Fogel, E. J. (1961). Clinical effects of fluphenazine dihydrochloride in chronic schizophrenia. *J. Neuropsychiat.* **3**, 105–111.

McLaughlin, B. E., et al. (1964). Chemotherapy for emotionally disturbed children: A follow-up report. *Diseases Nervous System* **25**, 735–738.

Mercier, J., et al. (1963). Contribution a l'etude pharmacologique de la fluphenazine (4,3,2 (trifluoromethyl) 10 phenothiazinyl-propyl-piperazine ethanol). I. Etude psychopharmacologique. *Arch. Intern. Pharmacodyn.* **145**, 450–478.

Michaux, M. H., et al. (1964). Phenothiazines in the treatment of newly admitted state hospital patients: Global comparison of eight compounds in terms of an outcome index. *Current Therap. Res.* **6**, 331–339. (Prolixin.)

Millar, J. (1963). A trial of fluphenazine in schizophrenia. *Brit. J. Psychiat.* **109**, 428–432.

Moore, L. E. (1963). Fluphenazine in the treatment of hospitalized mental patients. *Am. J. Psychiat.* **119**, 987–988. (Prolixin.)

Morrow, L. E. (1961). Fluphenazine in private psychiatric practice. *Am. J. Psychiat.* **117**, 1031–1032. (Prolixin.)

Morrow, L. E. (1961). Fluphenazine as a psychotherapeutic agent in private psychiatric practice. A clinical report. *Psychosomatics* **2**, 382–386.

Morrow, L. E. (1964). Fluphenazine in the long-term treatment of non-hospitalized psychiatric patients. *Am. J. Psychiat.* **120**, 1008–1010. (Prolixin.)

Mukasa, H., Ichihara, T., Matsuoko, S., and Akiyama, K. (1961). Clinical psychological studies on the effects of fluphenazine. *Brain Nerve (Tokyo)* **13**, No. 6, 431–442; *Psychopharmacol. Abstr.* **1**, 313.

Nesbitt, R. E. L., Jr. (1962). Nausea and vomiting of pregnancy. *In* "Current Therapy" (H. F. Conn, ed.), pp. 600–601. Saunders, Philadelphia, Pennsylvania. (Permitil.)

Niswander, G. D., and Karagan, I. (1959). Clinical experience with fluphenazine. *Diseases Nervous System* **20**, 403–405.

Nomura, A., et al. (1961). Clinical study of fluphenazine (Sevinol) in mental illness. *Seishin Igaku* **3**, No. 3, 239–242; *Psychopharmacol. Abstr.* **1**, 114.

Pennington, V. M. (1964). Ten years' progress in psychotropic medication. *Illinois Med. J.* **126**, 553–558. (Prolixin.)

Price, J. J., et al. (1964). Therapy of emesis gravidarum: A double blind study of fluphenazine with pyridoxine. *Penna. Med. J.* **67**, 37–40. [Naustat (fluphenazine and pyridoxine).]

A.3. FLUPHENAZINE

Price, J. J. (1961). Clinical evaluation of fluphenazine (Permitil) in obstetrics and gynaecology. *Med. Proc. S. Africa* **7**, 404–405.

Proctor, R. C. (1960). Results with fluphenazine in anxiety and tension. *Diseases Nervous System* **21**, 283–285.

Ravaris, C. L., et al. (1965). A controlled study of fluphenazine enanthate in chronic schizophrenic patients. *Diseases Nervous System* **26**, 33–39. (Prolixin.)

Rebucci, G. G. (1962). L'azione di un nuove derivato fenotiazinico la fluphenazine-sulle manifestazioni extrapiramidal di tipo ipercinetico. *Giorn. Psichiat. Neuropatol.* **15**, 269–282; *Psychopharmacol. Abstr.* **2**, No. 6, 449.

Reznikoff, L. (1960). The use of fluphenazine (Prolixin) in rehabilitation of chronic schizophrenic patients. *Am. J. Psychiat.* **117**, 457–458.

Riccitelli, M. L. (1964). Modern concepts in the management of anxiety and depression in the aged and infirm. *J. Am. Geriat. Soc.* **12**, 652–657.

Robie, T. R. (1960). Chemotherapy in melancholia. *Diseases Nervous System* **21**, Pt. 2, 124–129.

Robie, T. R. (1960). Drugs and organic therapy in depression. *Psychosomatics.* **1**, 161–166,

Robie, T. R. (1960). Anxiety amelioration, a dual approach. *Diseases Nervous System* **21**, 588–590.

Rodman, M. J. (1960). Where we stand today with tranquilizers. *R.N.* **23**, 45–49 and 88.

Roebuck, B. E. (1962). Treatment of ambulatory patients with fluphenazine dihydrochloride. *Virginia Med. Monthly* **89**, 22–26.

Rossi, G. V. (1964). The psychotherapeutic agents. *Am. J. Pharm.* **136**, 6–24.

Russ, J. D. (1961). Fluphenazine (Prolixin) suppositories as an antiemetic agent in pediatric patients. *Current Therap. Res.* **3**, 520–525.

Sainz, A. (1961). Comparison of the clinical effects of carphenazine and fluphenazine in chronic schizophrenics. *Diseases Nervous System* **22**, Suppl., 77–79.

Sainz, A. (1964). Phenothiazines in the management of stress and anxiety. *Psychosomatics* **5**, 167–173.

Sales, E. (1960). Flufenazina en el tratamiento de la ansiedad asociada a diversas afecciones medicas. *Med. Cir.* **23**, 255–258.

Santos, F. T. (1962). Fluphenazine and pyridoxine in nausea and vomiting of pregnancy. *M.D.* **11**, 474–480. (Pregnidox.)

Scardino, A. (1962). The management of pruritus by oral treatment: A controlled clinical study. *J. Am. Osteopath. Assoc.* **61**, 987–989.

Schiele, B. C. (1962). Newer drugs for mental illness; a review. *J. Am. Med. Assoc.* **181**, 126–133.

Seris, H., et al. (1964). L'action du fluphenazine (Moditen) sur le temps de reaction et le temps de reponse totale. Paper presented at the Soc. Franc. Physiol. et Med. Aeronaut. et Cosmonaut. March 20, 1964; *Presse Med.* **72**, 1827 (abstr.).

Shawver, J. R., Scarborough, J. S., and Frank, T. V. (1962). Comparison of chlorpromazine with fluphenazine dihydrochloride in treatment of schizophrenics. *Diseases Nervous System* **23**, 392–395.

Sigwald, J., Comte, C., and Juge, D. (1962). Neuroleptic drugs. *World Neurol.* **3**, 78–94.

Simpson, G. M., et al. (1965). Studies on a second long-acting fluphenazine. *Am. J. Psychiat.* **121**, 784–787.

Sines, L. K., and Hamlon, J. S. (1960). Clinical evaluation of a new phenothiazine in chronic psychiatric patients. *Diseases Nervous System* **21**, 86–90.

Sotelo, D., et al. (1963). Fluphenazine for chronic psychotic patients. *Western Med.* **4**, 90–91, (Prolixin.)

Stanton, J. B. (1962). The action of a new phenothiazine derivative, fluphenazine, on hyperkinetic extrapyramidal manifestations. *Giorn. Psichiat. Neuropatol.* **90**, 269–282; (1963). *World Med.* **33**, 122 (abstr.).

Strang, W. C., et al. (1962). Use of fluphenazine in an acute and intensive treatment center. *Current Therap. Res.* **4**, Suppl., 218–223.

Stratas, N. E. (1962). Fluphenazine in chronic refractory schizophrenics. *Am. J. Psychiat.* **119**, 72. (Prolixin.)

Suarez-Gonzalez, R. (1959–1960). Flufenazina (Sevinol) en los estados medicos de ansiedad *Med. Cir.* **23**, 259–268.

Sweeney, R. E. (1963). Oral treatment of skeletal muscle spasm: A double-blind clinical study. *Current Therap. Res.* **5**, 305–309. (Orpitil.)

Takahata, C., et al. (1961). Experience with fluphenazine in treatment of psychiatric and neurological diseases. *Shinyo* **14**, No. 4, 544–552; *Psychopharmacol. Abstr.* **1**, 117–118.

Talso, P. J., et al. (1965). Combined therapy of hypertensive disease: An evaluation of the value of a phenothiazine derivative. *Appl. Therap.* **7**, 38–41.

Taylor, I. J. (1959). Clinical evaluation of a new phenothiazine tranquilizer, fluphenazine (Prolixin). *Am. J. Psychiat.* **116**, 457–458.

Tornetta, F. (1962). The effect of Prolixin on post-anesthetic vomiting in children: A controlled study. *Anesthesia Analgesia, Current Res.* **41**, 288–294.

Tuteur, W., et al. (1962). Tranquilizers and social obstacles. *Current Therap. Res.* **4**, Suppl., 206–212.

Ulett, G. A., et al. (1964). A study of the behavior and EEG patterns of patients receiving tranquilizers with and without the addition of chlordiazepoxide. *J. Neuropsychiat.* **5**, 558–565.

Vestre, N. D., et al. (1962). A comparison of fluphenazine, triflupromazine, and phenobarbital in the treatment of chronic schizophrenic patients: A double-blind controlled study. *J. Clin. Exptl. Psychopathol.* **23**, 149–159. (Prolixin.)

Viglioglia, P. A. (1963). Tratamiento dermatologico con una asociacion medicamentosa. *Dia Med.* **35**, 654–655. (Celestamine.)

Wachsmuth, R. (1962). Fluphenazine: More than just another psychotropic drug. *Nervenarzt* **33**, 466; (1963). *Drugs Made Germany* **6**, 57 (abstr.). (Lyogen.)

Wachsmuth, R. (1962). Probleme der psychiatrischen Pharmakotherapie und die Stellung des Fluphenazine in der Behandlung der Psychosen. *Arzneimittel- Forsch.* **16**, 87–95.

Wachsmuth, T. (1961). Uber die Behandlung psychotischer Patienten mit Fluphenazin. *Med. Klin. (Munich)* **56**, 396–398.

Waites, L., et al. (1963). Fluphenazine in management of disturbed mentally retarded children. *Diseases Nervous System* **24**, 113–114. (Prolixin.)

Warter, J. P., et al. (1963). Oral therapy of skeletal muscle spasm with combined orphenadrine-fluphenazine. *J. New Drugs* **3**, 317–320. (Orpitil.)

Welsh, A. L. (1964). The newer tranquilizing drugs. *Med. Clin. N. Am.* **48**, 459–481. (Permitil.)

Wissmer, B. (1964). Preliminary report on the action of fluphenazine in the treatment of functional digestive disorders. *Proc. Intern. Cong. Gastroenterol., Brussels*, 1964 6 pp. (Permitil.)

Wood, D. R. (1963). Miscellaneous drugs of interest to dentists. *Dental Clin. N. Am.* pp. 459–472. (Prolixin.)

Wortis, J. (1960). Physiological treatment. *Am. J. Psychiat.* **116**, 595–601.

Yoshimura, S. (1961). The clinical use of fluphenazine in schizophrenics. *Clin. Psychiat. (Tokyo)* **3**, No. 5, 421–424; *Psychopharmacol. Abstr.* **1**, 635.

Zeedick, J. F., et al. (1961). Evaluation of fluphenazine dihydrochloride (Prolixin) as a premedicating agent in surgical anesthesia. *Anesthesia Analgesia, Current Res.* **40**, 323–327.

Ziporyn, M., et al. (1964). The use of fluphenazine hydrochloride (Prolixin) in acute functional psychoses. *J. Neuropsychiat.* **5**, 297–299.

Zocchi, A., and Dimitri, K. (1961). Effects of fluphenazine dihydrochloride in state hospital patients. *Illinois Med. J.* **119**, 398–400.

~ A.4 ~
Mepazine

Chemical Papers

Clarke, E. G. C. (1957). Microchemical identification of some antihistamine drugs. *J. Pharm. Pharmacol.* **9**, 752–758.

Frahm, M., Fretwurst, E., and Soehring, K. (1956). Papierchromatographischer Nachweis einiger Phenothiazin-Derivate im Harn. (Demonstration by paper chromatography of some phenothiazine derivatives in the urine.) *Klin. Wochshr.* **34**, 1259–1262.

Meyer, F. (1957). Nachweis von Phenothiazin-Derivaten. *Arzneimittel-Forsch.* **7**, 296–298.

Neuhoff, E. W., and Auterhoff, H. (1955). Zur Analytik der Antihistamine; 4. Mitteilung. *Arch. Pharm.* **288**, No. 8–9, 400–407.

Schwerbrock, J. (1956). Ueber den Nachweis von Phenothiazinderivaten durch die Papierchromatographie. (Ossing) Institut fuer Gerichtliche Medizin der Westfaelischen Wilhelms-Universitaet Muenster. *Auszug aus der Inaugural-Dissertation, Muenster.*

Thieme, H. (1956). Zur Analytik einiger therapeutisch verwendeter Phenothiazinderivate. III. Mitt: Beitrag zur photometrischen Bestimmung. *Pharmazie* **11**, 725–726.

Biology and Pharmacology

Ahrens, A., and Witzleb, E. (1955). Ueber periphere Kreislaufwirkungen von zwei Phenothiazinderivaten. (Peripheral circulatory effects of two phenothiazine derivatives.) *Arch. Intern. Pharmacodyn.* **104**, 42–49.

Benstz, W. (1955). Stroemungscalorimetrische Untersuchungen zur Beeinflussung der peripheren Waermeabgabe und des Energieunsatzes durch synthetische Hibernatoren. (Blood stream calorimetry experiments on the influence of peripheral heat loss and energy change during artificial hibernation.) *Arch. Exptl. Pathol. Pharmakol.* **226**, No. 4, 377–382.

Benstz, W. (1956). Zur Wirkung synthetischer "Hibernatoren" auf die Serum—und Erythrocytencholinesterasen unter Beruecksichtigung gleichzeitiger Kreislaufanalysen. (On the effect of synthetic "hibernators" on the serum and erythrocyte cholinesterases with consideration of simultaneous circulation analyses.) *Klin. Wochschr.* **34**, 796.

von Bubnoff, N., Hoffman, D., Schmid, E., and Taugner, R. (1955). Zur sympatholytischen adrenolytischen und noradrenolytischen Wirkung der Phenothiazine. (The sympatholitic, adrenolytic and noradrenolytic action of phenothiazine.) *Arch. Exptl. Pathol. Pharmakol.* **224**, 443–451; *Excerpta Med. Sect. VI* **10**, 782. (1956). First presented at 21. Tagung Deut. Pharmacol. Ges., 1954, Saarbruecken.

Budde, H., and Witzleb, E. (1955). Zur Wirkung von Phenothiazinderivaten auf Strukturen im autonomen Nervensystem. (The effect of phenothiazine derivatives on structures in the autonomic nervous system.) *Arch. Intern. Pharmacodyn.* **101**, 126–138.

Frey, H. H. (1956). Versuche zur Beeinflussung der Thiobarbituratextrasystolie beim Hund. (Experiments to influence the thiobarbiturate extrasystole in the dog.) *Arzneimittel-Forsch.* **6**, 693–694, (1956). Rundschau; Kolloquien des Pharmakologischen Instituts der Universitaet Hamburg; Kolloquium ueber narkose und Anaesthesie.

Fromm, G. (1955). Tierexperimentelle Untersuchungen ueber den Einfluss einger laengeren Medikation des Phenothiazinderivats Pacatal auf die Bildung von komplementbindenden Antikoerpern. (Experimental investigations in animals of the influence of longer medication with the phenothiazine derivative Pacatal on the formation of complement-binding antibodies.) *Zhr. Immunitaeforsch.* **112**, 373–381.

Gadermann, E. (1956). Die Abhaengigkeit der Kreislaufwirkung verschiedener Phenothiazinderivaten vom Angriffspunkt und der vegetativen Ausgangslage. (Dependence of the circulatory effects of various phenothiazine derivatives on site of action and the autonomic outlet.) *Klin. Wochschr.* **34**, 311–316.

Gadermann, E., and Donat, K. (1954). Zur Beeinflussung der Irritabilitaet des Herzens in der Narkose. (The influence of cardiac excitability in narcosis.) *Klin. Wochschr.* **32**, 713–716.

Graham, R. C. B., Lu, F. C., and Allmark, M. G. (1957). Combined effect of tranquilizing drugs and alcohol on rats. *Federation Proc.* **16**, 302.

Henriksen, U., Huus, I., and Kopf, R. (1957). Zur Frage Resorption, Verteilung und Ausscheidung von Chlorpromazin und N-Methylpiperidyl-3-Methylphenothiazin. *Arch. Intern. Pharmacodyn.* **109**, 39–54.

Himwich, H. E., Rinaldi, F., and Willis, D. (1956). An examination of phenothiazine derivatives with comparisons of their effects on the alerting reaction, chemical structure, and therapeutic efficacy. *J. Nervous Mental Disease* **124**, 53–57.

Kleinsorge, H., Kovách, A. G. B., Menyhárt, J., Földi, M., Koltay, E., Erdélyi, A., Molnar, G., Jellinek, H., Christle, H., and Roesner, K. (1956). Experimentelle Beobachtungen ueber den Einfluss von Phenothiazinderivaten auf die Nierenfunktion. *Z. Ges. Exptl. Med.* **127**, 543.

Kopf, R. (1955). Phenothiazinderivaternes farmakologi med specielt henblik pa N-methylpiperidyl-3-methylphenothiazin (lacumin). (Pharmacology of phenothiazine derivatives with special reference to N-methylpiperidyl-3-methylphenothiazine (Lacumin R). *Nord. Med.* **54**, 1779–1782.

Kopf, R. (1956). Resorption, Verteilung und Ausscheidung von Phenothiazinderivaten. (Absorption, distribution and excretion of phenothiazine derivatives.) *Klin. Wochschr.* **34**, 455–456; (1956). Verhandlungen aerztlicher Gesellschaften: Medizinische Gesellschaft Keiel.

Kovach, A. G. B., Kleinsorge, H., Róheim, P., Trányi, M., and Roesner, K. (1957). Analytische Untersuchungen ueber die zentralen und peripheren Angriffspunkte des N-Methyl-piperidyl-(3)-methyl-phenothiazin im gekreuzten Kreislauf. *Arzneimittel-Forsch.* **7**, 292–296.

Laborit, H., and Huguenard, P. (1952). Technique actuelle de l'hibernation artificielle. *Presse med.* **60**, No. 68, 5.

Nádor, K., and Pórszász, J. (1956). Der Einfluss einiger Aminoketone auf Koerpertemperatur und Stoffwechsel und ihre Narkose-potenzierende Wirkung. *Arzneimittel-Forsch.* **6**, 696–698.

Nieschulz, O., Popendiker, K., and Sack, K. H. (1954). Pharmakologische Untersuchungun ueber N-Alkyl-piperidyl-phenothiazin derivate. (Pharmacological studies on N-alkylpiperidyl-phenothiazin derivates.) *Arzneimittel-Forsch.* **4**, 232–242.

Nieschulz, O., Popendiker, K., and Hoffman, I. (1955). Weitere pharmakologische Untersuchungen ueber N-Methyl-piperidyl-(3)-methyl-phenothiazin. *Arzneimittel-Forsch.* **5**, 680–695.

Nieschulz, O., Hoffman, I., and Popendiker, K. (1956). Pharmakologische Untersuchungen ueber N-Alkyl-piperidyl-phenothiazin-Derivate. 2. Mitt. (Pharmacologic investigations of N-alkyl-piperidyl-phenothiazine derivatives. 2nd communication.) *Arzneimittel-Forsch.* **6**, 651–660.

Nieschulz, O., Hoffman, I., Popendiker, K., and Schumacher, H. (1957). Pharmakologische

A.4. MEPAZINE

Untersuchungen ueber *N*-Methyl-piperidyl-(3)-methyl-phenothiazin. 3. Mitteilung. *Arzneimittel-Forsch.* **7**, 259–270.

Pórszász, J., Nádor, K., Gibiszer-Porszász, K., and Bacsó, I. (1957). Pharmakologie der Aminoketone. III. Vergleichende Untersuchungen mit Largactil (3-Dimethylaminopropyl-3-chlor-10-phenothiazin), Pacatal (*N*-methyl-piperidy-3-methyl-phenothiazin) und F-933 (1-piperidinomethyl-benzodioxan). (Pharmacology of the aminoketones. III. Comparative investigations with Largactil (3-dimethylaminopropyl-3-chlor-10-phenothiazine), Pacatal (*N*-methyl-piperidyl-3-methyl-phenothiazine) and F-933 (1-piperidinomethyl-benzodioxane.) *Acta Physiol. Acad. Sci. Hung.* No. 11, 95–107.

Ravina, A. (1957). Tranquillisants pour animaux. *Presse Med.* **65**, No. 53, 1263.

Rosenkilde, H., and Govier, W. M. (1957). *J. Pharmacol. Exptl. Therap.* **120**, 375–378.

Truitt, E. B. (1957). The tranquilizers. 1: pharmacology of the ataractic drugs. *In* "Present Status of Psychopharmacology" (Krantz, J. C. ed.) *Mod. Med. Minneapolis* **25**, 77.

Westerink, D. (1956). De farmacologie en toepassing der fenothiazinederivaten. (The pharmacology and application of the phenothiazine derivatives.) *Pharm. Weekblad* **91**, 113–125.

Wiemers, K. (1956). Ueber den Einfluss von Phenothiazinderivaten auf die Ischaemietoleranz des Kaninchenhirns. (Influence of phenothiazine derivatives on ischemia tolerance of the rabbit brain.) *Klin. Wochschr.* **34**, 112; (1955). Verhandlungen aerztlicher Gesellschaften, Med. Ges. Freiburg i. Br.

Wilhelmi, G. (1955). Ueber den Einfluss von Phenothiazinpraeparaten auf den Regenerationsvorgang bei Planarien und beim Axolotl. *Helv. Physiol. Acta* **13**, C40–C42. (Verhandlungen; comptes rendus.)

Wilhelmi, G. (1956). Ueber die wachstums- und entzuendungshemmenden Eigenschaften einiger Phenotiazine, Iminodibenzyle und Acridine. *Arch. Exptl. Pathol. Pharmakol.* **227**, No. 6, 497–508.

Witzleb, E., and Budde, H. (1955). Zur Wirkung von Phenothiazinderivaten auf die Dynamik u. Energetik des Warmblueterherzens. (Effect of phenothiazine derivatives on the dynamics and metabolism of the heart of warm-blooded animals.) *Arch. Intern. Pharmacodyn.* **104**, 33–41.

Zakusov, V. V., and Kaverina, N. V. (1956). Farmakologiya koronarnoge krovoobrashcheniya. *Sov. Med.* **10**, 3–8.

Side Effects

Apter, J., and Rinsley, D. B. (1957). *Clin. Exptl. Psychopathol.* **18**, 335–341.

Burkitt, E. A., and Rixon, P. E. (1957). Pacatal. *Brit. Med. J.* I. 464. (Correspondence.)

Feldman, P. E., Bertone, J., and Panthel, H. (1957). Fatal agranulocytosis during treatment with Pacatal. *Am. J. Psychiat.* **113**, 842–843. (Case reports.)

Gadermann, E., and Donat, K. (1955). Vergleichende Untersuchungen zur Toxizitaet verschiedener Phenothiazinderivate. (Investigations on the toxicity of various phenothiazine derivatives.) *Arch. Intern. Pharmacodyn.* **102**, 85–95.

Gore, C. P., and Biezanek, A. (1956). Agranulocytosis during treatment with Pacatal. *Lancet* II, 1081.

Hiob, J., and Hippius, H. (1955). Ueberempfindlichkeitserscheinungen der Haut durch Megaphen. (Hypersensitivity of the skin to Megaphen.) *Aerztl. Wochschr.* **10**, 501–504.

Hiob, J., and Hippius, H. (1955). Agranulocytose nach Behandlung mit Phenothiazinderivaten. (Agranulocytosis after treatment with phenothiazine derivatives.) *Aerztl. Wochschr.* **10**, 924–925.

Hutchinson, J. T. (1956). Toxic reactions to Pacatal. *Lancet* II, 1216. (Letters to the Editor.)

Jores, A., and Droste, R. (1956). Der Tod im Status asthmaticus. (Death in status asthmaticus.) *Aerztl. Wochschr.* **11**, 39–41.
Kline, N. S. (1956). Pacatal. *Am. J. Psychiat.* **113**, 565. (Correspondence.)
Koenig, J., and Klippel, R. (1957). Zur chronischen Toxizitaet. (Chronic toxicity; pathologic-anatomic investigations on the dog.) *Med. Monatsschr.* **11**, 20–22.
Kopf, R. (1956). Beeinflussung der Leukozytenzahl durch Phenothiazinderivate. (Influence of phenothiazine derivatives on the leucocyte count.) *Arzneimittel-Forsch.* **6**, 220–222.
Pick, F. J. (1957). Agranulocytosis due to "Pacatal" *Brit. Med. J.* No. 5053,1111. (Correspondence.)
Wenderoth, H., and Lennartz, H. (1955). Agranulocytose nach Phenothiazine. (Agranulocytosis after phenothiazine.) *Med. Klin.* (*Munich*) **50**, 818–820; Review of the same case: Wenderoth, H. (1956). Agranulocytosis during treatment with Pacatal. *Lancet* II, 1312–1313. (Letters to the Editor.)
Werenberg, H. (1955). Lacuminterapi ved svaere sindsygdomme. *Nord. Med.* **54**, 1787–1789.
Young, J. H. (1957). New drugs in psychiatry. *J. Lancet* **77**, 301–306.

Clinical Papers

Aronski, A., Janiakowna, J., Leligdowicz, A., and Rogalski, E. (1956). O rownoczesnym stosowaniu pochodnych fenotiazyny i kwasu barbiturowego w leczeniu snem przeduzonym. (Simultaneous application of phenothiazines and barbituric acid in the prolonged therapeutic sleep.) *Polski Tygod. Lekar.* No. 11, 516.
Aronski, A. (1957). Klinische Erfahrungen mit der Anwendung von Pacatal in der Herzchirurgie. *Anaesthesist* **6**, 329–330.
Ayd, F. J. (1957). A clinical evaluation of Pacatal. *Diseases Nervous System* **18**, 4, No. 142.
Benkoe, S., Abrandi, E., and Vargha, M. (1956). Vegetativ krizis kezelése hibernáló szerekkel. (Therapy of autonomic crisis with hibernation-inducing agents.) *Orv. Hetilap* **97**, 1195–1197.
Bennett, I. F. (1957). The tranquilizers; part II. *J. Am. Pharm. Assoc., Pract. Pharm. Ed.* **18**, 547–549. (In 4 parts.)
Bowes, H. A. (1956). The ataractic drugs: The present position of chlorpromazine, Frenquel, Pacatal and Reserpine in the psychiatric hospital. *Am. J. Psychiat.* **113**, 530–539.
Braceland, F. J., Grinker, R. R., and Meduna, L. J. (1957). *Mod. Med.* (*Minneapolis*) **25**, 190–230.
Braun, M. (1957). Treatment of psychoses with a combination of Pacatal and Thorazine. *Am. J. Psychiat.* **114**, 460. (Clinical notes.)
Braun, M. (1957). Pacatal. *Am. J. Psychiat.* **113**, 838–839. (Clinical notes.)
Broglie, M. (1956). Der Phenothiazinechlaf in der inneren Medizin. *Medizinische* No. 46, 1628–1632.
Broglie, M. (1955). Schlaftherapie innerer Krankheiten. (Therapeutic sleep in internal medicine.) *Therap. Gegenwart* **94**, 281–287.
Bruckman, N., Kitchener, M., Saunders, J. C., and Kline, N. S. (1957). Mepazine (Pacatal); further report. *Am. J. Psychiat.* **114**, 262–263.
Bucceri, M. A., Richardson, J., and Rovenstine, E. A. (1958). Preliminary observations on Pacatal in anesthesia. *N.Y. State J. Med.* **58**, 63–65.
Budde, H., and Witzleb, E. (1954). Zur Atemwirkung einiger neuroplegischer Substanzen. (The respiratory effects of some neuroplegic substances.) *Verhandl. Deut. Ges. Inn. Med.* **60**, 790–793. Review: (1954). *Klin. Wochschr.* **32**, 758; (1954). Verhandlungen aerztlicher Gesellschaften: 60. Tagung. Deut. Ges. Inn. Med. Muench.
Carr, C. J., and Kinnard, W. J. (1957). The phrenotropic agents. *Interns. Record Med.* **170**, 493–504.

Davies, J. J., Huggins, D. H., and Wolkenstein, C. F. (1956). Pacatal in anaesthesia. *Can. Anaesthesial. Soc. J.* **3**, 3.
Davies, J. J., Huggins, D. H. M., and Wolkenstein, C. F. (1956). Pacatal in anaesthesia; a preliminary report. Presented at the meeting of the Western Division, Canadian Anaesthetists Society, Vancouver, B.C. April 5–7, 1956. *Can. Anaesthesiol. Soc. J.* **3**, 224–234.
Dechene, J. P. (1957). Pharmacologic hibernation in lung surgery for the tuberculous patient. *Can. Anaesthesiol. Soc. J.* **4**, 60–65.
Denber, H. C. B. (1958). Ineffectiveness of mepazine (Pacatal). *Am. J. Psychiat.* **114**, 656.
Donat, K. (1955). Zur Verhuetung von Rhythmusstoerrungen des Herzens bei operativen Eingriffen. (Prevention of arrythmia in surgical intervention.) *Anaesthesist* **4**, 65–68.
Donat, K. (1954). Die endovasale Anaesthesie des Herzens mit einem neuen Phenothiazinderivat und ihre Ansendungsmoeglichkeiten. (Endovasal anesthesia of the heart with a new phenothiazine and its possible applications.) Presented at the 44th Tagung Ges. Inn. Med., Bremen, July, 1954.
Donat, K. (1957). Zur Beeinflussung von Funktionsstoerungen des Herzens und Fehlsteuerungen des vegetativen Nervensystems. *Deut. Med. Wochschr.* **82**, 382–386.
Feldman, P. E. (1957). Clinical evaluation of Pacatal. *Am. J. Psychiat.* **114**, 143–146.
Feldman, P. E. (1957). A comparative study of various ataractic drugs. *Am. J. Psychiat.* **113**, 589–594.
Fernandez-Bastidas, M. A. (1957). Veintiseis casos de toxemia tratados con un nuevo derivado de la Fenotiazina. *Rev. Colombiana Obstet. Ginecol.* **8**, 67–76.
Flipse, M. J. (1957). Pacatal in office practice. *Clin. Med.* **4**, 1237–1241.
Friese, K. H. (1956). Vorlaeufige Erfahrungen bei der Behandlung psychiatrischer Kranker mit Phenothiazinen. (Early results in phenothiazine therapy in psychiatry.) *Medizinische* No. 19, 734–735.
Gadermann, E. (1955). Experimentelle und Klinische Erfahrungen mit Phenothiazinderivaten. (Experimental and clinical experiences with phenothiazine derivatives.) *Kongressber.* 44, *Tagung Nordwest. Ges. Inn. Med.*, Hamburg, 1955 pp. 55–56.
Gillie, A. K. (1957). The use of Pacatal in low-grade mental defectives. *J. Mental Sci.* **103**, 402–405.
Grobschedl, A., and Hyden, H. (1956). Vegetativum und Chirurgie der Lungentuberkulose. (Autonomic nervous system and surgery in tuberculosis of the lung.) *Zentr. Chir.* **81**, 791–796.
Hartmann, K., Hiob, J., and Hippius, H. (1955). Zur vergleichenden Psychopathologie der Schock und Phenothiazinwirkungen. *Fortsch. Neurol. Psychiat.* **23**, 354–366.
Hecker, W. C., and Berg, H. (1955). Zur allgemeinen Operationsvorbereitung und Nachbehandlung im Kindesalter. (On the general pre- and post-operative treatment in childhood.) *Chirurg.* **26**, 193–196.
Hellmann, R. (1955). Ueber erste Versuche mit der Pacatal-Vorbehandlung bei Inactin-Aethernarkosen in der Gynaekologie. (First trial of pre-treatment with pacatal in inactin-ether narcosis in gynecology.) *Zentr. Gynaekol.* **77**, No. 51, 2018–2023.
Hellmann, R. (1956). Zur Psychologisierung der Geburtshilfe. (Psychology in obstetrics.) *Zentr. Gynaekol.* **78**, 1665–1671.
Hiob, J., and Hippius, H. (1955). Ueber die Behandlung von Psychosen mit dem Phenothiazinderivat "Pacatal". (The treatment of psychoses with the phenothiazine derivative "Pacatal".) *Med. Klin. (Munich)* **50**, 1746–1748.
Hohmann, G. (1956). Erfahrungen mit Thiogenal; kurze Mitteilung. (Experiences with Thiogenal; short report.) *Anaesthesist* **5**, 9–10.
Horatz, K. (1953). Ueberblick ueber den heutigen Stand der modernen Anaesthesis. (A general review of present attitudes in modern anesthesiology.) Deutsche Gesellschaft fur Kiefer -und Gesichtschirugie, Duesseldorf, Vortrag Sept. 19, 1953.

A.4. MEPAZINE

Horatz, K. (1954). Die Vorteile der potenzierten Narkose mit Abkuenhlung. (Advantages of potentiated narcosis with hypothermia.) *Kaeltetechnik* (Sonderheft) pp. 28–31.

Horatz, K. (1954). Die potenzierte Narkose ohne und mit Unterkuehlung; ihre Vorteile, Grenzen und Gefahren. (Potentiated narcosis with and without hypothermia; their advantages, limitations and dangers.) *Muench. Med. Wochschr.* **96**, 426–429.

Horatz, K. (1954). Die potenzierte Narkose mit dem Phenothiazine-Koerper P 391. (Potentiated narcosis with the phenothiazine P 391.) *Anaesthesist* **3**, 193–195.

Horatz, K. (1955). Die Lokalanaesthesie in der aerztlichen Praxis. (Local anesthesia in medical practice.) *Deut. Med. J.* **6**, 444–446.

Horatz, K. (1955). Wie hoch ist der Bedarf an Infusionsfluessigkeit bei grossen Operationen zur Aufrechterhaltung der Kreislaufstabilitaet; Erfahrungen bei 1742 Eingriffen in Allgemeinnarkose. *Anaesthesist* **4**, 123–126.

Kleinsorge, H. (1953). Erfahrungen mit der Schlaftherapie innerer Erkrankungen. *Med. Monatsschr.* **11**, 760.

Kleinsorge, H. (1954). Kreislauf-und Stoffwechselprobleme bei Anwendung von Phenothiazinderivaten in der Schlaftherapie. (Circulatory and metabolic problems in connection with use of phenothiazines in therapeutic sleep.) *Aerztl. Wochschr.* **9**, 271–274.

Kleinsorge, H., and Roesner, K. (1954). Zur Schlaftherapie. (Therapeutic sleep.) *Neuralmedizin* **2**, 5–15.

Kleinsorge, H., and Roesner, K. (1954). Theorie und Technik der Schlaftherapie. *Deut. Gesundheitsw.* **9**, 211–218.

Kleinsorge, H., and Roesner, K. (1956). Primenenie proizvodnykh fenotiazinapdlia terapii snom. (Application of phenothiazine derivatives in therapeutic sleep.) *Zh. Nevropatol. i psikhiat R.* **56**, No. **4**, 296–299.

Kleinsorge, H., and Roesner, K. (1956). Therapie mit den sogenannten Winterschlafmitteln (Phenothiazinderivaten) beim status asthmaticus. (Therapy with the so-called hibernation agents (phenothiazine derivatives) in status asthmaticus.) *Allergie Asthma* **2**, 173–175.

Kleinsorge, H., and Roesner, K. (1956). Schlaftherapie mit Phenothiazinderivaten. (Therapeutic sleep with phenothiazine derivatives.) *Therap. Gegenwart* **95**, 441–446.

Kleinsorge, H., Roesner, K., and Wittig, H. H. (1955). Klinische und experimentelle Beobachtungen bei Anwendung von Phenothiazinderivaten. *Med. Klin. (Munich)* **50**, 1451–1454.

Kline, N. S., and Jacob, G. M. (1955). Use of Pacatal (N-methyl piperidyl-(3)-methylphenothiazine) in psychiatric patients. *Am. J. Psychiat.* **112**, 1, No. 63.

Kopf, R. (1957). Zur Frage der Alkoholpotenzierung durch Phenothiazine. *Arch. Intern. Pharmacodyn.* **110**, 56–64.

Krall, J. (1955). Die thorakale Angiographie beim Bronchialcarcinom. (Thoracic angiography in bronchial carcinoma.) *Thoraxchirurgie* **3**, 121–138.

Krzanowski, M., and Rogers, M. (1957). Pacatal. *Brit. Med. J.* I, 463–464. (Correspondence.)

Leiberman, D. M., and Vaughan, G. F. (1957). The use of some new pharmacological agents in psychiatry. *J. Mental Sci.* **103**, 110–118.

Lienau, C. (1957). Heilschlafbehandlung mit Pacatal bei Alkoholismus und Morphinismus. *Muench. Med. Wochschr.* **99**, No. 3, 80.

Lomas, J. (1957). Treatment of schizophrenia; Pacatal and chlorpromazine compared. *Brit. Med. J.* II, 78–80.

MacGregor, J. (1956). "Pacatal"; a clinical trial of a new ataractic drug. *S. African Med. J.* **30**, 1108–1111.

Magistris, F. (1956). Hibernationsprobleme im Hinblick auf ein neuses Phenothiazinderivat (Pacatal). (Problems of hibernation with regard to a new phenothiazine derivative, Pacatal.) *Wien. Med. Wochschr.* **106**, 86–90.

Mathewson, H. S. (1957). Analgesia and the pharmacology of pain. *J. Lancet* **77**, 387–389.

Mignault, G. (1957). Two years' experience using the phenothiazine amine derivatives in anaesthesia and artificial hibernation with special mention of the new derivative "Pacatal". *Can. Anaesthesiol. Soc. J.* **4**, 37–42.

Mitchell, P. H., Sykes, P., and King. A. (1957). Effects of "Pacatal" on symptoms in chronic psychotic female in-patients. *Brit. Med. J.* I, 204–207.

Ohling, C., and Muender, H. W. (1954). Narkoseerfahrungen mit Inactin-Flaxedil in der mittleren Chirurgie. (Experiments with inactin-flaxedil anesthesia in average surgery.) *Zentr. Chir.* **79**, No. 43, 1827–1832.

Ohling, A. C., and Muender, H. W. (1956). Intravenoese Narkose mit Muskelerschlaffung ung Blutdrucksenkung. (Intravenous narcosis with muscle relaxation and blood-pressure lowering.) *Zentr. Chir.* **81**, 1392–1398.

Roesner, K. (1954). Schlaf-oder Daemmerkur, Heilschlaf, Schlaftherapie und kuenstlicher Winterschlaf. *Landarzt* **30**, No. 24, 642–646.

Rohardt, H. (1955). Praktische Erfahrungen mit den Phenothiazinderivaten in der Chirurgie. *Med. Klin. (Munich)* **50**, 1611–1613.

Rollenhagen, J. E., and Scherer, G. (1957). Indikationen der Phenothiazinderivate in der Chirurgie. *Medizinische* No. 40, 1458–1460.

Rudy, L. H., Himwich, H. E., and Tasher, D. C. (1957). Clinical evaluation of two phenothiazine compounds, promazine and mepazine. *Am. J. Psychiat.* **113**, 979–983.

Sangowicz, J., and Gauthier, J. (1956). Resumé d'une étude clinique sur Pacatal et Medomine, portant respectivement sur 40 Cas. *Union Med. Can.* **85**, 1170–1171.

Sarwer-Foner, G. J., and Koranyi, E. K. (1957). The clinical investigation of Pacatal in open psychiatric settings. *Can. Med. Assoc. J.* **77**, 450–459.

Schneeweiss, J., and Gassmann, W. (1956). Zur Pathogenese und Therapie der Neuritis diabetica. (On the pathogenesis and therapy of neuritis diabetica.) *Deut. Med. J.* **7**, 649–651.

Schulz, H. P. (1957). Beitrag zur Behandlung des Parkinsonismus; die Beeinflussung des parkinsonistischen Tremors durch Pacatal. *Medizinische* No. 31–32, 1131–1133.

Seitz, D. (1956). Die Schlafbehandlung mit Phenothiazinen in der Neurologie. (Therapeutic sleep induced by phenothiazines in neurology.) *Nervenarzt* **27**, 19–23.

Seyffert, H. M. (1955). Die Wirkung von Phenothiazinderivaten bei multipler Sklerose. (The effect of phenothiazine derivatives on multiple sclerosis.) *Muench. Med. Wochschr.* **97**, 1623–1625.

Simpson, R. W. (1957). Pacatal. *Brit. Med. J.* I, 464. (Correspondence.)

Simpson, R. W. (1957). The effects of Pacatal on chronic mental illness. *J. Mental Sci.* **103**, 610–613.

Soehring, K. (1957). Der gegenwartige Stand der Praemedikation in Klinik und Praxis. *Arzneimittel-Forsch.* **7**, 634–635; (1957). Rundschau; Kolloquien des Pharmacologischen Instituts der Universitaet Hamburg; Kolloquium ueber narkose und Anaesthesie.

Stoll, B. A. (1957). New drugs for irradiation sickness. *Radiology* **68**, 380–385.

Thorpe, J. G., and Baker, A. A. (1956). A research method to assess a new tranquilizing drug. Pacatal in deteriorated psychotic patients. *J. Mental Sci.* **102**, 790–795.

Watrous, W. G. (1957). Promethazine in clinical anesthesia. *Anesthesia Analgesia, Current Res.* **36**, 38–45.

Werenberg, H. (1955). Lacumin therapy in severe mental disorders. *Nord. Med.* **54**, 1787.

Williams, H. (1957). Pacatal in anaesthesia. Impressions from 200 cases. *New Zealand Med. J.* **56**, 41–43.

A.5
Methdilazine

A.M.A. Council on Drugs. (1956). New drugs and developments in therapeutics. *J. Am. Med. Assoc.* **175**, 1170–1171.

Arbesman, C. E., and Ehrenreich, R. J. (1961). New drugs in the treatment of allergies. *N. Y. J. Med.* **61**, 219–229.

Borofsky, L. G. (1959). The use of methdilazine hydrochloride in electroencephalography of children. *Am. J. Diseases Children* **98**, 566.

Bouhuys, A. (1963). Prevention of Monday dyspnea in byssinosis: A controlled trial with an antihistamine drug. *Clin. Pharmacol. Therap.* **4**, 311–314.

Crawford, L. V., and Grogan, F. T. (1960). Clinical evaluation of methdilazine hydrochloride, a new antihistamine, using double-blind and placebo control. *J. Tenn. State Med. Assoc.* **53**, 307–310.

Crepea, S. B. (1960). Data on tacaryl and forhistal. *J. Allergy* **31**, 283–284.

Dobkin, A. R., and Palko, D. (1960). The antisialogogue effect of phenothiazine derivatives: Comparison of promaine, levomepromazine, trifluoperazine, proclorperazine, methdilazine and prothipendyl. *Anesthesiology* **21**, 260–262.

Dobkin, A. B. (1960). Protentiation of thiopental anesthesia by derivatives and analogues of phenothiazine. *Anesthesiology* **21**, 292–296.

Dornette, W. H. L., Poe, M. F., Cavallaro, R. J., and Sheffield, W.E. (1962). A doubleblind study of Tacaryl as a narcotic potentiator when used for preliminary medication. *Anesthesia Analgesia, Current Res.* **41**, 32–36.

Eisenberg, B. C., and Salkin, D. (1962). The management of allergic emergencies. *Med. Clin. N. Am.* **46**, 459–472.

Friend, D. G. (1961). Method for evaluating antipruritic agents. *Clin. Pharmacol. Therap.* **2**, 605–609.

Frohman, I. P. (1962). Methdilazine hydrochloride in pruritic dermatoses: A double-blind evaluation in general office practice. *Med. Times* **90**, 25–28.

General Practitioner Clinical Trials (1961). Variations of a cough syrup. *Practitioner* **187**, 362–366.

Grater, W. C. (1963). Clinical determination of the dose response curve of methdilazine hydrochloride in allergic disorders. *Clin. Med.* **70**, 82–87.

Howell, C. M., Jr. (1960). Evaluation of methdilazine hydrochloride as an antipruritic agent. *N. Carolina Med. J.* **21**, 194–195.

Lish, P. M., and McKinney, G. R. (1963). Pharmacology of methdilazine. II. Some determinants and limits of action on vascular permeability and inflammation in model systems. *J. Lab. Clin. Med.* **61**, 1015–1026.

Lish, P. M., Albert, J. R., Peters, E. L., and Allen, L. E. (1960). Pharmacology of methdilazine. *Arch. Intern. Pharmacodyn.* **129**, 77–107.

Lubowe, I. I. (1962). A clinical evaluation of a new antipruritic. *Current Therap. Res.* **4**, 64–66.

McKinney, G. R., and Lish, P. M. (1960). The effects of methdilazine HCl (Tacaryl$_R$) and sodium salicylate on ultraviolet light-induced erythema in guinea pigs. *Pharmacologist* **2**, 75.

Mead Johnson & Company. (1960). Tacaryl. *U.S. Offic. Gaz., U.S. Pat. Office* **752**, TM31.

Mead Johnson & Company. (1960). Tacaryl. The antihistamine methdilazine HCl with sustained action; tablets 8 Mg. and also syrup (Rx), (chemical name). *Mod. Drugs* pp. 1903, 1906.

Mead Johnson & Company. (1959). Tacaryl; antihistamine. *U.S. Offic. Gaz., U.S. Pat. Office* **749**, TM90.

Mead Johnson Laboratories (Canada). (1962). Tuscopine; balanced formulation containing noscapine, glyceryl guaiacolate, pseudoephedrine, methdilazine hydrochloride (Tacaryl). *Can. Med. Assoc. J.* **86**, outside back cover.

Miller, J. (1962). A double-blind, placebo-controlled crossover study of methdilazine hydrochloride in the management of hay fever. *Current Therap. Res.* **4**, 568–571.

Mock, D. C., Jr. (1963). Controlled evaluation of two antihistamine compounds using nasal engorgement as an index of response. *J. Allergy* **34**, 432–438.

Rawitz, W. E., and Merksamer, D. (1962). Evaluation of methdilazine hydrochloride in therapy of allergic rhinitis. *Current Therap. Res.* **4**, 564–567.

Smith, M. A., and Curwen, M. P. (1961). Controlled trials of two oral antipruritic drugs, trimeprazine and methdilazine. *Brit. J. Dermatol.* **73**, 351–358.

Spoto, A. P., and Sierker, H. O. (1960). Treatment of allergic disorders with methdilazine. *Ann. Allergy* **18**, 761–764.

Taylor, C., Gardier, R. W., Stoelting, V. K., and Dallas, M. E. (1962). Clinical investigation of a new phenothiazine compound, methdilazine. *Clin. Pharm. Therap.* **3**, 593–598.

Toriya, K., Asai, E., Ueno, K., and Mori, R. (1962). Experience in the use of Tacaryl in so-called allergic rhinitis. *Otolaryngology* **34**, 777–784. (Japanese.)

Wahner, H. W., and Peters, G. A. (1960). An evaluation of some newer antihistaminic drugs against pollinosis. *Proc. Staff Meetings Mayo Clin.* **35**, 161–169.

Weikel, J. H., Jr., and Lish, P. M. (1959). Some important aspects of the pharmacology of methdilazine. *Pharmacologist* **1**, 64.

Weikel, J. H., Jr., Wheeler, A. G., and Joiner, P. D. (1960). Metabolic fate and toxicology of methdilazine 10-(1-methyl-3-pyrrolidylmethyl) phenothiazine. *Toxicol. Appl. Pharmacol.* **2**, 68–82.

Wu, Y. H., and Feldkamp. R. F. (1961). Pyrrolidines. III. 10-(1-substituted 3-pyrrolidinylmethyl phenothiazines). *J. Org. Chem.* **26**, 1529–1530.

~ A.6 ~
Methoxypromazine

Allgen, L. G., Jonsson, B., Rappe, A., and Dahlbom, R. (1959). On the urinary elimination of methoxypromazine in man. *Experientia* **15**, 318–319.
Apfeldorf, M., *et al.* (1960). Methoxypromazine in chronic schizophrenia. *Am. J. Psychiat.* **117**, 72–73.
Apt, L. (1960). Complications of phenothiazine tranquilizers: ocular side effects. *Survey Ophthalmol.* **5**, 550–555.
Ayd, F. J., Jr. (1960). Current status of major tranquilizers. *J. Med. Soc. New Jersey* **57**, 4–14.
Ayd, F. J., Jr. (1960). Tranquilizers and the ambulatory geriatric patient. *J. Am. Geriat. Soc.* **8**, 909–914.
Ayd, F. J., Jr. (1961). Phenothiazine tranquilizers: eight years of development. *Med. Clin. N. Am.* **45**, 1027–1040.
Ayd, F. J., Jr. (1961). A survey of drug-induced extrapyramidal reactions. *J. Am. Med. Assoc.* **175**, 1053–1060.
Ayd, F. J., Jr. (1964). Uses and side effects of phenothiazines. *Mind (London)* **1**, 326–348; *Mod. Med. (Minneapolis)* **32**, 110–113.
Azima, H., Durost, H., and Cahn, C. (1958). Vesprin and Mopazine: two new phenotropic substances. *Am. J. Psychiat.* **114**, 747.
Bajaj, J. S. (1961). Psychopharmaceuticals. *Punjab Med. J.* **11**, 25–32.
Baker, W. W. (1961). Pharmacology of the central nervous system. *Prog. Neurol. Psychiat.* **16**, 95–123.
Beckman, H. (1961). "Pharmacology. The Nature, Action and Use of Drugs", 2nd ed. pp. 280, 287, 419, 420, 600, and 709–711. Saunders, Philadelphia, Pennsylvania.
Bellville, J. W. (1964). Antiemetic agents. *In* "Drugs of Choice 1964–1965". (W. Modell ed.), pp. 324–337. Mosby, St. Louis, Missouri.
Benson, W. M., and Schiele, B. C. (1960). Current status of tranquilizing and antidepressive drugs. *J. Lancet* **80**, 579–592.
Benson, W. M., and Schiele, B. C. (1962). The major tranquilizers. *In* "Tranquilizing and Antidepressive Drugs", Thomas, Springfield, Illinois. pp. 12, 13, 18, and 21.
Bodi, T., *et al.* (1960). Methoxypromazine maleate in cases of psychoneurosis. *Postgrad. Med.* **27**, 541–547.
Bodi, T., *et al.* (1960). Tentone in psychoneurosis. *Current Med. Dig.* **27**, 139–140.
Borel, C. B., and Dechosal, F. (1957). Therapeutic trials with 2 phenothiazine derivatives: RP 4632 (Mopazine) and RP 6140 (Stemetil). *Ann. Med.-Psychol.* **115**, 526–529.
Bradley, P. B., and Hance, A. J. (1957). The effect of chlorpromazine and methopromazine on the electrical activity of the brain in the cat. *Electroencephalog. Clin. Neurophysiol.* **9**, 191–215.
Brett, R. J. (1961). A note on the tranquilizers. *Rocky Mt. Med. J.* **58**, 34–35 and 59–60.
Burns, R. P. (1961). Ocular side effects of systemic medication. *Northwest Med.* **60**, 1083–1092.
Cahn, J., Georges, G., and Pierre, R. (1957). Etude pharmacologique d'un Nouveau Derive de la Phenothiazine, le 4632 RP ou Methopromazine. *Compt. Rend. Soc. Biol.* **151**, 2082–2084.
Carver, M. J. (1963). Differential effects of phenothiazines on hexose phosphate dehydrogenases. *Biochem. Pharmacol.* **12**, 19–24.

A.6. METHOXYPROMAZINE

Cattell, J. P., and Malitz, S. (1960). Revised survey of selected psychopharmacological agents. *Am. J. Psychiat.* **117**, 449–453.

Concise Directory of Psychic Drugs. (1960). *Med. World News* **1**, 12–13. (Editorial.)

Courvoisier, S., Ducrot, R., Fournel, J., and Julou, L. (1957). Propriete Pharmacodynamique de la Methopromazine, Nouveau Neuroleptique Apparente a la Chlorpromazine. (Pharmacodynamic properties of methopromazine; new neuroleptic related to chlorpromazine.) *Compt. Rend. Soc. Biol.* **151**, 689–692.

Current Concepts in Therapy. (1961). Complications from psychotherapeutic drugs. *New Engl. J. Med.* **264**, 399–400. (Editorial.)

Delay, J., et al. (1956). Clinical trial of methopromazine; comparison with chlorpromazine. Presented at the 54th Congress of Psychiatrists and Neurologists of France, Bordeaux, Sept. 1956.

Delay, J., et al. (1956). A new neuroleptic phenothiazine: Methopromazine (4632 R.P.), Presented at the 54th Congress of Psychiatrists and Neurologists of France, Bordeaux, Sept. 1956.

Foltz, L. M. (1962). Critical evaluation of tranquilizers. *J. Kentucky Med. Assoc.* **60**, 733–738.

Freeman, J. T. (1963). "Clinical Principles and Drugs in the Aging", pp. 485. Thomas, Springfield, Illinois.

Freyhan, F. A. (1959). Therapeutic implications of differential effects of new Phenothiazine compounds. *Am. J. Psychiat.* **115**, 577–585.

Friend, D. D. (1960). The phenothiazines. *Clin. Pharmacol. Therap.* **1**, 5–10.

Friend, D. G. (1964). Sedatives and tranquilizers in general medical practice. *In* "Drugs of Choice 1964–1965", (W. Modell, ed.), pp. 266–279. Mosby, St. Louis, Missouri.

Gosline, E., Walters, C. J., and Saunders, J. C. (1959). Clinical report on methoxypromazine. A new phenothiazine. *Am. J. Psychiat.* **116**, 939.

Gray, W. D., Osterberg, A. C., Rauh, C. E., and Hill, R. T. (1960). The behavioral and other pharmacodynamic actions of methoxypromazine [TENTONE (R)]; a tranquilizing agent. *Arch. Intern. Pharmacodyn.* **125**, 101–120.

Hukuji, G. (1962). The present situation of tranquilizers (in Japanese). *Rinsho Naika Shonika* **17**, 427.

Hurst, L. A. (1961). Tranquilizers and psycho-energizers. *Med. Proc.* (*Johannesburg*) **6**, 158–163.

Jourdan, F., Duchene-Marullaz, P., et al. (1958). Methopromazine, Appareil Cardio-Vasculaire et Systeme Nerveux Vegetatif. *Compt. Rend. Soc. Biol.* **152**, 91–93.

Kato, L., and Gozsy, B. (1961). Differential and quantitative affinity of psychoactive drugs to mucopolysaccharides. *Indian J. Med. Res.* **49**, 788–798.

Kato, L., et al. (1962). Attempt to classify psychotropic drugs, based on their affinity to mucopolysaccharides *in vivo*. *J. Clin. Exptl. Psychopathol.* **23**, 75–90.

Khozen, N., et al. (1962). The mammotropic effect of tranquilizing drugs. *Arch. Intern. Pharmacodyn.* **141**, 291–305.

Kline, N. S. (1960). Psychopharmaceuticals; uses and abuses. *Postgrad. Med.* **27**, 620–629.

Kline, N. S. (1961). The use of psychopharmaceuticals in office practice. *Med. Clin. N. Am.* **45**, 1677–1684.

Levinsky, W. J. (1961). Current therapy of common medical problems, the psychotherapeutic agent. *Delaware State Med. J.* **33**, 72–76.

Levy, L., and Ban, T. (1962). Phenothiazine drugs and the general practioner. *Can. Med. Assoc. J.* **86**, 415–417.

Lifshitz, K., and Kline, N. S. (1963). Psychopharmacology of the aged. *In* "Clinical Principles and Drugs in the Ageing". (J. T. Freeman, ed.), pp. 421–457. Thomas, Springfield, Illinois.

Martin, G. J., Brendel, R., and Beiler, J. M. (1956). Physiological effects of phenothiazine derivatives. *Arzneimittel-Forsch.* **6**, 408–409.

Editorial (1959). A mild phenothiazine for office practice. *Med. Sci. Publ., Army Med. Serv. Grad. School, Walter Reed Army Med. Center* **5**, 815–816.

Editorial (1960). New and nonofficial drugs; methoxypromazine maleate. *J. Am. Med. Assoc.* **172**, 1519–1520.
Editorial (1963). Neuropsychiatric disorders. *Year Book Drug Therapy* 1962–1963, 330–366.
Rossie, G. V. (1960). Psychotherapeutic drugs. *Am. J. Pharm.* **132**, 86–97.
Schafer, W. B. (1961). The actions and pediatric uses of Ataractic drugs. *Los Angeles Child Hosp. Med. Bull.* **8**, 75–80.
Schiele, B. C. (1962). Newer drugs for mental illness. *J. Am. Med. Assoc.* **181**, 126–133.
Scott, G. T. (1959). Melanophore dispersing action of ataraxic drugs. *Biol. Bull.* **117**, 400 (abstr.).
Scott, G. T., and Nading, L. K. (1961). Relative effectiveness of phenothiazine tranquilizing drugs causing release of MSH. *Proc. Soc. Exptl. Biol. Med.* **106**, 88–90.
Societye des Usines Chimiques Rhone-Poulenc. (1955). Derivatives of phenothiazine. *British Patent* 724, 217.
Sulman, F. G. (1959). The mechanism of the "Push and Pull" principle. II. Endocrine effects of hypothalamus depressants of the phenothiazine group. *Arch. Intern. Pharmacodyn.* **118**, 298–307.
Tice, L. F. (1960). New drugs of 1959. *Am. J. Pharm.* **132**, 46–77.
Viaud, P. (1954). Les Amines Derivees de la Phenothiazine. *J. Pharm. Pharmacol.* **6**, 361–389.

∼ A.7 ∼
Perphenazine

Chemical Papers

Anders, M. W., *et al.* (1962). Gas chromatography of some pharmacologically active phenothiazines. *J. Chromatog.* **7**, 258–260.
Cares, R. M., *et al.* (1963). Comparative review of the structure and side-effects of newer psychotropic agents. *Diseases Nervous System* **24**, Pt. 2, 92–105.
Cooper, T. B., *et al.* (1963). Iodoamino acid distribution in the serum of schizophrenic patients receiving Perphenazine. *Life Sci.* **7**, 527–531.
Eagleson, D. A. (1963). Paper chromatographic differentiation of some important phenothiazines encountered in toxicology. *Am. J. Clin. Pathol.* **39**, 648–651.
Forrest, F. M., *et al.* (1959). A rapid, semi-quantitative urine color test for piperazine-linked phenothiazine drugs (Compazine, Trilafon and analogous compounds). *Am. J. Psychiat.* **116**, 549–551.
Forrest, F. M., *et al.* (1961). Review of rapid urine tests for phenothiazine and related drugs. *Am. J. Psychiat.* **118**, 300–307.
Forrest, I. S., *et al.* (1960). Urine color test for the detection of phenothiazine compounds. *Clin. Chem.* **6**, 11–15.
Gothelf, B., *et al.* (1963). Quantitative colorimetric method and extraction procedure for determination of chlorpromazine in animal tissues. *Intern. J. Neuropharmacol.* **2**, 95–99.
Gold, S., *et al.* (1962). Phenothiazines in urine. *J. Mental Sci.* **108**, 88–94.
Heffelfinger, J. C., *et al.* (1960). False negative urine tests in surveys for phenylketonuria. *Pediatrics* **25**, 1086–1087.
Hetzel, C. A. (1961). Method for the estimation of phenothiazine derivatives in urine and blood. *Clin. Chem.* **7**, 130–135.
Heymann, J. J., *et al.* (1960). The estimation of phenothiazines using chemically impregnated paper strips. *Am. J. Psychiat.* **116**, 1108–1109.
Hoffer, A., *et al.* (1961). The presence of unidentified substances in the urine of psychiatric patients. *J. Neuropsychiat.* **2**, 331–362.
Hollister, L. E., *et al.* (1960). Abnormal symptoms, signs, and laboratory tests during treatment with phenothiazine derivatives. *Clin. Pharmacol. Therap.* **1**, 284–283.
Janssen, P. A. J., *et al.* (1959). Chemistry and pharmacology of CNS depressants related to 4-(4-hydroxy-4-phenylpiperidino) butyrophenone. Part I.—Synthesis and screening data in mice. *J. Med. Pharm. Chem.* **1**, 281–297.
Jucker, E. (1961). Chemie der psychotropen Pharmaka. *Chimia (Aarau)* **15**, 267–294.
Kabasakalian, P., *et al.* (1959). Polarographic oxidation of phenothiazine tranquilizers. *Anal. Chem.* **31**, 431.
Lever, P. G., *et al.* (1964). Observations on phenothiazine concentrates and diluting agents. *Am. J. Psychiat.* **120**, 1000–1002.
Mellinger, T. J., *et al.* (1962). Chromatography and electrophoresis of phenothiazine drugs. *J. Pharm. Sci.* **51**, 1169–1173.
Parker, K. D., *et al.* (1962). Separation and identification of tranquilizers by gas chromatography. *Anal. Chem.* **34**, 757–760.
Parkes, M. W. (1961). Tranquilizers. *Progr. Med. Chem.* **1**, 72–131.

Paulus, W., et al. (1963). Dunnschichtchromatographische Untersuchungen einiger Phaenothiazine und ahnlich wirkender Stoffe. *Arzneimittel-Forsch.* **13**, 609–610. (Decentan.)
Rajeswaran, P., et al. (1961). Tranquilizing and related drugs: Properties for their identification (Part I). *Bull. Narcotics, U.N. Dept. Social Affairs* **13**, 15–37.
Rajeswaran, P., et al. (1961). Tranquilizing and related drugs: Properties for their identification (Part II). *Bull. Narcotics, U.N. Dept. Social Affairs* **13**, 21–32.
Rajeswaran, P., et al. (1962). Tranquilizing and related drugs: Properties for their identification (Part III). *Bull. Narcotics, U.N. Dept. Social Affairs* **14**, 19–33.
Sobolewski, G., et al. (1960). A scheme for the rapid identification in urine of commonly used sedatives, hypnotics and tranquilizers. *Clin. Chem.* **6**, 153–161.
Sunshine, I. (1963). Use of thin layer chromatography in the diagnosis of poisoning. *Am. J. Clin. Pathol.* **40**, 576–582.
Varcerkova, J., et al. (1962). Uber den papierchromatographischen Nachweis der Antihistaminica und Ataractica durch Umkehrphasenchromatographie im System Petroleum-Athanol/Wasser/Ammoniak. *Pharmazie* **17**, 22–29.
Vacerkova, J., et al. (1962). Uber das papierchromatographische verhalten der Antihistaminica, Ataractica und Gangliopiegica in Zusammenhang mit der Konstitution. *J. Chromatog.* **7**, 527–534.
Yung, D. K., et al. (1963). Identification and differentiation of some phenothiazine-type tranquilizers. *J. Pharm. Sci.* **52**, 365–370.

Biology and Pharmacology

Bennett, J. L., et al. (1961). Five phenothiazine derivatives; evaluation and toxicity studies. *Arch. Gen. Psychiat.* **4**, 413–418.
Bhargava, K. P., et al. (1963). Anti-emetic activity of phenothiazines in relation to their chemical structure. *Brit. J. Pharmacol.* **21**, 436–440.
Biel, J. H., et al. (1962). Cholinergic blockade as an approach to the development of new psychotropic agents. *Ann. N.Y. Acad. Sci.* **96**, 251–262.
Blumberg, H., et al. (1959). High activity of potent analgesics on conditioned rat tranquilizer tests. *Proc. Soc. Exptl. Biol. Med.* **101**, 594–596.
Borsy, J., et al. (1960). A method of assaying tranquilizing drugs based on the inhibition of orientational hypermotility. *Arch. Intern. Pharmacodyn.* **124**, 180–190.
Brown, D. A., et al. (1964). The effects of some centrally-acting drugs on ganglionic transmission in the cat. *Brit. J. Pharmacol.* **23**, 241–256.
Burkman, A. M. (1961). Antagonism of apomorphine by chlorinated phenothiazines. *J. Pharm. Sci.* **50**, 156–160.
Burkman, A. M. (1962). Relationship of relative inhibitor potency to magnitude of challenge. I. Phenothiazine suppression of pecking syndromes of varying intensity. *Arch. Intern. Pharmacodyn.* **137**, 404–409.
Burkman, A. M. (1961). Relative potencies of some phenothiazines as pecking syndrome inhibitors. *J. Pharm. Sci.* **50**, 771–773.
Chow, M. I. (1959). Effect of monoamine oxidase inhibitors on experimental convulsions. *Federation Proc.* **18**, 1485.
Cook, L., et al. (1960). The interaction of drugs and behavior. *Neuropsychopharmacology*, **2**, 77–92.
Cook, L., et al. (1962). Drug effects on the behavior of animals. *Ann. N.Y. Acad. Sci.* **96**, 315–335.
Cranston, E. M. (1961). Anti-estrus drugs on substrus of ovariectomized C_3H mice. *Proc. Soc. Exptl. Biol. Med.* **106**, 514–518.

Cranswick, E. H., et al. (1964). Perphenazine and thyroid function. Am J. Psychiat. **120**, 1133–1134.
Danon, A., et al. (1963). Stimulation of prolactin secretion by perphenazine in pituitary hypothalamus organ culture. Proc. Soc. Exptl. Biol. Med. **114**, 366–368.
Decsi, L. (1961). Further studies on the metabolic background of tranquilizing drug action Psychopharmacolgia **2**, 224–242.
Delay, J., et al. (1960). Effects correcteurs et protecteurs de l'acide adenosine-t-triphosphorique vis-a-vis des syndromes neurologiques. Compt. Rend. Soc. Biol. **153**, 1177–1181.
DiMascio, A., et al. (1963). The psychopharmacology of phenothiazine compounds: A comparative study of the effects of chlorpromazine, promethazine, trifluoperazine and perphenazine in normal males. J. Nervous Mental Disease **136**, 15–28.
DiMascio, A., et al. (1963). The psychopharmacology of phenothiazine compounds: A comparative study of the effects of chlorpromazine, promethazine, trifluoperazine, and perphenazine in normal males. II: Results and discussion. J. Nervous Mental Disease **136**, 168–186.
Dobkin, A. B., et al. (1959). The effect of perphenazine on epinephrine-induced cardiac arrhythmias in dogs: I. Anaesthesia with fluothane, and fluothane-ether azeotrope. Can. Anaesthesiol. Soc. J. **6**, 243–250.
Dobkin, A. B., et al. (1959). The effect of perphenazine on epinephrine-induced cardiac arrhythmias in dogs. II. Anaesthesia with cyclopropane, chloroform and trichlorethylene. Can. Anaesthesiol. Soc. J. **6**, 251–262.
Dobkin, A. B., et al. (1962). The effect of SA 97, perphenazine and hydroxyzine on epinephrine-induced cardiac arrhythmias during methoxyflurane anaesthesia in dogs. Can. Anaesthesiol. Soc. J. **9**, 36–41.
Domino, E. F., et al. (1963). Effects of various drugs on a conditioned avoidance response in dogs resistant to extinction. J. Pharmacol. Exptl. Therap. **141**, 92–99.
Donnelly, J., et al. (1958). Similarities in the psychosomatic effects of insulin and chlorpromazine: A theoretical formulation. Dig. Neurol. Psychiat. **26**, 382.
Eckhardt, E. T., et al. (1962). The effect of phenothiazine derivatives on the disappearance of sulfobromothalein from mouse plasma. J. Pharmacol. Exptl. Therap. **138**, 387–391.
Eisler, M., et al. (1958). Effect of certain tranquilizers on gonadotrophin release in rats. Federation Proc. **17**, 366.
Ekström, N. A., et al. (1962). A method for quantitative determination of the inhibitory effect on the conditioned avoidance response of mice. Arzneimittel-Forsch. **12**, 1208–1209.
Emmerson, J. L., et al. (1963). Metabolism of phenothiazine drugs. J. Pharm. Sci. **52**, 411–419.
Enelow, A. J. (1964). A brief review of clinical psychopharmacology. Ariz. Med. **21**, 161–163.
Ernsting, M. J. E., et al. (1960). Biochemical studies on psychotropic drugs—I. The effect of psychotropic drugs of α-aminobutyric acid and glutamic acid in brain tissue. J. Neurochem. **5**, 121–127.
Evans, W. O. (1961). A new technique for the investigation of some analgesic drugs on reflexive behavior in the rat. Psychopharmacologia **2**, Fasc. 5, 318–325.
Fish, B. (1960). Drug therapy in child psychiatry: Pharmacological aspects. Comprehensive Psychiat. **1**, 212–227.
Gans, J. H. (1958). The pharmacology of preanesthetic agents. Cornell Vet. **48**, 300–304.
Gatti, G. L., et al. (1960). The technique of the "pole climbing response". Effect of various types of drugs on the latency-period and flight reaction of the rat. Neuropsychopharmacology **2**, 147–150.
Gatti, G. L., et al. (1961). The pole climbing response technique and its modifications designed to determine latency periods and climbing speeds of rats treated with psychotropic drugs. Sci. Rept. Ist. Super Sanita. **1**, 503–512.
Gold, E. M., et al. (1960). Comparative effects of certain non-narcotic central nervous

system analgesics and muscle relaxants on the pituitary adrenocortical system. *Ann. N.Y. Acad. Sci.* **86**, 178–190.

Gordon, M., *et al.* (1957). A biochemical evaluation of the activity of certain tranquilizers and their relationship to hormonal function. *Am. J. Psychiat.* **114**, 201–205.

Gottschalk, L. A., *et al.* (1960). Effects of perphenazine on verbal behavior patterns. A contribution to the problem of measuring the psychologic effects of psychoactive drugs. *Arch. Gen. Psychiat.* **6**, 632–639.

Grossman, S. P. (1961). Effects of chlorpromazine and perphenazine on bar-pressing performance in an approach-avoidance conflict. *J. Comp. Physiol. Psychol.* **54**, 517–521.

Guttman, H. N., *et al.* (1963). Evaluation of phenothiazines as membrane permeability alterants. Paper presented at 47th Annual Meeting, Atlantic City, New Jersey, April 16–20, 1963; (1963); *Federation Proc.* **22**, 569 (abstr.).

Guttman, H. N., *et al.* (1963). Protozoa as pharmacological tools: The phenothiazine tranquilizers. *Trans. N.Y. Acad. Sci.* [2] **26**, 75–89.

Hendley, C. D. (1957). Effect of Sch 3940 and methylpentynyl carbamate on electrical activity of the brain: comparison with other CNS depressants. *Federation Proc.* **16**, 306.

High, J. P., *et al.* (1962). Pharmacology of fluphenazine (Prolixin). *Toxicol. Appl. Pharmacol.* **2**, 540–552.

Hoffmeister, F. (1961). Ver gleichende elektroencephalographische Untersuchungen einiger Phenothiazin-Derivate an wachen Katzen und Kaninchen. *Psychopharmacologia.* **2**, Fasc. 1, 27–46.

Hollister, L. E., *et al.* (1959). Serum oxidase activity in chronic schizophrenics treated with tranquilizing drugs. *Am. J. Psychiat.* **116**, 553–554.

Hotovy, R., *et al.* (1960). Die pharmakologischen Eigenschaften des Perphenazinsulfoxyds. *Arzneimittel-Forsch.* **10**, 638–650.

Huang, C. L., *et al.* (1964). Perphenazine (Trilafon) metabolism in psychotic patients. *Arch. Gen. Psychiat.* **10**, 639–646.

Huang, C. L., *et al.* (1961). Preliminary report on the metabolism of perphenazine (Trilafon) in psychotic patients. Paper presented at 13th Annual Meeting American Association Clinical Chemists, Aug. 28–31, 1961; *Clin. Chem.* **7**, 574 (abstr.).

Irwin, S., *et al.* (1957). Chlorpiprozine, a new tranquilizer: Comparison with chlorpromazine in the mouse, rat, cat, dog, and monkey. *J. Pharmacol. Exptl. Therap.* **119**, 154–155.

Irwin, S., *et al.* (1959). Perphenazine (Trilafon), a new potent tranquilizer and antiemetic: I. Behavior profile, acute toxicity and behavioral mode of action. *Arch. Intern. Pharmacodyn.* **118**, 358–374.

Irwin, S. (1958). Factors influencing acquisition of avoidance behavior and sensitivity to drugs. *Federation Proc.* **17**, 380.

Irwin, S., *et al.* (1960). Conditioned locomotor response with drug as the unconditioned stimulus: Individual differences. *Neuropsychopharmacology* **2**, 151–157.

Irwin, S. (1959). Comparative potency of phenothiazine tranquilizers in suppressing avoidance and locomotor behavior: its implications. Paper presented at the Miami meeting of the American Society for Pharmacology and Experimental Therapeutics, Inc., Aug. 31–Sept. 3, 1959; (1959). *Pharmacologist* **1**, 51.

Irwin, S. (1961). Correlation in rats between the locomotor and avoidance suppressant potencies of eight phenothiazine tranquilizers. *Arch. Intern. Pharmacodyn.* **132**, 279–286.

Irwin, S. (1962). Influence of experimental variables on the rate of tolerance development to chlorpromazine and perphenazine. *Federation Proc.* **21**, 419.

Jacobsen, E. (1958). The pharmacological classification of central nervous depressants. *J. Pharm. Pharmacol.* **10**, 273–294.

Jacobsen, E. (1959). The comparative pharmacology of some psychotropic drugs. *Bull. World Health Organ.* **21**, No. 4 and 5, 411–493.

Jamin, G., *et al.* (1959). Effect of centrally acting drugs upon muscular exercise in rats. *Can. J. Biochem. Physiol.* **37**, 417–423.

Janssen, P. A. J., et al. (1960). Effects of various drugs on isolation-induced fighting behavior of male mice. *J. Pharmacol. Exptl. Therap.* **129**, 471–475.

Jarrett, R. J. (1963). Some endocrine effects of two phenothiazine derivatives, chlorpromazine and perphenazine, in the female mouse. *Brit. J. Pharmacol.* **20**, 497–506.

Katona, F. (1962). Physiological effect of phenothiazines on some invertebrate animals. *U.S. Dept. Health Educ. & Welfare, Psychopharmacol. Serv. Center Bull.* **2**, 77–79.

Khazan, N., et al. (1962). The mammotropic effect of tranquillizing drugs. *Arch. Intern. Pharmacodyn.* **136**, 291–305.

Khazan, N., et al. (1963). ADH-like effect of tranquilizers in amphibians. *Proc. Soc. Exptl. Biol. Med.* **112**, 490–494.

Kivalo, E., et al. (1960). The effect of perphenazine on the ACTH release induced by neurotropic stress. *Psychopharmacologia* **1**, Fasc. 4, 288–293.

Knapp, W., et al. (1957). Some general observations involving tranquilized cockerels. *Southeastern Vet.* **9**, 13–14.

Kothari, N. J., et al. (1961). Effect of phenothiazines and hydrazines on pituitary-adrenal-cortical-response. *Psychopharmacologia* **2**, Fasc. 1, 22–26.

Lespagnol, A. (1960). La phenothiazine et ses derives. Aspects chimiques e pharmacodyn amiques. *Bull. Soc. Chim. France* **7**, 1291–1299.

Lukemeyer, J. W. (1963). Studies on the antimicrobial properties of perphenazine. Thesis (121 pp.) submitted to faculty of the Graduate School, Indiana University, June, 1963.

McKenna, J. M., et al. (1964). Perphenazine (Trilafon) and chlorpromazine in experimental shock. *Federation Proc.* **17**, 393.

Mayer, G., et al. (1961). Action de la perphenazine chez la Ratte, variations de l'etat hormonal suivant les doses administrees. *Compt. Rend. Soc. Biol.* **155**, 1285–1288.

Mechner, F., et al. (1961). A procedure for observing the time course of drug effects of operant behavior. *Federation Proc.* **20**, Pt. 1, 397 (abstr.).

Milne, J. (1959). The analysis of phenothiazine derivatives with tranquilizing properties. *J. Am. Pharm. Assoc. Sci. Ed.* **48**, 117–122.

Minakami, A., et al. (1961). Effect of various tranquilizers on the conditioned escape action of rat. *Japan. J. Pharm. Chem.* **22**, No. 2, 47; *Psychopharmacol. Abstr.* **1**, 670.

Minchin, R. L. H., et al. (1964). Comparison of psycho-therapeutic and anthelmintic activities. *Brit. J. Psychiat.* **110**, 411–414.

Mockle, J. A. (1960). Aspects pharmacologique et therapeutique des derives de la phenothiazine. *Can. Pharm. J.* **93**, 25, 54–56, and 58.

Morpurgo, C. (1962). Influence of phenothiazine derivatives on the accumulation of brain amines induced by monoamine oxidase inhibitors. *Biochem. Pharmacol.* **11**, 967–972.

Morpurgo, C., et al. (1964). Influence of antiparkinson drugs and amphetamine on some pharmacological effects of phenothiazine derivatives used as neuroleptics. *Psychopharmacologia* **6**, Fasc. 3, 178–191.

Myers, H. M., et al. (1963). Pharmacology of the sedative-hypnotic and tranquilizing drugs. *Dental Clin. N. Am.* pp. 489–502.

Oltman, J. E., et al. (1963). Protein-bound iodine in patients receiving perphenazine. *J. Am. Med. Assoc.* **185**, 726–727.

Oltman, J. E., et al. (1964). Further report on protein-bound iodine in patients receiving perphenazine. *Am. J. Psychiat.* **121**, 176–178.

Peng, M. T. (1963). Locus of emetic action of epinephrine and dopa in dogs. *J. Pharmacol. Exptl. Therap.* **139**, 345–349.

Pevaroff, S. B., et al. (1963). Circulatory effects of intravenous trimethobenzamide hydrochloride, perphenazine, and prochlorperazine. *J. Oral Surg. Anaesthesia Hosp. Dental Serv.* **21**, 24–29.

Plotnikoff, N. P. (1961). Drug resistance due to inbreeding. *Science* **134**, 1881–1882.

Plotnikoff, N. P. (1963). Effect of neurotropic drugs on a non-conditioned avoidance response. *Arch. Intern. Pharmacodyn.* **145**, 430–439.

Plotnikoff, N. P. (1963). Effect of psychoactive drugs on escape from audiogenic seizures. *Arch. Intern. Pharmacodyn.* **145**, 413–420.
Purshottam, N. (1962). Effects of tranquilizers on induced ovulation in mice. *Am. J. Obstet. Gynecol.* **83**, 1405–1409.
Purshottam, N., et al. (1961). Induced ovulation in the mouse and the measurement of its inhibition. *Fertility Sterility* **12**, 346–352.
Quadbeck, G. (1960). Zusammenhang zwischen Blut-Hirnschranken-Beeinflussung und klinischer Wirksamkeit neuroplegischer substanzen. *Med. Exptl.* **2**, No. 2–4, 192–198. (Decentan.)
Quadbeck, G. (1962). Effects of phenothiazine derivatives on blood brain barrier system. *U.S. Dept. Health, Educ. & Welfare. Psychopharmacol. Serv. Center Bull.* **2**, 83–84.
Quinton, R. M. (1963). The increase in the toxicity of yohimbine induced by imipramine and other drugs in mice. *Brit. J. Pharmacol.* **21**, 51–66.
Rafaelsen, O. J. (1959). Action of chlorpromazine and some other phenothiazine derivatives on the carbohydrate metabolism of isolated rat diaphragm and spinal cord. *Acta Psychiat. Neurol. Scand.* **38**, Suppl. 136, 73–77.
Rafaelsen, O. J. (1961). Action of phenothiazine derivatives on carbohydrate uptake of isolated rat diaphragm and isolated rat spinal cord. *Psychopharmacologia* **2**, Fasc. 3, 185–196.
Rocha E Silva, M., et al. (1963). Antagonists of bradykinin. *Med. Exptl.* **8**, 287–295.
Rosenkilde, H. (1957). A comparison of the anti-emetic effect of various tranquilizers. *J. Pharmacol. Exptl. Therap.* **119**, 180.
Rosenkilde, H., et al. (1957). A comparison of some phenothiazine derivatives in inhibiting apomorphine-induced emesis. *J. Pharmacol. Exptl. Therap.* **120**, 375–378.
Roth, F. E. (1957). Autonomic and cardiovascular studies on chlorpiprozine, a new tranquilizer. *J. Pharmacol. Exptl. Therap.* **119**, 181.
Roth, F. E., et al. (1958). Perphenazine (Trilafon) and chlorpromazine in experimental shock. *Proc. Soc. Exptl. Biol. Med.* **99**, 157–160.
Scheidy, S. F., et al. (1958). Tranquilizing drugs in veterinary practice. *Cornell Vet.* **48**, 331–347.
Scott, G. T., et al. (1961). Relative effectiveness of phenothiazine tranquilizing drugs causing release of MSH. *Proc. Soc. Exptl. Biol. Med.* **106**, 88–90.
Shurtleff, D., et al. (1962). The effects of some phenothiazine derivatives on the discrimination of auditory clicks. *Psychopharmacologia* **3**, Fasc. 3, 153–165.
Siou, G. (1958). Etude chez le rat de quelques substances dites (tranquillisantes) a l'aide d'un test d'agressivite. *J. Physiol. (Paris)* **50**, 507–509.
Steiner, W. G., et al. (1963). An electroencephalographic study of the blocking action of selected tranquilizers as a function of terminal methyl amine group. *Biochem. Pharmacol.* **12**, 687–691.
Steiner, W. G., et al. (1963). Effects of antidepressant drugs on limbic structures of rabbit. *J. Nervous Mental Disease* **137**, 277–284.
Steiner, W. G., et al. (1963). An electroencephalographic study of some structural aspects of D-amphetamine antagonism in phenothiazine and related compounds. *Intern. J. Neuropharmacol.* **2**, 327–335.
Symchowicz, S., et al. (1962). The distribution and excretion of radioactivity after administration of 35S-labelled perphenazine (Trilafon). *Biochem. Pharmacol.* **11**, 417–422.
Symchowicz, S., et al. (1962). Short communications. The metabolism of 35S-labelled perphenazine (Trilafon). *Biochem. Pharmacol.* **11**, 499–501.
Taeschler, M., et al. (1960). Zur Bedeutung vershiedoner pharmakodynamischer Eigenschaften dor Phenothiazinderivate fur ihre klinische Wirksamkeit. *Psychiat. Neurol.* **139**, 85–104.
Tedeschi, D. H., et al. (1961). Central serotonin antagonist activity of a number of phenothiazines. *Arch. Intern. Pharmacodyn.* **132**, 172–179.

Truitt, E. B. (1958). Some pharmacologic correlations of the chemotherapy of mental disease. *J. Nervous Mental Disease* **126**, 184–210.
Unger, H. R., et al. (1959). The efficacy of Trilafon in potentiating Bonamine motion sickness prophylaxis in dogs. *U.S. Air Force, School Aviation Med.* **59-78**, 1–4.
Velardo, J. T. (1958). Induction of pseudopregnancy in adult rats with Trilafon, a highly potent tranquilizer. *Fertility Sterility* **9**, 60–66.
Wallace, G. D., et al. (1960). Restraint of chimpanzees with perphenazine. *J. Am. Vet. Med. Assoc.* **136**, 222–224.
Wang, S. C. (1958). Perphenazine, a potent antiemetic. *Federation Proc.* **17**, 417.
Wang, S. C. (1958). Perphenazine, a potent and effective antiemetic. *J. Pharmacol. Exptl. Therap.* **123**, 306–310.
Weaver, L. C., et al. (1964). Effect of antiemetics and other compounds on protoveratrine induced emesis in dogs. *J. Pharm. Sci.* **53**, 417–420.
Wert, E. B. (1961). Pregancy tests. *J. Am. Med. Assoc.* **177**, 279.
Winbury, M. M., et al. (1958). Suppression of cyclopropane-epinephrine arrhythmias in dogs by four phenothiazine derivatives. *Anesthesiology* **19**, 743–751.
Wyant, G. M. (1962). A comparative study of eleven antiemetic drugs in dogs. *Can. Anaesthesiol. Soc. J.* **9**, 399–407.

Side Effects

Adler, E. (1960). Dystonic reaction to perphenazine (Trilafon). *Med. J. Australia* **47**, No. 1, 707.
Amdisen, A. (1964). Drug-produced obesity; experiences with chloromazine, perphenazine and clopenthixol. *Danish Med. Bull.* **2**, No. 6, 182–189.
Anderson, J. H., et al. (1961). The complications and side effects of the phenothiazine ataraxics. A review of 178 clinical series of 10 phenothiazine derivates. *Bol. Assoc. Med. Puerto Rico* **53**, 123–151.
Appel, K. E., et al. (1959). The practical value of tranquilizers and their dangers. *J. Omaha Mid-West Clin. Soc.* **20**, 3–10.
Apt, L. (1960). Complications of phenothiazine tranquilizers: ocular side effects. *Surv. Ophthalmol.* **5**, 550–555.
Arneson, G. A. (1961). The risk of the new psychotropic drugs. *J. Louisiana State Med. Soc.* **113**, 372–376.
Ask, O. (1960). Considerations sur la dermatite de contact provoquee par les derives de la phenothiazine. *Therapie* **15**, No. 2, 266–269; (1961). *Excerpta Med. Sect. XIII* **15**, 198 (abstr.).
Ayd, F. J., Jr. (1960). Drug-induced extrapyramidal reactions: their clinical manifestations and treatment with Akineton. *Psychosomatics* **1**, 143–150.
Ayd, F. J., Jr. (1961). A survey of drug-induced extra-pyramidal reactions. *J. Am. Med. Assoc.* **175**, 1054–1060.
Ayd, F. J., Jr. (1963). Uses and side effects of phenothiazines. *Mind* **1**, 326–348; (1964). *Appl. Therap.* **6**, 301 and 303.
Barnett, A. M. (1960). Dystonic reaction to perphenazine (Trilafon). *S. African Med. J.* **34**, 134.
Ben-David, M., et al. (1965). Production of lactation by non-sedative phenothiazine derivatives. *Proc. Soc. Exptl. Biol. Med.* **118**, 265–270.
Bergmann, F., et al. (1962). Comparison of the influence of graded doses of phenothiazines and pentobarbitone on central nystagmus. *Exptl. Neurol.* **5**, 210–217.
Berkowitz, D., et al. (1961). Occurrence of jaundice during treatment with perphenazine and beta-phenyliso-prophylhydrazine. *Am. J. Digest. Diseases* **6**, 160–165.

Berry, R. V., et al. (1958). An ususual complication following the use of Trilafon in children. *U.S. Armed Forces Med. J.* **9**, 745–749.
Bickerstaff, E. R., et al. (1960). Oculogyric crises with phenothiazine derivatives. *Brit. Med. J.* I., 647. (Fentazin.)
Blom, S., et al. (1961). Comparison between akathisia developing on treatment with phenothiazine derivatives and the restless legs syndrome. *Acta Med. Scand.* **170**, 689–694.
Bloom, J. B., et al. (1965). Effect on the liver of long-term tranquilizing medication. *Am. J. Psychiat.* **121**, 788–797.
Boyd, W. D. (1959). Dystonic reaction to perphenazine. Correspondence. *Brit. Med. J.* I, 859. (Fentazin.)
Bruns, W. T. (1959). Potential side-reactions of tranquilizing agents. *Wisconsin Med. J.* **58**, 356 and 374.
Burns, R. P. (1961). Ocular side effects of systemic medication. *Northwest Med.* **2**, 1083–1092.
Cain, H. D., et al. (1960). Phenothiazine ataraxics. Extrapyramidal reactions. *Calif. Med.* **93**, 24–27.
Campbell, F. A. (1961). Suicidal attempt by overdose of perphenazine (Fentazin, Trilafon). *J. Irish Med. Assoc.* **48**, 116; *Psychopharmacol. Abstr.* **1**, 123.
Cann, H. M., et al. (1960). Accidental ingestion and overdosage involving psychopharmacologic drugs. *New Engl. J. Med.* **263**, 719–724.
Cannistra, F., et al. (1959). Perphenazine in obstetrics. Evaluation of its use to replace an analgesic. *Obstet. Gynecol.* **14**, 337–341.
Cares, R. M., et al. (1961). A survey of side-effects and/or toxicity of newer psychopharmacologic agents. *Diseases Nervous System* **22**, Pt. 2, 97–105.
Cattell, J. P. (1959). Psychopharmacological agents: a selective survey. Clinical notes. *Am. J. Psychiat.* **116**, 352–354.
Chicone, L. (1961). L'intoxication par les derives de la phenothiazine. Revue et rapport de 25 cas. *Union Med. Canada* **90**, No. 5, 469–474; *Psychopharmacol. Abstr.* **1**, 191.
Cilliers, A. J. (1959). Perphenazine poisonings: a case report. *Med. Proc. S. Africa* **6**, 93–95.
Cohen, H. (1960). Primary glutethimide addiction. *N.Y. J. Med.* **60**, 280–281.
Cohen, S. (1959). Clonic convulsions. Correspondence. *J. Am. Med. Assoc.* **169**, 2066.
Cohen, S., et al. (1964). Tranquilizers and suicide in the schizophrenic patient. *Arch. Gen. Psychiat.* **11**, 312–321.
Cohlan, S. Q. (1960). Convulsive seizures caused by phenothiazine tranquilizers. *Gen. Practitioner (Australia)* **21**, 136–137.
Cook, G. C., et al. (1965). Jaundice and its relation to therapeutic agents. *Lancet* I, 175–179.
Cranswick, D. H., et al. (1962). An abnormal thyroid finding produced by a phenothiazine. *J. Am. Med. Assoc.* **181**, 554–555.
de Glanville, H. (1961). Specific tranquilizer toxicity. Letters to the editor. *Lancet* II, 109–110.
Dietrichson, G. J. F., et al. (1962). Neck-face syndrome. *Tidsskr. Norske Laegeforen.* **82**, 213–214 and 208.
Dine, O. L., et al. (1959). Muscle spasms due to perphenazine (Trilafon). *New Zealand J. Med.* **58**, 377–378.
Druckman, R., et al. (1962). Chronic involuntary movements induced by phenothiazines. *J. Nervous Mental Diseases* **135**, 69–76.
Dubois, J. R., Jr. (1963). Neurologic complications of phenothiazine therapy. *Henry Ford Hosp. Med. Bull.* **11**, 59–63.
Ehrlich, R. M. (1959). A neurological complication in children on phenothiazine tranquillizers. *Can. Med. Assoc. J.* **81**, 241–243.
Erslov, A. J., et al. (1962). Detection and prevention of drug-induced blood dyscrasis. *J. Am. Med. Assoc.* **181**, 114–119.
Fairchild, R. C. (1960). Intoxications in children. *Med. Times* **88**, 1273–1274.
Fentem, P. H., et al. (1961). Fatal jaundice after administration of pheniprazine. *Brit. Med. J.* II, 1616–1617. (Fentazin.)

Flegenheimer, W. V. (1959). Dyskinesias following therapy with phenothiazine derivatives. *J. Mt. Sinai Hosp., N.Y.* **26**, 440–446.

Fout, L. R., et al. (1961). Neck-face syndrome; a report of severe reactions to phenothiazine drugs in four patients. *Ohio Med. J.* **57**, 405–406.

Frankau, I. M., et al. (1960). The treatment of drug-addiction. *Lancet* II, 1377–1379. (Fentazin.)

Freedman, D. X., et al. (1961). Factors that determine drug-induced akathisia. *Diseases Nervous System* **22**, Suppl., 69–76.

Freedman, D. X., et al. (1961). Thresholds for drug-induced akathisia. *Am. J. Psychiat.* **117**, 930–931.

Friedman, J. H., et al. (1961). An unusual central nervous system complication of perphenazine. A case report. *Diseases Nervous System* **22**, 398–400.

Goodman, D., et al. (1959). Contact dermatitis to phenothiazine drugs. *J. Invest. Dermatol.* **33**, 27–29.

Gowdey, C. W., et al. (1961). Parkinsonism and the use of tranquilizers. *Can. Psychiat. Assoc. J.* **6**, 79–87.

Graff, T. D., et al. (1959). Clonic convulsions after the oral use of perphenazine (Trilafon) Clinical notes. *J. Am. Med. Assoc.* **169**, 834–835.

Graham, G. K. (1959). Severe side reaction to therapeutic dosage of perphenazine. *New Engl. J. Med.* **260**, 1133.

Gross, M., et al. (1960). Discontinuation of treatment with ataractic drugs; a preliminary report. *Am. J. Psychiat.* **116**, 931–932.

Grunthal, E., et al. (1961). Uber Schadigung der Oliva inferior durch Chlorperphenazin (Trilafon). *Psychiat. Neurol.* **140**, 249–257; (1961). *Dig. Neurol. Psychiat.* **29**, 87 (abstr.).

Gruich, F. G. (1960). Drug reactions simulating extrapyramidal effects. *Obstet. Gynecol.* **16**, 618–620.

Haden, P. (1964). Gastrointestinal disturbances associated with withdrawal of ataractic drugs. *Can. Med. Assoc. J.* **91**, 974–975.

Herschel, P. (1959). The tranquilizing drugs: Unfavorable effects in children. *Kaiser Found. Med. Bull.* **7**, 61–73.

Hobday, J. D., et al. (1962). Unusual neonatal haemorrhage. *Brit. Med. J.* II, 193. (Fentazin.)

Hodgsson, J. E. (1959). Accurate pregnancy testing in tranquilized patients. *J. Am. Med. Assoc.* **170**, 1890–1892.

Hollister, L. E. (1958). Allergic reactions to tranquilizing drugs. *Ann. Internal Med.* **49**, 17–29.

Hollister, L. E. (1961). Current concepts in therapy. Complications from psychotherapeutic drugs. I. *New Engl. J. Med.* **264**, 291–293.

Hollister, L. E. (1961). Current concepts in therapy. Complications from psychotherapeutic drugs. III. Antidepressant drugs. *New Engl. J. Med.* **264**, 399–400.

Hollister, L. E. (1964). Adverse reactions to phenothiazines. *J. Am. Med. Assoc.* **189**, 311–313.

Hollister, L. E. (1964). Complications from psychotherapeutic drugs—1964. *Clin. Pharmacol. Therap.* **5**, 322–333.

Hooper, J. H., Jr., et al. (1961). Abnormal lactation associated with tranquilizing drug therapy. *J. Am. Med. Assoc.* **178**, 506–507.

Hunter, R., et al. (1964). An apparently irreversible syndrome of abnormal movements following phenothiazine medication. *Proc. Roy. Soc. Med.* **57**, 758–762.

Jacobziner, H., et al. (1958). Briefs on accidental chemical poisonings in New York City. Incident 7. *N.Y. State J. Med.* **58**, 4056–4057.

Jacobziner, H., et al. (1959). Accidental chemical poisonings in adults. Incident 5. *N.Y. State J. Med.* **59**, 2224–2225.

Jacobziner, H., et al. (1959). Tranquilizer and lye poisonings. Incident 4. Briefs on accidental chemical poisonings in New York City. *N.Y. State J. Med.* **59**, 4015–4016.

Jenkins, S. B. (1963). The use and abuse of phenothiazines in treatment of acute psychoses. *J. Natl. Med. Assoc.* **55**, 515–519.

Johnson, W. (1960). Toxic amblyopia from perphenazine (Fentazin). *J. Mental Sci.* **106**, 352–354.

Joyce, C. R. B. (1959). Consistent differences in individual reactions to drugs and dummies. *Brit. J. Pharmacol.* **14**, 512–521.

Karn, W. N., et al. (1959). Pharmacologically induced Parkinson like signs as index of therapeutic potential. *Diseases Nervous System* **20**, 119–122.

Karpas, C. M. (1960). Severe and fatal reactions to tranquilizers. Questions and answers. *J. Am. Med. Assoc.* **172**, 1872.

Kassler, H. M. (1964). The neck-face syndrome following the use of phenothiazine drugs. *Oral Surg., Oral Med., Oral Pathol.* **17**, 450–452.

Kaye, S. (1962). Simple reliable tests for some common poisons and drug overdosage. *Clin. Med.* **69**, 1971–1975.

Kennedy, B., et al. (1961). Phototoxic and photoallergic skin reactions resulting from modern drug therapy. *J. Louisiana State Med. Soc.* **113**, 365–371.

Keup, W. (1959). Effect of phenothiazine derivatives on liver function. *Disease Nervous System* **20**, 161–175.

Kirshbaum, B. A., et al. (1964). Photosensitization due to drugs; a review of some of the recent literature. *Am. J. Med. Sci.* **248**, 445–468.

Klett, C. J., et al. (1960). Weight changes during treatment with phenothiazine derivatives. *J. Neuropsychiat.* **2**, 102–108.

Kline, N. S. (1959). Psychopharmaceuticals: effects and side effects. *Bull. World Health Organ.* **21**, No. 4 and 5, 397–410.

Korst, D. R. (1959). Agranulocytosis caused by phenothiazine derivatives. *J. Am. Med. Assoc.* **170**, 2076–2081.

Kovan, R. A. (1958). Case reports. Acute anxiety from abuse of tranquilizing drugs. *J. Am. Osteopath. Assoc.* **57**, 596–598.

Kozinn, P. J., et al. (1960). Oculogyric crisis after a small dose of perphenazine. Case report of an eight-year-old girl. *J. Am. Med. Assoc.* **174**, 304–305.

Krogh, I., et al. (1960). Angranulocytose after behandling med phenothiazinderivater. *Ugeskrift Laeger* **122**, No. 25, 860–861; *Excerpta Med. Sect. VI.* **15**, 339 (abstr.).

Kurland, A. A., et al. (1960). The phenothiazine tranquilizers—their neurological complications and significance. *Psychosomatics* **1**, 192–194.

Larson, A. N., et al. (1959). A note on the clinical effects of perphenazine at very high dosages. *Am. J. Psychiat.* **116**, 456–457.

Lehmann, H. E. (1963). Use and abuse of phenothiazines. *Appl. Therap.* **5**, 1057–1060, 1062, 1067 and 1069.

Lerner, S., et al. (1962). Extrapyramidal reactions to prochlorperazine and perphenazine in same patient. *N.Y. State J. Med.* **62**, 2852–2853.

Lockey, S. D. (1964). Adverse reactions to drugs. *Penna. Med. J.* **67**, 45–51.

Lowance, M. I. (1960). Drug reactions: report of 150 cases. *Southern Med. J.* **53**, 850–852.

Lutz, J. F., et al. (1960). Extrapyramidal effects due to perphenazine (Trilafon). Report of 3 cases of stiffjaw sign. *Am. J. Obstet. Gynecol.* **79**, 296–298.

Mandel, W., et al. (1961). Withdrawal of maintenance antiparkinson drug in the phenothiazine-induced extrapyramidal reaction. *Am. J. Psychiat.* **118**, 350–351.

Marcus, S., et al. (1960). Trismus due to perphenazine (Trilafon) and proclorperazine (Compazine). *Calif. Med.* **92**, 226–228.

Martin, G. J. (1963). The biochemical basis of psychotherapeutics; part III. *J. Germantown Hosp.* **4**, 23–28.

Massey, L. W. (1965). Skin pigmentation, corneal and lens opacities with prolonged chlorpromazine treatment. *Can. Med. Assoc. J.* **92**, 186–187.

May, R. H. (1959). Catatonic-like states following phenothiazine therapy. *Am. J. Psychiat.* **115**, 1119–1120.
Melvin, K. E. W. (1962). Tetanus-like reactions to phenothiazine drugs. *New Zealand Med. J.* **61**, 90; (1963). *Clin. Med.* **70**, 978 (abstr.).
Middleton, G. D., et al. (1960). Hypotensive effect of perphenazine. *Brit. Med. J.* II, 1454–1455. (Fentazin.)
Montgomery, R. D. (1959). Acute dystonic reaction to perphenazine. *Brit. Med. J.* I, 215.
Moore, H. W. (1962). Toxicity of phenothiazine tranquillizers. *J. S. Carolina Med. Assoc.* **58**, 485–486.
Morpurgo, C. (1962). Effects of antiparkinson drugs on a phenothiazine-induced catatonic reaction. *Arch. Intern. Pharmacodyn.* **137**, 84–90.
Moya, F., et al. (1963). The effects of drugs used in labor on the fetus and newborn. *Clin. Pharmacol. Therap.* **4**, 628–653.
Nahunek, K. (1962). Die Behandlung Endogener Depressionen Mit Perphenazin Und Trihexyphenidyl. Beziehung Zur Extrapyramidalen Symptomatologie. *Acta Psychiat. Scand.* **38**, No. 2, 108–116.
Nahunek, K., et al. (1961). Therapeutic results with perphenazine in schizophrenic psychoses with reference to extrapyramidal symptomatology. *Cesk. Psychiat.* **57**, No. 4, 238–245; (1962). *Excerpta Med. Sect. VIII* **15**, 939 (abstr.).
Neghandi, D. B., et al. (1960). Acute dystonic reaction to perphenazine. Case reports. *E. African Med. J.* **37**, 295.
Neurotoxic effects accompanying poisoning from the phenothiazide tranquilizers. (1960). *Am. J. Hosp. Pharm.* **17**, 248.
Nour-Eldin, F. (1962). Unusual neonatal haemorrhage. *Brit. Med. J.* II, 411. (Fentazin.)
Oliver, H. R., et al. (1961). Complications in Trilafon therapy. *Diseases Nervous System* **22**, 32–34.
Ose, E. (1959). Promotion of infections by tranquilizers. Foreign letters. *Tidsskr. Norske Laegeforen. J. Am. Med. Assoc.* **172**, 262 (1960).
Paterson, A. S. (1959). Addiction to tranquillizers. Notes and queries. *Practitioner* **183**, 773.
Pisciotta, A. V., et al. (1958). Agranulocytosis following administration of phenothiazine derivatives. *Am. J. Med.* **25**, 210–223.
Popper, H., et al. (1965). Drug-induced liver disease; a penalty for progress. *Arch. Internal Med.* **115**, 128–136.
Preston, J. (1959). Central nervous system reactions to small doses of tranquilizers. Report of one death. *Am. Practitioner Dig. Treat.* **10**, 627–630.
Proctor, R. C. (1960). The use and abuse of tranquilizing drugs. *J. Tenn. State Med. Assoc.* **53**, 295–299.
Reboton, J., Jr., et al. (1962). Pigmentary retinopathy and irido-cycloplegia in psychiatric patients. *J. Neuropsychiat.* **3**, 311–316.
Rectem, V., et al. (1960). Intoxications accidentelles au Trilafon. *Acta. Paediat. Belg.* **14**, Fasc. 1, 47–49.
Richard, J. (1961). Reactions d'intolerance a la perphenazine chez l'enfant. *Acta. Pediat. Belg.* **15**, No. 1, 38–43; *Psychopharmacol. Abstr.* **1**, 192.
Robinson, A. S. (1960). "Neck-face syndrome" related to phenothiazine drugs. *J. Am. Med. Assoc.* **173**, 504–506.
Rodman, M. J. (1962). Drug poisonings. *R.N.* **25**, 68–74.
Rodman, M. J. (1962). New drugs for headache. *R.N.* **25**, 47–52, 64 and 66.
Rodman, M. J. (1964). Management in drug abuse and addiction. *R.N.* **27**, 59–64 and 77–79.
Rose, T. F. (1958). The use and abuse of the tranquilizers. *Can. Med. Assoc. J.* **78**, 144–148.
Sandford, J. R. (1959). Dystonic reaction to perphenazine. Correspondence. *Brit. Med. J.* I, 859.

Satanove, A. (1965). Pigmentation due to phenothiazines in high and prolonged dosage. *J. Am. Med. Assoc.* **191**, 263–268.
Saunders, J. C., *et al.* (1964). Phenothiazine effect on human antibody synthesis. *Brit. J. Psychiat.* **110**, 84–89.
Sensitivity to perphenazine. (1962). *Brit. Med. J.* II, 496.
Shafer, S., *et al.* (1962). Extrapyramidal effects of tranquillisers. *Lancet* I, 221–222. (Fentazin.)
Shanon, J. (1959). Neuromuscular symptoms simulating conversion hysteria caused by perphenazine (Trilafon). *Diseases Nervous System* **20**, 24–26.
Shanon, J., *et al.* (1957). An interesting reaction to a tranquilizer: tonic seizures with perphenazine (Trilafon). *Am. J. Psychiat.* **114**, 556.
Shaw, C. C., *et al.* (1959). Treacherous tranquilizers. *Anesthesia Analgesia, Current Res.* **38**, 319–327.
Shaw, C. C., *et al.* (1959). Treacherous tranquilizers. *Am. J. Med. Sci.* **237**, 141–150.
Shaw, E. B. (1958). Convulsive seizures following phenothiazine tranquilizers. *Pediatrics* **22**, 175–176.
Shaw, E. B., *et al.* (1959). Phenothiazine tranquilizers as a cause of severe seizures. *Pediatrics* **23**, 485–492.
Sherman, S., *et al.* (1960). Oculogyric crisis induced by phenothiazine drugs. *Diseases Nervous System* **21**, 333–334.
Shidemann, F. E. (1961). Toxicity of the phenothiazines. *Wisconsin Med. J.* **60**, 487–488.
Shield, J. A. (1958). Tranquilizers. Uses and abuses. *Virginia Med. Monthly* **85**, 111–117.
Simpson, G. M. (1961). Uneventful trifluoperazine (Stelazine) therapy after previous granulocytic depression. *J. Mental Sci.* **107**, 258–260.
Simpson, G. M., *et al.* (1964). Phenothiazine-produced extra-pyramidal system disturbance. *Arch. Gen. Psychiat.* **10**, 199–208.
Smith, M. J., *et al.* (1961). Severe extrapyramidal reaction to perphenazine treated with diphenhydramine. *New Engl. J. Med.* **264**, 396–397.
Smith, M. J., *et al.* (1962). Acute dystonic reactions to phenothiazines and response to antihistamines. *Diseases Nervous System* **23**, 466–468.
Spira, H. (1958). Uses and limitations of tranquilizing drugs in the treatment of psychiatric illness. *J. Med. Assoc. Alabama* **27**, 261–267.
Straube, W., *et al.* (1962). The long-term treatment of extrapyramidal hyperkinesias with perphenazine. *Nervenarzt* **33**, 549–553. (Decentan.)
Sykes, P. (1960). Severe reactions to fentazine in mental deficiency practice. *J. Mental Sci.* **106**, 1584–1586.
Taeschler, M., *et al.* (1961). Inhibition of emotional reactions by phenothiazine tranquillizers. *Nature* **190**, 1014–1015.
Thrower, J. C. (1963). Iatrogenic effect of drugs and anesthesia. *J. S. Carolina Med. Assoc.* **59**, 1–6.
Tranquilizer poisonings. July 1959 through Dec. 1960. (1963). *J. Iowa State Med. Soc.* **53**, 302–304.
Uhrbrand, L., *et al.* (1960). Reversible and irreversible dyskinesia after treatment with perphenazine, chlorpromazine, reserpine and electroconvulsive therapy. *Psychopharmacologia* **1**, Fasc. 5, 408–418.
Vates, T. S., *et al.* (1960). Acute extrapyramidal syndromes following the use of phenothiazine derivatives. *Med. Ann. District Columbia* **29**, 670–673.
Watson, J. (1960). Dystonic reaction to perphenazine (Trilafon). *Med. J. Australia* **47**, No. 1, 541–542.
Weekley, R. D., *et al.* (1960). Pigmentary retinopathy in patients receiving high doses of a new phenothiazine. *Arch. Ophthalmol.* **64**, 65–76.
Weintraub, W. (1962). The clinical use and misuse of tranquilizers. *Maryland Med. J.* **11**, 286–289.

Witton, K. (1961). Orthostatic hypotension secondary to psychotropic disorders; treatment with emphasis on parenteral Ritalin. *Diseases Nervous System* **23**, 189–192.
Wood, T. E., et al. (1961). Neurologic manifestations of phenothiazine toxicity. *Bull. Mason Clin.* **15**, 115–119.

Clinical Papers

Abrahamson, I. A., Sr., et al. (1959). Cataract surgery. (Modern concepts.) *Eye, Ear, Nose, Throat Monthly* **38**, 52–55.
Adelson, D., et al. (1962). A study of phenothiazines with male and female chronically ill schizophrenic patients. *J. Nervous Mental Disease* **134**, 543–554.
Aita, J. A. (1962). Maternal neurologic complications in pregnancy. *Nebraska State Med. J.* **47**, 280–285.
Aivazian, G. H. (1962). Pharmacotherapy in child psychiatry. *Memphis Med. J.* **37**, 201–205.
Albert, C. A., et al. (1959). The place of perphenazine (Trilafon) in anesthesia. *Med. Ann. District Columbia* **28**, 552–555.
Altschule, M. D. (1960). Drug action and psychological function. *J. Neuropsychiat.* **2**, 71–75.
American Medical Association. (1958). Council on drugs. Psychotherapeutic drugs. *J. Am. Med. Assoc.* **166**, 1040–1041.
Anderson, G., et al. (1959). Effect of Trilafon on nausea and vomiting during labor. *Obstet. Gynecol.* **13**, 504–505.
Angst, J. (1960). Begleiterscheinungen und Nebenwirkungen moderner Psychopharmaka. *Praxis (Bern)* **49**, 506–511.
Annesley, P. T. (1959). Fentazin (perphenazine) in chronic schizophrenia. *Med. Press* **2**, 461–462.
Antos, R. J. (1960). Use of perphenazine orally or parenterally among nonpsychotic patients. *Southwestern Med.* **41**, 463–464.
Appel, S. H., et al. (1958). Tranquilizing drugs: an approach to the chemotherapy of mental disease. *Bull. Tufts-New Engl. Med. Center* **4**, 22–35.
Archer, J. S., et al. (1962). Phenothiazine tranquilizers in anesthesia. Review, with report on fluphenazine. *N.Y. State J. Med.* **62**, 828–833.
Atkinson, R. P. (1959). Depressive episodes. *Gen. Practitioner, (Australia)* **20**, 111–119.
Ayd, F. J., Jr. (1957). A clinical appraisal of Trilafon. *Am. J. Psychiat.* **114**, 554–555.
Ayd, F. J., Jr. (1957). Tranquilizing drugs in private practice. *N.Y. State J. Med.* **57**, 1742–1747.
Ayd, F. J., Jr. (1957). Treatment of ambulatory and hospitalized psychiatric patients with Trilafon. *Diseases Nervous System* **18**, 394–397.
Ayd, F. J., Jr. (1957). The treatment of anxiety, agitation and excitement in the aged. A preliminary report on Trilafon. *J. Am. Geriat. Soc.* **5**, 92–96.
Ayd, F. J., Jr. (1958). The art of treatment with tranquilizing drugs. *Ohio Gen. Practitioner* **10**, 10–11 and 19.
Ayd, F. J. (1959). Clinical indications and toxicity of prolonged perphenazine therapy. *New Engl. J. Med.* **261**, 172–174.
Ayd, F. J., Jr. (1959). Fluphenazine: its spectrum of therapeutic application and clinical results in psychiatric patients. *Current Therap. Res.* **1**, 41–48.
Ayd, F. J., Jr. (1960). Current status of major tranquilizers. *J. Med. Soc. New Jersey* **57**, 4–14.
Ayd, F. J. (1960). Tranquilizers and the ambulatory geriatric patient. *J. Am. Geriat. Soc.* **8**, 909–914.
Ayd, F. J., Jr. (1963). Prolonged perphenazine therapy and thyroid function. *Am. J. Psychiat.* **120**, 592–594.

Ayd, F. J., Jr. (1964). Perphenazine: a reappraisal after eight years. *Diseases Nervous System* **25**, 311–317.
Ayd, F. J., Jr., *et al.* (1959). Treatment of depressive states in ambulatory patients. *Diseases Nervous System* **20**, 34–37.
Ban, T. A., *et al.* (1961). The stimulating effect of RP 8228 on inactive psychiatric patients. *J. Neuropsychiat.* **3**, 91–95.
Barbour, J. P., Jr. (1963). Maintenance therapy of chronic psychotics with perphenazine. *Am. J. Psychiat.* **120**, 176–177.
Barr, M. (1961). Antiemetic agents. *Apothecary* **73**, 17–18, 20 and 37.
Barsa, J. A. (1960). Combination drug therapy in psychiatry. *Am. J. Psychiat.* **117**, 448–449.
Barsa, J. A., *et al.* (1961). Fluphenazine use with chronic psychotic patients. *Diseases Nervous System* **23**, 211–212.
Bartholomew, A. A. (1963). Perphenazine (Trilafon) in the immediate management of acutely disturbed chronic alcoholics. *Med. J. Australia* **1**, 812–814.
Bellville, J. W. (1961). Postanesthetic nausea and vomiting. *Anesthesiology* **22**, 773–780.
Bellville, J. W., *et al.* (1960). Postoperative nausea and vomiting. V. Antiemetic efficacy of trimethobenzamide and perphenazine. *Clin. Pharmacol. Therap.* **1**, 590–595.
Bellville, J. W., *et al.* (1964). Postoperative nausea and vomiting IV: factors related to postoperative nausea and vomiting. *Anesthesiology* **21**, 186–193.
Bennett, I. F. (1957). The tranquilizers. *J. Am. Pharm. Assoc. Pract. Ed.* **18**, 547–549.
Bennett, I. F. (1957). The tranquilizers. Part IV. *J. Am. Pharm. Assoc. Pract. Ed.* **18**, 714–716.
Benson, W. M., *et al.* (1962). Current status of tranquilizing and antidepressive drugs. *J. Lancet* **80**, 579–592.
Bente, D., *et al.* (1960). EEG-Veränderungen unter chronischer Medikation von Piperazinyl-Phenothiazin-Derivaten. *Med. Exptl.* **2**, No. 2–4, 132–137. (Decentan.)
Bhargava, K. P., *et al.* (1964). Tranquillizing and hypotensive activities of twelve phenothiazines. *Brit. J. Pharmacol.* **22**, 154–161.
Birnberg, C. H., *et al.* (1959). Perphenazine suppositories in nausea and vomiting of pregnancy. *Am. J. Obstet. Gynecol.* **77**, 438–441.
Bjerkelund, C., *et al.* (1964). Perphenazine (Trilafon) in the prophylaxis of nausea and vomiting following acute myocardial infarct. 14 pp. with 11 tables.
Black, J. (1960). Phenothiazines as antiemetics and tranquilizers. *J. Med. Assoc. Alabama* **29**, 492–500.
Blackburn, H. L., *et al.* (1961). Behavioral effects of interrupting and resuming tranquilizing medication among schizophrenics. *J. Nervous Mental Disease* **133**, 303–308.
Blair, D. (1963). Drugs for depression. *Brit. Med. J.* I, 945. (Fentazin.)
Bleuler, M. (1964). Neue Therapiemoglichkeiten im Vergleich zu alten in der Psychiatrie. *Deut. Med. Wochschr.* **89**, 501–506.
Bobon, J., *et al.* (1960). Present status of neuroleptic therapy. *Rev. Med. Liege* **16**, No. 23, 694–699.
Bordeleau, J. M., *et al.* (1963). Evaluation of perphenazine in the treatment of Haitian psychotics. *Can. Psychiat. Assoc. J.* **8**, 111–115.
Böszörmenyi, Z. (1961). A frenolon es perphenazin a psychiatriai gyakorlatban. *Ideggyogy. Szemle* **14**, No. 8, 247–256; *Psychopharmacol. Abstr.* **1**, 613.
Bovet, D. (1959). Tranquilizing drugs. *Gazz. Chim. Ital.* **89**, 232–264.
Bowes, H. A. (1964). Some experiences with a combination of amitriptyline and perphenazine in severe psychiatric syndromes. *Psychosomatics* **5**, 44–47.
Bowes, H. A., *et al.* (1963). Office psychopharmacology. *Psychosomatics* **4**, 22–26. (Trilafon, Etrafon.)
Bowman, K. M. (1959). Alcoholism and geriatrics. *Am. J. Psychiat.* **115**, 619–623.
Bowman, K. M. (1960). Alcoholism. *Am. J. Psychiat.* **116**, 626–628.

Braceland, F. J. (1958). The phrenotropic drugs in mental illness. *J. Mich. Med. Soc.* **57**, 1696–1701.
Braceland, F. J. (1964). Drugs effective in emotional disorders. *Postgrad. Med.* **35**, 237–242.
Braceland, F. J., et al. (1957). Use of drugs in the treatment of neuroses and in the office management of psychoses. *Mod. Med. Minneapolis* **25**, 190–193, 196, 198–200, 203, 205, 207, 211–12, 215–217, 219, 221, 223–225, 227 and 230.
Braly, B. E., et al. (1961). The use of intramuscular perphenazine to control postoperative vomiting, a report of 2,794 cases. *Am. J. Surg.* **102**, 120–123.
Bruni, L. (1958). L'uso della perfenazina in dermatologia. *Minerva Med.* **49**, Suppl. 39, 2004–2007.
Bucove, A. (1964). Postpartum psychoses in the male. *Bull. N.Y. Acad. Med.* **40**, 961–971.
Buki, R. A. (1964). The use of psychotropic drugs in the rehabilitation of sex-deviated criminals. *Am. J. Psychiat.* **120**, 1170–1175. (Etrafon.)
Caffey, E. M., Jr. (1961). Experiences with large scale interhospital cooperative research in chemotherapy. *Am. J. Psychiat.* **117**, 713–719.
Caffey, E. M., Jr. (1962). The use of drugs in outpatient and inpatient psychiatric practice. *Virginia Med. Monthly* **89**, 55–59.
Cahn, C. H., et al. (1957). Perphenazine. Observations on the clinical effects of a new tranquillizing agent in psychotic conditions. *Can. Psychiat. Assoc. J.* **2**, 104–112.
Callahan, J. D., et al. (1960). Objective measures in psychopharmacology base-line observations. *Missouri Med.* **57**, 714–718.
Callens, M. (1958). Note préliminaire sur l'emploi de perphénazine ("Trilafon" Schering) dans les psychoses graves. *Acta Neurol. Psychiat. Belg.* **58**, 925–933.
Campden-Main, B. C., et al. (1962). American psychiatry: Current practices and views in psychopharmacology. *Diseases Nervous System* **23**, 135–140.
Capparell, H. V. (1962). Drug therapy in mental illness. *Penna. Med. J.* **65**, 899–905.
Carr, C. J., et al. (1957). The phrenotropic agents. *Intern. Record Med.* **170**, 493–504.
Cater, M. (1961). Tranquilizer for cesarean section. *Mod. Vet. Pract.* **42**, 54–55.
Casey, J. F., et al. (1960). Treatment of schizophrenic reactions with phenothiazine derivatives. A comparative study of chlorpromazine, triflupromazine, mepazine, prochlorperazine, perphenazine, and phenobarbital. *Am. J. Psychiat.* **117**, 97–105.
Cattell, J. P., et al. (1960). Revised survey of selected psychopharmacological agents. *Am. J. Psychiat.* **117**, 449–453.
Chapple, E. D., et al. (1963). The measurement of activity patterns of schizophrenic patients. *J. Nervous Mental Disease* **137**, 258–267.
Chieffi, A. (1960). Die medikamentöse Behandlung der kindlichen Neurosen. *Hippokrates* **31**, No. 24, 839; (1961). *Med. Klin. (Munich)* **56**, IX (abstr.).
Cihak, D. (1958–1959). Tranquilizers for large animals. *Iowa State Coll. Vet.* **21**, 25–26.
Coffee, H. L. (1964). Combined amitriptyline and perphenazine in combined depression and anxiety. *J. Med. Assoc. Georgia* **53**, 107–109. (Etrafon.)
Cohen, A. I. (1959). Perphenazine in allergic conditions. *Intern. Record Med.* **172**, 33–36.
Cohen, A. I. (1960). Trancopal in the treatment of musculoskeletal conditions and symptoms of allergy: report on 1391 patients. *Current Therap. Res.* **2**, 374–378.
Cohen, H., et al. (1958). Trilafon in the treatment of chronically psychotic hospitalized patients. *Am. J. Psychiat.* **115**, 452–454.
Cohen, I. M. (1958). Use of drugs in treating the emotionally disturbed patient. *Med. Ann. District Columbia* **26**, 292–297.
Collins, J. A., et al. (1960). A comparative quantitative study of antiwhealing drugs in man. *Appl. Therap.* **2**, 609–618.
Conger, C. W., et al. (1961). Control of postoperative nausea and vomiting. A double blind study of perphenazine (Trilafon) in two hundred and thirty-six patients. *Ohio Med. J.* **57**, 897–899.

Conway, S., et al. (1960). Perphenazine in Huntington's chorea. (Letters to the editor.) Lancet II, 982.
Cranswick, E. H., et al. (1963). Perphenazine and thyroid function. *J. Am. Med. Assoc.* **186**, 1102.
Culpepper, W. S. (1963). Headache: a second look by the general physician. *Postgrad. Med.* **33**, 311–315.
Cummins, A. J. (1958). Nausea and vomiting. The physiology of symptoms (III). *Am. J. Digest. Diseases* **3**, 710–721.
Cutolo, L. C., et al. (1959). Effect of perphenazine on postoperative emesis. *A.M.A. Arch. Surg.* **79**, 666–669.
Cutting, W., et al. (1958). Drugs affecting the psyche. *Kaiser Found. Med. Bull.* **6**, 128–137.
Cwynar, S., et al. (1962). Evaluation of the drug Trilafon produced by the Ferrosan Company according to experiences of the psychiatric clinic of the Academy of Medicine in Lodz. *Neurol. Neurochir. Psychiat. Polon.* **12**, 751–752.
Dack, G. M. (1960). Current status of therapy in microbial food poisoning. Report to the Council on Drugs. *J. Am. Med. Assoc.* **172**, 929–932.
Dale, P. W. (1961). Current concepts in therapy. Medical management of mental problems in the aged. *New Engl. J. Med.* **265**, 84–86.
Dandiya, P. C., et al. (1963). Studies on central nervous system depressants. Influence of some tranquillizing agents on morphine analgesia. *Arch. Intern. Pharmacodyn.* **141**, 223–232.
Darling, H. F. (1958). Use of perphenazine in 100 hospitalized patients. *Diseases Nervous System* **19**, 428–429.
Darling, H. F., et al. (1960). Fluphenazine: comparative studies. *Diseases Nervous System* **21**, 409–413.
Davies, T. S. (1959). Dystonic reaction to perphenazine. *Brit. Med. J.* I, 368.
Deming, Q., et al. (1959). Tranquilizing drugs. Combined staff clinic. *Am. J. Med.* **27**, 767–780.
Dickson, R. J. (1958). Preliminary report on Trilafon in radiation sickness. *Radiology* **70**, 259–260.
DiPalma, J. R. (1963). The basic pharmacologic principles underlying the use of sedatives and tranquilizers. *Clin. Pediat.* **2**, 225–232.
Dobkin, A. B. (1958). Efficacy of ataractic drugs in clinical anaesthesia: A review. *Can. Anaesthesiol. Soc. J.* **5**, 177–208.
Dobkin, A. B. (1959). Perphenazine in clinical anesthesia. *Can. Anaesthesiol. Soc. J.* **6**, 341–346.
Dobkin, A. B., et al. (1960). The antisialogogue effect of phenothiazine derivatives. *Brit. J. Anaesthesia* **32**, 57–59.
Dobkin, A. B., et al. (1960). Double blind study of phenothiazines used in pre-anaesthetic medication: a clinical evaluation of promethazine (Phenergan), promazine (Sparine), proclorperazine (Stemetil), and levomepromazine (Nozinan). *Can. Anaesthesiol. Soc. J.* **7**, 158–168.
Domino, E. F. (1962). Human pharmacology of tranquillizing drugs. *Clin. Pharmacol. Therap.* **3**, 599–664.
Dorfman, W. (1963). Combined drug treatment. *Am. J. Psychiat.* **120**, 275–276. (Etrafon, Triavil.)
Dorfman, W. (1963). Recent advances in psychopharmacology. *Diseases Nervous System* **24**, 694–697.
Dorfman, W. (1964). Current concepts of depression, part V; treatment of depression. *Psychosomatics* **5**, 7–13.
Dorfman, W. (1964). Some experiences in "total" treatment of patients with emotional illness. *Psychosomat. Med.* **5**, 351–354.
Doust, J. W. L., et al. (1962). Acute effects of ataractic drugs on spontaneous autonomic and

metabolic oscillating systems in schizophrenic and other psychiatric patients. *Can. Psychiat. Assoc. J.* **7**, 76–89.
Downing, J. G. (1960). Dermatologic therapy. *Med. Times* **88**, 789–796.
Dundas, E., et al. (1961). Inhibition of experimental skin wheal by some ataractic and antihistaminic drugs. *J. Allergy* **32**, 1–7.
Dundee, J. W., et al. (1961). The effects of premedication with phenothiazine derivatives on the course of methohexitone anaesthesia. *Brit. J. Anaesthesia* **33**, 382–396.
Dundee, J. W., et al. (1962). The phenothiazines. *Brit. J. Anaesthesia* **34**, 247–250.
Dundee, J. W., et al. (1964). Clinical studies of induction agents. X: The effect of phenothiazine premedication on thiopentone anaesthesia. *Brit. J. Anaesthesia* **36**, 106–109.
Dzikowski, H. (1961). Treatment by perphenazine in psychiatry in the light of personal clinical experiments. *Neurol. Neurochir. Psychiat. Polon.* **11**, No. 5, 705–711; (1963). *Excerpta Med., Sect. VIII* **16**, 169 (abstr.).
Ebaugh, F. G. (1958). Uses and abuses of tranquilizing drugs. *Dallas Med. J.* **44**, 602–608.
Edds, G. T. (1957). Tranquilizers . . . a summary. *Rocky Mt. Vet.* **5**, 28–30.
Eichner, E. (1960). Premenstrual tension syndrome and primary dysmenorrhea. *West Va. Med. J.* **56**, 1–8.
Eisenberg, B. C. (1958). Relief of allergic symptoms with tranquilizers in combination with other drugs. *Clin. Med.* **5**, 897–898, 900, and 902–904.
Eisenberg, L., et al. (1961). The effectiveness of psychotherapy alone and in conjunction with perphenazine or placebo in the treatment of neurotic and hyperkinetic children. *Am. J. Psychiat.* **117**, 1088–1093.
Enelow, A. J. (1965). Drug treatment of psychotic patients in general medical practice. *Calif. Med.* **102**, 1–4.
England, A. C., Jr. (1959). The management of Parkinson's disease. Treatment in internal medicine. *A.M.A. Arch. Internal Med.* **104**, 439–468.
English, D. C. (1961). A comparative study of antidepressants in balanced therapy. *Am. J. Psychiat.* **117**, 865–872.
Ernst, E. M. (1958). Perphenazine in nausea and vomiting and anxiety states. *Penna. Med. J.* **61**, 355–359.
Ernst, E. M. (1963). Anxiety and depression. Treatment in general practice. *Penna. Med. J.* **66**, 43–45. (Etrafon.)
Esser, A. H., et al. (1965). Productivity of chronic schizophrenics in a sheltered workshop; a quantitative evaluation of the effects of drug therapy. *Comprehensive Psychiat.* **6**, 41–50.
Exton-Smith, A. N. (1962). Tranquillizers and sedatives in the elderly. *Practitioner* **188**, 732–738.
Fanburg, S. J. (1959). Ancillary therapy of dermatoses with perphenazine. *J. Med. Soc. New Jersey* **56**, 332–334.
Fekete, G., et al. (1963). Dilatation coronaire produite par des derives de la phenothiazine. *Presse Med.* **71**, 1191 (abstr.)
Feldman, P. E. (1957). Ataractics. A study of the current status of tranquilizing drugs. *J. Kansas Med. Soc.* **58**, 658–661.
Ferreira, M. J., et al. (1961). A perphenazina em cirurgia. *Anais Paulistas Med. Cir.* **82**, 1–11.
Foltz, L. M. (1962). Critical evaluation of tranquilizers. *J. Kentucky Med. Assoc.* **60**, 733–738.
Forrest, F. M., et al. (1964). Drug maintenance problems of rehabilitated mental patients: The current drug dosage "merry-go-round". *Am. J. Psychiat.* **121**, 33–40.
Fox, V. (1960). The management of alcoholism. *J. Med. Assoc. Alabama* **29**, 501–505.
Freedman, A. M. (1958). Drug therapy in behavior disorders. *Pediat. Clin. N. Am.* **5**, 573–594.
Freyhan, F. A. (1959). Therapeutic implications of differential effects of new phenothiazine compounds. *Am. J. Psychiat.* **115**, 577–585.
Friedman, A. P. (1958). Treatment of headache. *Med. Clin. N. Am.* **42**, 659–676.
Friedman, A. P. (1959). Migraine and other common headaches. *World-Wide Abstr.* **2**, 10–20.

Friedman, A. P. (1960). Chronic headache. *Med. Times* **88**, 889–901.
Friedman, A. P. (1960). Evaluation of nonnarcotic chemical agents in headaches. *A. N.Y. Acad. Sci.* **86**, 216–225.
Friedman, A. P. (1961). Headache as a problem for the general practitioner. *Med. Clin. N. Am.* **45**, 1611–1624.
Friend, D. G. (1958). The tranquilizers. *Med. Clin. N. Am.* **42**, 1253–1268.
Friend, D. G. (1959). Current concepts in therapy. *New Engl. J. Med.* **260**, 1231–1232.
Friend, D. G. (1959). Current concepts in therapy. Tranquilizers. II. The phenothiazines I. *New Engl. J. Med.* **260**, 1028–1031.
Fromer, J. L. (1960). Dermatologic allergy VI. Critique and review of the recent literature. Progress in allergy. *Ann. Allergy* **18**, 292–337.
Fromm, H. R. (1958). Neue Arzneimittel. *Pharm. Ztg., Ver. Apotheker-Ztg.* **103**, 251–253.
Garner, H. H. (1959). Psychiatric aspects of surgery. *Ind. Med. Surg.* **28**, 351–361.
Garner, H. H. (1961). Psychiatry-office problems. Part VI. Treatment of alcoholism and drug addiction in the office. *Am. Practitioner Dig. Treat.* **12**, 21–25.
Gercke, H. (1958). Erfahrungen mit einem Perphenazin-Präparat in der Psychiatrie. *Therap. Gegenwart* **97**, 502–505. (Decentan.)
Gerz, H. O. (1962). The use of a phenothiazine compound in the rehabilitation of schizophrenic patients. *Am. J. Psychiat.* **119**, 167–168.
Gibbon, J. (1961). Some examples of the combined use of psychotropic agents. *Diseases Nervous System* **22**, Pt. 2, 81–85.
Giffen, M. B. (1961). Emotional dysfunction and the use of psychopharmacological drugs in a military theater. *Mil. Med.* **126**, 199–203.
Giorgio, D. J. (1960). Anti-emetics and tranquilizers in surgical patients. *J. Indiana State Med. Assoc.* **53**, 441–442.
Glaser, E. M., et al. (1959). Effect of drugs on motion sickness produced by short exposures to artificial waves. *Lancet* I, 853–856.
Goldman, D. (1958). The results of treatment of psychotic states with newer phenothiazine compounds effective in small doses. *Am. J. Med. Sci.* **235**, 67–77.
Goldman, L., et al. (1959). Corticosteroid therapy of the common chronic eczematous hand dermatitis. *Gen. Practitioner (Australia)* **20**, 85–91.
Goshen, C. E. (1960). Psychopharmacology reappraised. *Gen. Practitioner (Australia)* **21**, 106–114.
Gottschalk, L. A. (1960). Introspection and free association as experimental approaches to assessing subjective and behavioral effects of psychoactive drugs. *In* "Drugs and Behavior" (L. Uhr and J. G. Miller, eds.), pp. 587–590. Wiley, New York.
Graff, T. D., et al. (1959). Consciousness and pain during apparent surgical anesthesia. Report of a case. *J. Am. Med. Assoc.* **170**, 2069–2071.
Gran, L. (1962). Perphenazine in postoperative nausea and vomiting. *Tidsskr. Norskl Laegeforen.* **82**, 817; (1962). *J. Am. Med. Assoc.* **182**, 92 (abstr.).
Gready, T. G., et al. (1959). Intramuscular perphenazine in labor. *Am. J. Obstet. Gynecol.* **77**, 412–418.
Greenfield, A. R. (1961). Perphenazine in the management of acute alcoholic intoxication. *Current Therap. Res.* **3**, 217–220.
Greenfield, A. R. (1961). Use of phenothiazines in alcoholic agitation. *Med. Ann. District Columbia* **30**, 726–728.
Greenfield, A. R. (1963). Control of alcoholic agitation and depression. *Current Therap. Res.* **5**, 597. (Trilafon, Etrafon.)
Grimaldi, R. (1960). The clinical use of fluphenazine in pregnancy. *J. N.Y. Med. Coll., Flower Fifth Ave. Hosp.* **2**, 42–49.
Gross, H., et al. (1960). Klinische Probleme der Chlorperphenazin-Behandlung von Psychosen. *Muench. Med. Wochschr.* **102**, No. 12, 600–604. (Decentan.)

Gutierrez Caloca, R. (1958). La perfenazina en cardiologia. *Rev. Med. Cienc. Afines (Buenos Aires)* **17**, 143–148.
Haase, H. J. (1963). Möglichkeiten und Grenzen der Psychopharmakotherapie mit Tranquilizern und Neuroleptika. *Deut. Med. Wochschr.* **88**, 505–514.
Hampton, S. F. (1957). Emergency treatment of severe asthma. *Postgrad. Med.* **22**, 462–468.
Hanlon, T. E., et al. (1964). The comparative effectiveness of amitriptyline, perphenazine, and their combination in the treatment of chronic psychotic female patients. *J. New Drugs* **4**, 52–60. (Triavil.)
Haran, T. (1960). Perphenazine (Fentazin) in the management of chronic schizophrenia. *J. Irish Med. Assoc.* **66**, 135–138.
Harer, W. B. (1958). Tranquilizers in obstretrics and gynecology. *Obstet. Gynecol.* **11**, 273–279.
Harley, R. D., et al. (1959). Ataractic and antiemetic drugs in cataract surgery. *Am. J. Ophthalmol.* **47**, 177–185.
Harper, J., et al. (1964). The tranquillizers. *Practitioner* **192**, 5–11.
Haselhuhn, D. H., et al. (1959). Work in progress on antiemetics. *Caduceus* **7**, 2.
Hawke, W. A., et al. (1964). Tranquilizers. *Clin. Pediat.* **3**, 192–196.
Hayes, J. B. (1960). Dual action therapy in depressive symptoms. *J. Neuropsychiat.* **2**, 20–23.
Hayes, J. B., et al. (1959). Potentiation and facilitation of insulin coma therapy. *Am. J. Psychiat.* **116**, 164–165.
Heinrich, K., et al. (1960). Chlorperphenazin in der psychiatrischen und neurologischen Therapie. *Nervenarzt* **31**, 128–133. (Decentan.)
Herman, M. (1958). Anxiety and tension states. *Med. Clin. N. Am.* **723**, 32.
Herndon, R. W. (1960). Tranquilizers as pre-medication for local and general anesthesia in ambulatory patients. *J. Georgia State Dental Assoc.* **34**, D34–D42.
Hewitt, M. I. (1960). Which tranquilizer? *J. Indiana State Med. Assoc.* **53**, 1475–1483.
Heyns, M. H., et al. (1961). The use of anti-emetic drugs in anaesthesia. *S. African Med. J.* **35**, 241–242.
Himwich, H. E. (1959). Some drugs used in the treatment of metal disorders. *Am. J. Psychiat.* **115**, 756–759.
Himwich, H. E. (1959). The management of alcoholism. *Mod. Med. (Minneapolis)* **23**, 32.
Himwich, H. E. (1960). Some drugs useful in the treatment of emotional disorders-physiology, indications, and contraindications. *Am. Practitioner Dig. Treat.* **11**, 687–698.
Himwich, H. E. (1965). Psychoactive drugs. *Postgrad. Med.* **37**, 35–44.
Hinton, J. M. (1959). A comparison of perphenazine (Fentazin) sodium amylobarbitone and a placebo in anxious and depressed outpatients. *J. Mental Sci.* **105**, 872–877.
Hippius, H. (1960). Psychopharmaka und Pharmakotherapie der Psychosen. *Therap. Gegenwart* **99**, 413–419. (Decentan.)
Hockle, J. A. (1960). Aspects pharmacologique et therapeutique des derives de la phenothiazine. *Can. Pharm. J.* **93**, 25, 54–56, and 58.
Hodge, J. R. (1959). Akathisia: the syndrome of motor restlessness. *Am. J. Psychiat.* **116**, 337–338.
Hoffman, F. A., et al. (1960). Untersuchungen über das Verhalten des Jendrassik'schen Bahnungseffektes auf spinale Eigenreflexe unter neuroleptischer Medikation. *Med. Exptl.* **2**, No. 2–4, 126–131.
Hohman, L. B. (1962). Psychoses: Mental depression. *In* "Current Therapy" (H. F. Conn, ed.), pp. 544–546. Saunders, Philadelphia, Pennsylvania.
Hohman, L. B. (1963). Psychoses: Mental depression. *In* "Current Therapy" (H. F. Conn, ed.), pp. 548–550. Saunders, Philadelphia, Pennsylvania.
Hollister, L. E. (1958). The present status of tranquilizing drugs. *Calif. Med.* **89**, 1–6.
Hollister, L. E., et al. (1960). Trifluoperazine in chronic psychiatric patients. *J. Clin. Exptl. Psychopathol.* **21**, 15–24.

Hollister, L. E., et al. (1963). Perphenazine combined with amitryptiline in newly admitted schizophrenics. *Am. J. Psychiat.* **120**, 591–592. (Etrafon.)

Hordern, A. (1961). Psychiatry and the tranquilizers. *New Engl. J. Med.* **265**, 584–588.

Houston, F. J. (1962). Treatment of alcoholic delirium. *Can. Med. Assoc. J.* **87**, 1129.

Hsi-P'ing, C. (1961). Sedative and antiemetic action of a new neuroplegic drug, ethaperazine. *Farmakol. Toksikol.* **24**, No. 2, 140–145; *Psychopharmacol. Abstr.* **1**, 401.

Hughes, J. (1958). The treatment of the epileptic child. *J. Pediat.* **53**, 66–88.

Hurst, L. (1960). Phenothiazine derivatives in the treatment of schizophrenia. *J. Mental Sci.* **106**, 755–770.

Illberg, P. (1964). The use of perphenazine in the treatment of drug resistant schizophrenics. *Am. J. Psychiat.* **120**, 810–812.

Kalinowsky, L. B., et al. (1961). Pharmacotherapy. *In* "Somatic Treatments in Psychiatry" pp. 53–56. Grune & Stratton, New York.

Kant, F., et al. (1961). Ambulatory psychotherapy for the schizophrenic patient with the aid of drugs. *Diseases Nervous System* **22**, 45–48.

Kaplan, H. S. (1959). Tranquilizers in the office practice of medicine. *N.Y. State J. Med.* **59**, 2871–2887.

Karacan, I., et al. (1963). Evaluation of combined antidepressant and tranquilizing drug (amitriptyline-perphenazine) in the treatment of hospitalized chronic schizophrenic patients. *Am. J. Psychiat.* **120**, 500–501. (Triavil.)

Karliner, W. (1960). Use of psychopharmacological agents. Recent developments. *Am. Practitioner Dig. Treat.* **11**, 278–281.

Katzman, B. (1960). The menopausal syndrome. *Med. Times* **88**, 1185–1187.

Katzman, B. (1962). The use of perphenazine and trichlormethiazide for premenstrual tension. *Med. Times* **90**, 70–73.

Kennedy, D. R. (1957). Tranquilizers. The most talked about drugs on the market today. *Can. Pharm. J.* **90**, 44–45 and 52.

Kennedy, R. E., et al. (1961). An effective drug combination. *Am. J. Psychiat.* **118**, 547–548.

Kennedy, R. E., et al. (1963). Amitriptyline-perphenazine in the treatment of schizophrenia. *Am. J. Psychiat.* **119**, 1092–1093. (Triavil.)

King, J. H. (1957). Some aspects of geriatric ophthalmology. *Eye, Ear, Nose Throat Monthly* **36**, 667–672.

Kirsner, J. B. (1959). Current concepts on the medical management of ulcerative colitis. *J. Am. Med. Assoc.* **169**, 433–442.

Kirsner, J. B., et al. (1958). The irritable colon. *Gastroenterology* **34**, 491–501.

Klerman, G. L., et al. (1961). Psychological effects of piperazine phenothiazines. *Federation Proc.* **20**, Pt. 1, 393 (abstr.).

Klett, C. J., et al. (1960). A clinical trial of five phenothiazines using sequential analysis. *J. Clin. Exptl. Psychopathol.* **21**, 89–100.

Kline, E. E., et al. (1963). Clinical and experimental experiences with the tranquilizer drugs. *Illinois Vet.* pp. 14–18.

Kline, N. S. (1956). Says tranquilizers aid in handling of aged. *Drug Trade News* **31**, 55.

Kline, N. S. (1958). Clinical clues as to mode of action of the ataractic drugs. A round table. *Psychiat. Quart.* **32**, 41–84.

Kline, N. S. (1958). Psychopharmacology. *Progr. Neurol. Psychiat.* **13**, 441–463.

Kline, N. S. (1960). Psychopharmaceuticals: uses and abuses. *Postgrad. Med.* **27**, 620–629.

Kline, N. S. (1961). The use of psychopharmaceuticals in office practice. *Med. Clin. N. Am.* **45**, 1677–1684.

Kodahl, T. (1958). Trilafon. *Ugeskrift Ulaeger* **120**, 361–363.

Kofman, O. (1962). Treatment of alcoholic delirium. *Can. Med. Assoc. J.* **87**, 1129–1130.

Kofman, O. (1958). Experience with reserpine (Serpasil) and perphenazine (Trilafon) in acute alcoholic intoxications and alcoholic psychosis. *Can. Med. Assoc. J.* **79**, 988–991.

Koranyi, E. K., et al. (1960). Experimental sleep deprivation in schizophrenic patients. *A.M.A. Arch. Gen. Psychiat.* **2**, 534–544.
Kothari, N. J., et al. (1960). A comparison of perphenazine, proketazine, nialamide and MO-482, in chronic schizophrenics. *Am. J. Psychiat.* **117**, 358–360.
Kraines, S. H. (1960). Psychotropic drugs and the emotional circuit. *J. Neuropsychiat.* **2**, 55–65.
Kraines, S. H. (1963). A practical therapy for chronic alcoholic patients. *Memphis Mid-South Med. J.* **38**, 457–469.
Kraines, S. H. (1964). Psychotropic drugs in general practice. *Memphis Mid-South Med. J.* **39**, 9–27.
Kris, E. B. (1965). Psychiatric treatment of the aged. *Current Therap. Res.* **7**, 145–149.
Kris, E. B., et al. (1964). Combined perphenazine-amitriptyline as adjuvant therapy in psychiatric aftercare. *Am. J. Psychiat.* **121**, 498–501.
Krogh, I. (1958). Trilafonbehandling af 51 mandlige patienter. *Ugeskrift Laeger* **120**, 371–372.
Kupperman, H. S., et al. (1959). Contemporary therapy of the menopausal syndrome. *J. Am. Med. Assoc.* **171**, 1627–1637.
Kurland, A. A. (1962). The phenothiazine tranquilizers—10 years later (1962). *Current Therap. Res.* **4**, Suppl., 191–199.
Kurland, A. A., et al. (1961). The comparative effectiveness of six phenothiazine compounds, phenobarbital and inert placebo in the treatment of acutely ill patients: global measures of severity of illness. *J. Nervous Mental Disease* **133**, 1–18.
Kurland, A. A., et al. (1961). Comparative studies of the phenothiazine tranquilizers; methodological and logistical considerations. *J. Nervous Ment. Disease* **132**, 61–74.
Kurland, A. A., et al. (1959). Preadmission drug treatment of state psychiatric hospital patients. *Am. J. Psychiat.* **115**, 1028–1029.
Kurland, A. A., et al. (1962). The comparative effectiveness of six phenothiazine compounds, phenobarbital and inert placebo in the treatment of acutely ill patients: personality dimensions. *J. Nervous Mental Disease* **134**, 48–61.
Kurtz, P. L. (1958). The current status of the tranquillizing drugs. *Can. Med. Assoc. J.* **78**, 209–215.
LaBurt, H. A. (1959). Appraisal of drug therapy. *Diseases Nervous System* **20**, 93–96. (Sect. 2.)
Laffan, R. J., et al. (1961). Antiemetic action of fluphenazine (Prolixin) a comparison with other phenothiazines. *J. Pharmacol. Exptl. Therap.* **131**, 130–134.
Lai, G. (1963). Stimulation et sedation dans le traitement des etats depressifs. *Psychopharmacologia* **4**, No. 3, 206–220.
Landeen, F. H. (1961). Perphenazine as a prophylactic antiemetic in surgery. A double-blind study among 580 patients. *Am. Surgeon* **27**, No. 6, 462–468; (1961). *Psychopharmacol. Abstr.* **1**, 240.
Lander, E. W. (1959). The use of a tranquilizer drug in childbirth. *Southwestern Med.* **40**, 704–705.
Landman, M. E. (1959). New therapy in gastrointestinal disease. Preliminary report of 100 patients. *J. Med. Soc. New Jersey* **56**, 348–349.
Laricchia, R. (1958). Osservazioni sull-impiego di un nuovo derivato della fenotiazine, la perfenazine, nella pratica neuropsichiatrica. *Minerva Med.* **44**, Suppl. 39, 1993–1995.
Larson, A. N., et al. (1958). Clinical observations of the effects of perphenazine at high dosage levels with chronic psychiatric patients. Personal communication.
Leake, C. D. (1957). Mood-altering drugs. *Proc. Teachers' Seminar on Pharmacol.* pp. 139–154.
Lehmann, H. E. (1958). Tranquillizers and other psychotropic drugs in clinical practice. *Can. Med. Assoc. J.* **79**, 701–708.
Lehmann, H. E. (1961). New drugs in psychiatric therapy. *Can. Med. Assoc. J.* **85**, 1145–1151.
Lemere, F. (1959). Psychopharmaceutical drugs in general practice. *Med. Times* **87**, 1422–1425.

Leopold, I. H. (1961). Use of newer drugs in relation to ophthalmology. *Postgrad. Med.* **29**, 557–562.

Levinsky, W. J. (1961). Current therapy of common medical problems; the psychotherapeutic agent. *Delaware State Med. J.* **33**, 72–76.

Levy, L., et al. (1962). Phenothiazine drugs and the general practitioner. *Can. Med. Assoc. J.* **86**, 415–417.

Lewis, J. J. (1964). The classification of tranquillizers. *Practitioner* **192**, 12–22.

Lieser, H. (1960). Bedeutet Decentan in der psychiatrischen Therapie einen Fortschritt? *Med. Monatsschr.* **14**, No. 1, 18–22.

Lind, B. (1960). Control of postoperative vomiting with perphenazine (Trilafon). A double-blind study. *Acta Anaesthesiol. Scand.* **4**, 181–188.

Lindsay, D. S. (1960). The place of tranquillizer and antidepressant drugs in practice. *Can. Med. Assoc. J.* **81**, 1430–1432.

Liubimov, B. I. (1961). Experimental comparative evaluation of the activity of neuroplegic substances of the phenothiazine series. *Farmakol. i Toksikol.* **24**, No. 2, 136–140; (1961). *Psychopharmacol. Abstr.* **1**, 410.

Lloyd, D. N., et al. (1964). Sensory changes with phenothiazine medication in schizophrenic patients. *J. Nervous Mental Disease* **139**, 169–175.

Lundquist, G. (1961). Antidepressive drugs. *Nord. Psykiat. Tidskr.* **15**, No. 1, 41–67; (1961). *Psychopharmacol. Abstr.* **1**, 438.

Lynn, F. H., et al. (1960). The patient on a tranquillizing regimen. *Am. J. Nursing* **60**, 234–240.

McHardy, G., et al. (1959). Management of acute peptic ulcer; measures to prevent recurrence. *Postgrad. Med.* **25**, 668–676.

Mackmull, G. (1960). Team effort in the treatment of hemiplegia. *Clin. Med.* **7**, 1589–1598.

McLaughlin, B. E., et al. (1964). Clinical trials with amitriptyline and perphenazine among psychiatric outpatients. *Diseases Nervous System* **25**, 169–171. (Etrafon.)

McLaughlin, B. E., et al. (1964). Chemotherapy for emotionally disturbed children: a follow-up report. *Diseases Nervous System* **25**, 735–738.

Malitz, S., et al. (1959). Potentiation of extrapyramidal side-effects by dextro amphetamine (Dexedrine) in psychiatric subjects receiving a phenothiazine derivative (Trilafon). Paper presented at the New York Neurological Soc. and N.Y. Acad. of Med. Sect. of Neurol. and Psychiat., Feb. 10, 1959; *A.M.A. Arch. Neurol.* **1**, 322–333 (abstr.).

Mapp, Y., et al. (1962). Psycho-pharmacology. II: Tranquilizers and antipsychotic drugs. *Psychosomatics* **3**, 458–463.

Marangoni, B. A. (1957). Use of a new tranquilizer, perphenazine in 60 patients with anxiety and tension. *Am. Practitioner Dig. Treat.* **8**, 1959–1961.

Marks, J. (1963). Predrug behavior as a predictor of response to phenothiazines among schizophrenics. *J. Nervous Mental Disease* **137**, 597–601.

Mason-Browne, N. L. (1957). Perphenazine—a drug modifying consciousness. *Am. J. Psychiat.* **114**, 173–174.

Mason-Browne, N. L. (1958). Perphenazine in practice. *Can. Med. Assoc. J.* **79**, 985–988.

Mason-Browne, N. L., et al. (1957). Effect of perphenazine (Trilafon) on modification of crude consciousness. *Diseases Nervous System* **18**, 300–306.

Mathewson, H. S. (1957). Analgesia and the pharmacology of pain. *J. Lancet* **77**, 387–389.

Mattey, W. E. (1963). Combination therapy for relief of anxiety and depression. *Current Therap. Res.* **5**, 310–318. (Etrafon.)

Merskey, H., et al. (1961). An investigation of some therapeutic and physiological effects of perphenazine in Huntington's Chorea. *Psychopharmacologia* **2**, Fasc. 6, 436–445.

Michaux, M. H., et al. (1963). Combined psychotropic drug therapy. *Diseases Nervous System* **24**, 739–741.

Michaux, M. H., et al. (1964). Phenothiazines in the treatment of newly admitted state

hospital patients: global comparison of eight compounds in terms of an outcome index. *Current Therap. Res.* **6**, 331–339.
Middleton, T. F. (1958). Nausea and vomiting in pregnancy. *Postgrad. Med.* **24**, 699–701.
Milch, L. J., et al. (1959). Effectiveness of perphenazine and systral against motion sickness. *J. Appl. Physiol.* **14**, 245–246.
Mises, R., et al. (1963). Essai de la perphenazine chez l'enfant et l'adolescent. *Ann. Med. Psychol.* **121**, 89–92.
Mischler, J. E., et al. (1961). An evaluation of three ataractic and antiemetic agents for intra ocular surgery. A double-blind study of 182 cases. Preliminary report. *Eye, Ear, Nose Throat Monthly* **40**, 844–849.
Modern tranquilizers. (1961). Review for daily use by the general practitioner. *Gen. Practitioner* **24**, 18–21 and 26.
Mohr, H. (1958). Die Pharmakotherapie neuropsychiatrischer Erkrankungen mit Trilafon. *Praxis (Bern)* **47**, 37–41.
Mohr, H. (1958). Die Pharmakotherapie neuropsychiatrischer Erkrankungen mit Trilafon. *Med. Klin. (Munich)* **53**, IX–X.
Moldenhauer, B. (1960). Chlorperphenazin, in der Neuropsychiatrie. *Aerztl. Wochschr.* **15**, 163–167. (Decentan.)
Molling, P. A., et al. (1961). The impact of placebo and of perphenazine in committed delinquent boys. Paper presented at the 117th Annual Meeting, Summaries of Scientific Papers, Am. Psychiat. Assoc. Chicago, May 8–12, 1961; *Psychopharmacol. Abstr.* **1**, 371.
Molling, P. A., et al. (1962). Committed delinquent boys; the impact of perphenazine and of placebo. *Arch. Gen. Psychiat.* **7**, 70–76.
Moore, D. C., et al. (1958). Control of postoperative vomiting with perphenazine (Trilafon) a double blind study. *Anesthesiology* **19**, 72–74.
Moore, J., et al. (1961). Alterations in response to somatic pain associated with anaesthesia. VII: The effects of nine phenothiazine derivatives. *Brit. J. Anaesthesia* **33**, 422–431. (Fentazin.)
Moravec, C. L., et al. (1961). Relief of emotional stress. *Med. Times* **89**, 249–253.
Morgan, D. R., et al. (1958). A clinical appraisal of "Sparine," "Stemetil," "Trilafon" and "Marsilid." *Med. J. Australia* **45**, 696–700.
Mostert, J. W. (1963). "Imbretil" as a relaxant in anaesthesia. *S. African Med. J.* **37**, 328–330.
Munnell, E. W., et al. (1960). The control of pain in late gynecologic cancer. *Bull. Sloane Hosp.* **6**, 55–60.
Nakajima, H., et al. (1963). Die pharmakologische Therapie des schizophrenen Formenkreises. *Therap. Gegenwart* **102**, 665–672.
Naviau, J., et al. (1963). Essai de la perphenazine en therapeutique psychiatrique. *Ann. Med.-Psychol.* **121**, 98–104.
Nelson, R. M. (1959). "Tranquilization" of the heart with the ataractic drugs. *J. Thoracic Cardiovasc. Surg.* **38**, 610–617.
Nesbitt, R. E. L., Jr. (1962). Nausea and vomiting of pregnancy. *In* "Current Therapy" (H. F. Conn, ed.), pp. 600–601. Saunders, Philadelphia, Pennsylvania.
Nielsen, R. H. (1958). The use of perphenazine in ocular surgery. *Am. J. Ophthalmol.* **46**, 345–351.
Nilsson, G. L., et al. (1962). The general practicing physician and the phenothiazine tranquilizers. *Maryland Med. J.* **11**, 130–134.
Nunez Viscarra, K. L. (1961). Variaciones de la tiocianemia en enfermos mentales poraccion de la perfonazina. *Folia Clin. Intern.* **11**, No. 3, 148 and 156; *Psychopharmacol. Abstr.* **1**, 220.
O'Reilly, P. O., et al. (1957). Perphenazine (Trilafon) treatment of psychoses. *Can. Med. Assoc. J.* **77**, 952–955.
Ostfeld, A. M. (1960). Tranquillisers in general medical practice. *Triangle* **4**, 335–340.

O'Toole, C. P. (1962). Perphenazine as premedication. *Brit. Med. J.* II, 1471. (Fentazin.)
Overall, J. E., *et al.* (1963). Comparison of acetophenazine with perphenazine in schizophrenics: Demonstration of differential effects based on computer-derived diagnostic models. *Clin. Pharmacol. Therap.* **4**, 200–208.
Pakenham-Walsh, R. (1960). Perphenazine in Huntington's chorea. Letters to the editor. *Lancet* II, 982.
Papper, E. M. (1960). The proper use of tranquilizers in surgical patients. *Trans. Am. Acad. Ophthalmol.* **64**, 689–693.
Parish, F. A. (1958). Tension and anxiety in allergic and asthmatic patients. *Med. Times* **86**, 211–216.
Pearce, K. I. (1960). Elipten: A clinical evaluation of a new anticonvulsant; preliminary report. *Can. Med. Assoc. J.* **82**, 953–959.
Pearl, D. (1962). Phenothiazine effects in chronic schizophrenia. *J. Clin. Psychol.* **18**, 86–89.
Pennington, V. M. (1959). The phrenotropic action of Trilafon (perphenazine) in 323 neuropsychiatric patients. *Am. J. Psychiat.* **116**, 65–66.
Pennington, V. M. (1960). The psychotropic action of perphenazine in neuropsychiatric patients. *J. Mississippi Med. Assoc.* **1**, 243–248.
Pennington, V. M. (1962). Combined psychopharmaceutical treatment in 460 neuropsychiatric patients. *Am. J. Psychiat.* **118**, 935–937.
Pennington, V. M. (1964). Ten years' progress in psychotropic medication. *Illinois Med. J.* **126**, 553–558.
Pennington, V. M. (1964). The phrenotropic action of perphenazine-amitriptyline. *Am. J. Psychiat.* **120**, 1115–1116. (Etrafon.)
Pennington, V. M. (1964). Perphenazine, amitriptyline combination seems effective as antidepressant agent. Exhibit, Am. Med. Assoc., Clinical Convention; *Am. Med. Assoc.* **190**, 37 (abstr.).
Perk, D. (1963). Psychotropic drugs—their action and value. *S. African Med. J.* **44**, 194–197.
Perloff, M. M., *et al.* (1960). Anxiety or depression? A common diagnostic and therapeutic problem in general practice. *Clin. Med.* **7**, 2237, 2239–2240, 2242, 2244, 2249, 2251, and 2254.
Phillips, O. C., *et al.* (1958). The effect of Trilafon on postanesthetic nausea, retching and vomiting. A controlled study. *Current Res. Anesthesia Analgesia* **37**, 341–346.
Phillips, O. C., *et al.* (1960). The effects of Trilafon on post-anesthetic nausea, retching and vomiting: continued study. *Current Res. Anesthesia Analgesia* **39**, 38–45.
Phillips, O. C., *et al.* (1960). Trilafon analgesia during labor. *Obstet. Gynecol.* **15**, 182–187.
Piuck, C. L. (1963). Clinical impressions of hydroxyzine and other tranquilizers in a child guidance clinic. *Diseases Nervous System* **24**, 483–488.
Preisig, R., *et al.* (1958). Use of perphenazine in anxiety states and hyperemesis. Report of 135 cases. *Am. Practitioner Digest. Treat.* **9**, 740–744.
Proctor, C. D., *et al.* (1964). Extension of tranquilizer action by anticholinesterases. *Toxicol. Appl. Pharmacol.* **6**, 1–8.
Purkis, I. E., *et al.* (1963). The effectiveness of anti-emetic agents: a comparison of the antiemetic activity of trifluopromazine (Vesprin), perphenazine (Trilafon) and trifluoperazine (Stelazine) with that of dimenhydrinate (Gravol) in postanaesthetic vomiting. *Can. Anaesthesiol. Soc. J.* **10**, 539–549.
Quintero Lobo, F. (1962). Empleo de la perfenazine, adicionada al fenobarbital, en la premedicacion de la intervencion cesarea. *Rev. Clin. Matern. "David Restrepo"* **3**, 101–105.
Rappaport, H. (1963). Drugs and psychiatry. *Delaware Pharmacist* **17**, 12.
Rechtschaffen, A., *et al.* (1964). Schizophrenia and physiological indices of dreaming. *Arch. Gen. Psychiat.* **10**, 89–93.
Redmon, B. F. (1957). Tranquilizers—Some clinical results. *Southeastern Vet.* **9**, 34–35.

Rees, L. (1960). Drug treatment of disease. Chlorpromazine and allied phenothiazine derivatives. *Brit. Med. J.* II, 522–525.
Reiss, F. (1959). Trilafon (Perphenazine) as a tranquilizer in dermatoses. *Conn. State Med.* **23**, 22–24.
Riccitelli, M. L. (1964). Modern concepts in the management of anxiety and depression in the aged and infirm. *J. Am. Geriat. Soc.* **12**, 652–657.
Riding, J. E. (1963). The prevention of postoperative vomiting. *Brit. J. Anaesthesia* **35**, 180–188.
Riese, J. A. (1958). Prantal with phenobarbital or with Trilafon in gastrointestinal diseases. *Am. J. Gastroenterol.* **30**, 497–499.
Robbie, D. S. (1959). Post anaesthetic vomiting and anti-emetic drugs. *Anaesthesia* **14**, 349–354.
Roberts, H. (1960). Postoperative nausea and vomiting: the response to anti-emetic drugs with special reference to cyclizine and perphenazine. *Can. Anaesthesiol. Soc. J.* **7**, 116–126.
Robin, A. A. (1963). A retrospective controlled study of tranquillizers in long-stay patients. *J. Neurol. Neurosurg. Psychiat.* **26**, 262–264.
Rodman, M. J. (1957). Drugs for the "Age of Anxiety". *R.N.* **20**, 48–53, 90, and 93.
Rogina, V. (1962). Tranquillizers: success and problems. *Lijecnicki Vjesnik* **84**, 1042–1047.
Rondepierre, J. J., et al. (1963). La perphenazine, phenothiazine piperazines en therapeutique psychiatrique. *Presse Med.* **71**, 809–810.
Rondepierre, J. J. (1963). The use of perphenazine in the treatment of schizophrenic syndromes. 8 pp. (Manuscript.)
Ross, W. D. (1964). Neurocirculatory asthenia. *In* "Current Therapy" (H. F. Conn, ed.), p. 166. Saunders, Philadelphia, Pennsylvania.
Rossi, G. V. (1960). Psychotherapeutic drugs. *Am. J. Pharm.* **132**, 86–97.
Rossi, G. V. (1963). Review article; synergism; with special reference to central nervous system depressants. *J. Pharm. Sci.* **52**, 819–832.
Rossi, G. V. (1964). The psychotherapeutic agents. *Am. J. Pharm.* **136**, 6–24.
Rossi, G. V. (1964). L'anestesia con neurolettici derivati dalla fenotiazina VI.—idrossietil-piperazine-propil-N-cloro-fenotiazina (perfenazine). *Osped. Ital. Chir.* **10**, 701–707.
Roth, F. E., et al. (1959). Perphenazine (Trilafon), a new potent tranquilizer and antiemetic: II. General pharmacology. *Arch. Intern. Pharmacodyn.* **118**, 375–383.
Rothman, I. (1957). Psychopharmacology and hypnotism. *J. Am. Osteopathol. Assoc.* **57**, 201–204.
Roughead, P., et al. (1960). Clinical observations of the use of perphenazine (Fentazin) in mental hospital patients. *J. Mental Sci.* **106**, 571–580.
Rudolph, J. A., et al. (1959). Trilafon (perphenazine) and Meticorten (prednisone) as ancillary therapy in allergic conditions. *J. Florida Med. Assoc.* **45**, 1018–1020.
Sainz, A. (1964). Phenothiazines in the management of stress and anxiety. *Psychosomatics* **5**, 167–173.
Sakurai, T. (1961). Drug-therapy of neurosis. *J. Japan. Psychosomat. Soc.* **1**, No. 2, 72–79; *Psychopharmacol. Abstr.* **1**, 635.
Salzberger, G. J. (1964). Perphenazine treatment of patients with acute alcoholism or schizophrenia. *Clin. Med.* **71**, 1565–1570.
Sanchez-Medina, A. (1961). Empleo de la perfenazina a dosis minimas eficaces en psiquiatria. *Med. Cirg., Bogota* **25**, 169–177.
Sanger, M. D. (1962). The use of tranquilizers and antidepressants in allergy. *Ann. Allergy* **20**, 705–709.
Sannerstedt, R. (1961). Deparpreparat för oralt bruk. *Nord. Med.* **65**, 845–849.
Schiele, B. C. (1961). The selective use of antidepressive drugs in the treatment of depressive disorders. *J.-Lancet* **81**, 451–457.
Schiele, B. C. (1962). Newer drugs for mental illness; a review. *J. Am. Med. Assoc.* **181**, 126–133.

Schneider, P. B. (1958). Psycho-pharmacologie et medicaments tranquillisants. *Schweiz. Apotheker-Ztg.* **96**, 905–917.

Schopmans, A. (1958). Uber Perphenazinbehandling von Psychosen. *Med. Klin. (Munich)* **53**, 757–759. (Decentan.)

Schultz, S., *et al.* (1957). Perphenazine (Trilafon) therapy—A pilot study. *Can. Med. Assoc. J.* **77**, 1117–1118.

Scott, M. E. (1961). Tranquilizing drugs. A review of the history of man's search for the ideal tranquilizer is presented. *J. Med. Assoc. Georgia* **50**, 11–13.

Scurr, C. G., *et al.* (1958). Trials of perphenazine in the prevention of post-operative vomiting. *Brit. Med. J.* I, 922–923.

Seleny, F. L., *et al.* (1963). Observations on postoperative vomiting. *Can. Anaesthesiol. Soc. J.* **10**, 30–36.

Seevers, M. H. (1957). The "tranquilizers". *Univ. Mich. Med. Bull.* **23**, 338–340.

Settel, E. (1957). The use of perphenazine (Trilafon) to control anxiety and agitation in aged patients. *J. Am. Geriat. Soc.* **5**, 1003–1008.

Settel, E. (1958). Treatment of acute and chronic arthralgias with a tranquilizing agent (Trilafon) in addition to prednisone or prednisolone. *J. Am. Geriat. Soc.* **6**, 749–753.

Settel, E. (1961). Office management of senile agitation. *Med. Clin. N. Am.* **45**, 1605–1609.

Shanon, J. (1958). A dermatologic and psychiatric study of perphenazine (Trilafon) in dermatology. *A.M.A. Arch. Dermatatol.* **77**, 119–120.

Shapiro, A. K. (1964). Rational use of psychopharmaceutic agents. *N.Y. State J. Med.* **64** 1084–1095.

Sharpley, P., *et al.* (1964). Comparison of butaperazine and perphenazine: a double-blind controlled study. *Psychopharmacologia* **5**, No. 3, 209–216.

Shimazono, Y. (1964). On the effectiveness of chlorpromazine, reserpine and perphenazine on schizophrenic patients. 6 pp. with 4 tables.

Sigwald, J., *et al.* (1962). Neuroleptic drugs. *World Neurol.* **3**, 78–94.

Silverman, M., *et al.* (1959). A review of drugs in the elderly psychiatric patient. *N. Carolina Med. J.* **20**, 428–432.

Simon, J. L. (1958). Some experience with perphenazine, a new tranquilizer. *J. Louisiana State Med. Soc.* **110**, 196–199.

Simonsen, L. E., *et al.* (1962). Postoperative vomiting: A review and present status of treatment. *Can. Anaesthesiol. Soc. J.* **9**, 51–60.

Simonsen, M. (1964). Phenothiazine depressive reaction. *J. Neuropsychiat.* **5**, 259–265.

Sloane, R. B. (1960). Recent trends in psychiatric management. *Can. Med. Assoc. J.* **83**, 1084–1088.

Smith, J. A., *et al.* (1959). A graphic comparison of five phenothiazines. *Am. J. Psychiat.* **116**, 392–399.

Smith, J. A., *et al.* (1963). Choice of psychoactive drugs by psychiatric residents. *Diseases Nervous System* **24**, 310–313.

Smith, M. E. (1963). Perphenazine and amitriptyline as adjuncts to psychotherapy. *Am. J. Psychiat.* **120**, 76–77. (Etrafon.)

Soulairac, A. (1963). Un neuroleptique derive de la phenothiazine: la perphenazine. *Ann. Med.-Psychol.* **1**, 719–727.

Spengler, J. (1962). Medications de la sphere psychique. *Praxis (Bern)* **50**, 467; (1961). *Nouveautes. Med.* **11**, 10–13 (abstr.).

Sprogis, G. R. (1960). Perphenazine (Trilafon) suppositories in nausea and vomiting—a clinical study. *Ohio State Med. J.* **56**, 1644–1646.

Steinhilber, R. M. (1961). Current practices in general medicine. 21: An appraisal of tranquilizers. *Proc. Staff Meetings Mayo Clin.* **36**, 165–170.

Steinhilber, R. M. (1962). An appraisal of tranquilizers. *Anesthesia Analgesia* **41**, 377–380.

Steinhilber, R. M. (1962). Psychoses: schizophrenia. In "Current Therapy" (H. F. Conn, ed.), pp. 541–544. Saunders, Philadelphia, Pennsylvania.
Stephens, F. O., et al. (1961). An organization for outpatient surgery. Lancet I, 1042–1044.
Stevens, J. D. (1964). Psychopharmacology. *J. Neuropsychiat.* **5**, 566–576.
Stewart, B. L. (1959). Perphenazine in urology and surgery. *Am. Practitioner Dig. Treat.* **10**, 845–848.
Stewart, R. H. (1961). Phenothiazine derivatives in labor and delivery. A study of four drugs. *Obstet. Gynecol.* **17**, 701–713.
Sugiyama, H., et al. (1960). Perphenazine and reserpine as antiemetics for staphylococcal enterotoxin. *Proc. Soc. Exptl. Biol. Med.* **103**, 168–172.
Taber, R. I., Irwin, S., and Fox, J. A. (1964). Comparison of the enanthates of perphenazine and fluphenazine. Presented at the Fall Meeting of the Am. Soc. for Pharmacology and Exptl. Therap., Inc. Aug. 24–27, 1964; *Pharmacologist* **6**, 179 (abstr.).
Tanowitz, H., et al. (1959). Unidirectional regressional modified ECT vs. tranquilizers in chronic schizophrenics. *Diseases Nervous System* **20**, (Sect. 2), 132–141.
Taylor, I. J. (1958). Hospitalizing the psychiatric patient. *Maryland Med. J.* **7**, 297–300.
Taylor, I. J. (1958). Psychiatric aspects of chronic alcoholism. *Maryland Med. J.* **7**, 23–27.
Thal, N. (1958). Maintenance therapy for mental patients. *Postgrad. Med.* **24**, 638–647.
Thomas, J. W. (1960). Headaches as related to allergy. *West Va. Med. J.* **56**, 129–133.
Tolle, R. (1964). Phenothiazine—Überblick und Indikationen. *Med. Klin.* (*Munich*) **59**, 801–808.
Toms, E. C. (1961). A comparative study of selected tranquilizers in the treatment of psychiatric patients. *J. Nervous Mental Disease* **132**, 425–431.
Toogood, J. H. (1959). The effect of ataractic and antihistaminic drugs on the experimental skin wheal. *J. Allergy* **30**, 280.
Tuteur, W., et al. (1962). Tranquilizers and social obstacles. *Current Therap. Res.* **4**, Suppl., 206–212.
Wachsmuth, R. (1962). Dei Stellung des Fluphenazin in der Schizophreniebehandlung. In "Neurolepsie und Schizophrenie. Symposium at Universitäts—Nervenklinik, Mainz, 1962" (H. Kranz and K. Heinrich, eds.), pp. 145–152. Thieme, Stuttgart. (Decentan.)
Wachsmuth, R. (1962). Probleme der psychiatrischen Pharmakotherapie und die Stellung des Fluphenazins in der Behandlung der Psychosen. *Aerztl. Forsch.* **16**, 87–95.
Wagner, G. (1962). Die Entwicklung des Arzneischatses auf dem Gebiet der Sedativa und Hypnotica. *Pharm. Zentralhalle* **101**, 3–17.
Weinswig, M. (1962). Psychotherapeutic agents—Part II *Indiana Pharmacist* **44**, 91–92.
Weiss, I. I. (1958). Trilafon treatment in psychotics. *Am. J. Psychiat.* **114**, 1118–1119.
Weiss, I. I. (1959). Perphenazine treatment in psychotics. *J. Clin. Exptl. Psychopathol.* **20**, 44–52.
Weiss, S., et al. (1958). Symptomatic relief of nausea and vomiting with Trilafon (perphenazine). *Am. J. Gastroenterol.* **29**, 173–176.
Welsh, A. L. (1961). The treatment of psoriasis. *Family Physician* **1**, 33–39.
Welsh, A. L. (1964). The newer tranquilizing drugs. *Med. Clin. N. Am.* **48**, 459–481.
Werner, G. (1959). Tranquilizing drugs. Therapeutics. *Am. J. Med. Sci.* **237**, 631–650.
Whittaker, C. B., et al. (1963). Withdrawal of perphenazine in chronic schizophrenia. *Brit. J. Psychiat.* **109**, 422–427. (Fentazin.)
Wilcox, P. H. (1961). Electrostimulation therapy and drugs. (A future for computers.) *Diseases Nervous System* **22**, Sect. 2–Suppl., 50–54.
Williams, R. C., et al. (1958). Professional and therapeutic rationale of tranquilizers. *Vet. Med.* **53**, 127–130.
Wilson, W. P., et al. (1960). A sympotomatic analysis of the effects of perphenazine. *Diseases Nervous System* **21**, 340–346.

Wittich, F. W. (1959). Trilafon in allergy. A preliminary report. *Rev. Allergy Appl. Immunol.* **13**, 59–61.
Wood, L. A., *et al.* (1961). The effect of phenothiazines on the interactional behavior of schizophrenic patients. *Am. J. Psychiat.* **117**, 825–829.
Wortis, J. (1958). Physiological treatment. *Am. J. Psychiat.* **114**, 603–607.
Wortis, J. (1959). Physiological treatment. *Am. J. Psychiat.* **115**, 599–606.
Wortis, J. (1960). Physiological treatment. *Am. J. Psychiat.* **116**, 595–601.
Wortis, J. (1961). Physiological treatment. *Am. J. Psychiat.* **117**, 595–600.
Wortis, J. (1964) Psychopharmacology and physiological treatment. *Am. J. Psychiat.* **120**, 643–648.
Wortis, S. B. (1959). Some new chemotherapeutic agents reported useful in psychiatric practice. *Postgrad. Med.* **26**, 646–651.
Wright, R. L. D., *et al.* (1964). Value of continuous drug administration for chronic long-term mental hospital patients. *Can. Psychiat. Assoc. J.* **9**, 352–357.
Wright, W. (1959). Use of tranquilizers in dermatology. *J. Am. Med. Assoc.* **171**, 1642–1646,
Wunderlich, H. (1960). Über Phenothiazinbasen. Übersichten und originale. *Pharmazie* **15**, 149–154.
Yanof, Z. A. (1959). Practical considerations in the management of psychosomatic problems in general medicine. *Ohio State Med. J.* **55**, 1085–1090.
Yontef, R. (1958). Perphenazine as a tranquilizer in dermatoses. *J. Med. Soc. New Jersey* **55**, 18–20.

∽ A.8 ∽
Pipamazine

Ann. Meeting Brit. Med. Assoc., Oxford, England. Convention Report. *Appl. Therap.* **5**, 764, 766, 769, 1963.

Bellville, J. W. (1962). Antiemetic agents. *In* "Drugs of Choice 1962–1963" (W. Modell, ed.), pp. 314–28. Mosby, St. Louis, Missouri.

Bhargava, K. P., and Chandra, O. (1963). Anti-emetic activity of phenothiazines in relation to their chemical structure. *Brit. J. Pharmacol.* **21**, 436–440.

Bhargava, K. P., and Chandra, O. (1964). Tranquillizing and hypotensive activities of twelve phenothiazines. *Brit. J. Pharmacol.* **22**, 154–161.

Bhargava, K. P., and Jaitly, K. D. (1964). The effect of some phenothiazine tranquillizers on the oestrous cycle of albino mice. *Brit. J. Pharmacol.* **22**, 162–165.

Blatchford, E. (1961). Studies of anti-emetic drugs: A comparative study of Cyclizine (marzine R), pipamazine (mornidine R), trimethobenzamide (tigan R), and hyoscine. *Can. Anaesthesiol. Soc. J.* **8**, 159.

Cares, R. M., and Buckman, C. (1963). Comparative review of the structure and side-effects of newer psychotropic agents. *Diseases Nervous System* **24**, 92–105.

Chicoine, L. (1961). L'intoxication par les derives de la phenothiazine: Revue et rapport de 25 cas. *Union Med. Canada* **90**, 469–474.

Delgado, J. N., Cosgrove, F. P., and Isaacson, E. I. (1964). Phenothiazine derivatives. *Texas J. Med.* **60**, 315–318.

Denson, J. S., and Elesh, W. E. (1961). A double-blind study of a new antiemetic drug: SC-9387. *Anesthesia Analgesia, Current Res.* **40**, 430–436.

Dobkin, A. B. (1960). Potentiation of thiopentone anaesthesia: comparison of promethiazine, chlorpromazine, perphenazine, fluphenazine, thiopropazate, pipamezine and trifluopromazine. *Brit. J. Anaesthesia* **32**, 424.

Dobkin, A. B. (1964). Sedatives, analgesics, antidotes, and their interaction. A review. *Can. Anaesthiol. Soc. J.* **11**, 252–279.

Dobkin, A. B., Israel, J. S., and Criswick, V. G. (1962). Prolongation of thiopental anaesthesia with hydroxyzine, SA 97, thiethylperazine, and thioridazine. *Can. Anaesthesiol. Soc. J.* **9**, 342–346.

Dobkin, A. B., Woodworth, H., and Israel, J. S. (1962). The antisialogogue effect of hydroxyzine, thiethylperazine, and N'-p-chloro-benzylhydryl-N'-methyl homopiperazine (SA 97). *Can. Anaesthesiol. Soc. J.* **9**, 234–238.

Dundee, J. W., and Moore, J. (1962). The phenothiazines. *Brit. J. Anaesthesia* **34**, 247–250.

Dundee, J. W., Love, W. J., and Moore, J. (1963). Alterations in response to somatic pain associated with anaesthesia. XV. Further studies with phenothiazine derivatives and similar drugs. *Brit. J. Anaesthesia* **35**, 597–610.

Friend, D. G. (1960). The phenothiazines. *Clin. Pharmacol. Therap.* **1**, No. 1, 5–10.

Hollister, L. E. (1964). Adverse reactions to phenothiazines. *J. Am. Med. Assoc.* **189**, 311–313.

Lear, E., Suntay, R., Fisch, H. J., Chiron, A. E., and Pallin, I. M. (1961). Ataraxic drugs in preanesthetic medication: Blind studies in 1,852 patients. *Anesthesiology* **22**, 529–536.

Lewis, J. J. (1964). The classification of tranquillizers. *Practitioner* **192**, 12–22.

Lewis, R. A., and Gyang, F. N. (1965). Inhibition of sickling by phenothiazines. Comparison of derivatives. *Arch. Intern. Pharmacodyn.* **153**, 158–171.

McQueen, E. G. (1963). Toxic effects of phenothiazine tranquillizers. *New Zealand Med. J.* **62**, 460–462.

Moertel, C. G., Reitemeier, R. J., and Gage, R. P. (1963). A controlled clinical evaluation of antiemetic drugs. *J. Am. Med. Assoc.* **186**, 116–118.

Poison control centers. Tranquilizer poisonings (1959–1960). *J. Iowa Med. Soc.* **53**, 302–304.

Riding, J. E. (1960). Post-operative vomiting (abridged). *Proc. Roy. Soc. Med.* **53**, 671.

Rodman, M. J. (1963). Drugs for treating emotional mental illness. *R.N.* **26**, 67–74, 95.

Scott, E. E. (1963). Mycosis fungoides. *In* "Current Therapy 1963" (H. F. Conn, ed.), pp. 188–189. Saunders, Philadelphia, Pennsylvania.

Simonson, M. (1964). Phenothiazine depressive reaction. *J. Neuropsychiat.* **5**, 259–265.

Verrett, J., and McLaughlin, J., Jr. (1963). Teratogenic effects of rumple chick embryos. *J. Am. Med. Assoc.* **184**, 34.

Watson, G. I. (1963). Ancoloxin and fetal abnormalities. *Brit. Med. J.* **1**, 122. (Letter.)

Weaver, L. C., Rahdert, E., Richards, A. B., and Abreu, B. E. (1964). Effect of antiemetics and other compounds on protoveratrine induced emesis in dogs. *J. Pharm. Sci.* **53**, 417–420.

Welsh, A. L. (1964). The newer tranquilizing drugs. *Med. Clin. N. Am.* **48**, 459–481.

Wheatley, D. (1964). Drugs and the embryo (correspondence). *Brit. Med. J.* **1**, 630.

~ A.9 ~
Prochlorperazine

Chemical Papers

Arbasino, M., and Corona, G. L. (1964). La molecola della piperazina in recenti composti d'interesse farmacologico. (The piperazine molecule in recent compounds of pharmacological interest.) *Boll. Chimicofarm.* **103**, (4) 226–240.

Bhargava, K. P., and Chandra, O. (1963). Anti-emetic activity of phenothiazines in relation to their chemical structure. *Brit. J. Pharmacol.* **21** (3), 436–440.

Cerletti, A., *et al.* (1962). 3-Athyl-mercapto-10-(3'-(1''-methyl-piperazyl-4'')-propyl-1')-phenothiazin (Thiethylperazin), ein spezifisches Antiemeticum. Benziehungen zwischen Struktur und antiemetischer. Wirkung weiterer Phenothiazin-Derivate. (3-Ethylmercapto-10-(3'(1''-methylpiperazyl-4'')-propyl-1')-phenothiazine (thiethylperazine), a specific antiemetic agent; relation between structure and antiemetic effect of phenothiazine derivatives.) *Arzneimittel-Forsch.* **12** (10), 964–968.

Cochin, J., and Daly, J. W. (1963). The use of thin-layer chromatography for the analysis of drugs. Identification and isolation of phenothiazine tranquilizers and of antihistaminics in body fluids and tissues. *J. Pharmacol. Exptl. Therap.* **139** (2), 160–165.

Deviller, M. (1961). Methode simple de diagnose de quèlques phénothiazines substituées (Simple method for determining several substituted phenothiazines.) *Ann. Pharm. Franc* **19** (2), 131–135.

Eagleson, D. A. (1963). Paper chromatographic differentiation of some important phenothiazines encountered in toxicology. *Am. J. Clin. Pathol.* **39** (6), 648–651.

Eberhardt, H., *et al.* (1963). Der Nachweis von psychotropen Phenothiazin-Derivaten und ihrer Ausscheidungsprodukte mit Hilfe der Dünnschichtchromatographie. (Thin-layer chromatography of psychotropic phenothiazine derivatives and their excretion products.) *Arzneimittel-Forsch.* **13** (9), 804–805.

Forrest, F. M., and Forrest, I. S. (1963). Urine testing for phenothiazine and related drugs; its significance for achieving and maintaining rehabilitation of chronic mental patients. *Am. Arch. Rehabil. Therap.* **11**, 8–19.

Forrest, F. M., *et al.* (1959). A rapid, semi-quantitative urine color test for piperazine-linked phenothiazine drugs ("Compazine," Trilafon and analoguous compounds.) *Am. J. Psychiat.* **116** (6), 549–551.

Forrest, F. M., *et al.* (1961). Review of rapid urine tests for phenothiazines and related drugs. *Am. J. Psychiat.* **118** (4), 300–307.

Hamacher, J., and Hildebrandt, G. (1964). Zusammenhänge zwischen chemischer Konstitution und Herz-Kreislauf-Wirkung therapeutisch angewendeter Phenothiazin- und Thiaxanthen-Derivate. (Relationship between chemical structure and cardiovascular activity of therapeutic phenothiazine and thiaxanthene derivatives.) *Arzneimittel-Forsch.* **14** (9), 977–981.

Hetzel, C. A. (1961). Method for the estimation of phenothiazine derivatives in urine and blood. *Clin. Chem.* **7** (2), 130–135.

Jindal, M. N., *et al.* (1960). Structure activity relationship of chlorpromazine and related phenothiazine derivatives on pentobarbitone anaesthesia in mice. *Arch. Intern. Pharmacodyn.* **129** (1–2), 166–171.

Lazerte, G. D., and McMillin, T. J. (1964). False positive urine tests due to drugs. *Northwest. Med.* **63** (2), 106–108.

Levine, J., et al. (1961). Interference of indican in the estimation of phenothiazine. *Am. J. Psychiat.* **117** (8), 747–748.

Lucas, G. H., and Fabierkiewicz, C. (1963). Useful tests to identify phenothiazine tranquillizers. *J. Forensic Sci.* **8** (3), 462–476.

Lyons, L. E., and Mackie, J. C. (1963). Electron-donating properties of central sympathetic suppressants. *Nature* **197** (4867), 589.

Martin, H. F., et al. (1963). A method for calculating gas chromatographic relative retention values for high boiling phenothiazine derivatives. *Anal. Chem.* **35** (12), 1901–1904.

Masuda, Y., and Ikekawa, N. (1962). Gas chromatography of some synthetic drugs. *J. Pharm. Soc. Japan.* **82** (12), 1664–1666.

Mellinger, T. J., and Keeler, C. E. (1962). Chromatography and electrophoresis of phenothiazine drugs. *J. Pharm. Sci.* **51** (12), 1169–1173.

Mellinger, T. J., and Keeler, C. E. Spectrofluorometric identification of phenothiazine drugs. *Anal. Chem.* **35** (4), 554–558.

Milne, J. (1959). The analysis of phenothiazine derivatives with tranquilizing properties. *J. Am. Pharm. Assoc. Sci. Ed.* **48** (2), 117–122.

Paulus, W., et al. (1963). Dünnschichtchromatographische Untersuchungen einiger Phenothiazine und ähnlich wirkender Stoffe. (Thin-layer chromatography of some phenothiazines and compounds with similar action.) *Arzneimittel-Forsch.* **13** (7), 609–610.

Posner, H. S., and Forrest, F. M., et al. (1960). Urinary tests for piperazine-linked phenothiazines and for chlorpromazine. *Am. J. Psychiat.* **117** (6), 561–563.

Rogers, A. R. (1964). The influence of spectral slit width on the absorption of visible or ultra-violet light by pharmacopoeial substances. *J. Pharm. Pharmacol.* **16** (6), 433–434.

Schieser, D. W., and Tuck, L. D. (1962). Free radical studies by electron-spin resonance of some derivatives of phenothiazine. *J. Pharm. Sci.* **51** (7), 694–695.

Seeman, P. M., and Bialy, H. S. (1963). The surface activity of tranquilizers. *Biochem. Pharmacol.* **12** (10), 1181–1191.

Seno, S., et al. (1964). Thin-layer radiochromatographic study of prochlorperazine photodeterioration. *J. Pharm. Sci.* **53** (9), 1101–1103.

Tiwari, N. M., et al. (1960). Structure activity relationship of chlorpromazine and related phenothiazines of atropine-like activity on rabbit intestine. *Arch. Intern. Pharmacodyn. Therap.* **125** (3–4), 456–462.

Vesell, E. S. (1959). Urinary test for a metabolite of prochlorperazine. *New Engl. J. Med.* **260** (21), 1078.

Yung, D. K., and Pernarowski, M. (1963). Identification and differentiation of some phenothiazine-type tranquilizers. *J. Pharm. Sci.* **52** (4), 365–370.

Biology and Pharmacology

Bálint, G. (1964). Experimental comparison of the anaesthesia potentiating effect of Hydergin and some phenothiazine derivatives. *Acta Physiol. Acad. Sci. Hung.* **25** (3), 295–298.

Beaulnes, A., and Lavallee, M. (1964). Differential effects of some phenothiazine derivatives against calcium-induced ventricular arrhythmias in the isolated rabbit heart. *Can. J. Physiol. Pharmacol.* **42** (6), 845–853.

Benjamin, F. B., et al. (1957). Effect of a tranquilizing agent on galvanic skin response. *J. Appl. Physiol.* **11** (2), 216–218.

Bhargava, K. P., and Jaitly, K. D. (1964). The effect of some phenothiazine tranquillizers on the oestrous cycle of albino mice. *Brit. J. Pharmacol.* **22** (1), 162–165.

A.9. PROCHLORPERAZINE

Binet, P., and Decaud, J. (1962). Action de dérivés de la phénothiazine, de la thiophényl-pyridylamine et de l'iminodibenzyle sur la thermorégulation du rat. (Effect of derivatives of phenothiazine, thiophenylpyridylamine and iminodibenzyl on thermoregulation of the rat.) *Therapie* **17**, 1315–1319.

Blažek, J. (1963). Phenothiazinderivate in der Pharmazie. (Phenothiazines in pharmacy.) *Pharm. Praxis, Beilage Pharmazie* **5**, 85–90.

Boyd, E. M., and Cassell, W. A. (1957). Agents affecting apomorphine-induced vomiting. *J. Pharmacol. Exptl. Therap.* **119** (3), 390–394.

Brillhart, J. R. (1959). Tranquilizer interference in the Rana pipiens chorionic gonadotropin test. *Obstet. Gynecol.* **14** (5), 581–587

Broussolle, P., et al. (1959). Acces confuso-onirique dû à la prochlorpérrazine chez une cyclothymique. Considérations cliniques, électroencéphalographiques et thérapeutiques. (Severe confusion due to prochlorperazine in a cyclothymic. Clinical, electroencephalographic and therapeutic aspects.) *Ann. Med. Psychol.* **117** (1:1), 151–160.

Büchi, J. (1963). Emetica, Antiemetica und Mittel gegen Reisekrankheiten. (Emetics, antiemetics and anti-motion sickness compounds.) *Pharm. Acta Hely.* **38** (6), 321–337.

Burkman, A. M. (1961). Antagonism of apomorphine by chlorinated phenothiazines. *J. Pharm. Sci.* **50** (2), 156–160.

Burkman, A. M. (1961). Relative potencies of some phenothiazines as pecking syndrome inhibitors. *J. Pharm. Sci.* **50** (9), 771–773.

Burkman, A. M. (1962). Relationship of relative inhibitor potency to magnitude of challenge. I. Phenothiazine suppression of pecking syndromes of varying intensity. *Arch. Intern. Pharmacodyn.* **37** (3–4), 404–409.

Cook, L. (1958). The pharmacology of proclorperazine. *Psychiat. Res. Rept.* No. 9, pp. 1–4.

Cook, L., et al. (1958). Evaluation of the activity of a group of centrally acting agents. *J. Pharmacol. Exptl. Therap.* **122** (1), 14A–15A.

Cook, L., and Kelleher, R. T. (1962). Drugs effects on the behavior of animals. *Ann. N.Y. Acad. Sci.* **96** (1), 315–335.

Courvoisier, S., et al. (1957). Propriétés pharmacodynámiques générales de la prochlorpémazine (6.140 R.P.). (General pharmacodynamic properties of prochlorperazine (RP 6140)). *Compt. Rend. Soc. Biol.* **151** (6), 144–148.

Cuatico, W., et al. (1964). S^{35}-Prochlorperazine autoradiography of the central nervous system. *Federation Proc.* **23** (2), 129.

Cummins, A. J. (1960). Effect of prochlorperazine and of prochlorperazine-isopropamide on basal gastric secretion. *Am. J. Digest. Diseases* **5** (6), 523–528.

Cushman, P., and Hilton, J. G. (1963). Acute phenothiazine administration on pituitary-ACTH release and adrenal cortical function in the dog. *Clin. Res.* **11** (4), 403.

Cushman, P., Jr., and Hilton, J. G. (1964). Pituitary-adrenal function during acute prochlorperazine administration in the dog. *Am. J. Physiol.* **207** (6), 1374–1378.

Dandiya, P. C. (1963). Studies on central nervous system depressants. II. The action of some general nervous depressants on coaxially stimulated guinea pig's ileum. *Arch. Intern. Pharmacodyn.* **141** (1–2), 216–222.

Dandiya, P. C., and Menon, M. K. (1963). Studies on central nervous system depressants. III. Influence of some tranquilizing agents on morphine analgesia. *Arch. Intern. Pharmacodyn.* **141** (1–2), 23–32.

De Jaramillo, G. A. V., and Guth, P. S. (1963). A study of the localization of phenothiazines in dog brain. *Biochem. Pharmacol.* **12** (6), 525–532.

Delphaut, J., et al. (1963). Action de quelques phénothiazines sur l'agitation et l'hyperagitition provoquée par l'amphétamine et la cocaine de la Souris blanche. (Effect of various phenothiazines on activity and hyperactivity produced by amphetamine and cocaine in mice.) *Compt. Rend. Soc. Biol.* **157** (12), 2229–2232.

de Maria, F. J. (1965). The effect of some drugs on placental monoamine oxidase activity. *Can. Med. Assoc. J.* **92** (7), 351.
Deshpande, V. R., et al. (1963). Effect of chlorpromazine and prochlorperazine on the Metrazol induced convulsions in frogs. *Arch. Intern. Pharmacodyn.* **141** (3–4), 525–531.
Dhawan, B. N., et al. (1961). Antagonism of apomorphine-induced pecking in pigeons. *Brit. J. Pharmacol.* **16** (2), 137–145.
Diamond, E. F., and Limperis, N. M. (1961). Motility disturbances caused by prochlorperazine. *Illinois Med. J.* **120** (1), 34–35.
Dobkin, A. B. (1960). Potentiation of thiopental anesthesia by derivatives and analogues of phenothiazine. *Anesthesiology* **21** (3), 292–296.
Dobkin, A. B., and Palko, D. (1960). The antisialogogue effect of phenothiazine derivatives: Comparison of promaine, levomepromazine, trifluoperazine, proclorperazine, methdilazine and prothipendyl. *Anesthesiology* **21** (3), 260–262.
Domino, E. F. (1962). Human pharmacology of tranquilizing drugs. *Clin. Pharmacol. Therap.* **3** (5), 599–664.
Drill, V. A. (1963). Pharmacology of hepatotoxic agents. *Ann. N.Y. Acad. Sci.* **104** (3), 858–874.
Duchesnay, G. (1957). Action d'un dérivé de la phénothiazine (6140 R.P.) sur les centres des VIIIe et Xe paires craniennes. (The effect of a phenothiazine derivative (RP 6140) on the eighth and tenth cranial nerves.) Paper Presented at German Meeting of Therapeutics, Karlsruhe, September 6, 1957.
Ducrot, R., and Koetschet, P. (1956). Propriétés anti-émétiques d'un nouveau derivé de la phénothiazine la chloro-3 (*N*-methyl-piperazinyl-3′ propyl)-10 pheno-thiazine (R.P. 6140). (Antiemetic properties of a new phenothiazine derivative, the 2-chloro-10-(3-*N*-methylpiperazinylpropyl) phenothiazine (R.P. 6140-SKF 4657-I_2)). *20th Intern. Physiol. Congr. Brussels*, 1956. *Abstr. Commun.*, p. 258.
Dumont, C., et al. (1964). Sur une nouvelle méthode d'enregistrement de la motilité chez l'animal de laboratoire maintenu dans son milieu d'élévage—son application a l'étude de quelques agents modificateurs du comportement. [A new method for recording motility in the laboratory animal maintained in its natural habitat; its application to the study of some agents which affect behavior.] *Arch. Intern. Pharmacodyn.* **151** (1–2), 60–75.
Eckhardt, E. T., and Plaa, G. L. (1962). The effect of phenothiazine derivatives on the disappearance of sulfobromophthalein from mouse plasma. *J. Pharmacol. Exptl. Therap.* **138** (3), 387–391.
Elliott, R. C., and Quilliam, J. P. (1964). Some actions of centrally active and other drugs on the transmission of single nerve impulses through the isolated superior cervical ganglion preparation of the rabbit. *Brit. J. Pharmacol.* **23** (2), 222–240.
Fabius, A. J. M., and De Ruiter, H. (1964). Inhibition of lipase activity of lung and adipose tissue by phenothiazine derivatives. *Nature* **202**, (4939), 1336–1337.
Fish, B. (1960). Drug therapy in child psychiatry: Pharmacological aspects. *Comprehensive Psychiat.* **1** (4), 212–227.
Flanagan, T. L., et al. (1962). Excretion patterns of phenothiazine-S^{35} compounds in rats; effect of change in structure on metabolism. *J. Pharm. Sci.* **51** (10), 996–999.
Fowler, P. J., et al. (1964). The effects of various central nervous system stimulants and depressants on confinement motor activity. *Federation Proc.* **23** (2), 198.
Freeman, A. R., and Spirites, M. A. (1962). Effect of some phenothiazine derivatives on the hemolysis of red blood cells *in vitro*. *Biochem. Pharmacol.* **11**, 161–163.
Friedman, A. P. (1963). Studies in the pharmacotherapy of headache. *Neurology* **13** (3, Part 2), 27–33.
Gözsy, B., and Kátó, L. (1960). Investigations into the mechanism of action of neuroleptic drugs. *Arch. Internat. Pharmacodyn. Therap.* **128** (1–2), 75–81.

Göszy, B., and Kátó, L. (1962). Prévention de la réaction anaphylactique chez le rat. [Prevention of anaphylactic reaction in the rat.] *Compt. Rend. Soc. Biol.* **156** (3), 556–559.

Greenberg, R., and Sabelli, H. C. (1964). Drug effects on epinephrine release from rat adrenal medulla homogenates and granule preparations. *Proc. Soc. Exptl. Biol. Med.* **116** (3), 705–712.

Guttman, H. N., and Friedman, W. (1963). Protozoa as pharmacological tools: the phenothiazine tranquilizers. *Trans. N.Y. Acad. Sci.* **26** (1), 75–89.

Helper, E. W., *et al.* (1958). The effect of tranquilizing agents and related compounds on the succinoxidase system. *Arch. Biochem. Biophys.* **76** (2), 354–361.

Heyman, J. J. (1964). Nicotinamide metabolism in schizophrenics, drug addicts, and normals: the effect of psychotropic drugs and hormones. *Trans. N.Y. Acad. Sci.* **26** (3), 354–360.

Hollister, L. E., *et al.* (1959). Serum oxidase activity in chronic schizophrenics treated with tranquilizing drugs. *Am. J. Psychiat.* **116** (6), 553–554.

Irwin, S. (1961). Correlation in rats between the locomotor and avoidance suppressant potencies of eight phenothiazine tranquilizers. *Arch. Intern. Pharmacodyn.* **132** (3–4), 279–286.

Janssen, P. A., *et al.* (1960). Effects of various drugs on isolation-induced fighting behavior of male mice. *J. Pharmacol. Exptl. Therap.* **129** (4), 471–475.

Janssen, P. A., *et al.* (1960). Apomorphine-antagonism in rats. *Arzneimittel-Forsch.* **10** (12), 1003–1005.

Jindal, M. N., and Deshpande, V. R. (1961). Neuromuscular blockade by some phenothiazine derivatives. *Arch. Intern. Pharmacodyn.* **132** (3–4), 322–330.

Justin-Bescancon, L., and Laville, C. (1964). Action antiémétique du métoclopramide vis-à-vis de l'apomorphine et de l'hydergine. [Antiemetic action of metoclopramide towards apomorphine and hydergine.] *Compt. Rend. Soc. Biol.* **158** (4), 723–727.

Káto, L., and Gözsy, B. (1961). Differential and quantitative affinity of psychoactive drugs to mucopolysaccharides. *Indian J. Med. Res.* **49** (5), 788–798.

Káto, L., *et al.* (1962). Attempt to classify psychotropic drugs, based on their affinity to mucopolysaccharides *in vivo*. *J. Clin. Exptl. Psychopathol.* **23** (2), 75–90.

Ketchel, M. M., and Sturgis, S. H. (1959). Influence of prochlorperazine on hydrocortisone inhibition of *in vitro* leucocyte migration. *Proc. Soc. Exptl. Biol. Med.* **100** (2), 391–394.

Khazan, N., *et al.* (1962). The mammotropic effect of tranquilizing drugs. *Arch. Intern. Pharmacodyn.* **136** (3–4), 291–305.

Killam, E. K. (1962). Drug action on the brain-stem reticular formation. *Pharmacol. Rev.* **14**, 175–223.

Kopmann, E., and Hughes, F. W. (1958). Effects of glutamats on the potentiating action of certain ataratics. *Proc. Soc. Exptl. Biol. Med.* **97** (1), 83–85.

Krysicka-Doczkal, H., *et al.* (1963). Farmakologické vlastnosti prochlorperazinu. [Pharmacological properties of prochlorperazine.] *Cesk. Farm.* **12** (9), 445–447.

Lazarus, J., and Cooper, J. (1959). Oral prolonged action medicaments; their pharmaceutical control and therapeutic aspects. *J. Pharm. Pharmacol.* **11** (5), 257–290.

Le Breton, R., *et al.* (1962). De l'alcoolémie chez des malades en cours de traitement chimiotherapique. [Alcohol in the blood during chemotherapeutic treatment of patients.] *Ann. Med. Psychol.* **120** (1–4), 755–759.

Lecoq, R., *et al.* (1962). Recherches chronaximetriques sur l'action qu'exercent quelques psycholeptiques et psychotroniques sur les effets nerveux de l'alcool ethylique; conclusions pratiques. [Chronaximetric research on the action which psycholeptics and psychotonics exert on the nervous effects of ethyl alcohol; practical conclusions.] *Ann. Pharm. Franc.* **20** (7–8), 607–622.

Lehmann, H. E., and Csank, J. (1957). Differential screening of phrenotropic agents in man: Psychophysiologic test data. *J. Clin. Exptl. Psychopathol.* **18** (3), 222–235.

Lever, P. G., and Hague, J. R. (1964). Observations on phenothiazine concentrates and diluting agents. *Am. J. Psychiat.* **120** (10), 1000–1002.

Lipman, V. C., et al. (1963). Effect of anticholinergic psychotomimetics on motor activity and body temperature. *Arch. Intern. Pharmacodyn.* **146** (1–2), 174–191.

Longo, V. G. (1960). Action de la chlorpromazine, de la prochlorpémazine et de la levomepromazine sur l'electroencéphalogramme et sur le comportement du lapin. [Action of chlorpromazine, proclorpemazine and levomepromazine on electroencephalogram and behavior of rabbits.] *Electroencephalog. Clin. Neurophysiol.* **12** (3), 695–704.

Luzzatto, A., and Crema, A. (1960). Crisi masticatorie con scialorrea, spasmi tonici, tonicoclonici e rotazioni coatte in conigli sottoposti ad iniezione intracarotidea di un derivato fenotiazinico (proclorperazina). [Masticatory crises with sialorrhea, tonic and tonicoclonic spasms and forced rotations of rabbits given intracarotid injection of prochlorperazine, a phenothiazine derivative.] *Boll. Soc. Ital. Biol. Sper.* **36** (11), 557–560.

McIntosh, J. C., and Cooper, J. R. (1964). Function of N-acetyl aspartic acid in the brain: Effects of certain drugs. *Nature* **203** (4945), 658.

McKenna, O. C., and Angelakos, E. T. (1965). Distribution of catecholamines in various parts of the cat brain and some effects of phenothiazine treatment. *Federation Proc.* **24** (2), 194.

Macko, E., and Steelman, R. L. (1958). Acute, subacute, and chronic toxicity of prochlorperazine (2-chloro-10-[3'(N-methylpiperazinyl)-propyl]-phenothiazine) in mice, rats and dogs. *Federation Proc.* **17** (1), 390.

Maickel, R. P., et al. (1964). The effect of various drugs on the ability of cold-exposed rats to maintain normal body temperature. *Federation Proc.* **23** (2), 567.

Mao, T. S. S., et al. (1965). Inactivation of serum complement activity by phenothiazines. *Federation Proc.* **24** (2), 392.

Medina, H., et al. (1964). The effect of certain phenothiazines on the structure and metabolic activity of sarcosomes of guinea pig heart. *Biochem. Pharmacol.* **13** (3), 461–467.

Minchin, R. L. H., and Holdaway, I. (1964). Comparison of psycho-therapeutic and anthelmintic activities. *Brit. J. Psychiat.* **110** (466), 411–414.

Misurec, J., and Nahunek, K. (1964). Changes in photo-Metrazol (photo-myoclonic) threshold in treatment with some psycho-pharmacological drugs. *Electroencephalog. Clin. Neurophysiol.* **17** (5), 607.

Moya, F. (1962). Passage of drugs across the placentra. *Am. J. Obstet. Gynecol.* **84** (11) 1778–1798.

Murphy, E., et al. (1957). SKF 5137 (dl-N-[2:2-diphenyl-3-methyl-4-(N-morpholino)-butyrl]-pyrrolidine HCl), an analgetic: Potentiation of various effects in rats by chlorpromazine and prochlorperazine. *J. Pharmacol. Exptl. Therap.* **119** (2), 172–173. (Abstr.)

Phillips, B. M., and Miya, T. S. (1962). Excretion of S^{35} following administration of S^{35}-prochlorperazine to rats subjected to experimental stress. *Proc. Soc. Exptl. Biol. Med.* **109** (3), 576–577.

Phillips, B. M., and Miya, T. S. (1962). Disposition of S^{35}-prochlorperazine in the rat. *Pharmacologist* **4** (2), 170.

Phillips, B. M., and Miya, T. S. (1963). Disposition of S^{35}-prochlorperazine in the jaundiced rat. *Proc. Soc. Exptl. Biol. Med.* **112** (3), 706–708.

Phillips, B. M., and Miya, T. S. (1964). Disposition of S^{35}-prochlorperazine in the rat. *J. Pharm. Sci.* **53**, 1098–1101.

Plotnikoff, N. (1961). Drug resistance due to inbreeding. *Science* **134** (3493) 1881–1882.

Plotnikoff, N. (1963). Effect of neurotropic drugs on a non-conditioned avoidance response. *Arch. Intern. Pharmacodyn.* **145** (3–4), 430–439.

Potts, A. M. (1962). The concentration of phenothiazines in the eye of experimental animals. *Invest. Ophthalmol.* **1** (4), 522–530.

Purshottam, N., et al. (1961). Induced ovulation in the mouse and the measurement of its inhibition. *Fertility Sterility* **12** (4), 346–352.

Raevskii, K. S. (1961). Sravnitelnaya protivosudorozhnaya aktivnost' proizvodnykh fenotiazina pri eksperimentalnom elektroshoke. [Comparative anticonvulsant activity for various phenothiazine derivatives on experimental shock.] *Byul. Eksperim. Biol. i Med.* **51** (2), 64–68.
Raynaud, G., and Valette, G. (1963). Action des dérivés de la phénothiazine et de l'halopéridol sur la crise audiogéne de la souris. [Action of phenothiazine derivatives and haloperidol on audiogenic seizures in the mouse.] *Arch. Intern. Pharmacodyn.* **142** (3–4), 425–439.
Roizin, L. (1963). Mitrochondria (pleomorpho metabolosomes) as histometabolic gradients (effects of prochlorperazine on the rat brain as revealed by electron microscope). *Diseases Nervous System* **24** (4, Part 2), 61–66.
Roizin, L., et al. (1962). Clinical and tissue studies of prochlorperazine in rats and monkeys. *Psychopharmacol. Serv. Center Bull.* **2** (5), 81–83.
Rosen, E. (1963). Relationship of *in vitro* release to urinary recovery in man of a sustained-release preparation of S^{35}-prochlorperazine. *J. Pharm. Sci.* **52** (1), 98–100.
Rosenblum, W., and Zweifach, B. W. (1964). The effect of tranquilizers on the contractile response of cerebral arteries. *J. Pharmacol. Exptl. Therap.* **145** (1), 58–63.
Ryall, R. W. (1958). Effect of drugs on emotional behaviour in rats. *Nature* **182** (4649), 1606–1607.
Scott, G. T. (1962). Physiological action of psychoactive drugs on melanocytes in fish and frogs. *Psychopharmacol. Serv. Center Bull.* **2** (5), 58–62.
Scott, G. T., and Nading, L. K. (1961). Relative effectiveness of phenothiazine tranquilizing drugs causing release of MSH. *Proc. Soc. Exptl. Biol. Med.* **106** (1), 88–90.
Šedivec, V. (1964). The effect of psychotropic drugs on electrical brain activity. *Activatis Nervosa Super.* **6** (2), 204–205.
Sharma, P. L., and Arora, R. B. (1961). Antiarrhythmics. XII. Antiarrhythmic activity of some phenothiazine derivatives in experimental cardiac arrhythmias. *Indian J. Med. Res.* **49** (6), 1099–1112.
Shelley, W. B., and Juhlin, L. (1961). A new test for detecting anaphylactic sensitivity: The basophil reaction. *Nature* **191** (4793), 1056–1058.
Siva Sankar, D. V. (1961). Effect of psychopharmacological drugs on brain oxidative activity. *J. Neuropsychiat.* **3** (2), 123–125.
Slocum, Y. K. (1961). Serum transaminase tests for liver function on outpatients in follow-up clinic. *Am. J. Psychiat.* **118** (1), 75–76.
Steiner, W. G., and Himwich, H. E. (1963). Effects of antidepressant drugs on limbic structures of rabbit. *J. Nervous Mental Diseases* **137** (3), 277–284.
Stewart, J. (1962). Differential responses based on the physiological consequences of pharmacological agents. *Psychopharmacologia* **3** (2), 132–138.
Taeschler, M., and Cerletti, A. (1959). Differential analysis of the effects of phenothiazine-tranquilizers on emotional and motor behaviour in experimental animals. *Nature* **184** (4689), Suppl. 11, 823–824.
Takayanagi, I. (1964). Phenothiazine derivatives; relationship between peripheral and central actions. *Arzneimittel-Forsch.* **14** (6), 694–698.
Tedeschi, D. H., et al. (1958). Effects of various phenothiazines on minimal electroshock seizure threshold and spontaneous motor activity of mice. *J. Pharmacol. Exptl. Therap.* **123** (1), 35–38.
Tedeschi, D. H., et al. (1961). Central serotonin antagonist activity of a number of phenothiazines. *Arch. Intern. Pharmacodyn.* **132** (1–2), 172–179.
Tedeschi, D. H., et al. (1964). Effects of centrally acting drugs on confinement motor activity. *J. Pharm. Sci.* **53** (9), 1046–1050.
Tedeschi, R. E., et al. (1959). Effects of centrally active drugs on fighting behavior in mice. *J. Pharmacol. Exptl. Therap.* **125** (1), 28–34; (1958). *Abstr. in Federation Proc.* **17** (1), 414.

Teller, D. N., et al. (1965). Mescaline. XVI. Effect of chronic injections on binding of neuroleptics to mouse mitochondria, in vitro. Federation Proc. **24** (2), 301.

Tiwari, N. M., et al. (1960). Effect of tranquilising agents on water and saline-induced diuresis in rats. Arch. Intern. Pharmacodyn. Therap. **128** (3–4), 383–390.

Usdin, V. R., et al. (1961). Effects of psychotropic compounds on enzyme systems. I. Inhibition of human plasma and erythrocyte cholinesterases. II. In vitro inhibition of monoamine oxidase. Proc. Soc. Exptl. Biol. Med. **108** (2), 457–463.

Vallade, L., et al. (1959). Etude de l'action de la prochlorpémazine sur l'électrogénése céréorale. [Action of prochlorpemazine on cerebral electrogenesis.] Ann. Med. Psychol. **117** (2:4), 701–710.

Van Loon, E. J., et al. (1962). Canine hepatic secretion and urinary excretion of three S^{35}-labeled phenothiazines. Psychopharmacol. Serv. Center Bull. **2** (5), 56–57.

Van Loon, E. J., et al. (1964). Hepatic secretion and urinary excretion of three S^{35}-labeled phenothiazines in the dog. J. Pharm. Sci. **53** (10), 1211–1213.

Vasicka, A., and Kretchmer, H. E. (1959). The effect of prochlorperazine on uterine contractions; a clinical and experimental study. Obstet. Gynecol. **14** (4), 500–510.

Weil-Malherbe, H., and Posner, H. S. (1963). The effect of drugs on the release of epinephrine from adrenomedullary particles in vitro. J. Pharmacol. Exptl. Therap. **140** (1), 93–102.

White, R. P., and Westerbeke, E. J. (1962). Relationship between central anticholinergic actions and antiparkinson efficacy of phenothiazine derivatives. Intern. J. Neuropharmacol. **1**, 213–216.

Winsor, T. (1957). Control of conditioned responses of digital blood vessels. Clin. Res. Proc. **5** (1), 66.

Wyant, G. M. (1962). A comparative study of eleven anti-emetic drugs in dogs. Can. Anaesthesiol. Soc. J. **9** (5), 399–407.

Zakirov, U. B. (1961). Vliyanie meterazina na uslovnoreflektornayu deyatel 'nost'. [Effect of Meterazine on conditioned reflexes.] Farmakol. i Toksikol. **24** (3), 271–275.

Zakirov, Y. B. (1961). Protivorvotnoie i sedativnoie deistvie meterazina. (Antiemetic and sedative action of meterazine.) Farmakol. i Toksikol. **24** (4), 422–425.

Zakirov, U. B. (1964). K farmakologii meterazina. [Pharmacology of meterazine.] Farmakol. i Toksikol. **27** (5), 523–525.

Zakrzewska, F. (1963). Analiza kliniczna i elektromiograficzna zaburzeń ruchowych w przebiegu leczenia srodkami neuroleptycznymi. [Clinical and electromyographic analysis of motor disorders during treatment with neuroleptic compounds.] Neurol. Neurochir. Psychiat. Polon. **13**, 679–686.

Side Effects

Anderson, J. H., and Sanchez-Longo, L. P. (1961). The complications and side effects of the phenothiazine ataraxics: a review of 178 clinical series of 10 phenothiazine derivatives. Bol. Asoc. Med. Puerto Rico **53** (4), 123–151.

Anonymous. (1961). Extrapyramidal effects of tranquilisers. Lancet II (7208), 918–919.

Anselmo, R. S. (1962). Side effects of phenothiazine drugs; case report and literature review. Harper Hosp. Bull. **20** (1), 43–45.

Ayd, F. J., Jr. (1960). Drug-induced extrapyramidal reactions: their clinical manifestations and treatment with Akineton. Psychosomatics **1** (3), 143–150.

Ayd, F. J., Jr. (1961). A survey of drug-induced extrapyramidal reactions. J. Am. Med. Assoc. **175** (12), 1054–1060.

Bacon, G. A. (1964). Compounding of symptoms with prochlorperazine ("Compazine"). Wisconsin Med. J. **63** (10), 475–476.

Battiata, S. V., and O'Reilly, W. R. (1959). Untoward reactions following the use of prochlorperazine ("Compazine"): A report of two cases. *Clin. Proc. Children's Hosp.* **15** (6), 147–150.
Benjamin, F. B., et al. (1957). Effect of prochlorperazine on psychologic, psychomotor, and muscular performance. *U.S. Armed Forces Med. J.* **8** (10), 1433–1440.
Best, W. R. (1963). Drug-associated blood dyscrasias: Recent additions to the registry. *J. Am. Med. Assoc.* **185** (4), 286–290.
Bhaskaran, K., et al. (1962). Fatal bone-marrow aplasia complicating prochlorperazine therapy. *Am. J. Psychiat.* **119** (4), 373–374.
Blom, S., and Ekbom, K. A. (1961). Comparison between akathisia developing on treatment with phenothiazine derivatives and the restless legs syndrome. *Acta Med. Scand.* **170** (6), 689–694.
Bloom, J. B., et al. (1965). Effect on the liver of long-term tranquilizing medication. *Am. J. Psychiat.* **121** (8), 788–797.
Boissier, J.-R., and Simon, P. (1964). Equivalences expérimentales du syndrome neurologique des neuroleptiques. [Experimental equivalents of the neurological syndrome produced by neuroleptics.] *Encephale* **53**, Suppl., 109–122.
Braceland, F. J. (1963). Stimulants and tranquilizers—their use and abuse. *Bull. N.Y. Acad. Med.* **39** (10), 649–665.
Brody, I. A. (1959). Shock after administration of prochlorperazine in patient with pheochromocytoma: report of a case with spontaneous tumor destruction. *J. Am. Med. Assoc.* **169** (15), 1749–1752.
Broussolle, P., and Rosier, Y. (1959). Evolution des symptomes neurologiques dus aux neuroleptiques. [Evolution of neurologic symptoms caused by neuroleptics.] *Ann. Med. Psychol.* **117** (1/1), 140–151.
Bücher, W. H. (1959). Untoward neurological reactions to prochlorperazine. *Bull. Los Angeles Children's Hosp.* **6**, 77–81.
Cahen, R. L. (1964). Evaluation of the teratogenicity of drugs. *Clin. Pharmacol. Therap.* **5** (4), 480–514.
Cain, H. D., and Malcolm, M. (1960). Phenothiazine ataraxics; extrapyramidal reactions. *Calif. Med.* **93** (1), 24–28.
Cann, H. M., and Verhulst, H. L. (1960). Accidental ingestion and overdosage involving psychopharmacologic drugs. *New Engl. J. Med.* **263** (15), 719–724.
Cares, R. M., and Buckman, C. (1961). A survey of side-effects and/or toxicity of newer psychopharmacologic agents. *Diseases Nervous System* **22** (4), 97–106.
Cares, R. M., and Buckman, C. (1963). Comparative review of the structure and side-effects of newer psychotropic agents. *Diseases Nervous System* **24** (4), 92–105.
Castelnuovo-Tedesco, P., et al. (1963). Galactorrhea, headache and weight-gain during treatment with thioridazine. *Am. J. Psychiat.* **119** (12), 1178–1179.
Cawein, M. J., and Lappat, E. J. (1963). Toxic reactions of the hematopoietic system to chemical substances. *Southern Med. J.* **56** (6), 685–690.
Chaffin, D. S. (1964). Phenothiazine-induced acute psychotic reaction; the "psychotoxicity" of a drug. *Am. J. Psychiat.* **121** (1), 26–32.
Chamberlin, R. T., and Trembly, B. (1965). Dystonia phenothiazorum. *J. Maine Med. Assoc.* **56** (2), 30–31.
Chicoine, L. (1961). L'intoxication par les dérivés de la phénothiazine; revue et rapport de 25 cas. [Toxicity due to phenothiazine derivatives; review and report of twenty-five cases.] *Union Med. Canada* **90** (5), 469–474.
Cleveland, W. W., and Smith, G. F. (1958). Complications following the use of prochlorperazine ("Compazine") as an antiemetic. *A.M.A. J. Diseases Children* **96** (3), 284–287.
Cohlan, S. Q. (1960). Convulsive seizures caused by phenothiazine tranquilizers. *Gen. Practitioner* **21** (2), 136–137.

Collins, I. S. (1964). Hazards of drug therapy. *Med. J. Australia* **1** (7), 222–230.
Cook, G. C., and Sherlock, S. (1965). Jaundice and its relation to therapeutic agents. *Lancet* I (7378), 175–179.
Cornman, H. D., III. (1961). A parallel between the profile of clinical activity and the character of extrapyramidal activity of neuroleptics. "Extrapyramidal System and Neuroleptics," pp. 479–481. Editions psychiatriques, Montreal.
Cowger, M. L., and Labbe, R. F. (1965). Contraindications of biological-oxidation inhibitors in the treatment of porphyria. *Lancet* I (7376), 88–89.
Darling, H. F. (1959). Extrapyramidal symptoms of triflupromazine, mepazine, prochlorperazine. *Diseases Nervous System* **20** (12), 569–571.
Delay, J., et al. (1957). Similitude des accidents nerveux de la proclorperazine avec certains troubles post-encéphalitiques. [Similarity of neurological side effects of proclorperazine to certain postencephalitic disorders.] *Ann. Med. Psychol.* **115** (1:3), 506–310.
Delay, J., et al. (1957). Nouveaux types d'accidents nerveux dûs a un médicament neuroleptique, la prochlorpérazine. [New types of neurological side effects of prochlorperazine, a new neuroleptic agent.] *Ann. Med.-Psychol.* **115** (1:3), 510–519; *Presse Med.* **65** (36), 859 (abstr.).
Deller, D. J., et al. (1959). Jaundice during prochlorperazine therapy. *Brit. Med. J.* II (5142), 93.
Denber, H. C. B. (1958). Some preliminary results with a new phenothiazine derivative: Procloperazine. *Psychiat. Res. Rept.* No. 9, pp. 16–22.
Dickey, R. F., and Hartman, D. L. (1964). Photodermatitis induced by drugs. I. Contact photodermatitis. *Skin* **3** (6), 169–177.
Druckman, R., et al. (1962). Chronic involuntary movements induced by phenothiazines. *J. Nervous Mental Disease* **135** (1), 69–76.
Eckhardt, W. F., Jr. (1961). Cervical-lingual-masticator myoclonus; a reaction to prochlorperazine. *Conn. Med.* **25** (5), 284–286.
Editorial. (1965). Side effect of phenothiazines. *Can. Med. Assoc. J.* **92** (3), 135–136.
Ehrlich, R. M. (1959). A neurological complication in children on phenothiazine tranquilizers. *Can. Med. Assoc. J.* **81** (4), 241–243.
Epps, R. P., and Scott, R. B. (1961). Tranquilizers as a source of intoxication in children. *Med. Ann. District Columbia* **30** (6), 317–321.
Erslev, A. J. (1962). Detection and prevention of blood dyscrasias. *J. Am. Med. Assoc.* **181** (2), 114–119.
Favre-Tissot, M. (1963). Medication psycho-trope et anomalies du développement embryofoetal; a propos d'une enquête systématique chez 359 gestantes traitées par ces médications. [Psychotropic drugs and embryo-fetal abnormalities, with reference to systematic study of 359 pregnant women treated with these drugs.] *Thesis* Lyon, pp. 85–136.
Fischer, A., and Gottreich, N. S. (1960). Anemia as a complication of proclorperazine therapy. *Am. J. Psychiat.* **116** (10), 932–933.
Flegenheimer, W. V. (1959). Dyskinesias following therapy with phenothiazine derivatives. *J. Mt. Sinai Hosp.* **26**, 440–446.
Fournier, E. (1964). Intoxications par thymoleptiques et tranquillisants. [Intoxication by thymoleptics and tranquilizers.] *Gaz. Med. France* **71**, 2851-passim.
Freedman, D. X., and DeJong, J. (1961). Factors that determine drug-induced akathisia. *Diseases Nervous System* **22** (2), 69–76.
Freedman, D. X., and DeJong, J. (1961). Thresholds for drug-induced akathisia. *Am. J. Psychiat.* **117** (10), 930–931.
Freyhan, F. A. (1957). Psychomotilität, extra-pyramidale Syndrome und Wirkungsweisen neuroleptischer Therapien (Chlorpromazine, Reserpine, Proclorperazine). [Psychomotility, extrapyramidal syndromes and mechanism of action of neuroleptic therapies (chlorpromazine, reserpine, prochlorperazine).] *Nervenarzt* **28** (11), 504–509.

Frost, R. W., and Fraser, F. C. (1962). Drug therapy and congenital defects. *J. Am. Med. Assoc.* **182** (3), 319–320.
Gailitis, J., *et al.* (1960). Alarming neuromuscular reactions due to prochlorperazine. *Ann. Internal Med.* **52** (3), 538–543.
Gayral, L., *et al.* (1964). Troubles neuro-végétatifs latents au cours des cures par les neuroleptiques; incidents et accidents chez les enfants et les adolescents. [Latent autonomic disorders during neuroleptic treatment; incidents in children and adolescents.] *Encephale* **53**, Suppl., 175–179.
Goldsmith, R. W. (1959). Antidote for prochlorperazine intoxication in children. *J. Am. Med. Assoc.* **170** (3), 361.
Hollister, L. E. (1964). Adverse reactions to phenothiazines. *J. Am. Med. Assoc.* **189** (4), 311–313.
Grandell, A., and Ma, J. Y. (1959). Jaundice precipitated by prochlorperazine ("Compazine") in the treatment of alcoholic psychiatric disturbance. *J. Med. Soc. New Jersey* **56** (9), 553–554.
Haase, H. J. (1961). Extrapyramidal modification of fine movements—a "conditio sine qua non" of the fundamental therapeutic action of neuroleptic drugs. *Rev. Can. Biol.* **20**, 425–449.
Hartman, D. L., and Dickey, R. F. (1964). Photodermatitis induced by drugs. II. Photodermatitis medicamentosa. *Skin* **3** (7), 198-passim.
Himwich, H. E. (1965). Psychoactive drugs. *Postgrad. Med.* **37** (1), 35–44.
Hirsch, S., and Hirsch, D. L. (1961). Dystonic reactions produced by tranquilizers. *Am. J. Psychiat.* **117** (11), 1037–1038.
Hollister, L. E. (1957). Unexpected asphyxial death and tranquilizing drugs. *Am. J. Psychiat.* **114** (4), 366–367.
Hollister, L. E. (1961). Current concepts in therapy: Complications from psychotherapeutic drugs. *New Engl. J. Med.* **264** (6), 291–293.
Hollister, L. E. (1964). Complications from psychotherapeutic drugs—1964. *Clin. Pharmacol. Therap.* **5** (3), 322–333.
Hollister, L. E. (1965). Toxicity of psychotherapeutic drugs. *Practitioner* **194** (1159), 72–84.
Hollister, L. E., *et al.* (1960). Abnormal symptoms, signs, and laboratory tests during treatment with phenothiazine derivatives. *Clin. Pharmacol. Therap.* **1** (3), 284–293.
Holzel, A. (1965). Drug toxicity in children. *Practitioner* **194** (1159), 98–103.
Hooper, J. H., *et al.* (1961). Abnormal lactation associated with tranquilizing drug therapy. *J. Am. Med. Assoc.* **178** (5), 506–507.
Huang, L. C., and Yeh, Y. S. (1963). Side effects caused by phenothiazine tranquilizers. *Acta Paediat. Sinica* **4**, 245–250. (In Chinese.)
Hugeley, C. M., Jr. (1964). Drug-induced blood dyscrasias. II. Agranulocytosis. *J. Am. Med. Assoc.* **188** (9), 817–818.
Hunter, R., *et al.* (1964). An apparently irreversible syndrome of abnormal movements following phenothiazine medication. *Proc. Roy. Soc. Med.* **57** (8), 758–762.
Jabbour, J. T., *et al.* (1958). Severe neurological manifestations in four children receiving "Compazine" (prochlorperazine.) *J. Pediat.* **53** (2), 153–159.
Jacobziner, H., and Paybin, H. W. (1958). A case of accidental ingestion of "Compazine," (p. 1537) excerpt from ingestion accidents and their mode of occurrence. *N.Y. State J. Med.* **58** (9), 1535–1539.
Jacobziner, H., and Raybin, H. W. (1958). Briefs on accidental chemical poisonings in New York City. *N.Y. State J. Med.* **58** (21), 3500–3505.
Jacobziner, H., and Raybin, H. W. (1959). Poisonings with alarming symptoms. *N.Y. State J. Med.* **59** (18), 3460–3464.
Jacobziner, H., and Raybin, H. W. (1960). Briefs on accidental chemical poisonings in New York City. Parkinsonism due to overdosage of prochlorperazine. *N.Y. State J. Med.* **60** (6), 894.

Jacobziner, H., and Raybin, H. W. (1962). Accidental chemical poisonings. Intoxications due to tranquilizing drugs and plants. *N.Y. State J. Med.* **62** (19), 3130–3132.

Jacobziner, H., and Raybin, H. W. (1962). Prochlorperazine dimaleate poisoning. *N.Y. State J. Med.* **62** (23), 3804–3806.

Jenkins, S. B. (1963). The use and abuse of phenothiazines in treatment of acute psychoses. *J. Natl. Med. Assoc.* **55** (6), 515–519.

Kirshbaum, B. A., and Beerman, H. (1964). Photosensitization due to drugs; a review of some of the recent literature. *Am. J. Med. Sci.* **248** (4), 445–468.

Kistner, R. W. (1964). Hazards of obstetrical and gynecological drugs. *Ohio State Med. J.* **60** (12), 1125–1129.

Klett, C. J., and Caffey, E. M., Jr. (1960). Weight changes during treatment with phenothiazine derivatives. *J. Neuropsychiat.* **2** (2), 102–108.

Knox, J. M. (1963). Photosensitivity reactions in various diseases. *Postgrad. Med.* **33** (6), 564–570.

Knox, J. M. (1964). Photosensitivity—a common physical allergy. *Southern Med. J.* **57** (8), 904–908.

Kranes, A., and Clark, W. H., Jr. (1965). Fever, rash and jaundice in a twenty-two-year-old man. *New Engl. J. Med.* **272** (5), 254–259.

Lanzoni, V., et al. (1958). Circulatory effects of intravenous prochlorperazine ("Compazine") in humans. *Federation Proc.* **17** (1) 386.

Lerner, S., and Weiner, M. J. (1962). Extrapyramidal reactions to prochlorperazine and perphenazine in same patient. *N.Y. State J. Med.* **62** (17, Part I), 2852–2853.

Locket, S. (1963). Some observations on poisoning in children and poisoning by sleeping tablets and tranquilizers. *Anglo-Ger. Med. Rev.* **2** (1), 42–48.

Lockey, S. D. (1964). Adverse reactions to drugs. *Penna. Med. J.* **67** (8), 45–51.

Lutz, E. G., and Rotov, M. D. (1964). Angioneurotic edema of the tongue with phenothiazine administration; report of two cases. *Diseases Nervous System* **25** (7), 419–422.

McDonald, J. K. (1962). An unusual attempt at suicide. *Am. J. Psychiat.* **118** (8), 746.

McFarland, R. B. (1963). Fatal drug reaction associated with prochlorperazine ("Compazine"): Report of a case characterized by jaundice, thrombocytopenia, and agranulocytosis. *Am. J. Clin. Pathol.* **40** (3), 284–290.

McKeever, G. E. (1964). Tetanus vs drug reaction. *J. Am. Med. Assoc.* **188** (12), 1090.

McKown, C. H., et al. (1963). Overdosage effects and danger from tranquilizing drugs. *J. Am. Med. Assoc.* **185** (6), 425–430.

Mahoudeau, D., et al. (1957). Syndrome pseudo-tétanique transitoire consécutif a l'absorption d'un dérivé de la phénothiazine. [Transitory pseudo-tetanic syndrome following absorption of a phenothiazine derivative.] *Bull. Soc. Med. Hop. (Paris)* **73**, 123–127.

Mahrer, P. R., et al. (1958). Atropine-like poisoning due to tranquilizing agents. *Am. J. Psychiat.* **115** (4), 337–339.

Mandel, W., and Oliver, W. A. (1961). Withdrawal of maintenance antiparkinson drug in the phenothiazine-induced extrapyramidal reaction. *Am. J. Psychiat.* **118** (4), 350–351.

Marcus, S., et al. (1960). Trismus due to perphenazine (Trilafon) and prochlorperazine ("Compazine"). *Calif. Med.* **92** (3), 226–228.

Marzuoli, U., et al. (1965). Sindrome extrapiramidale con crisi oculogire subentranti da terapia proclorpemazinica; a proposito di un caso. [Extrapyramidal syndrome with oculogyric crises during treatment with prochlorperazine; case report.] *Minerva Med.* **56** (3–4), 87–90.

Mason, S. R., et al. (1959). Acute, transitory, severe central nervous system toxicity following administration of prochlorperazine. *N.Y. State J. Med.* **59** (10), 2037–2040.

Massonnat, J., and Arroyo, H. (1958). Accident d'intolérance grave a la prochlorpérazine (6140 PP). [Severe intolerance reaction to prochlorperazine (RP 6140).] *Presse Med.* **66** (42), 963.

Meister, G. S. (1958). Correspondence regarding neurological manifestation due to "Compazine." *J. Pediat.* **53** (4), 507.
Mercer, J. K. (1964). Accidental administration of "Compazine." *Illinois Med. J.* **126** (1), 47–48.
Moore, H. W. (1962). Toxicity of phenothiazine tranquilizers. *J. S. Carolina Med. Assoc.* **58**, 485–486.
Moya, F., and Thorndike, V. (1963). The effects of drugs used in labor on the fetus and newborn. *Clin. Pharmacol. Therap.* **4** (5), 628–653.
Nehlil, J. (1963). Les accidents des neuroleptiques. [Complications of neuroleptics.] *Clinique (Paris)* **58**, 595–599.
Nelson, N. M. (1959). Toxic hazards. Severe neurologic reactions to antiemetics. *New Engl. J. Med.* **260** (25), 1296–1298.
O'Hara, V. S. (1958). Extrapyramidal reactions in patients receiving prochlorperazine. *New Engl. J. Med.* **259** (17), 826–828.
Paulson, G. (1960). Procyclidine for dystonia caused by phenothiazine derivatives. *Diseases Nervous System* **21** (8), 447–448.
Pellerat, J., and Rives, H. (1960). Frequence des accidents cutanes induits par les neuroleptiques chez les malades mentaux. [Incidence of cutaneous side effects due to neuroleptics in mental patients.] *Bull. Soc. Franc. Dermatol. Syphilig.* pp. 838–839.
Pellerat, J., and Rives, H. (1961). A propos des photosensibilisations dues aux dérivés de la phenothiazine. [Photosensitization due to phenothiazine derivatives.] *Rev. Soc. Franc. Allergie* pp. 184–185.
Perez-Semper, L. M. (1960). Neuromuscular reactions secondary to the administration of prochlorperazine: some notes on diagnosis and management. *Am. Practitioner* **11** (11), 962–963.
Perlmutter, M., and Cohn, H. (1964). Myxedema crisis of pituitary or thyroid origin. *Am. J. Med.* **36** (6), 883–892.
Pisciotta, A. V., *et al.* (1958). Agranulocytosis following administration of phenothiazine derivatives. *Am. J. Med.* **25** (2), 210–223.
Plachta, A. (1965). Asphyxia relatively inherent to tranquilization; review of the literature and report of seven cases. *Arch. Gen. Psychiat.* **12** (2), 152–158.
Plummer, H. B., *et al.* (1960). Tetanus-like reactions to prochlorperazine. *J. Am. Med. Assoc.* **172** (6), 600.
Pokras, N. M., and Kingsbury, B. C., Jr. (1963). Extrapyramidal reactions to prochlorperazine and similar antiemetic drugs. *Oral Surg., Oral Med., Oral Pathol.* **16**, 1261–1265.
Potts, A. M. (1962). Retinotoxic and choroidotoxic substances; The Jonas S. Friendenwald Memorial Lecture. *Invest. Ophthalmol.* **1** (3), 290–303.
Potts, A. M. (1962). Uveal pigment and phenothiazine compounds. *Trans. Am. Ophthalmol. Soc.* **60**, 517–552.
Potts, A. M. (1964). The reaction of uveal pigment *in vitro* with polycyclic compounds. *Invest. Ophthalmol.* **3** (4), 405–416.
Rabinowitz, P., and Friedman, I. S. (1961). Drug-induced lactation in uremia. *J. Clin. Endocrinol. Metab.* **21** (11), 1489–1493.
Ravin, L. J., *et al.* (1958). A note on the photosensitivity of phenothiazine derivatives. *J. Am. Pharm. Assoc., Sci. Ed.* **47** (10), 760.
Reboson, J. Jr., *et al.* (1962). Pigmentary retinopathy and irido-cycloplegia in psychiatric patients. *J. Neuropsychiat.* **3** (5), 311–316.
Ritota, M. C., and Sanowski, R. (1964). Acute intermittent porphyria. *J. Med. Soc. New Jersey* **61** (3), 101–103.
Rodriguez-Ferrera, J. C. (1964). Acciones toxicas de los psicofarmacos. [Toxic effects of psychotropic drugs.] *Med. Clin. (Barcelona)* **42**, 125–128.
Rogers, J. B. (1963). The grimacing syndrome: A report of two cases. *Practitioner* **190** (1135), 132–133.

Rosati, D. (1964). Hypotensive side effects of phenothiazine and their management. *Diseases Nervous System* **25** (6), 366–369.

Rudersdorf, H. E. (1963). Drug-induced depression of central nervous system. *J. Am. Med. Assoc.* **186** (2), 174.

Sarwer-Foner, G. J. (1960). Recognition and management of drug-induced extrapyramidal reactions and "paradoxical" behavioural reactions in psychiatry. *Can. Med. Assoc. J.* **83** (7), 312–318.

Satanove, A. (1965). Pigmentation due to phenothiazines in high and prolonged dosage. *J. Am. Med. Assoc.* **191** (4), 263–268.

Scime, I. A., and Tallant, E. J. (1959). Tetanus-like reactions to prochlorperazine ("Compazine"); report of eight cases exhibiting extrapyramidal disturbances after small doses. *J. Am. Med. Assoc.* **171** (13), 1813–1817.

Shaw, E. B. (1960). Side reactions from tranquilizing drugs. *Pediat. Clin. N. Am.* **7** (2), 257–267.

Shaw, E. B., et al. (1959). Phenothiazine tranquilizers as a cause of severe seizures. *Pediatrics* **23** (3), 485–492.

Sherlock, S. (1962). Jaundice. *Brit. Med. J.* I (5289), 1359–1366.

Sigwald, J., et al. (1959). Les accidents neurologiques des medications neuroleptiques. [Neurological side effects of neuroleptic medications.] *Rev. Neurol.* **100**, 553–595.

Sigwald, J., et al. (1959). Quatre cas de dyskinesie facio-bucco-linguo-masticatrice à évolution prolongée secondaireé un traitement par les neuroleptiques. [Four cases of facio-bucco-linguo-masticatory dyskinesia of prolonged evolution accessory to neuroleptic treatment.] *Rev. Neurol.* **100**, 751–755.

Silver, M. L., et al. (1960). Special toxic effects of prochlorperazine ("Compazine") on cervico-facial musculature. *Rhode Island Med. J.* **43** (6), 383–384.

Simonson, M. (1964). Phenothiazine depressive reaction. *J. Neuropsychiat.* **5** (5), 259–265.

Sirnes, T. B. (1963). Drug induced extrapyramidal reactions. *Acta Neurol. Scand.* **39**, Suppl. 4, 209–217.

Smith, M. J., and Denner, J. L. (1962). Acute dystonic reactions to phenothiazines and response to antihistamines. *Diseases Nervous System* **23** (8), 466–468.

Smithy, G., and Homburger, F. (1957). Prochlorperazine for the treatment of nausea and vomiting in patients with advanced cancer and other chronic diseases. *New Engl. J. Med.* **256** (1), 27–28.

Sobel, A. M. (1960). Treatment of extrapyramidal reactions to phenothiazine derivatives. *U.S. Armed Forces Med. J.* **11** (12), 1446–1450.

Solomon, F. A., Jr., and Campagna, F. A. (1959). Jaundice due to prochlorperazine ("Compazine"), *Am. J. Med.* **27** (5), 840–843.

Spellberg, M. A. (1964). Intrahepatic cholestasis vs. postheptatic jaundice; methods of diagnosis with a note on hypercholesteremic xanthomatosis in a patient with chlorpromazine cholestasis. *Med. Clin. N. Am.* **48** (1), 53–65.

Symposium. (1961). Iatrogenically induced liver disease. *Bull. N.Y. Acad. Med.* **37** (11), 767–787.

Tysk, L. (1964). Some effects of stimulants and depressants on central inhibition as manifested in retinal rivalry. *Acta Psychiat. Scand.* **40** (2), 160–170.

Vates, T. S., and Masucci, E. F. (1960). Acute extrapyramidal syndromes following the use of phenothiazine derivatives. *Med. Ann. District Columbia* **29** (12), 670–673.

Verhulst, H. L., and Crotty, J. J. (1962). Tranquilizers. *Natl. Clearinghouse Poison Control Center* pp. 1–8.

Vilkin, M. I. (1963). Extrapyramidal side effects of trifluoperazine. *J. Neuropsychiat.* **4** (4), 236–239.

Waldman, S. (1963). Unusual manifestations associated with a phenothiazine-induced dystonic reaction. *Psychosomatics* **4** (3), 173–174.

Yasuna, E. (1962). Acute myopia associated with prochlorperazine ("Compazine") therapy. *Am. J. Ophthalmol.* **54**, 793–796.
Waugh, W. H., and Metts, J. C., Jr. (1960). Severe extrapyramidal motor activity induced by prochlorperazine; its relief by the intravenous injection of diphenydramine. *New Engl. J. Med.* **262** (7), 353–354.
Weinstein, A., et al. (1959). Cholestasis due to prochlorperazine. *J. Am. Med. Assoc.* **170** (14), 1663–1664.
Winfield, M. E. (1960). Transient hemiballism. *Ann. Internal Med.* **53** (4), 822–827.

Clinical Papers

Achaintre, A., et al. (1957). Les nouvelles phénothiazines dans le traitement de la schizophrénie. [New phenothiazines in the treatment of schizophrenia.] Paper Presented at International Psychiatric Congress, Zürich, September, 1957.
Adelson, D., and Epstein, L. J. (1962). A study of phenothiazines with male and female chronically ill schizophrenic patients. *J. Nervous Mental Disease* **134** (6), 543–554.
Ainslie, J. D. (1961). The use of newer psychiatric drugs in medical practice; their specificity of action in relation to target symptoms and dynamic situation. *J. Florida Med. Assoc.* **47** (8), 901–906.
Altschule, M. D., and Brem, J. (1963). Periodic psychosis of puberty. *Am. J. Psychiat.* **119** (12), 1176–1178.
Anonymous. (1963). Drugs in the treatment of Méniere's disease. *Brit. Med. J.* I (5347), 1719–1721.
Anonymous. (1964). Choice of drugs for emotional disorders. *Med. Letter* **6** (12), 45–46.
Archer, J. S., and Hicks, R. G. (1962). Phenothiazine subgroups. *N.Y. State J. Med.* **62** (23), 3769–3772.
Ayd, F. J., Jr. (1960). Tranquilizers and the ambulatory geriatric patient. *J. Am. Geriat. Soc.* **8** (12), 909–914.
Ayd, F. J., Jr. (1963). The phenothiazine tranquilizers: A re-evaluation after ten years experience. *Mind* **1**, 326-passim.
Bagans, J. A., et al. (1957). The therapeutic experiment: Observations on the meaning of controls and on biologic variation resulting from the treatment situation. *J. Lab. Clin. Med.* **49** (2), 282–285.
Baron, S. H., and Fisher, S. (1962). Use of psychotropic drug prescriptions in a prepaid group practice plan. *Public Health Rept. U.S.* **77** (10), 871–881.
Barsa, J. A. (1958). Use of chlorpromazine combined with prochlorperazine. *Am. J. Psychiat.* **114** (12), 1112–1113.
Batterman, R. C., et al. Clinical re-evaluation of daytime sedatives. *Postgrad. Med.* **26**, 502–509. (1959).
Bennett, J. L., and Kooi, K. A. (1961). Five phenothiazine derivatives; evaluation and toxicity studies. *Arch. Gen. Psychiat.* **4** (4), 413–418.
Berman, H. H., et al. (1958). Prochlorperazine as an antiemetic in the severely retarded child. *AMA. Diseases Children* **95** (2), 146–149.
Bhargava, K. P., and Chandra, O. (1964). Tranquillizing and hypotensive activities of twelve phenothiazines. *Brit. J. Pharmacol.* **22** (1), 154–161.
Bhaskaran, K., et al. (1962). Fatal bone-marrow aplasia complicating prochlorperazine therapy. *Am. J. Psychiat.* **119** (4), 373–374.
Blackburn, H. L., and Allen, J. L. (1961). Behavioral effects of interrupting and resuming tranquilizing medication among schizophrenics. *J. Nervous Mental Disease* **133** (4), 303–308.
Borel, C. B., et al. (1957). Essais thérapeutiques avec deux dérivés des phénotiazines, 4632 R.P. (mopazine) et le 6140 R.P. (stémetil). [Therapeutic trials with two phenothiazine

derivatives, RP 4632 (mopazine) and RP 6140 (Stemetil).] *Ann. Med. Psychol.* **115** (1:3), 526–529.
Bowman, P. W., and Blumberg, E. (1958). Ataractic therapy of hyperactive, mentally retarded patients. *J. Maine Med. Assoc.* **49** (7), 272–273.
Bowen, E. H., Jr. (1959). Some recent drugs useful in anesthesiology. *Anesthesia Analgesia, Current Res.* **38** (1), 14–20.
Boyd, E. M. (1957). Antiemetic action of prochlorperazine. *Can. Med. Assoc. J.* **76** (4), 286–289.
Braceland, F. J. (1964). Drugs effective in emotional disorders. *Postgrad. Med.* **35** (3), 237–242.
Braun, M., *et al.* (1959). A synergistic action of prochlorperazine and mepazine in two cases of schizophrenia. *J. Clin. Exptl. Psychopathol.* **20** (2), 144–146.
Brill, N. Q., *et al.* (1964). Controlled study of psychiatric outpatient treatment. *Arch. Gen. Psychiat.* **10**, 581–595.
Broussole, P., and Dubon, P. (1956). Premier bilan des effets cliniques d'un nouveau. neuroleptique. (First report on clinical effects of a new neuroleptic.) *Ann. Med. Psychol*, **2** (3), 512.
Broussolle, P., *et al.* (1960). L'emploi de la prochlorpémazine en pratique psychiatrique. [Use of prochlorpemazine in practical psychiatry.] *Ann. Med. Psychol.* **118** (1:2), 277–287.
Broussolle, P., *et al.* (1957). La prochlorperazine en psychiatrie, expérience tirés de 240 cures. [Prochlorperazine in psychiatry, experience in 240 cases.] *Presse Med.* **65** (73), 1628–1631.
Buge, M. A., *et al.* (1964). Ya-t-il un traitement de la schizophrénie? [Is there a treatment for schizophrenia?] *Presse Med.* **72** (22), 1311–1313.
Burstein, P. N., *et al.* (1964). Ruptured berry aneurysm during pregnancy; successful repair under hypothermia. *Obstet. Gynecol.* **24** (3), 463–467.
Caffey, E. M., Jr. (1961). Experiences with large scale interhopsital cooperative research in chemotherapy. *Am. J. Psychiat.* **117** (8), 713–719.
Capparell, H. V. (1962). Drug therapy in mental illness. *Penna. Med. J.* **65** (8), 899–905.
Carter, C. H. (1959). Prochlorperazine in emotionally disturbed, mentally defective children. *Southern Med. J.* **52** (2), 174–178.
Casey, J. F., *et al.* (1960). Treatment of schizophrenic reactions with phenothiazine derivatives. A comparative study of chlorpromazine, triflupromazine, mepazine, prochlorperazine, perphenazine, and phenobarbital. *Am. J. Psychiat.* **117** (2), 97–105.
Chatterji, N. N. (1962). Treatment of chronic schizophrenia with prochlorperazine. *J. Indian Med. Assoc.* **38** (5), 225–226.
Christian, C. D., and Paulson, G. (1958). Severe motility disturbance after small doses of prochlorperazine. *New Engl. J. Med.* **259** (17), 828–830.
Conner, P. K., and Meyer, J. H. (1959). Preliminary clinical observations on a potential antiemetic agent, prochlorperazine ("Compazine"). *Antibiot. Med. Clin. Therap.* **4** (9), 508–514.
Conway, C. F., Jr. (1960). Tranquilizers: Their use and abuse. *Trans. Studies Coll. Physicians Phila.* **28** (1), 38–45.
Cornman, H. D., III (1962). Clinical use of the phenothiazine derivatives in general practice. *In* "Psychosomatic Medicine". First Hahnemann Symposium (J. H. Nodine and J. H. Moyer, eds.), pp. 461–464. Lea & Febiger, Philadelphia, Pennsylvania.
Council on Drugs. (1958). Prochlorperazine. *J. Am. Med. Assoc.* **167** (4), 468–469.
Cox, E. M., and Lougheed, J. C. (1962). Pre- and postoperative use of prochlorperazine. *J. Tenn. State Med. Assoc.* **55** (4), 154–155.
Craft, M. J. (1959). Tranquillizers, a latin square trial. *J. Mental Sci.* **105** (439), 482–488.
Craft, M. (1959). Mental disorder in the defective; the use of tranquilizers. *Am. J. Mental Deficiency* **64** (1), 63–71.
Culpepper, W. S. (1963). Headache: a second look by the general physician. *Postgrad. Med.* **33** (4), 311–315.

Cytryn, L., et al. (1960). The effectiveness of tranquilizing drugs plus supportive psychotherapy in treating behavior disorders of children: A double-blind study of eighty outpatients. *Am. J. Orthopsychiat.* **30**, 113–129.
Daeschner, G. L., et al. (1958). Treatment of nausea and vomiting in children with prochlorperazine. *J. Pediat.* **53** (2), 148–152.
Dalsgaard-Nielsen, T. (1960). Prochlorperazine in the prophylaxis of migraine. *Lancet* II (7155), 877.
De Gannes, L., and Bricaire, H. (1957). Les accidents nerveux d'un nouvel antiémétique (6140 RP). [Neurological side effects of a new antiemetic (6140 RP).] *Presse Med.* **65** (22), 499.
Delay, J., et al. (1957). Le syndrome excito-moteur provoqué par les médicaments neuroleptiques. [Motor excitation caused by neuroleptic drugs.] *Presse Med.* **65** (79), 1771–1774.
Denham, J. (1958). The use of prochlorperazine (Stemetil) in chronic psychotic disorders. *J. Mental. Sci.* **104** (437), 1190–1194.
Dichiara, J. B. (1963). Utilización de la proclorperazina en psiquiatría; cinco años de experiencias clinicas; communicacion previa. [Use of prochlorperazine in psychiatry; five years of clinical experience; preliminary communication.] *Dia. Med.* **34**, 2201–2203.
Dillon, H., and Leopold, R. L. (1961). Children and the post-concussion syndrome. *J. Am. Med. Assoc.* **175** (2), 86–92.
Dransfield, G. A. (1958). A clinical trial comparing prochlorperazine (Stemetil) with chlorpromazine (Largactil) in the treatment of chronic psychotic patients. *J. Mental Sci.* **104** (437), 1183–1189.
Dubois, J. R. (1963). Neurologic complications of phenothiazine therapy. *Henry Ford Hosp. Med. Bull.* **11** (1), 59–63.
Dundee, J. W., et al. (1963). Alterations in response to somatic pain associated with anaesthesia. XV. Further studies with phenothiazine derivatives and similar drugs. *Brit. J. Anaesthesia* **35**, 597–610.
Dymond, S. C. (1963). Treatment of Méniere's disease. *Brit. Med. J.* I (5323), 124–125.
Eckstam, E. E. (1959). Prochlorperazine as a pre- and postoperative adjunct: report of a pilot study with follow-up. *Wisconsin Med. J.* **58** (7), 357–360.
Eiduson, S., et al. (1960). A study of fast (tablet) vs. slow-release ("Spansule") forms of "Compazine." *Trans. 4th Res. Conf. Chemotherap. Psychiat., VA Washington, D.C.* **4**, 248–250.
Eisenberg, L. (1964). Role of drugs in treating disturbed children. *Children* **2** (5), 167–173.
Ekbom, K. A. (1960). Restless legs syndrome. *Neurology* **10**, 868–873.
Ellard, J. (1963). Psychotropic drugs in general practice. *Med. J. Australia* II (19), 773–777.
Enelow, A. J. (1965). Drug treatment of psychotic patients in general medical practice. *Calif. Med.* **102** (1), 1–4.
Farber, S., and Vawter, G. F. (1961). Clinical pathological conference: The Children's Hospital Medical Center, Boston, Mass. *J. Pediat.* **58** (3), 424–432.
Faurbye, A., et al. (1964). Neurological symptoms in pharmacotherapy of psychoses. *Acta Physiol. Scand.* **40** (i), 10–27.
Ferster, C. B., and DeMyer, M. K. (1961). Increased performances of an autistic child with prochlorperazine administration. *J. Exptl. Anal. Behavior* **4** (1), 84.
Fish, B. (1960). Drug therapy in child psychiatry: Psychological aspects. *Comprehensive Psychiat.* **1** (1), 55–61.
Fish, F. (1964). The influence of tranquillisers on the Leonhard schizophrenic syndromes. *Encephale* **53**, Suppl., 245–249.
Freed, H., and Frignito, N. (1961). Tranquilizers in child psychiatry: Current status on drugs, particularly phenothiazines. *Penna. Psychiat. Quart.* **1** (4), 39–48.
Freed, H., et al. (1959). Reading disability: A new therapeutic approach and its implications. *J. Clin. Exptl. Psychopathol.* **20** (3), 251–259.

Freyhan, F. A. (1958). The neuroleptic action and effectiveness of prochlorperazine in psychiatric disorders. *Psychiat. Res. Rept.* No. 9, pp. 32–45.

Freyhan, F. A. (1959). Therapeutic implications of differential effects of new phenothiazine compounds. *Am. J. Psychiat.* **115** (7), 577–585.

Friend, D. G., and McLemore, G. A., Jr. (1957). Antiemetic properties of a new chlorphenothiazine derivative, proclorperazine. *AMA. Arch. Internal Med.* **99** (5), 732–735.

Frierson, B. D. (1958). A preliminary evaluation of prochlorperazine ("Compazine") in chronically disturbed psychotic patients. *J. Nervous Mental Disease* **126** (6), 585–586.

Galbraith, A. J., *et al.* (1959). Stemetil in the treatment of chronic psychotics. *J. Mental Sci.* **105** (438), 256–259.

Gatto, L. E. (1965). Better drugs and responses in the field of psychiatry. *Southern Med. J.* **58** (1), 21–23.

Gerson, I. M., *et al.* (1964). Clinical trial of a potentiated diketopiperazine derivative as a psychopharmacological agent for the treatment of psychotic patients. *Am. J. Psychiat.* **121** (2), 179–181.

Ghosh, M., *et al.* (1965). Therapy of toxoplasmosis uveitis. *Am. J. Ophthalmol.* **59** (1), 55–61.

Goldman, D. (1958). The results of treatment of psychotic states with newer phenothiazine compounds effective in small doses. *Am. J. Med. Sci.* **235** (1), 67–77.

Goldman, D. (1958). Effect of prochlorperazine ("Compazine") on psychotic states. *Psychiat. Res. Rept.* No. 9, pp. 23–31.

Goldman, D. (1961). Psychodynamic observations in psychopharmacology. *Psychosomatics* **2** (5), 379–381.

Gonzalez, J. R., and Imahara, J. K. (1964). Electroshock therapy with the phenothiazines and reserpine; a survey and report. *Am. J. Psychiat.* **121** (3), 253–256.

Gorham, D. R., and Overall, J. E. (1960). Drug-action profiles based on an abbreviated. psychiatric rating scale. *J. Nervous Mental Disease* **131** (6), 528–535.

Gray, W. D. (1957). An appraisal of a new antiemetic drug: Prochlorperazine. *Intern. Record Med.* **170** (8), 469–472.

Green, M. A. (1962). Tranquilizers in allergy. *Postgrad. Med.* **32** (5), 497–501.

Griffin, P. J. (1962). Methocarbamol in neuromuscular reactions to phenothiazine derivatives. *Gen. Practitioner* **26** (6), 110–111.

Grinspoon, L., and Greenblatt, M. (1963). Pharmacotherapy combined with other treatment methods. *Comprehensive Psychiat.* **4** (4), 256–262.

Gross, M., *et al.* (1960). Discontinuation of treatment with ataractic drugs; a preliminary report. *Am. J. Psychiat.* **116** (10), 931–932.

Gross, M., *et al.* (1963). The repetitive administration of two psychological tests during withdrawal from ataractic drugs. *J. Nervous Mental Disease* **173** (6), 574–576.

Hagenbach, C. (1960). Prochlorperazine in the prophylaxis of migraine. *Practitioner* **184** (1102), 503–506.

Hamilton, M., *et al.* (1963). A controlled trial on the value of prochlorperazine, trifluoperazine and intensive group treatment. *Brit. J. Psychiat.* **109** (461), 510–522.

Hanlon, T. E., *et al.* (1959). Chlorpromazine, triflupromazine, and prochlorperazine in chronic psychosis. *AMA Arch. Gen. Psychiat.* **1** (2), 223–227.

Hanlon, T. E., *et al.* (1965). The comparative effectiveness of eight phenothiazines. *Psychopharmacologia* **7** (2), 89–106.

Harley, R. D., and Mishler, J. E. (1959). Ataractic and antiemetic drugs in cataract surgery. *Am. J. Ophthalmol.* **47** (2), 177–185.

Hasse, H. J. (1963). Moglichkeiten und Grenzen der Psychopharmakotherapie mit Tranquilizern und Neuroleptika. [Possibilities and limitations of psychopharmacotherapy with tranquilizers and neuroleptics.] *Deut. Med. Wochschr.* **88** (11), 505–514.

Hawke, W. A., and McGreal, D. A. (1964). Tranquilizers. *Clin. Pediat. (Phila.)* **3** (4), 192–196

Himwich, H. E. (1960). Some drugs useful in the treatment of emotional disorders; physiology indications, and contraindications. *Am. Practitioner* **11** (8), 687–696.

Holman, W.-T. (1958). High dosage "Compazine" in chronic schizophrenia. *Diseases Nervous System* **19** (7), 309–310.
Hopkins, C. E., and Geppert, T. V. (1958). Vomiting in infancy and early childhood: Treatment with prochlorperazine. *J. Pediat.* **52** (6), 687–689.
Hordern, A. (1961). Psychiatry and the tranquilizers. *New Engl. J. Med.* **265** (12). 584–588; *ibid.* **265** (13), 634–638.
Hordern, A. and Somerville, D. M. (1962). The general practitioner and psychiatric drug Treatment. *Med. J. Australia* **49** (1), 404–411.
Howat, D. D. C. (1960). Anti-emetic drugs in anaesthesia: A double blind trial of two phenothiazine derivatives. *Anaesthesia* **15** (3), 289–297.
Hurst, L. (1960). Phenothiazine derivatives in the treatment of schizophrenia. *J. Mental Sci.* **106** (443), 755–770.
Illingworth, R. S., and Harvey, C. C. (1960). Prevention of migraine in children by prochlorperazine. *Lancet* I (7116), 132.
Jacoby, M. G., et al. (1958). Applicability of sustained-release psychopharmacologic agents to psychiatric treatment. *Diseases Nervous System* **19** (10), 431–434.
Jenkins, S. B., and Samborski, A. H. (1964). Symptom specificity of anti-psychotic drugs. *J. Michigan State Med. Soc.* **63** (3), 187–193.
Jucker, E. (1962). Recent advances in the field of psychotropic drugs. *J. Sci. Ind. Res. (India)* **21A** (9), 415–423.
Judah, L. N., et al. (1961). Results of simultaneous abrupt withdrawal of ataraxics in 500 chronic psychotic patients. *Am. J. Psychiat.* **118** (2), 156–158.
Kappelman, M. D. (1962). Prochlorperazine in labor and delivery. *Obstet. Gynecol.* **19** (1), 118–120.
Karakashian, N. A., et al. (1958). Anesthesia in cataract surgery. *J. Intern. Coll. Surgeons* **29** (4), 449–452.
Kelly, E. L., et al. (1958). Personality differences and continued meprobamate and prochlorperazine administration. *AMA Arch. Neurol. Psychiat.* **80** (2), 241–246.
Kelly, E. L., et al. (1958). Continued meprobamate and prochlorperazine administration and behavior. *AMA Arch. Neurol. Psychiat.* **80** (2), 247–252.
Kennon, L., and Chen, K. (1962). Probability and complexation: A new approach. *J. Pharm. Sci.* **51** (12), 1149–1151.
King, P. D., and Weinberger, W. (1959). Comparison of prochlorperazine and chlorpromazine in hospitalized chronic schizophrenics. *Am. J. Psychiat.* **115** (11), 1026–1027.
Kissen, M. D. (1960). Treatment of acute and chronic alcoholism; a controlled evaluation *Pennsa. Med. J.* **63** (11), 1642–1645.
Klatzko, M. (1958). Porphyria treated with prochlorperazine. *New Engl. J. Med.* **259** (13), 635–636.
Klein, D. F., and Fink, M. (1962). Behavioral reaction patterns with phenothiazines. *Arch. Gen. Psychiat.* **7** (6), 449–459.
Klett, C. J., and Lasky, J. J. (1960). A clinical trial of five phenothiazines using sequential analysis. *J. Clin. Exptl. Psychopathol.* **21** (2), 89–100.
Kline, N. S. (1961). The use of psychopharmaceuticals in office practice. *Med. Clin. N. Am.* **45** (6), 1677–1684.
Kline, N. S., and Simpson, G. M. (1964). A long-acting phenothiazine in office practice. *Am. J. Psychiat.* **120** (10), 1012–1014.
Kline, N. S., et al. (1958). The use of prochlorperazine ("Compazine") in a variety of psychiatric conditions. *Psychiat. Res. Rept.* No. 9, pp. 5–15.
Koegler, R. R. (1965). Drugs, neurosis and the family physician. *Calif. Med.* **102** (1), 5–8.
Koegler, R. R., et al. (1964). A psychiatric clinic evaluates brief-contact therapy. *Mental Hosp.* **15** (10), 564-passim.
Kraines, S. H. (1964). Psychotropic drugs in general practice. *Memphis Med. J.* **39** (1), 9-passim.

Kris, E. B. (1965). Psychiatric treatment of the aged. *Current Therap. Res.* **7** (2), 145–149.
Kurland, A., et al. (1961). Comparative studies of the phenothiazine tranquilizers: methodological and logistical considerations. *J. Nervous Mental Diseases* **132** (1), 61–74.
Lambert, P.-A. (1964). Essai de systématisation des associations de neuroleptiques. [Trial systemization of neuroleptic combinations.] *Encephale* **53**, Suppl., 262–275.
Lamphier, T. A. (1959). The use of prochlorperazine in surgery. *J. Maine Med. Assoc.* **50** (1), 8 and 20.
Lamphier, T. A. (1960). "Compazine"; its routine preoperative and postoperative value. *J. Intern. Coll. Surgeons* **33** (1), 24–28.
Lapolla, A., and Nash, L. R. (1965). A comparative clinical study of prochlorperazine, SKF 4579, perphenazine, triflupromazine, chlorpromazine, and reserpine. *Clin. Med.* **72** (3), 495–503.
Lease, S. (1959). Electroshock therapy and tranquilizing drugs. *J. Am. Med. Assoc.* **170** (15), 1791–1795.
Lease, S. (1957). An evaluation of prochlorparazine in the ambulatory treatment of psychiatric patients. *Intern. Record Med.* **170** (10), 599–602.
Lecks, H. I., et al. (1962). Drug therapy of asthma. *Clin. Pediat. (Phila.)* **1** (2), 125–129.
Lecomte, G., et al. (1957). Efficacité de la prochlorpérazine à doses modéraés dans les états d'excitation. [Efficacy of prochlorperazine at moderate doses in states of excitation.] *Ann. Med.-Psychol.* **115** (1:5), 922–928.
Lloyd, D. M., and Newbrough, J. R. (1964). Sensory changes with phenothiazine medication in schizophrenic patients. *J. Nervous Mental Disease* **139** (2), 169–175.
Lourie, R. S. (1964). Psychoactive drugs in pediatrics. *Pediatrics* **34** (5), 691–693.
Love, W. R. (1963). Treatment of anogenital pruritus. *Ohio State Med. J.* **59** (9), 907–909.
McAfooa, L. G., Jr. (1957). Prochlorperazine ("Compazine") in emotional disturbances. *Diseases Nervous System* **18** (11), 430–433.
McGuigan, J. E., et al. (1960). Comparison of chloramphenicol, oxytetracycline, and prochlorperazine in salmonella gastroenteritis. *U.S. Armed Forces Med. J.* **11** (11), 1288–1293.
McLaughlin, B. E., et al. (1964). Chemotherapy for emotionally disturbed children: A follow-up report. *Diseases Nervous System* **25** (12), 735–738.
Mapp, Y., and Nodine, J. H. (1962). Psychopharmacology. II. Tranquilizers and antipsychotic drugs. *Psychosomatics* **3** (6), 458–463.
Markham, C. H. (1964). Diseases of the basal ganglia. *Mind.* **2** (1), 6–9.
Marks, J. (1962). Current views on psychotropic drugs. *New Zealand Med. J.* **61**, 391–397.
Marks, J. (1963). Predrug behavior as a predictor of response to phenothiazines among schizophrenics. *J. Nervous Mental Disease* **137** (6), 597–601.
Maurel, H., et al. (1960). Pratique psychiatrique hospitalière de la thiopropérazine; comparaison avec la prochlorpémazine. [Hospital, psychiatric practice with thioproperazine; comparison with prochlorpemazine.] *Ann. Med.-Psychol.* **118** (1:5), 978–983.
May, R. H. (1959). Catatonic-like states following phenothiazine therapy. *Am. J. Psychiat.* **115** (12), 1119–1120.
Mendel, W. M. (1958). Observations on the comparative effects of tranquilizers on patients previously treated with prochlorperazine. *Am. J. Psychiat.* **115** (5), 466–467.
Michaux, M. H., et al. (1964). Phenothiazines in the treatment of newly admitted state hospital patients: Global comparison of eight compounds in terms of an outcome index. *Current Therap. Res.* **6** (5), 331–339.
Miller, J. G. (1962). Objective measurements of the effects of drugs on driver behavior. *J. Am. Med. Assoc.* **179** (12), 940–943.
Milne, H. B., and Berliner, F. (1958). A clinical trial of Stemetil (prochlorperazine). *J. Mental Sci.* **104** (436), 873–879.
Milne, H. B., and Fowler, D. B. (1960). A clinical trial of Largactil (chlorpromazine), Stemetil (prochlorperazine) and Veractil (methotrimeprazine). *J. Mental Sci.* **106** (444), 1105–1110.

Mitchell, A. C., et al. (1959). Effects of prochlorperazine therapy on educability in disturbed mentally retarded adolescents. *Am. J. Mental Deficiency* **64** (1), 57–62.
Moertel, C. G., et al. (1963). A controlled clinical evaluation of antiemetic drugs. *J. Am. Med. Assoc.* **186** (2), 116–118.
Mounier-Kuhn, P., et al. (1957). Traitement des vertiges par le 6140 R.P. [Treatment of vertigo with RP 6140.] *J. Franc. Otorhinolaringol.* **6** (4), 673–676.
Moyer, J. H. (1957). Effective antiemetic agents. *Med. Clin. N. Am.* **41** (2), 405–432.
Noble, R. C., and Castner, C. W. (1958). Evaluation of prochlorperazine and a prochlorperazine-chlorpromazine combination in disturbed patients. *Diseases Nervous System* **19** (12), 531–533.
Nodine, J. H. (1962). Psychopharmacology. I. General principles. *Psychosomatics* **3** (5), 351–364.
Olmsted, K. E. P. (1963). Care of the patient with cataract; pre- and postoperative. *N.Y. J. Med.* **63** (12), 1799–1804.
Overall, J. E., and Gorham, D. R. (1960). Factor space D^2 analysis applied to the study of changes in schizophrenic symptomatology during chemotherapy. *J. Clin. Exptl. Psychopathol.* **21** (3), 187–195.
Packenstoe, G. S. (1959). Prochlorperazine in airsickness. *Penna. Med. J.* **62** (9), 1341–1343.
Peikes, I. L. (1957). Nausea and vomiting of pregnancy treated with a sustained release form of prochlorperazine. *Clin. Med.* **4** (11), 1385–1387.
Pennington, V. M. (1959). Prochlorperazine in the treatment of the schizophrenias. *Am. J. Psychiat.* **115** (9), 820–821.
Pennington, V. M. (1959). Clinical results of prochlorperazine. *Med. Times* **87** (11), 1432–1437.
Pennington, V. M. (1964). Ten year's progress in psychotropic medication. *Illinois Med. J.* **126** (5), 553–558.
Pilkington, T. L. (1959). Prochlorperazine (Stemetil) in mental deficiency. *J. Mental Sci.* **105** (438), 215–219.
Price, M. J. (1958). The treatment of nausea and vomiting of pregnancy with prochlorperazine. *Med. Ann. District Columbia* **27** (3), 123–125.
Rajotte, P., and Denber, H. C. B. (1963). Long-term community follow-up of formerly hospitalized psychotic patients. *J. Nervous Mental Diseases* **136** (5), 445–454.
Rajotte, P., et al. (1965). Etude comparative de la butapérazine et de la prochlorpérazine chez le schizophrène chronique. [Comparative study of butaperazine and prochlorperazine in the chronic schizophrenic.] *Can. Psychiat. Assoc. J.* **10** (1), 25–34.
Rees, L. (1962). The value and limitations of psychotropic drugs in psychiatric treatment. *Anglo-Ger. Med. Rev.* **1** (4), 448–459.
Rees, L. (1963). Indications for the use of drugs in the treatment of psychiatric disorders. *Postgrad. Med. J.* **39** (447), 48–52.
Reeves, J. E. (1957). Successful prochlorperazine therapy following chlorpromazine-induced jaundice. *Calif. Med.* **87** 338–339.
Riccitelli, M. L. (1964). Modern concepts in the management of anxiety and depression in the aged and infirm. *J. Am. Geriat. Soc.* **12** (7), 652–657.
Rickels, K., et al. (1959). Evaluation of tranquilizing drugs in medical outpatients; meprobamate, prochlorperazine, amobarbital sodium, and placebo. *J. Am. Med. Assoc.* **171** (12), 1649–1656.
Riesenman, F. R., and Pettit, M. B. (1959). Clinical efficacy of proclorperazine ("Compazine") in mental illness. *Am. J. Psychiat.* **115** (11), 1032–1033.
Robb, H. P. (1960). A comparison between prochlorperazine and chlorpromazine in mental deficiency. *J. Mental Sci.* **106** (445), 1413–1416.
Robbie, D. S. (1959). Post-anaesthetic vomiting and anti-emetic drugs. *Anaesthesia* **14** (4), 349–354.

Robin, A. A. (1963). The effect of tranquilizers on some aspects of the treatment of long stay patients. *Am. J. Psychiat.* **119** (11), 1076–1081.

Rogers, G. A. (1959). Alcoholism treated with prochlorperazine. *J. Med. Soc. New Jersey* **56** (5), 247–250.

Rosenkilde, H., and Govier, W. M. (1957). A comparison of some phenothiazine derivatives in inhibiting apomorphine-induced emesis. *J. Pharmacol. Exptl. Therap.* **120** (3), 375–378.

Rossi, G. V. (1963). Synergism: With special reference to central nervous system depressants. *J. Pharm. Sci.* **52** (9), 819–832.

Rossi, G. V. (1964). The psychotherapeutic agents. *Am. J. Pharm.* **136** (1), 6–24.

Rothstein, C., and Lacerva, S. P. (1959). Prochlorperazine in a psychotic geriatric group. *J. Maine Med. Assoc.* **50** (1), 4–7.

Rothstein, C., *et al.* (1962). Discontinuation of maintenance dosages of ataractic drugs on a psychiatric continued treatment ward. *J. Nervous Mental Disease* **134** (6), 555–560.

Sainsbury, P., and Lucas, C. J. (1959). Sequential methods applied to the study of prochlorperazine. *Brit. Med. J.* II (5154), 737–740.

St. Laurent, J., *et al.* (1962). Treatment of psychiatric patients with a phenothiazine derivative (prochlorperazine) with special reference to after care. *Am. J. Psychiat.* **118** (10), 938–940.

Salzberger, G. J. (1964). Experiences, concepts and some results with drugs in geriatric patients. *Diseases Nervous System* **25** (11), 670–673.

Sandberg, F. (1959). A comparative quantitative study of the central depressant effect of seven clinically used phenothiazine derivatives. *Arzneimittel-Forsch.* **9** (4), 203–206.

Sanger, M. D. (1962). The use of tranquilizers and antidepressants in allergy. *Ann. Allergy* **20** (11), 705–709.

Senekyj, J. P. (1960). Management of feeding problems in aged, disturbed patients. *J. Am. Geriat. Soc.* **8** (7), 537–539.

Settel, E. (1957). Treatment of anxiety and agitation with prochlorperazine in geriatric patients. *J. Am. Geriat. Soc.* **5** (10), 827–831.

Schaefer, J. F. (1959). Prochlorperazine; clinical evaluation. *Am. Practitioner* **10** (4), 647–649.

Schneider, J., *et al.* (1963). Die Modifikationen des EEG unter der Behandlung mit Psychopharmaka. Langzeituntersuchungen an Geisteskranken. [EEG modifications during treatment with psychotropic compounds; long-term studies in mental patients.] *Nervenarzt* **34** (12), 521–530.

Shapiro, A. K. (1964). Rational use of psychopharmaceutic agents. *N.Y. State J. Med.* **64** (9), 1084–1095.

Shaw, E. B., *et al.* (1959). Phenothiazine tranquilizers as a cause of severe seizures. *Pediatrics* **23** (3), 485–492.

Shubin, H., and Sherson, J. (1959). Prochlorperazine in the management of restive aged patients. *J. Am. Geriat. Soc.* **7** (5), 405–407.

Shubin, H., *et al.* (1958). Prochlorperazine ("Compazine") as an aid in the treatment of pulmonary tuberculosis. *Antiobiot. Med. Clin. Therap.* **5** (5), 305–309.

Sittampalam, A., and Abeywardane, A. L. (1962). A double blind placebo controlled trial of Stemetil (prochlorperazine) on chronic hospitalised schizophrenics. *Ceylon Med. J.* **7**, 97–101.

Smith, C. W., and Thomas, C. G. (1962). Prochlorperazine for emotional distress associated with cardiovascular disease. *Staff Bull. Harrisburg Hosp.* **10** (1), 14–18.

Smith-e-Incas, J., *et al.* (1961). Use of sustained release prochlorperazine therapy in the treatment of severely disturbed mental patients. *J. Natl. Med. Assoc.* **53** (3), 288–290.

Solan, M. J. (1959). Prochlorperazine and irradiation sickness. *Brit. Med. J.* II (5159), 1068–1069.

South-East Region (Scotland) Therapeutic Trials Committee. (1961). Controlled trial of prochlorperazine (Stemetil) in schizophrenia. *J. Mental Sci.* **107** (448), 514–522.

Southworth, H. (1964). The doctor's bag. *Clin. Pharmacol. Therap.* **5** (6, Part 1), 773–778.
Splitter, S. R. (1960). Treatment of the anxious patient in general office practice. *J. Clin. Exptl. Psychopathol.* **21** (2), 106–113.
Stevens, J. D. (1964). Psychopharmacology. *J. Neuropsychiat.* **5** (8), 566–576.
Stearns, P. E., and Sahhar, F. H. (1959). Prochlorperazine in the treatment of patients with severe mental deficiency. *Northwest Med.* **58** (8), 1106–1109.
Stevenson, L. E. (1961). A note on anorectics. *Med. Ann. District Columbia* **30** (7), 409–410.
Stewart, R. H. (1961). Phenothiazine derivatives in labor and delivery; a study of four drugs. *Obstet. Gynecol.* **17** (6), 701–713.
Staskiewicz, T. A. (1959). Screening patients for ataractic therapy; use of a hyperventilation test. *Am. Practitioner* **10** (4), 642–645.
Sullivan, C. L. (1958). Prochlorperazine for the treatment of nausea and vomiting of early pregnancy. *New Engl. J. Med.* **258** (5), 232–234.
Sundby, P., and Lien, J. B. (1959). Prochlorperazine and chlorpromazine; a comparative clinical trial. *Acta Psychiat. Neurol. Scand.* **34**, Suppl. 136, 82–88.
Sylvester, W. R. (1964). Nausea and vomiting in pregnancy; comparative evaluation of therapy with hydroxyzine and prochlorperazine in routine office practice. *Southwestern Med.* **45**, 52–55.
Symposium. (1957). Prochlorperazine in the treatment of mental disorders (Brentwood Conference, California). Monograph from Diseases Nervous System 1957.
Tanner, H., et al. (1963). Long-term progress of hospitalized schizophrenic patients on ataractic drugs. *J. Neuropsychiat.* **4** (5), 321–330.
Thimann, J., and Gauthier, J. W. (1959). Control of acute alcoholism with prochlorperazine; preliminary report. *New Engl. J. Med.* **260** (18), 915–917.
Toll, N. (1958). Deaner an adjunct for treatment of schizoid and schizophrenic patients. *Am. J. Psychiat.* **115** (4), 366–367.
Tolle, R. (1962). Uber zwei Piperazinderivate des Phenothiazins. (Two piperazine derivatives of phenothiazine.) *Nervenarzt* **33** (10), 457–462.
Toms, E. C. (1961). A comparative study of selected tranquilizers in the treatment of psychiatric patients. *J. Nervous Mental Disease* **132** (5), 425–431.
Tuft, H. S. (1959). Prochlorperazine as an aid in the treatment of bronchial asthma. *Ann. Allergy* **17** (2), 224–229.
Vischer, T. J. (1957). Clinical study of prochlorperazine, a new tranquilizer for the treatment of nonhospitalized psychoneurotic patients. *New Engl. J. Med.* **256** (1), 26–273.
Viukari, M. (1964). Psykotrooppisilla lääkkeillä poliklinisessä käytossä saatuja tuloksia [Psychotropic drugs in out-patient treatment.] *Duodecim* **80**, 400–404.
Weatherall, M. (1962). Tranquilizers. *Brit. Med. J.* I (5287), 1219–1224.
Welsh, A. L. (1964). The newer tranquilizing drugs. *Med. Clin. N. Am.* **48** (2), 459–481.
Wennersten, J. R. (1956). Office treatment of pain and psychic stress: The use of a new tranquilizing agent. *Clin. Med.* **3** (12), 1179–1183.
Wennersten, J. R. (1961). Management of restive aged patients in office practice. *J. Am. Geriat. Soc.* **9** (8), 694–698.
Wetterholm, B., et al. (1959). Some experiences with prochlorperazine. *Svenska Lakartidn.* No. 37, 2512.
Wheeler, W. L., Jr., et al. (1959). The use of prochlorperazine in seasickness. *Ind. Med. Surg.* **28** (9), 405–406.
Whitman, R. M. (1963). Symposium on sleep and dreams. II. Drugs, dreams and the experimental subject. *Can. Psychiat. Assoc. J.* **8** (6), 395–399.
Whittier, J. R., et al. (1959). Drug use-rate in a state hospital. *Am. J. Psychiat.* **116** (2), 169–171.
Wilcox, F. (1958). Prochlorperazine in hospitalized and private psychiatric patients. *Diseases Nervous System* **19** (3), 118–121.

Wilder, J. (1962). "Compazine" suppositories. *Am. J. Psychiat.* **119** (1), 84–85.

Wilson, I. C., *et al.* (1961). A double-blind trial to investigate the effects of "Thorazine" (Largactil, chlorpromazine), "Compazine" (Stemetil, prochlorperazine) and "Stelazine" (trifluoperazine) in pananoid schizophrenia. *J. Mental Sci.* **107** (446), 90–99.

Winkelman, N. W., Jr. (1959). Evaluation of two ataractic agents. Experience of one year with prochlorperazine and of seven months with benactyzine. *Diseases Nervous System* **20** (1), 27–30.

Wolf, J. W. (1962). The irritable colon syndrome: treatment with chlorpromazine and other phenothiazine drugs. *Missouri Med.* **59** (6), 495-passim.

Wood, C. D., *et al.* (1965). Review of antimotion sickness drugs from 1954–1964. *Aerospace Med.* **36** (1), 1–4.

Wright, W. (1959). Use of tranquilizers in dermatology. *J. Am. Med. Assoc.* **171** (12), 1642–1646.

Zakusov, V. V. (1964). Novye psikhofarmakologichesie sredstva; obzor. [New psychopharmacological compounds; review.] *Farmakol i. Toksikol.* **27** (1), 107–121.

Zelenik, J. S. (1964). Management of pain in labor. *Postgrad. Med.* **36** (4), 348–353.

~ A.10 ~
Promazine

Chemical Papers

Baumler, J., and Rippstein, S. (1961). Thin-layer chromatography as a quick method for the analysis of drugs. *Pharm. Acta. Helv.* **36**, 382–388 (in German, English summary).

Beckett, A. H., and Curry, S. H. (1963). Spectroscopic studies of the reaction of hydroxylated promazines and related compounds with sulphuric acid. *J. Pharm. Pharmacol.* **15**, 246–252; *Pharm. J.* **191**, 284.

Bickel, M. H., Sulser, F., and Brodie, B. B. (1963). Conversion of tranquilizers to antidepressants by removal of one N-methyl group. *Life Sci.* pp. 247–253.

Calo, A., Mariani, A., and Mariani-Marelli, O. (1958). Separation of phenothiazine derivatives. *Pharm. Acta Helv.* **33**, 126–131 (in French).

Cavatorta, L. (1959). Assay of promazine and its separation from chlorpromazine and promethazine. *J. Pharm. Pharmacol.* **11**, 49–53.

Clarke, E. G. C. (1957). Microchemical identification of some antihistamine drugs. *J. Pharm. Pharmacol.* **9**, 752–758.

Cusic, J. W. (1900). Method for producing aromatic aminoalkyl amines. U.S. Patent 2,687,414.

Eagleson, D. A. (1963). Paper chromatographic differentiation of some important phenothiazines encountered in toxicology. *Am. J. Clin. Pathol.* **39**, 648–651.

Eberhardt, H., Lerbs, O. W., and Freundt, K. J. (1963). Demonstration by thin layer chromatography of psychotropic phenothiazine derivatives in human urine. *Arzneimittel-Forsch.* **13**, 804–805 (in German, English summary).

Eiduson, S., and Wallace, R. D. (1958). Method for determination of phenothiazines in urine. *Federation Proc.* **17**, Part 1, 1441.

Emmerson, J. L., and Miya, T. S. (1963). Metabolism of phenothiazine drugs. *J. Pharm. Sci.* **52**, 411–419.

Forrest, F. M., Forrest, I. S., and Mason, A. S. (1958). Rapid urinary test for chlorpromazine, promazine and Pacatal: A supplementary report. *Am. J. Psychiat.* **114**, 931–932.

Forrest, F. M., Forrest, I. S., and Mason, A. S. (1961). Review of rapid urine tests for phenothiazine and related drugs. *Am. J. Psychiat.* **118**, 300–307.

Forrest, I. S., and Forrest, F. M. (1960). Urine color test for the detection of phenothiazine compounds. *Clin. Chem.* **6**, 11–15.

Gold, S., Griffiths, P. D., and Huntsman, R. G. (1962). Phenothiazines in urine. *J. Mental Sci.* **108**, 88–93.

Hetzel, C. A. (1961). Method for the estimation of phenothiazine derivatives in urine and blood. *Clin. Chem.* **7**, 130–135.

Heyman, J. J., Almudevar, M., and Merlis, S. (1959). A modification of the Forrest test for phenothiazines. *Am. J. Psychiat.* **116**, 259–260.

Janssen, P. A., J., and Niemegeers, C. J. E. (1959). Chemistry and pharmacology of compounds related to 4-(4-hydroxy-4-phenyl-piperidino)-butyrophenone. II. Inhibition of apomorphine vomiting in dogs. *Arzneimittel-Frosch.* **9**, 765–767.

Janssen, P. A. J., Van de Westeringh, C., Jageneau, A. H. M., Demoen, P. J. A., Hermans B. K. F., Van Daele, G. H. P., Schellekens, K. H. L., Van der Eycken, C. A. M., and

Niemegeers, C. J. E. (1959). Chemistry and pharmacology of CNS depressants related to 4-(4-hydroxy-4-phenylpiperidino)butyrophenone. Part I. Synthesis and screening data in mice. *J. Med. Pharm. Chem.* **1**, 281–297.

Mellinger, T. J., and Keeler, C. E. (1962). Chromatography and electrophoresis of phenothiazine drugs. *J. Pharm. Sci.* **51**, 1169–1173.

Petersen, P. V., Lassen, N., Holm, T., Kopf, R., and Moller Nielsen, I. (1958). Chemistry and pharmacological action of some thiaxanthene analogues of chlorpromazine, promazine and mepazine. *Arzneimittel-Forsch.* **8**, 395–397 (in German).

Pollack, B. (1958). The validity of the Forrest reagent test for the detection of chlorpromazine or other phenothiazines in the urine. *Am. J. Psychiat.* **115**, 77–78.

Rhone-Poulenc. (1959). Phenothiazine derivative. Belgian Patent 579,286; Derwent Belgian Patents Report 60A, C4.

Rhone-Poulenc. (1959). Prolonged effect promazine. Belgian Patent 579,356; Derwent Belgian Patents Report 60A, C8.

Rhone-Poulenc. (1946). Procedure for the preparation of phenothiazine derivatives. French Patent 917,595.

Ross, G., Weinstein, I. V., and Kabakow, B. (1958). Influence of phenothiazine and some of its derivatives on the determination of 5-hydroxy-indoleacetic acid in urine. *Clin. Chem.* **4**, 66–76.

Ryan, J. A. (1959). A colorimetric assay for unoxidized phenothiazine derivatives: a new complex salt. *J. Am. Pharm. Assoc., Sci. Ed.* **48**, 240–243.

Sorby, D. L., and Plein, E. M. (1961). Adsorption of phenothiazine derivatives by kaolin, talc, and Norit. *J. Pharm. Sci.* **50**, 355.

Street, H. V. (1962). The rapid separation of drugs and poisons by high temperature reversed phase paper chromatography. 2. Phenothiazine tranquilizers and imipramine. *Acta Pharmacol. Toxicol.* **19**, 312–324.

Vilallonga, F., Fried, E., Izquierdo, J. A. (1961). Promazine, promethazine, diethazine and imipramine at the air—0.1 M HCl interface. *Arch. Intern. Pharmacodyn.* **130**, 260–265.

Wiser, R., Knebel, C., Seifter, J. (1960). The determination of promazine in biological materials. *Pharmacologist* **2**, 83.

Young, D. K., and Pernarowski, M. (1963). Identification and differentiation of some phenothiazine-type tranquilizers. *J. Pharm. Sci.* **52**, 365–370.

Biology and Pharmacology

Arrigoni-Martelli, E., and Kramer, M. (1959). Pharmacological study of a new phenothiazine derivative: Perphenazine. *Arch. Intern. Pharmacodynamie* **119**, 311–333 (in Italian).

Barnes, T. C. (1960). Relationship of chemical structure to central nervous system effects of tranquilizing and anticonvulsant drugs. *J. Am. Pharm. Assoc., Sci. Ed.* **49**, 415–417.

Begany, A. J., Seifter, J., Pless, H. H., deV. Huber, R., and Bruce, W. F. (1956). Tranquilizing effect of phenothiazines in cats and rabbits. *Federation Proc.* Part 1, **15**, 1302.

Bieter, R. N. (1957). Pharmacology of the tranquilizing drugs. *Minn. Med.* **40**, 222–226.

Brillhart, J. R. (1959). Tranquilizer interference in the Rana pipiens chorionic gonadotropin test. *Obstet. Gynecol.* **14**, 581–587.

Burton, R. M., Burton, N. O., Kaplan, N. O., Goldin, A., Leitenberg, M., Humphreys, S. R., and Sodd, M. A. (1958). Effect of reserpine and promazine on diphosphopyridine nucleotide synthesis in liver. *Science* **127**, 30–32.

Carver, M. J., and Roesky, N. (1959). Phenothiazine derivatives as inhibitors of the glucose oxidative pathway in human erythrocytes. *Experientia* **15**, 138–139.

Citterio, C. (1958). Appearance and disappearance times of promazine in human organism. *Lavoro Neuropsichiat.* **22**, 530–544; *Chem. Abstr.* **53**, 984i.

Citterio, C. (1958). Influence of promazine on the blood sugar curve after glucose administration in normal individuals and in patients with schizophrenia. *Lavoro Neuropsichiat.* **23**, 107–114 (in Italian); *Chem. Abstr.* **53**, 8443f.

Clifford, D. H. (1957). Effect of preanesthetic medication with chlorpromazine, meperidine, and promazine on pentobarbital anesthesia in the cat. *J. Am. Vet. Med. Assoc.* **131**, 415–419.

Cunningham, J. A. (1959). A report on the use of promazine hydrochloride in equine practice. *Vet. Record* **71**, 395–397.

D'Angelo, C., Mastrogiovanni, P. D., Bellucci, O., Benincasa Stagni, E. (1958). Observations on some biological changes caused by chlorpromazine and promazine in the human organism. *Acta Neurol.* **13**, 302–309.

Dews, P. B. (1958). Effect of chlorpromazine and promazine on performance on a mixed schedule of reinforcement. *J. Exptl. Anal. Behavior* **1**, 73–82; *Biol. Abstr.* **33**, 37697.

Dolivo, M., and Maillard, J. M. (1961). Pharmacology of psycho- and neurotropic medicaments. *Helv. Med. Acta* **28**, 339–366 (in French, English summary).

Duhm, B., Koester, L., Maul, W., and Medenwald, H. (1958). Metabolism and retention of Verophen in the body of the rat. *Z. Naturforsch.* **13b**, 756–757.

Ehrmantraut, W. R., Shea, J. G., Tickten, H. E., Fazekas, J. F. (1957). Influence of promazine and methylphenidate on cerebral hemodynamics and metabolism. *AMA Arch. Internal Med.* **100**, 66–69.

Fedorov, N. A. (1957). Course of distribution and elimination of S^{35}-promazine in rats and rabbits following different methods of administration. *Uch. Zap. Mosk. Gos. Univ.* **6**, 197–204 (in Russian); *Chem. Abstr.* **53**, 5505i.

Fedorov, N. A. (1958). Distribution of S^{35}-labeled aminazine and promazine. *Zh. Nevropatol. Psikhiat.* **58**, 137–148 (in Russian).

Foote, R. H. (1959). Effect of promazine and chlorpromazine on the motility and fertility of bovine semen. (Abstract of paper presented at 54th Annual Meeting of American Dairy Science Assoc., Univ. of Illinois, Urbana, June 15–17, 1959.) *J. Dairy Sci.* **42**, 932.

Fox, C. L., Jr., Einbinder, J. M., and Nelson, C. T. (1958). Comparative inhibition of anaphylaxis in mice by steroids, tranquilizers and other drugs. *Am. J. Physiol.* **192**, 241–246.

Foxworthy, D. L., and Lehman, R. M. (1957). False-positive frog tests due to promazine hydrochloride (Sparine). *Obstet. Gynecol.* **10**, 385–387.

Frada, G., and Gucciardi, G. (1959). Further investigations on the effect of neuroplegic drugs in experimental phosphoric ester poisoning. *Med. Lavoro* **50**, 83–90 (in Italian).

Garren, H. W., and Hill, C. H. (1957). Effects of continually feeding tranquilizing agents to young white leghorns. *Poultry Sci.* **26**, 1386–1387.

Geller, I., and Seifter, J. (1959). The effects of promazine and Phenergan on multiple schedule reinforcement performance in the albino rat. *Federation Proc.* **18**, Part 1, 1549.

Glassman, J. M., Rauzzino, F., and Seifter, J. (1958). Phenothiazines: antiemetic, antihistaminic properties and responses to analeptic agents. *J. Pharmacol. Exptl. Therap.* **112**, 25A.

Goldenberg, H., Fishman, V., Heaton, A., Burnett, R. (1964). A detailed evaluation of promazine metabolism. *Proc. Soc. Exptl. Biol. Med.* **115**, 1044–1051.

Gorman, T. N. (1959). Promazine hydrochloride in equine practice. *J. Am. Vet. Med. Assoc.* **134**, 464–466.

Grahan, R. C. B., Lu, F. C., and Allmark, M. G. (1957). Combined effect of tranquilizing drugs and alcohol on rats. *Federation Proc.* **16**, Part 1, 1291.

Greer, F. G. (1958). Promazine hydrochloride in canine practice. *Vet. Record* **70**, 137.

Grenell, R. G. (1957). Mechanisms of action of psychotherapeutic and related drugs. *Ann. N.Y. Acad. Sci.* **66**, 826–835.

Guttman, H. N., and Friedman, W. (1963). Protozoa as pharmacological tools—the phenothiazine tranquilizers. *Trans. N.Y. Acad. Sci.* **26**, 75–89.

Haynes, F. A., and Perryman, B. S. (1958). Temporary alleviation of cannibalism in a Staffordshire Terrier bitch. *Mod. Vet. Pract.* **39**, 54–55.

Hosko, M. J., Gore, E. M., Tislow, R., and Seifter, J. (1957). Taming effect of promazine in the rhesus monkey. *J. Pharmacol. Exptl. Therap.* **119**, 153.

Janssen, P. A. J., Jageneau, A. H., and Niemegeers, G. J. E. (1960). Effects of various drugs on isolation-induced fighting behavior of male mice. *J. Pharmacol. Exptl. Therap.* **129**, 471–475.

Kamada, P. H. (1962). Studies on the anti-arrhythmic action of phenothiazine derivatives. II. *Japan Circulation J.* **26**, 1015–1019; *Excerpta Med. Sect. XVIII*, **7**, 2095.

Kanig, K. (1961). Biochemical and pharmacological basis for modern psychiatric pharmacotherapy. *Deut. Med. J.* **12**, 517–524. (in German).

Keplinger, M. I., Lanier, G. E., and Deichmann, W. B. (1959). Effects of environmental temperature on the acute toxicity of a number of compounds in rats. *Toxicol. Appl. Pharmacol.* **1**, 156–161; *Chem. Abstr.* **53**, 13417i.

Lagerspetz, K., and Tirri, R. (1963). The induction of physiological tolerance to promazine in mice. III. Respiratory enzymes in the brain in induced tolerance. *Ann. Med. Exptl. Biol. Fenniae (Helsinki)* **41**, 315–318.

Lank, R. B., and Kingrey, B. W. (1959). Electrocardiography of tranquilized cattle. *J. Am. Vet. Med. Assoc.* **134**, 437–439.

Lasagne, L., and McCann, W. P. (1957). Effect of "tranquilizing" drugs on amphetamine toxicity in aggregated mice. *Science* **125**, 1241–1242.

Laurence, D. R., and Webster, R. A. (1958). The activity of a variety of chemical compounds against experimental tetanus. *Brit. J. Pharmacol.* **13**, 334–338.

Leary, R. W., and Stynes, A. J. (1959). Tranquilizer effects in the social status, motivation, and learning of monkeys. *AMA Arch. Gen. Psychiat.* **1**, 499–505.

Low, H. (1959). The effects of promazines on mitochondrial adenosine triphosphatase reactions. *Biochim. Biophys. Acta* **32**, 11–18.

Lundvall, R. L. (1959). An unusual case of anaphylaxis in a pony. *Vet. Med.* **54**, 236–237.

Millican, R. C., and Rhodes, C. J. (1958). Relative effectiveness of certain phenothiazine derivatives against death from shock produced in mice by tourniquet trauma. *J. Pharmacol. Exptl. Therap.* **122**, 255–261.

Oelkers, H.-A. (1960). Betta splendens as a model for the differentiation of psychotropic drugs. *Arzneimittel-Forsch.* **10**, 392–395 (in German, English summary).

Opitz, K. (1962). Metabolic effects of psychotropic drugs. III. *Arzneimittel-Forsch.* **12**, 618–626 (in German, English summary).

Posner, H. S., Culpan, R., and Levine, J. (1963). Quantification and probable structure, in human urine, of the nonphenolic and phenolic metabolites of chlorpromazine. *J. Pharmacol. Exptl. Therap.* **141**, 377–391; *Federation Proc.* **22**, 540 (abstr.).

Raker, C. W., and Sayers, A. C. (1959). Promazine as a preanesthetic agent in horses. *J. Am. Vet. Med. Assoc.* **134**, 23–24.

Rosen, H., Blumenthal, A., Nead, M. H., Tislow, R., and Seifter, J. (1957). Gastric juice studies in rats. *Federation Proc.* **16**, Part 1, 1418.

Rosenkilde, H. (1957). Comparison of the anti-emetic effect of various tranquilizers. *J. Pharmacol. Exptl. Therap.* **119**, 180–181.

Sanchez, J. (1956). Use of a new phenothiazine derivative in the treatment of acute alcoholism. *Rev. Sanidad Policia (Lima, Peru)* **16**, 350–360 (in Spanish); *Excerpta Med. Sect. VIII* **10**, 3021.

Scheidy, S. F. (1960). Tranquilizers in veterinary medicine. *Veterinarian* **20**, 102–105.

Scheidy, S. F., and McNally, R. S. (1958). Tranquilizing drugs in veterinary practice. *Cornell Vet.* **48**, 331–347.

Scott, G. T., and Nading, L. K. (1961). Relative effectiveness of phenothiazine tranquilizing drugs causing release of MSH. *Proc. Soc. Exptl. Biol. Med.* **106**, 88–90; *Anat. Record* **138**, 382.

Seifter, J., Glassman, J. M., and Rauzzino, F. (1957). Pharmacological properties of promazine. *J. Pharmacol. Exptl. Therap.* **119**, 183.
Skorobogatov, V. I. (1963). Effects of phenothiazine derivatives on cerebrocortical bioelectric activity in rabbits. *Farmakol. i. Toksikol.* **26**, 414–418; *Chem. Abstr.* **60**, 2228a.
Silvestrini, B., and Maffii, G. (1959). Effects of chlorpromazine, promazine, diethazine, reserpine, hydroxyzine and morphine upon some mono- and polysynaptic motor reflexes. *J. Pharm. Pharmacol.* **11**, 224–233.
Siou, G., and Brunaud, M. (1958). Study in the rat of several substances said to be tranquilizing with the aid of a test for aggressiveness. *J. Physiol. (Paris)* **50**, 507–509; *Chem. Abstr.* **53**, 9456i.
Smith, J. A., Carver, M. J., and Helper, E. W. (1958). Effect of tranquilizing drugs on enzyme systems. *J. Psychiat.* **114**, 1011–1014.
Smith, W. P., Papper, S., and Rosenbaum, J. D. (1958). Inhibition of antidiuretic hormone activity as the mechanism of promazine-induced diuresis. *Clin. Res.* **6**, 289.
Spector, W. G., and Willoughby, D. A. (1963). The antagonism of substances that increase vascular permeability in the rat. *J. Pathol. Bacteriol.* **86**, 487–496.
Staib, I., Oehmig, H., Mossdorf, G., Drings, P., and Baldamus, C. (1963). Changes of cardiac output by premedication and various anesthetics (studies on human beings). *Arzneimittel-Forsch.* **13**, 628–633 (in German, English summary).
Stone, C. A., Porter, C. C., Stavosski, J. M., Ludden, C. T., and Totaro, J. A. (1964). Antagonism of certain effects of catecholamine-depleting agents by antidepressant and related drugs. *J. Pharmacol. Exptl. Therap.* **144**, 196–204.
Tedeschi, D. H., Benigni, J. P., Elder, C. J., Yeager, J. C., and Flanigan, J. V. (1958). Effects of various phenothiazines on electro-shock seizure threshold and spontaneous motor activity of mice. *J. Pharmacol. Exptl. Therap.* **123**, 35–38.
Tedeschi, D. H., Tedeschi, R. E., and Fellows, E. J. (1961). Central serotonin antagonist activity of a number of phenothiazines. *Arch. Intern. Pharmacodyn.* **132**, 172–179.
Tiwari, N. M., Sharma, M. L., Gupta, S. K., and Dashputra, P. G. (1960). Structure activity relationship of chlorpromazine and related phenothiazines of atropine like activity on rabbit intestine. *Arch. Intern. Pharmacodyn.* **125**, 456–462.
Tobe, B. A., and Goldman, B. S. (1963). The metabolism of the volatile amines. IV. The role of drugs in the pathogenesis of hepatic encephalopathy. *Can. Med. Assoc. J.* **89**, 874–880.
Truitt, E. B., Jr. (1958). Some pharmacologic correlations on the chemotherapy of mental disease. *J. Nervous Mental Disease* **126**, 184–210.
Viaud, P. (1954). The aminoderivatives of phenothiazine. *J. Pharm. Pharmacol.* **6**, 361–389 (in French).
Walkenstein, S. S., and Seifter, J. (1958). Fate, distribution and excretion of promazine. *Federation Proc.* **17**, Part I, 1646.
Walkenstein, S. S., and Seifter, J. (1959). Fate, distribution and excretion of S^{35} promazine. *J. Pharmacol. Exptl. Therap.* **125**, 283–286.
Weberlein, M. K., McClumpha, C. A., Brengle, L. A., Lickfeldt, W. E., and Dawson, H. A. (1959). Promazine in canine medicine. *J. Am. Vet. Med. Assoc.* **134**, 518–519.
Wilson, W. P., and Glotfelty, J. S. (1958). Effect of intravenous promazine on arousal responses in man. *Diseases Nervous System* **19**, 307–309.
Wirth, W. (1958). On the pharmacological action of promazine. *Arzneimittel-Forsch.* **8**, 507–511 (in German).
Wirth, W., Gosswald, R., and Vater, W. (1959). On the pharmacology of acylated phenothiazine compounds. *Arch. Intern. Pharmacodyn.* **123**, 78–114 (in German, English summary).
Yoshitani, H. (1963). Antiarrhythmic action of phenothiazine derivatives. III. The relation between chemical structure and antiarrhythmic action and side effects as well as clinical results. *Japan Circulation J. (English Edn.)* **27**, 487–498; *Chem. Abstr.* **60**, 2219h.

Zourlas, P. A. (1964). *In vitro* and *in vivo* effects of sparine (promazine hydrochloride) on human uterine contractility. *Am. J. Obstet. Gynecol.* **88**, 770–773.

Side Effects

Amias, A. G., and Fairbairn, D. (1963). Foetal death after pethidine and promazine. *Brit. Med. J.* II, 432–433.

Anderson, J. H., and Sanchez-Longo, L. P. (1961). The complications and side effects of the phenothiazine ataraxics: A review of 178 clinical series of 10 phenothiazine derivatives. *Bol. Soc. Med. Puerto Rico* **53**, 123–151.

Arterberry, S. D., Bonifaci, R. S., Nash, E. S., and Quimby, G. E. (1962). Potentiation of phosphorus insecticides by phenothiazine derivatives. *J. Am. Med. Assoc.* **182**, 848–850.

Ask, O. (1960). Considerations on contact dermatitis produced by phenothiazine derivatives. *Therapie* **15**, 266–269 (in French).

Ayd, F. J. (1960). Drug-induced extrapyramidal reactions: Their clinical manifestations and treatment with Akineton. *Psychosomatics* **1**, 143–149.

Bennett, N. M. (1963). Drug-induced agranulocytosis and septicaemia. *Med. J. Australia* pp. 575–597.

Best, W. R. (1963). Drug-associated blood dyscrasias. *J. Am. Med. Assoc.* **185**, 286–290.

Block, M. A. (1956). Medical treatment of alcoholism. *J. Am. Med. Assoc.* **162**, 1610–1619.

Borkowski, W. J., and Kohlmeyer, W. A. (1959). Convulsive seizures under promazine medication. *Virginia Med. Monthly* **86**, 213–216.

Buckmaster, J. F. (1957). Toxicity of "Sparine". *Brit. Med. J.* I, 1242.

Burns, R. P. (1961). Ocular side effects of systemic medication. *Northwest Med.* **60**, 1083–1092.

Cares, R. M., and Buckman, C. (1961). A survey of side effects and/or toxicity of newer psychopharmacologic agents. *Diseases Nervous System* **22**, 97–106.

Chirico, A., Carfagno, S., and Lytel, F. (1957). Agranulocytosis after promazine therapy. Report of a case. *New Engl. J. Med.* **256**, 899–900.

Clink, H. M. (1963). Foetal death after promazine and pethidine. (Correspondence.) *Brit. Med. J.* II, 684.

Cohlan, S. Q. (1960). Convulsive seizures caused by phenothiazine tranquilizers. *Gen. Practitioner* **21**, 136–137.

Conchubhair, S. Ua (1959). Death following treatment with promazine hydrochloride. *J. Irish Med. Assoc.* **44**, 117–119.

Cook, I., Melrose, A. G., and Roy, J. R. (1957). Agranulocytosis with recovery during promazine therapy. *Brit. Med. J.* II, 276.

Council on Drugs (1957). Blood dyscrasias associated with promazine hydrochloride therapy. *J. Am. Med. Assoc.* **165**, 685–686.

Darling, H. F. (1959). Acute toxic hypertension due to triflupromazine: Report of a case. *Am. J. Psychiat.* **115**, 1123.

Deacon W. W. (1961). Gangrene following the use of promazine. *Anaesthesia* **16**, 479–482.

De Jonge, J. H., and Wartena, S. (1960). Agranulocytosis after the use of promazine. *Ned. Tijdschr. Geneesk.* **104**, 427–429 (in Dutch, English summary).

Donaldson, I. A. (1963). Collapse after pethidine and promazine. *Brit. Med. J.* II, 1592.

Dowling, W. F., and Hunt, T. R., Jr. (1964). Hyperpyrexia during promazine therapy. *Southwestern Med.* **45**, 152–153.

Earle, B. V. (1957). Fatal agranulocytosis due to promazine hydrochloride. *Lancet* II, 925–926.

Fazekas, J. F., Shea, J. G., Ehrmantraut, W. R., and Alman, R. W. (1957). Convulsant action of phenothiazine derivatives. *J. Am. Med. Assoc.* **165**, 1241–1245.
Fromer, J. L. (1959). Dermatologic allergy V: Critique and review of the recent literature. *Ann. Allergy* **17**, 76–110.
Glaser, G. L., and Adams, D. A. (1958). Agranulocytosis associated with promazine administration: Report of three cases. *Ann. Internal Med.* **48**, 372–379.
Goodman, D., and Cahn, M. M. (1959). Contact dermatitis to phenothiazine drugs. *J. Invest. Dermatol.* **33**, 27–29.
Grondin, P., Bellemare, J.-L., Groulx, G., Saint Pierre, R. (1960). A case of gangrene of the hand following the intravenous injection of promazine (Sparine). *Laval Med.* **30**, 149–154 (in French).
Hall, L. W., and Stevenson, D. E. (1960). Effects of ataractic drugs on the blood-pressure and heart-rate of dogs. *Nature* **187**, 696–697.
Hamelberg, W. (1959). Arterial thrombosis after drug therapy (correspondence). *J. Am. Med. Assoc.* **169**, 746.
Hankoff, L. D., Kaye, H. E., Engelhardt, D. M., and Freedman, N. (1957). Convulsions complicating ataractic therapy; their incidence and theoretical implications. *N.Y. State J. Med.* **57**, 2967–2972.
Hatori, S., and Sato, K. (1961). Leucocytosis due to tranquilizers. *Clin. Psychiat. (Tokyo)* **3**, 275–280 (in Japanese).
Letter to the editor: False-positive pregnancy tests caused by Sparine and Thorazine. *Am. J. Clin. Pathol.* **31**, 466.
Hilbert, G. H. (1958). False positive pregnancy tests caused by Sparine and Thorazine. *J. Florida Med. Assoc.* **45**, 655–657.
Hindle, W., and Negus, D. (1960). Promazine overdosage. (Correspondence.) *Brit. Med. J.* I, 1507.
Hippius, H. (1960). Therapeutically undesirable effects of modern drugs. Part I. Phenothiazine derivatives and related compounds. *Internist* **1**, 453–460 (in German).
Hippius, H., and Kanig, K. (1958). Agranulocytoses occurring during neuropsychiatric phenothiazine therapy. *Aerztl. Wochschr.* **13**, 501–507 (in German).
Hollister, L. E. (1958). Allergic reactions to tranquilizing drugs. *Ann. Internal Med.* **49**, 17–29.
Hollister, L. E. (1964). Complications from psychotherapeutic drugs–1964. *Clin. Pharmacol. Therap.* **5**, 322–333.
Holmes, J. R., and Barg, P. (1959). Fatal agranulocytosis during promazine therapy. *Can. Med. Assoc. J.* **81**, 384.
Huguley, C. M., Jr. (1964). Drug-induced blood dyscrasias. II. Agranulocytosis. *J. Am. Med. Assoc.* **188**, 817–818.
Kaplan, N. M. (1959). Hypotension as a complication of promazine therapy. *AMA Arch. Internal Med.* **103**, 219–223.
Kemp, J. A. (1957). Jaundice occurring during administration of promazine. *Gastroenterology* **32**, 937–938.
Korn, R. J., Rock, W., and Zimmerman, H. J. (1958). Studies of hepatic function in patient receiving promazine. *Am. J. Med. Sci.* **235**, 431–436.
Kreisle, J. E. (1959). Agranulocytosis during promazine (Sparine) therapy. Report of a case. *Texas State J. Med.* **55**, 297–300.
Kurtzke, J. F. (1957). Seizures with promazine; preliminary report. *J. Nervous Mental Disease* **125**, 119–125.
McLean, D. D., Martin, A. R., Ellingson, R. J., and Smith, J. A. (1958). Seizures during therapy with phenothiazine derivatives. *Am. J. Psychiat.* **114**, 934–935.
May, R. H. (1959). Catatonic-like states following phenothiazine therapy. *Am. J. Psychiat.* **115**, 1119–1120.

Michaelson, A. K. (1959). Severe leukemoid reaction after promazine-induced agranulocytosis. *J. Florida Med. Assoc.* **45**, 1418–1419.
Moore, E. A. (1957). Toxicity of promazine hydrochloride (correspondence). *Brit. Med. J.* I, 1529.
O'Meara, D. J. P. (1963). Foetal death after pethidine and promazine (correspondence). *Brit. Med. J.* II, 749.
Opinsky, M., Serbin, A. F., and Rosenfeld, J. E. (1958). Arterial thrombosis with gangrene after use of promazine (Sparine) hydrochloride. *J. Am. Med. Assoc.* **168**, 1224–1225.
Pisciotta, A. V., Ebbe, S., Lennon, E. J., Metzger, G. O., and Madison, F. W. (1958). Agranulocytosis following administration of phenothiazine derivatives. *Am. J. Med.* **25**, 210–223.
Preziosi, P. (1958). Disorders caused by toxicity or intolerance of promazine. *Riforma Med.* **72**, 874–875 (in Italian).
Reinert, R. E. (1959). EEG changes with promazine. *Am. J. Psychiat.* **115**, 742–743.
Reinhart, M. J., Silverstein, B. S., and Cross, T. N. (1957). A case of agranulocytosis following Sparine administration. *Am. J. Psychiat.* **114**, 462–463.
Root, B. (1959). Arterial thrombosis after drug therapy (correspondence). *J. Am. Med. Assoc.* **169**, 746.
Rummele, W. (1959). Clinical experience with promazine. *Schweiz. Med. Wochschr.* **89**, 299–302 (in German, English summary).
Shell, J. H., Jr., McIntyre, D. B., Jr., Castellano, J. (1959). Gangrene after use of gamma-dimethylamino-n-propyl phenothiazine hydrochloride (promazine): A case report. *Am. J. Obstet. Gynecol.* **78**, 1219–1220.
Shideman, F. E. (1961). Toxicity of the phenothiazines. *Wisconsin Med. J.* **60**, 487–488.
Spillane, J. D. (1964). Drug-induced neurological disorders. *Proc. Roy. Soc. Med.* **57**, 135–140.
Sutherland, J. M. (1963). Observations on relationships between drug therapy and neonatal jaundice. *Ann. N.Y. Acad. Sci.* **111**, 461–471.
Talle, O. S., and Hardy, E. C. (1959). Oral side-actions accompanying promazine and chlorpromazine. *VA Dept. Med. Surg. Trans. 3rd Res. Conf. Chemotherapy Psychiat.*, 1958 **3**, 150–158.
Taylor, D. E. E., Hart, F. D., and Burley, D. (1964). Suicide in south London. An analysis of the admissions for attempted suicide in one medical unit of a general hospital. *Practitioner* **192**, 251–256.
Vann, D. (1959). Promazine-iproniazid: A brief report. *Am. J. Psychiat.* **115**, 824.
Voegele, G. E., and May, R. H. (1957). Epileptiform seizures under promazine therapy: Occurrence in two cases without history of former seizures. *Am. J. Psychiat.* **113**, 655–656.
Waitzkin, L. (1957). Hepatic dysfunction during promazine therapy. *New Eng. J. Med.* **257**, 276–277.
Winfield, D. L., and Aivazian, G. H. (1958). EEG changes associated with intensive Sparine therapy. *Electroencephalog. Clin. Neurophysiol.* **10**, 575.
Winfield, D. L., and Aivazian, G. H. (1959). EEG changes associated with intensive promazine therapy. *Am. Practitioner Dig. Treat.* **10**, 1182–1188.
Witton, K. (1961). Orthostatic hypotension secondary to psychotropic drugs. Treatment with emphasis on parenteral Ritalin. *Diseases Nervous System* **22**, 189–192.
Witton, K. (1961). Severe and fatal reactions to tranquilizers. (Questions and Answers.) *J. Am. Med. Assoc.* **175**, 175–176.
Woodward, D. J., and Solomon, J. D. (1956). Fatal agranulocytosis occurring during promazine (Sparine) therapy. *J. Am. Med. Assoc.* **162**, 1308–1309.
Zimmerman, H. J. (1963). Drugs and the liver. *Disease-A-Month* **1963**, 1–46.
Zineifler, A. J. (1960). Agranulocytosis and jaundice during therapy with meprobamate and promazine. *New Engl. J. Med.* **262**, 1229–1231.

Clinical Papers

Agresti, E. (1960). On the therapy of chronic psychopaths with promazine hydrochloride. *Rass. Studi Psychiat.* **49**, 612–617 (in Italian).

Ahnefeld, F. W. (1960). Phenothiazine medication with minimal side effects in surgery. *Anaesthesist* **9**, 230–232 (in German).

Aivazian, G. H., and Reese, H. C., Jr. (1959). Clinical evaluation of promazine therapy for schizophrenia. *Diseases Nervous System* **20**, 472–476.

Albanese, B. (1958). Promazine in the treatment of psychopathic epileptics. *Rass. Neuropsichiat. Sci. Affini* **12**, 320–322. (in Italian).

Acosta Gainza, J. A. (1960). Promazine and surgery. *Dia. Med.* **32**, 476–480 (in Spanish).

Atkinson, R. P. (1957). Clinical experiences with promazine (Sparine). *Lahey Clin. Bull.* **10**, 149–154.

Ayd, F. J., Jr. (1957). Tranquilizing drugs in private practice. *N.Y. State J. Med.* **57**, 1742–1747.

Ayd, F. J. (1961). Phenothiazine tranquilizers: Eight years of development. *Med. Clin. N. Am.* **45**, 1027–1040.

Azima, H., and Durost, H. (1957). Effects of promazine in mental syndromes. *Can. Med. Assoc. J.* **76**, 442–446.

Azima, H., and Durost, H. (1957). Comparison of the effects of promazine and chlorpromazine in mental syndromes. *Can. Med. Assoc. J.* **77**, 671–675.

Barsa, J. A., and Kline, N. S. (1957). Promazine in chronic schizophrenic patients. *Am. J. Psychiat.* **113**, 654.

Becker, G. S., and Israel, P. (1961). Integrated drug and psychotherapy in the treatment of alcoholism. *Quart. J. Studies Alc.* **22**, 610–633.

Benda, H. (1958). Promazine in mental deficiency. *Psychiat. Quart.* **32**, 449.

Bolton, R. N., and Benson, R. C. (1958). Use of promazine and meperidine in labor. *Western J. Surg., Obstet. Gynecol.* **66**, 253–257.

Bergin, J. T. F., and Bergin, M. (1958). Use of Sparine in low-grade mental defectives. *J. Irish Med. Assoc.* **42**, 29–30.

Bianchetti, L., and Amasio, C. (1959). Clinical investigations in the pharmacological study of promazine. *Minerva Anestesiol.* **25**, 71–74 (in Italian).

Black, J. (1960). Phenothiazines as antiemetics and tranquilizers. *J. Med. Assoc. State Alabama* **29**, 492–500.

Blaya, M. (1961). Critical study of the phenothiazine derivatives. *Arquiv. Neuro-Psiquiat.* **19**, 35–40 (in Portuguese, English summary).

Bleiching, E. P., and Bopp, K. P. (1958). Clinical experiences with a new phenothiazine derivative. *Medizinische* No. 41, 1631–1632 (in German).

Bosio, S. (1959). Results and considerations on the use of Talofen (promazine base) in premedication and potentiation of anesthesia. *Minerva Anestesiol.* **25**, 84–88.

Bovet-Dubois, N. (1961). Study of the indications of promazine in children's neuropsychiatry. *Praxis (Berne)* **50**, 653–656 (in French).

Bruck, M. A. (1958). Electroencephalographic changes in chronic schizophrenics under chemotherapy. *Am. J. Psychiat.* **114**, 945.

Bryant, M. E. (1958). Treatment of alcoholics by hypnosis. *Brit. J. Med. Hypn.* **9**, 40–42.

Burdine, W. E., Shipley, T. E., and Papas, A. T. (1957). Studies on the use of promazine in acute and chronic nervous and mental disturbances. *J. Med. Assoc. Georgia* **46**, 171–173.

Caballero, A. (1958). Promazine in obstetric analgesia. *Acta Ginecol. (Madrid)* **9**, 205–220 (in Spanish); *Excerpta Med. Sect. X* **12**, 968.

Campbell, A. J. M., and Henderson, J. (1959). A case of severe chorea gravidarum treated with promazine (Sparine). *Scot. Med. J.* **4**, 128–129.

Carter, C. H. (1960). Promazine therapy in emotionally disturbed patients. *Diseases Nervous System* **21**, 278–281.
Casey, J. F., Bennett, I. F., Lindley, C. J., Hollister, L. E., Gordon, M. H., and Springer, N. N. (1960). Drug therapy in schizophrenia. *AMA Arch. Gen. Psychiat.* **2**, 210–220.
Chassan, J. B. (1959). A statistical description of a clinical trial of promazine. *Psychiat. Quart.* **33**, 700–714.
Chicata, M. A., Almuda, M., and Mori, G. (1957). Experiences with promazine in the acute psychiatric syndromes. *Rev. Neuro-Psiquiat. (Lima)* **20**, 475–489 (in Spanish); *Ann. Med.-Psychol.* **1**, 251 (abstr.).
Clifford, D. H. (1958). Observations on effect of preanesthetic medication with meperidine and promazine on barbiturate anesthesia in an ocelot and a leopard. *J. Am. Vet. Med. Assoc.* **133**, 459–463.
Cobo, M. S., and Salce, G. M. (1959). Analgesia with promazine comparison of two methods. *Medico* **9**, 49–54 (in Spanish).
Cohen, S. (1961). Treatment of acute alcoholism. *Can. Med. Assoc. J.* **84**, 950–952.
Conrad, V. K. (1960). Advantages and disadvantages of psychopharmacological drugs in the hands of the practicing physician. *Wien. Med. Wochschr.* **110**, 951–956 (in German).
Craft, M. J. (1959). Tranquilizers, a Latin square trial. *J. Mental Sci.* **105**, 482–488.
Creel, F. L., and Woodward, D. J. (1958). Experiences in the use of promazine in hospitalized chronic psychotic patients. *J. Clin. Exptl. Psychopathol. Quart. Rev. Psychiat. Neurol.* **19**, 319–322.
Dameno, R., and Aparicio, N. E. (1960). Promazine in neonatal pathology. *Semana Med. (Buenos Aires)* **117**, 1500–1504, and 1517 (in Spanish).
Daniels, D. H., and Ohler, R. L. (1959). A study of delirium tremens with review of cases. *J. Maine Med. Assoc.* **50**, 255–261.
Daston, P. G. (1959). Effect of two phenothiazine drugs on concentrative attention span of chronic schizophrenics. *J. Clin. Psychol.* **15**, 106–109.
Davis, M. G. (1957). Obstetric analgesia with promazine. *J. Am. Osteopath. Assoc.* **57**, 255–256.
Deberdt, R. (1959). The treatment of acute psychiatric disorders with promazine. *Belg. Tijdschr. Chir. Geneesk.* **12**, 592–601 (in Dutch).
Dickhaut, H. H., and Pyrkoseh, W. (1958). The treatment of mental diseases. *Nervenarzt* **29**, 367–370 (in German).
Dobkin, A. B., and Purkin, N. (1960). Double-blind study of phenothiazines used in preanesthetic medication; a clinical evaluation of promethazine (Phenergan), promazine (Sparine), prochlorperazine (Stemetil), and levomepromazine (Nozinan). *Can. Anaesthesiol. Soc. J.* **7**, 156–169.
Edisen, C. B., and Samuels, A. S. (1958). Effects of promazine on psychiatric symptoms. *J. Louisiana State Med. Soc.* **110**, 164–169.
Ehrmantrat, W. R., Negron, M. C., Kleh, J., and Fazekas, J. F. (1959). Effects of combinations of psychopharmacologic agents. *Am. J. Med. Sci.* **238**, 412–416.
Emanuelli, H. (1958). The use of the hydrochloride of dimethylaminopropyl-N-phenothiazine in anesthesiology. *Acta Anesthesiol.* **9**, 115–119 (in Italian).
Engelhardt, D. M., Freedman, N., Hankoff, L. D., Glick, B. S., Kaye, H. E., and Buckwald, J. (1959). The treatment of schizophrenic out-patients with promazine and reserpine. *Psychiat. Quart.* **33**, 102–114.
Engelhardt, D. M., Freedman, N., Glick, B. S., Hankoff, L. D., Mann, D., and Margolis, R. (1960). Prevention of psychiatric hospitalization with use of psychopharmacological agents. *J. Am. Med. Assoc.* **173**, 147–149.
Engelhardt, D. M., Freedman, N., Hankoff, L. D., Mann, D., and Margolis, R. (1960). Changes of social behavior in chronic schizophrenic outpatients under phenothiazine treatment. *Comprehensive Psychiat.* **1**, 313–316.

England, A. C., Jr., and Schwab, R. S. (1959). The management of Parkinson's disease. *AMA Arch. Internal Med.* **104**, 439–468.
Erwin, H. J. (1958). Treatment of chronic psychoses with promazine. *J. Natl. Med. Assoc.* **50**, 338–340.
Esen, F. M., and Durling, D. (1957). The treatment of fourteen mentally retarded boys with Sparine. *Arch. Pediat.* **74**, 471–474.
Fazekas, J. F., Shea, J. G., and Sullivan, P. D., Jr. (1956). Ataractics in medical practice. *Gen. Practitioner* **14**, 75–81.
Fazekas, J. F., Schultz, J. D., Sullivan, P. D., and Shea, J. G. (1956). Management of acutely disturbed patients with promazine (Sparine). *J. Am. Med. Assoc.* **161**, 46–49.
Feldman, D. J. (1957). Drug therapy of chronic alcoholism. *Med. Clin. N. Am.* **41**, 381–392.
Figurelli, F. A. (1958). Delirium tremens: Reduction of mortality and morbidity with promazine. *J. Am. Med. Assoc.* **166**, 747–750.
Fink, L., and Vlavianos, G. (1958). Subjective evaluation of promazine therapy. *Psychiat. Quart.* **32**, 532–537.
Fink, L., and Vlavianos, G. (1958). Clinical impressions of the response to promazine therapy. *Am. J. Psychiat.* **114**, 1031–1032.
Fitzpatrick, M. J., De Blois, J. A., Jr., and Kushner, D. H. (1960). Barbiturate- and non-barbiturate-managed labors. A controlled study of promazine in the predelivery regimen. *Med. Ann. District Columbia* **29**, 326–332.
Fleming, B. G., Spencer, A. M., and Whitelaw, E. M. (1959). A controlled comparative investigation of the effects of promazine, chlorpromazine, and a placebo in chronic psychosis. *J. Mental Sci.* **105**, 349–358.
Fox, V. (1956). Management of acute alcoholism; experience with an additional series of 61 cases. *Am. Practitioner Dig. Treat.* **7**, 1461–1464.
Fox, V. (1960). The management of alcoholism. *J. Med. Assoc. State Alabama* **29**, 501–505.
Fox, V., and Smith, M. A. (1959). Evaluation of a chemopsychotherapeutic program for the rehabilitation of alcoholics. Observations over a two-year period. *Quart. J. Studies Alc.* **20**, 767–780.
Frain, M. K. (1957). Promazine treatment of chronic psychoses in 100 hospitalized patients. *J. Nervous Mental Disease* **125**, 529–533.
Frain, M. K. (1959). The quieting effect of meporbamate-Sparine on psychotic patients. *J. Louisiana State Med. Soc.* **111**, 308–310.
Freedman, N., Warshaw, L., Engelhardt, D. M., Blumenthal, I. J., and Hankoff, L. D. (1959). The effect of various therapies upon fecal incontinence in chronic schizophrenic patients. *J. Nervous Mental Disease* **128**, 562–565.
Freedman, N., Engelhardt, D. M., Hankoff, L. D., Schwartz, S., and Zobel, H. (1961). Patterns of verbal group participation in the drug treatment of chronic schizophrenic patients. *Intern. J. Group Psychotherap.* **11**, 60–73.
Gallini, R. (1957). Promazine, an improvement in neuroplegic therapy of internal disease. *Policlin., Rome Sez. Prat.* **64**, 621–629 (in Italian).
Galvan, C. A., Arredondo, R. L., and Deanda, L. B. (1960). Therapeutic use of phenothiazine derivatives in gynecology and obstetrics. *Ginecol. Obstet. (Mex.)* **15**, 283–300 (in Spanish).
Gerron, G., and Bourdo, S. (1960). Jaundice secondary to promazine, and an analysis of possible cross sensitivities between phenothiazine derivatives. *Gastroenterology* **38**, 87–90.
Gibbon, J. (1961). Some examples of the combined use of psychotropic agents. *Diseases Nervous System* **22**, 81–85.
Giffen, M. G. (1961). Emotional dysfunction and the use of psychopharmcological drugs in a military theater. *Mil. Med.* **126**, 199–203.
Gilberti, A. (1957). Combined promazine-meprobamate therapy in certain psychiatric conditions. *Giorn. Med. Marca Trevigiana* **15**, 255–261 (in Italian).

Gilmore, T. H., and Shatin, L. (1959). Quantitative comparison of clinical effectiveness of chlorpromazine and promazine. *J. Mental Sci.* **105**, 508–510.

Giorgio, D. J. (1960). Anti-emetics and tranquilizers in surgical patients. *J. Indiana State Med. Assoc.* **53**, 441–442.

Godfrey, L., Kissen, M. D., and Downs, T. M. (1958). Treatment of the acute alcohol-withdrawal syndrome. *Quart. J. Studies Alc.* **19**, 118–124.

Goldman, H. I. (1958). Outpatient treatment of the post alcoholic syndrome. *J. Am. Med. Assoc.* **167**, 2069–2071.

Gonder, T. A. (1957). Management of the paranoid schizophrenic with promazine. *Med. Ann. District Columbia* **26**, 542.

Graffeo, A. J. (1958). Promazine and azacylonol in the treatment of chronic psychotics. *N.Y. State J. Med.* **58**, 2056–2057.

Graffeo, A. J. (1960). Three years of treatment of chronic hospitalized psychotic individuals with promazine (Sparine). *Am. J. Psychiat.* **116**, 842.

Griffin, E. L., and Clement, J. E. (1960). The use of promazine and levallorphan to improve obstetric sedation. *Southern Med. J.* **53**, 655–658.

Gruenwald, F., Hanlon, T. E., Wachsler, S., and Kurland, A. A. (1960). A comparative study of promazine and triflupromazine in the treatment of acute alcoholism. *Diseases Nervous System* **21**, 32–38.

Guerrieri, S., Maritano, M., and Riffero, D. (1959). The use of promazine in practical anesthesiology. *Minerva Anesthesiol.* **25**, 320–322 (in Italian).

Gutersohn, M. T., and Reed, W. B. (1957). Clinical study of promazine hydrochloride. *J. Osteopathy* **64**, 21–23.

Hankoff, L. D., Engelhardt, D. M., Freedman, N., Mann, D., and Margolis, R. (1960). Denial of illness in schizophrenic outpatients; effects of psychopharmacological treatment. *Arch. Gen. Psychiat.* **3**, 657–664.

Hargreaves, M. A. (1961). An evaluation of the double-blind trial as a method of assessing promazine (Sparine) in the treatment of chronic psychotic patients. *J. Mental Sci.* **107**, 529–537.

Heaton-Ward, W. A., and Jancar, J. (1959). Promazine (Sparine) in the treatment of severe behavior disorders of mental defectives. *J. Midland Mental Deficiency Soc.* **5**, 43–47.

Himwich, H. E., Rinaldi, F., and Willis, D. (1956). Examination of phenothiazine derivatives with comparisons of their effects on the alerting reaction, chemical structure and therapeutic efficacy. *J. Nervous Mental Disease* **124**, 53–57.

Hochuli, E. (1961). Promazine, a new phenothiazine derivative in obstetrics. *Therap. Umschau* **18**, 299–302 (in German).

Hoffman, V. (1962). Treatment of spastic-hypertrophic pyloric stenosis with promazine and Eumydrine. *Muench. Med. Wochschr.* **104**, 463–465 (in German, English summary).

Hollister, L. E., and Glazener, F. S. (1960). Withdrawal reactions from meprobamate, alone and combined with promazine: a controlled study. *Psychopharmacologia* **1**, 336–341.

Horwitz, H. (1960). Prozine in organic disease. *Illinois Med. J.* **118**, 301–302.

Janssen, G., Stalmmler, H. G., and Heuter, W. (1959). The action and therapeutic use of Verophen in pediatric medicine. *Arkive. Kinderheilk.* **159**, 156–162 (in German, English summary).

Jauregui, F. B. (1959). Sedation and analgesia during labor using promazine and Pethidine. *Rev. Col. Med. Guatemala* **10**, 102–104 (in Spanish).

Anonymous. (1957). Promazine and chlorpromazine in mental syndromes. *J. Am. Med. Assoc.* **165**, 1619.

Kagan, G. (1959). Psychoneuroses in general practice. *Practitioner* **182**, 498–500.

Kenny, S. (1963). Anaesthesia and ophthalmology. *Brit. J. Anaesthesia* **35**, 317–321.

Kent, E. A., and Gitman, L. (1957). Promazine for emotionally disturbed, chronically ill, institutionalized aged. *Geriatrics* **12**, 647–652.

Kinross-Wright, V. J., and Morrison, S. B. (1958). Critical study of promazine therapy. *J. Clin. Exptl. Psychopathol. Quart. Rev. Psychiat. Neurol.* **19**, 219–225.
Kjenaas, E. A., and McHugh, R. B. (1960). The effect of promazine (Sparine) on patients with chronic schizophrenia. *Minn. Med.* **43**, 25–30.
Kleh, J., Ehrmantraut, W., and Fazekas, J. F. (1957). Choice of psychotropic drugs for prolonged therapy of neuropsychiatric disorder. *Proc. Intern. Symp. Psychotropic Drugs*, Milan p. 515.
Klein, D. F., and Fink, M. (1962). Behavioral reaction patterns with phenothiazines. *Arch. Gen. Psychiat.* **7**, 449–459.
Kuntze, C. D., and Sison, P. (1957). New adjunct to analgesia and sedation in labor: Preliminary report of results with promazine hydrochloride by intravenous injection. *Am. J. Obstet. Gynecol.* **74**, 498–504.
Lagae, J. (1963). Hiccough. *Belg. Tijdschr. Geneesk.* **18**, 31–33; *Psychopharmacol. Abstr.* **2**, 1423.
Lampshire, E. L. (1959). Balanced medication. *J. Dent. Children* **26**, 25–31.
Laties, V. G., Lasagna, L., Gross, G. M., Hitchman, I. L., and Flores, J. (1958). Controlled trial of chlorpromazine and promazine in the management of delirium tremens. *Quart. J. Studies Alc.* **19**, 238–243.
Lesse, S. (1957). Evaluation of promazine hydrochloride in psychiatric practice. *Am. J. Psychiat.* **113**, 984–987.
Lesse, S. (1959). Electroshock therapy and tranquilizing drugs. *J. Am. Med. Assoc.* **170**, 1791–1795.
Leube, H. (1960). Definition of the areas where Megaphen and Verophen are indicated. *Med. Welt* **12**, 644–645 (in German).
Levin, A. (1962). Ambulatory treatment of alcoholism. *Dia Med.* **34**, 1560–1561. (in Spanish).
Loewinthian, L. (1959). Analgesia in obstetrics: A recommended method. *Am. Practitioner Dig. Treat.* **10**, 1368–1370.
Luke, H. B. (1959). Promazine in the management of the tuberculous, mentally-ill patient. *Psychiat. Quart.* **33**, 422–428.
Maier, R. A., and Fox, V. (1958). Forced therapy of probated alcoholics. *Med. Times* **86**, 1051–1054.
Malitz, S. (1959). The use of modern pharmacologic agents in psychiatric disorders. *J. Chronic Diseases* **9**, 278–291.
Mangun, C. W., and Webb, W. W. (1956). Promazine hydrochloride in the treatment of chronic catatonic schizophrenics. *J. Nervous Mental Disease* **123**, 553–556.
Martins, A. F., Goes, J. de S., Jr., and Strasburg, O. (1959). Promazine in labor. *Rev. Paulista Med.* **54**, 177–181 (in Portuguese, English summary).
Szmyd, L., McCall, C. M., and Enright, E. T. (1959). Tranquilizing drugs in oral surgery. *School Aviation Med. USAF, Randolph AFB, Texas* **58**, No. 31.
McFaul, I. E., and Kohutiak, V. (1961). Control of hyperactivity in psychoses, alcoholism and drug addiction. *Med. Times* **89**, 290–293.
McGuire, T. F., and Leary, F. J. (1958). Tranquilizing drugs and stress tolerance. *Am. J. Public Health* **48**, 578–584.
Santayana Medrano, R. A. (1959). Analgesia in labor. *Rev. Med. Cubana* **70**, 32–33 (in Spanish).
Mehrotra, A. N. (1961). A long-acting phenothiazine in the management of geriatric patients. *Med. Press* 1961, 563–565.
Merlis, S., and Turner, W. J. (1961). Drug evaluation and practical psychiatric therapeutics. *J. Am. Med. Assoc.* **177**, 38–42.
Mitchell, E. H. (1956). Treatment of acute alcoholism with promazine (Sparine). *J. Am. Med. Assoc.* **161**, 44–45.
Moessner, G. F. (1959). Clinical evaluation of meprobamate-promazine combination for control of nausea and vomiting in pregnancy. *Western J. Surg. Obstet. Gynecol.* **67**, 180–182.

Morgen, D. R., and Van Leent, J. P. (1958). Clinical appraisal of "Sparine," "Stemetil," "Trilafon," and "Marsilid". *Med. J. Australia* **2**, 696–700.

Nelson, A. J. (1958). Promazine: A clinical note. *Vet. Med.* **53**, 356–360.

Neumann, W. (1957). Ataractic treatment in a private hospital; preliminary report of promazine in acute and chronic psychiatric patients. *N.Y. State J. Med.* **57**, 2963–2966.

Nunziata, I., and Sanguinetti, H. (1960). Use of promazine in anesthesiology. *Semana Med. (Buenos Aires)* **117**, 395–396, 422 (in Spanish).

Oswald, W. (1959). Meprobamate-promazine for treatment of psychosomatic illness in general practice. *Intern. Record Med.* **172**, 743–752.

Pesce, G., and Rugiero, G. (1958). Promazine as a preanesthetic medication. *Policlin. Sez. Prat. (Rome)* **65**, 620–622 (in Italian).

Palmer, L. S., and Apolito, A. (1958). Oral treatment of chronically ill mental patients with promazine. *N.Y. State J. Med.* **58**, 1294–1296.

Pardera, G. (1957). Notes on liver function test in mental patients treated with promazine. *Riv. Patol. Nervosa Mentale* **78**, 1106–1108 (in Italian).

Parks, R. V. (1958). Treatment of office patients with Prozine. *Intern. Record Med.* **171**, 678–684.

Perlstein, M. A., Himwich, H. E., Rowley, J. D., and Toman, J. (1957). Use of tranquilizing drugs in children—a Symposium. *Quart. Rev. Pediat.* **12**, 176–177.

Peterson, L. W., and Haynes, C. E. (1958). Premedication and sedation for the surgical patient. *J. Oral Surg.* **16**, 131–136.

Plazak, D. J. (1957). Case of corticotropic hormone-induced psychosis treated with promazine hydrochloride. *Mil. Med.* **120**, 99–101.

Plotz, E. J. (1961). Pregnancy tests (Questions and Answers). *J. Am. Med. Assoc.* **176**, 475.

Ponzi, A., and Tiengo, M. (1958). The use of promazine in obstetric and gynecologic surgery. *Minerva Anestesiol.* **24**, 402–403 (in Italian).

Ponzi, A., Tiengo, M., and Zuccoli, G. (1958). Theoretical considerations on the use of promazine in anesthesia and recovery after anesthesia. *Minerva Anestesiol.* **24**, 400–402 (in Italian).

Prescod, H. J., and Townley, M. C. (1957). Management of chronically disturbed patients with Sparine. *J. Mich. State Med. Soc.* **56**, 1273–1274.

Questions and Answers. (1959). Tranquilizers and operative management. *J. Am. Med. Assoc.* **171**, 1761–1762.

Raker, C. W., and English, B. (1959). Promazine: Its pharmacological and clinical effects in horses. *J. Am. Vet. Med. Assoc.* **134**, 19–23.

Rappeport, J. (1958). Treatment of acute alcoholic intoxication. *Current Med. Dig.* **25**, 57–62.

Rathod, N. H. (1961). Experience with promazine. *Am. J. Psychiat.* **118**, 504–508.

Remvig, J., and Schwsinger, F. (1962). A new hypnotic for senile confusion. *Ugeskrift Laeger* **124**, 1441–1442; *Excerpta Med. Sect. XX* **5**, 938.

Resek, F. (1957). Experiences with promazine in daily practice, report of 77 diverse cases. *Am. Practitioner Dig. Treat.* **8**, 1409–1414.

Rio, J. A. (1960). Clinical experience with promazine. *Semana Med. (Buenos Aires)* **116**, 1249–1250, 1264 (in Spanish).

Robertson, R. B. (1958). Control of symptoms in the chronic psychoses with concentrated liquid promazine. *Mil. Med.* **123**, 108–112.

Robertson, R. B. (1960). Clinical experience with a meprobamate-promazine combination in psychiatric practice. *Diseases Nervous System* **21**, 165–168.

Rojas, D. A. (1960). Promazine hydrochloride in the sedation, control, and correction of labor. *Prensa Med. Arg.* **47**, 945–946 (in Spanish).

Rolo, A. (1957). Promazine for management of the drug abstinence syndrome; rapid withdrawal of meperidine in a severely addicted patient. *N.Y. State J. Med.* **57**, 2701–2702.

Rolo, A. (1962). Drug withdrawal with promazine hydrochloride. *N.Y. State J. Med.* **62**, 1429–1431.
Ross, I. S. (1958). Promazine modification of reflex rigidity in a decerebrate child. *AMA J. Dis. Children* **95**, 534–537.
Rudy, L. H., Himwich, H. E., and Rinaldi, F. (1958). A clinical evaluation of psychopharmacological agents in the management of disturbed, mentally defective patients. *Am. J. Mental Deficiency* **62**, 855–860; *Excerpta Med. Sect. VIII*, 12, 2597.
Rudy, L. H., Himwich, H. E., and Tasher, D. C. (1957). Clinical evaluation of two phenothiazine compounds, promazine and mepazine. *Am. J. Psychiat.* **113**, 979–983.
Sahl, H. G. (1957). Management of the emotional factor in the practice of internal medicine. *Am. Practitioner Dig. Treat.* **8**, 1381–1385.
Salzberger, G. J. (1964). Management of alcoholism with promazine. *Diseases Nervous System* **25**, 33–37.
Sanchez Garcia, J. (1957). Promazine in acute alcoholic intoxication. *Rev. Neuro-Psiquiat. (Lima)* **20**, 575–580 (in Spanish); (1959). *Ann. Med. Psychol.* **1**, 246 (abstr. in French).
Sanudo, F. W., Marrero, R. U., and Carro, A. H. (1960). Promazine in clinical surgery. *Dia Med.* **32**, 688–690 (in Spanish).
De Senarclens, F. (1961). The effect of chlorpromazine and promazine on childbirth. *Gynaecologia* **151**, 165–173 (in French, English summary).
Schapperle, O., and Schindewolf, G. (1959). Promazine treatment in psychiatry. *Nervenarzt* **30**, 31–34. (in German).
Scheckel, C. L., and Boff, E. (1964). Behavioral effects of interacting imipramine and other drugs with d-amphetamine, cocaine, and tetrabenazine. *Psychopharmacologia* **5**, 198–208.
Schulman, J. L., and Sister Mary Clarinda (1964). The effect of promazine on the activity level of retarded children. *Pediatrics* **33**, 271–275.
Schyma, A. (1960). Pre- and postoperative medication with promazine hydrochloride (Protactyl). *Med. Welt* **52/53**, 2781–8 (1960) (in German).
Scott, J. (1960). Postoperative psychosis in the aged. *Ami J. Surg.* **100**, 38–42.
Settel, E. (1957). Treatment of the agitated senile patient with promazine. *Gen. Practitioner* **16**, 107–110.
Settel, E. (1958). Promazine in the treatment of the discharged, agitated, senile patient. *Intern. Record Med.* **171**, 272–276.
Shapiro, D. M. (1960). Premedication in cataract surgery. *N.Y. Physician Am. Med.* **55**.
Shaw, D. L., and Page, J. A. (1960). A three-year review of the pharmacologic properties and clinical performance of promazine. *Current Therap. Res.* **2**, 199–226.
Shea, J. G., Ehrmantraut, W. R., Ticktin, H. E., Sullivan, P. D., Jr., and Fazekas, J. F. (1956). Use of promazine in the management of medical emergencies. *Mil. Med.* **119**, 221–227.
Sibilio, J. P., Andrew, G., Dart, D., Moore, K. B., and Stehman, V. A. (1957). Treatment of chronic schizophrenia with promazine hydrochloride. *AMA Arch. Neurol. Psychiat.* **78**, 419–424.
Sibilio, J. P., Andrew, G., Dart, D., Moore, K. B., and Stehman, V. A. (1959). Effects of promazine hydrochloride on attention in chronic schizophrenia. *AMA Arch. Neurol. Psychiat.* **81**, 114–120.
Simpson, R. W., and Jesson, J. G. (1958). The effects of promazine (Sparine) in chronic schizophrenia. *J. Mental Sci.* **104**, 1199–1202.
Singer, G. M. (1959). Effects of promazine and a total-push program on the intellectual functioning of paranoid schizophrenics. *Dissertation Abstr.* **19**, 2153–2154.
Smith, A. P. (1959). The management of emotional disorders by the general practitioner. *J. Natl. Med. Assoc.* **51**. 288–291.
Smith, J. A., Warner, R., Wolford, J. A., and Rutherford, A. (1957). Tranquilizing medication in the aged mentally ill. *Geriatrics* **12**, 549–553.

Smith, J. A., Gouldman, C., Rutherford, A., and Wolford, J. C. (1959). Comparison of two phenothiazine derivatives and a barbiturate in chronic schizophrenia. *AMA Arch. Neurol. Psychiat.* **81**, 97–99.

Smigel, J. O. (1957). "Mood" therapy in the aged. Differential approaches to recent therapy. *Med. Times* **85**, 149–158.

Splitter, S. R. (1961). Treatment of office patients in a general practice with a meprobamate-promazine combination. *Intern. Record Med.* **174**, 289–296.

Sprague, L. D. (1957). Predelivery sedation with promazine. *Obstet. Gynecol.* **9**, 633–641.

Stewart, R. H. (1961). Phenothiazine derivatives in labor and delivery. A study of four drugs. *Obstet. Gynecol.* **17**, 701–713.

Stewart, R. J. (1962). Promazine in labor and delivery. *Rocky Mt. Med. J.* **59**, 41–43.

Stratas, N. E., and Schmidt, K. T. (1960). Initial therapy of the alcoholic. *Virginia Med. Monthly* **87**, 154–155.

Siverdlow, M., and Cockings, E. C. (1958). Pethidine-promazine supplementation of regional analgesia. *Brit. J. Anaesthesia* **30**, 375–376.

Siverdlow, M., and Nabi, G. F. O. (1959). The supplementation of regional analgesia. *Brit. J. Anaesthesiol.* **31**. 543–551.

Thal, N. (1958). Maintenance therapy for mental patients. *Postgrad. Med.* **24**, 638–647.

Therien, R. C. (1958). Practical aspects of newer and older anesthetic agents. *Nebraska State Med. J.* **43**, 9–12.

Thomas, D. W., and Freedman, D. X. (1964). Treatment of the alcohol withdrawal syndrome. Comparison of promazine and paraldehyde. *J. Am. Med. Assoc.* **188**, 316–318.

Turitto, P. (1957). A new combination of drugs in the treatment of postoperative vomiting. *Atti Accad. Fisiocrit. Siena, Sez. Med. Fis.* **4**, 456–460 (in Italian).

Ungerleider, J. T. (1958). Alcohol, convulsions and tranquilizers: A clinical and electroencephalographic study. *J. Nervous Mental Disease* **127**, 518–527.

Urquhart, R., and Forrest, A. D. (1959). Clinical trial of promazine hydrochloride and acetylpromazine in chronic schizophrenic patients. *J. Mental Sci.* **105**, 260–264.

Van Gasse, J. J. (1958). Counselling and ataraxia; an effective combination in the management of alcoholics. *Clin. Med.* **5**, 177–181.

Vergani, O., and Aldeghi, E. (1957). First results in the therapeutic use of promazine in children with neuropsychiatric disturbances. *Minerva Pediat.* **9**, 467–470; *J. Am. Med. Assoc.* **165**, 890 (abstr.).

Vlavianos, B., and Fink, L. (1959). Promazine and combined promazine-meprobamate treatment of hospitalized psychotic patients. *Am. J. Psychiat.* **116**, 168–169.

Votava, Z., Benesova, O., and Metysova, J. (1958). The potentiating action of certain derivatives of phenothiazine on the duration and depth of the narcosis of thiopental. *J. Physiol. (Paris)* **50**, 563–565; **63**; *Chem. Abstr.* **53**, 9457f.

Vyas, K. J. (1962). Treatment of vomiting in children with promazine hydrochloride. *Indian J. Pediat.* **29**, 232–234.

Wagner, H. (1960). Clinical results with promazine (Verophen). *Med. Klin. (Munich)* **55**, 388–390 (in German).

Walker, A. (1956). The new ataractic drugs. *Prensa Med. Arg.* **43**, 2667–2669 (in Spanish).

Wearing, M. P., and Love, E. J. (1964). Effect of analgesic, amnesic, and anesthetic drugs on the newborn. *Am. J. Obstet. Gynecol.* **88**, 298–301.

Wegryn, S. P., and Marks, R. A. (1958). Promazine, meperidine and spinal anesthesia for labor and delivery. *J. Am. Med. Assoc.* **167**, 1918–1921.

Weinman, B. S. (1959). Changes in fine-motor performance induced by drug therapy and a high activity ward program: An investigation of the effects of a tranquilizing drug, promazine hydrochloride, upon the fine-motor functions of hospitalized male chronic paranoid schizophrenics under a high and low activity ward program. *Dissertation Abstr.* **19**, 2158.

White, P. T., Demyer, W., and Demyer, M. (1964). EEG abnormalities in early childhood schizophrenia. A double-blind study of psychiatrically disturbed and normal children during promazine sedation. *Am. J. Psychiat.* **120**, 950–958.

Whittier, J. R., Korenyi, C. D., Diamond, O., Tomlinson, P. J., La Burt, H. A. (1959). Drug use-rate in a state hospital. *Am. J. Psychiat.* **116**, 169–171.

Wolf, J. W. (1962). The irritable colon syndrome. *Missouri Med.* **59**, 495–498, and 503.

Wortis, J. (1958). Physiological treatment. *Am. J. Psychiat.* **114**, 603–607.

Zuccoli, G., and Tiengo, M. (1958). Promazine for preanesthetic medication in pediatric surgery. *Minerva Anestesiol.* **24**, 403 (in Italian).

~ A.11 ~
Propiomazine

Akre, T., and Lingjaerde, O. (1960). Propiomazine (propavan)—a new hypnotic and sedative of the phenothiazine group. A double blind study with propiomazine, promethazine and placebo. *Tidsskr. Norske Laegeforen* **80**, 1108–1113 (in Norwegian, English summary).

Aston, R., Sekino, E., Greifenstein, F. E. (1962). Quantitation of drug effects upon conditioned avoidance behavior in the rat. *Toxicol. Appl. Pharmacol.* **4**, 393–401.

Brunaud, M., Segal, V., Navarro, J., and Aurousseau, M. (1959). Comparative study of the pharmacodynamic properties of propiomazine (1678 CB) and promethazine. *Arch. Intern. Pharmacodyn.* **119**, 367–388 (in French).

Brunson, J. G., Kalina, R. E., and Eckman, P. L. (1959). Studies on experimental shock. Effects of vasopressor amines and phenothiazine derivatives. *Am. J. Pathol.* **35**, 1149–1167.

Dobkin, A. B. (1960). Potentiation of thiopental anesthesia by derivatives and analogues of phenothiazine. *Anesthesiology* **21**, 292–296.

Gatling, R. R. (1962). The effects of sympathomimetic agents on the chick embryo. *Am. J. Pathol.* **40**, 113–127.

Glisson, C. S., and Carter, P. (1961). The use of propiomazine (largon) in obstetrical analgesia. A preliminary report. *Bull. Fulton County Med. Soc.* **35**, 17–19, and 43.

Grimaldi, R. D. (1962). Propiomazine, an adjuvant for obstetric analgesia. *Anesthesia Analgesia, Current Res.* **41**, 487–496.

Hormia, A. (1961). Methodological problems in research on psychopharmacological therapy in the light of tests with propiomazine. *Finska Lakaresallskapet* **105**, 15–25 (in Swedish).

Kolodny, A. L. (1962). Interrelation of mood change and analgesic response—analgesic therapy with and without phenothiazine agents. *Current Therap. Res.* **4**, 37—43.

Krakowski, A. J. (1962). Propiomazine for control of insomnia in nervous disorders. *Am. J. Psychiat.* **119**, 461–462.

Lear, E., Chiron, A. E., and Pallin, I. M. (1963). Propiomazine hydrochloride in preanesthetic medication. *N.Y. State J. Med.* **63**, 409–414.

Liang, H. S., Dodd, R. B., and Debruine, P. H. (1962). A study on the analgesic action of propiomazine and morphine with a method for assessment of pain in man. *Anesthesiology* **23**, 154–155 (abstr. of a paper presented on the work in progress program, Ann. Meeting of the Am. Soc. Anesthesiologist, Los Angeles, Oct. 24–6, 1961).

Markello, R. and King, B. D. (1966). Effect of propiomazine on respiration and circulation. *Anesthesiology*, **27**, 21.

Moore, J., and Dundee, J. W. (1962). Alterations in response to somatic pain associated with anaesthesia. XII. Further studies with atropine. *Brit. J. Anaesthesia* **34**, 712–716.

Powe, C. E., Fromhagen, C., and Cavanagh, D. (1962). Propiomazine hydrochloride in obstetrical analgesia. *J. Am. Med. Assoc.* **181**, 290–294.

Sadove, M. S. (1961). Propiomazine hydrochloride—a useful new phenothiazine compound. *Chicago Med.* **64**, 21–24.

Sadove, M. S., Kobak, A. J., and Kobak, A. J., Jr. (1962). A combination of new agents for predelivery medication. *Obstet. Gynecol.* **19**, 784–789.

Schwartz, M. R. R., Derouaux, G., and Ghyzens, C. (1961). The place of calcium propiomazine in internal medicine. *Scalpel* **114**, 603–609 (in French).

Smith, B. E., Modell, J. H., Pino, D. M., and Timmes, J. J. (1962). Intravenous propiomazine for supplementation of anesthesia in bronchoscopy. *J. Thoracic Cardiovascular Surg.* **43**, 333–337.

Stetson, J. B., and Jessup, G. V. S. (1963). Oral premedication in children—attempts to use largon[R]. *Anesthesia Analgesia, Current Res.* **42**, 97–108.

Tomenius, G. (1959). Clinical trial of 10-(alpha-dimethylaminopropionyl)phenothiazine methobromide. *Svenska Lakartidn.* **56**, 3100–3106; *Excerpta Med. Sect. VI* **15**, 1167.

Ullery, J. C., and Bair, J. R. (1962). Maternal-fetal effects of propiomazine-meperidine analgesia. *Am. J. Obstet. Gynecol.* **84**, 1051–1056.

Usdin, E., and Usdin, V. R. (1961). Effects of psychotropic compounds on enzyme systems. II. *In vitro* inhibition of monoamine oxidase. *Proc. Soc. Exptl. Biol. Med.* **108**, 461–463.

⁓ A.12 ⁓
Prothipendyl

Barre, C., and Lalanne, F. (1962). Dominal bei neurologischen und psychiatrischen Symptomen von Alterspatienten. *Semaine Hop. Paris Suppl. Med. Monde.* **38**, 690.

Barthel, J. H., and Gerber, K. W. (1960). Erfahrungen mit einer kombinierten Neuroleptika-Anwendung zur Therapie von Psychosen. *Med. Monatsschr.* **14**, 304.

Baruk, H., and Launay, J. (1962). Die Wirkung von Prothipendyl-HCl auf das psychomotorische Verhalten von Affen. Ein Vergleich mit der Wirkung von Chlorpromazin. *Ann. Med.-Psychol.* **120**, 638.

Baruk, H., and Launay, J. (1962). Thiophenylpyridylamin-Derivate: Prothipendyl; Wirkung von Prothipendyl-HCl auf das psychomotorische Verhalten von Affen. Vergleich mit der Wirkung von Chlorpromazin. *Ann. Moreau Tours* **1**, 136.

Bastie, J., Villeneuve-Leguevaque, G., Lafforgue, J., and Sageloly, ... (1962). Über 40 Kuren in der klinischen Psychiatrie. *Toulouse Med.* **63**, 893.

Baumann, P., and Simon, L. (1961). Einige Angaben über die Differentialdiagnostik der endotoxischen Tremoren und deren Beeinflussung. *Ideggyogy. Szemle* **14**, 324.

Baumann, P., and Simon, L. (1961). Einige Daten zur Differentialdiagnostik und Beeinflussung der endotoxischen Tremoren. *Proc. 7th Intern. Kongr. Neurol. Rome* 10./15.9.

Birke, E. R. (1961). Unruhezustande entpersonlichter altender Menschen. *Münch. Med. Wochschr.* **103**, 1018 and 1068.

Bolland, G., Hofmann, U., Völkner, E., and Straubing, S. (1960). Untersuchungen über psychophysische Einflüsse von Prothipendyl. *Deut. Med. J.* **11**, 340.

Bonfils, S., Dubrasquet, M., Lambling, A., and Michel, A. (1962). Derivate von Phenothiazin und Iminodibenzyl; Verhältnis zwischen Dosis und Wirksamkeit gegenüber experimentell durch einen Zwang erzeugten Ulcera. *Soc. Franc. Therap. Pharmacodyn.* **19**, 12; (1963). *Presse Med.* **71**, 428; (1963). *Therapie* **18**, 373.

Bonnet, J., et. al. (1961). Therapeutische Versuche mit Dominal im Rahmen einiger dermatologischer Syndrome. *Semaines Hop. Paris* **37**, 2411.

Börger, H. H. (1959). Prämedikation vor chirurgischen Eingriffen. *Aerztl. Praxis* **11**, 346.

Bourgeois, M. C. (1961). Klinische Prüfung von LG 206 (Dominal) bei Verwendung zur Prämedikation einer Serie von 90 chirurgischen Eingriffen. *Semaine Hop. Therap.* **37**, 554.

Bousquet, J., Javal, J., and Sapir, M. (1962). Prüfung eines Psychopharmakons, Dominal, in der psychosomatischen Medizin (Klinische Prüfung und Teste). *Semaine Hop. Therap.* **38**, 133.

Camatte, R., and Sarles, H. (1961). Behandlung von Verdauungsstörungen allergischer Genese mit Prothipendyl (Dominal). *Semaine Hop. Paris* **37**, 2989.

Carrère, J., Fournier, J., and Nicaise, H. (1961). Klinische Prüfung des Prothipendyl-HCl. *Ann. Med.-Psychol.* **119**, 197.

Cattan, R., and Cohen, M. (1962). Neurovegetative Störungen bei Colitis und ihre Behandlung. *Semaine Hop.* (Paris) **38**, 1220.

Cohen, M. (1963). Die Indikationen von Dominal in der Gastro-Enterologie. *Esprit Med. Pharmaceut.* **58**, 14.

Cohen, S., Ditman, K. S., Mooney, H. B., and Whittlesey, J. R. B. Prothipendyl (Timovan) in der Behandlung des Alkoholismus: Vorläufiger Bericht. *J. New Drugs* **1**, 235.

Constantin, B., Blanc, J. E., and Campocasso, J. (1962). Die Rolle von Prothipendyl in der Neuroleptanalgesie. *Rev. Agressiol.* **3**, Special, 39.

Constantin, B., Blanc, J. F., and Bernard, Y. (1962). Kombination von Xylocain und Dominal bei der Neuroleptanalgesie. *1st European Kongr. Anaesthesiol. Wien*, 1962.

Cousin, J. P. (1961). Die Stellung eines neuen Neuroleptikums, des Dominal, in der neuropsychiatrischen Therapie. *Therap. Semaine Hop.* **37**, 544; *J. Med. Chir. Prat.* **132**, 873.

Cristol, J. (1962). Prüfung von Prothipendyl-HCl in der Narkose-Prämedikation. *Anesthesie Analgesie Reanimation* **19**, 551.

Davison, J. R., Goulder, R. V. H., Sills. O, A., and Young, M. J. (1962). Eine klinische Beurteilung eines neuen Azaphenothiazin (Tolnate) zur Behandlung agitierter Patienten. *Brit. J. Clin. Pract.* **16**, 781.

Delaporte, J. C., and Soule, M. (1963). Klinische Prüfung von Prothipendyl (Dominal) in der Kinderpsychiatrie. *Vie Med. (Paris)* **44**, (Med. Therap.) 119.

Deligne, P., and Cahn, J. (1961). Prüfung einer neuen Art von Neuroleptanalgesie: Die Kombination von Dominal-Palfium. *Rev. Agressiol.* **2**, 371.

Demétrio, J. T., and Lagana, R. E. (1961). Antiemetische Wirkung eines neuen Neuroplegikums, des Chlorhydrat von Prothipendyl (Dominal). *Fichario Med.-Terap. Labofarma* **23** (95), 1.

Diehr, A. (1959). Untersuchungen mit einem neuen Psychosedativum in der Poliklinik. *Medizinische* **38**, 1766.

Dietel, K., and Dietel, V. (1958). Erste Erfahrungen mit Dominal, einem Thipendyl-Derivat, im Kindesalter. *Deut. Med. J.* **9**, 594.

Dietel V., and Kunze, C. (1960). Uber die Wirkung einer Thipendyl-Verbindung auf die Konzentrationsfahigkeit von Schulkindern. *Therap. Gegenwert* **99**, 392.

Dorn, H. (1960). Behandlung der konstitutionellen Neurodermitis mit dem Thipendyl-Derivat Dominal forte. *Z. Haut-Geschlechtskrankh.* **28**, 256.

Dumon, G., Dumon-Legré, M., and Laugier, J. (1961). Die Prüfung von Prothipendyl-Ampullen (Dominal) in der Prämedikation der Bronchoskopie. *Thérap. Semaine Hop.* **37**, 639.

Dumon, G., Dumon-Legré, M., and Laugier, J. (1962). Prothipendyl-Ampullen (Dominal) in der Prämedikation vor Bronchoskopien. *Provence Med.* **30**, 35.

Dyrssen, K., Hellgren, K., and Reis, G. V. (1960). Behandlung der muskulären Hypertonie mit Prothipendyl (Azacon). *Opuscula Med.* **5**, 225.

Dyrssen, K., and Reis, G. V. (1961). Die Behandlung von muskulären Hypertoniezuständen und Hyperkinesien mit Prothipendyl (Azacon). *Svenska Lakartidn.* **58**, 3364.

Edelstein, E. L., and Assael, M. (1962). Ataraktische Wirkung von Prothipendyl bei Krankenhauspatienten. *Diseases Nervous System* **23**, 163.

Enge, S., and Lechner, H. (1960). Ein tierexperimenteller Beitrag zur Wirkungsweise der Psychopharmaka. *Wien. Z. Nervenheilk. Grenzg.* **17**, 309.

Faure, L., Constantin, B., and Vuaroqueaux, M. (1962). Verwendung der Kombination Dominal + Palfium in der Geburtshilfe. Vorläufige Notiz. *Hopital (Paris)* **50**, 155.

Fladung, H. (1962). Psychosedative Maßnahmen in der werksärztlichen Praxis. *Arztl. Praxis* **14**, 507.

Gaillard, L., and Brugière, P. (1962). Verwendung von Dominal zur Prämedikation in der Kinderheilkunde. *Semaine Hop. Ann. Pediat.* **38**, 1170/262.

Gazaix, M. (1962). Dominal in der Allgemeinmedizin. Prüfung bei 25 Häftlingen des Gefängnisses Nizza in Vergleich zu 25 Kontrollpersonen, die mit Placebos behandelt wurden. *Semaine Hop. Paris* **38**, 700.

Goethe, H. (1958). Zur Methodik der experimentellen Prüfung antikinetotischer Pharmaka am Beispiel zweier Thipendylverbindungen. *Arzneimittel-Forsch.* **8**, 605.

Guyonnaud, M. (1961) Erste klinische Prüfung eines neuroplegischen Arzneimittels (Dominal). *J. Med. Chir. Prat.* **132**, 443.

Hartel, J. (1961). Erfahrungen mit einem Thipendyl-Derivat zur Erleichterung und Verkürzung der Geburt. *Zentr. Gynaekol.* **83**, 1061.

Hasse, G. F. (1959). Erfahrungen mit der Wirksamkeit einer neuen Thipendyl-Verbindung (Dominal forte) zur Anaesthesie-Vorbereitung in Chirurgie und Gynäkologie. *Muench. Med. Wochschr.* **101**, 1017.

Hawthorn, E., and Conti, V. (1962). Psychosomatische Schmerzen in der Rheumatologie und ihre Behandlung durch Dominal. *Therap. Semaine Hop.* **38**, 346.

Heyden, A. H. (1960). Narkosevorbereitung in Praxis und kleinerem Krankenhaus. *Aerztl. Praxis* **7**, 257.

Hift, S., and Kryspin-Exner, K. (1958). Prothipendyl-hydrochlorid, ein neues Neuroleptikum. *Wien. Med. Wochschr.* **108**, 664.

Hoffmann, R. (1960). Prä- und postoperative Behandlung mit Dominal forte, einem Thipendyl-Derivat bei gynäkologischen Eingriffen. *Med. Monatsschr.* **14**, 378.

Hook, G. (1960). Dominal in der werksärztlichen Praxis. *Homburg-Inform. Werksarzt* **7**, 174.

Horai, Z., Tsujimoto, H., and Yokoi, S. (1961). Die Behandlung innerer Krankheiten mit Timovan. *Clin. Rep. d. Fa. Nippon Shinyaku Ltd.* No. 1.

Horai, Z., Tsujimoto, and Yokoi, S. (1962). Die Verwendung von Thiophenylpyridylamin-HCl (Timovan) bei inneren Krankheiten. *Intern. Med. Pediat.* **17**, 407.

Hormia, M., and Hormia, A. (1961). Wirkung von Prothipendyl auf das Leberparenchym der weißen Ratte. *Ann. Med. Exptl. Biol. Fenniae* **39**, 374.

Huguenard, P., and Leger, P. (1960). Klinische Untersuchungen mit Dominal oder LG 206, einem Neuroplegikum. *Rev. Agressiol.* **1**, 627.

Huguenard, P., and Léger, P. (1961). Prüfung eines neuen Neuroplegikums: Dominal, in der Anaesthesie. *Therap. Semaine Hop.* **37**, Hors serie Juin, 47; *J. Med. Chir. Prat.* **132**, 731.

Hutschenreuter, K., and Pitzler, K. (1958). Klinische Erfahrungen mit einem neuen Neuroleptikum (Dominal forte) in der Chirurgie. *Med. Klin. (Munich)* **53**, 1415.

Hyvert, M., Chambon, J., and Coubronne, M. (1962). Klinische Erfahrungen mit einem neuen *Neuroleptikum. Genie Med.* **14**, 177, 21.

Izac, L. (1961). Prüfung von Dominal bei neuropsychiatrischen Zuständen. *Semaine Hop. Paris Suppl. Med. Monde* **37**, 784.

Jessel, H. J. (1960). Erfahrungen mit Prothipendyl in der Psychiatrie. *Deut. Med. Wochschr.* **85**, 192; (1960). *Ger. Med. Monthly* **5**, 127.

Jude, J.-P., Gatineaux, J.-M., and Maupome, J. J. (1963). Dominal bei psychisch debilen Kindern. *Ann. Med.-Psychol.* **121**, 588.

Jude, G., and Pavilla, J. (1962). Klinische Untersuchungen mit einem nicht kataleptisch wirkenden Neuroleptikum, Dominal, bei Alterspatienten. *Semaine Hop. Paris Suppl. Med. Monde* **38**, 626.

Juhlin, L., and Skogh, M. (1960). Die Wirkung von peroral verabreichtem Prothipendyl (Azacon) auf den *Juckreiz;* klinische Prüfung im doppelten Blindversuch. *Svenska Lakartidn.* **57**, 3078.

Koranyi, E. K., Smith, R. L., and Sarwer-Foner, G. J. (1958). Klinische Beurteilung von D 206, einem neuen Pyridylamin. *Med. Serv. J.* **14**, 130.

Koššak, O. (1961). Prothipendyl-Hydrochlorid als Neuroleptikum in der Chirurgie und Anaesthesiologie. *Med. Arch. (Sarajevo)* **15**, 37.

Krupp, H. (1961). Ambulante Therapie vegetativer Störungen. *Aerztl. Praxis* **13**, 714.

Kurka, P. (1959). Klinische Erfahrungen mit Prothipendyl (Dominal forte) in der Narkose-Prämedikation. *Wien. Klin. Wochschr.* **71**, 533.

Küster, H. (1958). Klinische Erfahrungen mit psychosedativer und neuroleptischer Therapie. *Aerztl. Praxis* **10**, 1085.

Küttler, R. (1958). Klinische Erfahrungen mit Dominal forte in der Chirurgie. *Med. Monatsschr.* **12**, 612.

Lefevre, P., Marinacce, G., and Lauzier, B. (1962). Ergebnisse, beobachtet in der psychiatrischen Therapie vom Chlorhydrat des Prothipendyl. *Gaz. Med. France* **69**, 157.

Lehoczky, T., and Halasy, M. (1962). *Neurologische Beobachtungen* und Untersuchungsergebnisse bei Anwendung von Prothipendyl (Dominal). *Med. Welt* **3**, 154.
Lerman, L. H. (1962). Tolnate (Prothipendyl-HCl.) als *postoperatives Antiemetikum* nach opthalmologischen Eingriffen. 1*st European Kongr. Anaesthesiol. Wien*, 1962.
Linke, H. (1958). Klinische Erfahrungen mit dem neuen Thiophenylpyridylamin-Derivat Dominal forte. *Muench. Med. Wochschr.* **100**, 969.
Linke, H. (1959). Klinische Beobachtungen und Untersuchungsergebnisse mit dem Neuroleptikum Dominal forte. *Fortschr. Med.* **77**, 133.
Longuet, Y. J., Durupt, M., and Coignet, J. L. (1962). Klinische Ergebnisse bei Verwendung von Prothipendyl-HCl in der Anaesthesiologie. *Semaine Hop. Paris Suppl. Med. Monde* **38**, 533.
Loos, M. (1962). Psychosedierung als modifizierte Form der *Heilschlaftherapie* psychasthenischer Versagenszustände. *Med. Welt* **46**, 2445.
MacLean, J. G. (1961). Behandlung von *Akne* mit Prothipendyl. *Can. Med. Assoc. J.* **84**, 427.
Mahon, R., and Trebesses, G. (1962). Verwendung eines neuen Psycholeptikums in der *Geburtshilfe*: Das Prothipendyl-HCl (Dominal). Soc. Natl. Gynecol. Obstet. France, Bordeaux; *Bull. Federation Soc. Gynecol. Obstet. Langue Franc.* **14**, 685.
Maisler, A. (1962). Klinische Prüfung eines neuen Neuroleptikums in der Dermatologie. *Semaine Hop. Paris* **38**, 139.
Malinas, Y., and Volmat, R. (1962). Die schweren *Schwangerschaftserbrechen*: Behandlung mit Prothipendyl (Dominal). (Klinische Prüfung von 2 Fällen). *Vie Med. Paris* **43**, 129.
Mans, J., Cornil, M., and Ajzenberg, D. (1962). Ergebnisse einer einjährigen Prüfung eines neuen Neuroleptikums: Dominal in der Psychiatrie. *Thérap. Semaine Hop.* **38**, 34.
Matsuda, K., Okuda, O. Wada, K., and Bokuba, F. (1961). Erfahrungen bei der Verwendung von Timovan (Prothipendyl-HCl) in der Psychiatrie. *J. New Remedies Clin.* **10**, 57.
Meißner, F. (1961). Die *Prämedikation im Kindes- und Säuglingsalter. Zentr. Chir.* **86**, 1081.
Messmer, E. (1960). Die Anwendung von Prothipendyl zur Behandlung unruhiger, schlafgestörter Zerebralsklerotiker. *Med. Welt* **48**, 2571.
Michaux, L., Duché, D. J., and Pringuet, G. (1962). Klinische Prüfung des Prothipendyl in der Kinderpsychiatrie. *Rev. Neuropsychiat. Infantile* **10**, 139.
Monroziès, M., and Fournie, J. (1962). Die Verwendung von Dominal in der *praktischen Geburtshilfe* während der Austreibungsperiode. *Toulouse Med.* **63**, 1047.
Mouren, P., Serratrice, G., Soulayrol, R. G., and Arditti, M. Prüfung eines Thiophenylpyridylamin-Derivates in der *neuropsychiatrischen Klinik*: Prothipendyl-HCl oder Dominal, ein neues Neuroleptikum. *Thérap. Semaine Hop.* **37**, 845.
Nakamura, T., Hatasa, K., Sofa, K., and Tsukahara, H. (1961). Erfahrungen mit Timovan (Thipendyl-Derivat) bei Kinderkrankheiten. *Japan. J. Pediat.* **14**, 100.
Nehlil, J., Métral, S., and Rouyer, ... (1962). Prothipendyl-HCl in der praktischen Psychiatrie. *Ann. Med.-Psychol.* **120**, 959. (1962).
Nelken, S., Bernadin, D., Moine, C., and Bousquet, G. (1962). Prüfung eines neuen Neuroleptikums in der Behandlung des *Schwangerschaftserbrechens* und der *Schwangerschaftstoxikose*: Prothipendyl-HCl oder Dominal (37 Beobachtungen). Soc. Natl. Gynec. Obstet. France, Lyon; *Bull. Federation Soc. Gynecol. Obstet. Franc.* **14**, 711.
Neuschaefer-Rube, R. (1959). Erfahrungen mit Dominal forte in der inneren Medizin. *Therap. Cegenwart.* **98**, 228.
Nüßgen, W. (1959). Erfahrungen mit Prothipendyl in der *Prämedikation. Anaesthesist* **8**, 14.
O'Connor, A., and MacIntyre, I. M. (1963). Kontrollierter klinischer Versuch mit Prothipendyl-HCl (Tolnate) zur Prämedikation. *J. Roy. Nav. Med. Serv.* **49**, 28.
Ota, T., Sumioka, K., and Kizu, Y. (1961). Erfahrungen bei der klinischen Verwendung von D 206 (Timovan) in der Gynäkologie und Geburtshilfe. *Clin. Rept. d. Fa. Nippon Shinyaku Lt.* **1**, 19.
Pelon, J. C., and Roger, A. (1962). Die Kombination LG 206 (Dominal)-Pyrrolamidol in der Anaesthesie. *Anesthesie Analgesie Reanimation* **19**, 539.

Piéri, J., Casalonga, L., Battesti, I. (1961). Therapeutische Ergebnisse von *N*-(3-Dimethylaminopropyl)-thiophenyl-pyridylamin-HCl in der allgemeinen Medizin. *Therap. Semaine Hop.* **37**, 940.

Plasse, G., Goirand, R., Casalta, E., Martin-Laval, J., and Ayme, Y. (1962). Dominal in der Geburtshilfe. *Semaine Hop. Paris* **38**, 611.

Pommé, B., Planche, R., and Yermia, H. (1962). Klinische Untersuchungen eines neuen Psycholeptikums, Dominal in der *Psychiatrie* (über 90 Beobachtungen). *Lyon Med.* **207**, 715.

Puech, J. (1961). Positive Effekte und Nebenwirkungen der Neuroleptika. Vorläufige Ergebnisse mit Prothipendyl in der Psychiatrie. *Semaine Hop. Paris* **37**, 3353.

Quandt, J., Hoin, L. V., and Schliep, H. (1958). Bemerkungen zur Behandlung mit Phenothiazin-Verbindungen innerhalb der *Psychiatrie* unter besonderer Berücksichtigung eines neuartigen Thiopenhylpyridylamin-Derivates. *Monatsschr. Psychiat. Neurol.* **135**, 197.

Querci, M., and Amasio, C. (1958). Betrachtungen über die Wirkungen eines neuen Mittels: Dominal (D 206). *Minerva Anestesiol.* **24**, 443.

Rebattu, J. P., *et al.*, and Chirat, P. (1962). Verwendung von Prothipendyl-Ampullen (Dominal) zur Vorbereitung von *Endoskopien unter Lokalanaesthesie* in der Oto-Rhino-Laryngologie. *J. Franc. Oto-rhinolaryngol.* **11**, 455.

Reboul, J., Delorme, G., and Mas, J. P. (1962). Wirkung eines neuen Neuroleptikums, Dominal, auf Schmerzen bei Neoplasmen. *Semaine Hop. Paris* **38**, 2237.

v. Reis, G. (1961). Prothipendyl zur Behandlung der *muskulären Hypertonie und Hyperkinesie*. Prid. 7th Intern. Kongr. Neurol. Rom 1961.

Richter, H. R., and Müller, H. R. (1959). Zur Beeinflussung *extrapyramidaler Bewegungsstörungen* durch ein neues Neuroplegikum der Thiophenylpyridylamin-Reihe (Prothipendyl, "Dominal forte" Homburg). *Schweiz. Med. Wochschr.* **89**, 794.

Rivoire, J., and Morin, A. (1962). Behandlung des *Pruritus bei Dermatosen* mit dem Chlorhydrat des Prothipendyl. *Lyon. Med.* **207**, 705.

Rondepierre, J. J., and Ropert, R. (1961). Unsere Erfahrungen mit Prothipendyl-Chlorhydrat (Dominal) in der Psychiatrie. *Therap. Semaine Hop.* **37**, 735.

Rondepierre, J. J., and Ropert, R. (1961). *Experimentelle und klinische Verabreichung* eines neuen Neuroleptikums, das Chlorhydrat des *N*-(3-Dimethyl-aminopropyl)-thiophenylpyridylamin oder Dominal. *Therap. Semaine Hop.* **37**, Hors serie Juin, 78; *J. Med. Chir. Prat.* **132**, 587.

Sabathié, M. (1963). Einführung von Prothipendyl (Dominal) in unsere praktische Anaesthesiologie. *Ann. Anesthesiol. Franc.* **4**, 75.

Saint-André, M. P. (1962). Drei Fälle von *Psoriasis guttata*, deren akute Erscheinungen durch *N*-(3-Dimethylamino-propyl)-thiophenyl-pyridylamin-HCl oder Dominal schnell abblaßten. Soc. de Dermatologie et de syphiligraphie, Marseille; *Bull. Soc. Franc. Dermatol. Syphiligraph.* **69**, 806.

Sauvan, R., Mercier, J. N., and Deschamps de Paillette, E. (1962). Prüfung eines neuen Neuroleptikums, Dominal, in der kardiovaskulären Therapie. *Semaine Hop. Paris Suppl. Med. Monde* **38**, 596.

Scharf, R. (1960). Wirkungen einer Thipendyl-Verbindung auf den Kreislauf. *Arzneimittel-Forsch.* **10**, 1005.

Schiemann, W. (1959). Uber die intern-klinische Anwendung von Psychosedativa und Neuroleptika. *Aerztl. Wochschr.* **14**, 505.

v. Schlichtegrell, A. (1958). *Zentrale und periphere Dämpfungswirkungen* in der Reihe der Thiophenylpyridylamin-Derivate. *Arzneimittel-Forsch.* **8**, 489.

Scholler, K. L. (1958). Erfahrungen mit dem Thipendyl-Derivat Dominal forte als Sedativum und Neuroleptikum in der Neurochirurgie. *Aerztl. Wochschr.* **13**, 1045.

Schönherr, W. (1958). Uber die Wirkung einer neuen Thipendyl-Verbindung in der Geburtshilfe. *Medizinische.* **37**, 1458.

Schuler, A., and Klebe, H. (1962). Synthesen von 4 Aza-Phenothiazinen; 4-Aza-Phenothiazine und deren 10-Aminoalkyl-Derivate. *Ann. Chem.* **653**, 172.

Schuppius, A. (1959). Untersuchungen über die *Beeinflussung des Geburtsverlaufes* durch ein Neuroleptikum mit Hilfe der Tokographie. *Medizinische* **45**, 2185.

Schütz, A. (1961). Psychisch bedingte Unruhezustände in der allgemeinen Praxis. *Landarzt* **6**, 229.

Stärck, G. (1958). Erfahrungen in der inneren Medizin mit dem Thipendyl-Derivat Dominal forte. *Med. Monatsschr.* **12**, 745.

Storch, H. H. (1958). Untersuchungen über die *Prämedikation* mit neuen vegetativ dämpfenden Mitteln. *Inaug. Dissertation Heidelberg.*

Tanaka, A. (1961). Erfahrungen mit Timovan—D 206. *Clin. Rep. d. Fa. Nippon Shinyaku Ltd.* **1**, 15.

Trebesses, M. G. (1963). Verwendung eines Psycholeptikums, Dominal, in der Geburtshilfe. *J. Med. Bordeaux* **140**, 299.

Uddenberg, C. E., and Lundgren, B. (1959). Prüfung von Azacon an Patienten einer psychiatrischen Klinik. *Svenska lakartidn.* **56**, 3272.

Vague, J., and Miller, J. (1962). Klinische Prüfung von Dominal 10 bei Anomalien des Körpergewichtes und vegetativen Dystonien. *Sud. Med. (Marseille)* **97**, (11), 111.

Valentin, H. (1958). Klinische Erfahrungen mit einer neuen Thipendyl-Verbindung in der Geburtshilfe und Gynäkologie. *Med. Klin. (Munich)* **53**, 1570.

Vogt, U. (1962). *Prämedikation* vor Eingriffen im Hals-Nasen-Ohren-Bereich. *HNO-Wegweiser* **10**, 249.

Volkstädt, H., and Bünte, H. (1959). Uber die Anwendung eines neuen Neuroleptikums in der Chirurgie. *Therap. Gegenwert.* **98**, 443.

Volmat, R., and Beaudouin, J. L. (1961). Erste klinische Versuche in der *Psychiatrie* mit einem neuen Neuroleptikum, das nicht zu den Phenpthiazinen gehört: Prothipendyl oder Dominal. *Sem. Hop. Paris* **37**, 2910; 1962. *J. Med. Chir. Prat.* **133**, 11.

Volmat, R., and Robert, R. (1962). Dominal in der medizinischen Allgemeinpraxis. *Sem. Hop. Paris Suppl. Med. Monde* **38**, 855.

Widmann, H., and Eckle, U. (1961). Chlorpromazin und Leukopenie, Prothipendyl und Leukozytose. *Med. Welt* **15**, 797.

Wolf, G. (1963). Die Behandlung von Unruhezuständen von Kindern in der Allgemeinpraxis. *Aerztl. Praxis* **15**, 1954.

Yozawa, R., Saito, K., Hosoi, Y., Yonezawa, T., Okamura, H., Segawa, H., and Chiba, M., Jr. (1961). Uber die Wirkung von D 206 bei der Prämedikation. *Japan. J. Anesthesiol. (Masui)* **10**, 197.

Zara, M. (1962). Dominal in der Geburtshilfe und Allgemeinmedizin. *Sem. Hop. Paris, Suppl. Med. Monde* **38**, 176.

~ A.13 ~
Thiethylperazine

Adriani, J., et al. (1962). Postanesthetic vomiting. *Am. J. Surg.* **103**, 2–5.

Alwyn, J. E. S. (1962). Hyperemesis gravidarum and its management with thiethylperazine (Torecan): A preliminary report. *Med. J. Australia* **49**, 339–341.

Austin, L. F. G. (1962). Clinical trials in obstetrics. *New Zealand Med. J.* **61**, 601–603.

Barone, G., et al. (1961). Esperienze Cliniche su un Nuovo Farmaco ad Azione Antiemetica. Clinical experiences with a new drug of antiemetic effect. *Gazz. Intern. Med. Chir.* **66**, 1835–1842.

Boissier, J. R., and Pagny, J. (1962). Etude Pharmacologique d'une Phenothiazine Neuroleptique, la Thiethylperazine ou GS 95 (Torecan). III. Action Antivomitive—Discussion generale. (Pharmacological study of thiethylperazine or GS 95 (Torecan). A neuroleptic phenothiazine derivative. III. Antiemetic effect—general discussion.) *Med. Exptl.* **6**, 320–326.

Boissier, J. R., et al. (1962). Etude Pharmacologique d'une Phenothiazine Neuroleptique, la Thiethylperazine (Torecan). II. Action Potentialisa-Trice des Hypnotiques. Activite Adenolytique. Pharmacological investigation of thiethylperazine (Torecan). A neuroleptic phenothiazine derivative. II. Potentiation of hypnotic drugs. Adrenolytic effects. *Med. Exptl.* **6**, 136–142.

Boissier, J. R., et al. (1961). Etude Pharmacologique d'une Phénothiazine Neuroleptique la Thiethylpérazine (Torecan). (Pharmacological investigation of thiethylperazine (Torecan) a Neuroleptic phenothiazine derivative.) *Med. Exptl.* **4**, 145–150.

Browne, D. C., and Sparks, R. D. (1960). Nausea and vomiting—study of thiethylperazine. Scientific Exhibit, American Medical Association Clinical Meeting, Washington, D.C., Nov. 28 to Dec. 2, 1960.

Browne, D. C., and Sparks, R. D. (1961). Nausea and vomiting, study of thiethylperazine. Scientific Exhibit, American College of Gastroenterology, Cleveland, Ohio, October 23–26, 1961.

Browne, D. C., and Sparks, R. (1961). Vomiting mechanism: A clinical study of thiethylperazine. *Southern Med. J.* **54**, 953–961.

Bruggisser, R. (1961). Die Behandlung von Brechzuständen in der Inneren Medizin. (Treatment of vomiting in internal medicine.) *Praxis (Bern)* **50**, 127–129.

Cerletti, A., et al. (1962). 3-Aethyl-mercapto-10-[3'-(1''-methyl-piperazyl-4'')-propyl-1]-Phenothiazin (Thiethylperazin), Ein Spezifisches Antiemeticum (3-ethyl-mercapto-10-[3'-(1''-methyl-piperazyl-4'')-propyl-1']-phenothiazine (Thiethylperazine), a specific antiemetic drug. (Relationships between structure and antiemetic activity of further phenothiazine derivatives.) *Arzneimittel-Forsch.* **12**, 964–968.

Chinellato, F. (1960). Ricerche Sperimentali sul Comportamento della Funzione Vestibolare dopo Somministrazione di Alcuni Farmaci. I. Un derivato della Fenothiazina. (Experimental investigations of the effect of certain drugs on vestibular function. I. A phenothiazine derivative.) *Boll. Soc. Ital. Biol. Sper.* **36**, 931–932.

Codiga, V. A. (1961). A new antiemetic for the treatment of nausea and vomiting associated with Roentgen therapy. *Intern. Record Med.* **174**, 375–379.

Cox, J., and Collins, J. H. (1962). Nausea and vomiting: Control by thiethylperazine. *Current Therap. Res.* **4**, 178–181.

De Bonis, B. (1961). Valutazione Clinica del Torecan, Nuovo Antiemetico, in Anestesia. (Clinical evaluation of Torecan. A new antiemetic, in anaesthesiology.) *Acta Anaesthesiol.* **12**, 363–373.

Dobkin, A. B., et al. (1963). Circulatory response to tilt with hydroxyzine, thiethylperazine maleate, SA 97, and perphenazine. *Anesthesia Analgesia Current Res.* **42**, 225.

Downs, H. S., et al. (1962). The antiemetic efficacy of thiethylperazine upon post-operative nausea and vomiting. *Surg., Gynecol. Obstet.* **115**, 604–608.

Eerola, R. (1962). Effect of thiethylperazine on postoperative vomiting. *1st European Congr. Anaesthesiol. World Federation Soc. Anaesthesiologists, Wien.* **3**, 174.

Guth, P. S., and De Jaramillo, G. A. V. (1962). Phenothiazine distribution in mammalian brain. *Federation Proc.* **21**, 178.

Lumio, J. S. (1962). Kokemuksia Tietylperatsiinin Vaikutuksesta Huimaustiloihin. (Evaluation of the effect of thiethylperazine in vertigo.) *Duodecim* **78**, 127–129.

Maritano, M., et al. (1960). Profilassi e Terapia del Vomito. (Prophylaxis and therapy of vomiting.) *Minerva Anestesiol.* **26**, 343–345.

North, W. C., et al. (1963). Factors concerned with postoperative emesis and its prevention with thiethylperazine. *J. Am. Med. Assoc.* **183**, 656.

Parkinson, R. P. (1962). Thiethylperazine in nausea and vomiting. *Gen. Practitioner* **25**, 6.

Pasquale, A., and Bruno, F. (1960). La Terapia del Vomito. (Therapy of vomiting.) *Minerva Med.* **52**, 2642–2645.

Priver, M. S., and Boros, H. H. (1962). Nausea and vomiting of pregnancy. A clinical note on the use of thiethylperazine as a safe and effective antiemetic. *Western Med.* **3**, 94.

Rasario, G. M. (1962). Su di un Nuovo Comsoto Fenotiazinico ad Attivita Antiemetica ed Antivertiginosa. (A new phenothiazine derivative of antiemetic and antivertiginous action.) *Riforma Med.* **76**, 99–101.

Rubin, W. (1962). Vertigo in otolaryngology. Experimental and clinical study. Scientific Exhibit. American Academy of General Practice, Las Vegas, Nevada, April 9–12, 1962.

Seltzer, A. P. (1963). Precaution urged in use of thiethylperazine maleate in ear, nose, and throat therapy. *E.E.N.T. Dig.* **25**, 53.

Sparks, R. D., Browne, D. C., and Ferrans, V. J. (1962). Thiethylperazine: effect on postoperative vomiting and localization in the central nervous system by fluorescence technics. *Am. J. Gastroenteral.* **37**, 404–414.

Taylor, C., and Soelting, V. K. (1963). Thiethylperazine: a clinical investigation of a new anti-emetic drug. *Can. Anaesthesiol. Soc. J.* **10**, 57.

Tellesson, W. G. (1962). Thiethylperazine and PAS therapy for tuberculosis. *Med. J. Australia* **49**, 849.

Vinciguerra, G. (1961). Esperienze sull'azione anticinetosica del Torecan (GS 95 Sandoz). (Experiences on the action of Torecan in kinesia.) *Inform. Med. (Genoa)* **16**, 94–96.

Wyant, G. M. (1962). A comparative study of eleven anti-emetic drugs in dogs. *Can. Anaesthesiol. Soc. J.* **9**, 399–407.

Zehnder, K., et al. (1962). The metabolism of thiethylperazine (Torecan). *Biochem. Pharmacol.* **11**, 551–556.

∽ A.14 ∽
Thiopropazate

Ainslie, J. D. (1961). The use of newer psychiatric drugs in medical practice: Their specificity of action in relation to target symptoms and dynamic situation. *J. Florida Med. Assoc.* **47**, 901.
Archer, J. S., and Hicks, R. G. (1962). Phenothiazine subgroups. *N.Y. State J. Med.* **62**, 3769–3772.
Ayd, F. J., Jr. (1959). The use of tranquilizing medications in general practice. *J. Indiana Med. Assoc.* **52**, 516.
Ayd, F. J. (1960). Current status of major tranquilizers. *J. Med. Soc. New Jersey* **57**, 4.
Ayd, F. J., Jr. (1960). Tranquilizers and the ambulatory geriatric patient. *J. Am. Geriat.* **8**, 909.
Ayd, F. J., Jr. (1961). Phenothiazine tranquilizers: Eight years of development. *Med. Clin. N. Am.* **45**, 1027–1040.
Ayd. F. J., Jr. (1961). A survey of drug-induced extrapyramidal reactions. *J. Am. Med. Assoc.* **175**, 1054.
Ayd, F. J., Bianco, E., Zullo, L. (1959). Treatment of depressive states in ambulatory patients. *Diseases Nervous System* **20**, 34.
Barsa, J. A. (1960). Combination drug therapy in psychiatry. (Clinical notes.) *Am. J. Psychiat.* **117**, 448.
Bennett, I. F. (1959). Clinical studies with phenothiazine derivatives in psychiatry. *In* "Effect of Pharmacologic Agents on the Nervous System" (F. J. Braceland, ed.), pp. 266–284. Williams & Wilkins, Baltimore, Maryland.
Benson, W. M., and Schiele, B. C. (1960). Current status of tranquilizing and antidepressive drugs. *J.-Lancet* **80**, 579.
Bianchi, R. G., and Craig, R. L. (1960). The effect of certain tranquilizers on intrabiliary pressure of cholecystectomized dogs. *Am. J. Digest. Diseases* **5**, 419.
Black, J. (1960). Phenothiazines as antiemetics and tranquilizers. *J. Med. Assoc. Alabama* **29**, 492.
Bourne, W. A. (1960). Sedation and analgesia in inoperable cancer. *Practitioner* **184**, 541.
Brett, R. J. (1961). A note on the tranquilizers. *Rocky Mt. Med. J.* **58**, 34–35 and 59–60.
Cain, H. D., and Malcolm, M. (1960). Phenothiazine atraxics-extrapyramidal reactions. *Calif. Med.* **93**, 24.
Capparell, H. V. (1962). Drug therapy in mental illness. *Penna. Med. J.* **65**, 899–905.
Carstairs, G. M. (1961). Advances in psychological medicine. *Practitioner* **187**, 495–504.
Cattell, J. P. (1959). Psychopharmacological agents: A selective survey. (Clinical notes.) *Am. J. Psychiat.* **116**, 352.
Cattell, J. P., and Malitz, S. (1960). Revised survey of selected psychopharmacological agents. *Am. J. Psychiat.* **117**, 449.
Chicoine, L. (1961). L'intoxication par les derives de la phenothiazine: Revue et rapport de 25 cas. *Union Med. Canada* **90**, 469–474.
Collins, J. A., Gowdey, C. W., Toogood, J. H., and Wanklin, J. M. (1960). A comparative quantitative study of antiwhealing drugs in man. *Appl. Therap.* **2**, 609.
Council on Drugs (1961). New drugs and developments in therapeutics: Drugs for mental illness (A Council on Drugs' Digest). *J. Am. Med. Assoc.* **177**, 245–246.

Dale, P. W. (1961). Current concepts in therapy: Medical management of mental problems in the aged. *New Engl. J. Med.* **265**, 84–86.
Darling, H. F. (1961). Acetophenazine (Tindal) and thiopropazate (Dartal) in ambulatory psychoneurotic patients. *Am. J. Psychiat.* **118**, 358–359.
Denver, H. C. B. (1959). Side effects of phenothiazins. *In* "Psychopharmacology Frontiers (Proc. of the Psychopharmacology Symposium of the Second International Congress of Psychiatry)" (N. S. Kline, ed.), p. 61. Little, Brown, Boston, Massachusetts.
Dews, P. B., (1958). Drugs affecting behavior. *In* "Pharmacology in Medicine" (V. A. Drill, ed.), pp. 309–334. McGraw-Hill, New York.
Dobkin, A. B. (1960). Potentiation of thiopentone anaesthesia: Comparison of promethazine, chlorpromazine, perphenazine, fluphenazine, thiopropazate, pipamazine and triflupromazine. *Brit. J. Anaesthesia* **32**, 424.
Dobkin, A. B., and Purkin, N. (1960). The antisialogogue effect of phenothiazine derivatives. *Brit. J. Anaesthesia* **32**, 57.
Dobkin, A. B., Israel, J. S., and Criswick, V. G. (1962). Prolongation of thiopental anaesthesia with hydroxyzine, SA 97, thiethylperazine, and thioridazine. *Can. Anaesthesiol. Soc. J.* **9**, 342–346.
Dobkin, A. B., Woodworth, H., and Israel, J. S. (1962). The antisialogogue effect of hydroxyzine, thiethylperazine, and N'-p-chloro-benzylhydryl-N'-methyl homopiperazine (SA 97). *Can. Anaesthesiol. Soc. J.* **9**, 234–238.
Domino, E. F. (1962). Human pharmacology of tranquilizing drugs. *Clin. Pharmacol. Therap.* **3**, 599–664.
Edisen, C. B., and Samuels, A. S. Thiopropazate hydrochloride (Dartal) chemotherapy for emotional disorders: A clinical evaluation. *AMA Arch. Neurol. Psychiat.* **80**, 481.
Editorial. (1960). The tranquillisers. *J. Indian Med. Assoc.* **35**, 458–461.
Elia, C. J. (1963). Treatment of dizziness. *E.E.N.T. Dig.* **25**, 19–28.
Ferrand, P. T. (1958). Observations with Dartal in chronic psychoses: A study of seventy-one patients. *Minn. Med.* **41**, 853.
Ferrand, P. T., Peterson, G., and O'Neill, R. (1961). A follow-up study of discharged patients on thiopropazate dihydrochloride (Dartal) medication. *Minn. Med.* **44**, 103.
Flaherty, J. A. (1961). Permitil: An evaluation of its use in psychiatric outpatients. *Delaware State Med. J.* **33**, 217–224.
Flegenheim, W. V. (1959). Dyskinesias following therapy with phenothiazine derivatives. *J. Mt. Sinai Hosp.* **26**, 440.
Foltz, L. M. (1962). Critical evaluation of tranquilizers. *J. Kentucky Med. Assoc.* **60**, 733–738.
Forrest, F. M., Forrest, I. S., and Mason, A. S. (1959). A rapid, semi-quantitative urine color test for piperazine-linked phenothiazine drugs. *Am. J. Psychiat.* **116**, 549.
Forrest, F. M., Forrest, I. S., and Mason, A. S. (1961). Review of rapid urine tests for phenothiazine and related drugs. *Am. J. Psychiat.* **118**, 300–307.
Foss, G. L., and Simpson, S. L. (1959). Oral methyltestosterone and jaundice. *Brit. Med. J.* I, 259.
Friend, D. G. (1958). The tranquilizers. *Med. Clin. N. Am.* **42**, 1253.
Friend, D. G. (1959). Current concepts in therapy: Tranquilizers II. Phenothiazines 2. *New Engl. J. Med.* **260**, 1231.
Friend, D. G. (1960). Current drug therapy: The phenothiazines. *Clin. Pharmacol. Therap.* **1**, 5.
Friend, D. G. (1961). Current concepts in therapy: Tranquilizers III. Meprobamate, phenaglycodol and chlordiazepoxide. *New Engl. J. Med.* **264**, 870–873.
Fulghum, D. S., Smith, D., and Jernigan, E. (1960). Appraisal of Dartal in treatment of Huntington's chorea. *Diseases Nervous System* **21**, 46.
Gellman, V. (1962). Report from Poison Centre, Winnepeg Children's Hospital. The phenothiazine derivatives. *Manitoba Med. Rev.* **42**, 631–632.

Gold, M. I. (1959). Tranquilizing drugs: Classification and structural interrelations. *Am. Practitioner Dig. Treat.* **10**, 241.
Goodman, D., and Cahn, M. M. (1959). Contact dermatitis to phenothiazine drugs. *J. Invest. Dermatol.* **33**, 27.
Hamilton, L. D., and Bennett, J. L. (1962). Acetophenazine for hyperactive geriatric patients. *Geriatrics* **17**, 596–601.
Heaton-Ward, W. A., Carpenter, W. H. K., and Jancar, J. (1959). Appearance of Parkinsonism in mentally defective patients treated with Dartalan with the occurrence of oculogyric crises in identical twins. *Brit. Med. J.* II, 107.
Hewitt, M. I. (1960). Which tranquilizer? *J. Indiana State Med. Assoc.* **53**, 1475.
Hinwich, H. E. (1960). Some drugs useful in the treatment of emotional disorders-physiology, indications, and contraindications. *Am. Practitioner Dig. Treat.* **11**, 687.
Himwich, H. E. (1960). The management of alcoholism. *Mod. Med. Canada* **15**, 55.
Hock, C. W. (1959). Treatment of gastrointestinal disorders with an anticholinergic tranquilizer combination. *J. Med. Assoc. Georgia* **48**, 218.
Hohman, L. B. (1961). Mental depression. *In* "Current Therapy" (H. F. Conn, ed.), pp. 563–564. Saunders, Philadelphia, Pennsylvania.
Hohman, L. B. (1962). Psychoses: Mental depression. *In* "Current Therapy" (H. F. Conn, ed.), pp. 544–546. Saunders, Philadelphia, Pennsylvania.
Holden, J. C. (1960). Meprobamate as a routine sedative in geriatrics. *Scot. Med. J.* **5**, 526.
Hollister, L. D. (1961). Current concepts in therapy: Complications from psychotherapeutic drugs. I. *New England J. Med.* **264**, 291.
Hollister, L. E. (1958). The present status of tranquilizing drugs. *Calif. Med.* **89**, 1.
Hollister, L. E., Bennett, J. L., Kaim, S. C., and Kimball, I. Jr. (1963). Drug-induced EEG abnormalities as predictors of clinical response to thiopropazate and haloperidol. *Am. J. Psychiat.* **119**, 887–888.
Hordern, A. (1961). Medical progress: Psychiatry and the tranquilizers. *New Engl. J. Med.* **265**, 584–588.
Hordern, A. (1961). Psychiatry and the tranquilizers. *New Engl. J. Med.* **265**, 634–638.
Irwin, S. (1961). Correlation in rats between the locomotor and avoidance suppressant potencies of 8 phenothiazine tranquilizers. *Arch. Intern. Pharmacodyn.* **132**, 279–286.
Janssen, P. A. J. (1959). Chemistry and pharmacology of CNS depressants related to 4-(4-Hydroxy-4-phenylpiperidino)butyrophenone: Part I—Synthesis and screening data in mice. *J. Med. Pharm. Chem.* **1**, 281.
Kabat, H. (1959). Drug therapy of cerebellar ataxia and disorders of the basal ganglia, based on cerebellar-striatal antagonism. *Ann. Internal Med.* **50**, 1438.
Kabat, H., and McLeod, M. (1959). Neuromuscular dysfunction and treatment of athetosis. *Conn. State Med.* **23**, 710.
Kapalan, H. S. (1959). Tranquilizers in the office practice of medicine. *N.Y. State J. Med.* **59**, 2871.
Kaye, S. (1962). Simple, reliable tests for some common poisons and drug overdosage. *Clin. Med.* **69**, 1971–1972, 1974–1975.
Kennedy, B., O'Quinn, S., Perret, W. J., Tilley, J. C., and Henington, V. M. (1961). Phototoxic and photoallergic skin reactions resulting from modern drug therapy. *J. Louisiana State Med. Soc.* **113**, 365.
Kirsner, J. B. (1959). Ulcerative colitis. *In* "Current Therapy" (H. F. Conn, ed.), pp. 197–202. Saunders, Philadelphia, Pennsylvania.
Kirsner, J. G. (1959). Current concepts of the medical management of ulcerative colitis. *J. Am. Med. Assoc.* **169**, 433.
Kline, N. S. (Moderator). (1958). Clinical clues as to mode of action of the ataractic drugs: A round table. *Psychiat. Quart.* **32**, 41.
Kline, N. S. (1961). The use of psychopharmaceuticals in office practice. *Med. Clin. N. Am.* **45**, 1677–1684.

Klotz, M. (1959). The history and pharmacology of the atractic drugs. *Diseases Nervous System* **20**, 365.
Kollister, L. E. (1959). Drugs in emotional disorders: Past and present. *Ann. Internal Med.* **51**, 1032.
Kraines, S. H. (1960). Psychotropic drugs and the emotional circuit. *J. Neuropsychiat.* **2**, 55.
Laird, D., and Hope, J. (1959). Dartal in treatment of hospitalized schizophrenic patients. *Diseases Nervous System* **20**, 302.
Laurence, D. R., and Moulton, R. (1960). "Clinical Pharmacology." Little, Brown, Boston, Massachusetts.
LaVerne, A. A. (1961). Compendium of neuropsychopharmacology. *J. Neuropsychiat.* **2**, 375–384.
Law, D. H., Smith, F. W., Benson, G. D., and Sleisenger, M. H. (1959). Therapeutics: Drug therapy of gastrointestinal disease. *Am. J. Med. Sci.* **238**, 638.
Leiberman, D. M., and Vaughan, G. F. (1958). *Practitioner* **181**, 510.
Levinsky, W. J. (1961). Current therapy of common medical problems: The psychotherapeutic agent. *Delaware State Med. J.* **33**, 72.
Lichstein, J. (1959). Tranquilizers and gastric secretion. *J. Gasteroenterol.* **33**, 178.
McHardy, G. (1961). Diarrhea. *In* "Current Therapy" (H. F. Conn, ed.), pp. 223–224. Saunders, Philadelphia, Pennsylvania.
McHardy, G., McHardy, J., and Browne, D. (1959). Management of acute peptic ulcer; measures to prevent recurrence. *Postgrad. Med.* **25**, 668.
McLean, J. D. (1963). Psychopharmacological agents in general practice. *Nova Scotia Med. Bull.* **42**, 12–17.
Mathews, F. P. (1958). A clinical appraisal, Dartal. *Am. J. Psychiat.* **114**, 1034.
Mishler, J. E., and Harley, R. D. (1961). An evaluation of three ataractic and antiemetic agents for intraocular surgery. *Eye, Ear, Nose, Throat Monthly* **40**, 844–849.
Moravec, C. L., and Moravec, M. E. (1961). Relief of emotional stress. *Med. Times* **89**, 249.
Moser, R. H. (1961). Diseases of medical progress: Progress report. *Clin. Pharmacol. Therap.* **2**, 446–522.
Mozan, A. A. (1959). Chymotrypsin therapy of peptic ulcer results in 78 cases. *Postgrad. Med.* **26**, 542.
Pennington, V. M. (1962). Combined psychopharmaceutical treatment in 460 neuropsychiatric patients. *Am. J. Psychiat.* **118**, 935–937
Perloff, M. M., and Levick, L. J. (1960). Anxiety or depression? A common diagnostic and therapeutic problem in general practice. *Clin. Med.* **7**, 2237.
Phelps, M. E. (1959). Why and which tranquilizer. *J. Louisiana State Med. Soc.* **3**, 149.
Plotnikoff, N. P., and Washington, H. (1958). Bioassay of ataractics against lethal action of mescaline in mice. *Proc. Soc. Exptl. Biol. Med.* **98**, 660.
Reboton, J., Jr., Weekly, R. D., Bylenga, N. D., and May, R. H. (1962). Pigmentary retinopathy and irido-cycloplegia in psychiatric patients. *J. Neuropsychiat.* **3**, 311–316.
Rees, L. (1960). Drug treatment of disease: Chlorpromazine and allied phenothiazine derivatives. *Brit. Med. J.* II, 522.
Riccitelli, M. L. (1964). Modern concepts in management of anxiety in aged. *J. Am. Geriat. Soc.* **12**, 652.
Robinson, A. S. (1960). Neck-face syndrome related to phenothiazine drugs. *J. Am. Med. Assoc.* **173**, 504.
Rudolph, J. A., Rudolph, B. M. (1959). Trilafon (perphenazine) and meticorten (prednisone) as ancillary therapy in allergic conditions. *J. Florida Med. Assoc.* **45**, No. 9, 1018–1020.
Schaffner, F. H., and Chesrow, E. (1959). Cholestasis produced by the administration of norethandrolone. *Am. J. Med.* **26**, 249.

Schaumann, O. (1961). Beeinflussung verschiedener Wirkungen von Thiopropazat durch ein zentrales Stimulans. *Arzneimittel-Forsch.* **11**, 343–350.
Schaumann, W., and Kurbjuweit, H.-G. (1961). Beeinfussung der analgetischen Wirkung des Morphins durch Reserpin und Thiopropazat, Naunyn Schmiedeberg. *Arch. Exptl. Pathol. Pharmakol.* **241**, 346–355.
Scott, M. E. (1961). Tranquilizing drugs. *J. Med. Assoc. Georgia* **50**, 11.
Settel, E. (1959). Evaluation of an anticholinergic tranquilizer combinatic in gastrointestinal disorders. *Clin. Med.* **6**, 1227.
Shaw, C. C., and Felts, P. W. (1959). Treacherous tranquilizers. *Am. J. Med. Sci.* **141**, 237.
Shideman, F. E. (1961). Toxicity of the phenothiazines. *Wisconsin Med. J.* **60**, 487–488.
Sleisenger, M. H. (1959). Wohl, M. G. (ed.). Chronic dyspepsia: its relationship to sliding hiatus hernia and gastritis. *In* "Long-Term Illness: Management of the chronically ill Patient" (M. G. Wohl, ed.), pp. 263–267. Saunders, Philadelphia, Pennsylvania.
Smith, J. A., *et al.* (1959). A graphic comparison of five phenothiazines. *Am. J. Psychiat.* **116**, 392.
Souder, C. L. R. (1959). Treatment of Huntington's Chorea with thiopropazate: Case histories. *Delaware State Med. J.* **31**, 239.
Spaulding, W. B. (1962). Dangers in the use of some potent drugs. *Can. Med. Assoc. J.* **87**, 1275–1281.
Steinhilber, R. M. (1962). Psychoses: Schizophrenia. *In* "Current Therapy" (H. F. Conn, ed.), pp. 541–544. Saunders, Philadelphia, Pennsylvania.
Steinhilber, R. M. (1961). Current practices in general medicine. An appraisal of tranquilizers. *Proc. Staff Meetings Mayo Clin.* **36**, 165.
Steinhilber, R. M. (1961). Psychoses: Schizophrenia. *In* "Current Therapy" (H. F. Conn, ed.), pp. 560–563. Saunders, Philadelphia, Pennsylvania.
Stoll, B. A. (1962). Radiation sickness. An analysis of over 1,000 controlled drug trials. *Brit. Med. J.* II, 507–510.
Stone, G. C., Bernstein, B. M., Hambourger, W. E., and Drill, V. A. (1960). Behavioral and pharmacological studies of thiopropazate a potent tranquilizing agent. *Arch. Intern. Pharmacodyn.* **127**, 85.
Stone, C. A., Wenger, H. C., Ludden, C. T., Stavorski, J. M., and Ross C. A. (1961). Antiserotonin-antihistaminic properties of cyproheptadine. *J. Pharmacol. Exptl. Therap.* **131**, 73.
Tice, L. F. (1958). New drugs of 1957. *Drug Cosmetic Ind.* **82**, 454.
"Tranquilizing Drugs" (1959). Combined staff Clinics of the College of Physicians and Surgeons, Columbia University, and the Presbyterian Hospital, New York. *Am. J. Med.* **27**, 767.
Vaisberg, H., and Saunders, J. C. (1963). Treatment of dyskinesias including Huntington's Chorea with thiopropazate and R-1625. *Dis. Nerv. Sys.* **24**, 449–500.
Vates, T. S., and Masucci, E. F. (1960). Acute extrapyramidal syndromes following the use of phenothiazine derivatives. *Med. Ann. District Columbia* **29**. 670.
Werner, G. (1959). Therapeutics—tranquilizing drugs. *Am. J. Med. Sci.* **237**, 631.
Wilson, C. W. M., and Huby, P. M. (1961). An assessment of the responses to drugs acting on the central nervous system. *Clin. Pharmacol. Therap.* **2**, 587–598.
Witkin, L. B., Spitaletta, P., and Plummer, A. J. (1959). Effects of some central depressants on two simple reflexes in the mouse. *J. Pharmacol. Exptl. Therap.* **126**, 330.
Wortis, J. (1959). Review of psychiatric progress 1958: Physiological treatment. *Am. J. Psychiat.* **115**, 599.
Wortis, S. B. (1958). A list of some of the newer drugs used in psychiatric practice. *Am. J. Psychiat.* **114**, 169.

∽ A.15 ∽
Thioridazine

Chemical Papers

Eiduson, S., and Geller, E. (1963). The excretion and metabolism of S-35 labelled thioridazine in urine, blood, bile and feces. *Biochem. Pharmacol.* **12**, 1429.
Eiduson, S., *et al.* (1963). Thioridazine excretion pattern after single and multiple doses in a neuropsychiatric patient. *Biochem. Pharmacol.* **12**, 1437.
Forrest, F. M., *et al.* (1961). Review of rapid urine tests for phenothiazine and related drugs. *Am. J. Psychiat.* **118**, 300.
Forrest, I. A., *et al.* (1960). A rapid urine color test for thioridazine (Mellaril, TP-21, Sandoz). *Am. J. Psychiat.* **116**, 928.
Gold, S., *et al.* (1962). Phenothiazines in urine. *J. Mental Sci.* **108**, 88.
Ragland, J. B., *et al.* (1961). Spectrofluorimetric determination of phenothiazine tranquilizers in biological samples. *Federation Proc.* **20**, Part I, 397.
Rieder, H. P. (1960). Einige specktrophotometrische Charakteristika von Phenothiazin und Thioxanthenderivaten. (Some spectrophotometric characteristics of phenothiazine and thioxanthene derivatives.) *Med. Exptl.* **3**, 353.
Rutschmann, J., *et al.* (1961). 3-Methylthio-10-β-(1'-methyl-2'-piperidyl)-éthyl-phénothiazine (thioridazine, Melleril), étude du métobolisme chez le rat. (3-Methylthio-10-[β-(1'-Methyl-2'-Piperidyl)-Ethyl]-phenothiazine (thioridazine, Mellaril), study of its breakdown in rats.) *Chimia Aarau* **15**, 406.
Vacerkova, J., *et al.* (1962). Ueber den papierchromatographischen Nachweis der Antihistaminica und Ataractica durch Umkehrphasenchomatographie im System Petroleum-Aethanol/Wasser/Ammoniak. (On paper chromatographic determination of antihistamines and ataractics using phase reversal chromatography in a system petroleum/ethanol/water/ammonia.) *Pharmazie* **17**, 22.

Biology and Pharmacology

Boissier, J. R. (1959). L'apport de la pharmacologie experimentale á l'etude des neuroleptiques et des tranquillisants. (Report of the experimental pharmacology for the study of neuroleptics and tranquilizers.) *Actualites Pharmacol.* **12**, 1.
Boissier, J. R., and Pagny, J. (1960). Action antitussive de quelques phénothiazines. (Antitussive effect of some phenothiazines.) *Therapie* **15**, 97.
Boissier, J. R., and Simon, P. (1960). L'utilisation du test de la traction (Test de Julou-Courvoisier) pour l'etude des psycholeptiques. (The use of the traction test (Test of Julou-Courvoisier) for the study of psycholeptics.) *Therapie* **15**, 1170.
Bonfils, S., *et al.* (1963). Derives de la phenothiazine et de l'iminodibenzyle: relation dose efficacite vis-a-vis de l'ulcere. *Therapie* **18**, 373.
Cohen, S. (1963). Excretory patterns and clinical response to the tablet and prolonged action forms of thioridazine. *West Pharmacol. Soc.* **6**, 65.
Eckhardt, E. T., and Plaa, G. L. (1961). Effect of phenothiazines on hepatic blood flow in the mouse. *Pharmacologist* **3**, No. 2, 61.

Frommel, E., et al. (1960). De la pharmacodynamie differentielle des thymoanaleptiques et des substances "neuroleptiques" en experimentation animale. (Comparative pharmacodynamics of thymoanaleptics and "tranquilizing" agents in animal experiments.) *Therapie* **15**, 1175.

Haley, T. J., et al. (1959). A pharmacologic study of Mellaril, 2-methylmercapto-10-[2-(N-methyl-2-piperidyl) ethyl] phenothiazine hydrochloride. *Toxicol. Appl. Pharmacol.* **1**, 377.

Haley, T. J., et al. (1959). Pharmacological effects of Mellaril. *Federation Proc.* **18**, Part I, 399.

Haley, T. J., et al. (1960). Pharmacological comparison of chlorpromazine and Mellaril, 3-methylmercapto-10-[2-(N-methyl-2-piperdyl)-ethyl]-phenothiazine hydrochloride. *Arch. Intern. Pharmacodyn.* **124**, 455.

Heistad, G. T., and Torres, A. A. (1959). A mechanism for the effect of a tranquilizing drug on learned emotional responses. *Univ. Minn. Med. Bull.* **30**, 518.

Hoffman, F. A., and Bente, D. (1960). Untersuchungen über das Verhalten des Jendrassik'schen Bahnungseffektes auf spinale Eigenreflexe unter neuroleptischer Medikation. (Investigations on the behavior of Jendrassik's facilitation effect on spinal tendon reflexes under tranquilizing drugs.) *Med. Exptl.* **2**, 126.

Itil, T. (1961). Elektroencephalographische Befunde zur Klassifikation neuround thymoleptischer Medikamente. (EEG reaction for the classification of neuroleptic and thymoleptic drugs.) *Med. Exptl.* **5**, 347.

Keup, W. (1959). Influence of phenothiazines on liver function. *In* "Psychopharmacology Frontiers" (N.S. Kline, ed.), pp. 365–371. Little, Brown, Boston, Massachusetts.

Mayer, K. (1959). Klinische und pharmakopsychologische Untersuchungen zur therapeutischen Wirkungsweise von Phenothiazinen. (Clinical and pharmacopsychological studies on the thereapeutic mode of action of phenothiazines.) *Medizinische* pp. 733–736.

Mayer, K. (1960). Untersuchungsmethoden zur Beurteilung der Wirkung psychotroper substanzen. (Experimental methods for the evaluation of the effect of psychotropic drugs.) *Med. Exptl.* **2**, 90.

Meuwly, J. (1960). Wirkung von KS 33 und Melleril im tierversuch. (Effect of KS 33 and Mellaril in animal experiments.) *Therap. Umschau* **17**, 371.

Murphree, O. D., et al. (1962). Survival of offspring of rats administered phenothiazines during pregnancy. *J. Neuropsychiat.* **3**, 295.

Neve, H. K. (1961). The excretion of thioridazine (Mellaril, TP 21) in urine. *Acta Pharmacol. Toxicol.* **17**, 404.

Plaa, G. L., et al. (1960). Effect of thioridazine and chlorpromazine on rat liver hemodynamics. *Am. J. Physiol.* **199**, 793.

Plaa, G. L., et al. (1961). Effect of CCl_4 on certain aspects of thioridazine metobolism. *Federation Proc.* **20**, Part I, 171.

Purshottam, N. (1962). Effects of tranquilizers on induced ovulation in mice. *Am. J. Obstet. Gynecol.* **83**, 1405.

Swinyard, E. A., et al. (1959). Some neuropharmacological properties of thioridazine hydrochloride (Mellaril). *J. Pharmacol. Exptl. Therap.* **126**, 312.

Taeschler, M., and Cerletti, A. (1959). Differential analysis of the effects of phenothiazine-tranquilizers on emotional and motor behavior in experimental animals. *Nature* **184**, 823.

Taeschler, M., and Cerletti, A. (1959). Effets de quelques dérivés de la phénothiazine sur des reactions motrices et emotionnelles du rat. (Effect of some phenothiazine drivatives on motor and emotional reactions in rats.) *J. Physiol. (Paris)* **51**, 873.

Taeschler, M., and Cerletti, A. (1958). Zur Pharmakologie von Thioridazin, Melleril. (The pharmacology of thioridazine, Mellaril.) *Schweiz. Med. Wochschr.* **88**, 1216.

Tobik, S., and Czaicki, W. (1960). Leczenie wczesnego aespoiu poresekcyjnego (Dumping syndrom). (Treatment of the early syndrome after gastric resection, dumping syndrome.) *Polski Tygod. Lekar.* **15**, 1120.

Torres, A. A. (1961). Anxiety versus escape conditioning and tranquilizing. *J. Comp. Psychol.* **54**, 349.
Ulett, G. A., *et al.* (1961). Influence of chlordiazepoxide on drug-altered EEG patterns and behavior. *Med. Exptl.* **5**, 386.
Weidmann, H. (1961). Zur Pharmakologie psychotroper Wirkstoffe. (The pharmacology of psychotropic drugs.) *Schweiz. Arch. Tierheilk.* **103**, 191.
Wright, R. L. D., and Kyne, W. P. (1960). A clinical and experimental comparison of four anti-schizophrenic drugs. *Psychopharmacologia* **1**, 437.
Zehnder, K., *et al.* (1962). The metabolism of thioridazine (Mellaril) and one of its pyrrolidine analogues in the rat. *Biochem. Pharmacol.* **11**, 535.

Side Effects

Anderson, J. H., *et al.* (1961). The complications and side effects of the phenothiazine ataraxics. A review of 178 clinical series of 10 phenothiazine derivatives. *Bol. Asoc. Med. Puerto Rico* **53**, 3.
Appelbaum, A. (1963). An ophthalmoscopic study of patients under treatment with thioridazine. *Arch. Ophthalmol.* **69**, 578.
Bach, J. M., and Fleeson, W. (1960). Granulocyte suppression with thioridazine hydrochloride. *J. Am. Med. Assoc.* **173**, 793.
Block, S. L. (1962). Jaundice following thioridazine administration. *Am. J. Psychiat.* **119**, 77.
Blumberg, A. G., and Klein, D. F. (1961). Severe papilledema associated with drug therapy. *Am. J. Psychiat.* **118**, 168.
Bovi, A. (1963). Prove combinate di funzionalita epatica in un gruppo di soggetti trattati con tioridazina. (Application of a series of liver function tests in a group of persons treated with thioridazine.) *Rass. Studi Psichiat.* **52**, 312.
Castelnuovo-Tedesco, P., *et al.* (1963). Galactorrhea, headache and weight gain during treatment with thioridazine. *Am. J. Psychiat.* **119**, 1178.
Clein, L. (1962). Thioridazine and ejaculation. *Brit. Med. J.* II, 548–549.
Datshkovsky, J. (1961). Mellaril: Ejaculation disorders. *Am. J. Psychiat.* **118**, 564.
de Margerie, J. (1962). Ocular changes produced by a phenothiazine drug: Thioridazine. *Trans. Can. Ophthalmol. Soc.* **25**, 160.
Ehlers, H. (1963). Poisoning with psychopharmaca and barbiturate-free hypnotics. *Danish Med. Bull.* **10**, 117.
Enticknap, J. B., and Gordon, B. (1961). Suicide with thioridazine. *Brit. Med. J.* II, 522–523.
Freedman, D. X., and de Jong, J. (1961). Thresholds for drug-induced akathisia. *Am. J. Psychiat.* **117**, 930.
Freedman, D. X., and de Jong, J. (1961). Factors that determine drug-induced akathisia. *Diseases Nervous System* **22**, No. 2, Suppl. 69.
Freyhan, F. A. (1961). Loss of ejaculation during Mellaril treatment. *Am. J. Psychiat.* **118**, 171.
Furtado, D. (1959). Etude de la toxicité neurologique de deux nouveaux médicaments: l'imipramine et la thioridazine. (Study of the neurological toxicity of two new drugs: Imipramine and thioridazine.) *Rev. Neurol.* **100**, 763.
Guérin, A. (1960). Suicides au melleril et au nozinan. (Suicides with Mellaril and Nozinan.) *J. Med. Bordeaux* **137**, 748.
Guérin, A. (1960). Suicides au melleril et au nozinan. (Suicides with Mellaril and Nozinan.) *Ann. Med.-Psychol.* **118**/II, 353.
Heller, J. (1961). Another case of inhibition of ejaculation as a side effect of Mellaril. *Am. J. Psychiat.* **118**, 173.
Henne, M., Tonnel, M., and Henne, S. (1961). A propos des états mixtes, Une observation

de syndrome de Cotard maniaque. (Mixed manic states. Observation of a case of Cotard's syndrome.) *Ann. Med.-Psychol.* **119**/1, 318.
Heshe, J., et al. (1961). Retinabeskadigelse opstaet under thioridazinbehandling. (Retinopathy occurring during treatment with thioridazine.) *Nord. Psykiat. Tidskr.* **15**, 442.
Hollister, L. E. (1964). Adverse reactions to phenothiazines. *J. Am. Med. Assoc.* **189**, 311.
Hollister, L. E., and Barthel, C. A. (1959). Changes in the electroencephalogram during chronic administration of tranquilizing drugs. *Electroencephalog. Clin. Neurophysiol.* **11**, 792.
Jorgensen, F. (1962). Ejakulationshaemning under Mellerilbehandling. (Inhibition of ejaculation occurring during treatment with Mellaril.) *Ugeskrift Laeger* **124**, 565.
Kelly, H. G., et al. (1963). Thioridazine hydrochloride (Mellaril): Its effect on the electrocardiogram and a report of two fatalities with electrocardiographic abnormalities. *Can. Med. Assoc. J.* **89**, 546.
Keup, W. (1959). Effect of phenothiazine derivatives on liver function. *Diseases Nervous System* **20**, 161.
Madan, B. R. (1963). Some cardiovascular actions of thioridazine hydrochloride. *Arch. Intern. Pharmacodyn.* **144**, 299.
May, R. H. et al. (1960). Thioridazine therapy: Results and complications. *J. Nervous Mental Disease* **130**, 230.
Mayer, K. (1961). Thioridazinmedikation und Fahrtuchtigkeit. (Thioridazine administration and the ability to drive a car.) *Med. Exptl.* **5**, 186.
Morrison, S. B. (1960). Transient visual symptoms associated with Mellaril medication. *Am. J. Psychiat.* **116**, 1032.
Olsen, T. (1962). Ejakulationshaemning under Mellerilbehandling. (Inhibition of ejaculation during Mellaril medication.) *Ugeskrift Laeger* **124**, 871.
Pomme, B., et al. (1963). Troubles de la libido par chimiotherapie en practique psychiatrique. (Libido disorders precipitated by chemotherapy in psychiatry.) *Presse Med.* **71**, 1387.
Qureshi, M. S. (1962). Thioridazine and ejaculation. *Medicus (Karachi)* **15**, 39.
Rosati, D. (1964). Hypotensive side effects of phenothiazine and their management. *Diseases Nervous System* **25**, 366.
Shader, R. I. (1964). Sexual dysfunction associated with thioridazine hydrochloride. *J. Am. Med. Assoc.* **188**, 1007.
Shaw, R. K., et al. (1964). Agranulocytosis associated with thioridazine administration. *J. Am. Med. Assoc.* **187**, 614.
Singh, H. (1961). A case of inhibition of ejaculation as a side effect of Mellaril. *Am. J. Psychiat.* **117**, 1041.
Stratas, N. E., et al. (1963). A study of drug induced Parkinsonism. *Diseases Nervous System* **24**, 180.
Swanson, D. W. (1961). Hypotension associated with thioridazine HCl. *Am. J. Psychiat.* **117**, 834.
Taubel, D. E. (1962). Mellaril: Ejaculation disorders. *Am. J. Psychiat.* **119**, 87.
Waldrop, F. N., et al. (1961). A comparison of the therapeutic and toxic effects of thioridazine and chlorpromazine in chronic schizophrenic patients. *Comprehensive Psychiat.* **2**, 96.
Weekley, R. D., et al. (1960). Pigmentary retinopathy in patients receiving high doses of a new phenothiazine. *AMA Arch. Ophthalmol.* **64**, 65.
Wendkos, M. H. (1963). Thioridazine and electrocardiographic abnormalities. *Can. Med. Assoc. J.* **89**, 1297.
Williatte, P. (1961). Note sur un cas d'intoxication par le Melleril. (Note of a case of intoxication with Mellaril.) *J. Sci. Med. Lille* p. 597.
Witton, K. (1962). Sexual dysfunction secondary to Mellaril. *Diseases Nervous System* **23**, 175.
Zuckerman, F. (1962). Amenorrhea occurring during Mellaril treatment. *Am. J. Psychiat.* **118**, 947.

A.15. THIORIDAZINE

Clinical Papers

Aaronson, H. G., *et al.* (1962). Thioridazine hydrochloride in the treatment of a jaundiced psychotic patient. *J. Am. Med. Assoc.* **182**, 678

Alanen, Y. O. (1963). Skitsofrenian ja neuroosien välisistä rajatiloista. (Borderline cases between Schizophrenia and neurosis.) *Suomen Lääk. L.* **18**, 1179.

Alderton, H. R., and Hoddinott, B. A. (1964). A controlled study of the use of thioridazine in the treatment of hyperactive and aggressive children in a children's psychiatric hospital. *Can. Psychiat. Assoc. J.* **9**, 239.

Allen, M., *et al.* (1963). Thioridazine hydrochloride in the behavior disturbances of retarded children. *Am. J. Mental Deficiency* **68**, 63.

Alonso, V. (1961). Experiencias terapéuticas con Tioridazina en enfermos psicóticos. (Clinical experience with thioridazine in psychotic patients.) *Neurol.-Neurocir. Psiquiat. (Mex.)* **2**, 85.

Anastassopoulos, G., and Routsonis, C. (1961). Application de la thioridazine (Melleril) chez des malades ambulants psychotiques et psychonevrotiques. [Use of thioridazine (Mellaril) in psychotic and psychoneurotic out-patients.] *Galinos* **3**, 16.

Azima, H., *et al.* (1959). The effect of thioridazine (Mellaril) on mental syndromes. Comparison with chlorpromazine and promazine. *Can. Med. Assoc. J.* **31**, 549.

Bachmeyer, H. (1963). Schmerzlinderung in der Geburtshilfe. (Analgesia in obstetrics.) *Geburtsh. Frauenheilk.* **23**, 461.

Badham, J. N., *et al.* (1963). A trial of thioridazine in mental deficiency. *Brit. J. Psychiat.* **109**, 408.

Barindelli Irisarri, L. A., and Strazzarino, C. S. (1962). El Melleril en psiquiatria pediatrica. (Melleril in pediatric psychiatry.) *Rev. Psiquiat. Urug.* **27**, 57.

Barone, G., *et al.* (1959). La tioridazina in chirurgia generale. (Thioridazine in general surgery.) *Gazz. Intern. Med. Chir.* **64**, 3545.

Barsa, J. A., and Saunders, J. C. (1960). Thioridazine (Mellaril) in the treatment of chronic schizophrenics. *Am. J. Psychiat.* **116**, 1028.

Bartra, Vigo, V. A. (1962). La Tioridazina en el postoperatorio inmediato. (Thioridazine in the post operative period.) Thesis, Lima, Peru.

Barucci, M., and De Luca, P. L. (1960). Esperienze clinche con l'impiego della tioridazina in un gruppo di schizofrenici considerati irrecuperabili. (Clinical experiences with the use of thioridazine in a group of schizophrenics considered as incurable.) *Rass. Studi Psichiat.* **49**, 821.

Barucci, M., *et al.* (1962). Su una particolare fase di iperestesia emotiva osservata in alcuni schizofrenici durante il trattamento con tioridazina. (A special phase of heightened emotional sensitivity in a number of schizophrenics during treatment with thioridazine.) *Rass. Studi Psichiat.* **51**, 415.

Bastecky, J. (1962). Zkusenosti s lecbou mellerilem. (Experiences with Mellaril therapy.) *Cesk. Psychiat.* **58**, 413.

Bastecky, J. (1963). Pusobeni melleriulu na stabilizaci remise u endogennich depresi. (Effect of Mellaril on stabilisation of improvement in endogenous depression.) *Cesk. Psychiat.* **59**, 110.

Bauer, A. (1962). Klinische Erfahrungen mit Thioridazin (Melleril-Sandoz) anhand von 202 Fallen, zugleich ein Beitrag zur Problema-tik der Behandlung endogener Depressionen. (Clinical experiences with thioridazine (Melleril-Sandoz) in 202 cases, with a contribution on the problem of treatment of endogenous depressions.) *Nervenarzt* **33**, 321.

Belin, J. (1963). Trois ans d'experience des traitements par la thioridazine en medecine generale. (Three years' experience of treatment with thioridazine in general medical practice.) *J. Med. Lyon* **44**, 283.

Bellville, T. P., et al. (1963). A comparative study of thioridazine and carphenazine using sequential analysis. *Psychopharmacologia* **4**, 53.

Bercel, N. A. (1961). Clinical trial of thioridazine in private practice. *Am. Practitioner* **12**, 44.

Bergouignan, M., et al. (1960). Peut-on assigner des indications cliniques particulières aux diverses phenothiazines? Notre experience de la thioridazine. (Can particular clinical indications be assigned to various phenothiazines? Our experience with thioridazine.) *Ann. Med.-Psychol.* **118**, 923.

Bergouignan, M., et al. (1960). Resultats obtenus avec la thioridazine (TP-21 ou Melleril Sandoz) seule ou associee, dans quelques affections mentales. (Results obtained with thioridazine (TP-21 or Mellaril-Sandoz), alone or combined, in some mental disorders.) *Ann. Med.-Psychol.* **118**, 565.

Berguignan, M., et al. (1960). Une nouvelle phénothiazine, la thioridazine, au banc d'essai de la clinique psychiatrique. (Thioridazine, a new phenothiazine derivative: A trial in a psychiatric clinic.) *J. Med. Bordeaux* p. 376.

Bilikiewicz, A. (1961). Leczenie mellerylem w psychiatrii w świetle wlasnych doświadczén Klinicznych. (Mellaril treatment in psychiatry, personal clinical experiences.) *Neurol. Neurochir. Psychiat. Polan.* **11**, 131.

Bluestone, H. (1961). The treatment of anxiety in prison inmates. *Am. J. Psychiat.* **118**, 245.

Bonduelle, M., et al. (1961). La thioridazine en thérapeutique neurologique ambulatoire: Céphalées, impatiences. (Thioridazine for treatment in ambulant neurology: Headache and restless legs.) *Gaz. Med. Franc.* **68**, 1907.

Boissier, J. R. (1960). Neuroleptiques et catatonie expérimentale. (Tranquilizers and experimental catatonia.) *Therapie* **15**, 73.

Boissier, J. R., et al. (1959). Action pharmacologique d'un nouveau neuroleptique pheńothiazinique: la thioridazine (TP 21). (Pharmacologic action of thioridazine (TP 21); a new phenothiazine neuroleptic.) *Therapie* **14**, 793.

Brougher, J. C. (1960). The treatment of emotional disorders in obstetrics and gynecology with thioridazine. *Quart. Rev. Surg. Obstet. Gynecol.* **17**, 44.

Brunold, H. (1959). Erfahrunger mit einem neuen Phenothiazinderivat ("Melleril" Sandoz). (Experience with a new phenothiazine derivative (Melleril Sandoz).) *Therap. Umschau* **16**, 90.

Bunjac, M. (1961). Utilisation de la thioridazine chez les enfants inadaptes. (Use of thioridazine in problem children.) Thesis, Paris.

Burkard, M. (1962). Neue Wege zur Therapie der kindlichen Enuresis nocturna. (New ways to therapy of infantile enuresis nocturna.) *Med. Klin. (Munich)* **57**, 1226.

Caffey, E. M., et al. (1964). Discontinuation or reduction of chemotherapy in chronic schizophrenics. *J. Chronic Diseases* **17**, 347.

Cagnoni, G. (1961). Primi risultati dell'impiego della tioridazina nella gestante a termine ed in travaglio di parto. (First results of the use of thioridazine for pregant women at term and during labour.) *Attualita Ostet. Ginec.* **7**, 143.

Cajipe-Villegas, C. (1961). Clinical trial with Melleril on psychiatric patients. *Philippine J. Psychiat. Neurol.* **2**, 58.

Caldwell, W. G. (1960). The menopause. Understanding and treatment. *Med. Times* **88**, 1007.

Caldwell, W. G. (1961). Thioridazine in the emotional disorders of menopause. *Western Med.* **2**, 441.

Cavallé, A. (1960). Nuestros primeros ensayos con la tioridazina (TP-21). (Our first investigations with thioridazine (TP-21).) *Med. Clin. (Barcelona)* **34**, 289.

Chemin, J. (1962). Essai d'une prémédication tranquillisante en stomatologie par la thioridazine. (Attempts at tranquillizing premedication with thioridazine in stomatology.) *Cahiers Odonto-stomatol.* **12**, 33.

Cohen, S. (1958). TP-21, a new phenothiazine. *Am. J. Psychiat.* **115**, 358.

Cohen, S. (1964). Thioridazine (Mellaril)—a review. *Mind* **2**, 134.
Cohen, S., and Pillsbury, R. M. (1960). Psychopharmacology and the "deteriorated" schizophrenic patient. *Diseases Nervous System* **21**, 677.
Cole, J. O. (1964). Psychopharmacology Service Center Collaborative Study Group. Phenothiazine treatment in acute schizophrenia. *Arch. Gen. Psychiat.* **10**, 246.
Coltorti, M., and Di Simone, A. (1962). Valutazione terapeutica della tioridazina sulla base dei resultati ottenuti in 50 casi. (Evaluation, based on results in 50 cases, of the therapeutic effect of thioridazine.) *Minerva Med.* **53**, 3361.
Cotlenko, M. (1963). Traitement par les gouttes de thioridazine des troubles du caractere et des etats anxieux de l'enfant. (Treatment with thioridazine drops of character disorders and anxiety in children.) *Rev. Med. Franc.* **77**, Suppl. No. 2, 11.
Coullaut, R., et al. (1960). Nuestra experiencia con un nuevo derivado fenotiacinico (TP-21. Melleril) en la esquizofrenia. (Our experiences with a new phenothiazine derivative (TP-21. Mellaril) in schizophrenia.) *Bol. Cult. Consejo. Col. Med. Espana* **23**, 1.
Crawford, B. K. A. (1961). The treatment of non-european schizophrenic patients in a special unit with Mellaril. *Med. Proc.* **7**, 333.
Cuchí de la Cuesta, C. (1960). Ensayo clínico con el TP-21 o tioridazina en medicina interna. (Clinical examination of TP-21 (thioridazine) in internal medicine.) *Arch. Fac. Med. Zaragoza* **8**, 445.
Daggett, D. R., et al. (1962). Thioridazine in short term treatment of acute psychiatric disorders. *Clin. Med.* **69**, 927.
Daggett, D. R., et al. (1962). Thioridazine in short-term treatment of acute psychiatric disorders. *Minn. Med.* **45**, 9.
Damania, G. B., and Masani, K. R. (1961). Clinical evaluation of Mellaril—a new tranquillizer. *Indian J. Psychiat.* **3**, 95.
Dardenne, P., and Soleil-Ravoup, J. P. (1961). Effets de la thioridazine sur le comportement des femmes agees en milieu d'hospice. (Effects of thioridazine on the behavior of old-aged women in a hospital setting.) *Presse Med.* **69**, 826.
David, N. A., et al. (1960). Evaluation of thioridazine (Mellaril), a new phenothiazine, in the hospitalized patient. *Antibiot. Med. Clin. Therapy* **7**, 364.
Deberdt, R. (1961). Expériences avec la thioridazine (TP 21). (Experiences with thioridazine (TP 21).) *Acta Neurol. Belg.* **61**, 652.
D'Elia, G., and Rocco, P. G. (1963). Osservazione sulla utilizzazione di questionari nella sperimentazione clinico-farmacologica della tioridazina. (Use of questionnaires in a clinico-pharmacological trial of Melleril.) *Ann. Freniat.* **76**, 358.
Delay, J., et al. (1959). Essais clinques d'un nouveau neuroleptique, la thioridazine. (Clinical trial of a new tranquilizer, thioridazine.) *Ann. Med.-Psychol.* **117**, 724, T.1.
Delay, J., et al. (1959). Essais cliniques d'un nouveau neuroleptique, la thioridazine. (Clinical trials of a new tranquilizer, thioridazine.) *Presse Med.* **67**, 1213.
Destounis, N. (1963). Thioridazine and amenorrhea. *Am. J. Psychiat.* **120**, 188.
Dierks, M. (1963). A comparison of two phenothiazines in the treatment of schizophrenics *Am. J. Psychiat.* **119**, 775.
Diethelm, R., and Früh, A. (1961). Erfahrungen mit Melleril in der Kinderpsychiatrie. (Experience with Mellaril in pediatric psychiatry.) *Praxis (Bern)* **50**, 1364.
Ditman, K. S. (1961). Evaluation of drugs in the treatment of alcoholics. *Quart. J. Studies Alc.* **22**, 107.
Drwal, T., and Majczak, A. (1960). Próby leczenia chorych psychicznie benaktyzyna i melerylem. (Therapeutic trial of Benactyzine and Mellaril in mental patients.) *Polski Tygol. Lekar. Wiadomosci Lekar.* **13**, 349.
Editorial. (1960). Experimentelle Untersuchung psychoaktiver Pharmaka. (Experimental investigation of psychoactive drugs.) *Triangle* **4**, 244.
Flegel, H. (1962). Zur Dikumentation und Auswertung psychiatrisch-klinischer Verlaufs-

gegebenheiten fur die Erprobung von Psychopharmaka anlässlich Thioridazinmedikation. (On the documentation and evaluation of psychiatric-clinical courses for trial of psychopharmaca by using thioridazin medication.) *Nervenarzt* **33**, 112.

Floch, H. (1962). Essai de traitement symptomatique par la thioridazine de l'instabilite psychomotrice chez des enfants deficients mentaux. (Symptomatic treatment by thioridazine of psychomotor restlessness in mentally deficient children: A trial.) Thesis, Paris.

Flügel, F., et al. (1960). Zur Stellung des Thioridazins in der Pharmakotherapie depressiver Erkrankungen. (The status of thioridazine in the drug treatment of depressive diseases.) *Med. Exptl.* **2**, 153.

Foschi, F., and Monaci, G. (1962). Note sull'uso ospedaliero della tioridazina (Melleril) in malati acuti e cronici. (Remarks on the use of thioridazine (Melleril) in hospitalized patients, acute and chronic.) *Riv. Sper. Freniat.* **86**, 1039.

Frain, M. M. (1960). Preliminary report on Mellaril in epilepsy. *Am. J. Psychiat.* **117**, 547.

Freed, S. C. (1959). Thioridazine, a neuroleptic in general practice. *Intern. Record Med.* **172**, 644.

Geller, E., and Eiduson, S. (1960). Thioridazine excretion patterns after single and multiple doses. *Federation Proc.* **19**, 279.

Gomez-Reino and Filgueira, J., and Fernandez, V. L. (1962). Nuestras experiencias con el "Meleril" en la mania endogena y en las esquisofrenias paranoides cronicas. (Our experiences with Mellaril in endogenic mania and in chronic paranoid schizophrenia.) *Actas Luso-Espan. Neurol. Psyquiat. (Madrid)* **21**, 159.

Gorham, D. R., and Pokorny, A. D. (1964). Effects of a phenothiazine and/or group psychotherapy with schizophrenics. *Diseases Nervous System* **25**, 77.

Goswami, B. M. (1962). A clinical trial with thioridazine hydrochloride. *J. Indian Med. Assoc.* **39**, 25.

Gover, D. M. (1962). Thioridazine and chlorprothixene in the management of anxiety in tuberculous patients. *Am. Rev. Respirat. Diseases* **85**, 587.

Grenfell, R. F., et al. (1962). Antihypertensive drugs: A controlled evaluation. *J. Miss. Med. Assoc.* **3**, 93.

Gripwall, E. (1962). Ett nytt fenthiazinderivat—thioridazin. (Thioridazine, a new phenothiazine derivative.) *Nord. Med.* **68**, 1167.

Gross, H., et al. (1960). Thioridazin (Mellaril) ein neues Neuroleptikum für die Klinische und die ambulante Psychiatrie. (Thioridazine (Mellaril) a new tranquilizer for clinical and ambulant psychiatry.) *Wien. Med. Wochschr.* **110**, 844.

Gucciardi, G. (1960). Suff'effetto psicorilassante della tioridazina. (The psychorelaxant effect of thioridazine.) *Clin. Terap.* **18**, 103.

Guillerm, et al. (1961). Essai thérapeutique de la Thioridazine, Notes préliminaires. (Therapeutic trial with thioridazine. Preliminary report.) *Ouest Med.* **14**, 836.

Haug, J. O. (1959). Kontrollerte kliniske forsøk med thioridazin (Mellaril)—et nytt Phenothiazinderivat. (A controlled clinical trial of thioridazine (Mellaril), a new phenothiazine derivative.) *Tidsskr. Norske Laegeforen.* **79**, 317.

Haupt, F. J. G. (1960). A clinical trail of Mellaril (TP-21) in the treatment of mental disorders. *S. African Med. J.* **34**, 92.

Henne, M., et al. (1961). Resultats personnels de l'usage de thioridazine. Essais de fortes doses. (Experience with the use of thioridazine. Studies with high doses.) *Presse Med.* **69**, 995.

Herman, E., and Pleasure, H. (1963). Clinical evaluation of thioridazine and chlorpromazine in chronic schizophrenics. *Diseases Nervous System* **24**, 54.

Hirschmann, J. (1961). Phenothiazine in der Neurologie. (Phenothiazines in neurology.) *Med. Exptl.* **5**, 263.

Hoffet, H. (1962). Beitrag zur Behandlung der Depressionen, Typologische Gliederung depressiver Syndrome und somatotherapeutische Indikationsstellungen. (Contribution to the therapy of depressions. Typological classification of depressive syndromes and somatotherapeutic indications.) *Bibliotheca Psychiat. Neurol.* **115**, Fasc., 1–55.

Hofmann, G., and Kryspin-Exner, K. (1960). Klinische Erfahrungen mit einem neuen Neuroleptikum (TP-21, Melleril). (Clinical experiences with a new tranquilizer (TP-21, Mellaril).) *Wien. Med. Wochschr.* **110**, 897.

Hollister, L. E., and MacDonald, B. F. (1959). Thioridazine (Mellaril) in psychiatric patients. *Calif. Med.* **91**, 274.

Hollister, L. E., et al. (1960). Use of thioridazine for intensive treatment of schizophrenics refractory to other tranquilizing drugs. *J. Neurol. Psychiat.* **1**, 200.

Hollister, L. E., et al. (1963). Comparison of intramuscular and oral administration of chlorpromazine and thioridazine. *Arch. Intern. Pharmacodyn.* **144**, 571.

Hughes, W. (1961). A comparative evaluation of two phenothiazines in the management of chronic schizophrenia. *Can. Med. Assoc. J.* **84**, 268.

Jackson, E. B. (1961). Mellaril in the treatment of the geriatric patient. *Am. J. Psychiat.* **118**, 543.

Jacobs, R. (1962). Zur Therapie mit Melleretten in einem padopsychiatrischen Krankenhaus. (Therapy with Mellaril-10 in a paedopsychiatric hospital.) *Med. Welt* **1962**, 1427.

Jakab, I., and Muller, C. (1961). L'influence des produits pharmaceutiques sur l'expression graphique des aliénés. (Drug influences on graphic expression of psychiatric patients.) *Neuropsichiatria* **17**, 405.

Jancar, J. (1962). Mellarill and placebo in the treatment of severely subnormal patients. *J. Mental Subnorm.* **7**/1, 3.

Johnson, M. H., and Davies, J. R. (1963). Electroshock and thioridazine therapy in the presence of glaucoma. *Am. J. Psychiat.* **120**, 397.

Jones, A. L., et al. (1960). Use of thioridazine (Mellaril) in a variety of clinical settings. *Can. Med. Assoc. J.* **83**, 948.

Judah, L., et al. (1959). Psychiatric response of geriatric-psychiatric patients to Mellaril (TP-21 Sandoz). *Am. J. Psychiat.* **115**, 1118.

Kandic, B., and Grbesa, B. (1962). Osvrt na meleril (TP21) novi fenotijazinski derivat sa gledista njegove primene u psihijatriji (Review of Melleril (TP21). A new phenothiazine derivative, as regards its use in psychiatry.) *Vojnosanit. Pregled* **19**, 619.

Kateryniuk, N. (1961). Clinical study of thioridazine hydrochloride. *Diseases Nervous System* **22**, 149.

Kent, D. A. (1960). Thioridazine. *Brit. Med. J.* I, 1888.

Khakee, A., and Hess, G. F. (1960). Mellaril in the treatment of chronically disturbed patients: With special reference to reduced extrapyramidal complications. *Am. J. Psychiat.* **116**, 1029.

Kinross-Wright, J. (1959). Newer phenothiazine drugs in treatment of nervous disorders. *J. Am. Med. Assoc.* **170**, 1283.

Kinross-Wright, V. J. (1958). Evaluation of a new tranquilizing drug: Thioridazine. Scientific Exhibit Interim Meeting, Minneapolis, Minnesota, Dec. 2–5, 1958.

Kirchgraber, D. (1963). Klinik der Nebenerscheinungen eines "milden" und doch wirksamen neuroleptischen Mittels (Melleril). (Clinical aspects of the side effects of a "mild" but effective neuroleptic agent (Melleril).) *Schweiz. Arch. Neurol. Neurochir. Psychiat.* **91**, 412.

Kleibel, von F. (1961). Ein Weg zur Schmerzbekampfung bei Karzinomkranken. Klinische Prufung von Thioridazin (Melleril und Melleretten) an 251 Patienten. [A way to treat pains in patients with carcinonia. Clinical trial of thioridazine (Mellaril and Melleretten)—251 patients.] *Muench. Med. Wochschr.* **103**, 2341.

Kral, V. A. (1961). The use of thioridazine (Mellaril) in aged people. *Can. Med. Assoc. J.* **84**, 152.

Kristjansen, P., and Borup Svendsen, B. (1959). Mellerel-(Thioridazin-) behandling af langvarige psykoser. (Mellaril-(thioridazine) treatment in psychoses of long duration.) *Nord. Psykiat. Medlemsbl.* **13**, 80.

Kuberski, Z. (1961). Melleril zur Behandlung von Nervenkrankheiten bei Kindern. (Mellaril as therapy in nervous diseases of children.) *Praxis (Bern)*, **50**, 233.

Kuberski, Z. (1962). Proby leczenia plasawicy mniejszej melerylem. (Clinical trial with Melleril in chorea minor.) *Polski Tygod. Lekar. Wiadomosci Lekar.* **15**, 1273.

Lapolla, A. (1960). Therapeutic properties of a new phenothiazine in emotional stress. *Western Med.* **1**, 20.

Lasky, J. J., *et al.* (1962). Drug treatment of schizophrenic patients. A comparative evaluation of chlorpromazine, chlorprothixene, fluphenazine, reserpine, thioridazine and triflupromazine. *Diseases Nervous System* **23**, 698.

Lechner, H., *et al.* (1961). Psychopharmaca und Gehirnkreislauf. (Psychopharmaca and cerebral circulation.) *Med. Exptl.* **5**, 291.

Leder, S., and Urbański, I. (1960). Przypadek zaburzeń psychicznych w przebiegu rozsianego tocznia rumieniowatego. (Psychic disorders in a case of Lupus Erythematodes.) *Polski Tygod. Lekar.* **15**, 1418.

LeVann, L. J. (1961). Thioridazine (Mellaril) a psycho-sedative virtually free of side-effects. *Alberta Med. Bull.* **26**, 144.

Lichstein, J., and de Costa Mayer, J. (1962). Symptoms of autonomic imbalance and treatment in gastrointestinal dysfunction. *Am. Practitioner Dig. Treat.* **13**, 303.

Madan, B. R., and Pendse, V. K. (1963). Antiarrhythmic activity of thioridazine hydrochloride (Mellaril). *Am. J. Cardiol.* **11**, 78.

Magli, G. (1960). Un nuovo farmaco psico-rilassante nella pratica ostetrica. (A new psychorelaxant in obstetrical practice.) *Rass. Intern. Clin. Terap.* **40**, 950.

Majluf, E. (1961). La tioridacina en psiquiatria infantil. (Thioridazine in child psychiatry.) *Rev. Neuro-Psiquiat.* **24**, 291.

Manetti, P., and de Luca, P. L. (1962). Sull'impiego dell'orfenadrina in associazione con la tioridazina e con l'haloperidol. (On the use of orphenadrine together with thioridazine and with haloperidol.) *Rass. Studi Psichiat.* **51**, 419.

Mastrobuono, M. (1960). Contributo alla conoscenza di un nuovo neurolettico, il Melleril. (Contribution to clinical experience with a new tranquilizing drug, Mellaril.) *Riv. Sper. Freniat.* **84**, 477.

Mayer, K., and Oldenkott, P. (1960). Zur Behandlung der Trigeminusneuralgie mit zentral und peripher wirksamen Medikamenten. (Treatment of trigeminal neuralgia with central and peripheral effective drugs.) *Deut. Z. Nervenheilk.* **180**, 665.

Mayr, F., *et al.* (1962). Erfahrungen mit dem Phenothiazin-Derivat Melleril (Thioridazin) in der psychiatrischen Therapie. (Experiences with the phenothiazine derivative Mellaril (thioridazine) in psychiatric therapy.) *Wien. Med. Wochschr.* **112**, 366.

Michaux, M. H., *et al.* (1964). Phenothiazines in the treatment of newly admitted state hospital patients: global comparison of eight compounds in terms of an outcome index. *Current Therap. Res.* **6**, 331.

Micheletti, V., and Teti, V. (1959). Esperienze cliniche con un nuovo preparato fenotiazinico. (Clinical experiences with a new phenothiazine preparation.) *Riv. Sper. Freniat.* **83**, 1161.

Miller, J. (1960). Treatment of emotional problems in allergic disorders: A double-blind placebo-controlled study. *Psychosomatics* **1**, 1.

Monnerot, E., *et al.* (1962). Contribution a l'etude et a la mise en evidence de l'action originale ambivalente d' un neuroleptique majeur: la thioridazine (Mellaril). (Contribution to the study and evaluation of the ambivalent effect of a major tranquilizer: Thioridazine (Mellaril). *Ann. Med.-Psychol.* **121**, 137.

Mrozowski, J. (1962). Comparison of side effects and complications during treatment with Melleril (TP 21, "Sandoz") and chlorpromazine. *Polski. Tygod. Lekar.* **17**, 472.

Müller-Küppers, M. (1962). Kinderpsychiatrische Erfahrungen mit einem Neuroleptikum

(Thioridazin = Melleretten u. Melleril). (Experiences in child psychiatry with a new tranquilizer (Thioridazine = Mellaril).) *Muench. Med. Wochschr.* **104**, 2464.

Neuman, M. (1963). Tendances actuelles dans le traitement par les neuroleptiques en medecine generale. (Current trends in treatment with neuroleptics in general medicine.) *Gaz. Hop. (Paris)* **135**, 585.

Oettinger, L., and Simonds, R. (1962). The use of thioridazine in the office management of children's behavior disorders. *Med. Times (N.Y.)* **90**, 596.

Ollendorff, R. H. V. (1962). A trial of thioridazine (Mellaril) in the maintenance of chronic schizophrenics. *Brit. J. Clin. Pract.* **16**, 183.

Ostfeld, A. M. (1960). Tranquillizers in der Allgemeinpraxis. (Tranquillizers in general medical practice.) *Triangle* **4**, 335.

Overall, J. E., *et al.* (1964). Imipramine and thioridazine in depressed and schizophrenic patients. *J. Am. Med. Assoc.* **189**, 605.

Pasamanick, B., *et al.* (1964). Home vs hospital care for schizophrenics. *J. Am. Med. Assoc.* **187**, 177.

Pauig, P. M., *et al.* (1961). Thioridazine hydrochloride in the treatment of behavior disorders in epileptics. *Am. J. Psychiat.* **117**, 832.

Paulson, G., and Buffaloe, W. J. (1964). Use of thioridazine hydrochloride in epilepsy. *Diseases Nervous System* **25**, 243.

Péguiron, M. (1958). Essai d'un nouveau neuroleptique, le Melleril, en médecine ambulatoire. (Trial of a new tranquilizer, Mellaril, in medical out-patients.) *Praxis (Bern)* **47**, 1193.

Pennington, V. M. (1962). Combined psychopharmaceutical treatment in 460 neuropsychiatric patients. *Am. J. Psychiat.* **118**, 935.

Petit, J. M., *et al.* (1962). La thioridazine en thérapeutique psychiatrique. (Thioridazine in psychiatric therapy.) *Sud Med. Chir.* **98**, 926.

Petrilowitsch, N. (1961). Zur differenzierten Behandlung der Depressionszustande. (Differentiated treatment of depressive states.) *Med. Welt* **1961**. 2657.

Petrilowitsch, N. (1961). Ueber den Indikationsbereich des Thioridazin (Melleril-Sandoz) bei der Therapie depressiver Zustandsbilder. (The range of indications of thioridazine (Mellaril-Sandoz) for treatment of depressive states.) *Med. Exptl.* **5**, 247.

Piazzalunga, R. (1959). Osservazioni cliniche sull'effetto psicorilassante della tioridazine in medicina interna. (Clinical observations on the psychorelaxant effect of thioridazine in internal medicine.) *Clin. Terap.* **17**, 351.

Pincherle, M. (1959). Sull'impiego di un nuo psicorilassante (tioridazina) in medicina generale. (The use of a new psychorelaxant (Thioridazine) in general medicine.) *Bologna Med.* **5**, 835.

Pincherle, M. (1959). Esperienz cliniche con un nuovo neurolettico: la tioridazina. (Clinical experiences with thioridazine, a new neuroleptic.) *Arch. Psicol. Neurol. Psichiat.* **20**, 357.

Prado, H., *et al.* (1962). La psicoactividad del Melleril en medicina general. (Psychoactivity of Mellaril in general medicine.) *Neurol. Neurocir. Psiquiat. (Mex.)* **3**, 25.

Rance, A., *et al.* (1962). Sur l'action thérapeutique de la thioridazine (Melleril). (Therapeutic effect of thioridazin (Mellaril).) *Presse Med.* **70**, 300.

Rance, A., *et al.* (1962). Sur l'action thérapeutique de la thioridazine (Melleril). (The therapeutic effect of thioridazine (Mellaril).) *Sem. Hôp. (Paris)* **38**, 499.

Rance, A., and Mailet-Jurquet, R. J. (1961). Sur l'action thérapeutique de la thioridazine (Melleril). (The therapeutic effect of thioridazine (Mellaril).) *Ann. Med.-Psychol.* **119/11**, 985.

Rego, A. (1960). Algunas consideraciones sobre la asociación terapéutica de la tioridazina (Meleril) con los preparados reserpinicos y antidepresivos en el enfermo mental. (Studies on the combined use of thioridazine (Mellaril) with reserpine-like or antidepressive drugs in psychotics.) *Inform. Psiquiat.* **5**, 37.

Rémy, M. (1958). Essai d'un nouveau dérivé de la phénothiazine, le Mellaril, en clinique psychiatrique. (Trial of a new phenothiazine derivative, Mellaril, in clinical psychiatry.) *Schweiz. Med. Wochschr.* **88**, 1221.

Rémy, M. (1959). Essais comparés de quelques dérivés de la phénothiazine. (Comparative investigations of some phenothiazine derivatives.) *Schweiz. Arch. Neurol. Psychiat.* **84**, 297.

Rémy, M. (1959). Essais comparés de divers dérivés de la phénothiazine. (Comparative studies of various phenothiazine derivatives.) *Med. Hyg. (Geneve)* **17**, 81.

Rémy, M. (1961). Emploi prolongé des neuroleptiques en psychiatrie. Cing ans d'expériences cliniques avec le Melleril. (Prolonged treatment with tranquillizers in psychiatry. Five years clinical experience with Mellaril.) *Praxis (Bern)* **51**, 288.

Renard, P., et al. (1962). Essais cliniques de la thioridazine chez les enfants inadaptés d'âge scolaire. (Clinical trials with thioridazine in school-age children with adaptation difficulties.) *Presse Med.* **70**, 1416.

Renard, P., et al. (1962). Essais cliniques de la thioridazine chez les enfants inadaptés d'âge scolaire. (Clinical trials with thioridazine in school-age children with adaptation difficulties.) *Ann. Med.-Psychol.* **120**, 578.

Rentsch, M. (1960). Klinische Erfahrungen mit Thioridazin (Melleril) in der Padiatrie. (Clinical experiences with thioridazine (Mellaril) in pediatrics.) *Med. Hyg. (Geneve)* **18**, 140.

Richert, J. (1963). Ueber den Indikationsbereich des Thioridazins in der nervenärztlichen Praxis. (Range of indications for thioridazine in neuropsychiatric practice.) *Med. Welt* p. 973.

Rinsley, D. B. (1963). Thioridazine in the treatment of hospitalized adolescents. *Am. J. Psychiat.* **120**, 73.

Riser, M., et al. (1959). Frequence et aspects cliniques des accidents nerveux des nouvelles chimiotherapies neuroleptiques. (Frequency and clinical aspects of side effects of the new tranquilizing chemotherapy on the nervous system.) *Rev. Neurol.* **100**, 737.

Riser, M., et al. (1960). La thioridazine, médicament neuroleptique dérivé de la phenothiazine. (Thioridazine, a phenothiazine derivative, as neuroleptic drug.) *Presse Med.* **68**, 679.

Riser, M., et al. (1960). Traitement de la chorée de Huntington par la chlorpromazine (largactil) et par la thioridazine (melleril). (Treatment of Huntington's chorea with chlorpromazine (Largactil) and with thioridazine (Mellaril).) *Ann. Med.-Psychol.* **118**, 349.

Riser, M., et al. (1960). Notes sur quelques indications de la thioridazine. (Remarks on some indications of thioridazine.) *Ann. Med.-Psychol.* **118**, 558.

Roganti, M., and Barbieri, G. C. (1962). La sedazione preoperatoria nei cardiopatici e negli anziani. (Pre-operative sedation of cardiac and aged patients.) *Clin. Terap.* **22**, 795.

Romani, J. D. (1961). La place de la thioridazine (Melleril) en endocrinolgie—gynécologie. Syndrome prémenstruel, oedémes idiopathiques et ménopause. (The role of thioridazine in gynecological endocrinology, premenstrual syndrome, idiopathic oedema and climacterium.) *Gaz. Hop. (Paris)* **133**, 1557.

Rompel, H. (1963). Treatment of hebephrenic male Bantu schizophrenics with thioridazine (Mellaril). *Med. Proc.* **9**, 344.

Rotondi, A., et al. (1960). Esperienze cliniche con un nuovo preparato fenotiazinico: la tioridazina. (Clinical experience with a new phenothiazine derivative: Thioridazine.) *Ann. Neurol. Psichiat.* **54**, 269.

Saavedra, A., and Mariategui, J. (1960). La tioridacine en psiquiatria. (Thioridazine in psychiatry.) *Rev. Neuro-Psiquiat.* **22**, 585.

Sälde, H., and Walinder, J. (1962). Thioridazin, ett nytt fentiazinderivat vid kronisk schizofreni. (Thioridazine, a new phenothiazine-derivative for chronic schizophrenia.) *Svenska Lakartidn.* **59**, 1664.

Sanchez Longo, L. P., and Ifarraguerri, A. (1961). The control of aggressive behavior

in organic brain syndromes with the use of thioridazine. *Bol. Asoc. Med. Puerto Rico* **53**, 81.
Sandison, R. A. (1960). Thioridazine. *Brit. Med. J.* II, 65.
Sandison, R. A., et al. (1960). Clinical trials with Mellaril (TP-21) in the treatment of schizophrenia. A two-year study. *J. Mental Sci.* **106**, 732.
Sauter, R. (1959). Therapeutische Erfahrungen mit einem neuen Phenothiazinderivat. Melleril. (Therapeutic experiences with a new phenothiazine derivative, Mellaril.) *Praxis (Bern)* **48**, 140.
Savoldi, F., and Tosarelli, L. (1960). Sull'impiego di un nuovo neurolettico, il "Melleril", in terapie psichiatrica. (Use of a new tranquilizer "Mellaril" in psychiatric therapy.) *Gior. Psichiat. Neuropatol.* **88**, 195.
Savona, B. (1960). Dell'azione di un nuovo farmaco psicorilassante sulla gestante a termine. (Effect of a new psychorelaxant on pregnant women at term.) *Quadernl. Clin. Ostet. Ginecol.* **15**, 294.
Schiele, B. C., et al. (1961). A comparison of thioridazine, trifluoperazine, chlorpromazine, and placebo: A double-blind controlled study on the treatment of chronic, hospitalized, schizophrenic patients. *J. Clin. Exptl. Psychopathol.* **22**, 151.
Schnetzler, J. P., and Lamand, J. C. (1962). Association systématique de la thiopropérazine et de la thioridazine. A propos de 115 observations. (Routine combination of thioproperazine with thioridazine. Report of 115 cases.) *Ann. Med.-Psychol.* **120/11**, 123.
Schnetzler, J. P., and Lamand, J. C. (1962). La thioridazine dans le traitement des états dépressifs. (Thioridazine in the treatment of depression.) *Ann. Med.-Psychol.* **120**, 609.
Schopbach, R. R. (1961). The use of phenothiazines on a general hospital psychiatric service. *Henry Ford Hosp. Bull.* **9**, 369.
Seguin, J. (1960). Contribution à l'étude de l'action thérapeutique de "Melleril 50" en milieu hospitalier. (Contribution to the study of the therapeutic effect of "Mellaril 50" in hospitalized cases.) These, Paris.
Shaw, C. R., et al. (1963). Tranquilizer drugs in the treatment of emotionally disturbed children. I. Inpatients in a residential treatment center. *J. Am. Acad. Child Psychiat.* **2**, 725.
Sherman, S. (1961). A clinical evaluation of Mellaril. *Am. J. Psychiat.* **118**, 452.
Singh, H. (1963). Therapeutic use of thioridazine in premature ejaculcation. *Am. J. Psychiat.* **119**, 891.
Sloane, R. B., and Haden, P. (1961). Use of thioridazine (Mellaril) in psychological disorders. *Diseases Nervous System* **22**, 330.
Smelson, I. H., and Foy, J. L. (1962). Evaluation of injectable thioridazine in acute psychotic disorders. *Diseases Nervous System* **23**, 36.
Smith, J. A., et al. (1959). Effects of phenothiazines in chronic psychotics refractory to previous treatment. Scientific Exhibit. Am. Psychiat. Assoc., Philadelphia, Pennsylvania, April 27–30, 1959.
Somerville, D. M., et al. (1960). Phenothiazine side effects. Comparison of two major tranquilizers. *J. Mental Sci.* **106**, 1417.
Stabenau, J. R., and Grinols, D. R. (1964). A double-blind comparison of thioridazine and chlorpromazine. *Psychiat. Quart.* **38**, 42.
Stoerger, R. (1962). Zur neuroleptischen Behandlung endogener Psychosen. (Study on the treatment of endogenous psychoses with neuroleptics.) *Med. Monatsschr.* **16**, 155.
Svendsen, B. B., et al. (1961). Comparison of the effect of thioridazine and chlorpromazine on chronic schizophrenic psychosis using double blind technique. *Psychopharmacologia* **2**, 446.
Taeschler, M., and Cerletti, A. (1960). Zur Pharmakologie psychoaktiver Wirkstoffe. (Pharmacology of psychoactive agents.) *Muench. Med. Wochschr.* **102**, 1000.
Taeschler, M., and Cerletti, A. (1961). Inhibition of emotional reactions by phenothiazine tranquilizers. *Nature* **190**, 1014.

Taeschler, M., and Schlager, E. (1961). Psychopharmaka. 1. Mitteilung. (Psychopharmacological agents. 1st information.) *Schweiz. Apothekerztg.* **99**, 683.

Taeschler, M., et al. (1960). Zur bedeutung verschiedener pharmakodynamischer Eigenschaften der Phenothiazinderivat fur ihre klinische Wirksamkeit. (The significance of various pharmacodynamic properties of phenothiazine derivatives for their clinical effectiveness.) *Psychiat. Neurol.* **139**, 85.

Tomasi, A. M., et al. (1960). La terapia neurolettica nei cardiopatici organici e funzionali. (Neuroleptic treatment of patients with organic and functional cardiopathy.) *Boll. Soc. Ital. Cardiol.* **5**, 559.

Uddyback, O. T., and Chen, C. H. (1962). Thioridazine (Mellaril) on regressed schizophrenic patients. *Am. J. Psychiat.* **118**, 740.

van Rhijn, C. H. (1962). An evaluation of Mellaril by means of a controlled group. *Psychiat. Neurol. Neurochir.* **65**, 117.

Velasco, J. A., et al. (1961). Posibilidades del Meleril en la práctica pediátrica. (Value of Mellaril in pediatric practice.) *Rev. Espan. Pediat.* **27**, 77.

Vencovský, E., et al. (1959). Naše zkušenosti s léčbou psychos thiomethylphenothiazinem. (Předběžne sděleni.) (Our experiences with thiomethylphenothiazine in psychoses. Preliminary report.) *Pizen. Lekar. Sb.* **10**, 147.

Vencovský, E., et al. (1960). Použití Mellerilu v klinické praxi psychiatrické. (Use of Mellaril in clinical psychiatry.) *Cesk. Psychiat.* **56**, 411.

Vestre, N. D., et al. (1963). A comparison of the slow release and the regular forms of thioridazine: A double-blind controlled study in hospitalized psychiatric patients. *Current Therap. Res.* **5**, 183.

Wallinga, J. V. (1963). Use of a phenothiazine derivative, thioridazine, in the treatment of childhood emotional disorders. *Acta Paedopsychiat.* **30**, 211.

Warembourg, W., and Niquet, G. (1960). Essais d'un nouveau neuroleptique, la thioridazine ou Melleril. (Trials of a new tranquilizer, thioridazine or Mellaril.) *Mouvement Therap.* **5**, 99.

Weber, J. R. (1960). Melleril in der täglichen kinderpraxis. (Mellaril in the daily pediatric practice.) *Praxis (Bern)* **49**, 602.

Winnik, H. Z., et al. (1963). Therapeutic effects of thioridazine. *Diseases Nervous System* **24**, 551.

Wright, G. (1962). The treatment of non-hospitalized schizophrenics. *Am. J. Psychiat.* **119**, 261.

Wroblewski, F., and Block, S. L. (1962). Follow up of thioridazine administration. *Am. J. Psychiat.* **119**, 589.

Zaniboni, M., and Luzzago, C. (1960). Osservazioni cliniche sull'effetto psicorilassante della tioridazine in medicine pratica. (Clinical observations of the effect of thioridazine as a psychorelaxant in medical practice.) *Gazz. Med. Ital.* **119**, 204.

Zychiewicz-Krankowska, D., and Rogowska, J. (1961). Dotychczasowe wyniki leczenia psychoz melerylem. (Results so far obtained with Melleril in the treatment of psychoses.) *Polski Tygod. Lekar.* **16**, 476.

~ A.16 ~
Trifluoperazine

Chemical Papers

Barnes, T. C. (1960). Relationship of chemical structure to central nervous system effects of tranquilizing and anticonvulsant drugs. *J. Am. Pharm. Assoc. Sci. Ed.* **49** (7), 415–417.

Cares, R. M., and Buckman, C. (1963). Comparative review of the structure and side-effects of newer psychotropic agents. *Diseases Nervous System* **24** (4), 92–105.

Cochin, J., and Daly, J. W. (1963). The use of thin-layer chromatography for the analysis of drugs. Identification and isolation of phenothiazine tranquilizers and of antihistaminics in body fluids and tissues. *J. Pharmacol. Exptl. Therap.* **139** (2), 160–165.

Eagleson, D. A. (1963). Paper chromatographic differentiation of some important phenothiazines encountered in toxicology. *Am. J. Clin. Pathol.* **39** (6), 648–651.

Eckhardt, E. T., and Plaa, G. L. (1962). The effect of phenothiazine derivatives on the disappearance of sulfobromophthalein from mouse plasma. *J. Pharmacol. Exptl. Therap.* **138** (3), 387–391.

Forrest, F. M., and Forrest, I. S. (1963). Urine testing for phenothiazine and related drugs; its significance for achieving and maintaining rehabilitation of chronic mental patients. *Am. Arch. Rehabil. Therap.* **11**, 8–19.

Forrest, F. M., et al. (1959). A rapid, semi-quantitative urine color test for piperazine-linked phenothiazine drugs ("Compazine," trilafon and analoguous compounds). *Am. J. Psychiat.* **116** (6), 549–551.

Forrest, F. M., et al. (1961). Review of rapid urine tests for phenothiazine and related drugs. *Am. J. Psychiat.* **118** (4), 300–307.

Forrest, F. M., et al. (1963). Phenothiazines in urine. *Brit. J. Psychiat.* **109**, 447–449.

Hammarlund, E. R., et al. (1965). Additional sodium chloride equivalents and freezing point depressions for various medicinal solutions. *J. Pharm. Sci.* **54** (1), 160–162.

Horikawa, E. K., et al. (1960). Determination of fluoride ion in femurs of rats receiving organic fluoride. *J. Med. Pharm. Chem.* **2** (5), 541–551.

Jucker, E. (1963). Einige neuere Entwicklungen in der Chemie der Psychopharmaka. (New developments in the chemistry of psychotropic drugs.) *Angew. Chem.* **75** (12), 524–538.

Jucker, E. (1963). Some new developments in the chemistry of psychotherapeutic agents. *Angew. Chem.* **2** (9), 493–507.

Levine, J., et al. (1961). Interference of indican in the estimation of phenothiazine. *Am. J. Psychiat.* **117** (8), 747–748.

Lucas, G. H., and Fabierkiewicz, C. (1963). Useful tests to identify phenothiazine tranquillizers. *J. Forensic Sci.* **8** (3), 462–476.

Lyons, L. E., and Mackie, J. C. (1963). Electron-donating properties of central sympathetic suppressants. *Nature* **197** (4867), 589.

Margasínski, Z., et al. (1965). Rozdzial mieszanin pochodnych fenotiazyny metoda chromatografii cienkowarstowej. (Thin-layer chromatography of phenothiazine derivatives.) *Acta Polon. Pharm.* **21** (3), 253–255.

Martin, H. F., et al. (1963). A method for calculating gas chromatographic relative retention values for high boiling phenothiazine derivatives. *Anal. Chem.* **35** (12), 1901–1904.

Mellinger, T. J., and Keeler, C. E. (1962). Chromatography and electrophoresis of phenothiazine drugs. *J. Pharm. Sci.* **51** (12), 1169–1173.

Mellinger, T. J., and Keeler, C. E. (1963). Spectrofluorometric identification of phenothiazine drugs. *Anal. Chem.* **35** (4), 554–558.

Piette, L. H., and Forrest, I. S. (1962). Electron paramagnetic resonance studies of free radicals in the oxidation of drugs derived from phenothiazine *in vitro*. *Biochim. Biophys. Acta* **57** (2), 419–420.

Posner, H. S., and Levine, J. (1963). Inability to validate the urinary FPN test for phenothiazine drugs: Suggestions as to the cause of the discrepancy. *J. Nervous Mental Disease* **136** (6), 591–593.

Rogers, A. R. (1964). The influence of spectral slit width on the absorption of visible or ultra-violet light by pharmacopoeial substances. *J. Pharm. Pharmacol.* **16** (6), 433–434.

Seeman, P. M., and Bialy, H. S. (1963). The surface activity of tranquilizers. *Biochem. Pharmacol.* **12** (10), 1181–1191.

Sorby, D. L., and Plein, E. M. (1961). Adsorption of phenothiazine derivatives by kaolin, talc, and Norit. *J. Pharm. Sci.* **50** (4), 355.

Street, H. V. (1962). The rapid separation of drugs and poisons by high temperature reversed phase paper chromatography. 2. Phenothiazine tranquillizers and imipramine. *Acta Pharmacol. Toxicol.* **19** (4), 312–324.

Yung, D. K., and Pernarowski, M. (1963). Identification and differentiation of some phenothiazine-type tranquilizers. *J. Pharm. Sci.* **52** (4), 365–370.

Zografi, G., *et al.* (1964). Interfacial properties of phenothiazine derivatives. *J. Pharm. Sci.* **53** (5), 573–574.

Biology and Pharmacology

Arbasino, M., and Corona, G. L. (1964). La molecola della piperazina in recenti composti d'interesse farmacologico. [The piperazine molecule in recent compounds of pharmacological interest.] *Boll. Chimicofarm.* **103** (4), 226–240.

Arneson, G. A. (1964). Phenothiazine derivatives and glucose metabolism. *J. Neuropsychiat.* **5** (3), 181–185.

Ayd, F. J., Jr. (1959). Blood, urine and liver function studies in trifluoperazine-treated patients. *In* "Trifluoperazine" (J. H. Moyer, ed.), pp. 169–174. Lea & Febiger, Philadelphia, Pennsylvania.

Ben-David, M., *et al.* (1965). Production of lactation by non-sedative phenothiazine derivatives. *Proc. Soc. Exptl. Biol. Med.* **118** (1), 265–270.

Bennett, J. L., and Hamilton, L. D. (1961). Effects of chlorpromazine in combination with activating drugs on thyroid function tests. *J. Neuropsychiat.* **3** (2), 118–122.

Bhargava, K. P., and Jaitly, K. D. (1964). The effect of some phenothiazine tranquillizers on the oestrous cycle of albino mice. *Brit. J. Pharmacol.* **22** (1), 162–165.

Blažek, J. (1963). Phenothiazinderivate in der Pharmazie. [Phenothiazines in pharmacy.] *Pharm. Praxis, Beilage Pharmazie* **5**, 85–90.

Bloom, J. B., *et al.* (1965). Effect on the liver of long-term tranquilizing medication. *Am. J. Psychiat.* **121** (8), 788–797.

Brodie, D. A., and Valitski, L. S. (1963). Production of gastric hemorrhage in rats by multiple stresses. *Proc. Soc. Exptl. Biol. Med.* **113** (4), 998–1001.

Burkman, A. M. (1961). Relative potencies of some phenothiazines as pecking syndrome inhibitors. *J. Pharm. Sci.* **50** (9), 771–773.

Burton, R. M., *et al.* (1960). Interaction of nicotinamide with reserpine and chlorpromazine. III. Some effects on the diphosphopyridine nucleotide content in liver. *Arch. Intern. Pharmacodyn. Therap.* **128** (3–4), 260–275.

Chin, J. H., et al. (1964). Comparison of chlorpromazine, trifluoperazine, and pentobarbital on conditioned arousal to reticular stimulation. *Federation Proc.* **23** (2), 248.

Cook, L., and Kelleher, R. T. (1962). Drug effects on the behavior of animals. *Ann. N.Y. Acad. Sci.* **96** (1), 315–335.

Corne, S. J., et al. (1963). A method for assessing the effects of drugs on the central actions of 5-hydroxytryptamine. *Brit. J. Pharmacol.* **20** (1), 106–120.

Denber, H. C. B. (1961). Studies on mescaline. XI. Biochemical findings during the mescaline-induced state with observations on the blocking action of different psychotropic drugs. *Psychiat. Quart.* **35** (1), 18–48.

DiMascio, A., et al. (1963). The psychopharmacology of phenothiazine compounds: A comparative study of the effects of chlorpromazine, promethazine, trifluoperazine, and perphenazine in normal males. II. Results and discussion. *J. Nervous Mental Disease* **136** (2), 168–186.

Ditman, K. S. (1964). Drug immobilization of wild animals. *Mind* **2** (4), 103-passim.

Dobkin, A. B. (1960). Potentiation of thiopental anesthesia by derivatives and analogues of phenothiazine. *Anesthesiology* **21** (3), 292–296.

Elder, W. H. (1964). Chemical inhibitors of ovulation in the pigeon. *J. Wildlife Management* **28** (3), 556–575.

Emmerson, J. L., and Miya, T. S. (1963). Metabolism of phenothiazine drugs. *J. Pharm. Sci.* **52** (5), 411–419.

Flanagan, T. L., et al. (1962). Excretion patterns of phenothiazine-S^{35} compounds in rats; effect of change in structure on metabolism. *J. Pharm. Sci.* **51** (10), 996–999.

Forrest, I. S., and Forrest, F. M. (1964). Chlorpromazine and related phenothiazines: their metabolism. *Mind* **2** (2), 38-passim.

Fowler, P. J., et al. (1964). The effects of various central nervous system stimulants and depressants on confinement motor activity. *Federation Proc.* **23** (2), 198.

Freeman, A. R., and Spirtes, M. A. (1963). Effects of chlorpromazine on biological membranes. II. Chlorpromazine-induced changes in human erythrocytes. *Biochem. Pharmacol.* **12** (1), 47–53.

Gabay, S., and Harris, S. R. (1965). Biochemical interactions of phenothiazines. *Med. Tribune* **6** (38), 18.

Gabay, S., and Harris, S. R. (1965). Inhibition of d-amino acid oxidase by phenothiazines. *Federation Proc.* **24** (2), 581.

Gilbreath, J. C., et al. (1960). The effect of trifluoperazine and reserpine on reproductive efficiency in chickens. *Poultry Sci.* **39** (3), 735–739.

Glende, E. A., and Cornatzer, W. E. (1963). The effect of chlorpromazine, trifluoperazine and promethazine on brain sulfolipids. *J. Pharmacol. Exptl. Therap.* **139** (3), 377–382.

Guttman, H. N., and Friedman, W. (1963). Protozoa as pharmacological tools: The phenothiazine tranquilizers. *Trans. N.Y. Acad. Sci.* **26** (1), 75–89.

Hanson, H. M., and Stone, C. A. (1964). Antagonism of the antiavoidance effect of various classes of tranquilizing agents by anticholinergic drugs. *Pharmacologist* p. 179.

Harris, A. F., et al. (1960). Interaction of chlorpromazine with strandin. *Proc. Soc. Exptl. Biol. Med.* **104** (4), 542–547.

Hele, P. (1963). The interaction of phenothiazine derivatives and imipramine with polyphosphates of biological interest. *Biochim. Biophys. Acta* **76** (4), 647–649.

Heyman, J. J. (1964). Nicotinamide metabolism in schizophrenics, drug addicts, and normals: The effect of psychotropic drugs and hormones. *Trans. N.Y. Acad. Sci.* **26** (3), 354–360.

Hudson, R. D., and Domino, E. F. (1964). Comparative effects of three substituted phenothiazines on the patellar reflex and mean arterial blood pressure of the rabbit. *Arch. Intern. Pharmacodyn.* **147** (1–2), 36–42.

Irwin, S. (1961). Correlation in rats between the locomotor and avoidance suppressant

potencies of eight phenothiazine tranquilizers. *Arch. Intern. Pharmacodyn.* **132** (3–4), 279–286.
Jamieson, D., and Van Den Brenk, H. A. (1961). Relation of mast cell changes to hypothermia in the rat. *Biochem. Pharmacol.* **7** (1), 35–46.
Janssen, P. A. J., *et al.* (1960). Apomorphine-antagonism in rats. *Arzneimittel-Forsch.* **10** (12), 1003–1005.
Janssen, P. A. J., *et al.* (1965). Is it possible to predict the clinical effects of neuroleptic drugs (major tranquillizers) from animal data? I. "Neuroleptic activity spectra" for rats. *Arzneimittel-Forsch.* **15** (2), 104–117.
Kátó, L., and Gözsy, B. (1961). Differential and quantitative affinity of psychoactive drugs to mucopolysaccharides. *Indian J. Med. Res.* **49** (5), 788–798.
Kátó, L., *et al.* (1962). Attempt to classify psychotropic drugs, based on their affinity to mucopolysaccharides *in vivo*. *J. Clin. Exptl. Psychopathol.* **23** (2), 75–90.
Khazan, N., *et al.* (1962). The mammotropic effect of tranquilizing drugs. *Arch. Intern. Pharmacodyn.* **136** (3–4), 291–305.
Khazan, N., *et al.* (1963). ADH-like effect of tranquilizers in amphibians. *Proc. Soc. Exptl. Biol. Med.* **112** (2), 490–494.
Krista, L. M., *et al.* (1963). The influence of various drugs on the growth and beta-aminopropionitrile-induced dissecting aneurysm of turkeys. *Poultry Sci.* **42** (2), 522–526.
Krista, L. M., *et al.* (1963). Blood pressure and heart rate in the turkey as measured by the indirect method and their modifications by pharmacological agents. *Poultry Sci.* **42** (3), 646–652.
Leblanc, J., and Lemieux, L. (1961). Histamine and mental disease. *Med. Exptl.* **4** (4), 214–222.
Leibovich, F., and Maichak, A. (1962). Izmeneniya bioelektricheskoi aktivnosti kory golovnogo mozga u bolnih shizofrenii pod vliyaniem odokratnih priemov nebolshih doz Stelazina. [Changes in bioelectrical activity of brain in schizophrenics after single administration of small doses of "Stelazine".] *Zh. Nevropatol. i Psikhiat.* **62** (4), 585–593.
Lewis, R. A., and Gyang, F. N. (1965). Inhibition of sickling by phenothiazines; comparison of derivatives. *Arch. Intern. Pharmacodyn.* **153** (1), 158–171.
Lipman, V. C., *et al.* (1963). Effect of anticholinergic psychotomimetics on motor activity and body temperature. *Arch. Intern. Pharmacodyn.* **146** (1–2), 174–191.
Maickel, R. P., *et al.* (1964). The effect of various drugs on the ability of cold-exposed rats to maintain normal body temperature. *Federation Proc.* **23** (2), 567.
Minchin, R. L. H., and Holdaway, I. (1964). Comparison of psycho-therapeutic and anthelmintic activities. *Brit. J. Psychiat.* **110** (466), 411–414.
Morpurgo, C. (1962). Influence of phenothiazine derivatives on the accumulation of brain amines induced by monoamine oxidase inhibitors. *Biochem. Pharmacol.* **11**, 967–972.
Morpurgo, C., and Theobald, W. (1964). Influence of antiparkinson drugs and amphetamine on some pharmacological effects of phenothiazine derivatives used as neuroleptics. *Psychopharmacologia* **6** (3), 178–191.
Piazza, V., *et al.* (1964). Su alcune modificazioni indotte dalla trifluoperazina nell'ambito del chimismo acido gastrico. [Some changes in the chemistry of gastric acid induced by trifluoperazine.] *Clin. Terap.* **29** (6), 551–561.
Plotnikoff, N. (1963). Effect of neurotropic drugs on a non-conditioned avoidance response. *Arch. Intern. Pharmacodyn.* **145** (3–4), 430–439.
Plotnikoff, N. (1961). Drug resistance due to inbreeding. *Science* **134** (3493), 1881–1882.
Pscheidt, G. R., *et al.* (1964). Effects of psychotropic drug combinations on urinary constituents in the dog. *J. Neuropsychiat.* **5** (8), 502–508.
Psychoyos, A. (1963). A study of the hormonal requirements for ovum implantation in the rat, by means of delayed nidation-inducing substances (chlorpromazine, trifluoperazine). *J. Endocrinol.* **27** (3), 337–343.

Psychoyos, A., et al. (1963). Evolution de deux lots de foetus d'âge différent chez la ratte normale traitée par la trifluopérazine. Prolongation fonctionnelle des corps jaunes et rétention des premiers foetus in utero. [Evolution of two fetal lots of different ages in the normal rat treated with trifluoperazine. Functional prolongation of the yellow bodies and retention of the first fetus *in utero.*] *Compt. Rend.* **256** (23), 4980–4983.

Purshottam, N. (1962). Effects of tranquilizers on induced ovulation in mice. *Am. J. Obstet. Gynecol.* **83** (11), 1405–1409.

Purshottam, N., et al. (1961). Induced ovulation in the mouse and the measurement of its inhibition. *Fertility Sterility* **12** (4), 346–352.

Raevskii, K. S., et al. (1964). K farmakologii triftazina. [Pharmacology of Triphtazine.] *Zh. Nevropatol. i Psikhiat.* **64** (12), 1868–1876.

Rosenblum, W., and Zweifach, B. W. (1964). The effect of tranquilizers on the contractile response of cerebral arteries. *J. Pharmacol. Exptl. Therap.* **145** (1), 58–63.

Ruddell, J. S. (1963). An antagonist of suxamethonium bromide. *Lancet* I (7286), 889.

Scott, G. T. (1962). Physiological action of psychoactive drugs on melanocytes in fish and frogs. *Psychopharmacol. Serv. Center Bull.* **2** (5), 58–62.

Scott, G. T., and Nading, L. K. (1961). Relative effectiveness of phenothiazine tranquilizing drugs causing release of MSH. *Proc. Soc. Exptl. Biol. Med.* **106** (1), 88–90.

Shurtleff, D., et al. (1962). The effects of some phenothiazine derivatives on the discrimination of auditory clicks. *Psychopharmacologia* **3** (3), 153–165.

Sikharulidze, A. I. (1964). Vliyanie stelazina na vysshuyu nervnuyu deyatel "nost". [Effect of "Stelazine" on higher nervous activity.] *Farmakol. i Toksikse.* **27** (6). 656–658.

Slocum, Y. K. (1961). Serum transaminase tests for liver function on outpatients in follow-up clinic. *Am. J. Psychiat.* **118** (1), 75–76.

Smith, C. W., and Thomas, C. G. (1959). Gastric analyses before and after ingestion of trifluoperazine. *In* "Trifluoperazine" (J. H. Moyer, ed.), pp. 175–177. Lea & Febiger, Philadelphia, Pennsylvania.

Smith, R. L., et al. (1963). ACTH-hypersecretion induced by phenothiazine tranquilizers. *J. Pharmacol. Exptl. Therap.* **139** (2), 185–190.

Stanley, D. G., and Melki, S. (1963). Lactic dehydrogenase activity in schizophrenic patients. *Diseases Nervous System* **24** (10), 593–602.

Steiner, W. G., and Himwich, H. E. (1963). Effects of antidepressant drugs on limbic structures of rabbit. *J. Nervous Mental Disease* **137** (3), 277–284.

Stevens, J. D. (1964). Psychopharmacology. *J. Neuropsychiat.* **5** (8), 566–576.

Takayanagi, I. (1964). Phenothiazine derivatives; relationship between peripheral and central actions. *Arzneimittel-Forsch.* **14** (6), 694–698.

Tedeschi, D. H., et al. (1958). Effects of various phenothiazines on minimal electroshock seizure threshold and spontaneous motor activity of mice. *J. Pharmacol. Exptl. Therap.* **123** (1), 35–38.

Tedeschi, D. H., et al. (1958). Pharmacology of trifluoperazine. *In* "Trifluoperazine" (J. H. Moyer, ed.), p. 23–33. Lea & Febiger, Philadelphia, Pennsylvania.

Tedeschi, D. H., et al. (1959). The neuropharmacology of trifluoperazine: A potent psychotherapeutic agent. *Arch. Intern. Pharmacodyn. Therap.* **122** (1–2), 129–143.

Tedeschi, D. H., et al. (1959). Pharmacology of trifluoperazine. *In* "Trifluoperazine" (J. H. Moyer, ed.), pp. 157–168. Lea & Febiger, Philadelphia, Pennsylvania.

Tedeschi, D. H., et al. (1961). Central serotonin antagonist activity of a number of phenothiazines. *Arch. Intern. Pharmacodyn.* **132** (1–2), 172–179.

Tedeschi, D. H., et al. (1964). Effects of centrally acting drugs on confinement motor activity. *J. Pharm. Sci.* **53** (9), 1046–1050.

Tedeschi, R. E., et al. (1959). Effects of various centrally acting drugs on fighting behavior of mice. *J. Pharmacol. Exptl. Therap.* **125** (1), 28–34.

Tedeschi, R. E., et al. (1962). Neuropharmacology of tranylcypromine and trifluoperazine. *Can. Psychiat. Assoc. J.* **7**, Suppl. S55–S59.

Tejmar, J., et al. (1964). Our first experiences with time-interval reproduction test in psychiatry. *Activ Nervosa Super.* **6**, 66–67.
Usdin, V. R., et al. (1961). Effects of psychotropic compounds on enzyme systems. I. Inhibition of human plasma and erythrocyte cholinesterases. II. *In vitro* inhibition of monoamine oxidase. *Proc. Soc. Exptl. Biol. Med.* **108** (2), 457–463.
Van Loon, E. J., et al. (1962). Canine hepatic secretion and urinary excretion of three S^{35}-labeled phenothiazines. *Psychopharmacol. Serv. Center Bull.* **2** (5), 56–57.
Van Loon, E. J., et al. (1964). Hepatic secretion and urinary excretion of three S^{35}-labeled phenothiazines in the dog. *J. Pharm. Sci.* **53** (10), 1211–1213.
Vogt. M. (1965). Effect of drugs on metabolism of catecholamines in the brain. *Brit. Med. Bull.* **21** (1), 57–61.
Weil-Malherbe, H., and Posner, H. S. (1963). The effect of drugs on the release of epinephrine from adrenomedullary particles *in vitro*. *J. Pharmacol. Exptl. Therap.* **140** (1), 93–102.
Weil-Malherbe, H., and Posner, H. S. (1964). The biphasic effect of phenothiazines and reserpine on the release of epinephrine from adrenomedullary granules and its dependence on pH. *Biochem. Pharmacol.* **13** (5), 685–690.
White, R. P., and Westerbeke, E. J. (1962). Relationship between central anticholinergic actions and antiparkinson efficacy of phenothiazine derivatives. *Intern. J. Neuropharmacol.* **1**, 213–216.
Wyant, G. M. (1962). A comparative study of eleven anti-emetic drugs in dogs. *Can. Anaesthesiol. Soc. J.* **9** (5), 399–407.

Side Effects

Anderson, J. H., Sanchez-Longo, L. P. (1961). The complications and side effects of the phenothiazine ataraxics: a review of 178 clinical series of 10 phenothiazine derivatives *Bol. Asoc. Med. Puerto Rico* **53** (4), 123–151.
Anonymous. (1961). Extrapyramidal effects of tranquillisers. *Lancet* II (7208), 918–919.
Anonymous. (1962). Drugs and congenital malformations. *Can. Med. Assoc. J.* **87** (24), 1288–1290.
Anonymous. (1962). Trifluoperazine and teeth. *Brit. Med. J.* II (5311), 1071.
Ayd, F. J., Jr. (1960). Drug-induced extrapyramidal reactions: Their clinical manifestations and treatment with Akineton. *Psychosomatics* **1** (3), 143–150.
Ayd, F. J., Jr. (1961). A survey of drug-induced extrapyramidal reactions. *J. Am. Med. Assoc.* **175** (12), 1054–1060.
Bailey, B. H., and Kay, R. E. (1960). Prolonged phenothiazine hepatitis: Report of a case. *Am. J. Psychiat.* **117** (6), 557–558.
Ban, T. A., and St. Jean, A. (1964). The effect of phenothiazines on the electrocardiogram. *Can. Med. Assoc. J.* **91** (10), 537–540.
Barker, J. C., and Kerr, E. M. (1960). Overdose of trifluoperazine. *Lancet* II (7163), 1304.
Birge, H. L. (1964). Survey of recent contributions. 2. The increasing commentary on drugs as visual hazards. *Am. J. Med. Sci.* **247** (2), 226–230.
Boardman, R. H., et al. (1960). Overdose of trifluoperazine. *Lancet* II (7166), 1450–1451.
Brune, G. G., et al. (1962). Relevance of drug-induced extrapyramidal reactions to behavioral changes during neuroleptic treatment. I. Treatment with trifluoperazine singly and in combination with trihexyphenidyl. *Comprehensive Psychiat.* **3** (4), 227–234.
Caffey, E. M., Jr., and Klett, C. J. (1961). Side effects and laboratory findings during combined drug therapy of chronic schizophrenics. *Diseases Nervous System* **22** (7), 370–375.
Cahn, M. M., and Levy, E. J. (1958). Photosensitivity tests in subjects receiving trifluoperazine. *In* "Trifluoperazine" (J. H. Moyer, ed.), pp. 213–214. Lea & Febiger, Philadelphia, Pennsylvania.

Cares, R. M., and Buckman, C. (1961). A survey of side-effects and/or toxicity of newer psychopharmacologic agents. *Diseases Nervous System* **22** (4), 97–106.
Chicoine, L. (1961). L'intoxication par les dérivés de la phénothiazine; revue et rapport de 25 cas. [Toxicity due to phenothiazine derivatives; review and report of twenty-five cases.] *Union Med. Canada* **90** (5), 469–474.
Childers, R. T., Jr. (1962). Procyclidine and benztropine methanesulfonate compared in drug-induced extrapyramidal reactions. *Am. J. Psychiat.* **119** (5), 462–463.
Collins, I. S. (1964). Hazards of drug therapy. *Med. J. Australia* **1** (7), 222–230.
Corner, B. D. (1962). Congenital malformations; clinical considerations. *Med. J. Southwest* **77**, 46–52.
Cornman, H. D., III (1961). A parallel between the profile of clinical activity and the character of extrapyramidal activity of neuroleptics. "Extrapyramidal System and Neuroleptics", pp. 479–481. Editions psychiatriques, Montreal.
Davies, T. S. (1959). Dystonic reaction to trifluoperazine. *Brit. Med. J.* I (5132), 1301.
Dickey, R. F., and Hartman, D. L. (1964). Photodermatitis induced by drugs. I. Contact photodermatitis. *Skin* **3** (6), 169–177.
Doray, B. H. (1964). Medicaments donnés durant la gestation et aprés la naissance. Effets néfastes pour le foetus et le nouveau-né. [Drugs given during pregnancy and after birth. Untoward effects on fetus and newborn.] *Union Med. Canada* **93** (5), 555–560.
Dubois, J. R. (1963). Neurologic complications of phenothiazine therapy. *Henry Ford Hosp. Med. Bull.* **11** (1), 59–63.
Durlach, J., et al. (1962). Etude expérimentale et clinique des trouble du métabolisme de l'eau et du potassium au cours de traitements neuroleptiques. [Experimental and clinical study of disordered water and potassium metabolism during neuroleptic treatment.] *Anesthesie* **19** (3), 563–574.
Editorial. (1965). Side effect of phenothiazines. *Can. Med. Assoc. J.* **92** (3), 135–136.
Erslev, A. J., and Wintrobe, M. M. (1962). Detection and prevention of drug-induced dyscrasias. *J. Am. Med. Assoc.* **181** (2), 114–119.
Evans, J. H. (1965). Persistent oral dyskinesia in treatment with phenothiazine derivatives. *Lancet* I (7388), 458–460.
Fanning, W. J. (1961). Extrapyramidal symptoms associated with the administration of trifluoperazine: Report of a case treated with diphenydramine. *Can. Med. J.* **85** (27), 1459.
Feldman, P. E. (1958). Safety and toxicity of trifluoperazine. *In* "Trifluoperazine" (J. H. Moyer, ed.), pp. 206–212. Lea & Febiger, Philadelphia, Pennsylvania.
Flegenheimer, W. V. (1959). Dyskinesias following therapy with phenothiazine derivatives. *J. Mt. Sinai Hosp.* **26**, 440–446.
Fournier, E. (1964). Intoxications par thymoleptiques et tranquillisants. [Intoxication by thymoleptics and tranquilizers.] *Gaz. Med. France* **71**, 2851-passim.
Freyhan, F. A. (1958). Occurrence and management of extrapyramidal syndromes in psychiatric treatment with trifluoperazine. *In* "Trifluoperazine" (J. H. Moyer, ed.), pp. 195–205. Lea & Febiger, Philadelphia, Pennsylvania.
Gallant, D. M., et al. (1964). Withdrawal symptoms after abrupt cessation of anti-psychotic compounds; clinical confirmation of chronic schizophrenics. *Am. J. Psychiat.* **121** (5), 491–493.
Gordon, W. (1963). Photosensitivity; a report of cases and a clinical review. *S. African Med. J.* **37**, 1159–1162.
Haase, H. J. (1961). Extrapyramidal modification of fine movements—a "conditio sine qua non" of the fundamental therapeutic action of neuroleptic drugs. *Rev. Can. Biol.* **20**, 425–449.
Hall, G. (1963). A case of phocomelia of the upper limbs. *Australian Med. J.* I, 449–450.
Hartmann, K., and Hippius, H. (1959). Extrapyramidal-motorische Begleiteffekte der neuroleptischen therapie und ihre Behandlung. [Extrapyramidal motor side effects of neuroleptic therapy and their treatment.] *Aerztl. Wochschr.* **14**, 307–312.

Hays, G. B., et al. (1964). Slate-gray color in patients receiving chlorpromazine. *Arch. Dermatol.* **90** (5), 471–476.
Heninger, G. R., et al. (1964). Personality factors in variability of response to phenothiazines. *Am. Psychiat. Assoc. Sci. Proc.* pp. 210–211.
Hoaken, P. C. S. (1964). Jaundice during imipramine treatment. *Can. Med. Assoc. J.* **90** (24), 1367.
Hodge, J. R. (1959). Akathisia: The syndrome of motor restlessness. *Am. J. Psychiat.* **116** (4), 337–338.
Hollister, L. E. (1961). Current concepts in therapy; complications from psychotherapeutic drugs. *New Engl. J. Med.* **264** (6), 291–293.
Hollister, L. E. (1964). Adverse reactions to phenothiazines. *J. Am. Med. Assoc.* **189** (4), 311–313.
Hollister, L. E. (1964). Complications from psychotherapeutic drugs—1964. *Clin. Pharmacol. Therap.* **5** (3), 322–333.
Hollister, L. E. (1965). Toxicity of psychotherapeutic drugs. *Practitioner* **194** (1159), 72–84.
Hollister, L. E. (1965). Nervous system reactions to drugs. *Ann. N.Y. Acad. Sci.* **123** (1), 342–353.
Hooper, J. H., Jr., et al. (1961). Abnormal lactation associated with tranquilizing drug therapy. *J. Am. Med. Assoc.* **178** (5), 506–507.
Hudson, D. F., and Cornman, H. D., III (1959). Extrapyramidal symptoms associated with trifluoperazine therapy. *In* "Trifluoperazine" (J. H. Moyer, ed.), pp. 179–185. Lea & Febiger, Philadelphia, Pennsylvania.
Hunter, R., et al. (1964). A syndrome of abnormal movements and dementia in leucotomized patients treated with phenothiazines. *J. Neurol. Neurosurg. Psychiat.* **27** (3), 219–223.
Hunter, R., et al. (1964). An apparently irreversible syndrome of abnormal movements following phenothiazine medication. *Proc. Roy. Soc. Med.* **57** (8), 758–762.
Jacobziner, H., and Raybin, H. W. (1963). Phosphorus, trifluoperazine, and methyl alcohol intoxications. *N.Y. J. Med.* **63** (18), 2705–2707.
Johnson, F. P., et al. (1964). Sudden death of a catatonic patient receiving phenothiazines. *Am. J. Psychiat.* **121** (5), 504–507.
Joyston-Bechal, M. P. (1965). Persistent oral dyskinesia in treatment with phenothiazine derivatives. *Lancet* I (7385), 600–601.
Kane, F. J., Jr. (1963). Severe oral moniliasis complicating chlorpromazine therapy. *Am. J. Psychiat.* **119** (9), 890.
Kane, F. J., Jr., and Anderson, W. B. (1964). A fourth occurrence of oral moniliasis during tranquilizer therapy. *Am. J. Psychiat.* **120** (12), 1199–1200.
Kirshbaum, B. A., and Beerman, H. (1964). Photosensitization due to drugs; a review of some of the recent literature. *Am. J. Med. Sci.* **248** (4), 445–468.
Kistner, R. W., (1964). Hazards of obstetrical and gynecological drugs. *Ohio State Med. J.* **60** (12), 1125–1129.
Kohn, N., and Myerson, R. M. (1961). Cholestatic hepatitis associated with trifluoperazine. *New Engl. J. Med.* **264** (11), 549–550.
Kruse, W. (1960). Persistent muscular restlessness after phenothiazine treatment: Report of 3 cases. *Am. J. Psychiat.* **117** (2), 152–153.
Lang, A. W., and Moore, R. A. (1961). Acute toxic psychosis concurrent with phenothiazine therapy. *Am. J. Psychiat.* **117** (10), 939–940.
Lee, D. F., and Lucas, G. J. (1959). Acute intermittent porphyria treated with trifluoperazine. *U.S. Armed Forces Med. J.* **10** (10), 1242–1246.
Le Vann, L. J. (1963). Congenital abnormalities in children born in Alberta during 1961: A survey and a hypothesis. *Can. Med. Assoc. J.* **89** (3), 120–126.

Lichtigfeld, F. J. (1964). Drug induced parkinsonian syndrome in a case of tranquillizer poisoning. *Brit. J. Psychiat.* **110** (465), 226–227.
Lockey, S. D. (1964). Adverse reactions to drugs. *Penna. Med. J.* **67** (8), 45–51.
Lyons, J. A. (1965). Persistent oral dyskinesia in treatment with phenothiazine derivatives. *Lancet* I (7390), 868–869.
McGeer, P. L., et al. (1961). Drug-induced extrapyramidal reactions; treatment with diphenydramine hydrochloride and dihydroxyphenylalanine. *J. Am. Med. Assoc.* **177** (10), 665–670.
McKown, C. H., et al. (1963). Overdosage effects and danger from tranquilizing drugs. *J. Am. Med. Assoc.* **185** (6), 425–430.
Mandel, W., and Oliver, W. A. (1961). Withdrawal of maintenance antiparkinson drug in the phenothiazine-induced extrapyramidal reaction. *Am. J. Psychiat.* **118** (4), 350–351.
Mendels, J. (1964). Hypertension and tranylcypromine. *Am. J. Psychiat.* **121** (6), 595–597.
Middleton, P. McK., and Boulding, J. E. (1960). Suicide related to change of phenothiazine —a clinical note. *Can. Psychiat. Assoc. J.* **5** (1), 53–54.
Moriarity, A. J. (1963). Trifluoperazine and congenital malformations. *Can. Med. Assoc. J.* **88** (2), 97.
Morphew, J. A., and Barber, J. E. (1965). Peristent oral dyskinesia in treatment with phenothiazine derivatives. *Lancet* I (7386), 650.
Moulton, S. E., et al. (1961). Extrapyramidal side effects of trifluoperazine. *Proc. Staff Meetings Mayo Clin.* **36** (11), 268–270.
Paulson, G. (1960). Procyclidine for dystonia caued by phenothiazine derivatives. *Diseases Nervous System* **21** (8), 447–448.
Posner, H. S., et al. (1962). Cause of the odor of a schizophrenic patient. *Arch. Gen. Psychiat.* **7** (2), 108–113.
Potts, A. M. (1962). Uveal pigment and phenothiazine compounds. *Trans. Am. Ophthalmol. Soc.* **60**, 517–552.
Preston, J. (1959). Central nervous system reactions to small doses of tranquilizers. Report of one death. *Am. Practitioner* **10** (4), 627–630.
Price, L. B. (1963). Severe extrapyramidal seizure following ingestion of two milligrams of trifluoperazine ("Stelazine"). *J. Florida Med. Assoc.* **49** (8), 654–655.
Reboton, J., Jr., et al. (1962). Pigmentary retinopathy and irido-cycloplegia in psychiatric patients. *J. Neuropsychiat.* **3** (5), 311–316.
Reinhardt, D. J., III, et al. (1962). Serum cholesterol elevation with trifluoperazine ("Stelazine") therapy. *Delaware State Med. J.* **34** (11), 318–323.
Robinson, A. S. (1960). "Neck-face syndrome" related to phenothiazine drugs. *J. Am. Med. Assoc.* **173** (5), 504–506.
Rosin, A. J., and Exton-Smith, A. N. (1965). Peristent oral dyskinesia in treatment with phenothiazine derivatives. *Lancet* I (7386), 651.
Rovito, D. A., and Pirone, F. J. (1963). Acanthrocytosis associated with schizophrenia. *Am. J. Psychiat.* **120** (2), 182–185.
St. Jean, A., et al. (1964). Uses and abuses of antiparkinsonian medication. *Am. J. Psychiat.* **120** (8), 801–803.
Schrire, I. (1963). Trifluoperazine and foetal abnormalities. *Lancet* I (7273), 174.
Serpe, S. J., and Norins, A. L. (1961). Allergic purpura after administration of trifluoperazine. *N.Y. State J. Med.* **61** (20), 3517–3518.
Shafer, S., et al. (1962). Extrapyramidal effects of tranquillisers. *Lancet* I (7222), 221–222.
Sherlock, S. (1962). Jaundice. *Brit. Med. J.* I (5289), 1359–1366.
Sherman, S., et al. (1960). Oculogyric crisis induced by phenothiazine drugs. *Diseases Nervous System* **21** (6), 333–334.
Sigwald, J., et al. (1959). Les accidents neurologiques des medications neuroleptiques. [Neurological side effects of neuroleptic medications.] *Rev. Neurol.* **100**, 553–595.

Simonson, M. (1964). Phenothiazine depressive reaction. *J. Neuropsychiat.* **5** (5), 259–265.
Smith, D. R. (1964). Drug intoxication: Barbiturates and tranquilizers. *Appl. Therap.* **6** (3), 219–222.
Spellberg, M. A. (1964). Intrahepatic cholestasis vs. posthepatic jaundice: Methods of diagnosis with a note on hypercholesteremic xanthomatosis in a patient with chlorpromazine cholestasis. *Med. Clin. N. Am.* **48** (1), 53–65.
Twyman, J. B. (1963). Acute extrapyramidal reaction associated with trifluoperazine. *Virginia Med. Monthly* **90** (3), 132–133.
Vates, T. S., and Masucci, E. F. (1960). Acute extrapyramidal syndromes following the use of phenothiazine derivatives. *Med. Ann. District Columbia* **29** (12), 670–673.
Verhulst, H. L., and Crotty, J. J. (1962). Tranquilizers. *Natl. Clearinghouse Poison Control Center* pp. 1–8.
Vilkin, M. I. (1963). Extrapyramidal side effects of trifluoperazine. *J. Neuropscyhiat.* **4** (4), 236–239.
Walker, M. F. (1959). Simulation of tetanus by trifluoperazine overdosage. *Can. Med. Assoc. J.* **81** (2), 109–110.
Weicker, H. (1963). Teratogene substanzen. [Teratogenic substances.] *Med. Klin. (Munich)* **58** (50), 2032–2037.
Wheatley, D. (1964). Drugs and the embryo. *Brit. Med. J.* I (5383), 630.
Witton, K. (1961). Severe and fatal reactions to tranquilizers. *J. Am. Med. Assoc.* **175** (2), 175–176.
Worobec, T. (1965). Blood dyscrasias associated with antituberculosis and/or tranquilizing chemotherapy; a long-term clinical observation. *Diseases Chest* **47** (2), 208–217.

Clinical Papers

Ainslie, J. D. (1961). The use of newer psychiatric drugs in medical practice; their specificity of action in relation to target symptoms and dynamic situation. *J. Florida Med. Assoc.* **47** (8), 901–906.
Alexander, H. G. (1962). Electroconvulsive and non-convulsive stimulation combined with trifluoperazine in treating schizophrenic patients. *J. Neuropsychiat.* **3** (6), 388–389.
Allen, V. S. (1959). Trifluoperazine in the treatment of drug-resistant schizophrenics. *J. Clin. Exptl. Psychopathol.* **20** (3), 247–250.
Allen, V. S. (1960). One year's experience with trifluoperazine in treatment of chronic mental disorders. *J. Clin. Exptl. Psychopathol.* **21** (4), 285–292.
Allison, G. E. (1964). Psychiatry: Psychiatric drugs and the non-psychiatric practitioner. *Manitoba Med. Rev.* **44** (2), 102–106.
Altschuler, M. (1962). Massive doses of trifluoperazine in the treatment of compulsive rituals. *Am. J. Psychiat.* **119** (4), 367–368.
Anonymous. (1962). Stelazine. *Med. Letter* **4** (10), 38–39.
Anonymous. (1963). To-day's drugs: Tranquillizers. *Brit. Med. J.* II (5350), 163–164.
Anonymous. (1963). General practitioner clinical trials: Drugs in pregnancy survey. *Practitioner* **191** (1146), 775–780.
Anonymous. (1964). Choice of drugs for emotional disorders. *Med. Letter* **6** (12), 45–46.
Anonymous. (1965). Drug treatment of schizophrenia. *Brit. Med. J.* I (5435), 647–648.
Appleton, W. (1963). Massive doses of chlorpromazine: Effectiveness in controlling psychotic behavior. *Arch. Gen. Psychiat.* **9** (6), 586–592.
Archer, J. S., and Hicks, R. G. (1962). Phenothiazine subgroups. *N.Y. State J. Med.* **62** (23), 3769–3772.
Atkinson, R. M., and Rubin, R. T. (1964). Electroconvulsive treatment and severe cardiovascular disease. *Am. J. Psychiat.* **121** (3), 249–252.

Ayd, F. J., Jr. (1959). "Stelazine" therapy for the psychosomatic patient. *Clin. Med.* **6** (3), 387–392.
Ayd, F. J., Jr. (1959). Trifluoperazine therapy for everyday psychiatric problems. *Current Therap. Res.* **1** (1), 9 pp.
Ayd, F. J., Jr. (1963). The phenothiazine tranquilizers: A re-evaluation after ten years experience. *Mind* **1**, 326-passim.
Ayd, F. J., Jr. (1958). Treatment of neuroses with trifluoperazine; a preliminary report. *In* "Trifluoperazine" (J. H. Moyer, ed.), pp. 183–188. Lea & Febiger, Philadelphia, Pennsylvania.
Ayd, F. J., Jr. (1960). Tranquilizers and the ambulatory geriatric patient. *J. Am. Geriat. Soc.* **8** (12), 909–914.
Ballinger, C. M. (1959). Controlled tests of antiemetic drugs in volunteers. *In* "Trifluoperazine" (J. H. Moyer, ed.), pp. 137–143. Lea & Febiger, Philadelphia, Pennsylvania.
Baroody, N. B., and Baroody, W. G. (1959). Control of agitation and alcoholic hallucinosis with trifluoperazine; a prelininary report. *In* "Trifluoperazine" (J. H. Moyer, ed.), pp. 61–64. Lea & Febiger, Philadelphia, Pennsylvania.
Baroody, N. B., Jr., *et al.* (1960). Management of delirium tremens, preliminary observations with trifluoperazine. *J. Am. Med. Assoc.* **172** (12), 1284–1287.
Barron, A., *et al.* (1961). A "double blind" study comparing Ro 4-0403, trifluoperazine and a placebo in chronically ill mental patients. *Am. J. Psychiat.* **118** (4), 347–348.
Barsa, J. A., and Saunders, J. C. (1960). Trifluoperazine combined with chlorpromazine. *Am. J. Psychiat.* **116** (10), 925.
Barsa, J. A., *et al.* (1959). Trifluoperazine in the treatment of chronic schizophrenics. *Am. J. Psychiat.* **115** (9), 812.
Baruk, H., *et al.* (1963). Hallucinations et personnalité. Essais thérapeutiques par l'association de tranylcypromine et de phénothiazines pipérazinées et fluorées. [Hallucinations and personality. Therapeutic study of the combination of tranylcypromine and piperazine and fluorinated phenothiazines.] *Ann. Med. Psychol.* **121** (2/3), 437.
Bassino, P. G., and Piacquadio, A. (1964). Considerazioni cliniche su un nuovo farmaco nella medicazione preanestetica. [Clinical data on a new drug for preanesthetic medication.] *Minerva Anestiol.* **30**, 12–16.
Batt, J. C. (1959). A clinical trial of "Stelazine" in the treatment of chronic schizophrenia. *Postgrad. Med. J.* **35** (408), 571 and 573–574.
Beaudry, P., and Gibson, D. (1960). Effect of trifluoperazine on the behavior disorders of children with malignant emotional disturbances. *Am. J. Mental Deficiency* **64** (5), 823–826.
Bennett, J. L., and Hamilton, L. D. (1963). Sequential use of antidepressant drugs with chlorpromazine in chronic schizophrenia. *Psychiat. Quart.* **37** (1), 53–66.
Bensoussan, P. (1963). Bilan de plusieurs années d'emploi de la trifluopérazine en thérapeutique psychiatrique. [Results of several years' use of trifluopérazine in therapeutic psychiatry.] *Ann. Med. Psychol.* **121** (2/2), 250–255.
Bermudez, M. (1963). La trifluoperazina como antiemetico en el periodo postoperatorio immediato. [Trifluoperazine as an antiemetic in the immediate postoperative period.] *Semana Med.* (*Mex.*) No. 456.
Bethell, M. S., *et al.* (1961). Schizophrenia in general hospitals. *Brit. Med. J.* **11**, 453.
Bett, W. R. (1959). Phenothiazine derivatives in the treatment of mental disorders; a review of recent work. *Med. Proc.* **5**, 359–362.
Bett, W. R. (1960). The phenothiazines in psychiatry, with special reference to trifluoperazine ("Stelazine"): A review of the literature, *W. African Med. J.* **9**, 33–36.
Bhargava, K. P., and Chandra, O. (1963). Anti-emetic activity of phenothiazines in relation to their chemical structure. *Brit. J. Pharmacol.* **21** (3), 436–440.
Bhargava, K. P., and Chandra, O. (1964). Tranquillizing and hypotensive activities of twelve phenothiazines. *Brit. J. Pharmacol.* **22** (1), 154–161.

Bishop, M. P., et al. (1963). A comparison of SKF-7261 and trifluoperazine ("Stelazine") in the treatment of chronic schizophrenic patients. *J. Neuropsychiat.* **5** (1), 28–32.

Blachy, P. H., and Starr, A. (1964). Post-cardiotomy delirium. *Am. J. Psychiat.* **121** (4), 371–375.

Blackburn, H. L., and Allen, J. L. (1961). Behavioral effects of interrupting and resuming tranquilizing medication among schizophrenics. *J. Nervous Mental Disease* **133** (4), 303–308.

Blatchford, E., and Roberts, H. (1962). Intravenous trifluoperazine ("Stelazine") as a postoperative anti-emetic. *Can. Anaesthesiol. Soc. J.* **9** (4), 347–352.

Bordeleau, J.-M., and Gratton, L. (1958). Etude d'un nouveau neuroleptique: Le trifluoropérazine; rapport préliminaire. [Study of a new neuroleptic, trifluoroperazine; preliminary report.] *Union Med. Canada* **87** (12), 1552–1557.

Bordeleau, J.-M., and Gratton, L. (1959). Etude d'un puissant neuroleptique, la "Stelazine" (trifluoperazine). [Study of a potent neuroleptic, "Stelazine" (trifluoperazine).] *Union Med. Canada* **88** (7), 855–860.

Borg, G. (1964). Intryck från besök vid några olika typer av psykiatriska sjukhus i USA, speciellt California. [Impressions from visits to several different types of psychiatric hospitals in the USA, especially in California.] *Svenska Läkartidn.* **61** (29), 2192–2209.

Bowen, E. H., Jr. (1959). Some recent drugs useful in anesthesiology. *Anaesthesia Analgesia. Current Res.* **38** (1), 14–20.

Bowes, H. A., and Natarajan, R. (1963). Office psychopharmacology. *Psychosomatics* **4** (1), 22–26.

Braceland, F. J. (1964). Drugs effective in emotional disorders. *Postgrad. Med.* **35** (3), 237–242.

Bram, G. (1960). The treatment of psychoneurotic conditions with trifluoperazine. *Brit. J. Clin. Pract.* **14** (2), 107–109.

Bram, G. (1962). Treatment of psychoneurotic conditions with long acting trifluoperazine ("Stelazine"), *Spansule* capsules. *Brit. J. Clin. Pract.* **16** (2), 143–145.

Brooks, G. W. (1958). Definitive ataractic therapy in the rehabilitation of chronic schizophrenic patients; a preliminary report on the use of trifluoperazine. *In* "Trifluoperazine" pp. 54–61. Lea & Febiger, Philadelphia, Pennsylvania.

Brooks, G. W., and MacDonald, M. G. (1961). Effects of trifluoperazine in aged depressed female patients. *Am. J. Psychiat.* **117** (10), 932–933.

Broussolle, P., and Grunthaler, C. (1964). La trifluoperazine a doses filées en psychiatrie ambulatoire. [Trifluoperazine in small repeated doses in ambulatory psychiatry.] *Lyon Med.* **211**, 181-passim.

Broussolle, P., et al. (1962). La trifluoperazine, une phénothiazine fluorée et pipérazinée en psychiatrie hospitaliere. [Trifluoperazine, a fluorinated piperazine phenothiazine in hospital psychiatry.] *Presse Med.* **70** (8), 374–376.

Bucove, A. (1964). Posipartum psychoses in the male. *Bull. N.Y. Acad. Med.* **40** (12), 961–971.

Buffaloe, W. J., and Sandifer, M. G., Jr. (1961). A study of combined therapy with "Stelazine" and "Parnate" (SKF 385) in chronic anergic schizophrenics. *Am. J. Psychiat.* **117** (11), 1030–1031.

Buki, R. (1964). A treatment program for homosexuals. *Diseases Nervous System* **25** (5), 304–307.

Burt, O. P., and Bressler, F. D. (1961). Trifluoperazine in postoperative gynecological patients; a double-blind evaluation in 111 patients. *Ohio State Med. J.* **57** (9), 1008–1009.

Cacioppo, J., et al. (1961). A comparison between trifluoperazine and carphenazine in chronically ill schizophrenic in-patients. *Diseases Nervous System* **22** (2), 46–50.

Cahan, R. B. (1960). Efficacy of trifluoperazine in chronic mental illness. *Am. J. Psychiat.* **116** (9), 838–839.

Calwell, W. P. K., et al. (1964). A comparative study of oxypertine and trifluoperazine in chronic schizophrenia—a new application of the Wing rating scale. *Brit. J. Psychiat.* **110** (467), 520–530.

Capparell, H. V. (1962). Drug therapy in mental illness. *Penna. Med. J.* **65** (8), 899–905.
Carter, C. H. (1959). Trifluoperazine in the management of hyperactive, mentally defective children. *In* "Trifluoperazine" (J. H. Moyer, ed.), pp. 123–129. Lea & Febiger, Philadelphia, Pennsylvania.
Casey, J. F., *et al.* (1961). Combined drug therapy of chronic schizophrenics: Controlled evaluation of placebo, dextro-amphetamine, imipramine, isocarboxazid and trifluoperazine added to maintenance doses of chlorpromazine. *Am. J. Psychiat.* **117** (11), 997–1003.
Caso, A., *et al.* (1959). Observaciones sobre el uso de la trifluoperazine en la psiquiatrĭa de hospital. [Observations on the use of trifluoperazine in hospital psychiatry.] *Neurol. Neurochir. Psiquiat.* **1** (1), 23–29.
Cauffman, W. J., and Pauley, W. G. (1959). Trifluoperazine as an antiemetic in children. *In* "Trifluoperazine" pp. 149–156. Lea & Febiger, Philadelphia, Pennsylvania.
Chapple, E. D., *et al.* (1963). The measurement of activity patterns of schizophrenic patients. *J. Nervous Mental Diseases* **137** (3), 258–267.
Cheng, S. F., and Fogel, E. J. (1963). Trifluoperazine combined with amitriptyline in paranoid psychosis. *Am. J. Psychiat.* **119** (8), 780–781.
Childers, R. T., Jr. (1961). Controlling the chronically disturbed patient with massive phenothiazine therapy. *Am. J. Psychiat.* **118** (3), 246–247.
Childers, R. T., Jr. (1961). Response of schizophrenia to phenothiazines and placebo. *J. Clin. Exptl. Psychopathol.* **22** (4), 223–225.
Childers, R. T., Jr. (1962). Selective effectiveness of chlorpromazine and trifluoperazine in schizophrenia. *Diseases Nervous System* **23** (3), 156–157.
Childers, R. T., Jr. (1964). Comparison of four regimens in newly admitted female schizophrenics. *Am. J. Psychiat.* **120** (10), 1010–1011.
Childers, R. T., Jr., and Therrien, R. (1961). A comparison of the effectiveness of trifluoperazine and chlorpromazine in schizophrenia. *Am. J. Psychiat.* **118** (6), 552–554.
Cohen, J. J. (1959). Trifluoperazine in the menopausal syndrome. *In* "Trifluoperazine" pp. 116–121. Lea & Febiger, Philadelphia, Pennsylvania.
Cohen, N. H. (1962). The treatment of Huntington's chorea with trifluoperazine ("Stelazine"). *J. Nervous Mental Disease* **134** (1), 62–71.
Cohen, S., *et al.* (1958). Effect of trifluoperazine on some symptoms common among skid row alcoholics. *In* "Trifluoperazine" pp. 189–191. Lea & Febiger, Philadephia, Pennsylvania.
Cole, J. O. (1964). Therapeutic efficacy of antidepressant drugs; a review. *J. Am. Med. Assoc.* **190** (5), 448–455.
Coons, W. H., *et al.* (1962). Chlorpromazine, trifluoperazine and placebo with long-term mental hospital patients. *Can. Psychiat. Assoc. J.* **7** (4), 159–163.
Cornman, H. D., III (1962). Clinical use of the phenothiazine derivatives in general practice. *In* "Psychosomatic Medicine. First Hahnemann Symposium" (J. H. Nodine and J. H. Moyer, eds.), pp. 461–464. Lea & Febiger, Philadelphia, Pennsylvania.
Costa, J. S., and Hoffman, E. T. (1960). The use of trifluoperazine for acute alcoholism. *Med. Ann. District Columbia* **29** (10), 556–558.
Council on Drugs. (1961). New drugs and developments in therapeutics: Drugs for mental illness. *J. Am. Med. Assoc.* **177** (4), 245–246.
Crisp, A. H., and Roberts, F. J. (1963). The response of an adrenalectomized patient to ECT. *Am. J. Psychiat.* **119** (8), 784–785.
Danilenko, E. T. (1963). Klinicheskie i neirodinamicheskie sdvighi u boln'nykh schizofrenii pod vliyaniem lecheniya stelazinom. [Clinical and neurodynamic changes in schizophrenics treated with "Stelazine".] *Zh. Nevropatol. Psikhiat.* **63** (3), 424–430.
Danilenko, E. T. (1964). Primenenie stelazina dlya lecheniya bol'nykh shizofreniei v pozhilom vozraste. [Use of "Stelazine" in middle-aged schizophrenics.] *Zh. Nevropatol. i Psikhiat.* **64** (9), 1391–1395.

Davison, K. (1964). Episodic depersonalization; observations on 7 patients. *Brit. J. Psychiat.* **110** (467), 505–513.

Desrochers, J. L., and Schiffmann, W. (1961). Etude à court terme sur l'usage de la trifluopérazine contre les troubles du comportement chez l'enfant. [Short-term study on the use of trifluoperazine in behavior disorders in children.] *Union Med. Canada* **90** (4), 369–373.

Dierks, M. (1963). A comparison of two phenothiazines in the treatment of schizophrenics. *Am. J. Psychiat.* **119** (8), 775–776.

DiMascio, A., et al. (1963). The psychopharmacology of phenothiazine compounds: A comparative study of the effects of chlorpromazine, promethazine, trifluoperazine and perphenazine in normal males. I. Introduction, aims and methods. *J. Nervous Mental Disease* **136** (1), 15–28.

Dixit, Y. B., and Pathak, J. D. (1964). Assessment of mental alertness after administration of various phenothiazines. *J. Indian Med. Assoc.* **42**, 173–175.

Dobkin, A. B., and Palko, D. (1960). The antisialogogue effect of phenothiazine derivatives: Comparison of promaine, levomepromazine, trifluoperazine, proclorperazine, methdilazine and prothipendyl. *Anesthesiology* **21** (3), 260–262.

Donaldson, W. N. S. (1961). Trifluoperazine ("Stelazine") in the treatment of seasickness. *J. Roy. Nav. Med. Serv.* **47**, 100–103.

Doust, J. W., and Harrington, R. W. (1962). Acute effects of ataractic drugs on spontaneous autonomic and metabolic oscillating systems in schizophrenic and other psychiatric patients. *Can. Psychiat. Assoc. J.* **7** (2), 76–89.

Dundee, J. W., et al. (1963). Alterations in response to somatic pain associated with anaesthesia. XV. Further studies with phenothiazine derivatives and similar drugs. *Brit. J. Anaesthesia* **35**, 597–610.

Editorial. (1963). Phenmetrazine and trifluoperazine. *Med. J. Australia* I (1), 58.

Eilenberg, D., and Woods, L. W. (1962). Narcolepsy with psychosis: Report of two cases. *Proc. Staff Meetings Mayo Clin.* **37** (21), 561–566.

Ellard, J. (1963). Psychotropic drugs in general practice. *Med. J. Australia* **11** (19), 773–777.

Enelow, A. J. (1965). Drug treatment of psychotic patients in general medical practice. *Calif. Med.* **102** (1), 1–4.

Ernst, E. M. (1959). Trifluoperazine in anxiety and tension states. *Diseases Nervous System* **20** (7), 300–301.

Ernst, E. A. (1959). Trifluoperazine in the treatment of gastrointestinal tension states. In "Trifluoperazine" pp. 104–109. Lea & Febiger, Philadelphia, Pennsylvania.

Erdos, J. M., and Hillinger, J. (1960). Trifluoperazine in refractory schizophrenic patients. *Am. J. Psychiat.* **116** (11), 1026–1027.

Evangelakis, M. G. (1961). De-institutionalization of patients; the triad of trifluoperazine-group psychotherapy-adjunctive therapy. *Diseases Nervous System* **22** (1), 26–32.

Evans, D. A. P. (1963). Pharmacogenetics. *Am. J. Med.* **34** (5), 639–662.

Ext, H. J. (1960). Use of trifluoperazine in chronic psychotic patients. *Diseases Nervous System* **21** (3), 154–157.

Falardeau, I. F. (1959). Trifluoperazine as an adjunct in the management of emotional problems in the aged. In "Trifluoperazine" pp. 82–87. Lea & Febiger, Philadelphia, Pennsylvania.

Feinberg, I., et al. (1964). Sleep electroencephalographic and eye-movement patterns in schizophrenic patients. *Comprehensive Psychiat.* **5** (1), 44–53.

Feldman, P. E. (1958). An evaluation of trifluoperazine in chronic schizophrenia. In "Trifluoperazine" pp. 87–97. Lea & Febiger, Philadelphia, Pennsylvania.

Ferrero, R. G. A. (1961). Resultados terapeuticos de la trifluoperazina en las timopatias. [Therapeutic results with trifluoperazine in thymopathies.] *Semana Med. (Buenos Aires)* **118** (6), 250–252.

Fine, R. H. (1964). Clinical experience with trifluoperazine in the severely retarded. *J. Neuropsychiat.* **5** (6), 370–372.

Fischer, A. (1965). Effective psychopharmacology. *Calif. Med.* **102** (3), 217–221.

Fish, B. (1960). Drug therapy in child psychiatry: Pharmacological aspects. *Comprehensive Psychiat.* **1** (4), 212–227.

Fish, B. (1960). Drug therapy in child psychiatry: Psychological aspects. *Comprehensive Psychiat.* **1** (1), 55–61.

Fish, B. (1965). Psychiatric drugs: Evaluation of effects is improved. *Med. Tribune* **6** (31), 14.

Fisher, C., and Dement, W. C. (1963). Studies on the psychopathology of sleep and dreams. *Am. J. Psychiat.* **119** (12), 1160–1168.

Forrester, M. E. (1958). Disturbed chronic psychotic patients: Pilot trial of "Stelazine". *Brit. Med. J.* II (5088), 90–91.

Fouks, L., et al. (1962). Note sur l'utilisation clinique du 2145 T.H. [Clinical use of T.H. 2145.] *Ann. Med. Psychol.* **2** (4), 546–554.

Freed, H. (1958). On the combined use of trifluoperazine and electroshock therapy. In "Trifluoperazine" (J. H. Moyer, ed.), pp. 98–100. Lea & Febiger, Philadelphia, Pennsylvania.

Freed, H. (1961). The current status of the tranquilizers and of child analysis in child psychiatry. *Diseases Nervous System* **22** (8), 434–437.

Freed, H., and Frignito, N. (1961). Tranquilizers in child psychiatry: Current status on drugs, particularly phenothiazines. *Penna. Psychiat. Quart.* **1** (4), 39–48.

Galenko, V. E., and Kel'mishkeit, E. F. (1963). Lechenie stelazinom bolnyh paranoidnoi formoi shizofrenii. ["Stelazine" in treatment of paranoid schizophrenia.] *Zh. Nevropatol. i Psikhiat.* **63** (2), 269–274.

Garai, J. (1959). "Stelazine" in the treatment of schizophrenia. A preliminary report. *Med. Press* **241**, 473–475.

Garcia-Faure, M. A. (1962). Electroshock therapy and trifluoperazine in chronic schizophrenia. *Missouri Med.* **59** (3), 217-passim.

Gatto, L. E. (1965). Better drugs and responses in the field of psychiatry. *Southern Med. J.* **58** (1), 21–23.

Gearren, J. B. (1959). Trifluoperazine in emotionally disturbed office patients. *Diseases Nervous System* **20** (2), 66–68.

Gerson, I. M., et al. (1964). Clinical trial of a potentiated diketopiperazine derivative as a psychopharmacological agent for the treatment of psychotic patients. *Am. J. Psychiat.* **121** (2), 179–181.

Goddard, E. S. (1959). Trifluoperazine in psychoneurotic outpatients. *Can. Med. Assoc. J.* **81** (6), 467–470.

Goddard, E. S. (1959). Treatment of psychoneurotic patients in the general hospital. In "Trifluoperazine" pp. 21–27. Lea & Febiger, Philadelphia, Pennsylvania.

Goldman, D. (1958). Clinical experience with trifluoperazine; treatment of psychotic states. In "Trifluoperazine" pp. 71–86. Lea & Febiger, Philadelphia, Pennsylvania.

Goldman, D. (1962). The effect of "energizers" on neurotic patients. *Diseases Nervous System* **23** (11), 632–639.

Gonzalez, J. R. (1962). The first year's experience with a follow-up clinic for schizophrenics. *Penna. Psychiat. Quart.* **2** (1), 52–55.

Gonzalez, J. R., and Imahara, J. K. (1964). Electroshock therapy with the phenothiazines and reserpine; a survey and report. *Am. J. Psychiat.* **121** (3), 253–256.

Gordon, I. (1962). The backward patient—a new approach (preliminary report). *Penna. Psychiat. Quart.* **2** (2), 51–54.

Gottfries, C. G. (1963). Medikamentell behandling av migrän; ett meddelande med anledning av uppgifter i dagspressen. [Medical treatment of migraine; a report in connection with announcements in the lay press.] *Svenska Lakartidn.* **60** (21), 1555–1560.

Gratton, L., et al. (1962). Les syndromes hypermoteurs de l'enfant et ses réactions à la trifluoperazine. [Hypermotor syndrome in children and its response to trifluoperazine.] *Union Med. Canada* **91** (1), 23-31.

Gross-Gorton, V. E. (1963). Combined tranylcypromine-trifluoperazine therapy in newly admitted depressed patients. *Am. J. Psychiat.* **120** (4), 392-393.

Guerrant, J., et al. (1964). The blood-cerebrospinal fluid barrier in chronic schizophrenia and after trifluoperazine ("Stelazine") treatment. *J. Nervous Mental Disease* **139** (3), 222-231.

Guido, J. A., and Abe, G. Y. (1960). Trifluoperazine: A report of a clinical trial in backward psychotic patients. *Am. J. Psychiat.* **117** (5), 453-455.

Gunn, D. R. (1958). The role of trifluoperazine in the treatment of refractory mental patients. *In* "Trifluoperazine" pp. 47-53. Lea & Febiger, Philadelphia, Pennsylvania.

Gwynne, P. H., et al. (1962). Efficacy of trifluoperazine on withdrawal in chronic schizophrenia. *J. Nervous Mental Disease* **134** (5), 451-455.

Hacquard, M., et al. (1963). La trifluopérazine dans les psychoses chroniques. [Trifluoperazine in chronic psychoses.] *Ann. Med. Psychol.* **121** (1/4), 603.

Hamel, J. F. (1959). Control of anxiety-related symptoms with trifluoperazine. *In* "Trifluoperazine" pp. 110-115. Lea & Febiger, Philadelphia, Pennsylvania.

Hamilton, D., and Bennett, J. L. (1962). The use of trifluoperazine in geriatric patients with chronic brain syndrome. *J. Am. Geriat. Soc.* **10** (2), 140-147.

Hamilton, M., et al. (1963). A controlled trial on the value of prochlorperazine, trifluoperazine and intensive group treatment. *Brit. J. Psychiat.* **109** (461), 510-522.

Hanlon, T. E., et al. (1965). The comparative effectiveness of eight phenothiazines. *Psychopharmacologia* **7** (2), 89-106.

Harley, J. D., and Farrar, J. F. (1964). Maternal drug therapy and congenital cataracts. *Med. J. Australia* **1** (6), 212-213.

Hart, T. (1959). Ataractic drug therapy in the management of chronic alcoholics. *In* "Trifluoperazine" pp. 65-77. Lea & Febiger, Philadelphia, Pennsylvania.

Hasse, H. J. (1963). Möglichkeiten und Grenzen der Psychopharmakotherapie mit Tranquilizern und Neuroleptika. [Possibilities and limitations of psychopharmacotherapy with tranquilizers and neuroleptics.] *Deut. Med. Wochschr.* **88** (11), 505-514.

Hawke, W. A., and McGreal, D. A. (1964). Tranquilizers. *Clin. Pediat. (Phila.)* **3** (4), 192-196.

Hawks, D. V., and Silverstone, J. T. (1962). Drug treatment of Huntington's chorea. *Brit. Med. J.* II (5296), 52.

Haworth, K. W. (1958). Preliminary investigation of trifluoperazine in psychotic states. *In* "Trifluoperazine" pp. 120-124. Lea & Febiger, Philadelphia, Pennsylvania.

Heinrichs, E. H. (1964). Mental retardation. I. Definition, recognition, management and prevention. *S. Dakota J. Med. Pharm.* **17** (1), 26-32.

Heyman, J. J., et al. (1964). The use of nicotinamide test dose in the assessment of psychotropic drugs in schizophrenic patients. *J. Neuropsychiat.* **5** (4), 221-224.

Himwich, H. E. (1960). Some drugs useful in the treatment of emotional disorders—physiology, indications, and contraindications. *Am. Practitioner* **11** (8), 687-696.

Himwich, H. E. (1965). Psychoactive drugs. *Postgrad. Med.* **37** (1), 35-44.

Hofstatter, L., et al. (1964). The management of the mentally retarded by the family physician. *Southern Med. J.* **57** (3), 297-301.

Hollister, L. E., et al. (1960). Trifluoperazine in chronic psychiatric patients. *J. Clin. Exptl. Psychopathol.* **21** (1), 15-24.

Hollister, L. E., et al. (1960). Trifluoperazine in chronic psychiatric patients. *Trans. 4th Res. Conf. Chemotherap. Psychiat. VA Wash., D.C.* **4**, 201-204.

Honigfeld, G., et al. (1965). Behavioral improvement in the older schizophrenic patient; drug and social therapies. *J. Am. Geriat. Soc.* **13** (1), 57-72.

Hordern, A. (1961). Psychiatry and the tranquilizers. *New Engl. J. Med.* **265** (12), 584–588; ibid. **265** (13), 634–638.
Hordern, A., and Hamilton, M. (1963). Drugs and "moral treatment". *Brit. J. Psychiat.* **109** (461), 500–509.
Hordern, A., and Somerville, D. M. (1962). The general practitioner and psychiatric drug treatment. *Med. J. Australia* **49** (1), 404–411.
Hordern, A., and Somerville, D. M. (1963). Clinical trials in chronic schizophrenia. *Med. J. Australia* **1**, 40–43.
Hordern, A., et al. (1962). Does chronic schizophrenia respond to a combination of a neuroleptic and an antidepressant? *J. Nervous Mental Disease* **134** (4), 361–376.
Howell, R. J., et al. (1961). A comparison of fluphenazine, trifluoperazine and a placebo in the context of an active treatment unit. *J. Nervous Mental Disease* **132** (6), 522–530.
Hughes, W. (1961). A comparative evaluation of two phenothiazines in the management of chronic schizophrenia. *Can. Med. Assoc. J.* **84** (5), 251–254.
Hunter, H., and Stephenson, G. M. (1963). Chlorpromazine and trifluoperazine in the treatment of behavioural abnormalities in the severely subnormal child. *Brit. J. Psychiat.* **109** (460), 411–417.
Hurst, L. (1960). Phenothiazine derivatives in the treatment of schizophrenia. *J. Mental Sci.* **106** (443), 755–770.
Ibarra Medina, R. (1961). Trifluoperazina en pediatria. [Trifluoperazine in pediatrics.] *Semana Med. (Mex.)* **27** (349), 395–396.
Jenkins, S. B. (1963). The use and abuse of phenothiazines in treatment of acute psychoses. *J. Natl. Med. Assoc.* **55** (6), 515–519.
Jenkins, S. B., and Samborski, A. H. (1964). Symptom specificity of anti-psychotic drugs. *J. Mich. Med. Soc.* **63** (3), 187–193.
Jerums, N. (1963). Tratamiento combinado de insulina y trifluorperazina en las esquizofrenias. [Combined treatment with insulin and trifluoperazine in schizophrenia.] *Arch. Venezolanos Psiquiat. Neurol.* **9** (21), 25–29.
Johnson, W. A. (1963). Long-term trifluoperazine therapy in a schizophrenic patient. *Northwest Med.* **62** (11), 884.
Johnston, J. (1959). Trifluoperazine, a new phenothiazine in psychiatric practice. *S. African Practitioner* **6** 50–51.
Joseph, S. R. (1962). Combined antidepressant tranquilizer therapy in somatic and psychosomatic illnesses. *Ariz. Med.* **19** (11), 239–241.
Judah, L. N., et al. (1961). Results of simultaneous abrupt withdrawal of ataraxics in 500 chronic psychotic patients. *Am. J. Psychiat.* **118** (2), 156–158.
Kaminsky, A. R., et al. (1960). Trifuoperazina: ensayo clínico en terapéutica dermatológica. [Trifluoperazine: Clinical trial in therapeutic dermatology.] *Dia Med.* **32** (53), 1521-passim.
Kant, F., and Abele, H. B. (1961). Ambulatory psychotherapy for the schizophrenic patient with the aid of drugs. *Diseases Nervous System* **22** (1), 45–48.
Kateryniuk, N., and Morris, C. W. (1961). A clinical trial study of trifluoperazine. *Diseases Nervous System* **22** (11), 639–641.
Kennon, L., and Chen, K. (1962). Probability and complexation: A new approach. *J. Pharm. Sci.* **51** (12), 1149–1151.
Kinross-Wright, V. J. (1958). Trifluoperazine and schizophrenia. *In* "Trifluoperazine" pp. 62–70. Lea & Febiger, Philadelphia, Pennsylvania.
Kinross-Wright, J. (1959). Newer phenothiazine drugs in treatment of nervous disorders. *J. Am. Med. Assoc.* **170** (11), 1283–1288.
Klimczynski, J. J. (1958). Treatment of chronically ill psychotic patients with trifluoperazine: A preliminary report. *In* "Trifluoperazine" pp. 101–112. Lea & Febiger, Philadelphia, Pennsylvania.

Kline, N. S. (1961). The use of psychopharmaceuticals in office practice. *Med. Clin. N. Am.* **45** (6), 1677–1684.
Koegler, R. R., *et al.* (1964). A psychiatric clinic evaluates brief-contact therapy. *Mental Hosp.* **15** (10), 564-passim.
Kolodny, A. L. (1961). Evaluation of a tranquilizer in general practice. *Diseases Nervous System* **22** (3), 151–154.
Koresko, R. L., *et al.* (1963). "Dream time" in hallucinating and nonhallucinating schizophrenic patients. *Nature* **199** (4898), 1118–1119.
Kovitz, B. (1958). Management of psychotic tension symptoms with trifluoperazine; a preliminary report. *In* "Trifluoperazine," pp. 144–149. Lea & Febiger, Philadelphia, Pennsylvania.
Kraines, S. H. (1964). Psychotropic drugs in general practice. *Memphis Med. J.* **39** (1), 9-passim.
Kraines, S. H., *et al.* (1963). Evaluation of psychotropic drugs in private practice: A symposium. *Diseases Nervous System* **24** (3), 181–184.
Krawiecki, J. A., and Burns, J. W. (1959). Trifluoperazine in schizophrenia. *Brit. Med. J.* I (5136), 1532.
Kropach, K. (1959). The treatment of acutely agitated senile patients with trifluoperazine ("Stelazine"). *Brit. J. Clin. Pract.* **13** (12), 859–862.
Kropach, K. (1959). Trifluoperazine in schizophrenia. *Brit. Med. J.* I (5128), 1044–1045.
Kruse, W. (1958). Trifluoperazine in chronic and semichronic schizophrenia. *In* "Trifluoperazine," pp. 138–143. Lea & Febiger, Philadelphia, Pennsylvania.
Kruse, W. (1959). Effect of trifluoperazine on auditory hallucinations in schizophrenics. *Am. J. Psychiat.* **116** (4), 318–321.
Kruse, W. (1959). Experience with trifluoperazine in 110 female schizophrenics. *Am. J. Psychiat.* **115** (11), 1031.
Kruse, W. (1960). Trifluoperazine and tranylcypromine in chronic refractory schizophrenics. *Am. J. Psychiat.* **117** (6), 548–549.
Kruse, W. (1960). Die Wirkung des Trifluoperazins auf die Gehörstäuschungen Schizophrener. [Effect of trifluoperazine on auditory hallucinations in schizophrenics.] *Nervenarzt* **31** (4), 180–182.
Kutsenok, B. M., *et al.* (1964). Lechenie stelazinom dlitel'no boleyushchikh shizofrenei. ["Stelazine" in treatment of schizophrenia of long duration.] *Zh. Nevropatol. Psikhiat.* **64** (9), 1386–1390.
Lambert, P.-A. (1964). Essai de systématisation des associations de neuroleptiques. [Trial systemization of neuroleptic combinations.] *Encephale* **53**, Suppl., 262–275.
Langschmidt, E. H. (1959). A clinical trial of "Stelazine" in the treatment of mental disorders. *S. African Med. J.* **33** (31), 651–652.
Launay, J. (1963). Action de la trifluopérazine, 1 milligramme en cure ambulatoire dans le cadre d'une consultation industrielle. Association à la tranylcypromine. [Effect of trifluoperazine, 1 mg, in ambulatory treatment in an industrial dispensary. Combination with tranylcypromine.] *Ann. Med. Psychol.* **121** (2/3), 440–441.
Lawlis, M. G. (1958). A note on trifluoperazine in the management of hyperactive mentally retarded children. *In* "Trifluoperazine" pp. 180–182. Lea & Febiger, Philadelphia, Pennsylvania.
Lecomte, M. G., and Alcalay, R. (1963). Essai de comparaison entre la trifluopérazine et les autres neuroleptiques dans le traitement des schizophrénies anciennes et des délires chroniques. [Comparative study of trifluoperazine and other neuroleptics in the treatment of chronic schizophrenia and chronic delirium.] *Ann. Med. Psychol.* **121** (1/2), 252–256.
Léger, Y., *et al.* (1959). Evaluation clinique de la trifluopérazine. [Clinical evaluation of trifluoperazine.] *Can. Psychiat. Assoc. J.* **4** (4), 239–242.

Lehmann, H. E., and Knight, D. A. (1958). Psychophysiologic testing with a new phrenotropic drug. *In* "Trifluoperazine," pp. 34–35. Lea & Febiger, Philadelphia, Pennsylvania.
Lesse, S. (1961). Combined tranylcypromine-trifluoperazine therapy in the treatment of patients with agitated depressions. *Am. J. Psychiat.* **117** (11), 1038–1039.
Lesse, S. (1961). Combined use of tranylcypromine and trifluoperazine in ambulatory treatment of patients with agitated depressions; preliminary evaluation. *N.Y. State J. Med.* **61** (11), 1898–1903.
Lesse, S. (1962). The relative merits of tranylcypromine alone and tranylcypromine in combination with trifluoperazine in the treatment of patients with severe agitated depressions. *Am. J. Psychiat.* **118** (10), 934–935.
Le Vann, L. J. (1959). Trifluoperazine dihydrochloride: An effective tranquilizing agent for behavioural abnormalities in defective children. *Can. Med. Assoc. J.* **80** (2), 123–124.
Le Vann, L. J. (1959). The use of trifluoperazine as a tranquilizing agent in mentally defective children. *In* "Trifluoperazine," pp. 130–135. Lea & Febiger, Philadelphia, Pennsylvania.
Levinson, B. W., and Ginsburg, M. (1960). Chronic dements; a multifactorial therapeutic approach to their management. *Med. Proc.* **6**, 169–174.
Ling, G. M. (1962). Some effects of tranylcypromine and trifluoperazine on electrocortical activity (EEG activation). *Can. Psychiat. Assoc. J.* **7**, Suppl., S44–S54.
Lingl, F. A. (1964). Combined drug therapy compared with electric shock in psychotic depressions. *Am. J. Psychiat.* **120** (8), 808–810.
Lopez, J. A. N. (1964). Out patient treatment of acute schizophrenics. *Bol. Asoc. Med. Puerto Rico* **56** (1), 1–10.
Lourie, R. S. (1964). Psychoactive drugs in pediatrics. *Pediatrics* **34** (5), 691–693.
Lowther, G. H. (1960). Clinical experience with trifluoperazine in low-grade mental defectives. *Can. Med. Assoc. J.* **82** (23), 1158–1160.
Macdonald, R., and Watts, T. P. (1959). Trifluoperazine dihydrochloride ("Stelazine") in paranoid schizophrenia. *Brit. Med. J.* I (5121), 549–550.
Madgwick, J. R., and McNeill, D. L. (1959). Trifluoperazine in schizophrenia. *Brit. Med. J.* I (5128), 1045.
Madgwick, J. R., *et al.* (1958). "Stelazine" (trifluoperazine) a preliminary report on a clinical trial. *J. Mental Sci.* **104**, 1195–1198.
Maerz, J. C., *et al.* (1962). Psychosomatic disorders treated with trifluoperazine. *Psychosomatics* **111** (3), 220–222.
Mandel, W., and Evans, P. (1962). Comparison of butyrylperazine and trifluoperazine in chronic schizophrenic subjects. *Am. J. Psychiat.* **119** (1), 70–71.
Mandell, A. J. (1963). The psychologic management of coronary patients. *Gen. Practitioner* **27** (1), 82–91.
Mann, J. (1963). The initiation of treatment of unmanageable psychotics with intramuscular administration of trifluoperazine combined with chlorpromazine. *Am. J. Psychiat.* **120** (1). 74–76.
Mapp, Y., and Nodine, J. H. (1962). Psychopharmacology. II. Tranquilizers and antipsychotic drugs. *Psychosomatics* **3** (6), 458–463.
Marconi, M. (1962). La trifluoperazina: effetti farmacologici ed applicazioni cliniche. [Trifluoperazine: Pharmacological and clinical application.] *Minerva Med.* **53** (16), 566–574.
Margat, P., *et al.* (1963). Essai de la trifluopérazine. [Study of trifluoperazine.] *Ann. Med. Psychol.* **121** (2/1), 92–98.
Margolis, L. H. (1959). Intensive trifluoperazine therapy in office practice. *In* "Trifluoperazine," pp. 42–60. Lea & Febiger, Philadelphia, Pennsylvania.
Marjerrison, G., *et al.* (1962). Withdrawal of long-term phenothiazines from chronically hospitalized psychiatric patients. *Can. Psychiat. Assoc. J.* **9** (4), 290–298.

Markham, C. H. (1964). Diseases of the basal ganglia. *Mind* **2** (1), 6–9.
Markey, H. (1958). Patients with chronic schizophrenic reactions treated with trifluoperazine. *In* "Trifluoperazine" pp. 150–155. Lea & Febiger, Philadelphia, Pennsylvania.
Marks, J. (1962). Current views on psychotropic drugs. *New Zealand Med. J.* **61**, 391–397.
Marx, F. J. (1959). Adjunctive ataractic therapy in the treatment of functional and organic disorders. *In* "Trifluoperazine" pp. 89–95. Lea & Febiger, Philadelphia, Pennsylvania.
May, A. R., *et al.* (1959). Trifluoperazine ("Stelazine") in psychoneuroses. A clinical assessment. *J. Mental Sci.* **105** (441), 1059–1063.
May, P. R. A., and Tuma, A. H. (1964). The effect of psychotherapy and "Stelazine" on length of hospital stay, release rate and supplemental treatment of schizophrenic patients. *J. Nervous Mental Disease* **139** (4), 362–369.
May, P. R. A., and Tuma, A. H. (1965). Ataractic drugs and electroshock. *Intern. J. Neuropsychiat.* **1** (1), 84–89.
McLaughlin, B. E., *et al.* (1964). Chemotherapy for emotionally disturbed children: A follow-up report. *Diseases Nervous System* **25** (12), 735–738.
McLean, J. D. (1963). Psychopharmacological agents in general practice. *Nova Scotia Med. Bull.* **42** (1), 12–18.
McNeill, D. L. M., and Madgwick, J. R. A. (1961). A comparison of results in schizophrenics treated with (1) insulin, (2) trifluoperazine ("Stelazine"). *J. Mental Sci.* **107** (447), 297–299.
McNichol, R. W., and Seale, A. L. (1964). Treatment of outpatients with a combination of chlorpromazine and trifluoperazine. *Diseases Nervous System* **25** (4), 240–243.
McPeake, J. D., and DiMascio, A. (1964). Drug-personality interaction in the learning of a nonsense syllable task. *Psychol. Rept.* **15** (2), 405–406.
Medina, R. I. (1962). Trifluoperazina en pediatria. [Trifluoperazine in pediatrics.] *Semana Med.* (*Mex.*) pp. 395–396.
Meduna, L. J. (1964). The depression complex; a review of the history and treatment of twelve patients. *J. Neuropsychiat.* **5** (6), 373–385.
Melgar, M. C. (1962). Modificaciones del psicodiagnostico de Rorschach durante tratamientos realizados con "Stelazine" en esquizofrenicos cronicos. [Changes in psychodiagnosis with the Rorschach test during treatment of chronic schizophrenics with "Stelazine".] *Dia Med.* **34**, 130–133.
Meller, R. L. (1962). Treatment of depression with combined drug therapy. *Minn. Med.* **45** (1), 24–26.
Michaux, M. H., and Kurland, A. A. (1963). Combined psychotropic drug therapy. *Diseases Nervous System* **24** (12), 739–741.
Michaux, M. H., *et al.* (1964). Phenothiazines in the treatment of newly admitted state hospital patients: Global comparison of eight compounds in terms of an outcome index. *Current Therap. Res.* **6** (5), 331–339.
Milligan, W. L., *et al.* (1960). The treatment of psychotic patients; a clinical trial with trifluoperazine ("Stelazine"). *Med. Proc.* **6**, 109–112.
Moriarity, A., and Nance, M. R. (1963). Trifluoperazine and pregnancy. *Can. Med. Assoc. J.* **88** (7), 375–376.
Morton-Gore, N. (1964). Combined tranquillisation in the treatment of adolescents exhibiting the schizophrenic syndrome. *J. Mental Subnorm.* **18**, 53–62.
Moyer, J. H., and Conner, P. K. (1958). Clinical and laboratory observations on two trifluoromethyl phenothiazine derivatives. *J. Lab. Clin. Med.* **51** (2), 185–197.
Nadzharov, R. A. (1962). O lechenii Stelazinom kronicheskoi shizofrenii. [Treatment of chronic schizophrenia with "Stelazine".] *Zh. Nevropatol. i Psikhiat.* **62** (5), 740–745.
Nols, E. (1963). Etude clinique d'un neuroleptique majeur: la trifluopérazine, phénothiazine fluorée et pipérazinée. [Clinical study of a major neuroleptic: Trifluoperazine, a fluorinated piperazine phenothiazine.] *Ann. Med. Psychol.* **121** (2/4), 636.

Oakley, D. P. (1959). Trifluoperazine in schizophrenia. *Brit. Med. J.* I (5125), 862.
Obarrio y Rodolfo, J. M., *et al.* (1963). Estudios sobre una nueva asociacion medicamentosa. (Study of a new therapeutic combination.) *Semana Med. (Buenos Aires)* **123**, 71–73.
Ornstein, P. H. (1964). Evaluation of newer antidepressant drugs. *Gen. Practitioner* **30** (5), 91–95.
Ortega, R. A. (1959). La trifluoperazina en el tratamiento de diversas afecciones psicocutaneas. [Trifluoperazine in treatment of various psychocutaneous disorders.] *Semana Med. (Mex.)* **23** (290), 117-passim.
Oybir, F. (1962). Trifluoperazine in chronic, withdrawn schizophrenics. *Diseases Nervosa System* **23** (6), 348–350.
Pascual, F. T., *et al.* (1964). Combined antidepressant-tranquilizer regimen in depressed psychotics. *Bol. Asoc. Med. Puerto Rico* **56** (8), 291–298.
Payne, P. (1959). Trifluoperazine in treatment of the acutely ill psychotic. *Can. Med. Assoc. J.* **81** (1), 42–43.
Petersen, M. C. (1958). A clinical evaluation of trifluoperazine with particular reference to its effect upon depressed patients. *In* "Trifluoperazine," pp. 156–167. Lea & Febiger, Philadelphia, Pennsylvania.
Phillips, F. J., and Shoemaker, D. M. (1961). Trifluoperazine in anxiety associated with organic disorders. *Diseases Nervous System* **22** (9), 525–527.
Phillipson, R. (1960). A review of trifluoperazine ("Stelazine") in mental disease. *Irish J. Med. Sci.* **6**, 453–459.
Pochat, R., and Maddonni, O. (1961). Trifluoperazina en el tratamiento del enfermo alcoholico. [Trifluoperazine in treatment of alcoholism.] *Med. Panam.* **16** (4), 106–108.
Pollack, B. (1958). Clinical evaluation of trifluoperazine. *In* "Trifluoperazine" pp. 113–119. Lea & Febiger, Philadelphia, Pennsylvania.
Pollitt, J. (1963). The slowed-up patient. *Practitioner* **190** (1140), 747–751.
Prange, A. J., Jr. (1963). Recent advances in therapeutics: Psychoactive drugs. *N. Carolina Med. J.* **24** (2), 63–66.
Proctor, R. C. (1959). Clinical report of trifluoperazine, a longer-acting phenothiazine. *Clin. Med.* **6** (11), 2079-passim.
Proctor, R. C., and Gunn, C. G., Jr. (1959). Treatment of anxiety in hosiery mill workers. *In* "Trifluoperazine," pp. 28–36. Lea & Febiger, Philadelphia, Pennsylvania.
Prueter, G. W. (1959). Treatment of persistent nausea and vomiting of pregnancy with trifluoperazine. *In* "Trifluoperazine," pp. 144–148. Lea & Febiger, Philadelphia, Pennsylvania.
Prueter, G. W. (1959). Trifluoperazine in nausea and vomiting of pregancy. *Can. Med. Assoc. J.* **81** (1), 21–22.
Prueter, G. W. (1962). Combined tranylcypromine-trifluoperazine therapy in obstetrics and gynaecology. *Can. Psychiat. Assoc. J.* **7**, Suppl. S77–S83.
Rees, L. (1962). The value and limitations of psychotropic drugs in psychiatric treatment. *Anglo-Ger. Med. Rev.* **1** (4), 448–459.
Rees, L. (1963). Indications for the use of drugs in the treatment of psychiatric disorders. *Postgrad. Med. J.* **39** (447), 48–52.
Rettig, J. H., *et al.* (1958). A pilot study of trifluoperazine in mentally retarded patients. *In* "Trifluoperazine," pp. 173–179. Lea & Febiger, Philadelphia, Pennsylvania.
Reusch, J., *et al.* (1963). The acute nervous breakdown. *Arch. Gen. Psychiat.* **8** (2), 197–207.
Reznikoff, L. (1960). Experience with trifluoperazine in the treatment of 100 chronic anergic schizophrenic patients. *Am. J. Psychiat.* **116** (11), 1024–1026.
Richards, A. D. (1964). Attitude and drug acceptance. *Brit. J. Psychiat.* **110** (464), 46–52.
Rittelmeyer, L. F., Jr. (1965). Ten years of tranquilizers. *New Physician* **14** (4), 89–92.
Roberts, F. J. (1961). Single daily dose treatment of psychiatric patients with phenothiazine derivatives. *J. Mental Sci.* **107** (446), 104–108.

Robin, A. A. (1963). The effect of tranquillizers on some aspects of the treatment of long stay patients. *Am. J. Psychiat.* **119** (11), 1076–1081.
Roddy, L. R. (1960). Use of trifluoperazine in chronic psychoses. *Diseases Nervous System* **21** (9), 518–519.
Rogers, N. R. (1963). Trifluoperazine as a "mobilizing agent" in chronic withdrawn schizophrenics. *Diseases Nervous System* **24** (3), 162–166.
Rondepierre, J.-J., *et al.* (1963). La trifluopérazine á doses faibles; son emploi en service psychiatrique ouvert. [Low doses of trifluoperazine in an open psychiatric ward.] *Ann. Med. Psychol.* **121** (1/1), 96–100.
Rosati, D. (1962). Prolonged high dosage medication in chronic schizophrenia. *Am. J. Psychiat.* **119** (4), 360–361.
Ross, I. S. (1962). Chemotherapy compared with electroshock in 104 patients with relapsing psychiatric disorders. *Am. J. Psychiat.* **119** (3), 251–254.
Rossi, G. V. (1963). Synergism: With special reference to central nervous system depressants. *J. Pharm. Sci.* **52** (9), 819–832.
Rossi, G. V. (1964). The psychotherapeutic agents. *Am. J. Pharm.* **136** (1), 6–24.
Rowell, S. S., and Segall, M. L. (1960). The treatment of psychoneurotic conditions with trifluoperazine in general practice. *Practitioner* **184** (1100), 235–238.
Rubin, J. H. (1959). Trifluoperazine in the treatment of anxiety in patients with chronic chest disease. *In* "Trifluoperazine," pp. 96–103. Lea & Febiger, Philadelphia, Pennsylvania.
Rudy, L. H., *et al.* (1958). Trifluoperazine in the treatment of psychotic patients. *Am. J. Psychiat.* **115** (4), 364–365.
Rudy, L. H., *et al.* (1958). Triflupromazine and trifluoperazine: Two new tranquilizers. *Am. J. Psychiat.* **114** (8), 747–748.
Rudy, L. H., *et al.* (1958). Trifluoperazine in mentally defective patients. *In* "Trifluoperazine" (J. H. Moyer, ed.), pp. 169–172. Lea & Febiger, Philadelphia, Pennsylvania.
Rudy, L. H., *et al.* (1958). The use of trifluoperazine in the treatment of acute and chronic psychotic patients. *In* "Trifluoperazine," pp. 125–137. Lea & Febiger, Philadelphia, Pennsylvania.
Ruiz E. G., *et al.* (1959). Informe preliminar sobre el uso de la trifluoperazina en el tratamiento de psicosis y neurosis. [Preliminary report on the use of trifluoperazine in the treatment of psychosis and neurosis.] *Semana Med. (Mex.)* **22** (282), 311–315.
Sainz, A. (1964). Phenothiazines in the management of stress and anxiety. *Psychosomatics* **5** (3), 167–173.
Salzberger, G. J. (1963). Combined chlorpromazine and trifluoperazine on a readmission service. *Diseases Nervous System* **24** (9), 558–561.
Salzberger, G. J. (1964). Experiences, concepts and some results with drugs in geriatric patients. *Diseases Nervous System* **25** (11), 670–673.
Sanger, M. D. (1962). The use of tranquilizers and antidepressants in allergy. *Ann. Allergy* **20** (11), 705–709.
Sarwer-Foner, G. J., *et al.* (1959). Clinical investigation of trifluoperazine ("Stelazine") in open psychiatric settings. *Can. Med. Assoc. J.* **81** (9), 717–723.
Schiele, B. C. (1962). Newer drugs for mental illness: A review. *J. Am. Med. Assoc.* **181** (2), 126–133.
Schiele, B. C., *et al.* (1961). A comparison of thioridazine, trifluoperazine, chlorpromazine, and placebo: A double-blind controlled study on the treatment of chronic, hospitalized, schizophrenic patients. *J. Clin. Exptl. Psychopathol.* **22** (3), 151–162.
Schiele, B. C., *et al.* (1963). Treatment of hospitalized schizophrenics with trifluoperazine plus tranylcypromine: A double-blind controlled study. *Comprehensive Psychiat.* **4** (2), 66–79.
Schopbach, R. R. (1961). The use of phenothiazines on a general hospital psychiatric service. *Henry Ford Hosp. Med. Bull.* **9** (3), 369–373.
Scott, N. M., Jr. (1964). Gastrointestinal diseases of medical progress. *N.Y. J. Med.* **64** (5), 607–618.

Sexton, M. C. (1959). Use of trifluoperazine in chronic negro schizophrenics. *Am. J. Psychiat.* **115** (9), 821–822.
Shah, L. P., and Vahia, N. S. (1963). Drug treatment of psychoneurosis. *Bombay Hosp. J.* **5** (4), 1-passim.
Shapiro, A. K. (1964). Rational use of psychopharmaceutic agents. *N.Y. J. Med.* **64** (9), 1084–1095.
Sharpe, D. S. (1962). A controlled trial of trifluoperazine in the treatment of the mentally subnormal patient. *J. Mental Sci.* **108** (453), 220–224.
Sharpley, P., et al. (1964). A comparison of pargyline and tranylcypromine with and without the addition of trifluoperazine: A double-blind study. *Current Therap. Res.* **6** (5), 344–352.
Shaw, C. R., et al. (1963). Tranquilizer drugs in the treatment of emotionally disturbed children. I. Inpatients in a residential treatment center. *J. Am. Acad. Child Psychiat.* **2** (4), 725–742.
Sheth, S. (1963). Value of trifluoperazine in mental diseases. *Indian Pract.* **16** (7), 901–906.
Simpson, G. M. (1961). Uneventful trifluoperazine ("Stelazine") therapy after previous granulocytic depression. *J. Mental Sci.* **107** (447), 258–260.
Simpson, R. W., and Tolmie, J. B. (1962). A clinical assessment of trifluoperazine in psychotic illness. *Med. Proc.* **8**, 108–114.
Singer, K. (1963). Gilles de la Tourette's disease. *Am. J. Psychiat.* **120** (1), 80–81.
Sklar, E. (1959). The treatment of nausea and vomiting with trifluoperazine ("Stelazine"). *Brit. J. Clin. Pract.* **13** (7), 505.
Sluzki, C. E. (1961). Trifluoperazina en el tratamiento de delirios crónicos. [Trifluoperazine in the treatment of chronic delirium.] *Acta Neuropsiquiat. Arg.* **7**, 136–137.
Sluzki, C. E. (1962). Trifluoperacina en la esquizofrenia; estudio clínico acerca de la efectividad de la droga en psicoticos agudos y cronicos. [Trifluoperazine in schizophrenia; clinical study on the efficacy of the drug in acute and chronic psychotics.] *Med. Panam.* No. 2, 2–6.
Smith, J. A., et al. (1961). A comparison of results of controlled drug evaluations in two state hospitals. *Am. J. Psychiat.* **117** (9), 788–790.
Smith, J. A., et al. (1963). Tranquilizers and energizers—or neither? *Postgrad. Med.* **33** (4), 347–354.
Smith, J. A., et al. (1963). Choice of psychoactive drugs by psychiatric residents. *Diseases Nervous System* **24** (5), 310–313.
Smith Kline & French (Montreal). (1959). Trifluoperazine. *Can. Med. Assoc. J.* **80** (10), 835.
Smith, M. E., and Chassan, J. B. (1964). Comparisons of diazepam, chlorpromazine and trifluoperazine in a double-blind clinical investigation. *J. Neuropsychiat.* **5** (8), 593–600.
Smith-e-Incas, J., et al. (1960). Treatment of psychotic patients with trifluoperazine and trifluoperazine-chlorpromazine combination. *Can. Psychiat. Assoc. J.* **5** (3), 185–187.
Souder, F. R. (1959). Trifluoperazine in anxiety states. One year's clinical experience. *Antibiot. Med. Clin. Therapy.* **6** (12), 711–714.
Spicer, E. R., and Gysin, W. M. (1960). Use of trifluoperazine and discharge planning procedures in psychotic patients. *Nebraska State Med. J.* **45** (6), 313–315.
Stanley, W. J., and Walton, D. (1961). Trifluoperazine ("Stelazine") a controlled trial in chronic schizophrenia. *J. Mental Sci.* **107** (447), 250–257.
Stiller, R., and Glotzer, J. (1961). Trifluoperazine in the treatment of withdrawn catatonics. *Illinois Med. J.* **119** (5), 331–332.
Stoll, B. A. (1962). Radiation sickness. An analysis of over 1,000 controlled drug trials. *Brit. Med. J.* II (5303), 507–510.
Sulzer, E. S., and Schiele, B. C. (1962). The prediction of response to tranylcypromine plus trifluoperazine by the MMPI. *Am. J. Psychiat.* **119** (1), 69–70.
Talbot, D. R. (1964). Are tranquilizer combinations more effective than a single tranquilizer? *Am. J. Psychiat.* **121** (6), 597–600.

Tanner, H., et al. (1963). Long-term progress of hospitalized schizophrenic patients on ataractic drugs. *J. Neuropsychiat.* **4** (5), 321–330.

Terrell, M. S. (1962). Response to trifluoperazine and chlorpromazine, singly and in combination, in chronic, "backward" patients. *Diseases Nervous System* **23** (1), 41–48.

Tod, E. D. M. (1964). Puerperal depression; a prospective epidemiological study. *Lancet* II (7372), 1264–1266.

Tolan, E. J., and Peppel, H. H. (1959). Preliminary observations on trifluoperazine in schizophrenia. *Am. J. Psychiat.* **115** (10), 935.

Troshinsky, C. H., et al. (1962). Maintenance phenothiazines in aftercare of schizophrenic patients. *Penna. Psychiat. Quart.* **2** (4), 11–15.

Troyano-Rios, R., and Simon, J. L. (1960). Trifluoperazine, a potent tranquilizer. *Diseases Nervous System* **21** (5), 288–289.

Turnbull, T. A. (1959). A clinical trial in sea-sickness with trifluoperazine ("Stelazine"). *J. Roy. Nav. Med. Serv.* **45**, 132–135.

Vasconcellos, J. (1960). Clinical evaluation of trifluoperazine in maximum-security brain-damaged patients with severe behavioral disorders. *J. Clin. Exptl. Psychopathol.* **21** (1), 25–30.

Vézina, N. (1960). Evaluation clinique de la trifluopérazine en pédiatrie. [Clinical evaluation of trifluoperazine in pediatrics.] *Union Med. Canada* **89** (4), 436–444.

Videbech, T., and Ryberg, J. (1962). Kliniske erfaringer med trifluoperazine. [Clinical experiences with trifluoperazine.] *Ugrskrift Laeger* **124**, 1809–1810.

Vilkin, M. I. (1964). Comparative chemotherapeutic trial in treatment of chronic borderline patients. *Am. J. Psychiat.* **129** (10), 1004.

Vinař, O. (1964). Klinická psychofarmakologie v roce 1963. [Clinical psychopharmacology in 1963.] *Activatis Nervosa Super.* **6** (2), 129–159.

Vogt, A. H. (1961). The use of "Stelazine" and "Parnate" in chronic, withdrawn patients. *Am. J. Psychiat.* **118** (3), 256–257.

Walling, R. G. (1964). Depressions, their management and treatment. *J. Arkansas Med. Soc.* **60**, 361–363.

Wallis, G. G. (1958). Clinical trial of trifluoperazine in mental disorders. *J. Roy. Nav. Med. Serv.* **64**, 271–274.

Weatherall, M. (1962). Tranquillizers. *Brit. Med. J.* I (5287), 1219–1224.

Weckowicz, T. E., and Ward, T. F. (1960). Clinical trial of "Stelazine" on apathetic chronic schizophrenics. *J. Mental Sci.* **106** (444), 1008–1015.

Welsh, A. L. (1964). The newer tranquilizing drugs. *Med. Clin. N. Am.* **48** (2), 459–481.

Weston, F. K., and Loftus, A. P. T. (1961). A terminal double-blind trial of trifluoperazine ("Stelazine") in chronic schizophrenia. *Med. J. Australia* pp. 777–781.

Whiteley, J. S. (1961). The indications for combined treatment with trifluoperazine and amylobarbitone. *Brit. J. Clin. Pract.* **15** (7), 613–615.

Wilson, I. C., et al. (1961). A double-blind trial to investigate the effects of "Thorazine" (Largactil, chlorpromazine), "Compazine" (Stemetil, prochlorperazine) and "Stelazine" (trifluoperazine) in paranoid schizophrenia. *J. Mental Sci.* **107** (446), 90–99.

Wing, J. K., and Freudenberg, R. K. (1961). The response of severely ill chronic schizophrenic patients to social stimulation. *Am. J. Psychiat.* **118** (4), 311–322.

Winkleman, N. W., Jr. (1959). Some thoughts concerning trifluoperazine and its place in ataractic therapy. *In* "Trifluoperazine," pp. 78–81. Lea & Febiger, Philadelphia, Pennsylvania.

Winnik, H. Z., et al. (1962). Clinical trial of "Stelazine" treatment in schizophrenic psychosis refractory to alternative treatments. *Dapim Refuiim* **21** (3), 11–16.

Wood, C. D., et al. (1965). Review of antimotion sickness drugs from 1954–1964. *Aerospace Med.* **36** (1), 1–4.

Wortis, J. (1964). Psychopharmacology and physiological treatment. *Am. J. Psychiat.* **120** (7), 643–648.

Wright, R. L., and Kyne, W. P. (1960). A clinical and experimental comparison of four anti-schizophrenic drugs. *Psychopharmacologia* **1** (6), 437–449.

Wright, R. L. D., and Lynes, P. G. (1964). Value of continuous drug administration for chronic long-term mental hospital patients. *Can. Psychiat. Assoc. J.* **9** (4), 352–357.

Yohe, C. D. (1958). Office patients treated with trifluoperazine. *In* "Trifluoperazine," pp. 192–194. Lea & Febiger, Philadelphia, Pennsylvania.

Yohe, C. D. (1959). Psychiatric office patients treated with trifluoperazine. *In* "Trifluoperazine," pp. 37–41. Lea & Febiger, Philadelphia, Pennsylvania.

Zakusov, V. V. (1964). Novye psikhofarmakologichesie sredstva; obzor. [New psychopharmacological compounds; review.] *Farmakol. i Toksikol.* **27** (1), 107–121.

⌢ A.17 ⌢
Triflupromazine

Chemical Papers

Florey, K., and Restivo, A. R. (1958). A new synthesis of 10-(3-dimethylaminopropyl)-2-(trifluoromethyl) phenothiazine hydrochloride and 7-substituted derivatives. *J. Org. Chem.* **23**, 1018–1021.

Forrest, F. M., Forrest, I. S., and Mason, A. S. (1959). A rapid urine color test for triflupromazine (Vesprin). *Am. J. Psychiat.* **115**, 1114–1115.

Forrest, F. M., Forrest, I. S., and Mason, A. S. (1961). Review of rapid urine tests for phenothiazine and related drugs. *Am. J. Psychiat.* **118**, 300–307.

Forrest, I. S., and Forrest, F. M. (1960). Urine color test for the detection of phenothiazine compounds. *Clin. Chem.* **6**, 11–15.

Heyman, J. J., Almudevar, M., and Merlis, S. (1959). A modification of the Forrest test for phenothiazines. *Am. J. Psychiat.* **116**, 259–260.

Heyman, J. J., Bayne, B. and Merlis, S. (1960). The estimation of phenothiazines using chemically impregnated paper strips. *Am. J. Psychiat.* **116**, 1108–1109.

Smith, C. I., and Schlosser, A. (1958). Procedure for the estimation of Vesprin in biological fluids: Some results from its application in studies of the metabolism of Vesprin. *Monographs Therapy* **3**, 41–44.

Toler, C. S. (1960). Laboratory determinations during treatment with triflupromazine. *J. Louisiana State Med. Soc.* **112**, 298–300.

Yale, H. L. (1957). The development of a new ataractic agent, Vesprin, 10-(3-dimethylaminopropyl)-2-(trifluoromethyl) phenothiazine hydrochloride, and related compounds. *Monographs Therapy* **2**, 228–232.

Yale, H. L., Sowinski, F., and Bernstein, J. (1957). 10-(3-Dimethylaminopropyl)-2-(trifluoromethyl)-phenothiazine hydrochloride (Vesprin) and related compounds. I. *J. Am. Chem. Soc.* **79**, 4375–4389.

Biology and Pharmacology

Brillhart, J. R. (1959). Tranquilizer interference in the rana pipiens chorionic gonadotropin test. *Obstet. Gynecol.* **14**, 581–587.

Burke, J. C., Hassert, G. L., Jr., and High, J. P. (1956). The tranquilizing activity of 10-(3-dimethylaminopropyl)-2-(trifluoromethyl)-phenothiazine hydrochloride (MC 4703) and related phenothiazines in animals. *Am. Soc. Pharm. Exptl. Therap.*, Inc. Meeting, 1956; *J. Pharmacol. Exptl. Therap.* **119**, 136, 1957.

Fink, G. B., and Swinyard, E. A. (1959). Modification of maximal audiogenic and electroshock seizures in mice by psychopharmacologic drugs. *J. Pharmacol. Exptl. Therap.* **127**, 318–324.

Finnerty, F. A., Jr., and Buchholz, J. H. The cardiovascular dynamics of Vesprin. *Monographs Therapy* **2**, 210–213.

Gorham, D. R., and Overall, J. E. (1960). Drug-action profiles based on an abbreviated psychiatric rating scale. *J. Nervous Mental Diseases* **131**, 528–535.

Goshen, C. E. (1960). Psychopharmacology reappraised. *Gen. Practitioner* **21**, 106–113.

High, J. P., Hassert, G. L., Jr., Rubin, B., Piala, J. J., Burke, J. C., and Craver, B. N. (1960). Pharmacology of fluphenazine (Prolixin). *Toxicol. Appl. Pharmacol.* **2**, 540–552.
Jha, S. K., Lumb, W. V., and Johnston, R. F. (1961). Some effects of triflupromazine hydrochloride on goats. *Am. J. Vet. Res.* **22**, 915–920.
Jha, S. K., Lumb, W. V., and Johnston, R. F. (1961). Establishment of permanent carotid loops in goats. *Am. J. Vet. Res.* **22**, 948–949.
Piala, J. J., High, J. P., Greenspan, K., and Burke, J. C. (1957). Further laboratory observations on 10-(3-dimethylaminopropyl-2-(trifluoromethyl)-phenothiazine hydrochloride (MC 4703). *Am. Soc. Pharm. Exptl. Therap.*, Inc. Meeting, 1956; *J. Pharmacol. Exptl. Therap.* **119**, 176–177.
Piala, J. J., Hassert, G. L., Jr., High, J. P., and Burke, J. C. (1957). Pharmacology of Vesprin. *Monographs Therapy* **2**, 214–227.
Piala, J. J., High, J. P., Hassert, G. L., Jr., Burke, J. C., and Craver, B. N. (1959). Pharmacological and acute toxicological comparisons of triflupromazine and chlorpromazine. *J. Pharmacol. Exptl. Therap.* **127**, 55–65.
Scott, G. T., and Nading, L. K. (1961). Relative effectiveness of phenothiazine tranquilizing drugs causing release of MSH. *Proc. Soc. Exptl. Biol. Med.* **106**, 88–90.
Truitt, E. B., Jr. (1958). Some pharmacologic correlations of the chemotherapy of mental disease. *J. Nervous Mental Disease* **126**, 184–210.
Usdin, V. R., Su, S. C., and Usdin, E. (1961). Effects of psychotropic compounds on enzyme systems. I. Inhibition of human plasma and erythrocyte cholinesterases. *Proc. Soc. Exptl. Biol. Med.* **108**, 457–460.
Winbury, M. M., Haulser, L. M., Wolf, J. K., Klein, M. J., and Govier, W. M. (1958). Suppression of cyclopropane-epinephrine arrhythmias in dogs by four phenothiazine derivatives. *Anesthesiology* **19**, 743–751.

Side Effects

Anderson, J. H., and Sanchez-Longo, L. P. (1961). The complications and side effects of the phenothiazine ataraxics. A review of 178 clinical series of 10 phenothiazine derivatives. *Bol. Asoc. Med. Puerto Rico* **53**, 123–151.
Ayd, F. J., Jr. (1958). Fatal agranulocytosis due to triflupromazine hydrochloride. *Am. J. Psychiat.* **114**, 940.
Ayd, F. J., Jr. (1961). A survey of drug-induced extrapyramidal reactions. *J. Am. Med. Assoc.* **175**, 1054–1060.
Cahn, M. M., Levy, E. J., and Hamilton, W. L. (1957). The effect of Vesprin (MC 4703) in inducing photosensitivity reactions. *Monographs Therapy* **2**, 208–209.
Cain, H. D. and Malcolm, M. (1960). Phenothiazine ataraxics: Extrapyramidal reactions. *Calif. Med.* **93**, 24–28.
Cares, R. M., and Buckman, C. (1961). A survey of side-effects and/or toxicity of newer psychopharmacologic agents. *Diseases Nervous System* **22**, 97–106, Pt. 2.
Darling, H. P. (1959). Extrapyramidal symptoms of triflupromazine, mepazine, prochlorperazine. *Diseases Nervous System* **20**, 569–571.
Denzel, H. A. (1960). Clinical observations during the use of triflupromazine (Vesprin) in mental disorders with special regard to side reactions. *Wisconsin Med. J.* **59**, 315–317.
Goodman, D., and Cahn, M. M. (1959). Contact dermatitis to phenothiazine drugs. *J. Invest. Dermatol.* **33**, 27–29.
Klett, C. J., and Caffey, E. M. (1960). Weight changes during treatment with phenothiazine derivatives. *J. Neuropsychiat.* **2**, 102–108.
McKeever, G. E., and Alfidi, R. (1960). Tetanus-like dystonic reaction to triflupromazine hydrochloride. *J. Mich. State Med. Soc.* **59**, 1366–1368.
Preston, J. (1959). Central nervous system reactions to small doses of tranquilizers: Report of one death. *Am. Practitioner and Dig. Treat.* **10**, 627–630.

Clinical Papers

Adriani, J., Summers, F. W., and Antony, S. O. (1961). Is the prophylactic use of antiemetics in surgical patients justified? *J. Am. Med. Assoc.* **175**, 666–671.

Adriani, J., Arens, J., and Antony, S. O. (1962). Postanesthetic vomiting. *Am. J. Surg.* **103**, 2–5.

Ainslie, J. D. (1961). The use of newer psychiatric drugs in medical practice. *J. Florida Med. Assoc.* **47**, 901–906.

Anderson, E. (1958). Vesprin as an antiemetic particularly in pediatric patients. *Squibb Clin. Res. Notes* **1**, 1.

Ayd, F. J., Jr. (1960). Tranquilizers and the ambulatory geriatric patient. *J. Am. Geriat. Soc.* **8**, 909–914.

Ayd, F. J., Jr. (1960). Current status of major tranquilizers. *J. Med. Soc. New Jersey* **57**, 4–14.

Ayd, F. J., Jr. (1961). Phenothiazine tranquilizers: Eight years of development. *Med. Clin. N. Am.* **45**, 1027–1040.

Ayd, F. J., Jr., Goldman, D., Kline, N. S., Parsons, E. H., and Schiele, B. C. (1958). Panel discussion on tranquilizing drugs in the clinical management of mental disease in geriatric patients. *J. Am. Geriat. Soc.* **6**, 379–396.

Azima, H. (1957). The effects of Vesprin in mental syndromes: A preliminary report. *Monographs Therapy* **2**, 203–207.

Azima, H., Durost, H., and Cahn, C. (1958). Vesprin and Mopazine: Two new phenotropic substances. *Am. J. Psychiat.* **114**, 747.

Bair, H. V., Goldberg, B., and Leland, H. (1960). Mental retardation: Results with triflupromazine (Vesprin) in the treatment of mentally retarded children. *J. Kanas Med. Soc.* **61**, 386–389.

Barr, M. (1961). Aintiemetic agents. *Mid.-Atlantic Apoth.* **10**, 15–19.

Beiler, D. D. (1958). Case reports comparing Vesprin and other anti-nauseants. *Squibb Clin. Res. Notes* **1**, 4–5.

Bellville, J. W. (1958). Singultus treated with Vesprin. *Squibb Clin. Res. Notes* **1**, 5–6.

Bellville, J. W. (1961). Postanesthetic nausea and vomiting. *Anesthesiology* **22**, 773–780.

Bellville, J. W., Bross, I. D. J., and Howland, W. S. (1958). Antiemetic efficacy of triflupromazine and cyclizine. *Abstr. Fall Meeting Am. Soc. Pharmacol. Exptl. Therap.; Ann. Arbor, Mich.* 1958, 4.

Bellville, J. W., Bross, I. D. J., and Howland, W. S. (1959). The antiemetic efficacy of cyclizine (Marezine) and triflupromazine (Vesprin). *Anesthesiology* **20**, 761–766.

Bellville, J. W., Howland, W. S., Bross, I. D. J. (1960). Postoperative nausea and vomiting. *J. Am. Med. Assoc.* **172**, 1488–1493.

Bennett, I. F. (1959). Clinical studies with phenothiazine derivatives in psychiatry. *In* "The Effect of Pharmacologic Agents on the Nervous System" (F. J. Braceland, ed.), pp. 266–284. Williams & Wilkins, Baltimore, Maryland.

Benson, W. M., and Schiele, B. C. (1960). Current status of tranquilizing and antidepressive drugs. *J. Lancet* **80**, 579–592.

Blake, J. M., and Hayford, F. C. (1960). Use of triflupromazine hydrochloride for control of emetic reactions to nitrogen mustard therapy. *N.Y. State J. Med.* **60**, 2114–2117.

Bordeleau, J. M. (1960). Recent data on the neuroleptics. *Union Med. Canada* **89**, 192–196.

Bowman, H. W. (1959). Postoperative nausea and vomiting controlled with Vesprin. *Squibb Clin. Res. Notes* **2**, 7.

Bruckman, N. S., Saunders, J. C., and Kline, N. S. (1958). Triflupromazine (Vesprin) in the treatment of chronic schizophrenia. *Monographs Therapy* **3**, 24–27.

Burkhart, K. P. (1959). Vesprin in hyperemesis gravidarum. *Squibb Clin. Res. Notes* **2**, 7–8.
Burn, E. M. (1958). Clinical observations on the use of Vesprin emulsion in the care of the aged. *Monographs Therapy* **3**, 28–31.
Burstein, F. (1959). Anxiety and tension controlled with Vesprin. *Squibb Clin. Res. Notes* **2**, 2–3.
Cabrera Trigo, J. S. (1960). A phenothiazine derivative in laryngology and bronchoesophagology. *Dia Med.* **32**, 888.
Cahn, M. M., and Levy, E. J. The use of Vesprin in dermatology. *Monographs Therapy* **3**, 36–40.
Casey, J. F., Lasky, J. J., Klett, C. J., and Hollister, L. E. (1960). Treatment of schizophrenic reactions with phenothiazine derivatives: A comparative study of chlorpromazine, triflupromazine, mepazine, prochlorperazine, perphenazine, and phenobarbital. *Am. J. Psychiat.* **117**, 97–105.
Cattell, J. P. (1959). Psychopharmacological agents: A selective survey. *Am. J. Psychiat.* **116**, 352–354.
Cattell, J. P., and Malitz, S. (1960). Revised survey of selected psychopharmacological agents. *Am. J. Psychiat.* **117**, 449–453.
Coscarelli, L., and Caragliano, A. (1960). A clinical study of the management of surgical patients with triflupromazine. *Minerva Chir.* **15**, 530–538.
Council on Drugs (1961). New drugs and development in therapeutics. Drugs for mental illness. *J. Am. Med. Assoc.* **177**, 245–246.
Dale, P. W. (1961). Current concepts in therapy. Medical management of mental problems in the aged. *New Engl. J. Med.* **265**, 84–86.
Darling, H. F., Hess, G. H., Capistrano, A. C., and Hoerman, M. G. (1960). Fluphenazine comparative studies. *Diseases Nervous System* **21**, 409–413.
Dau, W. (1960). Premedication with Psyquil in stationary or ambulatory operations. *Med. Klin. (Munich)* **56**, 1595–1596.
Davies, J. I., and Hansen, J. M. (1959). Administration of Vesprin to 1520 patients prior to anesthesia. *Squibb Clin. Res. Notes* **2**, 5–7.
Davies, J. I., Hansen, J. M., and Angell, S. N. (1959). Triflupromazine (Vesprin) in anesthesia: A clinical evaluation. *Can. Anaesthesiol. Soc. J.* **6**, 375–384.
Davitti, L., and Pinoli, G. (1959). Therapeutic effects of trifluopromazine in obstetrics and gynaecology. *Minerva Med.* **11**, 1065–1068.
Deming, M. van N. (1958). Clinical evaluation of the antiemetic activity of Vesprin. *Squibb Clin. Res. Notes* **1**, 1.
Diamond, L. S., and Marks, J. B. (1960). Discontinuance of tranquilizers among chronic schizophrenic patients receiving maintenance dosage. *J. Nervous Mental Disease* **131**, 247–251.
Dobkin, A. B. (1960). Potentiation of thiopentone anaesthesia. *Brit. J. Anaesthesia* **32**, 424–426.
Dobkin, A. B., and Purkin, N. (1960). The antisialogogue effect of phenothiazine derivatives. *Brit. J. Anaesthesia* **32**, 57–59.
Dussik, K. T. (1960). The awakening from psychosis. *J. Neuropsychiat.* **2**, 41–48.
Ferguson, D. W., Hesser, R. N., James, G. T., and De Larios, A. T. (1958). The use of Vesprin in the rehabilitation of alcoholics. *Squibb Clin. Res. Notes* **1**, 6–7.
Fogel, S. H. (1959). Schizophrenia and other chronic psychotic disorders treated with Vesprin. *Squibb Clin. Res. Notes* **2**, 6.
Fox, V. (1958). Vesprin in the management of alcohol-withdrawal symptoms. *Monographs Therapy* **3**, 14–23.
Freed, H. (1957). Some preliminary observations on the use of Vesprin in children and adults. *Monographs Therapy* **2**, 197–202.
Freed, H. (1959). Dosage of Vesprin in children. *Squibb Clin. Res. Notes* **2**, 3–4.

Freed, H. (1961). The current status of the tranquilizers and of child analysis in child psychiatry. *Diseases Nervous System* **22**, 434–437.

Freedman, A. M. (1958). Drug therapy in behavior disorders. *Pediat. Clin. N. Am.* **5**, 573–594.

Freeman, A., and Bachman, L. (1959). Pediatric anesthesia: An evaluation of preoperative medication. *Anesthesia Analgesia Current Res.* **38**, 429–437.

Freyhan, F. A. (1959). Therapeutic implications of differential effects of new phenothiazine compounds. *Am. J. Psychiat.* **115**, 577–585.

Friend, D. G. (1958). The tranquilizers. *Med. Clin. N. Am.* **42**, 1253–1268.

Friend, D. G. (1960). The phenothiazines. *Clin. Pharmacol. Therap.* **1**, A5–A10.

Froke, L. B. (1959). Acute and chronic psychotic patients treated with Vesprin. *Squibb Clin. Res. Notes* **2**, 9–10.

Gallagher, W. J., and Pfeiffer, C. C. (1957). One year of Vesprin therapy in chronic schizophrenia. *Monographs Therapy* **2**, 188–196.

Giuffrida, S. (1960). Use of a new psychic-stabilizer (Vesprin) in obstetrics and gynecology. *Minverva Ginecol.* **12**, 43–46.

Goldman, D. (1957). Observations on the clinical use of Vesprin. *Monographs Therapy* **2**, 177–183.

Goldman, H. I. (1958). Vesprin in the treatment of the post-alcoholic syndrome. *Squibb Clin. Res. Notes* **1**, 6.

Goldman, D. (1958). The results of treatment of psychotic states with newer phenothiazine compounds effective in small doses. *Am. J. Med. Sci.* **235**, 67–77.

Goldman, H. I. (1959). Treatment of postalcoholic syndrome with triflupromazine hydrochloride. *J. Am. Med. Assoc.* **171**, 1502–1503.

Goldstein, B. (1959). Management of emorgence delirium with Vesprin. *Squibb Clin. Res. Notes* **1**, 3.

Gregoretti, L. (1960). First results in the treatment of chronic mental diseases with a new phenothiazine derivative: Trifluoropromazine. Clinical, therapeutic and psychopathological observations. *Rass. Neuropsichiat. Sci. Affini* **14**, 57–66.

Grillo, V. (1960). Vesprin in the treatment of neurodermatitis. *Minerva Dermatol.* **35**, 377–379.

Gruenwald, F., Hanlon, T. E., Wachsler, S., and Kurland, A. (1960). A comparative study of promazine and triflupromazine in the treatment of acute alcoholism. *Diseases Nervous System* **21**, 32–38.

Hanlon, T. E., Kurland, A. A., Esquibel, A. J., and Ota, K. Y. (1958). A comparative study of chlorpromazine and triflupromazine in the management of the chronic hospitalized psychotic patient. *J. Nervous Mental Disease* **127**, 17–20.

Hanlon, T. E., Ota, K. Y., Livchitz, C., and Kurland, A. A. (1959). Chlorpromazine, triflupromazine, and prochlorperazine in chronic psychosis. *AMA Arch. Gen. Psychiat.* **1**, 223–227.

Hecker, A. O., Wright, E. R., Harris, J. R., Philips, J. C., and Schiff, H. (1959). Comparative study of Vesprin and other tranquilizing agents. *Squibb Clin. Res. Notes* **2**, 5–6.

Hegarty, J. G. (1958). MC4703: A new phenothiazine derative. *J. Mental Sci.* **104**, 870–872.

Hegarty, J. G., and Dabbs, A. R. (1959). A controlled study of the effectiveness of trifluopromazine hydrochloride. *J. Mental Sci.* **105**, 811–814.

Herman, E., and Szulc-Kuberska, J. (1961). On the favorable effect of "wespryna" (Vesprin) on sympathetic and causalgic pain. *Polski Tygod. Lekars.* **16**, 96–98.

Herman, J. H., Baratz, B. H., and First, A. (1958). Use of Vesprin in obstetrical analgesia. A preliminary report. *J. Albert Einstein Med. Center* **6**, 145–148.

Heyns, M. H., and Jones, C. S. (1961). The use of anti-emetic drugs in anaesthesia. *S. African Med. J.* **35**, 241–242.

Hicks, R. G. (1958). Vesprin as a postoperative sedative. *Squibb Clin. Res. Notes* **1**, 4.

Himwich, H. E. (1959). Some drugs used in the treatment of mental disorders. *Am. J. Psychiat.* **115**, 756–759.

Himwich, H. E., Costa, E., Rinaldi, F., and Rudy, L. H. (1960). Triflupromazine and trifluoperazine in the treatment of disturbed mentally defective patients. *Am. J. Mental Deficiency* **64**, 711–712.

Hurst, L. (1960). Phenothiazine derivatives in the treatment of schizophrenia. *J. Mental Sci* **106**, 755–770.

Ilem, P. G., and Sainz, A. (1959). The psychiatric application of Vesprin. *Psychiat. Quart.* **33**, No. 1, 9–16.

Inga, E. F., and Bocci, U. (1960). Triflupromazine in the treatment of mental disorders. Clinical experience. *Riv. Sper. Freniat.* **84**, 755–758.

Jacoby, M. G. (1959). Treatment with high dosage triflupromazine. *Am. J. Psychiat.* **116**, 555–556.

Kaminsky, A., and Daitsch, J. (1958). Triflupromazine. Its use in dermatology. Special investigation in porphyria. *Prensa Med. Arg.* **45**, 2086–2089.

Kaplan, H. S. (1959). Tranquilizers in the office practice of medicine. *N.Y. State J. Med.* **59**, 2871–2887.

Kissen, M. D. (1958). The use of Vesprin in acute alcoholism during the period of alcohol withdrawal. *Monographs Therapy* **3**, 8–13.

Klatte, E. W. (1958). Control of alcohol-withdrawal symptoms by Vesprin. *Squibb Clin. Res. Notes* **1**, 7.

Klett, C. J., and Lasky, J. J. (1960). A clinical trial of five phenothiazines using sequential analysis. *J. Clin. Exptl. Psychopathol. Quart. Rev. Psychiat. Neurol.* **21**, 89–100.

Kline, N. S. (1959). Uses of reserpine, the newer phenothiazines, and iproniazid. *In* "The Effect of Pharmacologic Agents on the Nervous System" (F. J. Braceland, ed.), pp. 218–244. Williams & Wilkins, Baltimore, Maryland.

Kris, E. B. (1959). New dosage schedule for Vesprin in aftercare clinics and for anxiety and tension. *Squibb Clin. Res. Notes* **2**, 1.

Kurland, A. A. (1959). Chlorpromazine and triflupromazine in the management of chronic, female psychotics. *Squibb Clin. Res. Notes* **2**, 2.

Kurland, A. A., Hanlon, T. E., Tatom, M. H., Ota, K. Y., and Simopoulos, A. M. (1961). The comparative effectiveness of six phenothiazine compounds, phenobarbital and inert placebo in the treatment of acutely ill patients; global measures of severity of illness. *J. Nervous Mental Disease* **133**, 1–18.

Kurland, A. A., Hanlon, T. E., Tatom, M. H., and Simopoulos, A. M. (1961). Comparative studies of the phenothiazine tranquilizers: Methodological and logistical considerations. *J. Nervous Mental Diseases* **132**, 61–74.

Laconi, A., Cianchino, S., and Barberi, I. (1960). Triflupromazine for the management of certain symptoms of so-called radiation sickness. *Minerva Med.* **51**, 1823–1826.

Laffan, R. J., Papandrianox, D. P., Burke, J. C., and Craver, B. N. (1961). Antiemetic action of fluphenazine (Prolixin) a comparison with other phenothiazines. *J. Pharmacol. Exptl. Therap.* **131**, 130–134.

Langlykke, A. F. (1959). Triflupromazine hydrochloride. *In* "Handbook of Toxicology" (M. Gordon, ed.), Vol. IV. pp. 104–109. Saunders, Philadelphia, Pennsylvania.

Lapierre, J. (1961). Psychiatry and parkinsonism. *Montreal Med.* **13**, 23–28.

LaVerne, A. A. (1961). Compendium of neuropsychopharmacology. *J. Neuropsychiat.* **2**, 280–286.

Lear, E., Suntay, R., Chiron, A. E., Pallin, I. M., Fisch, H., and Abrams, G. (1959). Tranquilizers in anesthesia: Double-blind studies. I. Triflupromazine. *N.Y. State J. Med.* **59**, Pt. 1, 3220–3225.

Lear, E., Suntay, R., Fisch, H. J., Chiron, A. E., and Pallin, I. M. (1961). Ataraxic drugs in preanesthetic medication blind studies in 1,852 patients. *Anesthesiology* **22**, 529–536.

Leger, Y. (1958). Vesprin for the treatment of chronic schizophrenics. *Union Med. Canada* **87**, 831–833.

Leiberman, D. M., and Vaughan, G. F. (1958). Tranquilizers. *Practitioner* **181**, 510–516.

Levine, S., and Berg, M. D. (1959). Vesprin in the treatment of mentally regressed, female, psychotic patients. *Squibb Clin. Res. Notes* **2**, 7–8.

Libien, B. H. (1958). Antiemesis with Vesprin. *Squibb Clin. Res. Notes* **1**, 3.

Lynn, F. H., and Friedhoff, A. J. (1950). The patient on a tranquilizing regimen. *Am. J. Nursing* **60**, 234–240.

McCreight, D. W., Saez, A., and Freymuth, H. W. (1959). Vesprin in the treatment of chronic psychoses. *Squibb Clin. Res. Notes* **2**, 5.

McIntyre, J. W. (1960). Ataractics and the recovery room, with reference to triflupromazine. *Can. Anaesthesiol. Soc. J.* **7**, 176–178.

Magherini, G., and De Biase, G. (1960). Clinical observations on the treatment of some mental disorders with triflupromazine. *Rass. Studi Psichiat.* **49**, 1049–1056.

Markey, H. (1961). Lazarus, come forth. A program to help the patient with chronic psychosis return to living. *New Engl. J. Med.* **265**, 580–584.

Marques de Carvalho, H., Goncalves, J., Cardo, W. N., and Bairao, I. S. (1961). The use of triflupromazine in mental diseases. Clinical studies in 40 cases. *Hospital (Rio de Janeiro)* **60**, 101–120.

Mendel, W. M. (1958). Observations on the comparative effects of tranquilizers on patients previously treated with prochlorperazine. *Am. J. Psychiat.* **115**, 466–467.

Merlis, S., and Turner, W. J. (1961). Drug evaluation and practical psychiatric therapeutics. *J. Am. Med. Assoc.* **177**, 38–42.

Meyers, S. H., and Weiner, (1959). Preliminary report on triflupromazine (Vesprin). *Am. J. Psychiat.* **115**, 743.

Milne, J. (1959). The analysis of phenothiazine derivatives with tranquilizing properties. *J. Am. Pharm. Assoc. Sci. Ed.* **48**, 117–122.

Mitchell, E. H. (1958). Management of alcohol-withdrawal syndrome with Vesprin. *Squibb Clin. Res. Notes* **1**, 7–8.

Miura, T., Sato, K., Tominaga, J., and Satowa, H. (1960). Experiences in drug therapy with triflupromazine (Vesprin). *Diseases Nervous System* **21**, 700–701.

Morehouse, W. G., and Freed, J. E. (1958). Vesprin in the treatment of mental disease. *Monographs Therapy* **3**, 32–35.

Morgenstern, F. V., Funk, I. C., and Holt, W. L. (1960). Comparative short-term evaluation of triflupromazine hydrochloride, chlorpromazine hydrochloride, and placebo in acutely disturbed patients. *N.Y. State J. Med.* **60**, 254–258.

Nanarelli, V. (1958). Observations on treatment in psychiatric patients with triflupromazine. *Recent Progr. Med.* **24**, 3–7.

Natl. Inst. Mental Health. (1960). A concise directory of psychic drugs. *Med. World News*, **1**, 12–13.

Nieto, D. (1959). Trials with triflupromazine (Vesprin). *In* "Psychopharmacology Frontiers; Proc. Psychopharmacol. Symposium, Second Intern. Congr. Psychiat." (N. S. Kline, ed.), pp. 79–83. Little Brown, Boston, Massachusetts.

Niswander, G. D., Lind, S., and Schlesinger, J. (1957). Vesprin in the treatment of mental illness. *Monographs Therapy* **2**, 184–187.

O'Brien, C. F., and Anderson, C. W. G. (1959). Vesprin in the treatment of chronic mental illness. *J. Louisiana State Med. Soc.* **111**, 16–20.

O'Brien, C. F., and Anderson, C. W. G. (1959). Vesprin the treatment of schizophrenia, senile psychosis, and chronic brain syndrome. *Squibb Clin. Res. Notes* **2**, 2–3.

Orio, J. E. P. (1960). Triflupromazine. Its use as an antiemetic postoperatively, in connection of surgery in children (second infancy). *Cir. Panam.* **4**, 73–76.

Pennington, V. M. (1959). Clinical results of triflupromazine (Vesprin) in 132 psychotic patients. *Am. J. Psychiat.* **115**, 740–741.

Pennington V. M. (1959). Clinical trial of Vesprin in 132 psychotic female patients. *Squibb Clin. Res. Notes* **2**, 4.

Proctor, R. C. (1960). The use and abuse of tranquilizing drugs. *J. Tenn. State Med. Assoc.* **53**, 295–299.
Rebosolan, J. R. (1960). Use of triflupromazine hydrochloride in O.R.L. and endoscopies. *Prensa Med. Arg.* **48**, 2975–2978.
Redmon, B. F. (1957). Tranquilizers—some clinical results. *Southeastern Vet.* **9**, No. 2, 34–35.
Rees, L. (1960). Chlorpromazine and allied phenothiazine derivatives. *Brit. Med. J.* II, 522–525.
Reeves, J. E. (1958). Triflupromazine; a control study on ambulatory patients. *Postgrad. Med.* **24**, 687–690.
Reeves, J. E. (1959). Anxiety and tension treated with Vesprin. *Squibb Clin. Res. Notes* **2**, 1–2.
Reinhardt, R. F., Schiff, S. B., and Sinnett, E. R. (1959). The use of triflupromazine with iproniazid for the treatment of chronic schizophrenic patients. *Am. J. Psychiat.* **116**, 68–69.
Reshetylo, T. J. (1959). Vesprin in chronic schizophrenia. *Squibb Clin. Res. Notes* **2**, 11.
Roebuck, B. E., Chambers, J. L., and Williams, E. (1959). An evaluation of the therapeutic use of triflupromazine in mental disease. *J. Nervous Mental Disease* **129**, 184–192.
Roebuck, B. E., Chambers, J. L., and Williams, E. (1959). Vesprin, chlorpromazine, and a placebo in the treatment of mental disease. *Squibb Clin. Res. Notes* **2**, 1.
Rosarios, H. (1960). The use of trifluorpromazine in a clinic for out patients of psychiatry. *Dia Med. (Buenos Aires)* **32**, 292–294.
Rudy, L. H., Rinaldi, F., Costa, E., Himwich, H. E., Tuteur, W., and Glotzer, J. (1958). Triflupromazine and trifluoperazine: Two new tranquilizers. *Am. J. Psychiat.* **114**, 747–748.
Sainz, A., Bigelow, N., and Barwise. C. (1958). Rapid screening of phrenopraxic drugs. *Psychiat. Quart.* **32**, 273–280.
Sainz, A. (1959). Vesprin: The most effective broad-spectrum phrenopraxic. *Squibb Clin. Res. Notes* **2**, 11–12.
Schopfer, R. H. (1958). Clinical evaluation of Vesprin. *Squibb Clin. Res. Notes* **1**, 4.
Scott, M. E. (1961). Tranquilizing drugs. *J. Med. Assoc. Georgia* **50**, 11–13.
Schumann, R. M. (1959). Clinical trial of Vesprin in mentally defective patients. *Squibb Clin. Res. Notes* **2**, 8–9.
Sheiner, B. (1960). A preliminary report on postoperative use of Vesprin by drip method. *Anesthesia Analgesia, Current Res.* **39**, 435–437.
Slaroff, D. M. (1958). Control of radiation nausea by Vesprin. *Squibb Clin. Res. Notes* **1**, 2.
Sleeper, F. H. (1959). Vesprin in the management of patients with chronic psychoses. *Squibb Clin. Res. Notes* **2**, 9.
Smith, J. A., Christian, D., Rutherford, A., and Mansfield, E. (1958). A comparison of triflupromazine (Vesprin), chlorpromazine and placebo in 85 chronic patients. *Am. J. Psychiat.* **115**, 253–254.
Steinberg, A. (1959). Control of nausea and vomiting by Vesprin during nitrogen mustard therapy, radiation sickness, and other conditions. *Squibb Clin. Res. Notes* **2**, 9–10.
Steinberg, A. (1959). Singultus (hiccough) treated with Vesprin. *Squibb Clin. Res. Notes* **2**, 10.
Steinberg, A. (1960). Triflupromazine as a potent antiemetic agent in vomiting due to drug toxicity. *Postgrad. Med.* **28**, 62–66.
Stone, H. H. (1958). The use of Vesprin as an adjunct to the anesthetic management of the surgical patient. *Monographs Therapy* **3**, 1–7.
Stone, H. H. (1959). Preanesthetic sedation with Vesprin. *Squibb Clin. Res. Notes* **2**, 3–5.
Tame, C. (1960). Clinical trials of triflupromazine, particularly in psychoneuroses. *Gazz. Med. Ital.* **119**, 257–260.
Terry, J. A. C. (1961). The use of a new tranquilizer in domiciliary midwifery. *Practitioner* **186**, 619–621.

Utley, M. D. (1959). Preliminary results with Vesprin in emotionally disturbed patients. *Squibb Clin. Res. Notes* **2**, 10.

van der Veen, R. R. (1961). The use of triflupromazine: Case reports. *J. S. African Vet. Med. Assoc.* **32**, 97–98.

Walsh, G. P., Walton, D., and Black, D. A. (1959). The relative efficacy of "Vespral" and chlorpromazine in the treatment of a group of chronic schizophrenic patients. *J. Mental Sci.* **105**, 199–209.

Weber, C. E. (1959). Vesprin as an adjunct to obstetrical analgesia during labor. *Squibb Clin. Res. Notes* **2**, 8.

Welsh, A. L. (1958). Triflupromazine hydrochloride. *In* "Psychotherapeutic Drugs" pp. 22–26. Thomas, Springfield, Illinois.

Wentzler, J. D. (1958). Vesprin as an adjuvant to block anesthesia. *Squibb Clin. Res. Notes* **1**, 2–3.

Wentzler, J. D. (1959). Intravenous use of Vesprin as adjunctive medication to block anesthesia. *Squibb Clin. Res. Notes* **2**, 8–9.

Whittier, J. R., Diamond, O., Korenyi, C. D., Tomlinson, P. J., and LaBurt, H. A. (1959). Drug use-rate in a state hospital. *Am. J. Psychiat.* **116**, 169–171.

Widuch, M. (1959). Management of chronic brain syndrome with Vesprin emulsion, principally in children. *Squibb Clin. Res. Notes* **2**, 6–7.

Zeedick, J. F. (1960). Clinical investigation of triflupromazine hydrochloride (Vesprin) as a preanesthetic medication. *Anesthesia Analgesia, Current Res.* **39**, 283–286.

Zlotlow, M., and Paganini, A. E. (1957). Unilateral tremor in patients receiving Vesprin (triflupromazine). *Psychiat. Quart.* **31**, 762.

∼ A.18 ∼
Trimeprazine

Chemical Papers

Cochin, J., and Daly, J. W. (1963). The use of thin-layer chromatography for the analysis of drugs. Identification and isolation of phenothiazine tranquilizers and of antihistaminics in body fluids and tissues. *J. Pharmacol. Exptl. Therap.* **139** (2), 160–165.

Judah, J. D., and McLean, A. E. M. (1962). Action of antihistamine drugs in vitro. II. Ion movements and phosphoproteins in whole cells. *Biochem. Pharmacol.* **11**, 593–602.

Rosen, E., and Swintosky, J. V. (1960). Preparation of a ^{35}S-labelled trimeprazine tartrate sustained action product for its evaluation in man. *J. Pharm. Pharmacol.* **12**, Suppl., 237T–244T.

Seeman, P. M., and Bialy, H. S. (1963). The surface activity of tranquilizers. *Biochem. Pharmacol.* **12** (10), 1181–1191.

Sorby, D. L., and Plein, E. M. (1961). Adsorption of phenothiazine derivatives by kaolin, talc, and Norit. *J. Pharm. Sci.* **50** (4), 355.

Yung, D. K., and Pernarowski, M. (1963). Identification and differentiation of some phenothiazine-type tranquilizers. *J. Pharm. Sci.* **52** (4), 365–370.

Biology and Pharmacology

Alexander, L. (1958). Apparatus and method for the study of conditional reflexes in man. *AMA Arch. Neurol. Psychiat.* **80** (5), 629–649.

Alexander, L., and Horner, S. R. (1961). The effect of drugs on the conditional psychogalvanic reflex in man. *J. Neuropsychiat.* **2** (5), 246–261.

Anonymous. (1963). Antihistamines: Mechanism of action. *Brit. Med. J.* II (5373), 1642–1644.

Ben-David, M., *et al.* (1965). Production of lactation by non-sedative phenothiazine derivatives. *Proc. Soc. Exptl. Biol. Med.* **118** (1), 265–270.

Blazek, J. (1963). Phenothiazinderivate in der Pharmazie. [Phenothiazines in pharmacy.] *Pharm. Praxis, Beilage Pharmazie* **5**, 85–90.

Candlin, F. T. (1961). Use of trimeprazine in dogs and cats. *J. Am. Vet. Med. Assoc.* **139** (1), 120–121.

Carver, M. J. (1963). Differential effects of phenothiazines on hexose phosphate dehydrogenase. *Biochem. Pharmacol.* **12** (1), 19–24.

Courvoisier, S., *et al.* (1958). Propriétés pharmacologiques générales d'un nouveau dérivé de la phenothiazine. Neuroleptique puissant à action neurovégétative discréte, le chlorhydrate de (méthyl-2′-diméthylamino-3′ propyl-1′)-10 phénothiazine (6549 R.P.). [General pharmacological properties of a new derivative of phenothiazine. Potent neuroleptic with mild autonomic activity, 10-(3-dimethylamino-2-methylpropyl)phenothiazine, hydrochloride (R.P. 6549).] *Arch. Intern. Pharmacodyn.* **115** (1–2), 90–113.

Eckhardt, E. T., and Plaa, G. L. (1962). The effect of phenothiazine derivatives on the disappearance of sulfobromophthalein from mouse plasma. *J. Pharmacol. Exptl. Therap.* **138** (3), 387–391.

Flangan, T. L., *et al.* (1962). Excretion patterns of phenothiazine-S^{35} compounds in rats; effect of change in structure on metabolism. *J. Pharm. Sci.* **51** (10), 996–999.

Friend, D. G. (1961). Method for evaluating antipruritic agents: Studies on methdilazine. *Clin. Pharmacol. Therap.* **2** (5), 605–609.
Graham-Jones, O. (1964). Restraint and anaesthesia of some captive wild mammals. *Vet. Record* **76** (44), 1216–1248.
Hall, L. W., and Stevenson, D. E. (1960). Effects of ataractic drugs on the blood-pressure and heart-rate of dogs. *Nature* **187** (4738), 696–697.
Heimlich, K. R., *et al.* (1961). Evaluation of an oral sustained release dosage form of trimeprazine as measured by urinary excretion. *J. Pharm. Sci.* **50** (3), 213–215.
Herxheimer, H., and Stresemann, E. (1963). The effect of some new antihistamines on the anaphylactic microshock of the guinea-pig. *Brit. J. Pharmacol.* **21** (3), 414–418.
Hollister, L. E. (1963). Oral prolonged-action drugs. *J. Chronic Diseases* **16** (10), 1039–1041.
Jamieson, D., and Van Den Brenk, H. A. (1961). Relation of mast cell changes to hypothermia in the rat. *Biochem. Pharmacol.* **7** (1), 35–46.
Johnson, H. W., *et al.* (1960). Lactation with a phenothiazine derivative ("Temaril"): A case report. *Am. J. Obstet. Gynecol.* **80** (1), 124–127.
Johnson, P. C., and Masters, Y. F. (1962). Effect of sustained release on absorption and excretion of S^{35}-labeled trimeprazine tartrate. *J. Lab. Clin. Med.* **59** (6), 993–999.
Jones, R. S. (1963). Methylamphetamine as an antagonist of some tranquillising drugs in the horse. *Vet. Record* **75** (45), 1157–1159.
Kátó, L., and Gozsy, B. (1960). Effect of phenothiazine derivatives on dextran-induced edema. *J. Pharmacol. Exptl. Therap.* **129** (2), 231–236.
Kátó, L., and Gozsy, B. (1961). Improved method for quantitative evaluation of drug effects on dextran edema in the rat. *Toxicol. Appl. Pharmacol.* **3** (2), 145–152.
Laskin, D. M., and Kolodny, S. C. (1965). Inhibition of exudate production by anti-inflammatory drugs. *J. Oral Therap. Pharmacol.* **1** (4), 383–391.
Lecoq, R., *et al.* (1962). Recherches chronaximétriques sur l'action qu'exercent quelques psycholeptiques et psychotoniques sur les effets nerveux de l'alcool éthylique; conclusions pratiques. [Chronaximetric research on the action which psycholeptics and psychotonics exert on the nervous effects of ethyl alcohol; practical conclusions.] *Ann. Pharm. Franc.* **20** (7–8), 607–622.
Lin, T. H., *et al.* (1964). Effect of the site of release on the absorption of trimeprazine-S^{35} and penicillin G in dogs. *J. Pharm. Sci.* **53** (11), 1357–1359.
Rabinowitz, P., and Friedman, I. S. (1961). Drug-induced lactation in uremia. *J. Clin. Endocrinol. Metab.* **21** (11), 1489–1493.
Raynaud, G., and Valette, G. (1963). Action des dérivés de la phénothiazine et de l'halopéridol sur la crise audiogéne de la souris. [Action of phenothiazine derivatives and haloperidol on audiogenic seizures in the mouse.] *Arch. Intern. Pharmacodyn.* **142** (3–4), 425–439.
Rosenblum, W., and Zweifach, B. W. (1964). The effect of tranquilizers on the contractile response of cerebral arteries. *J. Pharmacol. Exptl. Therap.* **145** (1), 58–63.
Sicuteri, F., *et al.* (1960). Inhibition by lysergic acid derivatives of bronchospasm induced in guinea pigs by serotonin aerosol. *Med. Exptl.* **3** (2), 89–94.

Side Effects

Brachman, P. S., *et al.* (1959). Agranulocytosis induced by trimeprazine. *New Engl. J. Med.* **260** (3), 378–380.
Buisson, M. M., *et al.* (1962). A propos de crises d'épilepsie survenues au cours de traitements par le tartrate d'alimémazine (6549 R.P.) ou théraléne. [Epileptic attacks during treatment with alimémazine tartrate (RP 6549) or théraléne.] *Ann. Med.-Psychol.* **1** (4), 775–782.

Cares, R. M., and Buckman, C. (1963). Comparative review of the structure and side-effects of newer psychotropic agents. *Diseases Nervous System* **24** (4), 92–105.
Chicoine, L. (1961). L'intoxication par les dérivés de la phénothiazine; revue et rapport de 25 cas. [Toxicity due to phenothiazine derivatives; review and report of twenty-five cases.] *Union Med. Canada* **90** (5), 469–474.
Clendenning, W. E., et al. (1960). Trimeprazine agranulocytosis; report of a case. *Arch. Dermatol.* **82** (4), 533–536.
Favre-Tissot, M., et al. (1964). Psychopharmacologie et teratogenése bilan d'une premiére enquête clinique. [Psychopharmacology and teratogenesis; results of a first clinical questionnaire.] *Ann. Med. Psychol.* **122** (1/3), 389–400.
Fournier, E. (1964). Intoxications par thymoleptiques et tranquillisants. [Intoxication by thymoleptics and tranquilizers.] *Gaz. Med. France* **71**, 2851–passim.
Hartman, D. L., and Dickey, R. F. (1964). Photodermatitis induced by drugs. II. Photodermatitis medicamentosa. *Skin* **3** (7), 198-passim.
Hollister, L. E. (1964). Adverse reactions to phenothiazines. *J. Am. Med. Assoc.* **189** (4), 311–313.
Jacobziner, H., and Raybin, H. W. (1961). Briefs on accidental chemical poisonings in New York City: Imipramine hydrochloride, trimeprazine, and methapyrilene mixture ingestions. *N.Y. State J. Med.* **61** (16), 2811–2813.
Kirshbaum, B. A., and Beerman, H. (1964). Photosensitization due to drugs; a review of some of the recent literature. *Am. J. Med. Sci.* **248** (4), 445–468.
Knox, J. M. (1963). Photosensitivity reactions in various diseases. *Postgrad. Med.* **33** (6), 564–570.
Knox, J. M. (1964). Photosensitivity—a common physical allergy. *Southern Med. J.* **57** (8), 904–908.
Loo, P. P. (1964). Un cas d'intoxication par le Théralène. [One case of Theralene intoxication.] *Ann. Med.-Psychol.* **122** (2/1), 68–69.
Potts, A. M. (1964). The reaction of uveal pigment in vitro with polycyclic compounds. *Invest. Ophthalmol.* **3** (4), 405–416.
Sigal, C., and Mitchell, J. C. (1964). Essential cold urticaria; a potential cause of death while swimming. *Can. Med. Assoc. J.* **91** (11), 609–611.

Clinical Papers

Anderson, T. E., and Chalmers, D. (1959). A trial of trimeprazine in itching dermatoses. *Brit. J. Dermatol.* **71**, 214–218.
Anonymous. (1963). A new eruption of pregnancy. *Brit. Med. J.* I (5324), 138–139.
Anonymous. (1964). An antihistamine in measles. *Practitioner* **192** (1152), 814–816.
Anonymous. (1964). Today's drugs: Drugs for premedication. *Brit. Med. J.* II (5411), 737–739.
Armitage, P. (1963). Comparative trial of trimeprazine and amylobarbitone in pruritus. *Lancet* I (7281), 611.
Archer, J. S., and Hicks, R. G. (1962). Phenothiazine subgroups. *N.Y. State J. Med.* **62** (23), 3769–3772.
Ashur, M. E., and Farrar, R. H. (1959). Treatment of nighttime itching with a new oral antipruritic; a controlled study. *J. Am. Podiat. Assoc.* **49** (9), 393–396.
Ayd, F. J., Jr., et al. (1959). Trimeprazine therapy for physiologic and psychologic pruritus. *Southern Med. J.* **52** (12), 1554–1556.
Becker, S. W., Jr. (1965). Therapy of melanin hyperpigmentation. *Postgrad. Med.* **37** (2), 198–201.
Bell, B. T., et al. (1960). Use of trimeprazine to control pruritus in orthopedic surgery. *J. Am. Med. Assoc.* **174** (15), 1976–1977.

Binning, R., et al. (1962). Premedication for adenotonsillectomy. *Brit. J. Anaesthesia* **34**, 812–816.
Birch, C. A. (1964). Current therapeutics. CXCIV. The non-barbiturate sedatives. *Practitioner* **192** (1148), 290–296.
Bonafos, M., et al. (1964). Les associations alimémazine-dextromoramide et alimémazine-pethidine en anesthésiologie. Leur interêt au cours de l'anesthésie génêrale en urologie (a propos de 104 observations). [The combinations alimemazine-dextromoramide and alimemazine-pethidine in anesthesiology; their use during general anesthesia in urology (104 снзсз).] *Anesthesie Analgesie Reanimation* **21** (3), 413–419.
Borrie, P. (1959). Advances in the treatment of skin diseases. *Practitioner* **183** (1096), 419–424.
Brujis, R. G., et al. (1961). Antipruriginoso por via bucal. [Oral antipruritic.] *Dia Med.* **33** (31), 720-passim.
Callaway, J. L., and Olansky, S. (1959). Trimeprazine: An adjuvant in the management of itching dermatoses. *N. Carolina Med. J.* **18** (8), 320–321.
Cope, R. W. (1959). Vallergan. *Lancet* I (7071), 519.
Cope, R. W., and Glover, W. J. (1959). Trimeprazine tartrate for premedication of children. *Lancet* I (7078), 858–860.
Cornman, H. D., III. (1962). Clinical use of the phenothiazine derivatives in general practice. In "Psychosomatic Medicine. First Hahnemann Symposium" (J. H. Nodine and J. H. Moyer, eds.), pp. 461–464. Lea & Febiger, Philadelphia, Pennsylvania.
Council on Drugs. (1959). Trimeprazine tartrate ("Temaril"). *J. Am. Med. Assoc.* **171** (7), 893.
Dickstein, B. (1959). Trimeprazine for pruritus in children. *J. Albert Einstein Med. Center* **7** (2), 115–117.
Dougan, H. T. (1961). Treatment of the habitually hyperemotional child with trimeprazine; a clinical study. *Virginia Med. Monthly* **88** (5), 265–268.
Dubois, J. (1960). Essai du 6549 RP dans les dermatoses prurigineuses. [Study of RP 6549 in pruritus.] *Gaz. Sante Publ.* **27** (1).
Dundee, J. W., et al. (1963). Alterations in response to somatic pain associated with anaesthesia. XV. Further studies with phenothiazine derivatives and similar drugs. *Brit. J. Anaesthia* **35**, 597–610.
Editorial. (1964). Premedication for Ts and As. *Lancet* II (7373), 1327.
Epps, P. R., and Scott, R. B. (1959). The use of trimeprazine orally for the control of pruritus in children. *J. Natl. Med. Assoc.* **51** (4), 255–257.
Fraser, H. E. (1958). Trimeprazine—an antipruritic. *Bull. Assoc. Mil. Dermatol.* **7** (1), 12–13.
Gillet, G. B., and Keil, A. M. (1960). Trimeprazine tartrate in pediatric premedication; a preliminary communication. *Anaesthesia* **15** (2), 158–162.
Goldberg, L. C., and Diamond, A. (1958). An appraisal of a new antipruritic: Trimeprazine ("Temaril"). *Antibiot. Med. Clin. Therap.* **5** (9), 582–584.
Gould, A. H. (1962). Combined dexbrompheniramine-fluphenazine (Diperm Chronotab) in the oral treatment of pruritus. *J. New Drugs* **2** (3), 179–182.
Gould, A. H., and Neary, E. R. (1964). Newer developments in oral antipruritics. *Med. Clin. N. Am.* **48** (2), 411–419.
Gözsy, B., and Kátó, L. (1960). Investigations into the mechanism of action of neuroleptic drugs. *Arch. Intern. Pharmacodyn.* **128** (1–2), 75–81.
Grayson, L. D., and Shair, H. M. (1963). Atopic dermatitis. III. The correct choice of antihistamine agents. *Ann Allergy* **21** (3), 168–170.
Green, M. A. (1958). Clinical evaluation of a unique antiallergic drug—trimeprazine. *Ann. Allergy* **16** (6), 619–625.
Grieco, V. F. (1958). Evaluation of a new oral antipruritic. *Intern. Record Med.* **171** (10), 618–620.
Hare, P. J. (1963). Advances in the treatment of skin diseases. *Practitioner* **191** (1144), 426–430.

Hellier, F. F. (1963). A comparative trial of trimeprazine and amylobarbitone in pruritus. *Lancet* I (7279), 471–472.
Hudson, A. L. (1959). A new drug for control of itching—trimeprazine [1′-(3-dimethylamino-2-methylpropyl)-phenothiazine.] *Can. Med. Assoc. J.* **80** (2), 125.
Huguenard, P. (1959). Essais expérimentaux et cliniques avec l'alimemazine (6549 RP ou Théralène). [Experimental and clinical studies with alimémazine (RP 6549 or Theralene).] *Anesthesie* **26** (3), 484–509.
Joglekar, G. V., et al. (1963). Evaluation of antipruritic drugs in normal volunteers. *Clin. Pharmacol. Therap.* **4** (2), 197–199.
Kienhofer, R. F. (1961). Evaluation of an oral antipruritic. *Med. Times* **89** (4), 408–412.
Krause, H. (1960). Zur klinischen Behandlung des exsudativen Ekzems (Neurodermatitis). [Clinical treatment of exsudative eczema (Neurodermatitis).] *Z. Haut-Geschlechtskrankh.* **29** (9), 298–302.
Kristof, A. C., and Huot, J. M. (1960). Impression on Panectyl, a new antipruritic drug. *Manitoba Med. Rev.* **40** (7), 535–536.
Kristof, A. C., and Huot, J. M. (1961). Control of cough and dyspnea with trimeprazine. *Appl. Therap.* **3** (12), 974–977.
Kroll, C. (1961). Comparison of oral drugs in treatment of itching dermatoses. *Clin. Med.* **8** (7), 1351–1352.
Kropp, E. (1961). Pruritus und Antipruriginosa. (Pruritis and antipruritics.) *Med. Klin. (Munich)* **56** (8), 313–315.
Lambert, P.-A. (1964). Essai de systematisation des associations de neuroleptiques. (Trial systemization of neuroleptic combinations.) *Encephale* **53,** Suppl., 262–275.
Lear, E., et al. (1960). Antihistamine drugs in pre-anaesthetic medication; blind studies on 953 patients. *Brit. J. Anaesthesia* **32** (12), 582–589.
Lear, E., et al. (1961). Ataraxic drugs in preanesthetic medication; blind studies in 1,852 patients. *Anesthesiology* **22** (4), 529–536.
Lehmann, H. E., and Ban, T. A. (1964). Notes from the log-book of a psychopharmacological research unit. *Can. Psychiat. Assoc. J.* **9** (1), 28–32.
LeVan, P. (1958). The use of trimeprazine in the treatment of pruritic dermatoses. *Clin. Med.* **5** (8), 1077–1084.
Lincoln, C. S., et al. (1959). Treatment of itching, a preliminary report on results with a new oral antipruritic. *Calif. Med.* **90** (2), 126–127.
London, I. D. (1959). Trimeprazine, an oral antipruritic, a clinical and double-blind evaluation. *J. Med. Assoc. State Alabama* **28** (11), 342–345.
Love, W. R. (1963). Treatment of anogenital pruritus. *Ohio State Med. J.* **59** (9), 907–909.
McClellan, M. (1960). Antitussive effects of trimeprazine ("Temaril") in children. *Ohio State Med. J.* **56** (10), 1358–1359.
Miller, J. (1962). Antipruritic potency of a new antihistamine, dimethpyrindene: A comparative study with trimeprazine, a phenothiazine antihistamine. *Current Therap. Res.* **4** (4), 115–123.
Naviau, J., et al. (1961). Essai du tartrate d'alimémazine en thérapeutique psychiatrique; étude de cent quarante cas. [Alimemazine tartrate in therapeutic psychiatry; study of one hundred cases.] *Ann. Med.-Psychol.* **119** (1–3), 579–585.
Olansky, S. (1963). Clinical trial of an antihistamine for relief of pruritus. *Clin. Med.* **70** (9), 1657–1660.
Oldham, P. D. (1963). Trimeprazine and amylobarbitone in pruritus. *Lancet* I (7282), 666–667.
Panaccio, V. (1959). Etude d'un nouveau dérivé de la phenothiazine dans le traitement des dermatoses prurigineuses. [Study of a new phénothiazine derivative in treatment of pruritic dermatoses.] *Union Med. Canada* **88** (8), 964–966.
Panaccio, V. (1959). Trimeprazine, a new phenothiazine derivative for treatment of pruritic dermatoses. *Can. Med. Assoc. J.* **80** (11), 885–886.

Pittelkow, R. B. (1960). An evaluation of trimeprazine in pruritus. *Wisconsin Med. J.* **59** (6), 367–369.
Pittelkow, R. B. (1962). Pruritus, skin disorders, and trimeprazine. *Clin. Med.* **69** (4), 889–893.
Poole, R. F. (1960). Trimeprazine ("Temaril") as an antiemetic and antitussive in children. *N. Carolina Med. J.* **21** (6), 226–227.
Rafstedt, S. (1961). Theralen in pediatrics: New therapy for pruritus and agitation. *Svenska Läkartidn.* **58** (36), 2492.
Riccitelli, M. L. (1964). Modern concepts in the management of anxiety and depression in the aged and infirm. *J. Am. Geriat. Soc.* **12** (7), 652–657.
Roberts, R. B. (1959). Vallergan. *Lancet* I (7073), 630.
Robinson, R. C. V., and Robinson, H. M., Jr. (1958). Control of emotional tension in dermatoses. *Southern Med. J.* **51** (4), 509–513.
Roche, L., et al. (1963). Intérèt de l'alimemazine dans le traitement du délirium tremens. [Alimemazine in the treatment of delirium tremens.] *Lyon Med.* **209** (5), 255-passim.
Rossi, G. V. (1964). The psychotherapeutic agents. *Am. J. Pharm.* **136** (1), 6–24.
Salem, H., and Aviado, D. M. (1964). Antitussive drugs: With special reference to a new theory for the initiation of the cough reflex and the influence of bronchodilators. *Am. J. Med. Sci.* **247** (5), 585–600.
Sanner, J. C. (1958). Antipruritic therapy in chemical burns and dermatoses among coal miners. *Penna. Med. J.* **61** (12), 1632–1633.
Schmidt, B. B. (1960). Zur Anwendung neuer Phenothiazinpraparate in der Dermatologie. [Use of a new phenothiazine in dermatology.] *Therap. Gegenwart* **99** (10), 842–844.
Schoog-Lützenkirchen, A. (1961). Pruritusbehandlung mit Trimeprazin (Repeltin). [Treatment of pruritus with trimeprazine (Repeltin).] *Med. Welt* No. 11, 526–528.
Schubert, E. G. (1960). Erfahrungen mit dem oralen Antipruriginosum Repeltin. [Experiences with the oral antipruritic agent, Repeltin.] *Z. Haut-Geschlechtskrankh.* **28** (1), 25–26.
Seanor, H. E. (1961). Trimeprazine in pediatric practice; two years clinical experience. *N.Y. State J. Med.* **60** (9), 1537–1538.
Smith, H. (1959). Le Panéctyl en dermatologie. [Panectyl in dermatology.] *Union Med. Canada* **88**, 956–961.
Smith, M. A., and Curwen, M. P. (1961). Controlled trials of two oral antipruritic drugs, trimeprazine and methdilazine. *Brit. J. Dermatol.* **73**, 351–358.
Smith, P., Jr., et al. (1962). Double-blind crossover study of antipruritic effect of chlorcyclizine hydrochloride, trimeprazine, and a placebo. *Southern Med. J.* **55** (6), 643–645.
Taft, E. H., et al. (1960). Trimeprazine (Vallergan): Its assessment as an antipruritic. *Med. J. Australia* **2**, 208–210.
Trimpi, H. D. (1960). Effective plan for control of pruritus ani. *Disease Colon Rectum* **3** (2), 125–129.
Webster, R. A. (1961). Centrally acting muscle relaxants in tetanus. *Brit. J. Pharmacol.* **17** (3), 507–518.
Widlake, F. (1959). Vallergan. *Lancet* I (7069), 413.
Williams, P. L. (1958). A new oral antipruritic. *Northwest Med.* **57** (9), 1162–1164.
Wright, W. (1959). Use of tranquilizers in dermatology. *J. Am. Med. Assoc.* **171** (12), 1642–1646.
Zakusov, V. V. (1964). Novye psikhofarmakologichesie sredstva; obzor. [New psychopharmacological compounds; review.] *Farmakol. i Toksikol.* **27** (1), 107–121.
Zoila, A. R., et al. (1959). Le tartrate d'alimémazine (6549 RP) en thérapeutique psychiatrique. [Alimemazine tartrate (RP 6549) in therapeutic psychiatry.] *Presse Med.* **67** (23), 935–936.
Zoila, A. F., et al. (1959). Essai thérapeutique des états dépressifs par le tartrate d'alimémazine (6549 R.P.). [Treatment of depressive states with alimemazine tartrate (RP 6549).] *Ann. Med.-Psychol.* **117** (1:3), 557–564.

Appendix B
Meprobamate-like Agents Bibliographies
Compiled by MAXWELL GORDON

B.1	Phenaglycodol	477
B.2	Mephenoxalone	479
B.3	Promoxalone	481
B.4	Emylcamate	482
B.5	Hydroxyphenamate	483
B.6	Phenylpropanolcarbamate	484
B.7	Metaxalone	485
B.8	Methocarbamol	486
B.9	Oxanamide	490
B.10	Ectylurea	491
B.11	Methyprylone	492
B.12	Ethchlorvynol	497

~ B.1 ~
Phenaglycodol

Arora, R. B., and Sharma, P. L. (1958). Effectiveness of some anticonvulsant drugs in ventricular tachycardia resulting from acute myocardial infarction in the dog. *Indian J. Med. Res.* **46** (6), 802.

Balassi, G. P., and Blanda, F. (1959). Sulle possibilita d'impiego in campo ostetricoginecologico di un nuovo centrolettico psicopligico: il fenaglicodol. *Riv. Ostet. Ginecol. Prat. (Milano)* **41** (5), 496.

Berger, F. M., and Ludwig, B. J. (1964). Meprobamate and related compounds. *In* "Psychopharmacological Agents" (M. Gordon, ed.), Vol. 1, pp. 114. Academic Press, New York.

Bois Lambert, M. P. (1959). Un tranquillisateur nouveau: le phenaglycodol. *Arch. Hosp.* No. 29; (1958). *Union Med. Canada* **87**, 1213.

Boshes, L. D., and Doshay, L. J. (1964). Practical management of Parkinson's Disease. *Geriatrics* **19**, 644.

Carter, C. H. (1958). Phenaglycodol, an anticonvulsant effective in grand mal and petit mal seizures. *Antibiot. Chemotherapy* **5** (11), 675.

Cerri, O. (1958). Die Bestimmung von 2-p-chlorophenyl-3-methyl-2,3-butandiol (fenaglicodol). *Boll. Chim. Farm.* **97**, 261; (1958). *Pharm. Zentralhalle* **97**, 491.

Chin, L., and Swinyard, E. A. (1959). Pentylenetetrazol seizure threshold in meprobamate and phenaglycodol-treated mice. *J. Am. Pharm. Assoc., Sci. Ed.* **48** (1), 6.

Cohen, I. M. (1958). Use of drugs in treating the emotionally disturbed patient. *Med. Ann. District Columbia* **27**, 292.

Donati, A. (1958). L'azione clinica del 2-p-cloro-fenil-3-metil-2,3-butandiolo. *Minerva Med.* **49** (55), 2742.

Doshay, L. J. (1961). Treatment of Parkinson's disease. *New Engl. J. Med.* **264**, 988.

Friedman, A. P. (1960). Treatment of headache. *J. Occupational Med.* **2**, 268.

Friend, D. G. (1961). Current concepts in therapy. Tranquilizers. III. Meprobamate, phenaglycodol and chlordiazepoxide. *New Engl. J. Med.* **264**, 870.

angloff, H. (1959). Effect of phenaglycodol and meprobamate on spontaneous brain activity, evoked EEG arousal and recruitment in the cat. *J. Pharm. Exptl. Therap.* **126** (1), 30.

Grebe, R. M. (1959). "Handbook of Toxicology", Vol. IV (Tranquilizers). Saunders, Philadelphia, Pennsylvania.

Imberciadori, E. (1960). Primi Resultati Dell'impiego in Terapia Neuropsichiatrica del 2-p-chlorofenil-3-metil-2,3-butanediolo (Fenaglicodolo). *Minerva Med.* **51** (18), 757.

Kaisch, A. M., Fein, H. D., and Miller, J. W. (1959). Comparative effect of phenaglycodol, meprobamate and a placebo on the irritable colon; a double-blind study. *Am. J. Digest. Diseases* **4** (3), 229.

Kato, R. (1960). Induced increase of meprobamate metabolism in rats treated with phenobarbital or phenaglycodol. *Med. Exptl.* **3** (2), 95.

Kless, H. (1958). Psychotrope substanzen. *Arzneimittel-Forsch.* **8**, 623.

Kopmann, E., and Hughes, F. W. (1959). Potentiating effect of alcohol on tranquilizers and other central depressants. *AMA Arch. Gen. Psychiat.* **1**, 7.

Kugelmass, I. N. (1958). Phenaglycodol therapy in cerebral palsy. *Ann. N.Y. Acad. Sci.* **72** (8), 271.

Lehmann, H. W. (1958). Tranquilizers and other psychotropic drugs in clinical practice. *Can. Med. Assoc. J.* **79**, 701.

Lewis, J. J. (1963). Antidepressives and tranquilizers. *Pharm. J.* **191**, 85.

Luckenbach, F., and Micheletti, T. (1958). Sperimentazioni e Applicazioni Cliniche del 2-*p*-clorofenil-3-metil-2,3-butandiolo in Psichiatria. *Gazz. Med. Ital.* **117** (9), 373.

Maclure, J. G., Schanze, J. K., and Ferguson, J. H. (1959). Tranquilizers for gynecologic outpatients. *Obstet. Gynecol.* **13** (6), 760.

Murphy, H. W. (1964). Pinacol arrangement of phenaglycodol. I. *J. Pharm. Sci.* **53**, 298.

Quadrio, A. (1959). Alcune Osservazioni Sperimentali Sull'azione del Fenaglycodol Su Talune Funzione Psechiche. *Clin. Terap.* **16** (6), 583.

Tranquilizer poisonings. (1963). *Iowa State J. Med.* **53**, 302.

Tiengo, M. (1959). Impiego del 2-*p*-clorofenil-3-metil-2,3-butanodiolo in anestesia. *Minerva Anestesiol.* **25** (5), 215.

Vinegar, R., and Berger, F. M. (1959). Effect of certain tranquilizers on the reticuloendothelial system. *Proc. Soc. Exptl. Biol. Med.* **102**, 88.

Zukin, P., et al. (1959). Comparative effect of phenaglycodol and meprobamate on anxiety reactions. *J. Nervous Mental Disease* **129**, 193.

~ B.2 ~
Mephenoxalone

Abitol, H., Cabut, M. S., Ortiz, Guevara, R., and Grillo, S. A. (1962). Methoxadone and adrenolytic action. *Rev. Soc. Arg. Biol.* **38** (7/8), 253–257; (1964). *Chem. Abstr.* **61**, 936C.

American Cyanamid Co. (1963). Oxazolidin-2-ones. British Patent 938,424; (1964). *Chem. Abstr.* p. 4153E.

Canellas-Rodriguez, R. (1960). Clinical study of mephenoxalone in various syndromes of psychogenic etiology and psychiatric treatment. *Med. Espan.* **44**, 230–242.

Council on Drugs. (1963). New drugs and developments in therapeutics. *J. Am. Med. Assoc.* **183** (6), 469–470.

Daneman, E. A. (1964). Double blind study with diazepam, chlordiazepoxide, and placebo in the treatment of psychoneurotic anxiety. *J. Georgia Med. Assoc.* **53** (2), 55–58.

Denber, H. C. (1958). Note on methoxydone (AHR-233). *Am. J. Psychiat.* **115** (4), 360.

Dreyfuss, R. (1961). The practical application of a new cyclosedative in general medicine. *Praxis (Bern)* **50**, 548–552.

Editors. (1960). Methoxydone aids in neurospastic disease. *Med. Tribune* **1** (4), 16.

Editors. (1963). Mephenoxalone. *J. Am. Med. Assoc.* **185**, 300.

Fischer, E., and Szabo, J. L. (1960). Pharmacological investigation of 5-(o-methoxyphenoxymethyl)-2-oxazolidone. *Rev. Assoc. Med. Arg.* **74**. 82–83.

Fischer, E., and Tallaferro, A. (1960). Clinical trials of metoxadone. *Semana Med. (Buenos Aires)* **117**, 678–683.

Fischer, E., Szabo, J. L. J., and Stamburgo, M. (1960). Synergetic action of 2(o-methoxyphenoxymethyl)-5-oxazolidone on morphine, dihydro-codeine and aminopyrine analgesia. *Nature* **186** (4728), 893–894.

Friend, D. G. (1964). Sedatives and tranquilizers in general medical practice. In Modell, Walter, ed. "Drugs of Choice 1964–1965" (W. Modell, ed.), pp. 266–279. Mosby, Saint Louis, Missouri.

Furgiuele, A. R., Kinnard, W. J., and Buckley, J. P. (1961). Evaluation of certain psychopharmacological compounds. *J. Pharm. Sci.* **50** (3), 252–254.

Gordillo, R. (1963). Clinical study of mephenoxalone and tridihexetil chloride in peptic ulcer. *Rev. Col. Med. Guatemala* **14** (2), 53–55 (1964). *Biol. Abstr.* **45**, 24345 (in Spanish).

Gray, W. D., Osterberg, A. C., and Rauh, C. E. (1966). Neuropharmacological actions of mephenoxalone (Trepidone). *Arch. Intern. Pharmacodyn.* (in press).

Irikura, T., Masuzawa, K., Tada, M., and Uchida, H. (1963). Central nervous system depressants. I. Reaction of alcohols with carbonic acid derivatives and thermodynamic activity of the products. *Yakugaku Zasshi* **83**, 1175–1179; (1964). *Chem. Abstr.* **60**, 10664F.

Krumholz, W. V., Sheppard, C., and Merlis, S. (1964). Studies with aspirin: Psychopharmacologic and methodologic considerations. *Clin. Pharmacol. Therap.* **5** (6), (1), 691–694.

LaVeck, G. D., and Buckley, P. (1961). The use of psychopharmacologic agents in retarded children with behaviour disorders. *J. Chronic Diseases* **13** (2), 174–183.

Levine, I. M., Jossmann, P. B., Yood, B., DeAngelis, V., and Friend, D. G. (1960). The evaluation of neurospasmolytic agents in man by objective means. *Ann. N.Y. Acad Sci.* **86** (1), 208–215.

Lunsford, C. D. (1959). 5-(o-methoxyphenoxy)-2-oxazolidone. U.S. Patent 2,895,960.

Lunsford, C. D. (1963). Oxazolidones. A. H. Robins Co., Inc. German Patent 1,152,417; (1964). *Chem. Abstr.* **60**, 527F.

Lunsford, C. D. (1963). 5-(o-Alkoxyphenoxymethyl)-2-oxazolidones. A. H. Robins Co., Inc. German Patent 1,157,627; (1964). *Chem. Abstr.* **61**, 9281G.

Lunsford, C. D., Mays, R. P., Richman, J. A., Jr., and Murphy, P. S. (1960). 5-aryloxymethyl-2-oxazolidinones. *J. Am. Chem. Soc.* **82** (5), 1166–1171.

Martinez, M., and Salas, E. A. (1960). Contribution to the study of 5(o-methoxyphenoxymethyl)-2-oxazolidone. *Semana Med. (Buenos Aires)* **116**, 466–468.

Martinez, M., and Salas, E. A. (1960). Use of a new tranquilizing agent: 5(o-methoxyphenoxymethyl)-2-oxazolidone. *Semana Med. (Buenos Aires)* **117**, 1142–1147.

Milies, E., and Monti, M. (1962). Pharmacologic study of a new tranquilizer 5-(o-methoxyphenoxymethyl)-2-oxazolidinone. *Acta Neurol. Latinoam.* **8** (1), 58–62 (in Spanish); (1964). *Biol. Abstr.* **45**, 55923.

Mooney, H. B., Cohen, S., Ditman, K. S., and MacAndrew, C. (1961). Methoxydone in the treatment of chronic alcoholics. *J. New Drugs* **1** (1), 35–38.

Muller, B. P., Tarpey, R. D., Giorgi, A. P., Mirone, L., and Rouke, F. L. (1964). Effects of alcohol and mephenoxalone on psychophysiological test performance. *Diseases Nervous System* **25** (6), 373–375.

Pares, J., and Längar, M. (1960). Note concerning (o-methoxyphenoxymethyl)-5-oxazolidone-2 or mephenoxalone. *Helv. Chim. Acta* **43** (6), 1862–1864.

Rossi, G. V. (1964). The psychotherapeutic agents. *Am. J. Pharm.* **136**, 6–24.

Shatin, L., and Gilmore, T. H. (1961). Methoxydone (AHR-233) in hospitalized non-psychotic patients. *Am. J. Psychol.* **117**, 833–834.

Sternieri, E., Giaroli, M., and Bernardi, M. (1963). Action of 5-[(o-methoxyphenoxy)methyl]-2-oxazolidinone on the reproductive capacity, the course of pregnancy, and embryogenesis in the rabbit. *Biochim. Biol. Sper.* **2** (3–4), 426; (1964). *Chem. Abstr.* **61**, 15213G.

Timberlake, W. H. (1961). The lack of effect of mephenoxalone or of meprobamate on spasticity. *Newton-Wellesley Med. Bull.* **13** (1), 11–16.

Welsh, A. L. (1964). The newer tranquilizing drugs. *Med. Clin. N. Am.* **48** (2), 459–481.

Wilson, C. V. (1963). Isocyanates. Part II. Reaction. *Org. Chem. Bull.* **35** (3), 1–5.

Yeary, R. A., Benish, R. A., Brahm, C. A., and Miller, D. L. (1964). Toxicity of mephenoxalone in newborn rats and dogs. *Toxicol. Appl. Pharmacol.* **6** (6), 642–652.

Zieher, L. M., and Fischer, E. (1960). Effect of metoxadone on the psychomotor activity of rats. *Rev. Assoc. Med. Arg.* **74**, 531–533.

∼ B.3 ∼
Promoxolane

Berger, F. M. (1951). *Arch. Intern. Pharmacodyn.* **85**, 474–483.
Berger, F. M., Boekelheide, V., and Tarbell, D. S. (1948). The pharmacological properties of some 2-substituted-4-hydroxymethyl-1,3-dioxolanes. *Science* **108**, 561.
Boines, G. J. (1951). The use of dimethylane in the management of certain symptoms of menopause. *Delaware State Med. J.* **23**, 41.
Boines, G. J. (1953). Management of the menopause. The use of dimethylane in certain symptoms: 15-month study. *Med. Times* **81**, 50.
Boines, G. J., and Horoschak, S. (1951). Dimethylane in the treatment of dysmenorrhea. *Delaware State Med. J.* **23**, 183.
Kissen, M. D., and Fortnum, W. G. (1954). *Am. Practitioner* **5**, 32.
Kissen, M. D., Yaskin, H. E., Robertson, H. F., and Morgan, D. R. (1951). A new adjuvant in postalcoholic psychomotor agitation. *Quart. J. Studies Alc.* **12**, 587.
Vivino, A. E., and Ritter, G. (1953). Treatment of dysmenorrhea with a dioxolane. *Med. Ann. District Columbia* **22**, 117.

~ B.4 ~
Emylcamate

Martens, S. (1960). Clinical trial of emylcamate, a new internuncial blocking tranquilizer. A double-blind study in alcoholic outpatients. *Quart. J. Stud. Alcohol* **21**, 223.

Melander, B. (1959). Emylcamate, a potent tranquilizing relaxant. *J. Med. Pharm. Chem.* **1**, 443.

Melander, B., Mouchard, A.-L., and von Kraemer, C.-G. (1959). Psychotechnical studies on Nuncital (Kabi), a new tranquilizer. *Münch. Med. Wochschr.* **101**, 2175 (1960). (In German).

Uhr, L., and Miller, J. G. (1966). Experimentally determined effects of emylcamate (Striatran) on performance, autonomic response, and subjective reactions under stress.

B.5
Hydroxyphenamate

Alexander, L. (1961). Effect of hydroxyphenamate on the conditional psychogalvanic reflex in man. *Diseases Nervous System* **22**, No. 9, 17.

Bastian, J. W., and Clements, G. R. (1961). Pharmacology and toxicology of hydroxyphenamate. *Diseases Nervous System* **22**, No. 9, 9.

Bossinger, C. D. (1961). Chemistry of hydroxyphenamate. *Diseases Nervous System* **22**, No. 9, 7.

Cahn, B. (1961). Effect of hydroxyphenamate in the treatment of mild and moderate anxiety states. *Diseases Nervous System* **22**, No. 9, 30.

Cahn, M. M., and Levy, E. (1961). Use of hydroxyphenamate (Listica) in dermatologic therapy. *Diseases Nervous System* **22**, No. 9, 47.

Eisenberg, B. C. (1961). Amelioration of allergic symptoms with a new tranquilizing drug (Listica). *Diseases Nervous System* **22**, No. 9, 25.

Friedman, A. P. (1961). Pharmacological approach to the treatment of headache. *Diseases Nervous System* **22**, No. 9, 36.

Gouldman, C., Lunde, F., and Davis, J. (1961). Clinical trial of hydroxyphenamate in alcoholic patients. *Diseases Nervous System* **22**, No. 9, 44.

Greenspan, E. B. (1961). Use of hydroxyphenamate in some forms of cardiovascular disease. *Diseases Nervous System* **22**, No. 9, 33.

McLaughlin, B. E., Harris, J., and Ryan, F. (1961). A double blind study involving Listica, Librium and Placebo as an adjunct to supportive psychotherapy in a psychiatric clinic. *Diseases Nervous System* **22**, No. 9, 41.

~ B.6 ~
Phenylpropanolcarbamate

Benmiloud, K. (1961). Comparaison des differents modes d'action des medicaments "somnifere" a l'aide de l'acetographie. *Med. Hyg. Geneva* **19**, 872.
Bram, G. (1962). Klinische und Doppelblindversuche mit MH 532 bei Spannungskopfschmerz. *Praxis (Bern)* **51**, 648.
Büch, O. (1959). Zur antiphlogistischen Wirkung von MH 532. *Arch. Intern. Pharmacodyn.* **123**, 140.
Burgermeister, J. J. (1959). Les medicaments dits tranquillisants. *Rev. Med. Suisse* **12**.
Dubs, R. (1961). Das Cervikalsyndrom in der täglichen Praxis. *Pract. Oto-Rhino-Laryngol.* **23**, 31.
Forstier, J. (1960). Note sur l'effect du MH 532 sur diverses affections rhumatismales. *Rev. Rhumat.* **27**, 227.
Forestier, J. (1960). Essais d'un nouveau decontractant en rhumatologie. *Presse Med.* **22**, 845.
Garrone, G. (1959). Etude clinique d'un nouveau relaxateur musculaire a action tranquillisante. *Neuro-Psychopharmacol.* p. 568.
Garrone, G. (1960). Les indications d'un nouveau medicament relaxateur de la musculature en psychiatrie ambulatoire. *Schweiz. Med. Wochschr.* **90**, 217.
Haglind, K. (1961). Behandlung muskulaerer Verspannungen mit Gamaquil. *Svenska Lakartidn.* **58**, 2390.
Harder, A. (1961). Klinische Erfahrungen mit Haloperidol unsw. *Praxis (Bern)* **50**, 868.
Ideström, C. M. (1962). Die Wirkkung von MH 532 verglichen mit Meprobamate und Placebo. *Psychopharmacologica* **3**, 15.
Jung, A. (1960). Rheumatherapie auf verschiedenen Ebenen. *Praxis (Bern)* **49**, 163.
Kostek, T. (1961). Uber die Wirkung des Gamaquil auf Grund von Beobachtung eines Suizidfalles. *Praxis (Bern)* **50**, 902.
Linke, H. (1960). Psychotrope Substanzen. *Muench. Med. Wochschr.* **21**.
Monnier, M. (1959). Elektrophysiologische Analyse der Wirkungen verschiedener Neuroleptika. *Schweiz. Med. Wochschr.* **89**, 430.
Spilborghs, G. (1962). Le carbamate de gamma-phenylpropyle dans le douleurs vertebrales. *Hospital (Span.)* **62**, 145.
Stille, G. (1962). Zentrale Muskelrelaxantien. *Arzneimittel-Forsch.* **12**, 340.
Surber, W. (1959). Eine neue Substanz mit muskelrelaxierenden und tranquillisierenden Eigenschaften. *Arzneimittel-Forsch.* **9**, 143.
Thevenoz, F. (1959). Etude d'un nouveau decontractant en pratique rhumatologique. *Med. Hyg. (Geneva)* p. 552.

⁓ B.7 ⁓
Metaxalone

Bruce, B. B., Turnbull, L., Newman, J. and Pitts, J. (1966). Metabolism of metaxalone. *J. Med. Chem.* **9**, 286.

Carroll, M. N., Jr., Luten, W. R., and Southward, R. W. (1961). Pharmacology of a new oxazolidinone with anticonvulsant, analgetic and muscle relaxant properties. *Arch. Intern. Pharmacodyn.* **130**, 280.

Carter, C. H. (1962). A new muscle relaxant. *Diseases Nervous System* **23**, 1.

Fathie, K. (1964). A second look at metaxalone. *Current Therap. Res.* **6**, 677.

Gucker, T. (1962). Rehabilitation in injuries of spinal cord. *J. Occupational Med.* **4**, 61.

Kurtzke, J. F., and Gylfe, J. (1962). A new muscle relaxant in spasticity. *Neurology* **12**, 343.

Lunsford, C. D., Mays, R. P., Richman, J. A., and Murphey, R. S. (1960). 5-Aryloxymethyl-2-oxazolidinones. *J. Am. Chem. Soc.* **52**, 1165.

Morey, L. W., and Crosby, A. R. (1963). A new skeletal muscle relaxant. *J. Am. Osteopath. Assoc.* **62**, 517.

~ B.8 ~
Methocarbamol

Barbeau, A. (1964). Une Erreur do Diagnostic. *Union Med. Canada* **93**, 1083–1085.

Bigazzi, G. F. (1960). Il metocarbamolo negli spastici da lesione traumatica midollare, [Methocarbamol in spastic states caused by spinal cord injuries.] *Gazz. Med. Ital.* **119**, 187–189.

Campbell, A. D., Coles, F. K., Eubank, L. L., and Huf, E. G. (1961). Distribution and metabolism of methocarbamol. *J. Pharmacol. Exptl. Therap.* **131**, 18–25.

Carpenter, E. B. (1958). Methocarbamol as a muscle relaxant: Its clinical evaluation in acute trauma and chronic neurological states. *Southern Med. J.* **51**, 627–630.

Chaiken, B. H., Tansey, W. A., and Jacobs, A. L. (1959). Tetanus: A current appraisal. *J. Med. Soc. New Jersey* **56**, 232.

Chasens, A. I. (1959). Methocarbamol (Robaxin) as an adjunct in the treatment of bruxism. *J. Dental Med.* **14**, 166–170.

Cock, T. C. (1961). Newer concepts in the management of tetanus. *Calif. Med.* **95**, 15.

Coodley, E. L. (1963). Clinical evaluation of combined orphenadrine-fluphenazine in acute and chronic musculoskeletal disorders. *Clin. Med.* **70**, 1843–1846.

Cooper, R. W. (1959). Clinical observations on the toxicity of boron hydrides in man. *Aviation Med.* p. 180.

Crandell, D. L., and Whitcher, C. E. (1960). Control of neuromuscular manifestations of severe systemic tetanus. *J. Am. Med. Assoc.* **172**, 15–19.

Crandell, D. L., Hollandsworth, L. C., and Whitcher, C. E. (1959). The role of the anaesthesiologist in the management of severe systemic tetanus. *Can. Anaesthesiol. Soc. J.* **6**, 24–31.

Crookshank, J. W. (1962). Muscle relaxants in acute back strains. *J. Louisiana State Med. Soc.* **114**, 272–274.

Estrada, E. (1960). Methocarbamol in the control of severe skeletal muscle spasms in small animals. *J. Am. Vet. Med. Assoc.* **137**, 585–588.

Estrada, E. (1962). Management of acute lead poisoning in dogs. *Mod. Vet. Practice* **43**, 73–74.

Feinman, J., and Sherman, J. (1961). A clinical evaluation of methocarbamol injectable in oral surgery. *N.Y. State Dental J.* **27**, No. 10, 501–502.

Feuer, S. G., Rosenbaum, I., and Baranowska, H. (1962). Methocarbamol injectable in treatment of acute and chronic muscle spasm. *N.Y. State J. Med.* **62**, No. 12.

Fields, A. (1960). Intra-arterial therapy. *Angiologia* **1**, 31–37.

Fitzgerald, W. J. (1960). Clinical evaluation of methocarbamol in relief of local pain following episiotomy and perineal repair. *Miss. Valley Med. J.* **82**, 46–47.

Flinchum, D. (1959). Closed treatment of herniated intervertebral lumbar discs. *J. Med. Assoc. Georgia* **48**, 461–464.

Flinchum, D. (1961). Musculoskeletal disorders amenable to treatment with intravenous methocarbamol. *Clin. Med.* **8**, No. 11.

Forsyth, H. F. (1958). Methocarbamol (Robaxin) in orthopedic conditions (preliminary report of 100 cases). *J. Am. Med. Assoc.* **167**, 163–168.

Griffin, P. J. (1962). Methocarbamol in neuromuscular reactions to phenothiazine derivatives. *Gen. Practitioner* **26**, No. 6.

Grisolia, A., and Thomson, J. E. M. (1959). A clinical study of 46 males with low-back disorders treated with methocarbamol. *Clin. Orthoped.* No. 13, 299–304.

Honet, J. C., Casey, T. V., and Runyan, J. W., Jr. (1959). False-positive urinary test for 5-hydroxyindoleacetic acid due to methocarbamol and mephenesin carbamate. *New Engl. J. Med.* **261**, 188–190.

Horen, W. P. (1963). Arachnidism in the United States. *J. Am. Med. Assoc.* **185**, No. 11.

Howell, T. H. (1959). The elderly rheumatic patient. *Practitioner* **183**, 727.

Hudgins, A. P. (1959). Clinical evaluation of methocarbamol. *Clin. Med.* **6**, 2321–2324.

Hudgins, A. P. (1961). Indications and techniques for vaginal repair. *Clin. Med.* **8**, 243–247.

Huf, E. C. (1961). Distribution and metabolism of methocarbamol. *J. Pharmacol. Exptl. Therap.* **131**, 17.

Huf, E. G., Coles, F. K., and Eubank, I. L. (1959). Comparative plasma levels of mephenesin, mephenesin carbamate and methocarbamol. *Proc. Soc. Exptl. Biol. Med.* **102**, 276–277.

Jones, J. H. (1965). Methocarbamol in Black Widow Spider poisoning; report of a case.

Kane, A. A., Edelman, E., Cavalino, L., and Eckert, B. (1962). A muscle relaxant for treating dislocation and fracture. *Western Med.* **3**, 180.

Korngold, H. W. (1960). Management of acute wryneck in children. *Mod. Med.* p. 116.

Kozma, J. J. (1964). Paralytic ileus due to methocarbamol. *Clin. Med.* **71**, 527.

Kunin, I. J. (1961). Methocarbamol in the treatment of temporomandibular joint syndrome. *Oral Surg., Oral Med., Oral Pathol.* **14**, 296–299.

LaFratta, C. W., and Porterfield, J. B. (1961). A review of the "Fibrositis" question. *Southern Med. J.* **54**, 1242–1247.

Lamphier, T. A. (1961). The role of intravenous methocarbamol in the treatment of muscle spasm. *J. Abdomenal Surg.* **3**, No. 2.

Lanzetta, A. (1959). A new skeletal muscle relaxant, methocarbamol, potentiates the action of certain non-barbiturate hypnotics. *Minerva Anestesiol.* **25**, 210–211.

Lessard, R., Potvin, A., and Morin, Y. (1960). The use of methocarbamol in tetanus. *Can. Med. Assoc. J.* **83**, 1199–1202.

Leventen, E. O., and Vaccarino, F. P. (1960). Intravenous methocarbamol in 100 orthopedic patients. *Current Therap. Res.* **2**, 497–500.

Levine, I. M. (1961). Muscle relaxants in neurospastic diseases. *Med. Clin. N. Am.* **45**, 1017–1026.

Lewis, W. B. (1959). Use of methocarbamol in orthopedics. *Calif. Med.* **90**, 26–28.

Li, J. R. (1960). Methocarbamol in the treatment of Black Widow Spider poisoning; report of a case. *J. Am. Med. Assoc.* **173**, 662.

Lofaro, J. J. (1961). Treatment of acute alcoholism with methocarbamol. *N.Y. State J. Med.* **61**, 897.

Lukasek, E. O. (1960). Management of a case of acute lead poisoning. *Gen. Practitioner* **22**, 82–84.

Mangiameli, S. (1960). L'uso di un miorilassante (metocarbamolo) nella minaccia di parto prematuro. [The use of a muscle relaxant (methocarbamol) in threatened premature labor.] *Riv. Ostetet. Ginececol. Prat.* **42**, 112–114.

Meyers, G. B., and Urbach, J. R. (1961). Methocarbamol for acute low back pain in industry. *Penna. Med. J.* **64**, 876.

Miglietta, O. E., and Lowenthal, M. (1962). Measurement of the stretch reflex response as an approach to the objective evaluation of a spasticity. *Arch. Phys. Med. Rehab.* pp. 62–68.

Minvielle-Uruchurtu, L. (1961). The value of muscle relaxants in the postoperative management of anorectal operations. *Diseases Colon Rectum* **4**, 27–31.

Mooney, H. B., Cohen, S., Ditman, K. S., and Whittlesey, J. R. B. (1961). Methocarbamol (Robaxin R.) in the treatment of alcoholics. *J. New Drugs* **1**, No. 6, 245–278.

Morgan, A. M., Truitt, E. B., Jr., and Little, J. M. (1957). Plasma levels of mephenesin, mephenesin carbamate, guiaiacol glyceryl ether, and methocarbamol (AHR-85) after oral and intravenous administration in the dog. *J. Am. Pharm. Assoc.* **46**, 374.

O'Dell, T. B. (1961). Experimental parameters in the elevation of analgesics. *Chicago Med.* **63**, 9–15, No. 42.

O'Doherty, D. S., and Shields, C. (1958). Methocarbamol—new agent in treatment of neurological and neuro-muscular diseases. *J. Am. Med. Assoc.* **167**, 160–163.

Parikh, P. M., and Mukherji, S. P. (1960). Bromometric estimation of methocarbamol. *Drug Standards* **28**, 48–50, No. 2

Park, H. W. (1958). Clinical results with methocarbamol, a new interneuronal blocking agent. *J. Am. Med. Assoc.* **167**, 168–172.

Park, H. W., and Hajek-Nichols, N. (1959). Clinical observations on the relation of muscular rigidity and tremor in idiopathic paralysis agitans. *Southern Med. J.* **52**, 1246–1248.

Perchuk, E., Weinreb, M., and Aksu, A. (1961). A new treatment for nocturnal leg cramps. *Angiology* **12**, 102–104.

Pizzoferrato, A., and Zanoli, S. (1959). Methocarbamol in orthopedics and traumatology. *Minerva Ortoped.* **10**, 249–269.

Plumb, C. S. (1958). Clinical evaluation of methocarbamol (Robaxin) in an industrial facility. *J. Lancet* **78**, 531–532.

Plummer, H. B., Harrison, T., and Trever, R. W. (1960). Tetanus-like reactions to prochlorperazine. *J. Am. Med. Assoc.* **172**, 600 (correspondence).

Poppen, J. L., and Flanagan, M. E. (1959). Use of methocarbamol for muscle spasm after lumbar and cervical laminectomies. *J. Am. Med. Assoc.* **171**, 298–299.

Rogers, E. J. (1961). Methocarbamol as adjunctive in comprehensive care of neuromuscular disability. *Clin. Med.* **8**, 701–705.

Rogers, E. J. (1963). Double-blind comparative study of diazepam and methocarbamol in treatment of skeletal muscle spasm. *Western Med.* **4**, 11–15.

Roszkowski, A. P. (1960). A pharmacological comparison of therapeutically useful centrally acting skeletal muscle relaxants. *J. Pharmacol. Exptl. Therap.* **129**, 75.

Russell, F. E. (1962). Muscle relaxants in Black Widow Spider (*Lactrodectus mactans*) poisoning. *Am. J. Med. Sci.* **243**, No. 2.

Ryan, R. E. (1960). A new agent for the symptomatic relief of myalgia of the head. *Clin. Med.* **7**, 323–326.

Sachs, J. M., and Sorensen, V. B. (1961). Preliminary report on the effects of parabromdylamine maleate and methocarbamol after oral surgical procedures. *J. Oral Surg., Anesthesiol. & Hosp. Dental Serv.* **19**, 147–149.

Santamarina, V., Lopetegui, A., and Amador, C. M. (1959). Experiencia con un neuvo relajante muscular el metocarbamol (Robaxin) en rheumatologia. [Experience with a new muscle relaxant, methocarbamol (Robaxin) in rheumatology.] *Rev. Med. Cuba* **70**, 77–78.

Schaubel, H. J. (1959). A proven muscle relaxant—Injectable Robaxin—in a new form. *Orthopedics* **1**, 274–275.

Shaftan, G. W., and Herbsman, H. (1964). Intravenous methocarbamol in reduction of shoulder dislocations. *J. Am. Med. Assoc.* **188**, No. 1.

Smith, H. M. S. (1959). Methocarbamol therapy in equine tetanus. *J. Am. Vet. Med. Assoc.* **134**, 282.

Smith, S. F., Jr. (1962). Management of tetanus. *Am. Practitioner* **13**, No. 6, 384–388.

Sobel, A. M. (1960). Treatment of extrapyramidal reactions to phenothiazine derivatives. *U.S. Armed Forces Med. J.* **11**, 1446–1450.

Steigmann, F. (1961). Muscle relaxants. *Am. J. Nursing* **61**, 49–51.

Stern, F. H. (1964). A controlled comparison of three muscle relaxant agents. *Clin. Medicine* **71**, 367.

Tamas, A. A. (1959). Symptomatology and treatment of boron hydride intoxication. *Aviation Med.* p. 205.
Taylor, O. C., Jr., and Wall, H. L. (1961). Tetanus. *Southwestern Med.* **2**, 122–124.
Thorn, R. P., and Malia, E. R. (1962). Clinical evaluation of Robaxin for posthemorrhoidectomy discomfort. *Anesthesia Analgesia, Current Res.* **41**, 335–337, No. 3.
Tronzo, R. G. (1961). Traumatic dislocation of the hip in a child; a problem in anesthetic management. *J. Am. Med. Assoc.* **176**, 526–527.
Tronzo, R. G. (1963). Reduction of dislocated shoulders using methocarbamol. *J. Am. Med. Assoc.* **184**, 110–112.
Truitt, E. B., Jr., and Patterson, R. B. (1957). Comparative hemolytic activity of mephenesin, guaiacol glyceryl ether and methocarbamol *in vitro* and *in vivo*. *Proc. Soc. Exptl. Biol. Med.* **95**, 422–424.
Truitt, E. B., Jr., and Little, J. M. (1958). A pharmacologic comparison of methocarbamol (AHR-85), the monocarbamate of 3-(o-methoxyphenoxy)-1, 2-propanediol with chemically related interneuronal depressant drugs. *J. Pharmacol. Exptl. Therap.* **122**, 239–246.
Turow, D. D. (1960). Methocarbamol in the management of labor. *Clin. Med.* **7**, 925–928.
Utterback, R. A. (1963). Methocarbamol in the therapy of tetanus. *Arch. Neurol.* **9**, 555–560.
Vazuka, F. A. (1958). Comparative effects of relaxant drugs on human skeletal muscle hyperactivity. *Neurology* **8**, 446–454.
Weiss, J., and Weiss, S. (1962). Methocarbamol in low-back pain: Clinical study. *J. Am. Osteopath. Assoc.* **62**, 142–144.
Zucker, A. H. (1959). Clinical results with methocarbamol in opiate withdrawal. *Am. J. Med. Sci.* **237**, 190–193.

~ B.9 ~
Oxanamide

Ayd, F. J., Jr. (1965). Quiactin: A new tranquilizer; preliminary report on experience in ambulatory patients. *Med. Times* (in press).

Coats, E. A., and Gray, R. W. (1957). Quiactin in the treatment of emotional and mental disorders. *Diseases Nervous System* **18**, 191–193.

Feuss, C. D., and Gragg, L., Jr. (1957). Quiactin: An adjunct in the treatment of chronic psychoses. *Diseases Nervous System* **18**, 29–33.

Feuss, C. D., Jr., and Ivanov, C. J. (1958). Quiactin as an outpatient drug. *Marquette Med. Rev.* **23**, 78–80.

Hock, C. W. (1957). Bentyl with Quiactin: A new antispasmodic tranquilizer combination. Scientific Exhibit, 51st Annual Meeting, Southern Medical Association, Miama Beach, Florida, November 11–14, 1957.

Kristofferson, A. B., and Cormack, R. H. (1958). Some effects of Quiactin on normal behavior. *Clin. Res.* **6**, 416.

McFarling, C., Smith, E. U., and Shideman, F. E. (1959). Effect of 2-ethyl-3-propyl-glycidamide (Quiactin) on tracking and complex reaction time. *Federation Proc.* **18**, 420.

Proctor, R. C. (1957). A part-time psychiatric program for a moderate sized industry. *Diseases Nervous System* **18**, 223–225.

Proctor, R. C. (1958). Psychodynamic drugs: A re-evaluation and report. *Diseases Nervous System* **19**, 265–268.

Warren, M. R., Thompson, C. R., and Werner, H. W. (1949). Pharmacological studies on the hypnotic, 2-ethyl-3-propylglycidamide. *J. Pharmacol. Exptl. Therap.* **96**, 209–212.

Welsh, A. L. (1958). "Psychotherapeutic Drugs", pp. 106–112. Thomas, Springfield, Illinois.

Woodhull, R. B. (1966). Quiactin: Adjunctive use of a new tranquilizer in obstetrics and gynecology. *Calif. Med.*

~ B.10 ~
Ectylurea

Asung, C. L., Charcowa, A. I., and Villa, A. P. (1957). A study of the nonhypnotic calmative effect of 2-ethylcrotonylurea (Nostyn) in children with behavior problems. *N.Y. State J. Med.* **57**, 1911–1914.

Baker, J. P. (1954). A controlled trial of ethylcrotonylurea. *J. Mental Sci.* **105**, 852–862.

Barron, A. R., Rudy, L. H., and Smith, J. A. (1961). Effect of drugs on "poor" treatment cases. *Diseases Nervous System* **22**, 692–694.

Bauer, H. G., Seegers, W., Krawzoff, M., and McGavack, T. H. (1958). A clinical evaluation of ectylurea (Nostyn). *N.Y. State J. Med.* **58**, 520–526.

Butler, T. C. (1964). The metabolic fate of carbromal (2-bromo-2-ethylbutyrylurea). *J. Pharmacol. Exptl. Therap.* **143**, 23–29.

Cass, L. J., and Frederik, W. S. (1961). A controlled clinical evaluation of the appetite suppressant, benzphetamine, with and without the tranquilizer, ectylurea. *Am. J. Gastroenterol.* **36**, 82–88.

Diamond, L. K., and Allen, F. H., Jr. (1959). Maternal medications vs. Neonatal jaundice (correspondence section). *New Engl. J. Med.* **260**, 393.

Dobkin, A. B. (1960). Drugs which stimulate affective behavior—part III. Comparison of the effect of picrotoxin, pentylenetetrazol, Bemigride, pipradrol, ectylurea, vanillic acid diethylamide and deanol. *Anaesthesia* **15**, 273–279.

Ferguson, J. T., and Linn, F. V. Z. (1956). A new compound for the symptomatic treatment of tension and anxiety: 2-ethylcrotonylurea (Nostyn). *Antibiot. Med. Clin. Therapy* **3**, 329–333.

Hochman, R., and Robbins, J. J. (1958). Jaundice due to ectylurea. *New Engl. J. Med.* **259**, 583–585.

Kaplan, H. S. (1959). Tranquilizers in the office practice of medicine. *N.Y. State J. Med.* **59**, 2871–2887.

McHardy, G., McHardy, R. J. Craighead, C., et al. (1959). Evaluation of some new anthelminthic, anticholinergic, hydrocholeretic, and antispasmodic drugs. *Southern Med. J.* **52**, 102–107.

Runge, T. M. (1963). Monamine oxidase inhibitors in colitis. *Am. J. Gastroenterol.* **39**, 69–73.

Rutzler, H. L. (1959). Remarks made at New York State Medical Society, Panel Discussion on Early Recognition of Psychiatric Conditions. *N.Y. State J. Med.* **59**, 263.

Utley, M. D. (1958). Use of ectylurea (Nostyn) in mentally retarded patients; preliminary report of effects of seizures and spasticity. *Mich. State Med. Soc. J.* **57**, 1712–1714.

~ B.11 ~
Methyprylone

Bastian, J. W. (1961). Classification of CNS drugs by a mouse screening battery. *Arch. Intern. Pharmacodyn.* **133** (3–4), 347–364.

Bell, J. D. (1959). The use of a non-barbiturate hypnotic, methyprylon ("Noludar") in general practice. *J. Irish Med. Assoc.* **45**, 82–83.

Berger, H. (1961). Addiction to methyprylon: Report of case of 24-year-old nurse with possible synergism with phenothiazine. *J. Am. Med. Assoc.* **177** (1), 63–65.

Bernhard, K., Brubacher, G., and Lutz, A. H. (1954). Synthese einiger ^{14}C-signierter Dioxo-diaethyl-hydro-pyridine und Untersuchungen ueber deren Verteilung, Verweilzeit und Ausscheidung bei der Ratte. *Helv. Chim. Acta* **37** (214), 1839–1856.

Bernhard, K., Brubacher, G., and Lutz, A. (1954). Untersuchungen ueber Verteilung und Ausscheidung als Sedativa wirksamer Derivativate des Hexa-und Tetrahydro-pyridins mit Hilfe von ^{14}C-Signierungen. *Helv. Physiol. Pharmacol. Acta* **12**, C12—C13.

Bernhard, K., Just, M., Lutz, A. H., and Vuilleumier, J. P. (1957). Ueber das Verhalten in 5-Stellung methylierter Dioxo-diaethylhydropyridine im Stoffwechsel. *Helv. Chim. Acta* **40** (53), 436–444.

Billow, B. W., Steinberg, M., Lupini, S. B., Rothman, H., Carey, R., Paley, S. S., and Martorella, F. J. (1960). Clinical experiences with methyprylon, a non-barbiturate sedative and hypnotic drug. *Intern. Record Med.* **173** (5), 288–292.

Billow, B. W., Whiteman, N., Carey, R., Cabodevilla, A., Barnes, L., Rothman, N., and Paley, S. S. (1962). Evaluation of methyprylon in chronic insomniac patients with various physical disorders. *J. Natl. Med. Assoc.* **54** (2), 248–250.

Borushek, S., and Gold, J. J. (1964). Commonly used medications that interfere with routine endocrine laboratory procedures. *Clin. Chem.* **10** (1), 41–52.

Brandman, O., Coniaris, J., and Keller, H. E. (1955). A new, mild sedative-hypnotic, a piperidine derivative (Noludar). *J. Med. Soc. New Jersey* **52** (5), 246–253.

Cass, L. J., Frederik, W. S., and Andosca, J. B. (1955). Methyprylon: A new sedative and hypnotic drug. *New Engl. J. Med.* **253**, 586–591.

Cattaneo, A. D. (1959). Esperienze con il Metiprilone ("Noludar", Roche) in 412 pazienti chirurgici. *Minerva Anestesiol.* **25**, 271–280.

Chapman, J. E., and Lewis, C. E. (1962). Briefs from poison control centers: Darvon, dieldrin and noludar. *J. Kansas Med. Soc.* **63**, 228–229.

Cernish, S. M., Gruber, C. M., and Kohlsteadt, K. G. (1956). Obtaining data by telephone. A clinical evaluation of hypnotic drugs. *Proc. Soc. Exptl. Biol. Med.* **93**, 162–164.

Chinchinian, H. (1959). Use of tranquilizer therapy in office practice. *Marquette. Med. Rev.* **24**, 230.

Cochin, J., and Daly, J. W. (1963). The use of thin-layer chromatography for the analysis of drugs. Isolation and identification of barbiturates and nonbarbiturate hypnotics from urine, blood and tissues. *J. Pharmacol. Exptl. Therap.* **139** (2), 154–159.

de Haen, P. (1963). Today & tomorrow: Therapeutic research in review. *Med. Sci.* **14** (1), 84–105.

Dobkin, A. B., and Wyant, G. M. (1957). Clinical evaluation of methyprylon (noludar) as a preanaesthetic sedative hypnotic. *Can. Anaesthesiol. Soc. J.* **4** (1), 27–36.

Dressler, A. (1959). Ein papierchromatographischer Nachweis von 2,4-Dioxo-3,3-diaethyl-5-methylpiperidin (Noludar, Methyprylon). *Arch. Toxikol.* **17** (4), 293–294.

Dressler, A. (1960). Nachweis und papierchromatographische Auftrennung der barbituratfreien Sedativa Benedorm (Persedon), Elrodorm (Doriden), Noludar, Sedulon, Valamin, Bromural und Adalin sowie Antipyrin, Phenacetin und Meprobamat. *Deut. Z. Ges. Gerichtl. Med.* **50**, 457–463.

Eberhardt, H., Freundt, K. J., and Langbein, J. W. (1962). Der duennschichtchromatographische Nachweis von Schlafmitteln als Reinsubstanzen und nach Koerperpassage. *Arzneimittel-Forsch.* **12** (11), 1087–1089.

Ehlers, H. (1963). Poisoning with psychopharmaca and barbiturate-free hypnotics. *Danish Med. Bull.* **10** (4), 117–121.

Erwin, V. G., and Heim, H. C. (1963). Effects of some hypnotic drugs on respiration and oxidative phosphorylation in rat brain. *J. Pharm. Sci.* **52** (8), 747–751.

Finckh, R., and Kugler, J. (1964). Eignung verschiedener Mittel fuer das Schlaf-Elektroencephalogramm. *Arzneimittel-Forsch.* **14** (8), 969–972.

Fink, G. B., and Juchau, M. R. (1964). Comparative neurotoxicity and antipentylenetetrazol activity of some piperidinediones. *J. Pharm. Sci.* **53** (3), 325–327.

Frahm, M., Gottesleben, A., and Soehring, K. (1963). Die Identifizierung von Schlafmitteln aus waessrigen Loesungen und Harn mit Hilfe der Duennschichtchromatographie. *Pharm. Acta Helv.* **38** (11), 785–804.

Frick, P., Reutter, F., and von Rechenberg, H. K. (1962). Hypovolaemischer Schock infolge Extravasation von Plasma in das Interstitium bei Schlafmittelintoxikationen. *Schweiz. Med. Wochschr.* **92** (35), 1061–1065.

Fujimori, Y., Honma, Y., and Kaneko, Y. (1959). Studies on the anticonvulsant action of methyprylon. *Hirosaki Med. J.* **10** (1), 120–127.

Glatt, M. M. (1957). Methyprylone (correspondence). *Brit. Med. J.* I, 164.

Glatt, M. M. (1959). Drug treatment of insomnia (correspondence). *Brit. Med. J.* I, 50–51.

Goerttler, K. (1962). Der "teratologische Grundversuch" am bruteten Huehnchenkeim, seine Moeglichkeiten und Grenzen. *Klin. Wochschr.* **40** (16), 809–812.

Gold, M. I. (1958). New nonbarbiturate sedative-hypnotics! A pharmacologic review. *Anesthesia Analgesia, Current Res.* **37** (6), 347–351.

Goode, P. (1960). A six-month continuous study of methyprylon in the geriatric psychiatric patient with insomnia. *N.Y. J. Med.* **60** (16). 2546–2550.

Graham, R. C. B., Lu, F. C., and Allmark, M. G. (1957). Combined effect of tranquilizing drugs and alcohol on rats. *Federation Proc.* **16** (Part 1), 302.

Granick, S. (1964). A test for detection of porphyria-inducing drugs. *J. Am. Med. Assoc.* **190** (5), 475.

Hagenbucher, J. T., and Kleh, J. (1962). Treatment of insomnia in geriatric patients: Double-blind study with methyprylon and pentobarbital. *J. Am. Geriat. Soc.* **10** (12), 1038–1040.

Heise, G. A., and Boff, E. (1962). Continuous avoidance as a base-line for measuring behavioral effects of drugs. *Psychopharmacologia* **3** (4), 264–282.

Herzog, M. (1955). Behandlung von Depressionen in der Allgemeinpraxis mit Noludar. *Therap. Umschau* **12** (6). 86–87.

Hoffer, A. (1958). Lack of potentiation of alcoholic excitement by methyprylon (noludar). *Can. Med. Assoc. J.* **79**, 191 and 217–218.

Horstmann, W. (1962). Efrahrungen mit einem barbituratfreien Schlaf- und Beruhigungsmittel bei jungen Kindern. Klinische und elektroenzephalographische Untersuchungen mit 2,4-Dioxo-3, 3-diaethyl-5-methylpiperidin (Noludar). *Muench. Med. Wochschr.* **104**, 603–608.

Hufford, A. R. (1956). Marplan—an approach to gastrointestinal spasm and hyperacidity. *Postgrad. Med.* **20**, 514–524.

Ivey, E. P. (1958). Methylphenidate hydrochloride therapy after attempted suicide: Review of the literature and report of a case. *J. Am. Med. Assoc.* **167** (17), 2071–2073.

Jacobziner, H., and Raybin, H. W. (1961). Briefs on accidental chemical poisonings in New York City from the poison control center, New York City Department of Health—meprobamate, aspirin, and methyprylon intoxications. *N.Y. J. Med.* **61**, 1935–1938.

Jacobziner, H., and Raybin, H. W. (1960). Aminophylline and other severe poisonings. *N.Y. J. Med.* **60**, 3300–3303.

Jensen, G. R. (1960). Addiction to "Noludar": A report of two cases. *New Zealand Med. J.* **59**, 431–432.

Kemper, H. (1955). Erfahrungen mit einem neuen Schlafmittel aus der Piperidinreihe in der Psychiatrie. *Deut. Med. Wochschr.* **80** (27/28), 1034–1035.

Kolowrat, F. (1956). Klinische Pruefung eines neuen Schlafmittels der Piperidinreihe. *Medizinische* No. 11, 387–388.

Koppanyi, T., and McDermott, T. F. (1962). Methyprylon as an intravenous anesthetic. *Federation Proc.* **21** (2), 330.

Krause, H. (1955). Klinische Erfahrungen mit einem neuen barbitursaeurefreien Schlafmittel ("Noludar"). *Schweiz. Med. Wochschr.* **85** (15), 355–356.

Kretschmer, W., Jr. (1957). Ein neuer Piperidin-Abkoemmling als Schlaf- und Beruhigungsmittel. *Therap. Gegenwaet.* **96** (7), 247–249.

Lange, H.-J. (1956). Noludar, ein neues Schlafmittel. *Med. Klin. (Munich)* **51** (8), 303–304.

Lasagna, L. (1956). A study of hypnotic drugs in patients with chronic diseases: Comparative efficacy of placebo; methylprylon (Noludar); meprobamate (Miltown, Equanil) pentobarbital; phenobarbital; secobarbital. *J. Chronic Diseases* **3** (2), 122–133.

le Riche, W. H., and van Belle, G. (1963). Clinical and statistical evaluation of six hypnotic agents. *Can. Med. Assoc. J.* **88** (16), 837–841.

Lienert, G. A. (1956). Vergleichende pharmako-psychologische Untersuchungen ueber Schlafmittelwirkungen und -nachwirkungen. *Medizinische* **45**, 1608–1614.

Lodge Patch, I. C., Eilenberg, M. D., and Hare, E. H. (1960). Ethinamate and methyprylon as hypnotics: a comparative trial. *J. Mental Sci.* **106** (445), 1455–1458.

Loughlin, E. H., Mullin, W. G., Schwimmer, J., and Schwimmer, M. (1955). Clinical studies on toxicity and on hypnotic and sedative effects of Ro 1-6463, Noludar (3,3-diethyl-2,4-dioxo-5-methylpiperidine). *Intern. Record Med.* **168** (2), 52–60.

MacGregor, A. G. (1960). The non-barbiturate sedatives. *Practitioner* **184**, 15–17.

MacKay, F. J., Hehre, F. W., and Green, N. M. (1958). The effect of methyprylon on respiration and the cardiovascular system of man. *Anesthesia Analgesia, Current Res.* **37** (4), 226–228.

Martin, F., and Chesni, Y. (1962). Research into the techniques for provoking EEG activation in the epileptic subject: Introduction of noludar-R-Roche, a non-barbiturate sedative and derived from piperidine (Methylprylon). *Electroencephalog. Clin. Neurophysiol.* **14** (5), 782.

Masciocchi, A. (1957). Sperimentazione clinica ed elettroencefalografica di tre nuovi ipnotici non barbiturici. *Riv. Pato. Nervoso Ment.* **78**, 920–940.

Mitchell, R. E., Jr. (1958). Effects of a new spasmolytic-sedative in the treatment of 50 consecutive hospitalized gastrointestinal cases. *Am. J. Gastroenterol.* **29**, 177–186.

Mussler, K. H., and Hubach, H. (1956). Ueber sedative und hypnotische Effekte eines Piperidin—abkommelings. *Deut. Med. J.* **7** (17), 651–652.

Nelemans, F. A., and Zelvelder, W. G. (1962). The clinical evaluation of hypnotics: Objective versus subjective method. *Arch. Intern. Pharmacodyn.* **140** (1–2), 231–236.

Paulus, W., and Goenechea, S. (1963). IR-Nachweis von Revonal und Noludar im Leichenmaterial. *Arch. Toxikol.* **20** (3), 194–196.

Pelikan, E. W., and Kensler, C. J. (1958). Sedatives: Their pharmacology and uses. *Med. Clin. N. Am.* **42**, 1217–1237.

Pellegrino, E. D., and Henderson, R. R. (1957). Clinical toxicity of methyprylon (Noludar): Case report and review of twenty-three cases. *J. Med. Soc. New Jersey* **54**, 515–518.

Pellmont, B., Studer, A., and Juergens, R. (1955). "Noludar," ein neues Schlafmittel der Piperidinreihe. *Schweiz. Med. Wochschr.* **85** (15), 350–354.
Penprase, W. G., and Biles, J. A. (1958). The use of microscopic and x-ray diffraction methods for the identification of sedatives and anticonvulsants. *J. Am. Pharm. Assoc.* **47** (7), 523–528.
Percheson, P. B., Carroll, J. J., and Screech, G. (1959). Ritalin (Methylphenidate): Clinical experiences. *Can. Anaesthesiol. Soc. J.* **6** (3), 277–282.
Peters, U. H. (1963). Chronische Methyprylon-Intoxikation und ihre Psychopathologie. *Arch. Psychiat. Nervenkrankh.* **204**, 342–348.
Pletscher, A. (1962). Thalidomide and methyprylone. *S. African Med. J.* **36**, 1024.
Prego Silva, L. E. (1957). Experiencia clinica con un nuevo derivado de la piperidina. *Arch. Uruguay Med. Cir. Especial. (Montevideo)* **50**, 26–30.
Pribilla, O. (1956). Ein Ausscheidungsprodukt nach Gaben von 2,4-Dioxo-3, 3-diaethyl-5-methyl-piperidin beim Menschen. *Arzneimittel-Forsch.* **6** (12) 756–760.
Pribilla, O. (1959). Studien zur Toxikologie der Schlafmittel aus der Tetrahydropyridin- und Piperidin-Reihe. *Arch. Toxikol.* **18** (1), 1–86.
Radnay, P. A. (1957). Noludar, a useful sedative-hypnotic drug. *Postgrad. Med.* **21** (6), 617–623.
Randall, L. O., Iliev, V., and Brandman, O. (1956). Metabolism of methyprylon. *Arch. Intern. Pharmacodyn.* **106** (4), 388–394.
Reidt, W. U. (1956). Fatal poisoning with methyprylon (noludar), a nonbarbiturate sedative. *New Engl. J. Med.* **255** (5), 231–232.
Reiser, P., Kay, L. L., Printz, S., Cherico, P., and Harris, S. B. (1963). Clinical trial with methyprylon in patients with chronic insomnia. *Clin. Med.* **70** (2), 395–399.
Rickels, K., and Bass, H. (1963). A comparative controlled clinical trial of seven hypnotic agents in medical and psychiatric in-patients. *Am. J. Med. Sci.* **245** (2), 142–152.
Riser, M., Riser, A., and Rascol, A. (1957). De l'action hypnogene d'un derive de la piperidine. *Bull. Soc. Med. Hop. (Paris)* **73** (22–24), 685.
Robie, T. R. (1960). Chemotherapy in melancholia. *Diseases Nervous System* **21**, 124–129.
Rutishauser, M. (1963). Beeinflussung des Kohlenhydratstoffwechsels des Rattenhirns durch Psychopharmaka mit sedativer Wirkung. *Arch. Exptl. Pathol. Pharmakol.* **245** (3), 396–413.
Salim, E. F., Manni, P. E., and Sinsheimer, J. E. (1964). Nonketol reduction of tetrazolium salts in pharmaceutical analysis. *J. Pharm. Sci.* **53** (4), 391–394.
Satge, P., and Commare, M. (1960). Essais cliniques, chez l'enfant, d'un nouveau sedatif: le methyprylon. *Vie Med.* **41**, 25–26 and 29.
Schaffer, A. I., and Seegers, W. (1956). Effects of methyprylon (noludar) and phenobarbital on the electrocardiogram. *J. Am. Geriat. Soc.* **4** (11), 1078–1079.
Schallek, W., Kuehn, A., and Seppelin, D. K. (1956). Central depressant effects of methyprylon. *J. Pharmacol. Exptl. Therap.* **118** (2), 139–147.
Schallek, W., Kuehn, A., and Seppelin, D. (1956). Effects of methyprylon (Noludar) (R) on the central nervous system of the dog. *Abstr. Commun., 20th Intern. Physiol. Cong., Brussels,* 1956 pp. 798–799.
Schmitt, W. (1955). Klinische Pruefung einer neuen Piperidin-Verbindung als Schlafmittel. *Med. Klin. (Munich)* **50** (29), 1223–1224.
Seitz, R., Trier, M., and Juergens, R. (1956). Agranulozytose durch Schlafmittel. Nebenwirkungen von Arzneimitteln auf Blut und Knochenmark. *Intern. Symp. Malmo* 1956 pp. 143–160.
Senay, E. C. (1956). The effects of methyprylon (Noludar) upon the electroencephalogram. Doctoral Thesis, Yale University, New Haven, Connecticut, 10 pp.
Shideman, F. E. (1958). Hypnotics and Sedatives. *Postgrad. Med.* **24**, 207–223.
Shideman, F. E. (1961). Clinical pharmacology of hypnotics and sedatives. *Clin. Pharmacol. Therap.* **2** (3), 313–344.

Shulman, A., and Laycock, G. M. (1959). Further aspects of the analeptic activity of bemegride. *Australian J. Exptl. Biol. Med. Sci.* **35**, 421–426.

Shulman, A., and Laycock, G. M. (1958). Bemegride analepsis. *Brit. Med. J.* I, 871.

Shulman, A., and Laycock, G. M. (1958). Bemegride analepsis to deep hypnosis induced by a variety of hypnotics. *Australian J. Exptl. Biol. Med. Sci.* **36**, 347–358.

Sigg, E. B., Holland, R., and Schneider, J. A. (1957). Non-barbiturate depressants: Effect on EEG and central polysynaptic mechanisms. *Federation Proc.* **16** (Part 1), 119.

Sigg, E. B., Holland, R., and Schneider, J. A. (1958). The influence of some nonbarbiturate depressants on central polysynaptic mechanisms. *Arch. Intern. Pharmacodyn.* **116** (3–4), 450–463.

Stacher, A., and Boehnel, L. (1957). Klinische Erfahrungen mit einem neuen Schlafmittel bzw. Sedativum der Piperidinreihe. *Wien Med. Wochschr.* **107** (4), 995–996.

Stanton, H. C., and Keasling, H. H. (1956). Comparison of noludar (Methyprylon) and pentobarbital on respiratory minute volume in rabbits. *Proc. Soc. Exptl. Biol. Med.* **93**, 555–557.

Stewart, J. S. (1956). Clinical trial of metyprylone, a piperidine hypnotic. *Brit. Med. J.* II, 1465–1467.

Thomas, R. L. (1956). Newer analgesics and hypnotics. *Anesthesiology* **5** (1), Suppl., 711–715.

Thomson, T. J. (1958). Clinical comparison of methyprylone and quinalbarbitone as hypnotics: Sequential analysis used. *Brit. Med. J.* II, 1140–1141.

Thueer, W. (1956). Traitement de l'insomnie par un nouvel hypnogene, le Noludar Roche. *Praxis (Bern)* **45** (1), 416–418.

Truitt, E. B., Jr. (1960). An experiment in pharmacology designed to teach the evaluation of subjective responses to drugs. *J. Med. Educ.* **35** (11), 1014–1016.

Uleri, G. (1958). Sull'impiego del Noludar come sedativo della vigilia. *Minerva Anestesiol.* **24**, 29–31.

Ullius, K. (1956). Klinische Erfahrungen mit "Noludar," einem neuen Schlafmittel aus der Piperidin-Reihe. *Fortschr. Med.* **74** (21), 556.

Velarde, N. N., and Harris, R. (1960). The effect of methyprylon on the sleep of residents of an old age institution: A double-blind study. *J. Am. Geriat. Soc.* **8** (4), 269–276.

Voelksen, W. (1960). Mikrochemische Nachweise der Hypnotica aus der Tetrahydropyridin- und Piperidinreihe. I. Farb- und Kristallreaktionen. *Pharm. Ztg., Ver. Apotheker-Ztg.* **105** (35), 1029–1031.

Vogler, K., and Kofler, M. (1956). Spontane Spaltung von 2,4-Dioxo-3,3-diaethyl-5-methylpiperidin in die optischen Antipoden. *Helv. Chim. Acta* **39** (165), 1387–1394.

Weber, H. (1955). Erfahrungen mit einem barbituratfroien Beruhigungs- und Schlafmittel in der Paediatrie. *Med. Klin. (Munich)* (45), 1909–1910.

Weiss, G. W. (1961). Case report: Effects of an overdose of methyprylon in a geriatric patient. *J. Am. Osteopath. Assoc.* **61** (2), 129–130.

Winfield, D. L. (1960). The use of methyprylon as an aid in obtaining electroencephalograms in alcoholics. *J. Nervous Mental Disease* **130** (1), 45–48.

Winfield, D. L., and Hughes, J. G. (1959). The use of noludar in pediatric electroencephalography. *Electroencephog. Clin. Neurophysiol.* **9** (4), 713–715.

Winne, D. (1962). Die Wirkung einiger Schlaf—und Narkosemittel bei roentgenbestrahlten Mausen. *Arch. Exptl. Pathol. Pharmakol.* **243** (3), 212–231.

Zambianchi, A. (1957). Osservazioni cliniche ed elettroencefalografiche sugli effetti di un sedativo-ipnotico privo di acido barbiturico (2,4 dicheto 3,3 dietil 5 metil piperidina). *Riv. Psichiat.* **50**, 505–510.

Zambianchi, A. (1958). Klinische und elektroencephalographische Beobachtungen ueber die Wirkungen eines barbituratfreien Beruhigungs- und Schlafmittels (Noludar Roche). *Zentr. Ges. Neurol. Psychol.* **145**, 295.

Zamparo, D. (1956). Aspetti elettroencefalografici del sonno indotto in soggetti psichiatrici con un nuovo ipnotico piperidinico. *Gazz. Med. Ital.* **115** (10), 324–327.

~ B.12 ~
Ethchlorvynol

Aycribb, J. B. (1964). Two cases of withdrawal from ethchlorvynol. *Am. J. Psychiat.* **120**, 1201.
Ban, T. A., and McGinnis, K. (1962). Comparative clinical study of two hypnotic drugs. *Can. Med. Assoc. J.* **87**, 816.
Barg, U., and Sokol, J. K. (1964). Ethchlorvynol compared with other hypnotics in urologic patients. *Western Med.* **5**, 154.
Blinder, S. (1964). A clinical study of ethchlorvynol in cardiac patients. *Current Therap. Res.* **6**, 373.
Blumenthal, M. D., and Reinhart, M. J. (1964). Psychosis and convulsions following withdrawal from ethchlorvynol. *J. Am. Med. Assoc.* **190**, 154.
Boros, H. H., and Priver, M. S. (1964). Ethchlorvynol as a sedative in labor. *Am. J. Obstet. Gynecol.* **89**, 1016.
Carter, C. H. (1959). Ethchlorvynol in the treatment of mixed grand and petit mal epilepsy. *Epilepsia* **1**, 1.
Cattaneo, A. D., Antole, R. M., and Traverso, G. (1964). Controlled clinical study of a drug with hypnotic and sedative action: Ethchlorvynol (Arvynol). *Minerva Anestesiol.* **30**, 7.
Essig, C. F. (1964). Addiction to nonbarbiturate sedative and tranquilizing drugs. *Clin. Pharmacol. Therap.* **5**, 334.
Gladstone, H. (1964). Placidyl therapy in orthopedic patients. *Am. J. Orthoped.* **68**.
Kelman, H. (1965). Addiction to inocuous drugs. *Med. Times* **93**, 155.
Kempe, H.-W. (1964). Experiences with ethchlorvynol in a women's clinic. *Deut. Med. J.* **15**, 181.
Lawrence, W. D. (1964). Double-blind evaluation of ethchlorvynol during labor. *Western Med.* **5**, 14.
le Riche, W. H., and Csima, A. (1964). A clinical evaluation of four hypnotic agents, using a Latin-square design. *Can. Med. Assoc. J.* **91**, 435.
Mathews, V., Lehmann, H. E., and Ban, T. A. (1964). A comparative study of thirteen hypnotic drugs. *Appl. Therap.* **6**, 806.
Rein, C. R., and Fleischmajer, R. (1957). The tranquilizing efficacy of ethchlorvynol (Placidyl) in dermatological therapy. *AMA Arch. Dermatol.* **75**, 438.
Schremly, J. A., and Solomon, P. (1964). Drug Abuse and Addiction. *J. Am. Med. Assoc.* **189**, 512.
Schwartz, F. R. (1957). Ethchlorvynol (Placidyl) as a sedative in dermatological practice. *AMA Arch. Dermatol.* **75**, 747.
Shubin, H., Anastasi, J. D., and Glaskin, A. (1964). The effectiveness of ethchlorvynol as a soporific. *J. Germantown Hosp.* **5**, 17.
Siegel, I. (1965). Dependency upon tranquilizers. *J. Am. Med. Assoc.* **191**, 352.
Siegler, P. E., Winstin, D., and Nodine, J. H. (1964). The effect of hypnotics on psychomotor performance. *Pharmacologist* **6**, 205.

Appendix C
Addenda to Volume I

C.1 Chlorprothixene 501
C.2 Clinical Applications of the Monoamine Oxidase Inhibitors (Hydrazines): Addendum 519
C.3 Biochemistry and Pharmacology of the Monoamine Oxidase Inhibitors (Hydrazines): Addendum 523

~ C.1 ~
Chlorprothixene

Chemical Papers

American Cyanamid Co. (1960). Dimethylaminopropylidinethioxanthenes. British Patent. 834,143; *Chem. Abstr.* **54**, 24811f.

Awe, W., and Schulze, N. (1962). Systematic analysis of antihistamines, phenothiazines and phenothiazine-like compounds. *Pharm. Ztg., Ver. Apotheker-Ztg.* **107**, 1333–1339; (1963) *Chem. Abstr.* **58**, 13715b.

Bente, D., Hippius, H., Poldinger, W., and Stach, K. (1964). Chemische Konstitution und klinische Wirkung von antidepressiven Pharmaka. *Arzneimittel-Forsch.* **14** (6a), 486–490.

Bonovicino, G. E., Arlt, H. G., Pearson, K. M., and Hardy, R. A., Jr. (1961). Tranquilizing agents: Xanthine- and thioxanthene-9γ,-propylamines and related compounds. *J. Org. Chem.* **26**, 2383–2392; *Chem. Abstr.* **55**, 27340i.

Cochin, J., and Daly, J. W. (1963). The use of thin-layer chromatography for the analysis of drugs. Identification and isolation of phenothiazine tranquilizers and antihistaminics in body fluids and tissues. *J. Pharmacol. Exptl. Therap.* **139**, 160–165; *Psychol. Abstr.* **3** (1), 101.

Cochin, J., and Daly, J. W. (1963). Use of thin-layer chromatography for the analysis of drugs. Isolation and identification of barbiturates and non-barbiturate hypnotics from urine, blood and tissues. *J. Pharmacol. Exptl. Therap.* **139**, 154–159; *Chem. Abstr.* **58**, 14428d.

Cochin, J., and Daly, J. W. (1963). The use of thin-layer chromatography for the analysis of drugs. Identification and isolation of phenothiazine tranquilizer and of antihistamines in body fluids and tissues. *J. Pharmacol. Exptl. Therap.* **139** (2), 160–165.

Dunitz, J. D., Eser, H., and Stricker, P. (1964). Die Konfiguration des physiologisch wirksamen 2-Chloro-9-(w-dimethylaminopropyliden)-thioxanthens. *Helv. Chim. Acta* **47** (7), 1897–1902.

Engelhardt, E. L. (1962). (to Merck & Co.). 10(w-Aminoalkylidine)-thioxanthines. U.S. Patent 3,046,283; *Chem. Abstr.* **57**, 16569c.

Ferrari, M., and Toth, C. E. (1962). Thin-layer chromatography of C^{14}-labeled dinitrophenylamino acids. *J. Chromatog.* **9**, 388–390.

Ferrari, M., and Toth, C. E. (1962). Thin-layer chromatography of urinary metabolites of chlorpromazine and related psychotropic drugs. *J. Chromatog.* **9**, 388–390; *Index Med.* **4** (3), S-462.

Gothelf, B., and Karczmar, A. G. (1963). Quantitative colorimetric method and extraction procedure for determination of chlorpromazine in animal tissues. *Intern. J. Neuropharmacol.* **2** (1/2), 95–99; *Chem. Abstr.* **60**, 16196f.

Hamacher, J., and Hildebrandt, G. (1964). Zusammenhange zwischen chemischer Konstitution und Herz-Kreislauf-Wirkung therapeutisch angewendeter Phenothiazin und Thiaxanthene-Derivative. [Inter relations between chemical constitution and cardiovascular activity of therapeutically used phenothiazine and thiaxanthene derivatives 1st report.] *Arzneimittel-Forsch.* **14** (9), 977–981.

Hoffmann-La Roche & Co., F., A.-G. (1962). Tricylcic compounds. Belgian Patent 613,363.

Hoffmann-La Roche & Co., F., A.-G. (1960). Geometric isomerization of halo-substituted 9-alkylidenethiaxanthenes. British Patent 881,488 (Appl. June 8, 1960); *Chem. Abstr.* **56**, 7282g.

Hoffmann-La Roche & Co., F., A.-G. (Doebel, K., Rey-Bellet, G., Schlapfer, R., and Spiegelberg, H.). (1958). Xanthine and thioxanthine derivatives. German Patent 1,044,103; *Chem. Abstr.* **55**, 2691e, f, g.

Holm, T. (1963). Preparation and properties of 1,1-diaryl-1,3-butadienes. *Acta Chem. Scand.* **18** (9), 2437–2443 (in English); *Chem. Abstr.* **60**, 9245b, f.

Kefalas, A/S. (1960). Substituted thioxanthenes and their acid addition salts. Danish Patent 88,606; *Chem. Abstr.* **55**, 5536g.

Kefalas, A/S. (1962). Xanthenes and thiaxanthenes. French Patent 1,309,813; *Derwent Fine Chem. Patents J.* **2** (51).

Maehly, A. C., and Linturi, M. K. (1962). Detection of drugs other than barbiturates in the routine method for barbiturate analysis. *Acta Chem. Scand.* **16**, 283–286; *Chem. Abstr.* **57**, 6024g.

Mellinger, T. J., and Keeler, C. E. (1962). Chromatography and electrophoresis of phenothiazine drugs. *J. Pharm. Sci.* **51**, 1169–1173; *Psychopharmacol. Abstr.* **2** (10), 2492.

Mellinger, T. J., and Keeler, C. E. (1963). Spectrofluormetric identification of phenothiazine drugs. *Anal. Chem.* **35**, 554–558; *Chem. Abstr.* **58**, 13721e.

Mellinger, T. J., Mellinger, E. M., and Smith, W. T. (1964). Urine tests for chlorprothixene. *Am. J. Psychiat.* **120** (11), 1111–1114.

Merck & Co., Inc. (1960). Thiaxanthene derivatives. British Patent 829,763; *Chem. Abstr.* **54**, 18555h.

Paulus, W., Hoch, W., and Keymer, R. (1963). Thin-layer chromatography of several phenothiazines and substances of similar activity. *Arzneimittel-Forsch.* **13** (7), 609–610.

Petersen, P. V., Lassen, N., Holm, T., Kopf, R., and Nielsen, I. M. (1958). Chemische Konstitution und pharmakologische Wirkung einiger Thiaxanthene-Analoge zu Chlorpromazin, Promazin und Mepazin. *Arzneimittel-Forsch.* **8**, 395–397.

Peterson, P. V., Larsen, N. O., and Holm, T. O. (1963). (to Kefalas, A/S, Copenhagen-Walby) 9-(Propene-3-ylidene-1), and 9-(3'-(N-hydroxyalkylpiperazino-N)-propylidene) xanthenes and thioxanthenes. U.S. Patent 3,116,291.

Schaeren, S. F., Schlaepfer, R., Spiegelberg, H., and Vaterlaus, B. P. (1963). (to Hoffman-La Roche Inc.) Isomerizing stereoisomeric xanthene and thioxanthene compounds with oxalic acid. U.S. Patent 3,113,137; *Chem. Abstr.* **60**, 5462f.

Schindler, O., Lehner, H., Michaelis, W., and Schmutz, J. (1963). Synthese einiger thioxanthen-derivate. *Helv. Chim. Acta* **46** (4), 1079–1108.

Schalapfer, R., and Spiegelberg, H. (1963). (to Hoffmann-La Roche, Inc.) Method of isomerizing basically substituted stereoisomeric thioxanthenes. U.S. Patent 3,115,502.

Sirnes, T. B. (1963). Thiaxanthene derivatives and similar substances. Chemistry and pharmacology of the substances. *Nord. Psykiat. Tidskr.* **27**, 52–68 (in Norwegian).

Sjoberg, K., and Tufvesson, G. (1963). Methods for determining the presence of tranquilizers and other new drugs in urine of dogs. *Acta Vet. Scand.* **4** (3), 209–220 (in English); *Chem. Abstr.* **60**, 5878b.

Sprague, J. M. (1962). (to Merck & Co., Inc.) 10-(w-Aminoalkyl-10-hydroxythiaxanthenes). U.S. Patent 3,047,580; *Chem. Abstr.* **58**, 1437h, 1438a.

Sprague, J. M., and Engelhardt, E. L. (1960). (to Merck & Co., Inc.) Thiaxanthenes. U.S. Patent 2,951,082; *Chem. Abstr.* **55**, 4538–4539.

Gomez de Uribe, F. (1961). Quimica, farmacologia y toxicologia del Truxil, tioxantenderivado psicoactivo. (Chemistry, pharmacology and toxicology of Truxil, psychoactive derivative of thioxanthene.) *Med. Farm. (Madrid)* **25**, 206–221.

Wander, A.-G., Dr. A. (1962). (by J. Schmutz). Thioxanthene derivatives. Swizz Patent 358,081; *Chem. Abstr.* **57**, 13731a.

Biology and Pharmacology

Allgen, L. G., Jonsson, B., Nauckhoff, B., Anderson, M. L., Huus, I., and Moller Nielsen, I. (1960). On the elimination of chlorprothixene in rat and man. *Experientia* **16**, 325.

Bartholini, G., Pletscher, A., and Gey, K. F. (1961). Diminution of 5-hydroxytryptamine in thrombocytes *in vitro* by chlorpromazine and related compounds. *Experientia* **17**, 541–542. *Chem. Abstr.* **56**, 14870h.

Benesova, O., and Trinerova, I. (1964). The effects of psychotropic drugs on the cholinergic and adrenergic system. *Intern. J. Neuropharmacol.* **3**, 473–478.

Bergmann, H. (1963). Sensitivity changes of the isolated guinea pig intestine by premedication, anesthesia and spasmolytics. *Klin. Med. (Wein)* **18**, 413–430 (Ger.).

Bibawi, E., Girgis, B., and Abu-Khatwa, H. (1963). Effect of hypnotics and psychotropic drugs on prothrombin level. *J. Egypt. Med. Assoc.* **46**, 933–936.

Bielicki, F., Czyzewski, K., and Skora, K. (1960). Accumulation of radioactive iodine in the thyroid gland after administration of certain drugs producing autonomic blockade. *Endokrynol. Polska* **13**, 73–79.

Bornmann, G. (1961). Zum Einfluss einiger psychotroper Substanzen auf Magen und Gallefluss. (The effect of some psychotropic drugs on gastric function and bile flow.) *Arzneimittel-Forsch.* **11** (2), 89–90.

Bouyard, P., and Du Cailar, J. (1960). Cardiovascular effects of Ro4–0403. Experimental study. *Agressologie* **3**, 249–251 (in French).

Bradley, N. W., and Jones, B. M., Jr. (1962). Effects of Taractan and Tranimal on beef steers being fattened in drylot. *Kentucky Agr. Expt. Sta. Progr. Rept.* **116**, 3–4; (1963). *Biol. Abstr.* **41** (3), 10932 (no abstract).

Burge, E. (1961). Einfluss von Tranquillizersubstanzen auf die Alkoholwirkung. (Influence of tranquilizers on the effects of alcohol.) *Hefte Unfallheilk.* **24** (66), 99–102.

Cahn, J., Herold, M., Alano, J., Vanholten-Bamberger, I., Mathis, P., and Georges, G. (1960). Pharmacological study of Ro4–0404. *Agressologie* **3**, 235–247 (in French).

Cahn, J., Alano, J., and Hauser, F. (1961). L'association Taractan-Librium, ou neuroleptataraxie. Etude experimentale des effets sur l'EEG et le comportement psychomoteur. (Neuroleptotaraxia, or the combination of Taractan with Librium. Experiments; study of effects on the EEG and on psychometer behavior.) *Presse Med.* **69** (41), 1764.

Cahn, J., Alano, J., and Hauser, F. (1962). The Taractan:Librium combination on neuroleptataraxia. Experimental study of its effects on the EEG and psychomotor behavior. *Agressologie* **3**, 153–158 (in French).

Cascio, G., Criscuoli, P. M., Palazzoadriano, M., and Zito, M. (1962). The central effect of the α-isomer of 2-chloro-9-(3-dimethylaminopropylidene) thioxanthene (chlorprothixene). Relation between dose and effects. *Acta Neurol. Naples* **17** (6), 553–580.

Corne, S. J., Pickering, R. W., and Warner, B. T. (1963). A method of assessing the effects of drugs on the central actions of 5-hydroxytryptamine. *Brit. J. Pharmacol.* **20**, 106–120; **58**, 9534c.

Cornu, F., and Sellei-Biro, K. (1960). The significance of changes in serum proteins during psychiatric pharmacotherapy. *Med. Exptl.* **3**, 161–168 (in German). *Chem. Abstr.* **55**, 10683b.

Cranston, E. M. (1963). Ineffectiveness of five compounds on spontaneous mammary tumors of mice. *Cancer Chemotherapy Rept.* **27**, 11–12.

Day, C. A., and Yen, H. C. Y. (1962). Antagonism of drug induced tremors. *Federation Proc.* **2**, 335 (Abstr.); *Psychol. Abstr.* **2** (5), 948.

Dobkin, A. B., and Israel, J. S., Byles, P. H., and Lee, P. K. Y. (1963). Chlorprothixene and amitriptylene: Interaction with thiopentone, circulatory effect and antisialogogue effect. *Brit. J. Anaesth.* **35**, 425.

Duplay, J., Maestraehlis, P., Fauche, et al. (1964). A recent series of 5 voluminous neurinomas of the acoustic nerve. Total ablation and cure. Reflections on the anesthetic technic. *Neurochirurgie* **10**, 198–204 (in French).

Eberhard, F., Wilke, G., and Ansorg, W. (1961). Uber den Schutz der Gewebsatmung durch antioxidantisch wirkame Psycopharmaka. (The protection of tissue respiration by psychopharmacological agents with antioxidant activity.) *Psychopharmacologia* **2** (3), 160–171.

Florez, J. (1963). Influence of chlorprothixene upon the effects of excitation of respiratory airways. *Biochem. Pharmacol.* **12**, Suppl., 240 (Abstr. 847).

Florez, J. (1964). Influence of chlorprothixene and codeine upon the response to excitation of respiratory airways. *Proc. 2nd Intern. Pharmacol. Meeting, Prague*, 1963, No. 11, 211–220.

Forrest, I. S., Quesada, F., and Deitchman, G. L. (1964). Unicellular organisms as model systems for the mode of action of phenothiazine and related drugs. *Proc. Western Pharmacol. Soc.* **7**, 42–44.

Frommel, E., Fleury, C., and Beguin, M. (1960). On the pharmacodynamics of a new neuroleptic: α-isomer of 2-chloro-9-(3-dimethylaminopropylidene)-thioxanthene HCl or Taractan. Action on the sleep centers, on motor excitation caused by nikethamide, on pentylenetetrazole, electroshock and pschomotor excitation due to amphetamine. *Compt. Rend. Soc. Biol.* **154**, 1182–1185 (in French).

Fromell, E., Fleury, C., and Beguin, M. (1960). (On the pharmacology of a new neuroleptic: The α-isomer of 2-chloro-9-(3-dimethylaminopropylidene)-thioxanthene, or Taractan. Anesthetic, hypothermic, antipyretic action and atropinic effect. *Compt. Rend. Soc. Biol.* **154**, 1401–1403 (in French).

Gemperle, M. (1963). Bronchospirometry in neuroleptic analgesia. *Anaesthesist* **12**, 357–358 (in German).

Gey, K. F., and Pletscher, A. (1961). Effect of chlorpromazine and chlorprothixene on monoamine metabolism in the rat brain. *Helv. Physiol. Pharmacol. Acta* **19**, C22–C24 (in German).

Gey, K. F., and Pletscher, A. (1961). Influence of chlorpromazine and chlorproxthixene on the cerebral metabolism of monoamines. *In* "Systeme extra-pyrimidal et neuroleptiques —system and neuroleptics" (J.-M. Bordeleau, ed.), pp. 175–180. Editions psychiatriques, Montreal.

Gey, K. F., and Pletscher, A. (1961). Influence of chlorpromazine and chlorprothixene on the cerebral metabolism of 5-hydroxytryptamine, norepenephrine and dopamine. *J. Pharmacol. Exptl. Therap.* **133**, 18–24.

Ginsberg, A., French, P., McManus, D., and Grieve, J. M. (1963). The use of tranquilliser in the transport of slaughter stock. *Vet. Record* **75** (39), 996–999.

Hafely, W., Hurlimann, A., and Thoenen, H. (1964). Apparently paradoxical modification of peripheral noradrenaline effects by several thymoleptic agents. *Helv. Physiol. Pharmacol. Acta* **22**, 15–33 (in German).

Haydu, G. G., Noreika, L., Sankar, D. E., and Sankar, D. V. S. (1963). Short-term effect of psychotropic drugs on platelets. *Arch. Gen. Psychiat.* **9** (5), 510–512.

Healey, L. A., Harrison, M., and Decker, J. L. (1964). Uricosuric effect of chlorprothixene. *Arthritis Rheumat.* **7** (6), 737 (abstr.).

Heise, G. A., and Boff, E. (1962). Continuous avoidance as a base-line for measuring behavioral effects of drugs. *Psychopharmacologia* **3** (4), 264–282 (in English); *Chem. Abstr.* **60**, 3377c.

Herr, F., Stewart, J., and Charest, M. P. (1961). Tranquilizers and antidepressants; a pharmacological comparison. *Biochim. Pharmacol.* **8** (1), 25–26 (Abstr.).

Herr, F., Stewart, J., and Charest, M. P. (1961). Tranquilizers and antidepressants, a pharmacological comparison. *Arch. Intern. Pharmacodyn.* **134**, 328–342 (in English); *Chem. Abstr.* **56**, 13498d.

Himwich, H. E., Morillo, A., and Steiner, W. G. (1962). Drugs affecting rhinencephalic structures. *J. Neuropsychiat.* **3**, Suppl. 1, S15–S26; *Psychopharmacol. Abstr.* **2** (10), 2244.

Hougs, W. (1960). Pharmacological studies on chlorprothixen. *Acta Anaesthesiol. Scand.*, Suppl. 6, 44.

Jonasson, J., Rosengren, E., and Waldeck, B. (1964). Effect of some pharmacologically active amines on the uptake of arylalkylamines by adrenal medullary granules. *Acta Physiol. Scand.* **60**, 136–140.

Kato, J., and Gozsy, B. (1961). Differential and quantitative affinity of psychoactive drugs to mucopolysaccharides. *Indian J. Med. Res.* **49**, 788–798; *Chem. Abstr.* **56**, 6613d.

Kemper, F. (1960). The effect of chlorprothixen on edema of the rat's paw. *Arzneimittel-Forsch.* **10**, 777–778 (in German).

Lachmann, J., and Bergmann, F. (1961). L'influence de quelques medicaments sur le nystagmus central et vestibulaire, ainsi que sur les troubles de l'equilibre chez le lapin. (The influence of certain drugs on central and vestibular nystagmus as well as on disorders of equilibrium in the rabbit.) *Confinia Neurol.* **21** (3), 272–281.

Lacroix, E., and Leusen, I. (1961). On the subject of some pharmacodynamic properties of a thiaxanthene derivative, α2-chloro-9-(3-dimethylaminopropylidene)-thiaxanthene (Ro4-0403). *Arch. Intern. Pharmacodyn.* **130**, 170–179 (in French).

Leau, O. (1963). Relation between blood concentration and therapeutic action. *Presse Med.* **71**, 1969–1972 (in French).

Lecoq, R., Chauchard, P., and Mazoue, H. (1964). Etude chromaximetrique experimentale de quelques agents isotropes et de leur action sur les effects nerveux de l'alcool ethylique. II. Neuroleptiques, tranquillisants et orthoneurotiques. *Therapie* **19** (4), 975–982.

Lehmann, H. E., Ban, T. A., Kato, G., et al. (1964). Potentiation of pharmacological and therapeutic action of phenothiazines by nylidrin (Arlidin). *Comprehensive Psychiat.* **5**, 36–43.

Levy, I. E. S. (1961). Quantitative variations of urinary neutral 17-ketosteroids in schizophrenics from the action of Taractan. *Rev. Fac. Farm. Bioquim.* **23** (89/90), 76–77; (1963). *Biol. Abstr.* **41** (2), 6247.

Locker, A., and Ellegast, H. (1964). Die Strahlenschutzwirkung neuer psychotroper Pharmaka. *Experientia* **20** (7), 389.

Logoluso, R., Serra, C., and Municchi, L. (1963). Influence of various monoamineoxidase (MAO) inhibitors on normal and pathological brain electrical activity. *Biochem. Pharmacol.* **12**, Suppl., 177 (Abstr. 622).

Long, R., and Lessin, A. W. (1962). Inhibition of 5-hydroxytryptamine uptake by platelets in vitro and in vivo. *Biochem. J.* **82**, 4P–5P; *Chem. Abstr.* **56**, 7942e.

Nalda Filipe, M. A. (1962). R-875 and its antidotes. Importance of the carbonic anhydrase inhibitors. *Rev. Espan. Anestesiol.* **3**, 113–135.

Nash, J. B., Emerson, G. A., Faust, J. A., and Sahyan, M. (1960). Comparative effects of thiaxanthene analogues on the conditioned response in the rat. *Federation Proc.* **19**, 24 (Abstr.).

Nieforth, K. A., and Robichaud, R. C. (1964). 2-Aminobenzenethiol derivatives as potential psychotherapeutics agents. II. *J. Pharm. Sci.* **53** (5), 529–531.

Nielsen, I. M., Hougs, W., Lassen, N., Holm, T., and Petersen, P. V. (1962). Central depressant activity of some thioxanthine derivatives. *Acta Pharmacol.* **19**, 87–100.

Optiz, K., and Loeser, A. (1962). Abolition of the hypoglycemic effect of anti-diabetic substances by neuroleptics. *Deut. Med. Wochschr.* **87**, 105–106.

Opitz, K. (1962). Metabolic effects of psychotropic substances. *Arzneimittel-Forsch.* **12**, 333–340, 525–531 and 618–626; *Chem. Abstr.* **57**, 11806c.

Opitz, K., and Loeser, A. (1962). Reduction of the hypoglycemic effect of antidiabetic substances by neuroleptic agents. *Deut. Med. Wochschr.* **87**, 105–106; *Chem. Abstr.* **56**, 10860e.

Peck, H. M., and McKinney, S. E. (1960). Hematologic alterations produced in the dog by the administration of 2-chloro-10-(3-dimethylaminopropylidene)-thiaxanthene. *Federation Proc.* **19** (1, Part I), 391 (Abstr.).

Pekkarinen, A., Tala, E., Sotaniemi, E., and Niemela, N. (1961). The neurogenic influence of dogs and cats on the corticosteroid content in rat plasma and the excretion of corticosteroids in guinea pigs' urine. The effect of psychopharmaca and anaesthetic. *Biochem. Pharmacol.* **8** (1), 129.

Pellmont, B., Steiner, F. A., Besendorf, H., Baechtold, H. P., and Laeuppi, E. (1960). Introduction to the pharmacology of Taractan, a neuroleptic with a special mechanism of action. *Schweiz. Med. Wochschr.* **90**, 598–599 (in German).

Pellmont, B., Steiner, F. A., Besendorf, H., Baechtold, H. P., and Laeuppi, E. (1960). On the pharmacology of "Taractan" a neuroleptic with special peculiarity of action. *Helv. Physiol. Pharmacol. Acta* **18**, 241–258 (in German).

Pletscher, A., and Gey, K. F. (1961). Interference with the permeation of aromatic monoamines and amino-acids in brain, a possible new type of drug action. *Biochem. Pharmacol.* **8** (1), 82 (abstr.).

Pletscher, A., Kunz, E., Staebler, H., and Gey, K. F. (1963). The uptake of tryptamine by brain *in vivo* and its alteration by drugs. *Biochem. Pharmacol.* **12**, 1065–1070.

Pletscher, A., and Gey, K. F. (1964). The effect of psychotropic drugs on the metabolism of exogenous dl-2-C_{14}-3,4-dihydroxyphenylalanine. *Med. Exptl.* **11**, 169–176; (1965).

Pujman, V. (1964). Action of chlorprothixene on L-VUFB and LA-VUFB leukemia strains. *Acta Unio Intern. Contra Cancrum* **20** (1—2), 243–244 (in English).

Pujman, V., Metysova, J., Cernochova, S., and Hampejzova, H. (1961). Effect of chlorprothixene on leukemia strains VUFB. *Naturwissenschaften* **48**, 625–626; *Chem. Abstr.* **56**, 10848c.

Pujman, V., Cernochova, S., Hampejsova, H., *et al.* (1963). The effect of chlorprothixene and 6-mercaptopurine on the LA VUFB mouse leukemia. *Neoplasma (Bratisl)* **10**, 365–370.

Quadbeck, G. (1960). Relation between effects on the blood-brain barrier and the clinical action of neuroplegic substances. *Med. Exptl.* **2**, 147–153; *Chem. Abstr.* **54**, 21461g.

Quadbeek, G. (1962). Effects of phenothiazine derivatives on blood brain barrier system. *Psychopharmacol. Serv. Center Bull.* **2**, 83–84.

Quinton, R. M. (1963). The increase in the toxicity of yohimbine induced by imipramine and other drugs in mice. *Brit. J. Pharmacol.* **21** (1), 51–66.

Sankar, D. V. S., Gold, E., Phipps, E., and Sankar, D. B. (1962). General metabolic studies on schizophrenic children. *Ann. N.Y. Acad. Sci.* **96** (Art. 1), 392–397.

Schutz, E. (1960). Action of psychotropic drugs on respiration and blood pressure of rats. *Arzneimittel-Forsch.* **10**, 958–959; *Chem. Abstr.* **55**, 8659a.

Sigg, E. B., Soffer, L., and Gyermek, L. (1963). Influence of imipramine and related psycyoactive agents on the effect of 5-hydroxytryptamine and catecholamines on the cat nictitating membrane. *J. Pharmacol. Exptl. Therap.* **142**, 13–20.

Stefko, P. L., and Zbinden, G. (1963). Effect of chlorpromazine, chlordiazepoxide, diazepam and chlorprothixene on bile flow and intrabiliary pressure in cholecystectomized dogs *Gastroenterology* **39** (4), 410–417.

Steiner, W. G., and Himwich, H. E. (1963). Effects of antidepressant drugs on limbic. structures of rabbit. *J. Nervous Mental Diseases* **137** (3), 277–284.

Studer, A. (1961). Einfluss von Pharmaka auf die Histochemie des Nebenieremarkes der Ratte. (Influence of drugs on the histochemistry of the adrenal medulla of the rat.) *Pathol. Microbiol.* **24** (2), 221–226.

Stumpf, W., Graul, E. H., and Ries, H. (1963). Die Wirking psychotroper Substanzen auf die Schilddrusenfunktion. (The effect of psychotropic substances on thyroid functions.) *Arzneimittel-Forsch.* **13** (8), 682–688.

Ulett, G. A., Heusler, A. F., Wood, V. I., and Ward, T. J. (1962). Mechanical and electronic techniques in the measurement of psychopharmacologic response. *In* "Psychosomatic Medicine. The First Hahnemann Symposium" (J. H. Nodine and J. H. Moyer, eds.), pp. 384–390. Lea & Febriger, Philadelphia, Pennsylvania. *Psychol. Abstr.* **2** (5), 801.

Usdin, E., and Usdin, V. R. (1961). Effects of psychotropic compounds on enzyme systems. II. In vitro inhibition of monoamine oxidase (MAO). *Proc. Soc. Exptl. Biol. Med.* **108**, 461–463; *Chem. Abstr.* **56**, 12233b.

Vidal Beretervide, K. (1961). Adquisiciones recientes en psicofarmacologia. [Recent progress in psychopharmacology.] *Acta Neuropsiquiat. Arg.* **7** (2), 104–105.

Zetler, G., Muller, W., and Warm, I. (1959). Jactatio capitis, a pharmacologically elicited stereotype motor reaction in the mouse. *Arch. Exptl. Pathol. Pharmakol.* **237**, 247–263; *Chem. Abstr.* **54**, 3735f.

Zetler, G., Mahler, K., and Daniel, F. (1960). Versuche zu einer pharmakologischen Differenzierung kataleptischer Wirkungen. *Arch. Exptl. Pathol.* **238** (4), 486–501.

Side Effects

Boris, A., and Stevenson, R. H. (1964). Effects of some psychotropic drugs upon urinary water output. *Proc. Soc. Exptl. Biol. Med.* **115**, 170–171.

Cares, R. M., and Buckman, C. (1963). Comparative review of the structure and side effects of newer psychotropic agents. *Diseases Nervous System* **24** (4, Sect. 2), 92–105.

Dietze, H. J. (1963). Dyskinetic syndrome associated with chlorprothixene. *Am. J. Psychiat.* **120**, 503–504.

Ditman, K. S. (1964). Inhibition of ejaculation by chlorprothixene. *Am. J. Psychiat.* **120** (10), 1004–1005.

Ehlers, H. (1963). Poisoning with psychopharmaca and barbiturate-free hypnotics. *Danish Med. Bull.* **10**, 117–121.

Fier, M., and Goldberg, M. A. (1964). Convulsive seizures in chlorprothixene overdose. *Am. J. Psychiat.* **121** (1), 76–77.

Freundt, K. J., Eberhardt, H., and Liebaldt, G. (1963). Fatal poisoning with chlorprothixene. *Deut. Z. Ges. Gerichtl. Med.* **54**, 297–303 (in German).

Grahmann, H., and Peters, V. H. (1962). Durch Psychopharmaka induzierte und provozierte Psychosen, ihre Psychopathologie und ihre therapeutische Bedeutung. (Psychoses induced and precipitated by psychopharmacological drugs, their psychopathology and therapeutic importance.) *Nervenzart* **33**, 398–430; *Psychopharmacol. Abstr.* **2** (10), 2308.

Haden, P. (1964). Gastrointestinal disturbances associated with withdrawal of ataractic drugs. *Can. Med. Assoc. J.* **91** (18), 974–975.

Hafner, H., and Kutscher, I. (1964). Complications during clinical therapy with psychopharmaea. *Aerztl. Forsch.* **18**, 18–36 (in German).

Haid, A. (1964). Case of lupus erythematosus caused by chlorprothixene (Truxal). *Ugeskrift Laeger* **126**, 1112–1114 (in Danish).

Hartviksen, K., and Steenfeldt-Foss, O. W. (1962). Polyneuritis, a new complication of chlorprothixene (Truxal) therapy. *Tidskr. Norskl. Laegeforen.* **82**, 1039–1041 (in Norwegian).

Hollister, L. E. (1961). Current concepts in therapy. Complications from psychotherapeutic drugs. II. *New Engl. J. Med.* **264** (7), 345–347.

Hollster, L. E. (1964). Complications from psychotherapeutic drugs. *Clin. Pharmacol. Therap.* **5** (3), 322–333.

Jacobsen, P. (1963). Causes of death in narcotic intoxication in recent years. *Danish Med. Bull.* **10**, 115–116.

Liebaldt, G. (1964). Suicid mit Chlorprothixen. *Arzneimittel-Forsch.* **14** (6a), 596–598.

Lund-Johansen, P. (1962). Shock after administration of phenothiazines in patients with pheochromocytoma. *Acta Med. Scand.* **172**, 525–529.

Marjerrison, G., Irvine, D., Stewart, C. N., *et al.* (1964). Withdrawal of long-term phenothiazines from chronically hospitalized psychiatric patients. *Can. Psychiat. Assoc. J.* **9**, 290–298.

Parada Bravo, F., and Maass Jensen, N. (1964). Acute poisonings by psychopharmacological agents in childhood. *Rev. Chile Pediat.* **35**, 314–323 (in Spanish).

Petersen, K. E. (1963). Poisoning with Truxal and Taractan in children. A case of sickness resembling codeine poisoning. *Ugeskrift Laeger* **125**, 1628–1629 (in Danish).

Plumb, R., and Joseph, S. (1964). Ingestion of a toxic overdose of chlorprothixene by a 3 year old. *J. Pediat.* **65** (3), 458–461.

Ravn, J. (1961). Suicide attempt with chlorprothixen (Truxal). *Nord. Med.* **65**, 507 and 509 (in Danish).

Ravn, J. (1961). Duch Psychopharmaka hervorgerufene schizophenie-anliche Zustandsbilder bei manischen Patienten. (Schizophrenia-like conditions induced by psychopharmacological agents in manic patients.) *Neuropsychopharmacology* **2**, 266–267.

Schwarz, K. (1961). Gruppenspezifische Ekzemreaktionen bei Largactil-Sensibilisierung. (Group-specific eczematous reactions in Largactil sensitization.) *Praxis (Bern)* **50**, (12) 311–314.

Sedman, G. (1963). Increased libido with chlorprothixene. *Brit. Med. J.* II (5363), 999–1000.

Simpson, G. M. (1964). Reactions following the intramuscular administration of chlorprothixene. *Am. J. Psychiat.* **120** (10), 1021–1023.

Steinicke, O., and Zachau-Christiansen, B. (1964). Phenothiazine and chlorprothixene poisoning in children. *Nord. Med.* **72**, 1027–1029 (in Danish).

Tesarova, O., *et al.* (1963). Changes in liver function during the course of chlorprothixene therapy. *Activatis Nervosa Super.* **5**, 204 (in Czech.).

Clinical Papers

Alanen, Yo. (1963). Borderline states between schizophrenia and neuroses. *Suomen Laak.* **18**, 1179–1193 (in Finnish).

Alapin, B. (1964). Treatment of depressive states with chlorprothixene. *Polski Tygod. Lekar.* **19**, 759–762 (in Polish); (1965).

Alby, J. M., and Schuller, E. (1961). Psychopharmacologie-psychosomatique. (Psychopharmacology-psychosomatism.) *Vie Med.* **42**, 125–130.

Alexander, L. (1961). Effects of psychotropic drugs on conditional response in man. *Neuropsychopharmacology* **2**, 93–123.

Alexander, L. (1961). Objective evaluation of antidepressant therapy by conditional reflex technique. *Diseases Nervous System* **22** (5), 14–23.

Alsen, M., and Frey, T. S. (1959). On the treatment of alcoholic psychosis with Truxal. *Svensko Lakartidn.* **54**, 3344–3351 (in Swedish).

Alvarez-Ude, F. (1961). Esquema de la clinica del cloroprotixeno. (Outline of the clinical use of chlorprothixene.) *Med. Farm. (Madrid)* **25**, 222–225.

Alvarez-Ude, F. (1961). Clinica del chorprotixeno. (Clinical use of chlorprothixene.) *Medicamenta* **35**, 266–274.

Anderssen, N., and Skjaeggestad, O. (1961). Truxal as a hypnotic. Research on Truxal and a placebo. *Nord. Psykiat. Tidskr.* **15**, 321–324 (in Danish).

Anjos, E. S. (1962). Chlorprothixene ambulatory psychiatry. *Hospital (Rio de Janeiro)* **62**, 739–745 (in Portuguese); *Index Med.* **4** (3), S-462.

Anton, A. (1961). Experiences with Truxal in institutional practice. *Med. Welt* **22**, 1221–1223 (in German).

Arnold, O. H. (1959). Clinical experiences with the neuroleptic Truxal. *Wien. Med. Wochschr.* **190** (46), 892–898 (in German).
Arnold, O. H., Bauer, H., and Cmyral, K. (1964). Klinische Erfahrungen mit einem neuen Diebeinzodiazinpin-Derivat als Anti-depressivum. *Arzneimittel-Forsch.* **14** (6a), 540–544.
Arnold, O. H. (1961). Fortschritte in der Behandlung der endogenenen Psychosen. (Progress in the treatment of endogenous psychoses.) *Wien. Klin. Wochschr.* **73** (29/30), 501–510.
Arnold, O. H., and Hoff, H. (1961). The role of biological treatment in comprehensive psychiatric management. *In* "Recent Advances in Biological Psychiatry" (J. Wortis, ed.), Vol. 3, pp. 12–29. Grune & Stratton, New York.
Bardoni, F. (1960). On the treatment of mental disorders with 2-chloro-9-(3'-dimethylaminopropylidene)-thioxanthene. Clinical note. *Rass. Studi Psichiat.* **49**, 608–610 (in Italian).
Barre, L., Madre-Corbery, J., and Renard, P. (1961). Cures with thioxanthene; study of its application with 44 mental patients. *Encephale* **50**, 563–577 (in French).
Barrier, G. (1961). Note on the use of Taractan in major digestive tract surgery. Apropos of 25 case reports. *Agressologie* **2**, 171–174 (in French).
Barron, A., Beckering, B., Rudy, L. H., and Smith, J. A. (1961). A "double blind" study comparing Ro4-0403, trifluoperazine and a placebo in chronically ill mental patient. *Am. J. Psychiat.* **118**, 347–348.
Barsa, J. A., and Sauners, J. C. (1964). Benzquinamide in the treatment of psychotic patients. *Diseases Nervous System* **25** (10), 620–623.
Barsa, J. M., and Saunders, J. C. (1962). Chlorprothixene in the treatment of psychotic patients. *Am. J. Psychiat.* **119**, 468–469.
Barsa, J. A., and Saunders, J. C. (1964). A double blind study of a new chlorprothixene preparation. *Am. J. Psychiat.* **121** (5), 493–494.
Bassino, P. G., Chiri, A., and Ghigo, A. (1963). Psychoplegia and anesthetic nerve blocks for surgical purposes. Experience with a recent psychoplegic drug. *Minerva Anestesiol.* **29**, 76–83 (in Italian).
Baumler, J. (1963). Psychopharmaka und deren Nachweis bei Miszbrauch. *Chimia (Aaran)* **17** (8), 257–262.
Becache, A., Broussolle, P., Lambert, P.-A., Achaintre, A., Beaujard, M., and Berthier, C. (1961). Nouvelles recherches therapeutiques en psychiatrie concernant le chlorprothixene (Ro4-0403 ou Taractan). (New therapeutic and psychiatric investigations of chlorprothixene (Ro4-0403 or Taractan).) *Ann. Med.-Psychol.* **119** (T.1) (3), 587 (abstr.).
Beck, D. (1962). Autonomic research, therapy and prognosis of exhaustion depressions. *Schweiz. Arch. Neurol. Psychiat.* **90**, 370–391 (in German); *Index Med.* **4** (3), S-462.
Bengel, T., and Uher, W. (1962). Medical alleviation of labor pains with a thioxanthene derivative. *Med. Klin. (Munich)* **57**, 62–64 (in German).
Bente, D., Englemeier, M. P., Heinrich, K., Hippius, H., and Schmitt, W. (1964). Zur Stellung eines neuartigen Dibenzodiazipen-Derivatives in der Pharmakotherapie depressiver Erkrankungen. *Arzneimittel-Forsch.* **14** (6a), 538–540.
Blumenthal, M., and Rilva, P. (1961). Experiences with Truxal in the treatment of chronic patients. *Nord. Psykiat. Tidskr.* **15**, 377–380 (in Swedish).
Boittelle, M. G., and Boittelle-Lentulo, C. (1959). A propos d'un nouveau neuroplegique, le Ro.04.403. (In connection with a new neuroplegic, Ro 04.403.) *Ann. Med. Psychol.* **117** 2, 515–518.
Boitelle, M. G., Boittelle-Lentulo, C., Horassius, M., and Peron, P. (1960). Indications therapeutiques psychiatriques du Taractan (Ro4-0403). *Ann. Med.-Psychol.* **118**, 559 (abstr.).
Brauchitsch, H. von, and Bukowczyk, A. (1962). On the problem of the use of chlorprothixen ("Taractan") in the psychiatric hospital. *Schweiz. Arch. Neurol. Pscychiat.* **90**, 104–117 (in German).

Brotto, M. (1961). Clinical evaluation of a new derivative of thioxanthene (Taractan). *Sistema Nervosa* **13**, 176–192 (in Italian).

Brzezinska, I., Laskowska, D., and Wierzbicki, T. (1964). Attempted chlorprothixene (Taraxan) therapy of amential and catatonic conditions. *Neurol. Neurochir. Psychiat. Polon.* **14**, 159–162 (in Polish).

Cahn, C. H. (1963). Effect of chlorprothixene in patients with paranoid symptoms. *Can. Med. Assoc. J.* **89**, 719–720.

Calanca, G. (1961). Tests de dessin au cours des traitements chimiotherapiques des psychoses. (Sketching tests during the course of chemotherapy of psychosis.) *Concours Med.* **83** (8), 1121.

Campanini, T., De Risio, C., and Valla, S. (1961). Therapeutic results obtained with Taractan in depression. *Riv. Sper. Freniat.* **85**, 264–268 (in Italian).

Cappelen, T., and Monrad, L. H. (1961). Clinical experiences with Truxal and Hibanil in chronic schizophrenia. A double blind experiment. *Tidsskr. Norske Laegeforen.* **81**, 486–488 and 491 (in Norwegian).

Chang, S. C. (1963). Treatment of agitated patients with chlorprothixene. *Am. J. Psychiat.* **120** (1), 71–72.

Chantraine, J., and Pairoux, R. (1960). Contribution clinique a l'etude du chlorprotixene. *Ann. Med.-Psychol.* **118** (Part 11), 513–515.

Chantrainc, J., and Pairoux, R. (1960). Clinical contribution to the study of chlorprothixene. *Acta Neurol. Belg.* **60**, 846–858 (in French).

Cheng, S. F., and Fogel, E. J. (1963). Trifluoperazine combined with amitriptyline in paranoid psychosis. *Am. J. Psychiat.* **119**, 780–781; *Psychol. Abstr.* **3** (1), 51.

Cirilli, M., Block, F., and Uhry, P. (1961). Treatment of delerium tremens by a new neuroplegic agent. *Clinique* **56**, 497 (in French).

Clerici Lorenzini, A., and Ghezzi, C. (1962). Clinical evaluation of the action of 2-chloro-9-(dimethylaminopropylidene)-thioxanthene. *Minerva Anestiol.* **28**, 439–444 (in Italian).

Cornu, F., and Hoffet, H. (1961). Clinical experience with Taractan. *Diseases Nervous System* **22**, 40–44.

Darling, H. F. (1961). Chlorprothixine (Taractan) and isocarboxazid (Marplan) in pschotic depressions. *Am. J. Psychiat.* **117**, 931–932.

Darling, H. F. (1961). Chlorprothixine (Taractan) in private practice. *Diseases Nervous System* **22**, 154–156.

Dechene, J. P., McClish, A., and Fugere, L. (1963). Study of a new neuroleptic drug in anesthesia-resuscitation. *Union Med. Canada* **92**, 432–436 (in French).

De Giacomo, V. (1963). New developments in antidepressive drug therapy. *Clin. European* **2**, 121–125 (in Italian).

Deligne, P. (1961). New neuroleptics (R-1625 or Haloperidol, MD-2028 or Halo-Anisone, Ro4-0403 or Taractan, and LG 206 or Dominal) in different types of anesthesia without narcosis or anesthesia in the waking state. Indications in neurosurgical anesthesiology. Place of analgesia in neuroleptanalgesia. *Agressologie* **2**, 363–370 (in French).

Deligne, P. (1961). Nonveaux neuroleptiques dans differents types d'anesthesie sans narcose ou d'anesthesie vigile. Place de l'analgesie dans la neuroleptanalgesie. (The new neuroleptics in different types of non-narcotizing anesthesia—i.e. in waking anesthesia. Indications in neurosurgical anesthesiology. The role of analgesia in neuroleptic analgesia.) *Presse Med.* **69** (41), 1763.

Demay-Laulan, M., Fournial, P., Demay, J., Abraham, A., Goasguen, J., Roudiere, J. J., and Schocron, G. (1960). Note concerning the use of a new neuroplegic agent, Ro4-0403, in character disorders of epileptics. *Ann. Med.-Psychol.* **118** (1), 333–336 (in French).

Demay-Laulan, M., Fornial, P., Demay, J., Abraham, A., Goasguen, J., Roudiere, J. J., and Schocron, G. (1960). Note concerning the use of a new neuroplegic drug: Ro4-0403. *J. Med. Bordeaux* **137**, 918–925 (in French).

Denber, H. C., Rajotte, P., and Ross, E. (1960). Some observations on the chemotherapy of depression: Results with "Taractan". *Comprehensive Psychiat.* **1**, 308–312.

Denys, W. J. (1963). Cyclic epilepsy. Principal factors which may explain it. Illustration by the case of a man in whom the comitiality was improved by chlorprothixene. *Acta Neurol. Psychiat. Belg.* **63**, 892–901 (in French).

De Souza Compos, J., and Pinto, O. F. (1961). Some clinical observations on derivatives of thioxanthene and of benzoquinolizine in psychiatry. *Hospital (Rio de Janeiro)* **59**, 367–374 (in Portuguese).

Doutriaux, J. (1964). Autonomic hypertonia or deficiency in psychological preparation: 2 cases. *Anesthesie Analgesie Reanimation* **21**, 493–502 (in French).

Doutriaux, J. (1962). Palfuim—Taractan combination in anesthesiology. *J. Sci. Med. Lille* **80**, 77–88 (in French).

Du Cailar, J., Attissom, Rioux, J., Herail, J., and Malaterre, J. (1960). Clinical trials in anesthesiology of a new neuroplegic derived from the thioxanthene series: Ro4-0403. *Agressologie* **3**, 255–266 (in French).

Du Cailar, J., and Malaterre, M. (1962). A new neuroplegic in anesthesiology: Ro 4-0403. *Acta Anaesthesiol. Belg.* **13** (1), 29–40 (in French); *Chem. Abstr.* **60**, 7346d.

Dundee, J. W., Love, W. J., and Moore, J. (1963). Alterations in response to somatic pain associated with anaesthesia. XV. Further studies with phenothiazine derivatives and similar drugs. *Brit. J. Anaesthesia* **35**, 597–610.

Eckman, F., and Immich, H. (1963). Neuroleptics and dyskinetic reactions. *Nervenarzt* **34**, 374–376 (in German).

Editors. (1960). Chlorprothixene ("Taractan"). Combined neuroleptic, thymoleptic and ataractic properties. *Chemotherapy Rev.* **1** (5), 160 and 174.

Editors. (1963). (Council on Drug). Evaluation of chlorprothixene (Taractan). *J. Am. Med. Assoc.* **186** (2), 144–145.

Editors. (1964). (Die Leseprobe). Chlorprothixenum (Taractan "Roche"). *Deut. Med. Wochschr.* **89** (3), XXV.

Editors. (1960). Neue Spezialitaten. *Klin. Wochschr.* **38** (7), 338.

Editor. (1961). To-day's drugs. Taractan. *Brit. Med. J.* I (5220), 203.

Editor. (1963). Today's drugs. Tranquillizers. *Brit. Med. J.* II (5350), 163–164.

Edrizzi, G. (1961). Psychotropic drugs in psychiatric therapy and results obtained with a recent psychopharmacological agent: Taractan-Ro4-0403/20. *Rass. Neuropsichiat.* **15**, 319–343 (in Italian).

Feldman, P. E. (1960). Clinical evaluation of chlorprothixene. *Am. J. Psychiat.* **116**, 929–930.

Feer, H., Fuchs, M., and Straessle, M. (1960). Clinical trials of chlorprothixene (taractan). *Schweiz. Med. Wochschr.* **90**, 600–602 (in German).

Feer, H. (1962). Schizophrenie und Blutkeislauf. (Schizophrenia and circulation.) *Psychopharmacologia* **1962** (3), 395–412; *Psychopharmacol. Abstr.* **2** (10), 2278.

Fischer, A. R. (1961). Psychopharmacology and heart therapy with special reference to Taractan. *Med. Welt* **47**, 2482–2483 (in German).

Fish, F. (1964). The influence of the tranquilizers on the Leonhard schizophrenic syndrome. *Encephale* **53**, Suppl., 245–249.

Flegel, H., Harling, H. O., and Woedl, H. (1961). Truxal in the psychiatric hospital and ambulant follow-up treatment. *Psychiat. Neurol.* **142**, 176–187 (in German).

Forcada Calvo, A. (1961). La combinacion Librium—Tarasan en el tratamiento de las depresiones. (The combination of Librium with Taractan in the treatment of depressions.) *Actas Luso-Espan. Neurol. Psyquiat. (Madrid)* **20**, Suppl., 195–196.

Fratello, U. (1963). The combination of R-875, Ro4-0403 and methyl-4-betahydroxyethylthiazole in urological surgery. *Riforma Med.* **77**, 463–465 (in Italian).

Fratello, V. (1963). The combination of R-875, Ro4-0403 and S.C.T.Z. in urological surgery. *Minerva Anestesiol.* **29**, 450–452 (in Italian).

Galeano Munoz, J., and Ramirez, F. (1961). Effectos, clinicos del Taractan. (Clinical effects of Taractan.) *Acta Neuropsiquiat. Arg.* **7** (2), 105–107.

Gallant, D. M. (1963). Clinical management of side effects and toxicity in psychopharmacologic therapy. *Bull. Tulane Univ. Med. Fac.* **22**, 179–186; *Psychol. Abstr.* **3** (1), 9.

Gayer, W. (1962). Beitrag zur Pramedikation bei Kindern. (Contribution to the premedication of children.) *Praxis (Bern)* **51**, 642–647; *Psychopharmacol. Abstr.* **2** (10), 2304.

Gayou, G. G., Brinitzer, W., Gibbon, J., and Goldschmidt, L. (1961). Clinical trial of chlorprothixene. *Am. J. Psychiat.* **118** (5), 460.

Gayus, I. K., and Blanchette, J. E. (1962). Effects of chlorprothixene in well-established schizophrenic reactions. *Am. J. Psychiat.* **119**, 180–183.

Geller, W. (1959). Klinische Erfahrungen mit N714 trans aus der Rheinischen Landesheilanstalt Bonn, Mannerabteilung. Referat eines Vortrags, gehalten anlasslich des Symposions am 20 Juni 1959 in Koln.

Geller, W. (1960). Therapeutic results with a neuroleptic Truxal. *Med. Klin. (Munich)* **55**, 554–557 (in German).

Grimmeisen, H. (1961). Experiences with neuroleptic Taractan in anesthesia and clinical practice. *Muench. Med. Wochschr.* **103**, 1923–1925 (in German).

Gross, H., and Kaltenbaeck, E. (1961). Taractan (chlorprothixene) as a neuroleptic drug in clinical psychiatry. *Diseases Nervous System* **22**, 502–507.

Gross, H., and Kaltenbaeck, E. (1961). Experiences with the thioxanthene derivative chlorprothixen (Taractan) in clinical psychiatry. *Wien. Klin. Wochschr.* **73**, 64–69 (in German).

Gnat, T., et al. (1963). Preliminary results of chlorprothixene therapy of mental patients. *Neurol. Neurochir. Psychiat. Polon.* **13**, 103–106 (in Polish).

Gomez de Uribe, F. (1961). Quimica, farmacologia y toxicologia del Truxil tioxanderivado psicoactivo. (Chemistry, pharmacology and toxicology of Truxil, a psychoactive derivative of thioxanthene.) *Medicamenta* **35**, 275–282.

Gover, D. M. (1962). Thioridazine and chlorprothixene in the management of anxiety in tuberculous patients. *Am. Rev. Respirat. Diseases* **85**, 587–590.

Gualandi, W. (1964). Neuroleptanalgesia in so-called "poor-risk" patients. *Minerva Anestesiol.* **30**, 261–267 (in Italian).

Hagopian, P. B., and Crossfield, R. M. (1963). Experiences with chlorprothixene in a state hospital. *Diseases Nervous System* **24** (6), 353–356.

Hagopian, P. B., and Crossfield, R. M. (1962). Experiences with chlorprothixene in a state hospital. *Am. J. Psychiat.* **119**, 466–468.

Halberkann, J. (1960). Die Erfahrungen mit dem neuartigen Psychopharmakon "Truxal". *Fortschr. Med.* **78**, 55–56.

Hansen, C. J. (1961). Rehabilitation problems in a psychiatric hospital. *Ugeskift Laeger* **123** (23), 796–804.

Hartung, M. L., Bente, D., and Schneewind, K. A. (1964). Vergleichende Untersuchungen uber die Wirkung antidepressiver und enuroleptischer Pharmaka auf die Konzentrationsleistung. *Arzneimittel-Forsch.* **14** (6a), 584–587.

Haydu, G. G. (1962). Schizophrenic behavior and aspects of psychopharmacology. *Ann. N.Y. Acad. Sci.* **96**, 160–169; *Chem. Abstr.* **56**, 13513b; *Psychol. Abstr.* **2** (5), 846.

Haydu, G. G., Brinitzer, W., Gibbon, J., and Goldschmidt, L. (1961). A clinical trial of chlorprothixene. *Am. J. Psychiat.* **118**, 460.

Heer, H. (1961). On the use of the psychopharmacological agent Truxal in urology. *Z. Urol.* **54**, 519–522 (in German).

Heinrich, J.-P., and Spielman, J.-P. (1961). Note sur l'utilisation en therapeutique psychiatrique d'un derive du thioxanthene, la Taractan. A propos de 97 observations. (Note on the utilization in psychiatric therapy of a derivative of thioxanthene, Taractan. Ninety-seven observations.) *Ann. Med.-Psychol.* **119** (2), 372 (abstr.).

Heinrich, K. (1961). Probleme und Ergebnisse der Therapie endogener Psychosen mit neuen psychotropen Substanzen. (Problems and results of therapy of endogenous psychoses with new psychotropic substances.) *Med. Welt* **1961** (7), 335–340.

Hoff, H., and Hofmann, G. (1963). The use of neuroleptics in psychiatric and general practice. *Wien. Med. Wochschr.* **113**, 269–275 (in German).

Hoffet, H., and Cornu, F. (1960). Clinical experience with the thioxanthene derivative Ro4-0403 (Taractan). *Schweiz. Med. Wochschr.* **90**, 602–607 (in German).

Hoffet, H. (1962). Beitrage zur Behandlung der Depressionen. Typologische Gliederung depressiver Syndrome und somatotherapeutische Indikationsstellungen. (Contribution to the treatment of depression. A classification of depressive syndromes and indications for somatic treatment.) *Bibliotheca Psychiat. Neurol.* (Fasc. 115): 1–55; *Psychol. Abstr.* **2** (4), 675.

Hohmann, G. (1963). On the technic of ataralgesia. *Anaesthesist* **12**, 26–27 (in German).

Hoshina, Y., Nozaki, H., and Tamiya, O. (1962). The clinical effect of chlorprothixene on depressive states. *Brain Nerve* **14**, 519–522 (in Japanese).

Hoyrup, E. (1960). Experiences with truxal. *Ugeskrift Laeger* **122**, 1146–1149 (in Danish).

Huerlimann, F. (1961). Postoperative pain control with "Taractan," a new thioxanthene derivative. *Praxis (Bern)* **50**, 223–225 (in German).

Hutchinson, J. T., and Smedberg, D. (1963). Treatment of depression: A comparative study of ECT and six drugs. *Brit. J. Psychiat.* **109**, 536–538; *Psychol. Abstr.* **3** (1), 37.

Jahnke, E., and Le Beau, E. (1961). Scopalamine, Zwangsjacke, oder Neuroleptika beim Delerium Tremens? (Scopolamine, straitjacket or neuroleptics in delerium tremens?) *Med. Welt* (29/30), 1525–1527.

Jensen, P. S., and Vestergard, C. (1960). Injection treatment with chlorprothixen compared with trilafon. *Ugeskrift Laeger* **122**, 1149–1150 (in Danish).

Jequier-Doge, E. (1961). Le medecin praticien et les thymoleptiques. (The medical practitioner and the thymoleptics.) *Praxis (Bern)* **50** (18), 471–475.

Jub, J. (1962). Clinical experiences with Taractan, a neuroleptic of the thioxanthine series. *Med. Welt* **34**, 1779–1781 (in German).

Kaartinen, M. (1962). Clinical experiences with chlorprothixene. *Nord. Med.* **68**, 1161–1164 (in Swedish).

Karabanow, O. (1963). Clinical experiences with chlorprothixene in psychiatric syndromes. *Appl. Therap.* **5**, 133–136.

Karn, W. N., Jr., Mead, B. T., and Fishman, J. J. (1961). Double-blind study of chlorprothixene (Taractan) a panpsychotropic agent. *J. New Drugs* **1**, 72–79.

Kaubish, V. K. (1961). Experience with Truxal in the treatment of mental patients. *Zh. Nevopatol. i Psikhiat.* **61**, 881–885 (in Russian).

Kielholz, P., Labhardt, F., Battegay, R., Rummele, W., and Feer, H. (1963). Therapie der Depressionen und der depressiven Krankheitszustande. *Deut. Med. Wochschr.* **88** (34), 1617–1624.

Kielholz, P., and Beck, D. (1962). Autonomic examinations and therapy of exhaustion depression. *Praxis (Bern)* **51**, 962–965 (in German).

Kielholz, P., and Beck, D. (1962). Diagnosis, autonomic tests, treatment and prognosis of exhaustion depressions. *Comprehensive Psychiat.* **3**, 8–14.

Kind, H., and Angst, J. (1964). Zur ambulanten und stationaren Behandlung depressiver Zustande mit einem Dibenzodiazepin-Derivat. *Arzneimittel-Forsch.* **14** (6a), 55–551.

Kohlmann, T., and Rett, A. (1964). Klinische and pharmakopsychologische Untersuchungen mit Truxal bei gehirngeschadigten Kindern. *Wien. Klin. Wochschr.* **76**, 789–794.

Korskjaer, G., Morch, R., and Sovso, H. (1961). Truxal as an adjuvant in the treatment of neurosis. *Nord. Psykiat. Tidskr.* **15**, 316–320 (in Danish).

Krakowski, A. J. (1963). Chlorprothixene in private psychiatric practice: A one-year follow-up. *J. New Drugs* **3** (2), 110–114.

Krakowski, A. J. (1962). Propiomazine for control of insomnia in nervous disorders. *Am. J. Psychiat.* **119**, 461–462; *Psychol. Abstr.* **2** (5), 852.
Krakowski, A. J. (1962). Taractan in private psychiatric practice. *Psychosomatics* **3**, 37–41.
Krueger, H. J., Schwarz, H., and Jueneman, H. J. (1964). Beitrag zur Therapie depressiver Krankheitszustuende. *Med. Klin. (Munich)* **59** (50), 1985–1987.
Kruse, W. (1960). Preliminary report on a new psychotropic compound (Ro4-0403/4). *Am. J. Psychiat.* **116**, 849–850.
Kurland, A. A., and Yazicioglu, E. (1961). Effect of chlorprothixene on schizophrenic patients. *Diseases Nervous System* **22**, 636–638.
Laane, C. L. (1961). Out-patient treatment with psychoactive drugs. *Tidskr. Norskl. Laegeforan.* **81** (15), 915–920.
Lai, G. (1963). Stimulation et sedation dans le traitement des etats depressifs. *Psychopharmacologia* **4** (3), 206–220.
Lambert, P. A. (1964). Trial systematization of neuroleptic combinations. *Encephale* **53**, Suppl., 262–275 (in French).
Lammers, H. J. (1962). Experiences with the psychopharmacological agent Truxal. *Therap. Gegenwert* **101**, 310–319 (in German).
Lasky, J. L., Klett, C. J., Caffey, E. M., Bennett, J. L., Rosenblum, M.P., and Hollister, L. E. (1962). Drug treatment of schizophrenic patients. A comparative evaluation of chlorpromazine, chlorprothixine, fluphenazine, reserpine, thioridazine and triflupromazine. *Diseases Nervous System* **23** (12), 698–706.
Lasky, J. J. (1961). Preliminary report on VA cooperative study number six: An evaluation of the effectiveness of chlorpromazine (Thorazine), chlorprothixen (Taractan), fluphenazine (Prolixin), reserpine (Serpasil), thioridazine (Mellaril) and triflupromazine (Vesprin) in treating newly admitted schizophrenic patients. *Trans. 6th Res. Conf. Coop. Chemotherapy Studies Psychiat. Broad Approaches to Mental Illness*, 1961. Dept. of Med. & Surg., Vet. Admin., pp. 27–29. Washington, D.C.
Levy, H. A., Bodi, T., Siegler, P. E., *et al.* (1963). Chlorprothixene: A new phenothiazine ataractic agent: Spectrum in the out patient therapy of psychoneurosis. *J. Neuropsychiat.* **5**, 138–142.
Lund, E. (1961). Taractan-Truxal-chlorprothixenum (INN). *Nord. Med.* **66**, 1063–1065 (in Danish).
Luria, E., and Slavich, A. (1961). Clinical trials with a derivative of the thioxanthene series (Ro4-0403). *Rass. Studi Psichiat.* **50**, 481–498 (in Italian).
Ma, J. Y., and Crandell, A. (1962). Clinical and laboratory evaluation of chlorprothixene in institutionalized patients. *J. New Drugs* **2**, 26–34.
Maculans, G. A. (1964). Comparison of diazepam, chlorprothixene and chlorpromazine in chronic schizophrenic patients. *Diseases Nervous System* **25** (3), 164–168.
McCance, I. (1964). Potentiation of hexobarbitone infused intravenously. *Arch. Intern. Pharmacodyn.* **148** (1–2), (in English); *Chem. Abstr.* **60**, 12542b.
McCray, W. E., Hawkins, W. A., Kirkpatrick, W. L., and McGovern, W. J. (1963). Long-term drug treatment of psychiatric out-patients. *Diseases Nervous System* **24** (3), 167–172.
Madalena, J. C. (1962). The use of chlorprothixen (Ro4-0403) in manic-depressive psychosis. *Hospital (Rio de Janeiro)* **61**, 381–382 (in Portuguese).
Maddox, P. F. (1963). Treatment of emotional disorders with chlorprothixene. *J. Neuropsychiat.* **5**, 92–95.
Madsen, E., and Ravn, J. (1959). Indledende forsog med behandling med et nyt pskofarmakon Truxal. *Nord. Psykiat. Tidskr.* **13**, 82–86.
Mall, G. (1959). Erfahrungen mit N714 trans an der Pfalzischen Nervenklinik Landeck. Referat eines Vortrags, gehalten anlaszlich des Symposions am 20 Juni 1959 in Koln.
Mallmann-Muhlberger, E. (1963). Report on experiences with Truxal therapy in 65 children. *Med. Welt* **28**, 1455–1458 (in German).

Aquado Matorras, A., Naida Felipe, M. A., Peraita Peraita, P., et al. (1964). Neuroleptoanalgesia associated with hyperventilation or with urea. Comparative study of some constants in neurosurgical patients. Rev. Espan. Oto Neuro Oftal. 23, 155–165 (in Spanish).
Matsunaga, F., et al. (1963). Tranquilizing agents in the therapy of gastrointestinal diseases. J. Therap. (Tokyo) 45, 1614–1622 (in Japanese).
Matthews, V., Lehmann, H. E., and Ban, T. A. (1964). A comparative study of thirteen hypnotic drugs. Appl. Therap. 6 (10), 806–809.
Masciocchi, A. (1960). Resultats therapeutiques avec Ro4-0403 (Taractan) dans un groupe de malades mentaux. Ann. Med.-Psychol. 118, 567.
Masciocchi, A. (1960). A new derivative of the thioxanthine series (Taractan) in psychiatric therapy. Rass. Studi Psichiat. 49, 1057–1084 (in Italian).
Masciocchi, A., and Marino, A. (1962). Taractan in the treatment of delirium tremens. Riv. Sper. Freniat. 86, 993–1016 (in Italian).
Mentzos, S. (1961). Clinical experiences with a new psychosedative of the thioxanthene series. Med. Welt 20, 1104–1106 (in German).
Metysova, J., Metys, J., and Votava, Z. (1963). Pharmakologische Eigenschaften einiger neuen Tranquilizers und antidepressiven Substanzen. Arch. Intern. Pharmacodyn. 144 (3–4), 481–513.
Molcan, J., Tesarova, O., Schmidt, P., Polak, L., and Payerova, J. (1962). (The problem of chlorprothixene therapy of mental disorders.) Bratislav. Lekarske Listy 42, 283–288 (in Czech.); (1963). Index Med. 4 (3), S-462.
Molcan, J., Tesarova, O., Schmidt, P., Polak, L., and Payerova, J. (1962). Our experience with chlorprothixene and changes of some biological indices during the course of therapy. Activatis Nervosa Super. 4, 224–225 (in Czech.).
Morsier, C. D, and Roth, G. (1961). First therapeutic results with a new tranquilizing agent, Ro4-0403. Schweiz. Arch. Neurol. Psychiat. 88, 113–116 (in French).
Mueller, D. (1961). On a new psychopharmacon (chlorprothixen) in the treatment of endogenous psychoses. Psychiat. Neurol. Med. Psychol. (Lpz.) 13, 184–193 (in German).
Munarini, D., and Bertolotti, P. (1960). Preliminary research in psychiatry with a derivative of the thioxanthene series (Taractan). Riv. Sper. Freniat. 84, 1072–1083 (in Italian).
Naerra, N., Petersen, C., and Staffeldt, I. (1960). Chlorprothixen for premedication. Acta Anaesthesiol. Scand. Suppl. 6, 51–53.
Narros Martin, G., and Carranza Sanchez, L. J. (1962). Taractan in some psychiatric entities. Rev. Clin. Espan. 85, 261–270 (in Spanish).
Neumann, H., and Peters, U. H. (1961). Neurere Gesichtspunkte bei der Behandlung des Delerium Tremens. (New points of view in the treatment of delirium tremens). Med. Welt 31, 1559–1563.
Neyen, H. (1963). Chlorprothixene, as an antipruritic agent in dermatology. Med Welt 19, 1882–1884 (in German).
Nielsen, I. M., Petersen, P. V., and Ravn, J. (1959). Truxal, a new Danish psychopharmacon. Ugeskrift Laeger 121, 1433–1440 (in Danish).
Nielsen, I. M., and Neuhold, K. (1959). The comparative pharmacology and toxicology of the trans isomer of 2-chloro-9-(3′-dimethylaminopropylidene)-thiaxanthene HCl (Chlorprothixene, N714 trans) and chlorpromazine. Acta Pharmacol. Toxicol. 15, 335–355.
Nieto, D., Palavicini, F. F., and Castellanos, G. (1959). Experiencias clinicas preliminares sobre el efecto ataraxico del producto 2-chloro-9-(dimetilaminopropiliden) tioxanteno. Neurol. Neurocir. Psquiat. 1, 30–31.
Oettinger, L. (1962). Chlorprothixene in the management of problem children. Diseases Nervous System 23 (10), 568–571.
Oltman, J. E., and Friedman, S. (1961). Preliminary report on Taractan. Am. J. Psychiat. 117, 1120–1121.

Panaijotopoulos, D., and Abraham, G. (1961). De l'emploi du chlorprothixene (Taractan) en clinique psychiatrique. (The use of chlorprothixene (Taractan) in clinical psychiatry.) *Med. Hyg. (Geneve)* **19**, 416–418.

Pilkington, T. L. (1961). The effects of Librium and Taractan on the behaviour of psychotically disturbed mentally retarded children. Second International Congress in Mental Retardation, Vienna, 1961.

Pilkington, T. L. (1961). Comparative effects of Librium and Taractan on behavior disorders of mentally retarded children. *Diseases Nervous System* **22**, 573–575.

Plas, R., and Naquet, R. (1959). Neurophysiological study of the psychosedative Ro4-0403. *Compt. Rend. Soc. Biol.* **153**, 1411–1415 (in French).

Poeldinger, W. (1960). A neuroleptic with antidepressive effect, "Taractan" (Ro4-0403). *Praxis (Bern)* **49**, 468–472 (in German).

Pomme, B., and Girard, J. (1960). Early clinical results of a new neuroleptic Ro4-0403. *Semaine Hop. Paris* **36**, 2390–2391 (in French).

Ravin, J. (1961). Chlorprothixene: A new psychotropic entity. *Am. J. Psychiat.* **118**, 227–231.

Ravn, J., and Kragh, E. R. (1963). Treatment of manic patients with chlorprothixene (Truxal) in comparisons with other treatment methods, with special reference to the duration of stabilization. *Acta Psychiat. Scand.* **39**, Suppl. 169, 139 (in German).

Ravn, J. (1963). Chlorprothixene (Truxal and Taractan). *Nord. Psykiat. Tidscrift.* **27**, 69–82 (in Danish).

Ravn, J. (1961). The combined treatment of endogenous depression with imipramine (Trofanil) and chlorprothixene (Truxal) with special reference to ambulant therapy. *Acta Psychiat. Scand.* **37**, Suppl. 162, 168–178.

Ravn, J. (1960). Treatment with a new psychopharmacon, Truxal. *Svenska Lakartidn.* **57**, 2760–2774 (in Swedish).

Ravn, J. (1959). Truxal, ein neuartiges Psychopharmakon. Referat eines Vortrags in der Psychiatr und Nervenklinik der Universitat Wien am 25.9.1959.

Ravn, J. (1960). Truxal, a new type of psychopharmacological agent. *Wien. Klin. Wochschr.* **72**, 192–196 (in German).

Regent, M., and Revil, M. (1960). Anesthesic generale sans narcotique. Experimentation clinique d'un "neuroplegique," le Ro4-0403. *Agressologie* **3**, 267–274.

Remvig, J., and Sonne, L. M. (1961). Chlorprothixene ("Truxal") compared to chlorpromazine. *Psychopharmacologia* **2**, 203–208.

Remvig, J. (1960). Sedation of convulsive attacks with high doses of chlorprothixen (Truxal). *Ugeskrift Laeger* **122**, 1152 (in Danish).

Reznikoff, L. (1961). Clinical observations of therapeutic effect of chlorprothixene (Taractan) in psychoses. *Am. J. Psychiat.* **118**, 348–350.

Romaszewska, K. (1962). Past results of Taractan therapy in psychiatry. *Neurol. Neurochir. Psychiat. Polon.* **12**, 415–420 (in Polish).

Rubinietz, H. (1962). Clinical experiences with Truxan in post-operative therapy. *Deut. Med. J.* **13**, 756–757; (1963). *Index Med.* **4** (5), S-1141.

Sanchez-Hernandez, J. A. (1962). Neurolepanalgesia. *Gac. Med. Mex.* **92**, 944–949 (in Spanish); (1963). *Index Med.* **4** (5), S-1141.

Sarno, A. (1964). On the treatment of bronchospastic states with a new preparation with "anti-amine" action. *Gazz. Intern. Med. Chir.* **69**, 1167–1172 (in Italian).

Scanlon, E. P., and May, A. E. (1963). A controlled trial of Taractan in chronic schizophrenia. *Brit. J. Psychiat.* **109** (460), 418–421.

Schmalzl, N. (1962). Experiences with Truxal in internal clinical medicine. *Muench. Med. Wochschr.* **104**, 2182–2184.

Schmied, J. (1960). Use of a new psychosedative "Taractan" in geriatrics. A therapeutic note. *Therap. Umschau* **17**, 263–264 (in German).

Schmittkamp, H. J. (1962). On the effect of thioxanthene derivative ("Taractan") in brain injuries. *Therap. Umschau* **19**, 1959–1961 (in German).

Schou, M. (1963). Normothymotics, "mood-normalizers": Are lithium and the imipramine drugs specific for affective disorders? *Brit. J. Psychiat.* **109** (463), 803–808.
Sedivec, V., et al. (1963). EEG findings during the course of therapy with several new psychopharmacological agents. *Activalis Nervosa Super.* **5**, 205 (in Czech.).
Sirnes, T. B. (1964). The most important psychopharmaca in general practice. *Tidsskr. Norskl Laegeforen.* **84**, 281–283.
Skajaa, T., and Koisselgaard, N. (1960). Effect of chlorpromazine and chlorprothixen on the external pancreatic secretion. *Acta Anaesthesiol. Scandinav.* Suppl. 6, 45–50.
Sladki, E., and Prusinski, A. (1961). Taractan in the treatment of neuroses. *Therap. Umschau* **18**, 462–467 (in German).
Soulairac, A., Halpern, B., Geier, S., Bruhnes, M., Frelot, C., Grisoni, F., and Ochonisky, J. (1961). Apropos of EEG control during experimentation with a new neuroplegic agent, Ro4-0403, in psychiatric practice. *Rev. Neurol.* **105**, 241–244 (in French).
Soulairac, A., Halpern, B., Ochonisky, J., Geier, S., Grisoni, F., Bruhnes, M., and Frelot, C. (1961). A sedative and anxiolytic neuroplegic agent, 2-chloro-9(α-dimethylamino-propylidene)-thioxanthene or Ro4-0403. *Ann. Med.-Psychol.* **119** (2), 73–98 (in French).
Stelter, E. (1962). On the effect of Taractan in predominantly chronic institutionalized patients. *Therap. Umschau* **19**, 249–252 (in German).
Stille, G. (1964). Zur pharmakologischen Prufung von Antidepressiva Am Beispiel eines Dibenzodiazepins. *Arzneimittel-Forsch.* **14** (6a), 534–537.
Stoewsand, D. (1961). Experiences with a thioxanthene preparation (Taractan) in psychiatry. *Med. Welt* **4**, 197–199 (in German).
Straand, A. (1960). Preliminary report on Truxal, a new psychopharmacon. *Tidskr. Norske Laegforen.* **80**, 918–921 (in Norwegian).
Sylvest, B. (1960). Truxal as an antihydrotic agent. *Ugeskrift Laeger* **122**, 1786–1788 (in Danish).
Svendsen, B. B., and Willadsen, J. (1963). The use of haloperidol (serenase (R)) in chlorprothixen resistant patients. *Acta Psychiat. Scand.* **39**, Suppl. 169, 351–355.
Tschudin, A. (1960). Experiences with a new psychopharmacological agent Truxal. *Praxis (Bern)* **49**, 840–846 (in German).
Tubaro, E. (1963). Drugs on display. *Boll. Chimicofarm.* **102**, 740–744 (in Italian).
Tusques, J., and Corman, M. (1960) Contribution to the study of the therapeutic effects 2-chloro-9-(α-dimethylaminopropylidine)-thioxanthene (Ro4-0403). *Ann. Med.-Psychol.* **118** (2), 733–744 (in French).
Ucko, F. A. (1962). Clinical experience with chlorprothixene, a new psychotherapeutic agent. *Diseases Nervous System* **23**, 453–455.
Uhde, C. (1961). Erfahrungen mit einen neuen Neuroleptikum. (Experiences with new neuroleptic.) *Therap. Gegenwart* **100** (5), 263–265.
Vallejo-Nagera, J. A., and Calvo, A. F. (1960). Influence sur la pschomotricite d'un nouveau derive tioxantene R4-0403. *Ann. Med. Psychol.* **118**, 559.
Van Herck, J. (1961). Clinical study of Ro4-0403 in neuroses and psychoses. *Acta Neurol. Psychiat. Belg.* **61**, 631–651 (in French).
Vencovsky, E., Sedivec, V., Peterova, E., and Baudis, P. (1961). Preliminary clinical trials with chlorprothixene. *Cesk. Psychiat.* **57**, 406–407 (in Czech.).
Vencovsky, E., Sedivec, V., Peterova, E., et al. (1964). Chlorprothixene in psychiatric work. *Cesk. Psychiat.* **60**, 240–245; (1965).
Vinar, O. (1963). New experiences in the use of psychotropic drugs. *Activitas Nervosa Super.* **5** (1), 93–105; *Biol. Abstr.* **43** (6, Pt. 1), 23655.
Votava, Z. (1961). Third statewide psychopharmacological seminar in Jesenik. *Casopis Lekaru Ceskych.* **100** (27–28), 888–890 (in Czech.).
Votava, Z., Metysova, J., and Souskova, M. (1961). Influence of a new group of tranquilizers, derivatives of dibenzosuberene, on the central nervous system. *Biochem. Pharmacol.* **8** (1), 16 (abstr.).

Wasik, A., and Kotschy, A. (1962). Taractan—a new neuroleptic drug in the treatment of mental and neurological diseases. *Neurol. Neurochir. Psychiat. Polon.* **12**, 603–607 (in Polish).

Welsh, A. L. (1964). The newer tranquilizing drugs. *Med. C. N. Am.* **48** (2), 459–481.

Werenberg, H. (1959). Truxal. *Ugeskrift Laeger* **121**, 1736–1737 (in Danish).

Wickstrom, L. (1961). Report on a half year's treatment of chronically ill psychiatric patients with MAO inhibitors. *Svenka Lakartidn.* **58** (10), 664–668.

Wortis, J. (1963). Psychopharmacology and physiological treatment. *Am. J. Psychiat.* **119** (7), 621–626.

Zuercher, H., and Guertler, J. (1962). Experiences in the use of "Taractan" in general practice. *Praxis (Bern)* **51**, 110–113 (in German).

~ C.2 ~
Clinical Applications of the Monoamine Oxidase Inhibitors (Hydrazines): Addendum

JOHN H. BIEL

Aldrich Chemical Company, Inc., Milwaukee, Wisconsin

I. Mental Depression	. . . .	519
II. Angina Pectoris	. . . .	519
III. Hypertension	. . . .	520
IV. Epilepsy	. . . .	520
V. Diabetes	. . . .	521
VI. Side Effects and Toxicity	. . . .	521
References	. . . .	521

I. MENTAL DEPRESSION

Additional clinical papers on the use of the "ether" analog of pheniprazine (Catron®; JB-516), α-methyl-β-phenoxyethylhydrazine (phenoxypropazine; Drazine®) indicate that 10 mg. (b.i.d.) of this drug brought about substantial improvement in both endogenous and reactive depressions with only minimal side effects after 3–4 weeks of continuous medication (Imlah, 1963; Leahy *et al.*, 1963).

II. ANGINA PECTORIS

Horwitz and Sjoerdsma (1963) found that both pargyline (Eutonyl®) and isocarboxazid (Marplan®) produced a significant increase in exercise tolerance and a decrease in blood pressure, heart rate and cardiac output in anginal patients subjected to standard treadmill exercise. The degree of improvement in angina correlated with the above parameters and led the authors to conclude that decreased cardiac work may account for the favorable effects of the monoamine oxidase inhibitors in some patients with angina pectoris.

III. Hypertension

Hemodynamic studies carried out in a series of essential and renal hypertensive patients with a clinically effective antihypertensive agent, 1-D,L-seryl-2-isopropylhydrazine (Ro 4–1038), led Maxwell et al. (1962) and Maxwell (1963) to the conclusion that the hypotensive effect of this agent was "attributable almost solely to a decreased peripheral resistance." Although postural hypotension was marked, there was nevertheless a significant decrease of the blood pressure in the supine position.

In forty-four patients who received an average daily dose of 13.7 mg for 6 weeks, the mean arterial pressure decreased from 143 to 127 mm Hg (-11.2%) in the supine position and from 143 to 114 mm Hg (-20%) in the standing position. The onset in blood pressure drop varied from 3 to 15 days; a maximum decrease was achieved after 4 to 22 days. Following discontinuance of therapy, the blood pressure returned to pre-drug levels within an average of 8 days.

After 4 to 6 weeks of therapy with Ro 4–1038 urinary tryptamine levels had risen from 1- to 10-fold. However, this increase did not correlate well with the decrease in the blood pressure of individual patients.

On a milligram basis, Ro 4–1038 was more potent than either iproniazid or pheniprazine. The drug appeared to be superior to reserpine and chlorthiazide as a blood pressure lowering agent in moderate to severe hypertension, but was less active than the ganglionic blocking drugs.

Side effects included mood elevation (62%), parasympatholytic action (45%), interference with sexual potency and ejaculation (26%), sweating (16%), mydriasis (11%), and decreased anginal pain (6%). There was no loss of red-green color vision.

On the basis of this study, the authors conclude that Ro 4–1038 is a "valuable adjunct in the treatment of hypertension" (Maxwell et al., 1962).

$$HOCH_2CH(NH_2)CONH-NHCH(CH_3)_2$$
Ro 4–1038

IV. Epilepsy

Nialamide appears to be a useful adjunct to other anticonvulsant drugs in the control of *major* motor seizures in severely epileptic patients. In *milder* cases (less than two convulsions per month), the drug often produced an *increased* seizure incidence. The authors suggest "that a positive correlation may exist between nialamide's efficacy in decreasing seizure incidence and the severity of the seizure disorder, or perhaps with the degree of brain damage or the amount of cortical damage relative to subcortical involvement" (Maire and LaVeck, 1963).

Seizures resulting from nialamide administration have also been reported by Cares and Buckman (1961) in a review on side effects and toxicity of the newer psychopharmacological agents.

V. Diabetes

In a preliminary study of thirty-five depressed diabetic patients Wickstrom and Petterson (1964) report a significant hypoglycemic action with pheniprazine and mebanazine (Actomol®: α- methylbenzylhydrazine).

Van Praag and Leijnse (1964) found that in depressed patients who improved on MAO inhibitors therapy (iproniazid, isocarboxazid, or phenelzine) clinical recovery was associated with a concomitant and statistically significant increase in glucose tolerance.

Cooper and Keddie (1964) described a diabetic patient who, while stabilized on insulin therapy, developed a severe hypoglycemia during treatment with mebanazine.

As a possible mode of action, it has been suggested (Barrett, 1965) that MAO inhibitors may interfere with a compensatory hyperglycemic adrenergic response to a fall in blood sugar.

Further work will be required to establish whether the hydrazine MAO inhibitors exert a true antidiabetogenic effect, and, if so, whether this is a function of the hydrazine structure or their potent MAO inhibitory properties or both.

VI. Side Effects and Toxicity

Griffith and Oblath (1962) carefully reviewed the reported incidence of hepatitis and jaundice in some 102 of 500,000 patients that had received iproniazid.

The authors conclude that because of (1) duplication in the reporting of many hepatitis cases, (2) misdiagnosis of a true viral hepatitis, and (3) the use of other concomitant or previous drug therapy, the incidence of iproniazid-induced hepatitis is probably much less than believed heretofore. They encourage the continued use ("with routine precaution") of this "exceptionally valuable class of drugs."

Hanson et al. (1964) review the subject of red-green color discrimination following prolonged therapy with pheniprazine (Catron; JB-516). These authors also describe a test in pigeons which may be used to uncover interference of a new drug with wavelength discrimination. Following the chronic administration of pheniprazine, four out of six pigeons tested developed a disruption in wavelength discrimination. Upon withdrawal of the drug, all four animals recovered their normal discrimination.

References

Barrett, A. M. (1965). In press.
Cares, R. M., and Buckman, C. (1961). *Diseases Nervous System* **22**, Suppl., 97.
Cooper, A. J., and Keddie, K. M. G. (1964). *Lancet* **I**, 1133.

Griffith, G. C., and Oblath, R. W. (1962). *Am. J. Med. Sci.* **244**, 593.
Hanson, H. M., Witoslawski, J. J., and Campbell, E. H. (1964). *Toxicol. Appl. Pharmacol.* **6**, 690–695.
Horwitz, D., and Sjoerdsma, A. (1963). *Ann. N. Y. Acad. Sci.* **107**, 1033.
Imlah, N. W. (1963). *Am. J. Psychol.* **119**, 1091.
Leahy, M. R., Rose, J. T., and Plowman, R. (1963). *Am. J. Psychol.* **119**, 986.
Maire, F. W., and LaVeck, G. D. (1963). *Diseases Nervous System* **24**, 1.
Maxwell, M. H. (1963). *Ann. N. Y. Acad. Sci.* **107**, 993.
Maxwell, M. H., Gonick, H. C., Scaduto, L., Pearce, M. L., and Kleeman, C. R. (1962). *Circulation* **26**, 1279.
Van Praag, H. M., and Leijnse, B. (1964). *Lancet* **II**, 103.
Wickstrom, L., and Petterson, K. (1964). *Lancet* **II**, 995.

∽ C.3 ∽
Biochemistry and Pharmacology of the Monoamine Oxidase Inhibitors (Hydrazines): Addendum

A. Horita

Department of Pharmacology, University of Washington School of Medicine, Seattle, Washington

I. Biochemical Properties of MAO and MAO Inhibitors	523
II. Factors Influencing MAO Inhibitors	525
III. MAO Inhibitors and Tissue Amines	526
IV. Other Biochemical Actions of the Hydrazine Inhibitors	526
V. Pharmacological Properties of MAO Inhibitors	527
VI. Interaction of MAO Inhibitors with Other Substances	528
VII. Miscellaneous Actions.	530
References	530

During the period between late 1962 and the present, interest in the hydrazine-type inhibitors of monoamine oxidase (MAO) as pharmacological agents and as tools in biochemistry and pharmacology has continued, as is evident from the numerous recent scientific articles and reviews (Blaschko, 1963; Zeller, 1963a; Zeller and Fouts, 1963; Sourkes and D'Iorio, 1963; Kopin, 1964). The second New York Academy of Sciences Conference (Conference on MAO inhibitors, 1963) probably was the highlight of this period. This Conference reflected the change in direction of emphasis in research and clinical applications of these agents. Not only were the changes evident in concepts of the possible role of MAO in biochemical and physiological functions, but also the number of types of inhibitors had increased significantly. More emphasis was now being placed on the nonhydrazine inhibitors, such as pargyline, tranylcypromine, and 2-methyl-3-piperidinopyrazine (W3207A).

I. Biochemical Properties of MAO and MAO Inhibitors

The number of investigations on the mechanism of MAO as well as of its inhibitors appears to be increasing. The exact nature of MAO itself is still unknown, but the purification and crystallization of plasma amine oxidase

(Yamada and Yasunobu, 1962) represents a beginning toward the understanding of the mechanism of action of the enzyme. The authors (1963) have also demonstrated that cupric copper and pyridoxal phosphate are prosthetic groups for this enzyme. Plasma amine oxidase, however, displays considerably different properties from MAO of other tissues. Sakamoto et al. (1963) compared purified beef liver mitochondrial MAO and plasma MAO and found considerable differences, such as the pH optima and inhibitor activities. Others have also purified liver MAO (Ganrot and Rosengren, 1962; Barbato and Abood, 1963). The latter authors demonstrated that the enzyme was metal-dependent, and from studies of its biochemical properties, suggested the presence of two MAO's in beef liver. Comparative studies of MAO in various tissues also suggest that each tissue contains a single distinctive major MAO (Oswald and Strittmatter, 1963). Other studies based on differential substrate and inhibitor activities point to the possibility of several deaminating enzymes in mitochondria (Chodera et al., 1964). The question as to whether MAO is a flavoenzyme is still unanswered. Direct evidence for the participation of a flavin is lacking, but studies with riboflavin-deficient rats indicate that after inhibition by iproniazid recovery of MAO activity proceeds at a slower rate than in control animals (Wiseman-Distler and Sourkes, 1963). It has also been found that these deficient rats are more susceptible to inhibitors of the enzyme. The finding of Gorkin et al. (1964) that proflavin was also an effective inhibitor of MAO in vitro suggests the possibility of a role of a flavin in MAO; however, the authors point out that other enzymes which do not appear to contain flavin are also inhibited by proflavin and related compounds.

The mechanism of the interaction between substrates or inhibitors with the active sites of MAO has been the basis of several important investigations. On the basis of substrate reactivity, Zeller (1963b) postulated two types of interactions between MAO and substrates: eutopic complexes which lead to degradation of the substrate, and dystopic complexes which do not. This concept was extended to the inhibitors of MAO as well, and the suggestion was made that inhibitors may be bound to the active site in an analagous manner as a substrate in forming the eutopic or dystopic complexes. Belleau and Moran (1963) observed the deterium isotope effect of α-d_2-tyramine and d_2-kynuramine on MAO and found the deuterated substrates to be deaminated at a slower rate than tyramine, which establishes the fact that α-hydrogen abstraction constitutes the rate limiting step in MAO activity. Their kinetic data also permitted them to postulate on the mechanism of the deaminating action of MAO as well as on the physical-chemical properties of enzyme inhibition by various agents. Also at the physical-chemical level, Bloom (1963) discussed the structure-activity relationships of the substrates and inhibitors of MAO. This article was especially pertinent in correlating structure and activity of arylalkylhydrazines on MAO, dopamine β-hydroxylase, and the adrenergic receptors. Smith et al. (1962) found N,N-dimethyltryptamine and N,N-dimethyltryptamine-N-oxide to be metabolized by a solubilized MAO preparation. Observing that the N-oxide was metabolized under anaerobic conditions, they investigated the possibility of the formation of such an intermediate in the MAO reaction. The results indicated that although the N-oxide was a unique substrate, it was not involved in the deamination of N,N-dimethyltryptamine. Continuing their work on MAO, these authors investigated the mechanism of anti-MAO action of iproniazid (Smith et al., 1963). They found that iproniazid was cleaved nonenzymatically to yield a potent volatile inhibitor. The cleavage occurred only in the presence of oxygen and was catalyzed by cyanide and by boiled tissue extracts. The authors suggested that the active product was either isopropylhydrazine or an oxidation product of isopropylhydrazine, and they considered the possibility of such a step in the mechanism of the irreversible inhibition of MAO by iproniazid and related hydrazine inhibitors. Similar results were obtained by Kory and Mingioli (1964) who discovered (independently of Smith et al.) the volatile inhibitor phenomenon. Their results on experiments with different hydrazine inhibitors, semicarbazide, agents that trap or inhibit the formation of the product, and inspection of the absorption spectra of the volatile substance led them to conclude that it was not a hydrazine derivative.

The concept of a transformation of iproniazid or other hydrazine inhibitors to active intermediates is not new, as has been discussed in the earlier reviews. Further support of this concept is seen in the work of M. Schwartz (1962) and of Koechlin et al. (1962). Seiden and Westley (1963) also indicated such a mechanism in the inhibition of brain MAO by iproniazid, but they postulated that MAO is involved in the conversion of iproniazid to isopropylhydrazine. Nair et al. (1962) demonstrated the rapid appearance of C^{14}-iproniazid in the brain of rats after its intravenous administration. The rate of iproniazid appearance did not coincide with the well-known delayed onset of brain MAO inhibition. The authors explain that although iproniazid reaches the brain cells rapidly, MAO inhibition requires the enzymatic cleavage of iproniazid to isopropylhydrazine. In his studies on inhibitory mechanisms, Green (1964) compared the similarities between cupric ion-catalyzed decomposition of hydrazine derivatives and the inhibition of MAO by these compounds. From these observations, he suggests the possibility that MAO may be a copper enzyme which reacts with the hydrazines in a similar manner as do free cupric ions.

II. Factors Influencing MAO Inhibitors

The apparent anti-MAO activity of the hydrazine compounds appears to depend upon several factors besides the intrinsic reactivity of the inhibitor with the enzyme (Green, 1962). The extent of inhibition depends upon the time of contact prior to substrate addition while the rate of inhibition decreases with increasing duration of contact. This fall in rate was attributed to the disappearance of free inhibitor from the incubation mixture. Horita (1963) also observed the rapid disappearance of anti-MAO activity in the supernatant fraction of homogenates after exposure to pheniprazine (β-phenylisopropylhydrazine) but not to iproniazid. Similar results were observed in the livers and brains of intact animals after administration of the drugs. Whereas anti-MAO activity of pheniprazine disappeared from the supernatant fraction within 1 hour of administration, that of iproniazid persisted for many hours. These results indicated that the rapid peak of anti-MAO activity of pheniprazine and the slow peak of iproniazid depended upon the rate of removal or inactivation of free inhibitor from the incubation mixture or the intact animal tissues. The interaction of the hydrazine inhibitors with tissue components led to an examination of various other hydrazine derivatives. Of these compounds, phenelzine exhibited an unusual property in that it was not only an irreversible inhibitor of MAO, but it also acted as a substrate of the enzyme prior to its exerting its inhibitory activity (Horita, 1965a).

Other substances which were found to influence the activity of the hydrazine-type MAO inhibitors included carbonyl containing compounds (Horita and Matsumoto, 1962), the red blood cell and its constituents (Horita, 1965b), and the interaction of the hydrazines with 1,2-naphthoquinone-4-sulfonate (M. Schwartz, 1962).

III. MAO Inhibitors and Tissue Amines

The relationship between MAO inhibition, tissue amine levels, and amine metabolism has been discussed in the original review. Further substantiation of the role of MAO in controlling levels of serotonin and catecholamines has been presented (Spector, 1963; McNeill and Reidel, 1964; Green *et al.*, 1962). However, the inability of MAO inhibitors to potentiate the pressor response of normetanephrine in the rat has raised the question of the role of MAO in the metabolism of this intermediate (Vanov, 1963). Several studies on the effect of MAO inhibitors on amine metabolism in man have also been reported. Ganrot *et al.* (1962, 1963) observed that iproniazid in ordinary therapeutic doses inhibited human brain and liver MAO and increased the concentration of monoamines. Rosen and Goodall (1962) infused DL-norepinephrine-2-C^{14} in adult males and observed that after treatment with iproniazid, there resulted an alteration in the metabolism of norepinephrine as a consequence of MAO inhibition.

IV. Other Biochemical Actions of the Hydrazine Inhibitors

Because of the high reactivity of hydrazine compounds, the possibility of their biological activity being related to some other action besides MAO inhibition needs to be considered. In addition to their anti-MAO property, many of these compounds possess inhibitory activity against diamineoxidase (Burkard *et al.*, 1962; Kobayashi and Okuyama, 1962). A number of hydrazine derivatives, including some known MAO inhibitors, were compared for their ability to inhibit aromatic amino-acid decarboxylase *in vivo*. Some of the benzylhydrazine and benzyloxyamine derivatives were highly effective inhibitors, but pheniprazine and iproniazid were active only in extremely high doses (Hansson *et al.*, 1964). Other actions of hydrazines which appeared to involve neither MAO nor monoamine synthesizing enzymes included the following: decreased liver aspartate transaminases and an increase in alanine transaminase in chick embryo (Koivusulo *et al.*, 1963), an increased susceptibility to breakdown of ribosomal particles of goat brain cortex slices (Datta and Ghosh, 1963), and alterations of the metabolic pattern of perfused brain *in vivo* in the presence of several MAO inhibitors in pharmacologically active doses (Geiger *et al.*, 1962).

V. Pharmacological Properties of MAO Inhibitors

The original interest in MAO inhibitors was in their ability to affect behavior and brain function, and most early investigations were concerned with the mechanisms of their actions on the central nervous system. In the past several years, the emphasis has shifted to their cardiovascular and autonomic actions although work in the central nervous system area still continues (Furgiuele *et al.*, 1962; Manchanda *et al.*, 1963).

The influence of MAO inhibitors on the cardiovascular or autonomic actions of biogenic amines has been studied, and, in general, the effects of amines that are substrates of MAO are potentiated (Johnson and Sellers, 1962; Mantegazza and Riva, 1963; Frey, 1963). Most of the MAO inhibitors also exert a hypotensive action in man, and attempts are currently being made to explain the mechanism of this effect. Most of the explanations are based on some non-MAO inhibitory action of these agents, such as the proposal that nialamide diminishes the availability of the adrenergic transmitter that would lead to a decrease in sympathetic nerve activity (Davey *et al.*, 1963). Gessa *et al.* (1963) have also attributed the hypotensive action of the MAO inhibitors to a bretylium-like action in that they were able to counteract the decline in heart norepinephrine produced by guanethidine and also prevented nerve impulses from releasing norepinephrine at sympathetic nerve endings. Similar conclusions have been formed by Gatgounis and Aycock (1963), who found that adrenomedullary responsiveness to nicotine and tetramethylammonium was significantly blocked by certain MAO inhibitors in dogs.

The possibility of MAO inhibitors exerting effects on binding and release of catecholamines that are unrelated to MAO inhibition has been raised by Kopin and Axelrod (1963). However, Kopin *et al.* (1964) recently proposed a new hypothesis based on MAO inhibition to explain the hypotensive action.

They found that upon administration of a MAO inhibitor to cats the superior cervical nerve and other sympathetically innervated structures increased in levels of octopamine (β-hydroxytyramine). On stimulation of these nerves, the octopamine was released with the natural transmitter. This release of octopamine would represent the liberation of a "false transmitter" and replaces part of the transmitter normally released, which results in decreased adrenergic activity. This is an interesting hypothesis and it represents a mechanism that is related to the anti-MAO property of these agents.

Other studies on the cardio-vascular action of MAO inhibitors include; pressor activity of pheniprazine in dogs (Boyer et al., 1963) and attenuation of cardiovascular responses to exercise after MAO inhibition in man (Goldberg et al., 1962). These authors suggest that the anti-anginal action of MAO inhibitors could be the result of such attenuation of the cardiovascular system.

The effect of phenylalkylhydrazines have also been investigated in the uterus and heart (Rudzik and Miller, 1963). Depending on the structure of the inhibitors, the catecholamines were either increased or decreased. Anderson and Ammann (1963), extending their work on the effects of MAO inhibitors on ganglionic transmission, demonstrated a reversible blockade of the neuromuscular transmission of the isolated rat phrenic nerve-diaphragm preparation. The ganglionic blocking activity of several MAO inhibitors also has been confirmed (Urquiaga et al., 1963).

VI. Interaction of MAO Inhibitors with Other Substances

The fact that interactions occur between MAO inhibitors and various substances is well known. This is also evident in man according to the recent review by Goldberg (1964). From an experimental standpoint, the interaction between MAO inhibitors and reserpine still remains an intriguing phenomenon, and its mechanism is still not completely understood. Upon administration of reserpine in an animal pretreated with a MAO inhibitor, the usual fall in biogenic amine levels of various tissues does not occur, although a number of pharmacological responses are seen.

For example, pheniprazine inhibits reserpine-induced gastric acid secretion, serotonin lowering, and lesion formation (Kim and Shore, 1963); the authors conclude that this protection is a local action of pheniprazine, possibly due to the presence of high free serotonin concentrations. Iproniazid, however, did not prevent the action of reserpine on gastric secretion in dogs with chronic Pavlov cannula (Leusen et al., 1963). MAO inhibitors reversed the reserpine-induced norepinephrine depleting action of the rat or rabbit heart (Matsuo, 1962; Bhagat, 1963), while Tachi et al. (1963) reported that iproniazid, but not pheniprazine or SKF 385, was able to reverse the depressant effects of reserpine on the isolated atria. The dose of iproniazid employed in the reversal of the blood pressure response to reserpine also appears to be important, for with smaller doses the reversal may be present, but with increased doses of iproniazid it may be abolished (Hull and Horita, 1964).

The influence of MAO inhibitors on release of biogenic amines by reserpine appears to occur at the level of the storage granules (Clementi and Zocche, 1963; Pellegrino de Iraldi and De Robertis, 1963). Whether the blockade of release is a function of MAO inhibition, and if so, how MAO is related to the action of reserpine is not clear. In addition to reserpine, the norepinephrine releasing agent, α-methyldopa, normally a sedative, when administered after a MAO inhibitor exhibits marked central excitation (Van Rossum and Hurkmans, 1963). The authors conclude that this excitation is caused by accumulation of free catecholamines that are liberated by the decarboxylation products of α-methyldopa.

Various MAO inhibitors have been found that affect the metabolism, and, therefore, the duration of action of a number of pharmacological agents. Depending on the inhibitor and the interval between the administration of the inhibitor and certain sedative agents, the duration of the action of the sedatives could be increased or decreased (Stock and Westermann, 1962; Serrone and Fujimoto, 1962). The anorexic and psychomotor activity of amphetamine was potentiated after iproniazid and pivaloylbenzylhydrazine, but the mechanism of this phenomenon is uncertain (Spengler, 1962). Chodera (1963) reported on the ability of iproniazid to potentiate the effect of morphine on body temperature of rats and to delay the onset of morphine tolerance. Whether this is related to the inhibition of MAO is not known. This is also true of the interaction between MAO inhibitors and metrazol in which the convulsant and lethal effects of the latter agent were potentiated (Sansone and Dell'omodarme, 1963).

Another interesting interaction involving metabolism was found by Van Praag and Leijnse (1962) and by Kirberger (1963). In patients who had been dosed orally with serotonin or 5-hydroxyindoleacetic acid (5HIAA), they found that pretreatment with iproniazid or isocarboxazid would cause a decrease in urinary 5HIAA, while with phenelzine or nialamide the decrease in 5HIAA occurred only after serotonin loading. The former two MAO inhibitors apparently affect the metabolism of 5HIAA as well as the degradation of serotonin (Kirberger, 1963). This apparent paradox was also demonstrable in rats that had been treated with iproniazid and loaded orally with 5HIAA (Leijnse and Van Praag, 1964). In these experiments the decrease in 5HIAA excretion was attributed to a delayed absorption of the acid from the intestinal tract.

While the above discussion dealt with compounds that were affected by the MAO inhibitors, several instances in which other drugs affected the action of the inhibitor have also been observed. The usual rise in brain levels of serotonin and norepinephrine in the rat after MAO inhibitor was antagonized by pretreatment with several phenothiazine derivatives or with pentobarbital. This antagonism was explained as being caused by the hypothermia produced by the phenothiazines for in similarly treated rats kept at 36° C, brain amine levels rose in the normal manner. Schwartz et al. (1963) concluded from their studies that the counteracting effects of chlorpromazine on MAO inhibitors resulted from an interference with the penetration of monoamines or their precursors through brain membranes.

The antagonism of the long-acting irreversible hydrazine compounds by the reversible inhibitors was described earlier as competition for the active sites of the enzyme. Certain inhibitors, however, such as iproniazid and tranylcypromine, were only poorly antagonized by harmine, while others like pheniprazine and phenelzine were essentially completely antagonized. A detailed study of these differences indicated that tissue concentrations of those irreversible inhibitors which were readily antagonized were present for shorter periods than the harmala alkaloids, while iproniazid and SKF 385 persisted in tissues in their active forms beyond the duration of the reversible inhibitors. After disappearance of the reversible compounds, the irreversible inhibitors were still present and exerted much of their typical anti-MAO action (Horita and Chinn, 1964). Pheniprazine is also effectively antagonized by the reversible MAO inhibitor and adrenergic neuron blocking agent, BW 392C60 (Kuntzman and Jacobson, 1963).

VII. Miscellaneous Actions

Highman and Maling (1962) continued their work on the neurotoxic actions of some of the arylalkylhydrazines. Prolonged administration of phenylisopropyl- and phenylisobutylhydrazine resulted in lesions of several areas of the brain of dogs, but not in cats, rabbits, or squirrel monkeys. The toxicity appeared not to be related to MAO inhibition since other MAO inhibitors did not produce similar lesions. The dog appears to be especially sensitive to the neurotoxic actions of the hydrazine compounds for similar observations were made with several new hydrazine-type MAO inhibitors (Palmer and Noel, 1963). The toxicity and the lethality of repeated injections of iproniazid and pargyline in rats were enhanced when treated simultaneously with desiccated thyroid (Carrier and Buday, 1963).

References

Anderson, E. G., and Ammann, A. (1963). *J. Pharmacol. Exptl. Therap.* **140**, 179.
Barbato, L. M., and Abood, L. G. (1963). *Biochim. Biophys. Acta* **67**, 531.
Belleau, B., and Moran, J. (1963). *Ann. N. Y. Acad. Sci.* **107**, 822.
Bhagat, B. (1963). *Arch. Intern. Pharmacodyn.* **146**, 65.
Blaschko, H. (1963). In "The Enzymes," (P. D. Boyer, H. Lardy and K. Myrbäck, eds.), Vol. 8, p. 337. Academic Press, New York.

C.3. HYDRAZINES ADDENDUM

Bloom, B. M. (1963). *Ann. N. Y. Acad. Sci.* **107**, 878.
Boyer, S., Jenkins, H., and Robinson, S. (1963). *J. Pharm. Sci.* **52**, 423.
Burkard, W. P., Gey, K. F., and Pletcher, A. (1962). *Biochem. Pharmacol.* **2**, 117.
Carrier, R. N., and Buday, P. V. (1963). *Arch. Intern. Pharmacodyn.* **145**, 18.
Chodera, A. (1963). *Arch. Intern. Pharmacodyn.* **144**, 362.
Chodera, A., Gorkin, V. Z., and Gridnieva, L. I. (1964). *Acta Biol. Med. Ger.* **13**, 101.
Clementi, F., and Zocche, G. P. (1963). *J. Cell Biol.* **17**, 587.
Conference on MAO Inhibitors (1963). *Ann. N. Y. Acad. Sci.* **107**, 809–1158.
Datta, R. K., and Ghosh, J. J. (1963). *Biochem. Pharmacol.* **12**, 1355.
Davey, M. J., Farmer, J. B., and Reinert, H. (1963). *Brit. J. Pharmacol.* **20**, 121.
Frey, H. H. (1963). *Acta Pharmacol. Toxicol.* **20**, 90.
Furgiuele, A. R., Kinnard, W. J., and Buckley, J. P. (1962). *J. Pharmacol. Exptl. Therap.* **137**, 356.
Ganrot, P. O., and Rosengren, E. (1962). *Med. Exptl.* **6**, 315.
Ganrot, P. O., Rosengren, E., and Gottfries, C. G. (1962). *Experientia* **18**, 260.
Ganrot, P. O., Gottfries, C. G., and Rosengren, E. (1963). *Acta Psychiat. Neurol. Scand.* **39**, Suppl. 169, 3.
Gatgounis, J., and Aycock, J. (1963). *J. Pharmacol. Exptl. Therap.* **141**, 50.
Geiger, A., Gombos, G., Otsuki, S., Aguilar, V., Gothelf, B., Scruggs, W., and Whitney, G. (1962). *Intern. J. Neuropharmacol.* **1**, 283.
Gessa, G. L., Cuenca, E., and Costa, E. (1963). *Ann. N. Y. Acad. Sci.* **107**, 935.
Goldberg, L. I. (1964). *J. Am. Med. Assoc.* **190**, 456.
Goldberg, L. I., Horwitz, D., and Sjoerdsma, A. (1962). *J. Pharmacol. Exptl. Therap.* **137**, 39.
Gorkin, V. Z., Komisarova, N. V., Lerman, M. I., and Vergovkina, I. V. (1964). *Biochem. Biophys. Res. Commun.* **15**, 383.
Green, A. L. (1962). *Biochem. J.* **84**, 217.
Green, A. L. (1964). *Biochem. Pharmacol.* **13**, 249.
Green, H., Sawyer, J. L., Erickson, R. W., and Cook, L. (1962). *Proc. Soc. Exptl. Biol. Med.* **109**, 347.
Hansson, E., Fleming, R. M., and Clark, W. G. (1964). *Intern. J. Neuropharmacol.* **3**, 177.
Highman, B., and Maling, H. M. (1962). *J. Pharmacol. Exptl. Therap.* **137**, 344.
Horita, A. (1965a). *Brit. J. Pharmacol.* **24**, 245.
Horita, A. (1965b). *Toxicol. Appl. Pharmacol.* **7**, 97.
Horita, A. (1963). *J. Pharmacol. Exptl. Therap.* **142**, 141.
Horita, A., and Chinn, C. (1964). *Biochem. Pharmacol.* **13**, 371.
Horita, A., and Matsumoto, C. (1962). *Life Sci.* **10**, 491.
Hull, L. J., and Horita, A. (1964). *Nature* 202, 604.
Johnson, G. E., and Sellers, E. A. (1962). *Can. J. Biochem. Physiol.* **40**, 632.
Kim, K. S., and Shore, P. A. (1963). *J. Pharmacol. Exptl. Therap.* **141**, 321.
Kirberger, E. (1963). *Nature* **197**, 1211.
Kobayashi, Y., and Okuyama, T. (1962). *Biochem. Pharmacol.* **2**, 929.
Koechlin, B., Schwartz, M. A., and Oberhaensli, W. (1962). *J. Pharmacol. Exptl. Therap.* **138**, 11.
Koivusalo, M., Pentilla, I., Raina, A., and Tenhunen, R. (1963). *Acta. Physiol. Scand.* **57**, 454.
Kopin, I. (1964). *Pharmacol. Rev.* **16**, 179.
Kopin, I., and Axelrod, J. (1963). *Ann. N. Y. Acad. Sci.* **107**, 848.
Kopin, I., Fischer, J., Musacchio, J., and Dale-Horst, W. (1964). *Proc. Natl. Acad. Sci. U.S.* **52**, 716.
Kory, M., and Mingioli, E. (1964). *Biochem. Pharmacol.* **13**, 577.
Kuntzman, R., and Jacobson, M. M. (1963). *J. Pharmacol. Exptl. Therap.* **141**, 166.
Leijnse, B., and Van Praag, H. M. (1964). *Arch. Intern. Pharmacodyn.* **150**, 582.
Leusen, I., Thoenen, H., and Lacroix, E. (1963). *Arch. Intern. Pharmacodyn.* **141**, 190.

McNeill, J. H., and Reidel, B. (1964). *Can. J. Physiol. Pharmacol.* **42**, 33.
Manchanda, S. K., Subberwal, U., Anano, B. R., and Singh, B. (1963). *Arch. Intern. Pharmacodyn.* **143**, 408.
Mantegazza, P., and Riva, M. (1963). *J. Pharm. Pharmacol.* **15**, 472.
Matsuo, T. (1962). *Japan. J. Pharmacol.* **12**, 62.
Nair, V., Lal, H., and Roth, L. J. (1962). *Intern. J. Neuropharmacol.* **1**, 361.
Oswald, E. O., and Strittmatter, C. F. (1963). *Proc. Soc. Exptl. Biol. Med.* **114**, 668.
Palmer, A. C., and Noel, P. R. (1963). *J. Pathol. Bacteriol.* **86**, 463.
Pellegrino de Iraldi, A., and De Robertis, E. (1963). *Intern. J. Neuropharmacol.* **2**, 321.
Rosen, L., and Goodall, M. (1962). *Am. J. Physiol.* **202**, 883.
Rudzik, A. D., and Miller, J. (1963). *J. Pharmacol. Exptl. Therap.* **139**, 69.
Sakamoto, Y., Ogawa, Y., and Hayashi, K. (1963). *J. Biochem. (Tokyo)* **54**, 292.
Sansone, M., and Dell'omodarme, G. (1963). *Arch. Intern. Pharmacodyn.* **144**, 392.
Schwartz, D. E., Burkard, W. P., Roth, M., Gey, K. F., and Pletscher, A. (1963). *Arch. Intern. Pharmacodyn.* **141**, 135.
Schwartz, M. (1962). *J. Pharmacol. Exptl. Therap.* **135**. 1.
Seiden, L. S., and Westley, J. (1963). *Arch. Intern. Pharmacodyn.* **146**, 145.
Serrone, D. M., and Fujimoto, J. M. (1962). *Biochem. Pharmacol.* **11**, 609.
Smith, T. E., Weissbach, H., and Udenfriend, S. (1962). *Biochemistry* **1**, 137.
Smith, T. E., Weissbach, H., and Udenfriend, S. (1963). *Biochemistry* **2**, 746.
Sourkes, T. L., and D'Iorio, A. (1963). *In* "Metabolic Inhibitors" (R. M. Hochster and J. H. Quastel, eds.), Vol. 2, pp. 79–98. Academic Press, New York.
Spector, S. (1963). *Ann. N. Y. Acad. Sci.* **107**, 856.
Spengler, J. (1962). *Arch. Exptl. Pathol. Pharmakol.* **244**, 153.
Stock, K., and Westermann, E. (1962). *Arch. Exptl. Pathol. Pharmakol.* **243**, 44.
Tachi, S., Nakatani, G., and Fujiwara, M. (1963). *Japan. J. Pharmacol.* **13**, 74.
Urquiaga, X., Villarreal, J., Alosno-de Florida, F., and Pardo, E. G. (1963). *Arch. Intern. Pharmacodyn.* **146**, 126.
Vanov, S. (1963). *Arch. Intern. Pharmacodyn.* **141**, 62.
Van Praag, H. M., and Leijnse, B. (1962). *Psychopharmacologia* **3**, 202.
Van Rossum, J. M., and Hurkmans, J. A. T. (1963). *J. Pharm. Pharmacol.* **15**, 493.
Wiseman-Distler, M. H., and Sourkes, T. L. (1963). *Can. J. Biochem. Physiol.* **41**, 57.
Yamada, H., and Yasunobu, K. (1962). *J. Biol. Chem.* **237**, 1511.
Yamada, H., and Yasunobu, K. (1963). *J. Biol. Chem.* **238**, 2669.
Zeller, E. A. (1963a). *In* "Metabolic Inhibitors" (R. M. Hochster and J. H. Quastel, eds.), Vol. 2, pp. 53–78. Academic Press, New York.
Zeller, E. A. (1963b). *Ann. N. Y. Acad. Sci.* **107**, 811.
Zeller, E. A., and Fouts, J. R. (1963). *Ann. Rev. Pharmacol.* **3**, 9.

Author Index

Numbers in italics indicate the pages on which completed references are listed.

A

Abe, C., 100, *193*
Abele, H. B., 151, *180*
Abernathy, R. S., 96, 98, *161*
Abood, L. G., 74, *161*, 524, *530*
Aborg, S., 160, *197*
Abraham, D., *281*
Abrams, J., 153, *161*
Abse, D. W., 152, *161*
Aceto, M. D., 49, *161*
Achaintre, A., 228, *231*
Acheson, G. H., *277*
Adachi, N., 74, *198*
Adam, H. M., 74, *161*
Adams, R. N., 140, *188*
Adamson, R. H., 138, *174*
Addison, W. P., 154, *182*
Adelson, D., 153, *161*
Ader, R., 47, *161*
Ades, F., 153, *170*
Adey, W. R., 270, *281*
Adlerová, E., 293, *301*
Adlerstein, A. M., 219, *247*
Adriani, J., 107, *161*
Aganyants, E. K., 47, *161*
Aghajanian, G., 74, *161*
Aguilar, V., 527, *531*
Ahlquist, R. P., 273, *277*
Ahrens, A., 91, 92, *161*
Ainslie, J. D., 151, *161*
Akagi, M., 289, *300*
Akerfeldt, S., 251, *277*
Albaum, H. G., 73, *161*
Albert, J., 159, *177*
Albert, S. N., 71, 74, 85, 92, 93, *172*, *173*
Albonetti, G., 219, 224, *242*
Aldeghi, E., 220, *231*
Aleksandrovskii, I. A., 218, *231*
Aleksandrovskij, Y. A., 219, *240*
Alemà, G., 65, *192*, 218, 224, *231*

Alertsen, A. R., 253, *282*
Alexander, F., 143, 161, *161*
Alexander, L., 47, *161*
Alexander, P., 270, *282*
Algeri, E. J., 160, *161*
Ali, A., 219, *244*
Allegranza, A., 217, 218, *233*
Allemand, H. L., 229, *238*
Allen, C. R., 84, *171*
Allen, D. E., 143, 147, *168*
Allen, J. L., 153, *164*
Alleva, P. M., 218, 224, *231*
Allewijn, A., 217, 227, *242*
Allgén, L. G., 135, 145, 147, 148, *162*
Alliot, B., 226, *234*
Alloiteau, J. J., 103, *162*
Alluaume, R., 38, 68, 96, *182*
Alman, R. W., 71, 92, *172*
Almudejar, M., 149, *178*
Alosno-de Florida, F., 528, *532*
Alstaedter, R., 60, *198*
Altman, J., 66, 113, 150, *162*
Altschule, M. D., 44, 70, *162*, 251, 260, 273, 277, 280, 281, 282
Amai, R. L. S., 283, *301*
Amati, G., 218, *231*
Amati-Sas, S., 220, *239*
Ammann, A., 528, *530*
Amneli, G., 219, *241*
Anano, B. R., 527, *532*
Andén, N. E., 81, *162*, 217, *231*
Andersen, E. W., 107, *179*
Andersen, P., 50, *192*, 227, *231*
Anderson, E. G., 528, *530*
Anderson, E. L., 32, *162*
Anderson, J. A., 161, *195*
Anderson, J. P., 160, *192*
Anderson, T. E., 151, *169*
Ando, M., 50, 82, *198*
Andrejew, A., 82, *162*

533

AUTHOR INDEX

Andreoli, F. A., 220, *247*
Angel, C., 252, *279*
Angeleri, F., 50, *167*
Angst, J., 225, *231*
Anguera, G., 91, 115, *170*
Anokhina-Itskova, I. P., 40, *162*
Ansell, G. B., 82, *162*
Ansorg, W., 73, *171*
Anton, A. H., 258, *277*
Antonio, A., 109, *190*
Antony, G. S., 156, *162*
Appel, J. B., 48, *173*
Appell, K. E., 273, *280*
Appiani, L., 220, 229, *231*
Arbus, 219, *238*
Archdeacon, J. W., 84, *162*
Archer, J. D., 45, 106, *162, 168*
Archer, S., 297, *300, 301*
Ardillo, L., 220, *231, 242*
Ardisson, J. L., 54, *171*
Arfel, G., 230, *248*
Argenta, G., 219, 224, *237*
Ariens, E. J., 81, *162*
Armitage, A. K., 60, 62, 68, 85, 86, 88, 107, 108, 110, *181*
Armitage, S. G., 153, *188*
Arnold, A., 297, *300*
Arnold, A. C., 115, *168*
Arnold, E. T., 67, *162*
Arnold, J., 226, *239*
Arnold, O. H., 94, *162*
Arnott, G., 219, *244*
Arnould, F., 219, 226, 227, 230, *244, 245*
Arnould, P., 105, *183*
Arnozis, J. H. R., 229, *231*
Aron, E., 98, 104, *162*
Aronsen, K. F., 67, *162*
Arora, R. B., 68, 85, 94, *162, 192*
Arosio, G., 229, *231*
Arroyo, H., 160, *185*
Arthurs, D., 219, 220, *231, 236*
Árvay, A., 101, *162*
Ashby, W., 82, *162*
Ashcroft, G. W., 151, *162*
Assael, M., 103, *181*
Aston, R., 44, 60, *162*
Atwood, J. M., 220, *239*
Aubertin, E., 161, *162*
Aubin, B., 220, *243*
Aubry, U., 229, *231*
Audet, J., 229, *231*
Audisio, M., 226, *235*, 295, *300*

Auge, 219, *247*
Auterhoff, H., 148, 149, *187*
Avram, M. M., 161, *184*
Avroutzki, G. Y., 226, *231*
Axelrod, J., 64, 65, 81, 84, *162*, 256, 258, 259, 266, 269, *277, 278, 280, 281, 282*, 527, *531*
Axelrod, S., 254, *281, 282*
Aycock, J., 527, *531*
Ayd, F., 220, *231*
Ayd, F. J., Jr., 114, 150, 156, 157, 158, 159, 160, *162, 163*
Ayers, W. J., 254, *281*
Azima, H., 72, 106, 152, *163, 183, 193*, 220, *231*

B

Baart, N., 82, *172*
Baccaglini, B., 218, *231*
Bach-Y-Rita, P., 57, *187*
Baciocchi, M., 218, *231*
Bacon, H. M., 158, *163*
Bättig, K., 42, *176*
Bagdon, R., 85, *186*
Bailey, R., 229, *237*
Bailly, R., 218, 224, *235*
Bain, W. A., 151, *163*
Bair, H. V., 154, *163*
Baker, A. A., 154, *195*
Baker, L., 53, *187*
Baker, R. A., 159, *176, 187*
Baker, W. W., 50, *163*
Balagot, R. C., 60, 67, *191*
Baldessarini, R. J., 261, *281*
Balducci, M., 218, *232*
Balestrieri, A., 51, *163*
Balf, C. L., 275, *278*
Balling, J., 224, *234*
Baltzly, R., 25, *163*
Bamdas, E. M., 129, *192*
Ban, T. A., 37, 159, *163, 180*, 218, 219, 224, 228, *232, 242, 247, 248*
Bandettini Di Poggio, U., 218, *232*
Bangham, A. D., 106, *163*
Barbato, L. M., 524, *530*
Barbeau, A., *277*
Barber, R., 298, *301*
Barclay, G., 261, *280*
Barberini, E., 224, *235*
Bardenat, C., 228, *232*
Bardis, Cl., 226, 227, *246*
Baré, Cl., 226, *244*

AUTHOR INDEX

Barila, T. G., 94, *190*
Barker, J. C., 161, *163*
Barker, P. A., 151, *162*
Barkov, N. K., 62, *163*
Barnes, B. A., 254, *280*
Barnes, C. D., 40, *178*
Barnes, J. H., 291, *301*
Barraclough, C. A., 103, *163*
Barre, R., 226, *243*
Barrett, A. M., 521, *521*
Barros Hurtado, A., 219, *245*
Barry, H., 45, 50, *163*
Barry, H., III, 43, *198*
Barry, J. J., Jr., 154, *163*
Barsa, J., 160, 161, *181*
Barsa, J. A., 156, 159, *163*
Bartholini, G., 79, *163*
Bartlett, N. G., 72, *167*
Bartlett, R. G., 75, *163*
Barton, N., 230, *248*
Baruk, H., 41, 94, *163*
Basmajian, J. V., 44, *163*
Basquin, R., 218, 224, *235*
Bass, H., 288, *301*
Basu, S. N., 101, *163*
Bates, T. J. N., 161, *171*
Baumm, C., 287, *301*
Baxter, C. F., 270, *281*
Bayer, K. F., 59, *165*
Bayerlein, L., 229, *244*
Bayne, B., 148, 149, *178*
Beal, J. A., 161, *163*
Bean, J. W., 93, 111, *163*
Beatty, C. H., 83, *188*
Beaudoin, G., 229, *231*
Beaven, M. A., 143, 144, 145, *163*
Beck, L., 220, *232*
Beck, L. V., 96, *163*
Becker, B., 91, *168*
Becker, K. L., 156, *163*
Beckett, A. H., 128, 143, 144, 145, 147, *163*
Beckett, P. G. S., 252, 253, 273, *278*, *279*, *280*
Beeler, E. C., 24, *163*
Béguin, M., 66, *174*, *196*, 217, *237*
Behn, W., 114, 145, 147, 148, *163*
Beiler, J. M., 121, *185*
Belkin, M., 77, *163*
Bell, M. R., 297, *300*
Bell, N. W., 273, *278*
Bellander-Löfvenberg, S., 284, *300*
Belleau, B., 524, *530*
Bellinzona, G. B., 32, *162*

Bello, H., 219, *242*
Belloni, F., 77, *164*
Benaron, H. B. W., 91, 114, *163*, *180*
Benayoun, C., 224, *232*
Benazet, J., 219, *238*
Benazon, D., 65, *168*
Benda, P., 53, *170*
Ben-David, M., 118, *181*
Benditt, E. P., 93, *163*
Benfey, B. G., 63, 81, *163*, *186*
Benington, F., 82, *168*
Benitte, A., 38, 68, 96, *180*, *182*
Bennett, G. M., 25, *163*
Bennett, H. D., 106, *181*
Bennett, I. F., 153, *167*
Bennett, J. L., 151, 153, 154, 155, 156, *163*, *183*, 219, 222, *239*, 298, *300*
Bennett, P. B., 284, 285, *300*
Benson, G. K., 103, *164*
Bensoussan, P. A., 94, *164*
Bente, D., 52, 151, *164*, *188*, 227, 228, *232*, *239*
Berard, E., 52, 56, 86, 91, 92, *168*, *195*
Berg, S. S., 29, *164*
Bergen, J. R., 254, *277*, *279*
Berger, F. M., 77, *196*
Berger, M., 82, 140, 141, 148, 149, *164*, 173
Berges, J., 41, 94, *163*
Bergh, N. P., 67, *162*
Bergman, P. S., 160, *185*
Bergmann, F., 55, *164*
Bergmann, H., 220, *232*, *241*
Bernard, A., 253, *282*
Bernaskiewicz, E., 219, *240*
Bernheim, M. L. C., 83, *164*
Bernsohn, J., 74, 82, *164*
Bernstein, J., 29, 128, *198*
Bernthsen, A., 3, 24, *164*
Berry, J. F., 82, *185*
Berry, K., 159, *176*, *188*
Berthier, C., 160, *166*
Berti, F., 229, *232*
Berti, T., 110, 112, 136, 139, 145, 147, 148, *164*
Bertini, F., 219, *238*
Bertlet, H. H., 268, 269, *277*
Bertolotti, P., 226, *232*
Bertrand, I., 67, *1͡*
Bès, A., 219, *238*
Besse, J. H., 109, *164*, 230, *248*
Bessman, S. P., 271, *278*
Besson, S., 139, *164*

Bhagat, B., 528, *530*
Bhargava, K. P., 47, 58, 103, 128, *164*, 217, *232*
Bhose, L., *164*
Bianchi, G., 218, *232*
Bianchi, R. G., 76, *164*
Bianco, M., 77, *164*
Bickel, M. H., *277*, 292, *300*
Bickelhaupt, F., 293, *301*
Bickford, R. G., 64, *192*
Bieberdorf, F. W., 115, *168*
Bielinski, C., 225, *247*
Bigelow, L. B., 260, *282*
Bilett, B., 270, *280*
Billon, J. P., 150, *164*
Binet, P., 68, *164*
Bishop, M. P., 153, *174*, 218, 219, 222, 223, *232*, *237*, *245*, 266, *279*
Bishop, R. H., Jr., 152, *178*
Bisiani, M., 229, *232*
Bissière, H., 226, *232*, *234*
Bister, W., 218, *232*
Blackburn, H. L., 153, *164*
Blacker, G. J., 76, *189*
Blacker, K. H., 114, *164*
Blackford Rogers, W. J., 220, *232*
Blair, J. H., 204, 231, *246*
Blanc, M., 226, *232*
Blandin, J., 218, *232*
Blaschko, H., 523, *530*
Blatteis, C., 96, *178*
Blazek, J., 5, 147, 149, 150, *164*
Blès, G., 218, *233*
Bloch, A., 229, *238*
Bloch, M., 59, *164*
Block, W., 112, 139, *164*
Blois, M. S., 159, *164*
Blok, J., 39, *165*
Blom, S., 158, *164*
Bloom, B. M., 524, *531*
Bloom, H. J., 59, *164*
Bloomfield, S., 62, *164*
Blough, D. S., 50, *164*
Blumberg, A. G., 155, *165*
Blumberg, H., 47, *165*
Bobon, J., 202, 204, 217, 218, 219, 221, 224, 225, 227, 228, 230, 231, *232*, *236*
Bocher, C. A., 147, *173*
Bodi, T., 220, 231, *244*
Böcher, W., 220, *232*
Boeles, J. T. F., 39, *165*
Boer, G. E., 94, *165*

Boey, J., 217, *247*
Bogaard, J. M., 217, *246*
Bogdansky, D. F., 91, *165*
Boger, W. P., 230, 254, *247*, *282*
Bohacek, N., 218, *232*
Bois, P., 109, *180*
Boissier, J. R., 42, *165*, 217, *232*, *233*
Boissier, P., 54, 86, 87, 91, 94, *180*
Boistel, J., 56, *168*
Boitard, J., 26, 32, *192*
Bonafede, V. I., 53, 68, *165*
Bonhoure, J., 218, 224, *232*, *233*, *236*
Bonomolo, A., 82, *165*
Bonvallet, M., 50, *178*
Bonvicino, G. E., 25, *165*
Bordeleau, J. M., 160, *165*
Borel, R. O., 219, *237*
Borenstein, P., 218, *233*
Borg, D. C., 140, *165*
Borghesi, R., 218, *233*
Boriani, A., 107, *165*
Borison, H. L., 57, 58, 59, *165*
Bornmann, G., 104, *165*
Bortnick, T. L., 151, *165*
Bose, B. C., 82, *165*
Boshes, B., 82, *164*
Bossier, J. R., 217, *232*, *233*
Bouchacourt, A., 226, *243*
Bouchard, J., 218, *233*
Bouchardy, M., 228, *241*
Boulding, J. E., *280*
Boulton, T. B., 67, *165*
Bourdillon, R. E., 260, 261, *277*
Bourgeois, M., 226, *232*
Bourgeois-Gavardin, M., 55, 57, 67, 71, 84, 85, 87, 89, 90, 93, 94, 113, *165*, *194*
Bourjala, 159, *188*
Bousquet, W. F., 132, *165*
Boutillier, 228, *247*
Bouvard, R. J. M., 226, 227, *233*
Bouvier, S., 228, *240*
Bovet, D., 46, 51, 52, *180*, *184*
Bower, W., 44, *162*
Bowes, H. A., 151, *165*
Boyajy, L. D., 50, *197*
Boyd, C. E., 57, 70, 71, *165*
Boyd, E. M., 41, 57, 70, 71, *165*
Boyd, E. S., 50, *165*
Boyer, W. P., 528, *531*
Bozzi, R., 218, *233*
Braceland, F. J., 151, *165*
Bradley, P. B., 46, 50, 51, 52, *165*, *181*

AUTHOR INDEX 537

Bradshaw, A. K., 84, *165*
Brady, J. V., 50, *168*
Brady, R. O., 64, *162*
Braganca, B. M., 276, *277*
Brambilla, G., 229, *233*
Brand, E. D., 57, 58, *165*
Brandborg, G., 158, *172*
Brandrup, E., 218, *233*
Brauer, W., 218, *234*
Brauner, F., 220, *233*
Brena, S., 101, *165, 185*
Brendel, R., 121, *185*
Brendel, W., 69, *165*
Breuninger, H., 94, *165*
Brewer, W. R., 148, *165*
Bricaire, H., 160, *170*
Bridge, C. J., 253, *282*
Bridge, E. M., 285, *300*
Brienta, A., 229, *235*
Brignon, J. J., 148, 149, *165*
Brill, H., 159, 160, 161, *165*
Brillhart, J. R., 103, *165*
Brilmayer, H., 74, *174*
Brindle, G. F., 230, *247*
Brink, N. G., 260, *280*
Brodie, B. B., 60, 61, 63, 67, 91, 134, 135, 138, 145, 147, *165, 180, 189, 191*, 262, 263, 266, *277, 278*, 292, 294, *300, 301*
Broitman, S., 77, *176*
Brooks, G. W., 160, *166*
Brosius, C. O., 253, *279*
Brossi, A., 294, *300*
Broussolle, P., 160, *166*, 226, 227, 228, *233*
Brown, A. S., 220, *233*
Brown, B. B., 41, 42, *166, 172*
Brown, H., 230, *248*
Brown, M. L., 261, *277*
Brown, N., 218, *234*
Brown, R. E., 152, *196*
Brown, R. K., 254, *280*
Brown, W. G., 106, *181*
Brown, W. L., 52, *166*
Browne, A. D. H., 67, *166*
Browne, I., 153, *184*
Bruce, C., 76, *189*
Brue, F., 74, *183*
Bruecke, F. T., 38, *166*
Bruland, H., 50, *192*
Brunaud, M., 87, 115, *166, 170*
Brunaud, S., 87, 115, *166, 170*

Brune, G. G., 261, 268, 269, *277, 278*
Brunhes, M., 219, *247*
Bruni, A., 218, *233*
Bruni, C., 111, *186*
Bruno, A., 217, *233*
Bruscha, W., 72, *166*
Bryk, B., 156, *166*
Bubnoff, M. V., 87, *166*
Buchel, L., 217, *233*
Bucher, W. H., 160, *166*
Buck, H. W., 285, *300*
Buckley, J. P., 42, *174*, 527, *531*
Buckman, C., 158, *166*, 520, *521*
Buday, P. V., 530, *531*
Budde, H., 56, 85, 93, *166, 197*
Budinsky, J., 139, *166*
Buffardi, R., 218, *233*
Bugard, P., 285, *300*
Buhr, G., 229, *239*
Buis, C., 218, *233*
Buisson, P. J. C., 26, *166*
Bukowczyk, A., 218, *234*
Bull, C., 268, 269, *277*
Bullard, R. W., 70, *181*
Bulle, P. H., 81, 109, *166*
Bulow, G., 141, *188*
Bumpus, F. M., 269, *278*
Buniatian, H. D., *278*
Bunney, W. E., 256, 262, 264, *278*
Burbridge, T. N., 61, 83, 160, *166, 181, 192, 195*
Burchfield, H. P., 145, *180*
Burgat, R., 228, *231*
Burger, A., 24, 158, *166*
Burgermeister, J. J., 218, *233*
Burkard, W. P., 527, 530, *531, 532*
Burke, J. C., 38, 119, 137, 139, 147, *166, 188, 193*
Burkman, A. M., 47, 58, *166*
Burnett, R., 136, *175*
Burns, J. H., 107, 110, *166*
Burns, J. J., 145, *168*
Burns, R. H., 153, *184*
Burton, P., 219, 226, 227, 230, *244, 245*
Burton, R. M., 65, 76, 81, *166*
Bury, J., 230, *232*
Buscaino, G. A., 268, *278*
Bush, H. J., 230, *247*
Bushrod, M. A., 82, *162*
Busse, W., 94, *166*
Butler, N. G. P., 92, *171*
Butler, W. M., 135, *186*

Buzard, J. A., 83, *166*
Bylenga, N. D., 159, *190*
Byles, P. H., 229, *236*

C

Cadenius, B., 228, *239*
Caffey, E. M., 153, *183*, 219, 222, *239*
Caffey, E. M., Jr., 153, 155, 156, *166*, *167*, *181*, 298, *300*
Cahen, R. L., 59, *166*
Cain, H. D., 160, *166*
Cain, J. B., 105, *186*
Cairns, R. J., 159, *166*
Calbeck, M. J., *280*
Caldonazzo, C., 218, *233*
Calhoun, D. W., 50, *194*
Calligari, G., 220, 229, *233*, *234*
Calo, A., 147, 148, *166*
Camanni, F., 65, *166*
Camba, R., 113, *166*
Cambareri, P., 229, *236*
Cameron, D. E., 151, *166*, *278*
Cameron, I. A., 218, *233*
Campan, L., 229, *234*
Campbell, E. H., 521, *522*
Campbell, F. L., 24, *166*
Campbell, J. A., 115, *184*
Camplo, J., 226, *233*
Cann, H. M., 160, *166*
Cantarow, A., 97, *170*
Capehart, J., 45, *170*
Capoore, H. S., 159, *166*
Caprini, G., 218, *231*, *233*
Capron, C., 219, *246*
Capron, H., 218, 219, *233*, *242*
Carbonell Cadenas De Llano, J., 218, *233*
Cardani, A. J., 218, *233*
Cardo, W. N., 218, *233*
Cardon, P. V., 260, *278*
Cardon, P. V., Jr., 155, *186*, 261, *281*
Cardoso, A. C. S. Q., 80, *166*
Cares, R. M., 158, *166*, 520, *521*
Carfagno, S. C., 158, *166*
Carignan, G., 229, *233*
Carini, A., 218, *235*
Carlini, E. A., 273, *278*

Carlisle, H. J., 83, *190*
Carlsson, A., 217, *233*
Carmichael, D. M., 114, *182*
Carneiro, J., 80, *166*
Caron, M., 218, *233*
Carpino Boeri, A., 229, *234*, *238*
Carr, C. J., 39, 41, 42, 132, *166*, *167*, *181*
Carranza Sanchez, L. J., 219, *243*
Carreras, M., 50, *167*
Carrier, R. N., 530, *531*
Carruthers, G. F., 96, *167*
Carson, R. P., 61, *167*
Carter, C. B., 62, *167*
Carter, C. H., 160, *167*
Carter, J. T., 154, *182*
Carter, W. W., 50, *172*
Carver, M. J., 82, *167*
Casaglia, G., 220, *234*
Cascella, G., 219, *245*
Casey, J. F., 153, 156, *167*
Cassell, W. A., 57, 70, 71, *165*
Castaigne, A., 69, 98, *167*
Castner, C. W., 154, 156, *167*, *187*
Casy, A. F., 128, *163*
Catania, A. C., 48, *190*
Catenacci, A. J., 85, *171*
Cathala, H. P., 54, 86, 89, 90, *167*, *189*
Cattan, F., 218, 224, *235*
Cauquis, G., 150, *164*
Caussade, L., 53, *167*
Caustier, M., 226, *234*
Cavanaugh, D. J., 135, 140, 147, 148, *167*
Cavatorta, L., 149, *167*
Cavicchi Sandri, G., 147, *167*
Celice, J., 72, 106, *167*
Cenacchi, G., 218, 224, *234*
Century, B., 82, *167*
Ceraso, O. L., 229, *234*, *236*, *237*
Cerletti, A., 41, 47, *194*, 266, *278*
Cesare, E. D., 86, *169*
Cession-Fossion, A., 217, *234*, *236*
Cetrullo, C., 229, *234*
Challas, G., 218, *234*
Chamberlain, T. J., 49, *167*, *278*
Chambers, J. L., 153, *190*
Chambon, Y., 98, 103, 114, *162*, *167*
Chancel, M., 219, *243*
Chandra, O., 47, 58, 128, *164*
Chang, C. C., 262, *278*
Chanoit, P., 153, *173*
Chapel, J. I., 218, *234*

AUTHOR INDEX 539

Chappell, J. S., 153, *168*
Chardon, G., 86, 87, *167*, *185*
Charest, M. P., 41, 60, 61, *178*
Charkey, L. W., 96, *197*
Charpentier, P., 26, 28, *167*
Chartan, F. B. E., 72, *167*
Chase, P. E., 229, *239*
Chata, M. K., 87, *193*
Chatagnon, C., 156, 158, *167*, 228, *234*
Chatagnon, P., 156, 158, *167*, 228, *234*
Chatonnet, J., 98, *167*
Chatten, L. G., 147, *186*
Chatterjee, A., 82, *170*
Chauchard, B., 56, 85, 86, 90, 91, *167*
Chauchard, P., 56, 85, 86, 90, 91, *167*
Chaudhury, M. R., 103, *167*
Chaudhury, R. R., 103, *167*
Chedid, L., 96, *167*
Chen, C. H., 219, *239*
Chen, G., 43, *167*, 217, *234*
Cherico, P., 287, *301*
Chesi, R., 220, *234*
Chesrow, E. J., 293, *300*
Chessin, M., 65, *167*
Cheymol, J., 69, 99, *167*
Chicoine, L., 158, 160, *167*
Chiesara, E., 61, *180*
Child, K. J., 61, *167*
Childers, R. T., Jr., 151, 154, 160, *167*
Chimion, D., 50, *182*
Chin, J. H., 38, 107, *167*
Chin, L., 148, *165*
Chinn, C., 530, *531*
Chinn, H. I., 59, 60, 67, 115, *167*, *168*, *177*
Chiron, A. E., 67, 152, *182*, *183*
Chmouliovsky, M., 217, *237*
Cho, M. H., 42, *168*, 229, *236*
Chodera, A., 524, 529, *531*
Chodoff, P., 217, 229, *234*
Chollot, M.-L., 81, *185*
Chorazy, M., 77, *168*
Chow, M. I., 40, *178*
Christensen, J., 139, *168*, *196*
Christensen, J. A., 76, 139, *168*
Chuen, N., 146, *168*
Chusid, J. G., 53, 108, *181*
Cianasi, G. C., 220, *243*
Cima, L., 112, 136, 139, 145, 147, 148, *164*
Cipriani, G., 219, 220, *234*, *238*
Citro, A., 220, 229, *233*, *234*
Citterio, C., 148, *168*

Civai, O., 220, *234*
Clare, N. T., 143, *168*
Clark, D. L., 153, 154, *184*
Clark, L. C., Jr., 82, *168*
Clark, L. D., 50, *174*
Clark, M. L., 153, *168*
Clark, R., 50, *168*
Clark, R. L., 128, *168*
Clark, W. G., 527, *531*
Clarke, C. A., 260, 261, *277*, *278*
Clarke, D., 145, *168*
Clawson, J., 59, *165*
Clement, A. J., 65, *168*
Clementi, F., 529, *531*
Clerc, N. A., 56, 86, 91, 92, *168*
Clerigo, J., 224, *245*
Clérigo Delgado, J., 229, *245*
Cliche, F., 91, *168*
Clink, D. W., 47, *161*
Clodi, P., 75, 106, *168*
Clos, M., 219, 223, 224, *234*, *237*
Clout, I. R., 156, *168*
Cochin, J., 147, *168*
Cochrane, L. S. G., 74, 82, *164*
Cocou, F., 101, *186*
Cohen, I. M., 61, 106, 114, *168*
Cohen, L., *281*
Cohen, M., 252, *279*
Cohen, P. H., 159, *193*
Cohen, S., 145, *172*, *184*
Coirault, R., 226, *234*
Cole, A. C. E., 107, *168*
Cole, I., 261, *280*
Cole, J. O., 151, *168*
Coleman, R., 66, *181*
Colinet, M., 230, *232*
Collard, J., 202, 204, 217, 218, 219, 221, 224, 225, 227, 228, 230, 231, *232*, *234*, *235*, *236*
Collier, H. B., 143, 147, *168*, *194*
Collins, I. S., 158, *168*
Collins, V. J., 97, *168*
Colombo, P. A., 229, *234*
Cols, B., 229, *238*, *244*
Combette, H., 219, *237*
Combrisson, J., 150, *164*
Comoy, P., 26, 32, *192*
Condousis, G. A., *300*
Cone, T. E., Jr., 60, 67, *177*
Conner, P. K., *168*
Conney, A. G., 145, *168*
Conqvist, S., 72, *168*

Constant, M. A., 91, *168*
Constantine, J. W., 298, *301*
Conte, C., 226, *235*, 295, *300*
Converse, J. M., 97, *178*
Cook, L., 3, 41, 44, 48, 49, 50, 57, 119, 121, 129, *162*, *168*, *174*, *176*, *180*, 526, *531*
Cook, W. A., 218, 225, *234*
Cooper, A. J., 521, *521*
Coppen, A., 268, *278*
Coppola, F., 218, *235*
Coppolino, C. A., 155, *168*
Cor, M., 226, *236*
Coraboeuf, E., 56, *168*
Corcoran, A. C., 65, 94, 108, *174*, *185*, 266, *281*
Cordier, P., 148, *168*
Corman, M., 228, *232*
Cornatzer, W. E., 74, *175*
Corne, S. J., 37, *168*
Corneli, R., 218, *234*
Cornman, H. D., III., 158, *169*
Correll, R. E., 50, *180*
Corrivault, G. W., 118, *179*
Corsetti, 228, *247*
Corssen, G., 84, *171*, 229, *234*
Cosar, C., 112, *169*
Cosmides, G. J., 134, 136, *189*
Cosnier, J., 75, *169*
Cossa, P., 218, 228, *234*
Costa, E., 50, 65, 93, *169*, 262, 263, *278*, 527, *531*
Costello, W. J., 147, *178*
Costiloe, J. P., 49, 153, *168*, *192*
Cotzias, G. C., 140, *165*
Couadau, A., 229, *234*
Couadau, H., 229, *234*
Coulonjou, R., 226, *243*
Court, J. H., 218, *234*
Courvoisier, S., 38, 45, 52, 55, 57, 60, 61, 62, 67, 68, 70, 71, 72, 74, 85, 86, 89, 90, 91, 92, 93, 96, 102, 104, 105, 107, 108, 110, 112, 113, *169*
Covington, C. M., 154, *167*
Craft, M., 218, *234*
Craig, J. C., 3, 134, 143, 147, *169*
Craig, P. N., 26, 29, 30, 31, 32, 33, 128, 129, *162*, *169*, *176*, *187*, *188*, *191*
Craig, R. L., 76, *164*
Cranston, E. M., 77, 103, *169*
Cranswick, E. H., 204, 231, *246*
Craver, B. N., 38, *188*

Cremer, J. E., 73, *169*
Cremonesi, E., 229, *234*
Crémiaux, A., 226, *234*
Creveling, C. R., 260, 262, 263, *278*, *282*
Creze, J., 114, *169*
Crimmin, W. R. C., 148, *183*
Crisp, A. H., 155, *169*
Criswick, V. G., 217, *236*
Crockett, J. T., 145, *172*, *184*
Cromley, W. H., 47, *174*
Croufer, F., 226, *239*
Crouse, F. R., 153, 154, *184*
Crul, J. F., 247, *247*
Csaba, B., 97, *194*
Csák, A. Z., 109, *177*
Csegedy, J., 70, 76, *177*
Cuello, V. J., 260, *280*
Cuenca, E., 527, *531*
Cullíer, R. E., 33, *190*
Culling, C. F. A., 159, *188*
Cullumbine, H., 60, *162*
Culpan, R., 134, 136, *189*
Cummins, J. F., 114, *174*
Cuningham, J. A., 158, *169*
Cuocolo, R., 220, 229, *234*
Curry, S. H., 147, *163*
Curtis, D. R., 271, *278*
Cusic, J. W., 30, 127, *169*
Cutler, R. P., 151, *169*
Cutting, W., 42, *190*
Cwynar, S., 218, *234*
Czajkowski, N. P., 253, *279*
Czyba, J. C., 118, *180*

D

Dabbaa, M., 218, *233*
daCruz, A., 82, *169*
Dagan, 218, *234*
Dagand, 219, *247*
Dahlbom, R., 26, 145, 147, *162*, *169*
Dahlen, P., *191*
Dahlstrom, W. G., 152, *161*
Daigneux-Delhez, R., 218, 225, *232*
Dale-Horst, W., 527, *531*
Daly, J. W., 147, *168*, 258, 262, 263, *278*
Daly, M., 157, *188*
Damasio, R., 226, *234*
Dandiya, P. C., 70, 105, *169*
Danese, C., 86, *169*

Danhof, I. E., 76, *169*
Danik, J. J., 218, *234*
Danjard, J., 219, 226, *234, 243*
Danon, A., 103, *181*
Darcourt, G., 228, *234*
Das, N. N., 41, 50, 51, *169*
Das, P. K., 94, *162*
Dasgupta, S. R., 41, 43, 45, 50, 51, 54, 55, 82, 91, 102, *169, 170, 176*
Dashputra, P. G., 110, 121, *195*
da Silva, A. M., 219, 220, *239, 246*
Daskalov, Z., 219, *247*
Datta, R. K., 527, *531*
Dauch, 218, 219, *234, 247*
Daumézon, G., 226, *235*, 295, *300*
D'Auria, C., 229, *237*
Davey, M. J., 527, *531*
David, M., 53, *170*, 227, *235*
David, N. A., 62, *167*
Davidson, G. M., 153, *170*
Davidson, J. D., 135, 145, 147, *170*
Davies, B. M., 218, 219, *235, 242*
Davies, J. I., 67, *170*
Davis, J. M., 256, 262, 264, *278*
Davis, M. A., 298, *301*
Davis, R. V., 73, *186*
Davis, W. M., 45, *170*
Davoli, P., 218, *235*
Dawkins, M. J. R., 82, *170*
Dawson, B., 154, *186*
Dawson, J. F., Jr., 68, 71, *170*
Dayton, H. B., 47, *165*
de Alberquerque Fortes, J. R., 218, *233*
Dean, E. F., 161, *193*
DeBakey, M. E., 96, *188*
De Bellis, V., 229, *235*
Deberdt, R., 226, 227, *235*
DeBias, D. A., 97, *170*
De Blasi, S., 229, *235*
de Bruyne-Mottard, 219, *236*
de Carvalho, H. M., 218, *233*
De Casi, A., 219, *242*
De Castro, G., 220, *243*
Decaud, J., 68, *164*
Decortis, A., 109, *170*
Decourt, P., 91, 115, *170*
Decsi, L., 262, *278*
Décsi, L., 47, 82, *170*
De Eds, F., 3, *170*
Deegan, J., 49, *180*
Degelman, J., 154, *163*
De Gennes, L., 160, *170*

De Haene, A., 218, *235*
De Jaramillo, G. A. V., 134, *170*
De Kornfeld, J. J., 62, *183*
Delage, J., 155, *170*
Delahunt, C. S., 298, *301*
De La Pena Regidor, P., 67, *195*
Delavalade, 226, *237*
Delay, J., 38, 64, 76, 91, 94, *170*, 218, 224, 226, *235*
Deleau, D., 217, *241*
deLeeuw, J., 99, *167*
de Leonardis, M., 229, *236*
De Lerma Penasco, J. L., 218, *235*
Delgado, J. C., 224, *245*
Del Guerciom, L. R. M., 230, *248*
Deligné, P., 220, 227, *235*
Dell, P., 50, *178*
Della Beffa, A., 218, 224, *235*
Della Pietra, V., 218, 224, *235*
Della Rovere, M., 218, 224, *235*
Dell'omodarme, G., 529, *532*
DeLong, S. L., 159, *165, 170*
Delphaut, J., 43, *170*
DeMaar, E. W. J., 50, *170, 185*
Delrée, C., 204, 230, *232*
De Maio, D., 218, *235*
Demaret, A., 202, 221, 227, 230, *232, 236*
Dembicki, E. L., 114, *197*
De Meyer, R., 217, *236*
Demoen, P. J. A. W., 205, 217, *235, 240*
De Mondragon, C., 218, *235*
Dempsey, H., 152, *196*
Denavit, M., 230, *248*
Denber, H. C. B., 64, 160, 161, *170*, 218, *235*
Denckla, W. D., 260, *282*
Deneau, P. A., 153, *184*
Denenberg, V. H., 47, *170*
Denham, J., 160, *170*
Denhoff, E., 155, *170*
Deniker, P., 38, 64, 76, 91, 94, *170*, 224, 226, *235*
Denis, R., 229, *231*
Denner, J. L., 160, *193*
Denstedt, O. R., 143, *177*
Depoutot, J.-C., 226, *240*
Deprez, M., 218, *235*
De Risio, C., 43, *170*
Dermenghem, J. F., 226, 227, *243, 246*
Dermott, R. V., 160, *192*
Déro, M., 228, *245*

De Robertis, E., 529, *532*
De Ropp, R. S., 80, *170*
De Ryck, A., 226, 227, *235*
De Santis, S., 229, *234*
De Senarclens, F., 152, *170*
Deshpande, V. R., 81, 83, 118, *170*, *180*
Desmettre, G., 228, *231*
Dessaigne, S., 45, 118, *186*
Destombes, N., 161, *183*
Deviller, M., 148, 149, *170*
De Vleeschhouwer, G. R., 44, *170*
de Waart, C., 82, *172*
de Wied, D., 100, 102, *170*, *188*
Dews, P. B., 47, 50, 154, *171*
Dézsi, Z., 70, 76, *177*
Dhawan, B. N., 47, 96, *171*, *176*
Dick, P., 218, 224, *233*, *236*
Dickey, R. F., 159, *177*
Dickler, D., 67, *182*
Di Cristo, G., 219, *236*
Diègo, M., 229, *234*
Dietrich, E. V., 217, *248*
Dille, J. M., 50, 64, *172*, *178*, 286, *301*
Dillon, T. E., 153, 154, *184*
Di Mascio, A., 155, *171*
Dimmling, T., 115, *171*
Dingell, J. V., 137, *171*
D'Iorio, A., 523, *532*
Di Palma, J. E., 85, 151, *171*
Di Piazza, P., 224, *236*
Distel, R., 56, *168*
DiStefano, A. O., 269, *278*
Diverres, J. C., 42, *165*
Divry, P., 202, 217, 219, 221, 230, 231, *236*
Dixon, H. H., 83, *188*
Dixon, R. L., 137, *171*
Dizon, M., 62, 91, 94, 106, 108, 111, 112, 114, 152, *181*, *187*
Dobkin, A. B., 52, 55, 56, 71, 72, 85, 89, 92, 104, *171*, 217, 229, *236*, *239*
Doenicke, A., 220, 229, *236*, *238*
Dohan, F. C., 270, *282*
Dohmen, H., 82, *162*
Dolley, M., 219, *236*
Domanowsky, K., 220, *236*
Domer, F. R., 57, *171*
Domino, E. F., 61, 84, 132, *167*, *171*, *179*, 217, 229, *234*
Donat, K., 94, *174*
Dongier, M., 220, *236*, *238*
Dongièr, S., 220, *236*, *238*

Donnadieu, A., 94, 103, *171*
Donnet, J. L., 226, *235*
Donnet, V., 54, 139, 148, *171*, *176*
Dony, J. G. H., 213, 217, 229, *240*
Dotevall, G., 161, *171*
Doty, B. A., 43, *171*
Doty, L. A., 43, *171*
Doty, R. W., 43, 46, *191*
Doughty, R. B., 151, *163*
Douglas, A. D. M., 161, *171*
Doussinet, P., 224, *236*
Dresse, A., 217, *234*, *236*, *241*, *246*
Drill, V. A., 59, 63, 64, *194*
Dripps, R. D., 84, *171*, 229, *239*
Drouet, J., 140, *182*
Drouin, M., 75, *169*
Druart, R., 161, *176*
Dryon, L., 217, *247*
Dubin, A., 76, *189*
Dubois, C., 224, *236*
DuBois, K. P., 76, *186*
Dubost, P., 139, 147, 148, 149, *171*
Du Cailar, J., 229, *236*, *240*
Ducamin, 228, *247*
Ducet, G., 82, *162*
Duchastel, Y., 277
Duché, D. J., 220, *236*
Duchene-Marullaz, P., 54, 86, 87, 91, 94, *180*
Ducommun, P., 100, *171*
Ducrot, R., 3, 38, 45, 52, 55, 57, 60, 61, 62, 67, 68, 70, 71, 72, 74, 85, 86, 89, 90, 91, 92, 93, 96, 102, 104, 105, 107, 108, 110, 113, *169*, *177*
Duff, R. S., 92, *171*
Duhm, B., 139, *171*
Dumont, L., 118, *180*
Duncan, C. J., 114, *181*
Duncan, W. A. M., 137, *171*
Dundas, E., 155, *171*
Dundee, J. W., 69, *171*
Dupontreue, J., 148, *168*
Dupuy, R., 219, 224, *242*
Duquesne, L. P., 226, *244*
Durost, H., 219, 220, *231*, *236*
Dusinsky, G., 147, 149, *171*
Dussartre, J., 218, *233*
Dussik, K. T., 160, *193*
Dustan, H. P., 266, *281*
Dye, E. N., 156, *171*
Dykyj, R., 220, 236
Dyrberg, V., 220, *236*

E

Eades, C. G., 52, *185*
Earl, C. J., 158, *179*
Eberhard, F., 73, *171*
Eberhardt, H., 147, *171*
Ebersberger, E. M., 66, *195*
Ebert, A. G., 137, *178*
Eby, R. Z., 47, *174*
Eccleston, E., 268, *278*
Eckhardt, E. T., 83, *171*
Eckle, U., 158, *197*
Eckmann, F., 225, *236*
Eddy, N. B., 62, *171*
Edgerton, W. H., 33, *171*
Edgren, R. A., 83, *171*
Edwards, C. G., 153, *174*
Edwards, R. E., 298, *300*
Eechaute, W., 294, *300*
Egdahl, R. H., 100, *171*
Eger, W., 139, 147, *171*
Eggers, G. W. N., Jr., 84, *171*
Ehringer, H., 65, *171*, *178*, *278*
Eichenberger, E., 217, *247*
Eiduson, B. T., 251, *278*
Eiduson, S., 144, 145, 147, 148, *171*, *172*, *184*, 251, *278*
Eisdorfer, I. B., 147, *172*, *196*
Ekbom, K. A., 158, *164*
Ekman, L., 135, 147, *162*
Elam, C. B., 52, *166*
Elder, J. T., Jr., 64, *172*
Elder, O., 229, *236*
Elder, R., 229, *234*
Eldred, S. H., 273, *278*
Eliakim, M., 84, 95, 156, *172*
Elias, L., 229, *244*
Elissalde, B., 218, 220, *235*, *242*
Ellen, P., 56, *184*
Ellenbogen, W. C., 147, *172*
Ellin, R. I., 258, *279*
Elliott, K. A. C., 270, 271, *278*
Ellis, P. P., 159, *172*
Ellman, G. L., 114, *164*
Ellsworth, J., 47, *170*
Ellsworth, R. B., 153, *185*
Elo, R., 67, *172*
Elödi, P., 82, 137, *197*
Emmelin, N., 87, 91, *172*
Emmerson, J. L., 132, 139, *172*
Endicott, N. A., 152, *172*
Engelhardt, D. M., 151, *172*, *177*

Engelmeier, M. P., 227, *232*
Engels, W., 115, *190*
Enoch, M. D., 219, *236*
Ensor, Ch. R., 217, *234*
Enticknap, J. B., 161, *172*
Entwistle, C., 219, *236*
Eperjessy, Á., 70, 76, *177*
Epps, R. P., 160, *172*
Epstein, E. J., 153, *161*
Erdei, P., 70, 76, *177*
Erdos, E. G., 82, *172*
Erickson, R. W., 526, *531*
Ernst, A. M., 261, *278*
Ernsting, M. J. E., 82, *172*
Erslev, A. J., 158, *172*
Ervin, F. R., 147, 148, *167*
Espagno, G., 99, *186*
Essen-Möller, C., 274, *278*
Esser, A. H., 261, *280*
Esserman, H. B., 143, *172*
Essig, C. F., 50, *172*
Estler, C. J., 80, *172*
Estrada, E., 161, *172*
Estren, S., 160, *185*
Etzensperger, P., 45, *186*
Eunike, S., 230, *248*
Evans, D. A. P., 158, *172*
Evans, W. J., 25, *172*
Evans, W. O., 42, *172*
Evarts, E., 153, *181*
Evarts, E. V., 64, *162*
Evrard, E., 219, *236*
Exton-Smith, A. N., 156, *179*
Ey, H., 226, *236*
Eynetten, A., 145, 147, *198*
Ezz, E. A., 96, *185*

F

Fabian, L. W., 94, *165*
Fabierkiewicz, C., 147, *184*
Fabisch, W., 52, *172*
Fadiga, E., 51, *163*
Faggioli, L., 218, *235*
Faguet, M. M., 115, *172*
Faidherbe, J., 220, *236*, *238*
Failla, E., 219, *236*
Fairley, H. B., 155, *172*
Fajardo, S. G., 219, *236*
Fallard, R., 26, 32, *192*
Fanchamps, A., 64, *177*

Fanning, W. J., 160, *172*
Farkas, T., 204, 231, *246*
Farmer, J. B., 527, *531*
Farrand, E. A., 91, 96, *193*
Fau, R., 158, *172*
Faulkner, P., *277*
Faurbye, A., 158, *172*, 261, *278*
Favier, M., 219, *236*
Favre-Tissot, M., 226, *236*
Fazekas, J. F., 44, 71, 91, 92, *172*, *190*, *192*
Fedorov, N. A., 139, 141, 145, 147, 148, *172*
Feigley, C. A., 252, *279*
Feins, N., 230, *248*
Feldberg, W., 57, *171*
Feldman, P. E., 156, 159, *172*
Feldman, R. G., 41, *172*
Feldman, R. S., 46, *172*
Feldman, S., 84, 95, *172*
Feldmann, H., 220, *236*
Feldstein, A. M., 259, 268, *278*
Feller, K., 53, 70, 71, 94, *172*, *173*
Fellman, J. H., 148, 149, *173*
Fellows, E. J., 47, 79, 132, 160, *174*, *194*, *195*
Fels, I. G., 141, 147, 148, *173*
Fenters, J. D., 69, *173*
Ferguson, J. T., 161, *173*
Fernandez Lagravere, T. A., 269, *278*
Féron, A., 219, *238*, *239*
Ferrant, 226, *237*
Ferrari, H., 229, *234*, *236*, *237*
Ferrari, H. A., 229, *237*
Ferraris, E., 229, *233*
Ferreira, L. F., 219, *242*
Ferrero, A., 229, *234*
Ferrero, M., 219, *237*
Ferri, G., 219, *242*
Ferro, J., 229, *236*
Ferro-Diaz, P., 219, 226, *241*
Ferro-Milone, F., 219, *237*
Ferster, C. B., 48, *173*
Ferutta, A. M., 219, *237*
Field, W. E., 217, *248*
Fierlafyn, E., 220, 228, *237*
Filk, H., 55, 70, 71
Filmer, D. B., 138, 139, *197*
Fina, G., 218, *235*
Findlay, G. M., 3, 24, *173*
Finerty, M., 115, *189*
Finger, K. F., *277*, 298, *301*

Fink, G. B., 44, 52, 60, 63, *173*
Fink, M., 52, *173*
Finke, J., 286, *300*
Finkelstein, B. A., 115, *175*
Finkelstein, M., 74, 85, 93, *173*
Fiorito, L., 218, 224, *231*
Fisch, H. J., 152, *183*
Fischer, E., 269, *278*
Fischer, J., 527, *531*
Fischer, R., 158, *173*
Fishbein, W. N., 271, *278*
Fishman, V., 136, 138, 143, 144, 147, *173*, *175*
Fitts, D. D., 150, *188*
Fiume, S., 219, 224, *237*
Flacke, W., 71, *173*
Flanagan, T. L., 139, 145, 147, *173*, *178*, *191*, *196*
Flandrin, P., 158, *172*
Flataker, L., 253, 254, *281*, *282*
Flegel, H., 219, 224, 227, *237*
Fleming, R. M., 527, *531*
Fleming, W. W., 285, *301*
Fleury, C., 60, 62, *174*, 217, *237*
Flohil, J. M., 218, *233*
Florentin, M., 94, 103, *171*
Florentin, M. M., 94, 103, *171*
Florio, D., 218, *235*
Foldes, F. F., 82, *172*, 229, *237*
Follin, S., 153, *173*
Fontan, C. R., 147, *188*
Fontan, V., 161, *173*
Font du Picard, Y., 217, *232*, *233*
Foote, R. H., 102, *173*
Forcher, P., 72, 106, *167*
Forfar, J. O., 275, *278*
Forni, R. B., 73, *188*
Forrest, F. M., 134, 135, 140, 141, 145, 146, 147, 148, 149, *173*
Forrest, I. S., 134, 135, 137, 140, 141, 145, 146, 147, 148, 149, *173*, *188*, *196*
Forrest, J., 217, *232*
Forster, E., 68, *185*
Forster, K. S., 158, *176*
Fortin, R., 91, *168*
Fossoul, C., 147, 148, 149, *174*
Foster, C. A., 86, 92, *174*
Fotherby, K., 98, *174*
Fouks, 226, *237*
Foulks, R. G., *280*
Fournel, J., 38, 45, 52, 55, 57, 60, 61, 62, 67, 68, 70, 71, 72, 74, 85, 86, 89, 90, 91, 92,

93, 96, 102, 104, 105, 107, 108, 110, *169*, *174*
Fournier, M., 156, 158, *167*
Fourny, L., 219, *237*
Fouts, J. R., 137, 138, 139, *171*, *174*, 523, *532*
Fowler, P. J., 47, *174*
Fox, R. P., 82, *168*
Fox, W., 219, 223, 224, *234*, *237*
Foy, J. L., 151, *193*
Frahm, M., 114, 145, 147, 148, *163*, *174*
Franchi, G., 114, 148, *174*
Franchini, C., 219, *237*
Franco, N., 52, 56, *195*
Franco-Browder, S., 65, 108, *174*, *185*
Frank, M. M., 251, 252, *278*, *282*
Frank, T. V., 153, *192*
Frankau, I. M., 152, *174*
Frankova, S., 260, *279*
Frascella, G., 218, *232*
Fraser, H. F., 153, *174*
Fraser, R. S., 84, *165*
Fratello, U., 229, *237*
Frederickson, D. S., 274, *282*
Frederickson, W. K., 154, *197*
Freed, H., 152, 154, 155, 160, *174*
Freedman, D. X., 57, *174*, 261, 266, 272, *278*, *279*
Freedman, N., 151, *172*, *177*
Freeman, A. R., 76, *174*
Freeman, H., 268, *277*, *278*, *279*
Frélot, Cl., 219, *247*
Frenken, F., *279*
Fretwurst, E., 114, 145, 147, 148, *163*, *174*
Freund, H. G., 153, *187*
Freund, R. B., 76, *174*
Freundt, K. J., 147, *171*
Frey, H. H., 527, *531*
Frey, R., 229, *237*, *241*
Freyhan, F. A., 160, *174*, 273, *280*
Friebel, H., 62, 68, 115, *174*
Frieden, E., 252, *281*
Friedgood, C. E., 69, *190*
Friedhoff, A. J., 219, 226, *239*, 254, 258, 260, 261, *278*, *279*, *298*, *300*
Friedman, W., 118, *176*, *187*
Friedrich, R., 220, *237*
Friend, D. G., 114, *174*
Frierson, B. D., 159, *172*
Frignito, N., 152, 155, 160, *174*
Frogel, M., 151, *174*
Frohman, E. E., 253, *278* , *279*

Frommel, E., 60, 62, 66, *174*, *196*, 217, *237*
Fruchart, G., 161, *183*
Fry, W., 49, 50, *174*, *180*
Fuentes, O. A., 229, *236*, *237*
Fujii, K., 26, 27, 28, *174*
Fujimoto, J. M., 76, *189*, 529, *532*
Fujimoto, M., 136, *174*
Fujita, K., 78, *174*
Fujiwara, M., 528, *532*
Fuks, Z., 78, *191*
Fukuda, M., 99, *193*
Fuller, J. L., 50, *174*
Furchgott, R. F., 258, *279*
Furgiuele, A. R., 42, *174*, 527, *531*
Furst, A., 42, *190*

G

Gaddum, J. E., 266, *279*
Gadermann, E., 94, *174*
Gadient, F., 293, *300*
Gago, M. I., 219, *242*
Gahagan, L. H., 94, *184*
Gailitis, J., 160, *174*
Gailliot, P., 26, *166*
Gaitz, C. M., 153, *174*
Galbraith, G. C., 153, *174*
Gale, P. H., 260, *280*
Galibert, P., 161, *176*
Galindez, L., 219, *237*
Gallant, D. M., 153, *174*, 218, 219, 222, 223, *232*, *237*, *245*, 266, *279*, *300*
Gallo, G., 83, *197*
Gangloff, H., 50, *174*
Ganrot, P. O., 524, 526, *531*
Ganshirt, H., 74, *174*
Gantt, W. H., 47, *175*
Garattini, S., 65, *169*
Garbus, J., 60, *194*
Garcia-Rill, T., 219, *242*
Gardner, L. C., 50, *165*
Gardner, M. J., 153, *174*
Gardocki, J. F., 217, *237*, *248*
Garetz, F. K., 144, *174*
Garner, R. J., 82, *174*
Garry, J. W., 219, *237*
Gartner, H., 77, *188*
Gass, G. H., 104, *188*
Gastager, H., 225, *237*
Gastaut, H., 220, *236*, *238*
Gastel, R., 145, *168*

Gatgounis, J., 527, *531*
Gati, T., 104, *175*
Gatti, G., 219, *238*
Gattuso, R., 219, *238*
Gaudechon, J., 26, *166*
Gavaudan, L., 219, *238*
Gavin, J. G., 298, *301*
Gawienowski, A. M., 153, *185*
Gay, J. L., 76, *186*
Gayet-Hallion, T., 67, *164*
Gayral, L., 220, 226, 227, *238*, *246*
Geier, S., 219, 226, *247*
Geiger, A., 527, *531*
Geiger, H., 115, *175*
Geissmann, P., 226, *238*, *240*, *246*
Gelfand, M., 107, *175*
Geller, E., 144, *171*, 251, *278*
Gellhorn, E., 50, *195*
Gemperle, M., 229, *238*
Gerandal, C., 218, *233*
Gerard, J., 140, *182*
Gerard, R. W., *278*
Geraud, J., 219, *238*
Gerle, B., 219, 221, *238*
German, E., 224, *238*
German, G. A., 255, *279*
Germanova, K. I., 129, *192*
Gernay, J. M., 204, 224, 230, *232*
Gerrard, R. W., 49, *167*
Gershon, S., 112, 158, *184*, 261, *277*
Gerster, P., 155, *175*
Gesler, R. M., 287, *301*
Gessa, G. L., 527, *531*
Gey, K. F., 65, 79, 80, 81, *163*, *175*, *189*, 527, 530, *531*, *532*
Geyer, N., 155, *183*, 217, 219, *238*, *241*
Ghatge, N., 143, *161*
Ghosh, J. J., 527, *531*
Giacobini, E., 219, *238*
Giaja, J., 68, 70, 71, *175*
Gianasi, G. C., 220, *238*
Giancola, J. N., 273, *277*
Gianfranchi, M., 229, *238*
Gianelli, A., 219, *238*
Gianni, A. M., 114, 148, *174*
Gianniotti, G., 218, 224, *231*, *245*
Giao, T., 95, *175*
Giarman, N. J., 57, 80, *174*, *191*, 261, 266, 272, *279*
Gibbons, A. J., 76, *176*
Gibbons, T. B., 106, *175*
Gibbs, J. J., 154, *175*

Giberti Rosadini, I., 218, *231*
Gibson, W. C., *280*
Gigee, W. R., 97, *189*
Gilbert, R. G. B., 52, 55, 56, 71, 72, 85, 89, 92, 104, *171*
Giles, J. K., 84, *162*
Gilgash, C. A., 154, *175*
Gillespie, J. S., 264, *279*
Gillet, G., 219, *238*
Gillett, E., 43, *175*
Gillette, J. R., 134, 135, 137, 145, 147, 148, 149, *165*, *171*, *175*, *180*
Gilman, H., 25, *175*
Giordano, G. B., 219, 220, *234*, *238*
Giro, C., 105, *175*
Gitlow, S. E., 264, *279*
Gittelman, R. K., 152, *175*
Giudicelli, J. F., 217, *233*
Gjerris, F., 219, *238*
Gjessing, L. R., 261, 262, *281*
Gjuriš, V., 84, 95, *194*
Glasky, A., 84, *175*
Glaviano, V. V., 57, 58, *175*
Glende, E. A., 74, *175*
Glick, B. S., 151, *175*
Gliedman, L. H., 47, *175*
Glotzer, J., 151, *195*
Glowinski, M., 114, 147, *175*
Gobble, I. F., 219, 223, 224, *234*, *237*
Goble, S. L., 159, *185*
Göschke, H., 83, *175*
Goethe, H., 294, *300*
Goetzl, F. R., 286, *300*
Gözsy, B., 37, 109, *176*, *180*, 217, *241*
Goffioul, F., 224, *232*
Gold, E., 79, *191*
Gold, S., 139, 148, *175*
Goldberg, L. I., 528, *531*
Goldberg, M. E., 65, *175*
Goldenberg, H., 136, 138, 143, 144, 147, *173*, *175*
Goldin, A., 65, *166*
Goldin, S., 260, *281*
Goldman, D., 52, 151, *175*, 219, *238*
Goldring, S., 50, *175*
Goldsmith, R. W., 160, *175*
Goldstein, L., *279*
Goldstein, M., 258, *279*
Goldwurm, G. F., 217, 218, 219, 224, *233*, *238*
Gombos, G., 527, *531*
Gomez de la Sierra, B., 285, *301*

Gonçalves, B., 229, *238*
Gonçalves, J. A., 218, 219, *233*, *238*
Goncz, R. M., 273, *277*, *281*, *282*
Gonick, H. C., 520, *522*
Gonzalez, R. C., 47, 49, *175*
Good, W. W., 153, *175*
Goodall, M., 258, *279*, *281*, 526, *532*
Goodman, L. S., 57, 58, *165*, 284, *301*
Gordon, B., 161, *172*
Gordon, H. L., 155, *175*
Gordon, M., 3, 24, 26, 30, 31, 32, 33, 121, 129, 160, *169*, *171*, *175*, *176*, *187*, *191*, 291, 296, *300*
Gordon, M. H., 153, *167*
Gordon, M. W., 138, *176*
Gordon, R. A., 67, 99, *196*, 229, *243*
Gorham, D. R., 153, 154, *176*
Gori, E. C., 224, *236*
Gorkin, V. Z., 524, *531*
Gosline, E., 160, 161, *181*
Gothhelf, B., 527, *531*
Gottfries, C. G., 526, *531*
Gottlieb, J. S., 252, 253, 273, *278*, *279*, *280*
Gottlieb, L. S., 77, *176*
Goudet, A., 115, *172*
Gould, G. N., 161, *195*
Gourovitch, I. Y., 226, *231*
Gouzon, B., 139, 148, *176*
Goverdhan, M., 218, *234*
Govier, W. M., 83, 94, 96, *171*, *191*, *197*
Gowdey, C. W., 47, 96, 158, *167*, *176*
Gowen, G. F., 152, *176*
Goyne, J. B., 154, *194*
Grabow, L., 229, *238*
Gradwell, B. G., 153, *185*
Gralnick, A., 152, *172*
Grandjean, E., 42, *176*
Grasset, A., 38, 76, *170*
Grassi, F., 224, *245*
Gratton, L., 160, *165*
Graupner, K. I., 160, *190*
Graux, P., 161, *176*
Graves, G. D., 159, *193*
Gray, L. C., 102, *173*
Grebennik, L. I., 139, 148, 149, *176*
Greeff, K., 63, *163*
Green, A. L., 525, *531*
Green, D. E., 134, *169*
Green, D. M., 53, *189*
Green, H., 526, *531*
Green, J. P., 273, *278*, *279*
Greenberg, L., 98, 118, *176*

Greenberg, R., 81, *176*
Greenberg, S. M., 82, 83, 101, *176*, *185*
Greenfield, L., 69, *187*
Greengard, O., 50, *184*
Greengard, P., 75, 110, *176*, *190*
Greenhill, J. P., 152, *197*
Greenwood, D. J. 253, *280*
Gregory, I. D. R., 159, *166*
Greifenstein, F. E., 44, *162*
Greig, M. E., 76, *176*
Greiner, A. C., 159, *176*, *187*
Grenat, R., 91, 115, *170*
Grenell, R. G., 74, *176*
Gridnieva, L. I., 524, *531*
Griffin, F., 158, *173*
Griffin, P. J., 160, *176*, 288, *300*
Griffith, G. C., 521, *522*
Griffiths, P. D., 139, 148, *175*
Grillo, M. A., 262, *279*
Grimmett, J. D., 153, *185*
Grindlay, J. H., 105, *186*
Grisanti, M., 218, *235*
Grisoni, F., 219, *247*
Grönroos, M., 103, *176*
Groesswald, R., 120, *197*
Grof, S., 260, *279*
Groh, G., 217, *238*
Grolleau, D., 229, *240*
Gromova, E. A., 107, *176*
Gross, H., 228, *238*, *279*
Grossi, E., 82, *176*
Grossman, S. P., 45, 49, *176*
Grosz, H. J., 98, *176*
Groth, C., 155, *175*
Grover, J., 148, *176*
Grüber, H., 225, *237*
Grüninger, B., 229, *238*
Gruenstein, M., 104, *192*
Grunebaum, H. U., 273, *277*
Grunthaler, C., 228, *233*
Gruvel, G., 229, *238*
Gruvel, M., 229, *238*
Guccione, I., 96, *178*
Gudzinowicz, B. J., 141, *189*
Guerin, A., 161, *176*
Guerrin, F., 105, *195*
Gürtner, Th., 220, 229, *236*, *238*
Guesle, J., 104, *162*
Guha, G., 45, *176*
Guilbert, P., 219, *238*
Guillemin, R., 66, *182*
Gujral, M. L., 60, 96, *176*

Gulick, W. L., 56, *192*
Gundy, G., 268, *278*
Gunn, C. G., Jr., 50, 51, *176*
Gunster, J. C., 217, *237*
Gupta, G. P., 47, *171*
Gupta, S. K., 72, 110, 121, *176*, *195*
Gurd, F. R. N., 96, *179*, 254, *280*
Gutbub, T., 226, *238*, *240*, *246*
Guth, P. S., 39, 75, 134, *170*, *176*, *193*
Gutman, J., 55, *164*
Gutmann, F., 150, *176*
Guttman, H. N., 118, *176*
Guyotat, J., 228, *238*
Guze, S. B., 154, *195*
Gwynne, P. H., 153, *177*
Gyermek, L., 95, 109, *177*
Gylys, I., 82, *164*

H

Haahti, E. O. A., 147, *195*
Haarstad, J., 161, *177*
Haase, H. J., 151, *177*, 199, 223, 224, 228, 230, *238*
Haber, B., 138, *181*
Haberlandt, W. F., 220, *238*
Hach, V., *300*
Hachon, 218, *234*
Hackstein, F. G., 151, *177*, 225, *238*
Haddad, R. K., 255, *279*
Haden, P., 153, *177*
Hadnagy, C., 70, 76, *177*
Haefely, W., *279*
Haeger, K., 67, *162*
Häkkinen, H. M., *279*
Hafner, H., 158, *177*
Hafs, H. D., 113, *177*
Hagans, J. A., 153, *168*
Hagenbucher, J. T., 287, *300*
Hagerty, R. J., 160, *177*
Halasy, M., 219, 220, *242*
Halasz, M. F., 47, *177*
Halberg, F., 96, 98, *161*
Haley, T. J., 41, 94, 96, *177*, *197*, 286, *300*
Hall, G. H., 76, *177*
Hall, L. W., 95, 114, 161, *177*
Hallam, K. J., 144, *182*
Haller, H. L., 24, *166*

Halloran, A. V., 154, *193*
Hallot, A., 26, 32, *192*
Halpern, B. N., 3, *177*, 219, *247*
Hamacher, J., 121, *177*
Hamburger, C., 98, 99, *177*
Hamilton, L. D., 154, 155, 156, *163*
Hamilton, R. W., 30, 127, *169*
Hammen, C. S., 74, 85, 93, *173*
Hammer, H., 229, *239*
Hampson, L-G., 96, *179*
Hance, A. J., 50, 51, 52, *165*
Handcock, K. A., 151, *166*
Handford, S. W., 60, 67, *177*
Handley, C. A., 69, 91, 94, 106, 111, 114, *187*
Handley, P., 226, *239*
Hankoff, L. D., 151, *172*, *177*, 219, *244*
Hanlon, T. E., 144, 151, 153, *182*, *186*
Hannah, E. E., 158, *169*
Hanrahan, G. E., 91, *183*
Hansen, G., 219, *241*
Hansen, S., 159, *188*, 261, 262, *281*
Hanson, H. M., 47, 50, *177*, *179*, 521, 522
Hanson, R. K., 138, *176*
Hansson, E., 143, *177*, 527, *531*
Hapke, H. J., 81, *177*
Hara, T., 145, *179*
Harder, A., 219, *239*
Hardinge, M. G., 63, *177*
Hardy, R. A., Jr., 25, *165*
Hardy, W. G., 77, *163*
Harfenist, M., 25, *163*
Harl, J. M., 38, 76, *170*
Harmos, G., 104, *175*
Harnell, H., 273, *280*
Harper, J., 39, *177*
Harper, P., 260, 261, *277*
Harpur, R. P., 143, *177*
Harreveld, A. V., 270, *281*
Harrington, R. W., 151, *184*
Harris, A. F., 83, 109, *177*
Harris, H., 275, *279*
Harris, L. S., 297, *300*
Harris, S. B., 287, *301*
Harris, T. D., 57, 58, *165*
Harrison, C. V., 156, *190*
Harrison, S. I., 154, *177*
Harrison, T., 160, *189*
Hart, E. R., 50, *185*
Hart, L. G., 137, *171*
Hartman, D. L., 159, *177*

Hartmann, H., 55, *197*
Hartung, M. L., 228, *239*
Hartung, W. H., 258, *279*
Harwood, C. T., 100, *177*
Harwood, P. D., 143, *177*
Hashimoto, K., 159, *177*
Hassert, G. L., Jr., 38, *188*
Hauschild, F., 55, *197*
Hausler, H. F., 55, 102, *169*
Hausler, L. M., 94, *197*
Hausman, M., 25, *187*
Hausner, M., *196*
Havens, L. L., 155, *171*
Haverback, B. J., 104, *177*
Haward, L. R. C., 151, *177*, 219, *239*
Hawkins, D. R., 153, 154, *177*
Hawkins, H. M., 153, *174*
Haworth, D. H., 155, *183*
Hayaishi, O., 258, *279*
Hayashi, K., 145, *179*, 524, *532*
Haynes, E. E., 145, 147, 148, *177*
Hays, G. B., 159, *177*
Hazard, R., 64, *177*
Hazel, M., 77, *176*
Hearst, E., 134, 136, *189*
Heath, R. G., 50, 52, *186*, 252, *279*
Heaton, A., 144, *173*
Heider, C., 69, *187*
Heilizer, F., 153, *177*
Heim, H. C., 82, *194*
Heimlich, K. R., 145, *178*
Heinrich, H., 227, *232*
Heinrich, K., 228, *239*
Heistad, G. T., 50, *178*
Hekimian, L. J., 219, 226, *239*, 298, *300*
Helrich, M., 220, *239*
Hemphill, R. E., 151, *178*
Henne, M., 161, *178*
Henne, S., 161, *178*
Henneman, D. H., 273, *277*
Henriksen, R. I., 147, *178*
Henriksen, U., 139, 148, *178*
Henschel, W. F., 229, *239*
Herbst, H., 3, 30, *192*
Herman, E. H., 40, *178*
Herman, L., 153, *188*
Hermans, B., 205, 217, *240*, *247*
Herndon, J. F., 82, 83, 101, *176*, *185*
Herold, W., 154, *163*
Herr, F., 41, 60, 61, *178*
Herrero Aldama, P., 218, *233*
Herschberg, A. D., 226, *234*

Herschberger, R., 71, 92, *187*
Hershey, S. G., 67, 84, 96, *178*, *184*
Hertting, G., 65, 81, 84, *162*
Herxheimer, H., 109, *178*
Hess, H., 154, *191*
Hess, S. M., 137, *178*, 258, *279*
Hetzel, C. A., 148, *178*
Heyck, H., 71, *178*
Heyman, J. J., 145, 148, 149, *178*
Hickens, M., 260, *280*
Hiebel, G., 50, *178*
Hiestand, W. A., 68, 69, 71, 72, *170*, *187*, *197*
Hift, S., 94, *162*
High, J. P., 38, 137, *166*, *188*
Highman, B., 530, *531*
Hilarp, N. A., 217, *233*
Hildebrandt, G., 121, *177*
Hilgers, H., 220, *239*
Hill, L. D., 106, *175*
Hill, S. R., Jr., 152, *196*
Himbert, J., 86, 89, 90, *189*
Himwich, H. E., 40, 65, *194*, 261, 268, 269, 276, *277*, *278*, *279*, *280*, *282*, 291, *301*
Hinz, J. E., 84, *188*
Hippius, H., 151, *178*, 227, *232*
Hirsch, D. L., 158, *178*
Hirsch, S., 158, *178*
Hiss, R. A., 48, *173*
Hoagland, H., 268, *277*, *278*, *279*
Hoagland, R. J., 152, *178*
Hodge, J. R., 160, *178*
Hodgetts, V. E., 77, *195*
Hoehn-Saric, R., 154, *178*
Hoerlein, U., 120, *197*
Hoffenberg, R., 152, *178*
Hoffer, A., 261, *280*, *281*
Hoffman, D., 87, *166*
Hoffman, M. M., 106, *193*
Hoffman, R. A., 69, *178*
Hoffmann, I., 5, 121, 139, *178*, *187*
Hoffmann, M., 229, *239*
Hofmann, S., 220, 229, *239*
Hohl, H. H., *278*
Holdaway, I., 118, *186*
Holden, R. H., 155, *170*
Holderness, M. C., 229, *239*
Holland, D., 158, *172*
Holliday, A. R., 50, *178*
Holliday, P. D., 273, *277*, *281*, *282*
Hollister, F. P., 219, *239*

Hollister, L. E., 72, 115, 145, 148, 153, 156, 158, 160, 161, *167*, *178*, *183*, *189*, 219, 222, *239*, 298, *300*
Holmstedt, B., *178*
Holstein, A. P., 219, *239*
Holzbauer, M., 54, 87, 89, 91, 98, 99, *178*
Holzman, W. H., 153, *175*
Holzmann, C., 25, *178*
Honigfeld, G., 219, *239*
Hooper, J. H., Jr., 152, *178*
Hoover, M. P., 152, *178*
Hopkin, D. A. B., 55, 161, *178*, *190*
Hopkins, G. W., 154, *193*
Hopkins, T. H., 103, *194*
Horanská, D., *196*
Horclois, R. J., 28, *178*
Hordern, A., 151, *178*
Horita, A., 526, 529, 530, *531*
Hormia, A., 97, *178*
Horn, L., 97, *178*
Horner, S. R., 47, *161*
Horning, E. C., 147, *195*
Hornykiewicz, O., 65, 81, *171*, *178*, *278*
Horovitz, Z. P., 40, *178*
Horton, J. M., 220, 229, *233*, *239*
Horváth, E., 77, 100, *182*
Horvath, S. M., 91, 96, *178*, *193*
Horwitt, M. K., 82, *167*
Horwitz, D., 519, *522*, 528, *531*
Hoskin, F. C. G., 82, *179*
Hospigliosi, L., 219, *243*
Houde, R. W., 67, *179*
Hougs, W., 107, *179*
Houillon, 219, *239*
Houser, E., 270, *282*
Howard, R. E., 76, *166*
Howlett, J. G., 106, *193*
Howorth, P. J. N., 261, *280*
Hoyon, A., 220, *246*
Hrdek, J., *179*
Hsi-Jui, W., 81, *179*
Huang, C. L., 140, 141, 143, 144, 147, *179*, *182*
Huang, S. H., 50, *175*
Hudson, R. D., 84, *179*
Hürlimann, A., *279*
Huestis, D. W., 106, *193*
Huete-Armijo, A., 156, *179*
Huggens, J., 299, *301*
Huggins, R., 91, 94, 106, 111, 114, *187*
Hughes, F. W., 47, 50, 62, *179*, *181*

Huguenard, P., 38, 68, 96, *162*
Huguet, P., 226, *235*, 295, *300*
Huidobro, F., 84, 86, 87, 88, 91, 104, 107, *179*
Hukuhara, T., 285, *300*
Hulak, S., 219, *239*
Hull, L. J., 529, *531*
Humbeeck, L., 219, *239*
Humphreys, S. R., 65, *166*
Humphries, O., 153, 155, *181*
Hunder, G., 96, *179*
Hundziak, M., 153, *177*
Hunkar, K., 80, *185*
Hunter, J. H., 30, *190*
Hunter, R., 158, *179*
Huntsman, R. G., 139, 148, *175*
Huntz, A., 70, 76, *177*
Huntzinger, J. A., 47, *179*
Hunziker, F., 217, *247*, 290, *300*
Huot, L., 118, *179*
Hurkmans, J. A. T., 529, *532*
Husa, W. J., 79, *197*
Hussey, L. M., 114, *179*
Hutchinson, E. D., 50, *165*
Huus, I., 139, 148, *178*
Huygens, J., 217, *246*
Hye, H. K. A., 74, *161*

I

Ichimary, S., 228, *241*
Ideström, C. M., 153, *179*, 228, *239*
Iizuka, R., 113, *197*
Imlah, N. W., 519, *522*
Immich, H., 225, *236*
Ingalls, G. W., 98, *176*
Ingalls, J. W., 118, *176*
Inglis, F. G., 96, *179*
Ingram, C. G., 66, *179*
Ingvar, D. H., 50, *179*, 217, *239*
Inouye, A., 266, *280*
Inscoe, J. K., 258, *278*
Invernizzi, G., 219, *238*
Irwin, S., 38, 41, 45, 46, *179*
Isaacs, B., 58, 59, *179*
Isbell, H., 153, *174*
Isenberg, I., 150, *180*

Israel, J. S., 229, *236*, *239*
Israel, L., 226, *238*, *239*
Itil, T., 52, *164*
Ito, T., 78, *174*
Ivy, A. C., 286, *300*
Iwamoto, S., 228, *239*
Iwasa, K., 145, *179*
Iwase, S., 78, *174*
Izquierdo, I., 45, *179*

J

Jackson, D., 69, *179*
Jackson, J., 47, *179*
Jackson, J. A., 50, *168*
Jacob, E., 219, *239*
Jacob, R. M., 30, *179*
Jacobs, R., 219, 225, *239*, *247*
Jacobsen, P., 24, *186*
Jacobson, M. M., 530, *531*
Jacobziner, H., 160, *179*
Jacques, G. R., 30, *179*
Jaeggi, F., 220, *239*
Jaffe, G. E., 32, *162*
Jageneau, A. H. M., 41, 58, *179*, 203, 205, 217, *240*, *246*, 299, *301*
Jain, M. S., 25, *182*
Jaiswal, C. L., 110, 121, *195*
Jaitly, K. D., 103, *164*
Jameson, D., 270, *282*
Jamieson, D., 69, *179*
Jancar, J., 220, *239*
Janeway, K. P., 32, *162*
Janke, W., 226, *239*
Jannsse, G. T., 229, *239*
Janssen, P. A. J., 41, 42, 58, 121, *179*, 199, 202, 203, 204, 205, 209, 211, 213, 214, 215, 217, 220, 223, 229, 230, *238*, *239*, *240*, *244*, *246*, *247*, 295, 296, 297, 299, *300*, *301*
Janssens, J., 96, *180*
Janz, D., 158, *179*
Jaquenoud, P., 229, *236*, *240*
Jarrett, R. J., 103, *180*
Jasmin, G., 109, *180*, *277*
Jason, M., 227, *242*
Jasper, H. H., 270, *278*
Jaulmes, C., 38, 68, 96, *180*, *182*
Jean, B., 219, *246*

Jenkins, H. J., 60, *184*, 528, *531*
Jenkins, R. L., 218, *234*
Jenkins, S. B., 78, 151, *180*
Jenney, E. H., 284, *300*
Jenny, B., 219, *236*
Jensen, O., 219, *240*
Jenson, R. E., 153, *187*
Jesdinski, H. J., 220, *248*
Jeter, W. S., 69, *173*
Jervett, A., 42, *172*
Jindal, M. N., 61, 83, 110, 121, *180*, *195*
Jinks, R., 102, *170*
Jönsson, B., 145, 147, *162*
Jóhannesson, T., 73, *180*
Johansson, M., 66, *180*
Johnson, D. E., 145, *180*
Johnson, G., 70, *169*
Johnson, G. E., 68, *180*, 527, *531*
Johnson, H. E., 65, *175*
Johnson, P. C., 145, *180*
Joiner, P. D., 139, 147, *196*
Jones, B. E., 52, *196*
Jones, C. J., 96, *180*
Jones, D. H., 72, *183*
Jones, D. J., III, 153, 154, *184*
Jones, L. M., 97, *180*
Jongkees, L. B. W., 60, *180*
Joseph, A. D., 72, *176*
Joseph, L., 160, *192*
Josephs, Z. M., 151, *180*
Jouany, J. M., 140, *182*
Jourdan, F., 54, 86, 87, 89, 91, 94, *180*
Jouvet, M., 50, 51, *176*
Joye, E., 217, *237*
Joynt, R. J., 41, *180*
Jucker, E., 204, 231, *240*, 283, 293, *300*
Judah, J. D., 75, 82, *170*, *180*
Judah, L. N., 151, 153, *174*, *180*
Judson, A. J., 154, *180*
Jünemann, H. J., 219, 228, *246*
Juillet, P., 228, *240*
Jullien, G., 111, *191*
Just, O. H., 229, *240*
Juszkiewicz, T., 97, *180*

K

Kaada, B. R., 50, *192*
Kabat, H., 219, *240*
Kácl, K., 147, *195*

Kaczynski, M., 219, *240*
Kaelber, W. W., 41, 50, *180*
Kafoe, W. F., 82, *172*
Kahen, I., *280*
Kahlson, G., 273, *280*
Kahn, D. R., 229, *234*
Kaiser, C., 32, *162*
Kajdi, L., 285, *300*
Kajikuri, H., 96, *180*
KaKimoto, Y., 261, *282*
Kakolewski, J., 217, *240*
Kalandarishvili, A. S., 151, *165*
Kalberer, F., 135, 138, 144, *180*, *191*, *198*
Kaldahl, T., 157, *188*
Kalinovskaya, R. Y., 155, *180*
Kalkoff, W., 86, 90, *180*
Kalliomäki, J. L., 103, *176*
Kalz, F., 152, *183*
Kamano, A., 138, *181*
Kamenskaia, V. M., 219, *240*
Kamio, K., 114, *194*
Kamm, J. J., 134, 135, 137, 147, 148, 149, *175*, *180*
Kammerer, T., 226, *240*
Kamphausen, H., 219, *240*
Kandaperredy-Tellier, C., 220, *240*
Kandaurova, Yu. N., 217, *240*
Kaneko, J., 228, *241*
Kant, F., 151, *180*
Kanter, S. L., 72, *178*
Kapferer, J. M., 220, *241*
Kaplan, N. O., 65, *166*
Karapetyan, M. G., 129, *192*
Karczmar, A. G., 56, 141, 147, 148, *173*, *184*
Karok, 45
Karoly, A. J., *180*
Karp, M., 91, *180*
Karpovich, J. A., 158, *180*
Karreman, G., 150, *180*
Kassay, G., 80, *185*
Kastner, H., 62, 68, 115, *174*
Katila, O., 226, *241*
Kátó, L., 37, 61, 109, *176*, *180*, 217, *241*
Kato, R., 61, *180*
Katoaka, K., 266, *280*
Katona, F., 119, *180*
Katsas, G. G., 160, *161*
Katscher, J., 228, *241*
Katz, R., 217, *248*
Kauffman, D., 218, *235*
Kaufman, M., 141, 147, 148, *173*

Kaufman, M. A., 113, 140, *190*
Kaufmann, M. J., 41, 84, *180*
Kautschitsch, J., 153, *177*
Kawakami, M., 50, *195*
Kawasaki, A., 139, *187*
Kawi, D., 219, *244*
Kay, L. L., 287, *301*
Kaye, H., 154, *191*
Kayser, C., 68, *185*
Keating, V., 99, *180*
Kečkeš, S., 84, 101, 102, *194*
Keddie, K. M. G., 521, *521*
Keeler, C. E., 147, *186*
Keéri-Szanto, M., 229, *231*, *233*, *241*
Keéri-Szanto, N., 229, *231*
Kehl, R., 118, *180*
Keitel, P., 223, *241*
Kelemen, K., 46, *180*
Keleti, T., 81, 137, 140, *197*
Kelleher, R. T., 48, 49, 50, *168*, *174*, *180*
Keller, C., 157, *189*
Kelly, F. E., 151, *196*
Kelly, F. H., 101, *185*
Kelly, R. E., 107, 108, *181*
Kelsey, J. R., Jr., 106, *181*
Kemali, D., 255, *279*, *280*
Kennon, L., 140, *190*
Kent, B., 62, 91, 94, 106, 108, 111, 112, 114, 152, *181*, *187*
Kent, D. A., 219, *241*
Kent, G., 76, *189*
Kepes, E. R., 229, *237*
Keranen, G. M., 66, *181*
Kern, R., 229, *241*
Kerr, E. M., 161, *163*
Kerr, M., 107, *161*
Kertész, L., 101, *162*
Kesner, R., 43, 114, *197*
Kessler, E. K., 153, *182*
Kety, S. S., 251, 260, 261, 264, 273, 274, 276, *278*, *280*, *281*, *282*
Key, B. J., 46, 50, 51, 64, *165*, *181*
Keyriläinen, T. O., 103, *176*
Khanna, B. K., 60, *176*
Khazan, N., 103, 118, *181*
Khera, S., 155, *183*
Kherdikar, P. R., 61, *180*
Khorsandian, R., 220, 231, *244*
Khouw, L. B., 83, *181*
Khrabrova, O. P., 96, *181*
Kidron, D. P., 95, *172*
Kiel, H., 227, *241*

AUTHOR INDEX

Kiger, J. G., 146, *181*
Kiger, J. L., 146, *181*
Killam, E. K., 50, *181*
Killam, K. F., 50, 57, *181*, *187*, 270, *281*
Kim, K. S., 528, *531*
Kimbell, I., 153, *174*, 219, 222, *239*, 298, *300*
Kimsey, L. R., 114, *197*
Kimura, T., 50, *181*
Kinbergen, B. A., 132, *181*
Kinberger, B., 145, 147, 148, 149, *181*
King, E. E., 50, 51, *176*
King, F. A., 42, *186*
King, P. D., 160, *181*
King, T. O., 44, *170*
Kingston, W. R., 158, *192*
Kinnard, W. J., 42, *174*, 527, *531*
Kinnard, W. J., Jr., 41, 42, *181*
Kinross-Wright, J. V., 103, 139, 147, *181*, *190*
Kipman, S. D., 226, *245*
Kirberger, E., 529, *531*
Kirk, P. L., 146, 147, *188*, *190*
Kirpekar, S. M., 82, *181*
Kirschner, M., 258, 264, *279*
Kirshner, N., 256, *280*
Kiseleva, N. A., 75, 83, *198*
Kiss, A., 70, 76, *177*
Kistner, R. W., 114, *181*
Kistner, S., 82, *181*
Kitay, J. I., *280*
Kivalo, E., 82, *181*, 219, *241*
Klatskin, G., 156, *181*
Klebe, H., 33, *192*
Kleeman, C. R., 520, *522*
Kleh, J., 287, *300*
Klein, F., 53, 94, *164*, *170*
Klein, M., 67, *184*
Klein, M. J., 94, *197*
Kleinsorge, H., 145, 147, 148, *181*
Klenk, E., 275, *280*
Klepping, J., 69, *194*
Klerman, G. L., 155, *171*
Klett, C. J., 153, 155, 156, *166*, *167*, *181*, *183*
Kline, N. S., 155, 160, 161, *181*, *193*, 261, *280*
Kloppenstein, M. H., 50, *194*
Klugman, S., 153, *181*
Knight, M., 113, *190*
Knight, R. W., 62, 91, 94, 106, 108, 111, 112, 114, 152, *181*, *187*
Knopp, W., 158, *173*
Knowles, R. R., 160, *174*

Knox, J. M., 159, *181*
Kobayashi, Y., 527, *531*
Koch, L., 287, *300*
Koch, R., 98, 100, *182*
Kochan, I., 115, *189*
Kochhar, K. S., 155, *181*
Koechlin, B., 525, *531*
Koella, W., *279*
Koester, L., 139, *171*
Koetschet, P., 38, 45, 52, 55, 57, 60, 61, 62, 67, 68, 70, 71, 72, 74, 85, 86, 89, 90, 91, 92, 93, 96, 102, 104, 105, 107, 108, 110, *169*
Koeze, T. H., 113, *181*
Kohl, H., 269, *277*
Kohl, H. H., 138, *181*
Kohler, C., 226, 227, *242*
Kohn, N. N., 156, *181*
Koivusalo, M., 527, *531*
Kok, K., 82, 139, 147, 148, *181*
Kollias, J., 70, *181*
Kolloff, H. G., 30, *190*
Kolosov, M. N., 129, *192*
Kolsky, M., 38, 45, 52, 55, 57, 60, 61, 62, 67, 68, 70, 71, 72, 74, 85, 86, 89, 90, 91, 92, 93, 96, 102, 104, 105, 107, 108, 110, *169*
Komisarova, N. V., 524, *531*
Kooi, K. A., 151, 154, *163*
Kopeloff, L. M., 53, 108, *181*
Kopeloff, N., 53, 108, *181*
Kopera, J., 60, 62, 68, 85, 86, 88, 107, 108, 110, *181*
Kopf, R., 139, 148, *178*
Kopin, I. J., 258, 262, 268, *277*, *280*, 523, 527, *531*
Kopin, I. L., 65, 84, *162*
Kopmann, E., 47, 50, *179*, *181*
Korduba, C. A., 143, *194*
Kornetsky, C., 153, 155, *181*, *182*, 273, *282*
Korneva, E. A., 54, 85, *182*
Kory, M., 525, *531*
Kosir, B., 149, *182*
Kosir, J., 149, *182*
Kotionis, A. Z., 148, 149, *182*
Kotkin, S., 67, *182*
Kovács, B. M., 77, 100, 101, *182*
Kovács, G. S., 77, 100, 101, *182*
Kovács, K., 77, 100, 101, *182*
Kovitz, B., 154, *182*
Kozák, J., 82, *182*
Kraines, S. H., 151, *182*
Krais, W., 77, 102, 114, *182*, *188*

Krall, A. R., 270, *280*
Kramer, E. R., 65, *167*
Kraus, B., 220, *241*
Krause, D., 87, 88, 90, *182*
Kreindler, A., 50, *182*
Kreis, W., 135, 152, *198*
Kreiskott, H., 120, *197*
Kretzschmar, E., 76, *192*
Kreuscher, H., 217, 229, *237*, *241*
Kris, E. B., 114, *182*
Krishna, S., 25, *182*
Kristjansen, P., 218, 219, 224, *233*, *241*
Krivoy, W. A., 44, 57, 66, *182*
Kroeger, D. C., 57, *182*
Krüger, H. J., 219, 228, *246*
Kruger, S., 78, *182*
Krupp, P., 50, *186*
Kuchler, A., 98, 100, *182*
Kuehl, F. A., 260, *280*
Kuehn, W. F., 217, *237*
Kuenssberg, E. V., 284, *300*
Kugelberg, J., 217, 220, *244*
Kugler, J., 229, *236*
Kuizenea, M. H., 3, *195*
Kulcsar, S., 103, *189*
Kulikov, L. S., 155, *182*
Kulling, R. K., 297, *300*
Kulonen, E., *279*
Kum-Tatt, L., 150, *182*
Kuntzman, R., 262, *278*, 530, *531*
Kunz, E., 204, 231, *246*
Kurland, A. A., 143, 144, 147, 151, 153, *179*, *182*, *186*, 219, 226, *241*
Kurogochi, Y., 74, 82, *198*
Kushner, D., 76, *189*
Kutin, V. P., 151, *182*
Kutscher, I., 158, *177*
Kuttner, R. E., 138, *176*
Kwang Yi Lee, P., 229, *236*
Kyne, W. P., 153, *198*

L

La Barre, J., 217, *241*
Labhardt, F., 219, *241*
Laborit, H., 38, 68, 74, 96, 140, *180*, *182*,*183*
Labrosse, E. H., 153, *185*, 260, *280*
Lacassagne, A., 77, *183*
Lacerda, N., 219, *238*
Lacomme, M., 114, *183*
Lacourt, J., 219, *241*

Lacroix, E., 294, *300*, 528, *531*
Ladinskaya, M. Y., 50, *183*
La Du, N., 145, *165*
Laffan, R., 137, *166*
Laffargue-Leugerinel, B., 220, *241*
Lafferty, J. J., 29, 30, 31, 33, 128, 129, *169*, *188*
Lagercrantz, C., 140, *183*
Lagocki, A. M., 219, *242*
Laine, 226, *237*
Lal, H., 525, *532*
L'Allemand, H., 69, *165*
Lamarche, M., 105, *183*
Lamb, V. E., 91, *180*
Lambert, P., 160, *166*
Lambert, P. A., 219, 228, *241*
Lambertsen, C. J., 155, *183*
Lamoureaux, L., 52, 55, 71, 72, 92, 104, *171*
Lampé, L., 101, *162*
Lampo, B., 220, *245*
Lancaster, N. P., 72, *183*
Lands, A. M., 119, *184*
Lang, N., 82, *182*
Lang, W. J., 261, *277*
Langer, R., 229, *241*
Langeron, L., 161, *183*
Langner, E., 228, *238*
Lanman, R. C., 78, *191*
Lanteri, G., 219, *238*
Laporte, J., 77, *183*
Larrostis-Bicheron, C., 219, *245*
Larson, A. G., 229, *241*
Larsson, S., 80, *183*
Lasagna, L., 62, 112, *183*
Lasky, J. J., 153, 156, *167*, *183*
Lassenius, B., 145, 147, 148, *181*, 219, *238*, 284, *300*
Lassner, J., 219, *241*
Latham, L. K., 252, 253, 273, *278* , *279*, *280*
Laties, V. G., 50, *183*, *197*
La Veck, G. D., 520, *522*
Lauber, H., 219, *237*
Lauener, H., 217, *247*, 290, *300*
Laüterback, C. G., 154, *175*
Launay, J., 41, 94, *163*
Laurans, J., 224, *241*
Laurence, D. R., 107, 108, *181*, *183*
Lausen, H. H., 73, *180*
Lavagna, J., 228, *234*
Lavallée, J. P., 229, *233*, *241*
Laveneziana, D., 229, *232*
Lavigne, S., 56, *168*

Lavitola, G., 219, *241*
Lawin, P., 229, *241*
Lawson, J. I. M., 220, *241*
Laxdal, O. E., 155, *183*
Lázár, I., 109, *177*
Lazarus, M., 143, *183*
Leach, B. E., 252, *279*
Leach, H., 148, *183*
Leahy, M. R., 293, *300*
Leandri, M., 111, *191*
Lear, E., 67, 152, *182*, *183*
Leary, R. W., 50, *183*
Leahy, M. R., 519, *522*
Leblanc, J., 118, *179*
LeBlanc, J., 69, 77, 97, *183*
LeBlanc, J. A., 69, 70, 72, 77, 97, *183*
Le Breton, R., 61, *183*
Lechat, P., 217, *241*
Lechner, H., 155, *183*, 217, *241*
Lechner, K., 65, 81, *171*, *178*
Lecoeur, J. L. J., 219, *241*
Lecomte, J., 109, *170*, 217, *236*, *241*, *246*
Lecoq, R., 228, *232*, *234*
Lecourt, P., 87, *166*
Leder, M., 139, *164*
Ledesma Jimeno, A., 219, *241*
Lee, C. Y., 107, *194*
Lee, H., 219, 224, 228, *236*, *248*
Lee, P. K. Y., 229, *236*
Lee, R., 160, *192*
Lees, H., 253, *279*, *280*
Lefever, H. E., Jr., 153, 154, *184*
Lefton, M., 153, *177*
Le Gaudu, J., Fr., 226, *241*
Le Goaziou, F., 220, *241*
Le Guen, C., 224, *241*
Lehembre, J., 224, *241*
Lehman, H., 275, *280*
Lehmann, H., 261, *280*
Lehmann, H. E., 37, 63, 91, *163*, *180*, *183*, 219, *242*, *247*
Lehoczki, T., 219, 220, *242*
Lehr, H., 102, 114, *182*
Léider, L. L., 144, 146, *174*, *183*
Leijnse, B., 521, *522*, 529, *531*, *532*
Leitenberg, M., 65, *166*
LeLorier, G., 114, *183*
Lemaire, E., 161, *183*
Leme, J. G., 111, *183*
Lemieux, M., 217, *238*, *241*
Lempérière, T., 218, 224, *235*
Lenke, D., 66, *183*

Leonard, T. J., 219, *237*
Leone, B. N., 219, *242*
Leopold, I. H., 91, 112, *188*
Lepage, C., 229, *233*
Lerbs, O. W., 147, *171*
Lerman, M. I., 524, *531*
Lesinski, J., 114, *183*
Leslie, N. H., 230, *245*
Leslie, S. A., 260, 261, *277*
Lessin, A. W., 69, 79, 82, *183*, *184*
Lester, B. M., 30, 31, 32, 129, *162*, *169*
Lester, E. P., 152, *183*
Leterrier, F., 74, *183*
Letienne, R., 52, 55, 71, 72, 92, 104, *171*
Leusen, I., 294, *300*, 528, *531*
Levassort, C., 69, *167*
Le Vay, M. K., 151, *184*
Lever, P. G., 160, *193*, 270, *280*
Lever, W. F., 254, *280*
Levi, P. G., 218, 224, *232*, *242*
Levi-Minzi, S., 224, *236*
Levin, M. J., 67, *191*
Levin, M. L., 153, *184*
Levine, D., 149, *184*
Levine, E. H., 111, *188*
Levine, J., 134, 136, 149, *184*, *189*
Levine, N. M., 76, *174*
Levine, S., 67, 154, *184*, *191*
Levitov, M. M., 129, *192*
Levitt, M., 256, *280*
Levrie, J., 226, *235*
Levy, H. A., 220, 229, *244*
Lévy, J., 217, *233*
Lewis, J. J., 24, 39, 82, *181*, *184*, 284, 296, *300*
Lewis, T. R., 297, *300*
Lewis, W. H., Jr., 94, *184*
Leyla, M., 219, *246*
Leyritz, M., 219, *242*
Liberson, W. T., 41, 56, *184*
Liljestrand, A., 159, *184*
Lillehei, R. C., 96, *184*
Limanski, M., 114, 147, *175*
Lin, T. H., 139, 144, 147, 148, *173*, *184*
Lindan, O., 82, *184*
Lindell, S. E., 66, *180*
Lindenmann, A., 293, *300*
Lindenmuth, W. W., 152, *176*
Lindlar, H., 294, *300*
Lindley, C. L., 153, *167*
Lindqvist, M., 217, *233*

Lindqvist, R., 219, *242*
Linford Rees, W. L., 219, *242*
Lingjaerde, O., 253, *282*
Lioanag, E. M., 224, *244*
Lipschutz, S., 26, 31, 32, 129, *187*
Lipton, B., 67, 84, *184*
Lisdky, A., 219, *247*
Litin, E. H., 152, *184*
Litteral, E. B., 67, 152, *184*, *194*
Livingston, S., 285, *300*
Llewellin, W. L., 45, *170*
Lods, J. C., 219, 224, *242*
Loeffler, K. O., 134, *169*
Loennecken, S. J., 94, *166*
Loeser, A., 55, 65, 70, 71, *173*, *188*
Loewe, S., 63, *184*
Loftus, T. A., 153, 154, *184*
Loguloso, E., 218, *232*
Lohrenz, J. G., 151, *166*
Long, J. P., 119, *184*
Long, R. F., 79, *184*
Longenhagen, J. B., 155, *183*
Longo, V. G., 51, 52, *184*
Longobardi, A., 160, *174*
Lorcy, P., 156, *167*
Loret, L., 219, *242*
Lorian, V., 115, *189*
Lorizio, A., 219, *237*
Lorr, M., *184*
Louars, 218, *234*
Lourenço, C. F. S., 229, *244*
Louw, J. H., 82, 152, *178*
Lovett, Doust, J. W., 151, *184*
Løvtrup, S., 82, *184*
Louw, J., 82, *162*
Low, H., 82, *184*
Lu, F. C., 62, 103, *167*, *185*
Lubin, G. T., 145, *184*
Luby, E. D., 253, *279*
Lucas, G. H., 147, *184*
Luciano, M., 219, *242*
Ludany, G., 104, *175*
Ludwig, P., 140, *188*
Luna, N. E., 219, *242*
Lundholm, L., 273, *280*
Lupulesco, A., 101, *186*
Luria, E., 219, *242*
Lutz, H., 229, *240*
Lutzenkirchen, A., 115, *184*
Luxembourger, C., 226, *242*
Lwoff, J. M., 217, *233*
Lyle, C. B., 159, *177*

Lyman, F. L., 274, *280*
Lynch, V. D., 49, *161*

M

Maass, A. R., 139, *173*, *191*, *196*, *198*
MacArthur, J. G., 58, 59, *179*
McBay, A. J., 160, *161*
Maccagnani, G., 219, 224, *232*, *242*
McCandless, R. F. J., 24, 160, *176*, 291, 296, *300*
McCann, W. P., 112, *183*
McCarthy, D. A., 153, *184*
McCaskill, M. R., 152, *190*
MacCasland, B. W., 154, *180*
McClanahan, W. S., 159, *195*
McCluskey, R. T., 83, *197*
McCormick, W. G., 96, *177*
McCourt, W. F., 153, *184*
McCulloh, E. F., 96, *177*
McCullough, W., 72, *195*
MacCusker, K., 219, 226, *241*
MacDonald, I. A., 219, *236*
McDonald, J. K., 160, 161, *184*
McDonald, R. K., 155, *184*
MacDonnell, D. R., 145, *178*
MacDougall, E. J., 151, *162*
McElroy, W. D., 74, *176*
McFarlane, J. R., 159, *170*
McFarlane, W. J. G., 159, *170*, *187*
McGeer, P. L., 260, *280*, *281*
McGinn, J. T., 161, *184*
McGough, E. C., 76, *189*
McGowan, St. W., 220, *241*
McGrath, W. R., 60, *184*
McIlwain, H., 50, *184*, 217, *242*
McIntyre, J. W. R., 84, 92, *165*, *171*, 230, *248*
MacIntyre, L., 261, 262, *281*
McIsaac, W. M., 269, 270, *280*
McKay, A. R., 47, *176*
McKay, J., 151, *197*
Mckenna, J. M., 96, *191*
Mackie, A., 143, *161*
Mackiewicz, J., 112, 158, *184*
Macko, E., 161, *184*
MacLachlan, I., 288, *301*
McLaughlan, J. M., 115, *184*
McLennan, H., *280*
MacMahon, H. E., 156, *196*
MacMillan, W. H., 97, *189*
McNair, D. M., *184*

McNeill, J. H., 526, *532*
McNichol, R. W., 156, *184*
McRae, C., 158, *192*
MacRae, W. R., 220, *233*
Madalena, J. C., 219, 224, *242*
Madedda, A., 219, *242*
Maderna, A., 220, *231*
Madjerek, Z., 53, 58, 59, 61, 67, 69, 90, *184*
Madjidi, A., 229, *237*, *241*, *242*
Madkour, M. K., 87, *193*
Madre, J. C., 226, *245*
Madsen, J. A., 284, *301*
Mäkelä, S., 82, *181*
Maer, M., 226, 227, *242*
Märki, F., 269, *280*
Maffii, G., 39, 50, *184*, *193*
Magee, J. T., 158, *166*
Magee, W. L., 74, 82, *185*
Magnier, P., 220, *242*
Mahfouz, M., 96, *185*
Mahoudeau, D., 220, *242*
Mahrer, P. R., 160, *185*
Maickel, R. P., 70, *185*
Maier, A., 68, *185*
Maier, C., 156, *191*
Mainardi, C., 220, *242*
Maire, F. W., 520, *522*
Maitron, 226, *242*
Malcolm, M., 160, *166*
Malhotra, C. L., 81, *185*
Maling, H. M., 530, *531*
Malleson, A., 268, *278*
Mallov, S., 98, *185*
Malmejac, J., 87, *185*
Malossi, M., 155, *185*
Manchanda, S. K., 527, *532*
Mandel, W., 158, *185*
Mandell, A. J., 83, *185*
Manganaro, D., 219, *242*
Manghi, E., 43, 56, *170*, *185*
Mann, D., 151, *172*, *177*
Mann, J. D., 260, *280*
Mann, J. S., 258, *277*
Mann, P. J. G., 279, *281*
Manni, C., 229, 230, *242*, *247*
Mannion, P. L., 67, *166*
Mantegazza, P., 527, *532*
Mapp, Y., 220, 231, *244*
Marchais, P., 227, *242*
Marconi, M., 39, *185*
Marcou, G., 229, *241*
Marcus, S., *185*

Margolis, G., 55, 57, 71, 84, 85, 87, 89, 90, 91, 93, 113, *165*, *172*, *175*, *177*
Margolis, L. H., 159, *185*
Margolis, R., 151, *175*, *177*
Mariani, A., 147, 148, *166*
Mariani, E., 82, *165*
Mariani Marelli, O., 147, 148, *166*
Marie, C., 219, *239*
Marijan, N., 95, *194*
Marino, A., 219, *243*
Marjanen, P., 103, *176*
Markovic-Giaja, L., 68, 70, 71, *175*
Marks, V., 152, *185*
Marocco, F., 101, *165*, *185*
Marquardt, P., 52, 84, 88, 91, *185*
Marquez, C., 219, *242*
Marrazzi, A. S., 47, 50, 64, *177*, *185*, *190*
Marriott, A. S., 217, *242*
Mars, G., 72, *185*
Marsboom, R., 217, 227, 230, *242*, *243*
Marshall, B. M., 229, 230, *243*, *247*
Marsico, V., 220, *243*
Martel, J., 151, *192*
Martens, S., 252, *279*
Martin, G. J., 121, *185*
Martin, G. Narros, 219, *243*
Martin, H. F., 141, *189*
Martin, R. C., 67, 84, 89, *194*
Martin, W. R., 50, 52, 81, 84, *170*, *185*
Martin-Dupont, C., 161, *162*
Mary, N. Y., 147, *169*
Masciocchi, A., 219, 224, *243*
Mashkovsky, M. D., 39, 107, *185*
Mason, A. S., 146, 148, 149, *173*
Mason, J. W., 100, *177*
Mason, M. M., 103, *189*
Mason-Browne, N. L., 154, *185*
Masquin, P., 226, *243*
Masse, G., 81, *185*
Massey, L. W. C., 159, *185*
Massie, S., 3, *185*
Masson, G. M. C., 65, 94, 108, *174*, *185*
Massonnat, J., 160, *185*
Master, R. S., 161, *185*
Masters, Y. F., 145, *180*
Masucci, E. F., 158, 161, *196*
Masurat, T., 82, 83, *176*, *185*
Matge, H., 224, *246*
Mathalone, M. B. R., 159, *185*
Máthé, V., 80, *185*
Mathis, 226, *237*
Mathues, J. K., 101, *185*

AUTHOR INDEX

Matsumoto, C., 526, *531*
Matsumoto, K., 268, 269, *277*
Matsuo, T., 528, *532*
Matsuyama, M., 78, *174*
Mattei, F., 148, *168*
Mattheeuws, D., 217, 227, *243*, *248*
Matthews, V., 219, *242*
Mattke, D., 228, 230, *238*, *243*
Mattocks, A. N., 258, *279*
Mauceri, J., 160, 161, *185*
Maul, W., 139, *171*
Maurel, H., 160, *166*
Maxwell, G. M., 275, *278*
Maxwell, M. H., 520, *522*
May, A. R., 153, *185*
May, R. H., 159, *190*
Mayer, S. W., 101, *185*
Maynert, E. W., 262, *281*
Mayr, F., 155, *183*, 217, 219, *238*, *241*
Mazurkiewicz, I. M., 62, *185*
Mazzarella, B., 229, *243*
Mazzoni, P., 229, *242*
Mead, B. T., 153, *185*
Medenwald, H., 139, *171*
Medveczky, L., 101, *162*
Medvedev, B. A., 107, *185*
Mefferd, R. B., 153, *185*
Megre Velloso, F., 224, *243*
Méhes, J., 82, *170*
Meidinger, F., 52, 54, *186*
Meier, R., 111, *186*
Meites, J., 103, *194*
Meisinger, M. A. P., 260, *280*
Mellinger, T. J., 147, *186*
Melotti, V., 218, *233*
Melville, K. I., 84, 85, 88, 93, *186*
Memoli, G., 229, *243*
Mendelsohn, F., 219, *244*
Mendelsohn, R. M., 153, *186*
Mendelson, J., 74, *176*
Mendigutia, C., 219, *243*
Menguy, R. B., 105, *186*
Mennear, J. H., 80, *186*
Mercier, J., 45, 53, 118, *186*
Meritt, D. A., 50, *165*
Merkle, F. H., 140, *186*
Merland, A., 220, *243*
Merlis, S., 145, 148, 149, *178*
Mesham, P. R., 69, *171*
Messer, M., 82, *186*
Messina, N., 220, *234*
Metcalf, J. S., 50, *175*

Metcalf, R. L., 24, *186*
Metts, J. C., 160, *196*
Meurice, E., 219, *243*
Meyer, F., 219, *239*, 298, *300*
Meyer, H. J., 53, *186*
Meyer, V., 24, *186*
Meyer-Burg, J., 53, *186*
Meyers, G. S., 298, *301*
Meyre, F., 147, *186*
Miachon, S., 217, *245*
Michaux, M. H., 151, 153, *182*, *186*
Michaux, R., 261, *281*
Michaux, W. W., 156, 184, 186, 226, *241*
Miche, F., 218, *233*
Mickle, W. A., 50, 52, *186*
Midenet, J., 228, *241*
Miech, G., 227, *247*
Miettinen, P., 230, *245*
Milani, B., 219, *243*
Milbled, G., 87, 161, *176*, *195*, 219, *244*
Milch, L. J., 73, *161*
Milcou, S. M., 101, *186*
Miles, B., 113, *190*
Milette, G., 228, *243*
Miletzky, O., 99, *186*
Millan, E., 230, *248*
Millar, R. A., 81, *186*
Miller, J., 528, *532*
Miller, J. K., 41, 70, 71, *165*
Miller, N. E., 45, 50, *163*, *176*
Miller, R. E., 47, *186*
Millican, R. C., 96, 97, *186*
Milligan, W. L., 156, *186*
Milne, H. B., 219, *243*
Milne, J. B., 147, *186*
Milne, J. J., 147, *186*
Milner, L., 220, *243*
Minami, M., 82, *198*
Minard, F. N., 73, *186*
Minchin, R. L. H., 118, *186*
Mingioli, E., 525, *531*
Miraillet, P., 228, *238*
Mirsky, A. F., 154, 155, *186*
Mirsky, I. A., 47, *186*
Mitchell, J. C., 42, *186*, 285, *300*
Mitchell, R. B., 115, *168*
Mitra, S. K., 161, *193*
Miura, T., 228, *243*
Mixon, B. M., Jr., 94, *190*
Miya, T. S., 42, 80, 132, 139, *172*, *186*, *188*, *196*
Miyahara, R. C., 229, *231*

AUTHOR INDEX

Mock, J., 287, *301*
Moe, R., 85, *186*
Moeschlin, S., 155, *175*
Moffitt, E. A., 154, *186*
Mohme-Lundholm, E., 273, *280*
Moldenhauer, B., 156, *166*
Molders, V., 219, *236*
Molinaroli, P., 230, *248*
Molinatti, G. M., 65, *166*
Monard, Y., 217, *234*
Monceaux, J. P., 219, *238*, *239*, *243*
Monnerot, E., 219, 226, *243*
Monnier, M., 50, *174*, *186*, 262, *281*
Monroe, B. L., 114, *187*
Monroe, R. R., 50, 52, *186*
Monteverdi, T., 219, 226, *243*
Montigneaux, P., 219, *243*
Moog, E., 65, *198*
Moon, L. E., Jr., 298, *300*
Mora, A., 149, *193*
Mora-Castaneda, F., 273, *277*
Moraczewski, A. S., 76, *186*
Moran, J., 229, *243*, 524, *530*
Moran, N. C., 85, 135, 147, *186*, *191*
Morand, P., 76, *186*
Morel, P., 226, *247*
Mori, F., 219, *244*
Moriarity, A. J., 114, *186*
Morin, G., 226, *243*
Morin, R., 82, *168*
Morin, Y., 219, *245*
Morocutti, C., 113, *186*
Morosini, C., 219, *243*
Morozova, T. N., 151, *187*
Morpurgo, C., 65, *187*, 217, *243*
Morpurgo, M., 72, *185*
Morrell, F., 53, *187*
Morris, G., 62, 71, 91, 92, 94, 106, 108, 111, 112, 114, 152, *181*, *187*
Morris, R. W., 41, 44, *168*
Morrow, W., 153, *187*
Morse, W. H., 154, *171*
Mortelmans, J., 217, 230, *242*, *243*
Mortier, D., 156, 158, *167*
Morton, M. E., 101, *185*
Moses, A. H., 102, *187*
Moss, C. S., 153, *187*
Mostert, J. W., 220, *243*
Motz, G., 154, *187*
Motzenbecker, F. P., 219, *239*
Mouille, P., 217, *232*
Mouton, P., 226, 227, *246*

Moyer, J. H., 38, 62, 69, 71, 91, 92, 94, 106, 108, 111, 112, 114, 152, *168*, *179*, *187*
Mráz, M., 97, *187*, *195*
Müller, C., 229, *240*
Mueller, H. F., 219, *243*
Müller, M. L., 227, *232*
Mukherjee, K. L., 43, 54, 82, *169*
Mulke, G., 71, *173*
Mullen, A. J., 153, *174*
Mundeleer, P., 220, *243*
Munkvad, I., 217, *243*, *245*
Munroe, J., 151, *169*
Murnane, J. P., 273, *277*
Murphree, H. B., 64, *187*, *279*, *284*, *300*
Murphree, O. D., 43, 114, 151, 153, *174*, *180*, *187*
Murphy, C. M., 24, *187*
Murphy, J. V., 47, *186*
Musacchio, J., 527, *531*
Muskus, A., 285, *301*
Myerson, R. M., 156, *181*

N

Nadeau, G., 145, 148, 149, *187*, *193*
Nading, L. K., 101, *192*
Nagatsu, T., 50, 82, *198*
Nair, V., 525, *532*
Nairn, R. C., 94, *185*
Nakayama, M., 109, *187*
Nakatani, G., 528, *532*
Nalda Felipe, M. A., 229, *243*
Namajuska, I., 74, 82, *164*
Nance, M. R., 114, *186*
Nanni Costa, P., 220, *238*, *243*
Nasmyth, P. A., 98, 99, *187*
Natarajan, R., 151, *165*
Nathan, H. A., 118, *187*
Nauta, W. T., 82, *172*
Naviau, J., 226, *244*
Naylor, L. Z., 159, *192*
Nayrac, P., 219, *244*
Negoesco, I., 101, *186*
Negwer, M., 3, 5, *187*, 288, *300*
Neimann, N., 53, *167*
Neller, K., 219, 227, *237*
Nellhaus, G., 148, *187*
Nelson, J. W., 39, 61, *168*, *190*
Nelson, N. M., 160, *187*
Nelson, R. D., 24, *187*

Nelson, R. M., 98, *187*
Nervacs, C., 140, *182*
Nesselhof, W. M., 222, 223, *237*
Netschey, A., 150, *176*
Neuhoff, E. W., 148, 149, *187*
Neuman, M., 5, 38, *187*
Neumann, H., 219, *244*
Neve, H. K., 145, 147, 148, *187*
Neverre, G., 87, *185*
Newman, J. H., 139, *173*
Newton, J. C., 159, *163*
Nezelof, C., 104, *162*
Ngai, S. H., 85, 89, *187*
Niaussat, P., 140, *182*
Nichols, J. E., 154, *167*
Nicholson, G. A., 159, *176*, *187*
Nicholson, J., 29, *164*
Nick, J., 219, *244*
Nickerson, M., 69, *192*, 264, *281*
Nicoll, C. S., 103, *194*
Nicolle, M. H., 219, *244*
Nicoletti, R. L., 229, *244*
Niemegeers, C. J. E., 41, 58, *179*, 202, 203, 204, 205, 209, 211, 213, 214, 215, 217, 229, *240*, *244*, 297, *300*
Nieschke, W., 220, *232*
Nieschulz, O., 5, 121, 139, *178*, *187*
Nigro, R. R., 229, *244*
Nikawitz, E. J., 32, *162*
Nikitina, G. M., 47, *187*
Nilsson, E., 217, 220, *239*, *244*
Nishi, K., 100, *193*
Nishigori, T., 228, *247*
Nishimura, T., 261, 262, *281*
Nishizono, M., 151, *187*
Nistri, M., 219, *244*
Nizard, I., 61, *183*
Noack, H., 114, *187*
Noble, R. C., 156, *187*
Noblin, C. D., 266, *279*
Nodiff, E. A., 25, 26, 29, 31, 32, 128, 129, *169*, *187*
Nodine, J. H., 153, *187*, 220, 231, *236*, *244*
Noel, P. R., 530, *532*
Noif, N., 161, *183*
Nols, E., 202, 217, 219, 231, *236*
Nomura, A., 228, *244*
Nondedeu, 218, *234*
Nordström, L., 217, 220, *244*
Norman, D., 72, *187*
Norton, J., 98, *176*
Noteboom, L., 261, *281*

Novick, W. J., 139, 147, *173*, *196*
Nowill, W. K., 55, 57, 71, 84, 85, 87, 89, 90, 91, 93, 113, *165*
Noyes, H. E., 98, *187*
Nuyts, A., 228, *244*

O

Oberhaensli, W., 525, *531*
Oblath, R. W., 521, *522*
Ochonisky, J., 219, 226, *247*
Odell, G. V., 147, *178*
Özer, F., 69, *195*
Ogasawara, J., 109, *187*
Ogasawara, K., 97, *187*
Ogawa, Y., 139, *187*, 524, *532*
Oger, J., 99, *167*
Oh, Y. H., 254, *281*
Ohler, E. A., 83, 100, *187*, *192*
Oishi, H., 147, *195*
Okasha, A., 219, *244*
Okayama, T., 527, *531*
Oketani, Y., 289, *300*
Olds, J., 57, *187*
Olds, M. E., 56, *187*
O'Leary, J. L., 50, *175*
Oles, M., 219, *244*
Olin, K., 160, *197*
Oliver, W. A., 158, *185*
Olivetti, M., 65, *166*
Ollendorff, H. V., 161, *187*
Olling, C. C. J., 100, *188*
Olmstead, M. P., 33, *188*
Olson, A., 153, *188*
Olson, K. J., 3, *195*
Olsson, O., 219, *244*
Omarova, V. A., 148, *188*
O'Mullane, E. J., 92, *174*
O'Neill, N. C., 154, *186*
Oosterbaan, W. M., 219, *244*
Oosterhuis, H. K., 82, *172*
Opitz, K., 65, 70, 80, 118, *188*
O'Regan, J. B., 224, *244*
O'Reilly, P. O., 224, *244*
Orgel, S. Z., 97, *188*
Orlans, F. B., 277
Orloff, M. K., 150, *188*
Ormond, R. E., 260, *280*
Orzack, M. H., 153, *181*

AUTHOR INDEX

Osaki, S., 252, *281*
Oskam, A. C. W., 217, 227, *244*
Osmond, H., *280*
Osmund, H., 261, *281*
Osswald, W., 72, *193*
Osterman, E., 284, *300*
Oswald, E. O., 524, *532*
Ota, K. Y., 151, 153, *182*, *186*
Otis, L. S., 45, *188*
Otsuki, S., 527, *531*
Ottenstein, B., 275, *281*
Otto-Servais, M., 217, *236*
Overall, J. E., 153, 154, *176*, 219, 222, *239*, 298, *300*
Overton, R. C., 96, *188*
Owen, J. E., 50, *196*
Owens, H. F., 291, *301*
Ozawa, T., 50, 82, *198*

P

Paasonen, M. K., 79, *188*
Pace, R., 153, 154, *177*
Pache, R., 226, *234*
Page, I. H., 266, 269, *278*, *281*
Pagliano, S., 219, *244*
Pagny, J., 217, *232*, *233*
Pagot, 226, *237*
Pakkenberg, H., 158, *172*
Palazzetti, P., 114, *188*, *195*
Paleologue, A., 219, *244*
Paley, H. M., *177*, 219, *244*
Pallin, I. M., 67, 152, *182*, *183*
Palmentieri, P., 229, *237*
Palmer, A. C., 530, *532*
Pancer, E., 219, *244*
Panjwani, M. H., 109, 160, *190*
Paoletti, P., 82, *176*
Paoletti, R., 82, *176*
Paoli, F., 218, *234*
Papachristou, C., 219, *245*
Paprocki, J., 224, *243*
Paquay, J., 219, 226, 227, 230, *244*, *245*
Pardo, E. G., 528, *532*
Pare, C. M. B., 264, 274, *281*
Paredes, A., 153, *168*
Parent, M., 229, *231*
Pariante, F., 224, *245*
Pariente, M., 226, *245*
Park, L. C., 261, *281*
Parker, C. A., 270, *282*

Parker, K. D., 147, *188*
Parkes, M. W., 69, *183*
Parkhurst, B. H., 273, *277*
Parmelee, E. T., 101, *185*
Parrish, A. E., 111, *188*
Pasananick, B., 153, *177*
Pascal, S., 139, 147, 148, 149, *171*
Paschkis, K. E., 83, 97, *170*, *191*
Pasqualini, G., 219, *242*
Pasternack, B., 153, 154, *177*
Pataky, I., 66, *188*
Patay, R., 109, *164*
Patel, M. A., 72, *176*
Patrick, R. W., 65, 84, *162*
Patton, R. E., 160, 161, *165*
Paul, S. D., 91, 112, *188*
Pauls, J. F., 47, *174*
Paulson, G., 160, *188*
Pavloff, A. M., 30, 31, 32, 33, 129, *162*, *169*, *188*
Pavlou-Karageorgiadou, A., 219, *245*
Pearce, M. L., 520, *522*
Pearl, D., 153, *188*
Pearl, J., 298, *300*
Pearson, J. W., 62, *183*
Peckham, W. D., 143, *194*
Pedrazzini, A., 229, *231*
Pedronetto, S., 229, *231*
Peigne, F., 218, *235*
Pelaz, E., 219, 220, 224, *245*
Pellegrino de Iraldi, A., 529, *532*
Pellerat, J., 159, *190*
Penman, A. S., 153, *186*
Penman, J., 59, *164*
Pennell, R. B., 277, *279*
Pennington, V. M. 156, *188*
Penrose, L. S., 274, *281*
Pentilla, I., 527, *531*
Pereira, F. B. L., 229, *245*
Perèz, R., 219, *243*
Pérez Sanfelix, J., 219, 224, 229, *245*
Périer, M., 219, *245*
Perini, U., 220, *245*
Perkins, M. E., 85, *186*
Perlin, S., 259, 273, *282*
Perlman, P. L., 143, *194*
Pernarowski, M., 146, *198*
Pernet, A., 229, *244*
Pevrin, G. M., *281*
Perrin, G. M., *281*
Perrin, J., 160, *166*, 219, 226, *245*, *246*
Perrot, 159, *188*

Perry, C., 115, *189*
Perry, T. L., 159, *188*, 258, 261, 262, 269, *281*
Peruzzo, L., 73, *188*
Pessolano, A. A., 128, *168*
Peters, J. E., 43, *187*
Peters, K., 76, 77, *188*
Peters, R. A., 83, *188*
Petersen, P. B., 158, *172*
Peterson, R. D., 83, *188*
Petersson, B., 219, *238*
Petrie, A., 154, *188*
Petri, G., 77, 100, 101, *182*
Petrod, S., 228, *231*
Petromilli, M., 220, *248*
Petterson, K., 521, *522*
Pettit, M., 153, *181*
Peyronnaud, G., 224, *236*
Pfeiffer, A. K., 66, *188*
Pfeiffer, C. C., 47, *193*, *279*, 284, *300*
Pfeiffer, C. J., 104, *188*
Pfeiffer, E., 121, *188*
Pfeiffer, W. M., 151, *188*, 227, *232*
Pfister, K., III, 128, *168*
Philipszoon, A. J., 60, *180*
Phillips, B. M., 139, *188*
Phipps, E., 79, *191*
Piala, J. J., 38, 119, *166*, *188*
Pica, M., 229, *234*
Picchioni, A. L., 148, *165*
Pichot, P., 218, 224, *235*
Pickering, R. W., 37, *168*
Pidevich, I. N., 79, *188*
Piéchaud, C., 229, *238*
Pierce, E. C., 84, *171*
Pierson, M., 53, *167*
Piette, L. H., 134, 140, 141, *169*, *188*
Piétte, Y., 53, *188*
Pigem, J. M., 219, 224, 229, *245*
Pihkanen, T., 226, *241*
Pilon, L., 153, *173*
Pinchard, A., 202, 217, 219, 224, 228, 230, 231, *232*, *236*
Pincus, G., 103, *189*
Pind, K., 261, *278*
Piret, J., 218, *235*
Piret-Pilachon, J., 219, *245*
Pisano, J. J., *281*
Pisciotta, A. V., 84, 157, *188*, *189*
Pittman, J. A., 287, *300*
Plaa, G. L., 76, *189*
Plas, F., 72, 106, *167*

Plein, E. M., 150, *193*
Pletscher, A., 65, 79, 80, 81, *163*, *175*, *189*, 527, 530, *531*, *532*
Plotnikoff, N. N., 53, *189*
Plotnikoff, N. P., 53, *189*
Plowman, R., 519, *522*
Plummer, A. J., 39, *197*
Plummer, H. B., 160, *189*
Pocidalo, J. J., 54, 86, 89, 90, 96, *167*, *189*
Podlewska, A., 114, *183*
Pöldinger, W., 220, 225, *231*, *245*
Pöntinen, P. J., 229, *245*
Poire, R., 228, *245*
Pokorny, A. D., 153, *174*
Polaczek-Kornecki, T., 229, *245*
Poland, N., 115, *189*
Poley, B. S., 159, *170*
Polezhaieva, A. I., 285, *300*
Polishuk, W. Z., 103, *189*
Polk, A., 145, *178*
Pollack, B., 156, *189*
Polley, E., 139, *196*
Pollin, W., 260, 261, *281*
Pomarede-Ravoir, A., 220, *245*
Pomerat, C. M., 115, *189*
Pontius, R., 71, 92, *187*
Popendiker, K., 5, 121, 139, *178*, *187*
Popovic, V., 71, *189*
Poppe, H., 139, 147, *171*
Popper, H., 76, *189*
Popper, M., 115, *189*
Porteus, S. D., 154, *189*
Posner, H. S., 132, 134, 136, 146, 147, 148, 149, *189*
Potter, L. T., 81, *162*, 266, *281*
Potts, A. M., 138, *189*
Poulsen, E., 44, *170*
Poyart, 226, *247*
Pozdnyakov, V. S., 53, *189*
Prasad, K., 81, *185*
Pratt, J. P., 219, 222, 223, *245*
Preston, J. B., 50, *189*
Pribyl, E. J., 283, *301*
Price, S., 141, *189*
Primo, C., 103, *181*
Printz, S., 287, *301*
Prinzhorn, G., 230, *245*
Procaccini, S., 218, *231*
Proctor, R. C., 285, *301*
Protiva, M., 5, *189*, 293, *301*
Prueter, G. W., *189*

AUTHOR INDEX

Prumm, E., 220, *245*
Pruneyre, A., 139, 148, *176*
Prusmack, J. J., 145, 148, *178*
Pscheidt, G. R., 268, 269, *277*
Puca, A., 219, *245*
Pullman, A., 150, *189*
Pullman, B., 150, *189*
Pungor, E., 147, 149, *189*
Puppel, H., 52, 84, 88, *185*
Purshottam, N., 103, *189*
Purtscheller, W., 220, *241*
Puyuelo, R., 220, *238*

Q

Quadbeck, G., 40, 78, *189*
Quandt, J., 290, *301*
Quastel, J. H., 74, 82, *184*, 274, *277*, *281*
Quinci, A., 219, *242*
Quinn, G., 63, *189*
Quinn, G. P., 75, *176*, *277*, 294, *301*
Quivy, D., 67, *164*

R

Raab, W., 97, *189*
Rabache, R., 161, *176*
Rabe, A., 255, *279*
Racinet, P., 227, *245*
Raevsky, K. S., 52, 64, *189*
Rafaelsen, O. J., 80, *189*
Raffel, S., 115, *189*
Ragland, J. B., 134, 139, 147, *181*, *190*
Rahmann, H., 115, *190*
Raina, A., 527, *531*
Rainaut, J., 161, *190*
Rainer, H., 24, *187*
Raitt, J. R., 39, *190*
Rajagopalan, V., 230, *245*
Rajapurkar, M. V., 109, 160, *190*
Rajeswaran, P., 146, *190*
Rajotte, P., 218, *235*
Rajsner, M., 293, *301*
Ramamurthi, B., 230, *245*
Rampal, C., 111, *191*
Randrup, A., 217, *245*
Rappe, A., 145, 147, *162*
Rasch, P. J., 158, *172*
Rascol, A., 219, *238*
Raskin, A., *184*
Rasper, A., 219, *237*

Ravaris, C. L., 137, *166*
Ravin, H. A., 275, *281*
Ravin, L. J., 140, *190*
Ray, H. N., 82, *170*
Ray, O. S., 64, *190*
Ray, T. S., 153, *168*
Raybaud, 228, *247*
Raybin, H. W., 160, *179*
Rayner, S., 72, *168*
Rea, E. L., 91, *190*
Read, A. E., 156, *190*
Read, G. W., 42, *190*
Reale, A., 229, *242*
Reboton, J., Jr., 159, *190*
Reckless, D., 55, *190*
Redeker, A. G., 114, *194*
Redfield, B. G., 258, *282*
Redick, T. F., 96, *163*, 252, *281*
Rees, K. R., 82, 106, *163*, *170*
Rees, L., 151, *190*
Reeves, R. L., 106, *175*
Register, U. D., 75, *163*
Reichle, C., 62, *174*
Reid, A. A., 63, *190*
Reid, W. B., 30, *190*
Reiff, H. E., 32, *162*
Reilly, J., 96, *190*
Reinert, H., 527, *531*
Reio, L., 135, 147, *162*
Reiser, P., 287, *301*
Remvig, J., 151, *190*
Renald, P., 219, *245*
Renier-Cornec, A., 64, *177*
Restaino, R. M., 273, *277*
Reuber, H. W., 147, *178*
Revita, D. M., 151, *180*
Revol, M. L., 217, *245*
Revzin, A. M., 262, *278*
Rey-Bellet, J., 224, *236*
Reyes, R. M., 60, *191*
Reynaud, R., 226, 227, *233*
Reynolds, G. S., 48, *190*
Reynolds, L. W., 139, 144, 147, 148, *173*, *184*
Reynolds, R. W., 83, *190*
Reznikoff, L., 160, *190*
Rhoades, M. V., 83, *191*
Rhodes, C. J., 96, 97, *186*
Riberi, A., 96, *180*
Rice, E. G., 82, 83, *176*, *185*
Richards, A. D., 151, *190*
Richards, F., 159, *190*

Richards, J. B., 100, *171*
Richardson, D. J., 94, *184*
Richardson, H. L., 160, *190*
Richardson, M. E., 160, *190*
Richman, A., 72, *163*
Richmond, M. R., 3, *195*
Richter, D., 273, *281*
Rickels, K., 287, 288, *301*
Rico, J. M., 95, *175*
Riddle, W. C., 48, *180*
Ridges, A. P., 260, 261, *277*
Ridgeway, E. R., 74, 85, 93, *173*
Riding, J. E., 220, *245*
Riedel, B. E., 146, *168*, 526, *532*
Rieder, H. P., 147, *190*
Riehl, J. L., 81, 84, *185*
Riess, W., 102, 114, *182*
Rieunau, J., 99, *186*
Rigal, J., 226, *234*
Riggi, F., 219, *245*
Riley, P. A., Jr., 94, *190*
Rinaldi, F., 50, *169*
Rinne, U. K., 82, *181*
Riopelle, A. J., 47, *193*
Riou, 226, *237*
Ripstein, C. B., 69, 96, *180*, *190*
Riser, M., 228, *245*
Risse, K. H., 120, *197*
Ritchie, J. M., 110, *190*
Ritschel, W., 76, *190*
Ritter, K., 70, 71, *173*
Riva, M., 527, *532*
Rives, H., 159, *190*
Rizzo, E. M., 72, *190*
Rizzuto, N., 219, *242*
Robb, H. P., 53, 152, *190*
Robbins, E. B., 50, *196*
Robelet, A., 87, 105, *195*
Robert, J., 226, *236*, *248*
Roberts, E., 270, *281*
Roberts, F. J., 155, *169*
Robertson, D. H., 107, *168*
Robertson, R. H., 151, *196*
Robin, A. A., 219, *236*
Robinson, A. E., 137, 143, 144, 145, *163*, *190*
Robinson, A. S., 160, *190*
Robinson, S., 528, *531*
Robison, G. A., 78, *182*
Rocha e Silva, M., 109, 111, *183*, *190*
Rodgers, C. D., 152, *190*
Rodig, O. R., 33, *190*
Rodler, H., 155, *183*, 217, *241*

Rodnight, R., 269, *281*
Rodriguez, C. F., 145, *180*
Roebuck, B. E., 153, *190*
Rogers, S., 62, 91, 94, 106, 108, 111, 112, 114, 152, *181*, *187*
Rogers, W. P., 143, *183*
Rohde, P., 156, *190*
Rohmer, F., 226, *238*
Roizin, L., 113, 114, 137, 139, 147, *190*, *196*
Romani, B., 219, *236*
Romanova, G. A., 107, *176*
Rome, H. P., 64, *192*
Romildo Bueno, J., 224, *245*
Ronchi, E., 218, 219, 224, *232*, *235*, *245*
Rondepierre, A., 151, *192*
Rondepierre, J. J., 61, *183*
Rondez, R., 156, *191*
Rondish, I. M., 139, 144, 147, *173*, *184*
Roos, B. E., 66, *180*, 217, *231*, 245
Ropert, M., 64, *170*
Ropert, R., 50, *183*
Rosa, J. J., 219, *245*
Rosadini, G., 218, 224, *231*, *245*
Rosadini, L., 224, *245*
Rosati, D., 151, *190*
Rose, J. T., 293, *300*, 519, *522*
Rose, R. F., 67, *191*
Rosemberger, 218, *233*
Rosen, E., 145, *190*
Rosen, L., 258, *279*, *281*, 526, *532*
Rosenberg, A. J., 82, *162*
Rosenberg, D. E., 153, *174*
Rosenberg, F., 70, *183*
Rosenberg, F. J., 109, *191*
Rosenblatt, S., 264, *281*
Rosenblum, M. P., 153, *183*
Rosengren, E., 273, *280*, 524, 526, *531*
Rosner, H., 154, *191*
Rosner, K., 145, 147, 148, *181*
Ross, G. S., 111, *197*
Ross, J. J., 139, *191*, *198*
Ross, S., 47, 83, *170*, *175*, *191*
Rossi, G., 220, *246*
Rossiter, R. J., 74, 82, *185*
Roth, F. E., 96, *191*
Roth, L. J., 525, *532*
Roth, M., 530, *532*
Rothballer, A. B., 262, *281*
Rothlin, E., 266, *278*
Rothschild, G. H., 49, *167*, *278*
Rothstein, C., 151, *191*

AUTHOR INDEX

Rotondi, A., 218, *234*
Rouleau, Y., 219, *246*
Rountree, C. B., 62, *179*
Roussel, A., 218, *233*
Roux, C., 155, *191*
Roux, G., 220, 226, 227, *238*, *246*
Rovati, A. L., 44, *170*
Rovetta, P., 219, 224, *246*
Rowley, D. A., 93, *163*
Roy, H., 153, *174*
Roy, S. K., 134, *169*
Roy, S. V., 147, *169*
Royer, R., 219, *246*
Rubin, A., 140, *191*
Rudolph, L. A., 288, *301*
Rudorfer, L., *177*
Rudy, L. H., 151, *193*
Rudzik, A. D., 528, *532*
Ruggerini, R., 219, 230, *246*
Ruiz, A. B., 219, *246*
Ruiz, D. C. A., 219, *246*
Rumpf, K., 228, *239*
Rupp, J. J., 83, *191*
Ruskin, 141, *179*
Russell, E. S., 152, *191*
Russo, S., 72, *190*
Rutledge, C. O., 153, *197*
Rutledge, L. T., 42, 46, *191*
Rutschmann, J., 135, 138, 144, *180*, *191*, *198*
Ruttner, J. R., 156, *191*
Ryall, R. W., 109, *191*
Ryan, J. A., 147, 149, *191*
Ryman, B. E., 76, *177*

S

Saarima, H. S., 99, *191*
Saarne, A., 220, *246*
Sabathié, M., 220, 229, *238*, *246*
Sabelli, H. C., 81, *176*
Sacco, J. J., 228, *243*
Sackler, A. M., 109, *191*
Sackler, R. R., 109, *191*
Sacks, N. Z., 160, 161, *191*
Sadove, M. S., 60, 67, *191*
Saggiomo, A. J., 30, 31, 33, *176*, *191*, *196*
Saifer, A., 109, *177*
Saifi, A. Q., 82, *165*
Sainz, A. A., 152, 160, *191*
Saito, S., 99, 100, *193*
Sakamoto, Y., 524, *532*
Salles, 219, *239*
Salvador, R. A., 65, 76, 81, *166*
Salzman, N. P., 135, 138, 147, *191*
Samborski, A. H., 78, *180*
Sámel, M., 101, *191*
Sams, W. M., 159, *191*
Samuels, A. S., 161, *191*, 220, *246*
Samulak, G., 224, *246*
Sanchez, F., 219, *246*
Sanchez-Ruis, L., 219, *245*
Sanders, B. E., 254, *281*, *282*
Sandifer, M. G., Jr., 151, 153, 154, *177*, *197*
Sandler, M. M., 264, 274, *281*
Sandoz, S. A., 290, 291, 292, 293, 298, *301*
Sands, F. L., 140, 143, 144, *179*
Sane, I., 261, *282*
Sanford, J. P., 98, *187*
Sankar, D. B., 79, *191*
Sankar, D. V. S., 79, *191*
Sansone, M., 529, *532*
Santaella, A., 224, *246*
Santiago Barrios, S., 219, *246*
Santorelli, G., 219, *241*
Santos, A. S., 157, *189*
Santos, M. R., 219, *237*
Sanz, J. J., 220, *245*
Sapeika, N., 83, *191*
Saradjieff, P., 219, *242*
Saravis, C. A., *280*
Sarcinelli, L., 229, *242*
Sargant, W., 156, *190*, *191*
Sarwer-Foner, G. J., 219, *246*
Satanove, A., 159, *191*
Sato, M., 229, *244*
Sato, R., 228, *246*
Satory, E., 66, *188*
Satter, P., 230, *248*
Saunders, J. C., 151, 156, 159, *163*, *191*, 204, 231, *246*
Sautet, J., 111, *191*
Savarie, P. J., 109, *191*
Savelli, A., 219, 228, *236*, *240*
Savlov, E. D., 96, *191*
Sawusch, R. H., 154, *177*
Sawyer, C. H., 103, *163*
Sawyer, J. L., 526, *531*
Saxena, P. N., 47, 60, 109, *171*, *176*, *191*
Sayre, D. F., 258, *277*
Scaduto, L., 520, *522*

Scarborough, J. S., 153, *192*
Schaff, G., 68, *185*
Schalch, W., 138, *191*
Schallek, W., 40, *191*
Schanberg, S. M., 80, *191*, 268, *281*
Schanker, L. S., 78, *191*
Schaper, W. K. A., 203, 217, *246*, 299, *301*
Schaub, Cl., 226, *247*
Schaumkell, K. W., 68, 77, 99, 101, *191*
Scheckel, C. L., *191*
Scheidy, S. F., 161, *184*
Scheie, H. G., 159, *165*
Scheinberg, P., 273, *282*
Schellekens, K. H. L., 202, 203, 204, 205, 211, 213, 214, 215, 217, 229, *240*, 297, *300*
Schellenberg, H., 77, *192*
Schellenberger, A., 229, *236*
Schenck, G. O., 140, *192*
Schenker, E., 3, 30, *192*
Scherrer, P., 226, 227, *246*
Schiavi, F., 230, *247*
Schiele, B. C., 151, 153, 156, 159, *186*, *192*, *195*
Schieser, D. W., 140, *192*
Schieve, J. F., 273, *282*
Schildkraut, J. J., 262, 264, *281*
Schlatzer, R. K., 33, *190*
Schlictegroll, A. V., 33, *192*
Schliep, H., 290, *301*
Schmid, E., 87, *166*
Schmid, K., 254, *280*
Schmid, W., 94, *165*
Schmidt, C. F., 273, *280*
Schmidt, D., 220, *232*
Schmidt, G., 275, *281*
Schmidt, H., Jr., 83, *192*
Schmidt-Ginzkey, J., 217, *237*
Schmidtke-Ruhnau, D., 87, 88, 90, *182*
Schmitleröw, C. G., 143, 161,*177*, *192*
Schmitt, H., 95, *192*, 217, *246*
Schmitt, H., 95, *192*, 217, *246*
Schmitt, J., 26, 32, *192*
Schmitt, W., 227, *232*
Schmitz, B., 220, *246*
Schmutz, J., 217, *247*, 290, *300*
Schnack, H., 75, 106, *168*
Schneckloth, R. E., 266, *281*
Schneewind, K. A., 228, *239*
Schneider, J., 219, *246*
Schneider, J. A., 49, 54, 62, *192*, 298, *301*
Schneider, K., 261, *281*
Schneider, P., 230, *246*
Schnider, O., 294, *300*
Schönbeck, M., 228, *238*, *246*
Schoenfeld, W. N., 49, *193*
Scholefield, P. G., 274, *281*
Scholz, O., 76, *192*
Schoog, M., 115, *184*
Schreiber, M. M., 159, *192*
Schreiner, K., 82, *198*
Schrire, I., 114, *192*
Schroeder, E., 219, *245*
Schubert, G., 220, *232*
Schueler, F. W., 78, *182*
Schültz, E., 95, *192*
Schuette, D. V., 56, *192*
Schulenberg, J. W., 297, *300*
Schuler, W. A., 29, 33, *192*
Schulte, J. W., 286, *301*
Schultz, E. L., 254, *280*
Schulz, R., 71, *173*
Schumacher, H., 52, 84, 88, *185*
Schuster, E. M., 82, *162*
Schwab, G., 286, *300*
Schwartz, C. S., 104, *188*
Schwartz, D. E., 530, *532*
Schwartz, E., 56, *184*
Schwartz, L., 67, *191*
Schwartz, M. A., 525, 526, *531*, *532*
Schwarz, B. E., 64, *192*
Schwarz, H., 219, 228, *246*
Schweder, N., 220, *246*
Schweich, M. J., 151, *192*
Schweigh, M., 219, *246*
Scime, I. A., 160, *192*
Scott, C. C., 65, *167*
Scott, G. T., 101, 118, *192*
Scott, R. B., 160, *172*
Scott, W. E. B., 69, *171*
Scriabine, A., 298, *301*
Scruggs, W., 527, *531*
Sčudlik, M., *196*
Seabra-Dinis, J., 219, *246*
Seager, L. D., 114, *187*
Seale, A. L., 156, *184*
Sedivec, V., 50, *192*
Seevers, M. H., 153, *184*
Ségal, J., 219, *237*
Seiden, L. S., 525, *532*
Seidlová, V., 293, *301*
Seifter, J., 63, 139, 147, *194*, *196*
Seignot, J.-N., 219, *246*
Sekino, E., 44, *162*

AUTHOR INDEX

Selbach, H., 50, *192*
Sellers, E. A., 70, *169*, 527, *531*
Semprevivo, A., 224, *235*
Sen, N. P., 260, *281*
Senf, E., 220, *232*
Senf, R., 253, *279*
Serbinenko, M. V., 38, 44, *192*
Sergio, C., 65, *192*
Serrone, D. M., 529, *532*
Setekleiv, J., 50, *192*
Settel, E., 298, *301*
Sevy, R. W., 83, 100, *187*, *192*
Sfondrini, E., 219, *243*
Sforza, I., 230, *246*
Shackcloth, P., 152, *185*
Shackelford, R. T., 152, *178*
Shafer, S., 160, *192*
Shaklee, A. B., 47, *192*
Shanor, S. P., 82, *172*
Sharma, M. L., 110, 121, *195*
Sharma, P. L., 68, 85, 94, *192*
Shatin, L., 153, *192*
Shaw, D. M., 268, *278*
Shaw, E., 265, 266, *282*
Shaw, E. B., 160, *192*
Shawver, J. R., 153, *192*
Shay, H., 104, *192*, *194*
Shchelkumov, E. L., 293, *301*
Shea, J., 91, *190*
Sheatz, G. C., 44, *192*
Sheldon, G. L., 59, *167*
Shelton, J., 222, *239*
Shelton, J. G., 158, *192*
Shemano, I., 69, *192*
Shemyakin, M. M., 129, *192*
Shenoy, K. G., 115, *184*
Shepp, B., 49, *175*
Sheppard, P. M., 260, 261, *277*
Sherif, M. A. F., 87, *193*
Sherlock S., 156, *190*
Sherman, L. J., 273, *278*
Sherman, S., 160, *193*
Shibusawa, K., 99, 100, *193*
Shields, D. R., 230, *247*
Shields, J., 50, *175*
Shinagawa, J., 266, *280*
Shirley, D. A., 24, 25, *175*, *193*
Shlyafer, T. P., 57, *193*
Shminke, G. A., 155, *193*
Shnol', S. E., 141, 147, *172*
Shore, P. A., 60, 61, *165*, 294, *301*, 528, *531*
Short, H. W., 69, *197*

Shotlander, V., 106, *163*
Shumacker, H. B., 96, *180*
Shvetsov, Y. B., 129, *192*
Shyster, M., 219, *242*
Sichel, C., 226, *240*
Siciliano, C., 230, *246*
Siddall, J. R., 159, *193*
Sidley, N. A., 49, *193*
Sidley, N. T., 153, *184*
Siegel, E. P., 269, 273, *277*
Siegel, M., *281*
Siegler, P. E., 220, 231, *244*
Sierens, G., 217, 227, *242*
Sieron, G., 114, 147, *175*
Siffermann, A., 219, 226, *245*, *246*
Sigalos, J., 219, *244*
Silver, S. L., 60, 61, *165*
Silvestrini, B., 39, *193*
Simmons, C., 258, *279*
Simoes, M. S., 72, *193*
Simon, A., 61, 83, *166*, *181*, *195*
Simon, P., 217, *232*, *233*
Simon, W., 154, *193*
Simonis, A. M., 81, *162*
Simopoulos, A. M., 151, 153, *182*
Simpson, G. M., 153, 155, *193*, 204, 231, *246*
Sims, J. A., 138, *176*
Sines, J. O., 47, 50, *193*
Sines, L. K., 47, 50, *193*
Singer, L., 226, *238*, *240*, *246*
Singh, B., 527, *532*
Singleton, A. R., 114, *193*
Sinha, B. N., 155, *193*
Sinha, G. B., 161, *193*
Sinigaglia, M. G., 82, *193*
Sironi, P. G., 230, *246*
Sivadjian, J., 224, *246*
Siva Sankar, D. V., 74, *193*
Sjoerdsma, A., 91, 104, 135, 145, 147, *170*, *177*, *194*, 256, 260, *280*, *282*, 519, *522*, 528, *531*
Skinner, B. E., 35, *193*
Skude, I. M., 82, *174*
Slabok, M., 41, *179*
Slap, J. W., 220, 231, *244*
Slocum, Y. K., 156, *193*
Slone, D., 275, *281*
Small, S. M., 149, *184*, 254, *281*
Smelson, H., 151, *193*
Smiles, S., 25, *172*, *197*
Smilevich, A. B., *193*
Smith, C. I., 139, 147, *193*

Smith, C. M., 107, *167*
Smith, E. E., 75, *193*
Smith, E. V. C., 254, *281*, *282*
Smith, J. A., 151, *193*
Smith, K., 76, *166*
Smith, L. E., 24, *166*
Smith, M. E., 298, *301*
Smith, M. J., 160, *193*
Smith, N. L., 24, 26, 29, *187*, *193*
Smith, P. K., 60, 67, *177*
Smith, R. P., 47, *193*
Smith, T. E., 524, 525, *532*
Snedeker, E. H., 80, *170*
Snow, H. L., 159, *197*
Snow, L., 287, *301*
Soares, P. M., 229, *244*
Sobel, A. M., 114, 160, *193*
Sobel, D. E., 114, 160, *193*
Sobolewski, G., 145, 148, 149, *187*, *193*
Soderberg, U., 50, *179*
Sodoyez, J. C., 217, *246*
Söderberg, U., 69, *193*
Söderholm, R., 230, *245*
Soehring, K., 147, 148, 152, *174*, *193*
Soep, H., 217, *246*
Soergel, W., 220, *246*
Sövik, O., 253, *282*
Sokoloff, L., 260, 273, *278*, *282*
Solime, F., 226, *232*
Solms, W., 94, *162*
Solomon, J. D., 189, *189*
Solomon, N., 69, *190*
Solomon, P., 149, 153, *184*
Solsona, M., 149, *193*
Soma, L. R., 230, *247*
Somazzi, D., 219, *244*
Somerville, D. M., 159, *193*
Somoza, C., 83, *197*
Songar, A., 219, *247*
Sonne, L. M., 151, *190*
Sorby, D. L., 150, *193*
Soucachet, P., 218, *232*
Sourkes, T. L., 274, 276, *282*, 523, 524, *532*
Soulairac, A., 219, 226, *247*
Søvsø, H., 227, *231*
Sowinski, F., 29, 128, *198*
Soyka, D., 217, *247*
Spampinato, N., 229, *234*
Spatharas, G., 219, *244*
Spector, S., 256, 262, *278*, *280*, 526, *532*
Spellberg, M. A., 156, *193*

Spencer, G., 274, *282*
Spencer, P. S. J., 217, *242*, *247*
Spencer, W. A., 74, 85, 93, *173*
Spengler, J., 529, *532*
Sperco, J. E., 149, *173*
Sperling, H. H., *185*
Spiegel, E. A., 50, *163*
Spiess, W., 220, 229, *236*, *238*
Spink, W. W., 96, 98, *161*, *179*
Spinkova, V., 147, 149, *164*
Spirtes, M. A., 39, 75, 76, *174*, *176*, *193*
Spitaletta, P., 39, *197*
Spitz, H., 154, *194*
Spratt, R. J., 161, *193*
Sprehe, D. J., 222, 223, *237*
Sprince, H., 270, *282*
Springer, N. N., 153, *167*
Spude, J., 268, 269, *277*
Spurr, C., 91, 94, 106, 111, 114, *187*
Spurr, G. B., 91, 96, *178*, *193*
Stacey, C. H., 106, *193*
Stacey, R. S., 274, *281*
Stach, K., 293, *301*
Stahelin, H., 138, *191*
Staib, A. H., 94, *173*
Staib, F., 115, *171*
Stanbury, J. B., 274, *282*
Stancati, G., 219, *236*
Staniszewski, K., 57, *194*
Stanwell, P. M., 152, *174*
Starbuck, W. C., 82, *194*
Stark, E., 97, *189*
Stastny, P., 96, *198*
Steele, C. A., 222, *237*, 266, *279*
Steenfeldt-Foss, O. W., 219, *247*
Stefanachi, L., 219, 224, *236*, *245*, 268, *278*
Stefko, P. L., 105, *194*
Stehlin, S., 53, *167*
Stein, K. E., 151, 156, *192*
Stein, L., 63, *194*
Steiner, M., 228, *245*
Steiner, W. G., 40, 65, *194*
Stejskal, Z., 5, 147, 149, *164*
Stell, B. S., 155, *194*
Stelter, E., 225, *247*
Stéphanopoli, M. J., 219, *237*
Stephen, C. R., 55, 57, 67, 71, 84, 85, 87, 89, 90, 91, 93, 94, 113, *165*, *194*
Steriade, M., 50, *182*
Sterling, M., 153, *175*
Stern, D. N., 70, *185*

Stern, P., 53, 58, 59, 61, 67, 69, 90, *184*
Sternberg, U., 154, *194*
Stevenson, D. E., 95, *177*
Stevenson, T. D., 91, 104, *177*, *194*
Stewart, J., 41, 42, 60, 61, *178*, *194*
Stewart, L., 114, *194*
Stille, G., 217, *247*
Stiller, R., 151, *195*
Stjärne, L., 262, *282*
St. Jean, A., 217, 219, *241*, *247*
Stock, K., 529, *532*
Stoianoffnenoff, S., 228, *245*
Stoll, B. A., 220, *247*
Stone, C. A., 294, *301*
Stone, D., 253, *282*
Stone, G. C., 50, *194*
Stonehill, E., 218, *232*
Strauss, H., 160, 161, *185*
Strecker, H. J., 82, *164*
Streicher, E., 60, *194*
Strittmatter, C. F., 524, *532*
Stucke, W., 219, *247*
Stucki, J. C., 109, *194*
Sturmer, E., 70, 71, *173*
Sturtevant, F. M., 59, 63, 64, *194*
Stynes, A. J., 50, *183*
Su, C., 107, *194*
Su, S.-C., 76, *195*
Subberwal, U., 527, *532*
Subra, 219, *247*
Suga, T., 289, *300*
Sugerman, A. A., 219, 228, *247*, *279*
Sulcová, M., 147, *195*
Sullivan, C. L., 114, *194*
Sullivan, W. N., 24, *166*
Sulman, F. G., 100, 101, 102, 103, 118, 159, *181*, *194*
Sulser, F., 91, *165*, 277, 292, *300*
Summerfield, A., 38, *194*
Sun, D. C. H., 104, *192*, *194*
Suntay, R., 152, *183*
Supek, Z., 84, 95, 101, 102, *194*
Suquet, M., 26, 32, *192*
Surrey, A. R., 287, *301*
Susini, R., 219, *244*
Sutherland, P., 61, *167*
Sutherland, V. C., 61, *166*, *195*
Suva, J., 74, *194*
Suzuki, M., 114, *194*
Sved, S., 82, *184*
Svedmyr, N., 273, *280*
Svendsen, B. B., 219, *247*
Swain, J. M., 152, *194*
Swales, W. E., 143, 147, *168*, *177*, *194*
Sweet, R. B., 229, *234*
Swinehart, L. A., 114, *194*
Swintosky, J. V., 140, 145, 146, *190*, *194*
Swinyard, E. A., 44, 52, 60, 63, *173*, 284, *301*
Sykes, T. F., 218, *232*
Symchowicz, S., 143, *194*
Szabó, E., 97, *194*
Szara, S., 259, 269, 270, *282*
Szatmari, A., 44, *163*
Szeely, E. G., 50, *163*
Szent-Györgyi, A., 150, *180*
Szilágyi, T., 97, *194*
Szobor, A., 219, *247*

T

Tabau, R., 147, *194*
Tachezy, R., 151, *194*
Tachi, S., 528, *532*
Taeschler, M., 41, 47, *194*
Tainter, M. L., 286, *301*
Tait, A., 39, *177*
Takabataki, T., 70, *185*
Takada, M., 289, *300*
Takayanagi, I., 121, *194*
Takeo, Y., 261, *282*
Takesada, H., 228, *241*
Takesada, M., 261, *282*
Talairach, J., 227, *235*
Tallant, E. J., 160, *192*
Talwalker, P. K., 103, *194*
Tanaka, K., 56, *194*
Tanche, M., 69, 98, *167*, *194*
Taques, L. C., 229, *244*
Tardieu, C., 86, 89, 90, 96, *189*
Tardy, J., 42, *165*
Tarkian, M., 220, *246*
Tasker, R. R., 230, *247*
Tate, M. R., 3, *169*
Taterka-Seiler, W., 101, *194*
Tatom, M. H., 151, 153, *182*
Tauchert, E., 139, *178*
Tautermann, P., *196*
Tavernier, J., 161, *162*
Taylor, D. B., 63, *194*
Taylor, R. M., 219, *236*
Taylor, W. L., 134, 136, *189*

Tedeschi, D. H., 3, 79, 121, 129, 132, 160, 176, *194*, *195*
Tedeschi, O. H., 47, *174*
Tedeschi, R. E., 3, 79, 121, 129, 132, 160, 176, *194*, *195*
Telford, I. R., 113, *181*
Telkka, A., 79, *195*
Telmosse, F., 229, *241*
Temkov, I., 219, *247*
Tenhunen, R., 527, *531*
Teodoru, C. V., 83, *177*
Terentios, E., 219, *244*
Terrace, H. S., 50, *195*
Terrassier, J., 230, *247*
Terrell, M. S., 156, *195*
Terry, L. L., 104, 135, 145, 147, *170*, *177*
Tervooren, U., 100, *196*
Terzian, H., 52, *195*
Terzioğlu, M., 69, *195*
Tewfik, G. I., 219, *244*, *247*
Thalmann, K., 145, 147, 148, *181*
Thannhauser, S. J., 275, *281*
Theret, C., 78, 101, *195*
Therrien, R., 151, 154, *167*
Thieme, H., 147, *195*
Thienpont, D., 217, 227, 230, *242*, *243*
Thoenen, H., 528, *531*
Thomalske, G., 219, *246*
Thomas, G., 41, *179*
Thomas, J. J., 217, *247*
Thomas, J. O., 3, *170*
Thomas, L., 56, 98, *184*, *195*
Thomas, R., 298, *301*
Thompson, C. R., 109, *194*, 285, *301*
Thompson, T., 49, *195*
Thompson, W. E., 153, *174*, *196*
Thoms, R. K., 49, *161*
Thornicroft, S., 158, *179*
Thorpe, J. G., 154, *195*
Thuillier, J., 64, *170*
Thuries, J., 227, *247*
Tiberi, F., 220, *248*
Timmermans, F. J. M., 230, *247*
Timmous, E., 222, *237*
Timsit, M., 219, *242*
Tinant, M., 219, 230, *244*, *245*
Tipton, D. L., Jr., 61, *195*
Tissier, M., 217, *233*
Tissot, R., 218, *233*
Tiwari, N. M., 61, 110, 121, *180*, *195*
Tiwaskar, H. V., 81, *170*
Tkachenko, K. N., 107, *176*

Tofte, F., 161, *195*
Tokizane, T., 50, *195*
Tokui, T., 145, *179*
Toledo, J. B., 228, *247*
Tollinchi, G., 226, *234*
Tomich, E. G., 61, *167*
Tomizawa, K., 100, *193*
Tompsett, S. L., 275, *278*
Toms, E. C., 153, 154, *195*
Toner, J. J., 57, *168*
Tong, H. K., 150, *182*
Toogood, J. H., 155, *171*
Torda, T. A. G., 229, *237*
Torelli, L., 230, *247*
Tornetta, F. J., 230, *247*
Torney, D., 47, *176*
Torres, A. A., 43, *195*
Torres-Acero Fernandez, J. M., 67, *195*
Torrigiani, G., 219, 224, *238*
Torrubia, H., 226, *233*
Torsello, R., 114, *188*, *195*
Touraine, J., 227, *247*
Tourlentes, T. T., 154, *195*, 269, *277*
Tourney, G., 253, *279*
Tournier, P., 96, *190*
Tousignant, A., 151, *180*
Tower, D. B., 271, *282*
Traub, L., 145, 148, *178*
Traugott, N. N., 155, *195*
Tredici, L. M., 159, *195*
Tréfouel, M. J., 115, *172*
Trendelenburg, U., 285, *301*
Trethowan, W. H., 224, *247*
Trever, R. W., 160, *189*
Trifogli, L., 229, 230, *242*, *247*
Trigos, G., 72, *195*
Triner, L., 97, *195*
Tripod, J., 111, *186*
Trizio, W., 229, *235*
Trop, D., 229, 230, *231*, *241*, *247*
Troughton, S. E., 161, *195*
True, C., 113, *190*
Truitt, E. B., Jr., 66, *195*
Trystram, D., 228, *240*
Tsuchimoto, T., 228, *247*
Tsujimoto, A., 74, 82, *198*
Tsujimura, Y., 82, *198*
Tuason, V. B., 154, *195*
Tuck, L. D., 140, *192*
Tucker, R. G., 161, *184*
Tufvesson, G., 161, *192*
Turner, A. W., 77, *195*

Turner, M., 52, 56, 86, 91, 92, *168*, *195*
Turner, N., 52, 56, *195*
Turnin, J., 220, *238*
Turunen, M., 67, *172*
Tuteur, W., 151, *195*
Tye, A., 39, *190*

U

Ualverde, J. M., 269, *277*
Udenfriend, S., 256, 260, *280*, *281*, *282*, 524, 525, *532*
Udsen, P., 217, *245*
Ullberg, S., 135, 147, *162*
Ullyot, G. E., 24, 29, 32, 128, *169*, *175*, *195*
Unna, K. R., 50, 81, 84, *170*, *185*
Uroić, B., 84, 95, *194*
Uroma, E., 254, *280*
Urquiaga, X., 528, *532*
Usdin, E., 76, *195*, 217, *247*, 283, *301*
Usdin, V. R., 76, *195*, 217, *247*
Uyeo, S., 147, *195*
Uyterschaut, P., 225, *247*

V

Vácerková, J., 147, *195*
Vaillant, G. E., 151, *195*
Valéry, B., 228, *234*
Vallade, B., 228, *247*
Vallat, J. N., 161, *195*
Vallin, J., 219, 224, *242*
Valzelli, L., 65, *169*
Van Daele, P., 205, 217, *240*, *247*
Vandam, L. D., 84, *171*
Van Den Brenck, H. A., 69, *179*
Vanden Heuval, W. J. A., 147, *195*
Van Der Hoeven, T., 266, *282*
Vanderbrook, M. J., 3, *195*
Van der Eycken, C., 205, 217, *240*, *247*
Vander Kamp, H., 153, *188*
Van der Spek, P. A. F., 219, *247*
Vandewater, S. L., 67, 99, *195*
Van de Westeringh, C., 205, 217, *240*, *247*
Van Ess, P. R., 24, *195*
Vanlerenverghe, J., 87, 105, *195*
Van Loon, E. J., 82, 83, 101, 139, 144, 147, *173*, *176*, *184*, *185*, *196*
Van Meter, W. G., 83, *192*, 291, *301*
Vanni, F., 217, 219, *238*, *245*
Van Nueten, J. M., 217, 229, *240*, *247*, 297, *300*
Vanov, S., 526, *532*
Van Praag, H. M., 521, *522*, 529, *531*, *532*
van Proosdij-Hartzema, E. G., 60, 69, 91, 108, 112, *196*
Van Rossum, J. M., 217, *247*, 529, *532*
Van Wijk, L., 219, *244*
Van Winkle, E., 254, 260, 261, 266, *278*, *282*
Vanzelli, U., 220, *247*
Varela, L. B., 219, *248*
Varesi, E. M., 230, *246*
Varraso, A., 224, *235*
Vates, T., 260, *278*
Vates, T. S., 153, 158, 161, *182*, *196*
Vauterin, C., 226, *248*
Vautrin, M., 224, *246*
Vazquez, A. J., 269, *278*
Veech, R. L., 260, *282*
Veghelyi, P. V., 152, *196*
Vejdélek, Z. J., 293, *301*
Venkataraman, K., 3, *196*
Venning, G. R., 217, *248*
Verbruggen, F. J., 217, 229, *240*, *244*, 297, *300*
Vercruysse, J., 217, 230, *242*, *243*
Verga, G., 77, *164*
Vergovkina, I. V., 524, *531*
Verhave, T., 50, *196*
Verhulst, H. L., 160, *166*
Verly, W. G., 261, *281*
Verstraete, A., 217, 227, *243*, *248*
Vesell, E. S., 148, *196*
Vestre, N. D., 151, 153, 156, *192*, *196*
Viaud, P., 121, *196*
Victor, M., 273, *277*, *282*
Vigne, J., 147, *194*
Vignot, P., 226, *243*
Vijayvargiya, R., 82, *165*
Villa, J. L., 226, *248*
Villarreal, J., 528, *532*
Villaverde, R., 270, *280*
Vinař, O., *196*
Vincent, J. D., 226, *232*
Vinegar, R., 77, *196*
Virtue, R. W., 52, *196*
Visentini, P., 76, *196*
Vitek, V., 260, *279*
Vitger, J., 225, *248*
Vivoli, G., 105, *196*
Vogel, G., 100 109, *196*
Vogt, M., 54, 87, 89, 91, 98, 99, *178*

Voigt, R., 151, *196*
Voisin, A., 98, *162*
Vojtechovsky, M., 260, *279*
Vojvodić, S., 101, 102, *194*
Volk, B. W., 109, *177*
Vol'pe, M. M., 148, *196*
Von Berger, G. P., 51, 52, *184*
von Eiff, A. W., 220, *248*
von Euler, U. S., 262, *282*
von Horn, L., 290, *301*
von Ledebur, I., 66, *174*, *196*
von Schlichtegroll, A., 290, *301*
Voss, T. J., 152, *178*
Votava, Z., 139, *166*
Vourc'h, G., 230, *248*
Vourlekis, A., 151, *196*
Vroom, F. Q., 152, *196*
Vyner, B. H., 144, *179*

W

Waaler, T., 149, *196*
Waalkes, T. P., 260, *282*
Wada, J. A., 46, *196*
Waddell, A. W., 143, 149, *161*, *196*
Waelkens, J., 220, 231, *248*
Waelsch, H., 82, *164*
Wagemaker, H., 93, *163*
Wagman, A. I., 47, *193*
Wagman, W., 47, *193*
Wagner, J., 226, *242*
Wagner, M., 226, *240*
Wagner, S. A., 50, *163*
Waitzkin, L., 156, *196*
Wakim, K. G., 66, 113, *162*
Walaas, O., 253, *282*
Waldeck, B., 217, *233*
Waldrop, F. N., 151, *196*
Walkenstein, S. S., 139, 147, *196*
Walker, M. F., 160, *196*
Walker, R. G., 151, *196*, 230, *248*
Wallace, G., 155, *168*
Wallace, R. D., 147, 148, *171*
Wallenstein, S. L., 67, *179*
Waller, M. B., 48, 49, 50, *174*, *196*
Waller, P. F., 49, *196*
Walsh, L., 164, *164*
Walter, C., 252, *281*
Walter, M., 294, *300*

Wambsganss, E., 220, *248*
Wang, S. C., 57, 58, 85, 89, *175*, *187*
Wanklin, J., 155, *171*
Ware, K., 153, *196*
Warecka, K., 92, *196*
Warner, B. T., 37, *168*
Warner, K. A., 253, *279*, *280*
Warnes, H., 219, 224, 228, *243*, *248*
Warren, M. R., 285, *301*
Warren, R. J., *196*
Wartel, R., 226, *239*
Wase, A. W., 76, 139, *168*, *196*
Watkins, J. C., 271, *278*
Watt, J., 159, *196*
Watts, T. P. S., 204, 231, *246*
Waugh, W. H., 160, *196*
Weatherall. M., 151, *196*
Weaver, J. E., 42, *196*
Webb, F. J., 25, *163*
Webb, W. G., 287, *301*
Weber, B., 140, *182*
Webster, R. A., 108, *183*, *196*
Wechsler, M. B., 137, 139, 147, 149, *173*, *196*
Weck, G., 220, *246*
Weekly, R. D., 159, *190*
Weidley, E. F., 41, 44, *168*
Weijlard, J., 128, *168*
Weikel, J. H., Jr., 139, 147, *196*
Weinberg, S. J., 94, *197*
Weinberger, W., 160, *181*
Weiner, A., 83, 100, *187*, *192*
Weinstein, B. J., 114, *164*
Weinstein, G. J., *184*
Weise, V. K., 155, *184*
Weiss, B., 50, *183*, *197*
Weissbach, H., 258, 260, *282*, 524, 525, *532*
Weissman, A., 298, *301*
Weitzman, E. D., 111, *197*
Welch, V. C., 152, *178*
Wellhöner, H. H., 55, *197*
Welsh, A. L., 151, *197*, 295, *301*
Weltman, A. S., 109, *191*
Wendel, H., 155, *183*
Wendel, O. W., 96, *197*
Wentzel, D. G., 153, *197*
Werboff, J., 43, 114, *197*
Werdinius, B., 217, *231*
Werner, G., 41, 43, 45, 50, 51, 54, 91, *169*, *176*
Werner, H. W., 285, *301*
Wert, E. B., 152, *197*
West, E. D., 156, *197*

West, E. S., 83, *188*
Westermann, E., 529, *532*
Westley, J., 525, *532*
Westling, H., 66, *180*
Wetterholm, B., 160, *197*
Wetterholm, D. H., 159, *197*
Wheeler, A. G., 139, 147, *196*
Wheeler, C. E., 159, *177*
Wheeler, K. W., 283, *301*
Whitby, L. G., 65, 84, *162*
White, D., 69, *179*
White, H. R., 151, *191*
White, R. P., 50, *197*
White, T., 84, *197*, 273, *282*
Whitehead, W. A., 153, *197*
Whiteley, J. S., 153, *185*
Whitney, G., 527, *531*
Whitton, L. K., 138, 139, *197*
Wickard, C. P., 152, *190*
Wickstrom, L., 521, *522*
Widmann, H., 158, *197*
Widmark, M., 219, *238*
Wiener, W., 159, *177*
Wiersma, C. A. G., 270, *281*
Wight, C. F., 25, *197*
Wilcox, F., 160, *197*
Wilens, S. L., 83, *197*
Wilhelmi, G., 78, *197*
Wilke, G., 73, 113, *171*, *197*
Wilken, G., 229, *239*
Wilkens, B., 154, *175*
Wilkin, M. O., 156, 158, *167*
Wilkins, J. H., 291, *301*
Wilkinson, J. L., 155, *197*
Willadsen, J., 219, *247*
Williams, B. H., 219, *247*
Williams, C. M., *280*
Williams, E., 153, *190*
Williams, J. A., 113, *177*
Williams, R. A., 151, *196*
Williams, R. J., 153, *185*
Willrich, K., 151, *193*
Wilson, G. M., 151, *197*
Wilson, I. C., 151, *197*
Wilson, J. D., *281*
Wilson, J. W., 33, *171*
Wilson, W. P., 273, *282*
Winbury, M. M., 94, *197*
Winckler, C., 230, *248*
Winkelbauer, R. G., 114, *197*
Winkelman, N. W., 150, 151, 161, *197*
Winkelmann, R. K., 66, 113, *162*

Winnik, H. Z., 100, 101, 102, 103, *181*, *194*
Winter, C. A., 253, 254, *281*, *282*
Winter, F. C., 159, *197*
Winter, W. D., 154, *197*
Winters, E. P., 79, *197*
Winters, W. D., 63, *194*
Winthrop, S. O., 298, *301*
Wintrobe, M. M., 158, *172*
Wirt, A. L., 154, *193*
Wirt, R. D., 154, *193*
Wirth, W., 62, 120, *197*
Wiseman-Distler, M. H., 524, *532*
Wislicki, L., 107, *197*
Witherspoon, J. D., 69, *197*
Witkin, L. B., 39, *197*
Witkop, B., 64, *162*, 258, 262, 263, 269, *278*, *280*
Witoslawski, J. J., 47, *179*, 521, *522*
Witt, F. W., 67, *191*
Witt, P. N., 41, 98, 151, *185*, *197*
Witt, R. W., 114, *193*
Wittenborn, I. P., 261, *280*
Witton, K. J., 155, *197*
Wittkower, E. D., 152, *183*
Witzleb, E., 56, 85, 91, 92, 93, *161*, *166*, *197*
Wohlgast, R., 140, *192*
Wojnicka, H., 219, *240*
Wolf, J. K., 94, *197*
Wolf, J. W., 152, *197*
Wolf, S., 153, *168*
Wollemann, M., 81, 82, 135, 137, 140, *197*
Wollman, S., 230, *248*
Woodford, R. B., 273, *280*
Woolley, D. W., 265, 266, *282*
Wortis, J., 151, *198*
Wortz, E. C., 52, *166*
Wretmark, G., 72, *168*
Wright, J. B., 30, *190*
Wright, R. L. D., 153, *198*
Wruble, L. D., 157, *198*
Wulfsohn, N. L., 229, *237*
Wunderlich, H., 121, *198*
Wurtman, R. J., 251, 252, 262, *278*, *282*
Wylie, D. W., 297, *300*, *301*
Wyngarden, J. B., 274, *282*
Wynne, R., 153, *181*
Wypych, M., 219, *240*

X

Xhonneux, R., 203, 217, *246*

Y

Yagi, K., 50, 82, *198*
Yakovleva, M. I., 54, 85, *182*
Yakson, Z. P., 157, *198*
Yakubovskaya, V. I., 75, 83, *198*
Yale, H., 29, 119, 128, 137, *166*, *178*, *198*
Yamada, H., 524, *532*
Yamamoto, I., 74, 82, *198*
Yamamoto, K., 139, *187*
Yamamoto, T., 100, *193*
Yamashita, T., 114, *194*
Yang, P. R., 82, *198*
Yanniris, M., 219, *245*
Yasuda, M., 114, *194*
Yasue, T., 97, *187*
Yasunobu, K., 524, *532*
Yelnosky, J., 217, *237*, *248*
Yhland, M., 140, *183*
Yim, G. K. W., 80, *186*
Yogodzinski, L. H., 25, *165*
Yoshitani, H., 94, *198*
Young, R. L., 139, *191*, *198*
Yung, D. K., 146, *198*
Yuwiler, A., 251, 268, *278*, *282*
Yvonneau, M., 226, *236*

Z

Zaccala, M., 219, *237*
Zakusov, V. V., 151, *198*
Zamcheck, N., 77, *176*
Zapata-Ortiz, V., 96, *198*
Zaratzian, V. L., 66, *181*
Zarembo, J. E., *196*
Zarrow, M. X., 69, *178*
Zattoni, J., 229, *234*
Zauder, H. L., 230, *248*
Zbinden, G., 85, 105, *186*, *194*
Zecca, C., 219, 230, *246*, *248*
Zegveld, C., 230, *248*
Zehnder, K., 135, *198*
Zeleba, M. S., 151, *198*
Zelený, A., 82, *182*
Zelickson, A. S., 159, *198*
Zeller, E. A., 268, *282*, 523, 524, *532*
Zeller, H. C., 159, *198*
Zeller, K., 230, *246*
Zeltzerman, I., 151, *191*
Zenitz, B. L., 119, *184*
Zerbe, H., 219, *248*
Zerbini, E., 220, *248*
Zetler, G., 65, *198*
Zielinski, J., 145, 147, *198*
Zierach, H. J., 229, *241*
Zimbardo, P. G., 43, *198*
Zimerman, C., 228, *247*
Zimmerman, G. R., 104, *198*
Zindler, M., 230, *248*
Zipf, H. F., 60, *198*
Zirkle, C. L., 30, 31, 32, 33, 129, *162*, *169*, *188*
Zocche, G. P., 229, *232*, 529, *531*
Zografi, G., 39, *198*
Zoller, E., 82, *198*
Zolnerkiek, P., 229, *244*
Zuckerman, E., 50, *182*
Zugliani, J. A., 230, *248*
Zweifach, B. W., 96, *178*
Zwirn, P., 54, *171*

Subject Index

Letters in parentheses followed by a page number indicate the first three letters of an author's name and the page of the Bibliographic Appendexes on which a complete reference is given.

A

Abitylguanide, influenza and, 110
Aceperone, 203
   adrenolytic potency, 215
   antiemesis and, 213
   pharmacological effects of, 216
   potency of, 210, 211, 214
Acepromazine,
   emesis and, 58
   proprietary names for, 12
   tetanus and, 108
Acetabuton, clinical use of, 231
Acetabutone, structure of, 203
2-Acetaminofluorene,
   carcinogenicity, chlorpromazine and, 78
Acetate,
   incorporation, chlorpromazine and, 73, 76
Acetazin, 12
Acethylpromazin, 12
Acetophenazine, 21
   adolescent schizophrenia and, (Dar) 306
   ambulatory schizophrenic adults and, (Dar) 306
   anxiety reactions and, (Rob) 306
   biology and pharmacology of, 305
   cardiac patients and, (Tor) 307
   chemistry of, 305
   clinical use of, 306
   elderly psychotics and, (Wit) 307
   fighting behavior in mice and, (Kni) 305
   hyperactive geriatric patients and, (Ham) 306
   paranoid symptomatology and, (She) 307
   side effects of, 305
Acetopromazin, 12
Acetylcholine,
   activity, chlorpromazine and, 65, 90, 91
   chlorpromazine and, 40, 105
   cortical, chlorpromazine and, 56
   psychopharmacological agents and, 34
   role in central nervous system, 272

Acetylcholinesterase, chlorpromazine and, 82
2-Acetyl-10-(3'-dimethylamino-1'-propyl)-phenothiazine, 12
ω-N-Acetylhistamine, 272
2-Acetyl-10-(2'', N^1-hydroxyethyl-N^2,3'-piperazinyl-1'-propyl)phenothiazine, 21
2-Acetyl-10-{3'-[4-(2-hydroxyethyl)piperidino]propyl}-phenothiazine, 22
N-Acetylnormetanephrine, 257, 258
Acetylpromazin, 12
Acetylpromazine, gall bladder and, 105
N-Acetylserotonin, formation of, 266, 267
Aconitase, chlorpromazine and, 83
Aconitine,
   effects, chlorpromazine and, 93
Action potential, chlorpromazine and, 56
Acute cases, chlorpromazine and, 151
Adazine, 9
Addiction,
   methyprylon and, (Ber) 492, (Jen) 494
   ethchlorvynol and, (Ess) 497
Adenosine monophosphate, chlorpromazine and, 93
Adenosine triphosphatase, chlorpromazine and, 39, 47, 74, 82
Adenosine triphosphate,
   brain, chlorpromazine and, 73
   utilization, chlorpromazine and, 83
S-Adenosylmethionine,
   dopamine metabolism and, 261
   indole amine metabolism and, 269
Adrenal cortical hormones, chlorpromazine and, 70
Adrenalectomy,
   chlorpromazine and, 75, 100
   electro shock threshold and, 53
Adrenal gland,
   ascorbic acid, chlorpromazine and, 83
   weight, chlorpromazine and, 99, 103, 113
Adrenaline, *see also* Epinephrine,
   effects, chlorpromazine and, 50, 71, 99
   milk ejection and, 103

Adrenergic agents,
    blocking, chlorpromazine and, 84–86
Adrenochrome, schizophrenia and, 258–260
Adrenocorticotropic hormone,
    chlorpromazine and, 98–99
    perphenazine and, (Kiv) 339
    psychosis, promazine and, (Pla) 402
Adrenolutin, schizophrenia and, 258–260
Adrenolytic activity,
    neuroleptic potency and, 210, 214–215
    phenothiazines, 5
        structure and, 122–123
Adrenolytic agents, blood pressure and, 94
Affect,
    impeded, chlorpromazine and, 152
Affective behavior, ectylurea and, (Dob) 491
Affective states, norepinephrine and, 264
Aftercare, maintenance phenothiazines in, (Tro) 458
Age, response to phenothiazines and, 71
Aged,
    anxiety in,
        thiopropazote and, (Ric) 419
    depressed, trifluperazine and, (Bro) 446
    prochlorperazine and, (Shu) 386
    psychotic, acetophenazine and, (Wit) 307
    thioridazine and, (Dar) 427
    trifluperazine and, (Fal) 448
Aggressive behavior,
    chlorpromazine and, 38, 40, 49
    fluanisone and, 227
    haloperidol and, 218
    insect, drugs and, 118
    psychopharmacological agent testing and, 34
    rat, promazine and, (Sio) 393
    urinary indoles and, 268
Agitation,
    benperidol and, 228–229
    chlorpromazine and, 151, 152
    chlorprothixene and, (Cha) 510
    droperidol and, 230
    fluanisone and, 226
    methylperidol and, 225
    psychomotor, haloperidol and, 218, 220, 221
    senile, promazine and, (Set) 403
Agranulocytosis, see also Granulocytes
    chlorpromazine and, 157–158
    fatal,
        mepazine and, (Fel) 325
        promazine and, (Ear) 394

Agranulocytosis, fatal—*continued*
    promazine and, (Ben) 394, (Chi) 394, (Pis) 396, (Woo) 396
    thioridazine and, (Sha) 424
    triflupromazine and, (Ayd) 461
    trimeprazine and, (Bra) 470
Ahistan, 5
Akathisia,
    haloperidol and, 220, 221
    thioridazine and, (Fre) 423
    trifluperidol and, 222, 224
Akinesia, chlorpromazine and, 41
Akineton, 296
Alanine,
    levels,
        amphetamine and, 80
        chlorpromazine and, 80
        methoxypromazine and, 80
Albumin,
    labeled, capillary permeability to, 95
Alcohol,
    activity, chlorpromazine and, 61–62
    approach-avoidance training and, 45
    hallucinosis,
        trifluoperazine and, (Bar) 445
        intoxication, perphenazine and, (Gre) 352
    metabolism, chlorpromazine and, 83
    promazine and, (Gor) 391
    withdrawal syndrome, promazine and, (God) 400
Alcoholics,
    hydroxyphenamate and, (Gou) 483
    methocarbamol and, (Moo) 487
    perphenazine and, (Bar) 348
    promazine and, (Bry) 397
Alcoholism,
    acute,
        methocarbamol and, (Lof) 487
        promazine and, (Coh) 398, (Fox) 399
        trifluoperazine and, (Cos) 447
        chlorpromazine and, 152
    chronic,
        promazine and, (Fel) 399
        trifluoperazine and, (Har) 450
        methocarbamol and, (Moo) 487
        perphenazine and, (Sal) 359
        prochlorperazine and, (Rog) 386
        promazine and, (Bor) 394, (San) 392
        thiopropazote and, (Him) 418
Aldehyde oxidase, catecholamine oxidase and, 258

Aldol, 295
Alimemazin, 10
Alimenazine, 10
Alkaloids,
  emesis, chlorpromazine and, 59
Allergan, 7
Allergy,
  dermatologic, promazine and, (Fro) 395
  methdilazine and, (Gra) 330, (Spo) 331
  perphenazine and, (Coh) 349, (Rud) 359
  promazine and, (Hol) 395)
  trifluoperazine and, (San) 456
Alloxan diabetes, drug metabolism and, 137
Aloperidin, 200
Alpha waves, chlorpromazine and, 50
Amblyopia, perphenazine and, (Joh) 344
Amenorrhea,
  chlorpromazine and, 102–103, 159
  thioridazine and, (Des) 427, (Zuc) 424
Amimethylene, 294
Aminazin, 6
Amines,
  endogenous, mental disease and, 255–273
Amino acid(s),
  formation, chlorpromazine and, 80
  metabolism, chlorpromazine and, 80–81
Amino acid decarboxylases, chlorpromazine and, 79
D-Amino acid oxidase, chlorpromazine and, 82
γ-Aminobutyric acid,
  brain metabolism and, 270, 271
  distribution, chlorpromazine and, 82
  Krebs cycle and, 271
Aminoisobutyric acid,
  uptake, chlorpromazine and, 138
Aminopromazin, proprietary names for, 15
Aminopromazine, mammary glands and, 103
Aminopyrine,
  activity, chlorpromazine and, 62
  adaptive metabolism of, 146
  arthritic response and, 100
  blood pressure and, 94
  metabolism, microsomes and, 138
p-Aminosalicylic acid, phenothiazine tests and, 150
Amiperone, structure of, 202
Amitryptylene, serotonin and, 65, 79
Amniotic cells, chlorpromazine and, 78
Amobarbital,
  activity, chlorpromazine and, 60
  conditioned response and, 48
  yohimbine activity and, 65

Ampazine, 8
Amphactil, 6
Amphedroxyn, 286
Amphenidone, proprietary name and use of, 287
Amphetamine, 283
  brain amino acids and, 80
  conditioned response and, 46, 48
  diethyltryptamine and, 66
  drug testing and, 35
  electroencephalographic effects, chlorpromazine and, 51
  leukemia and, 78
  norepinephrine and, 262–264
  pressor effect, chlorpromazine and, 84
  proprietary name and use of, 285
  serotonin and, 79
  toxicity,
    chlorpromazine and, 63, 112
    promazine and, (Las) 392
  tremor and, 57
d-Amphetamine,
  chlorpromazine and, 156
  evaluation of, 42
Ampliactil, 6
Amplictil, 6
Amylobarbitone, trifluoperazine and, (Whi) 458.
Analgesia,
  chlorpromazine and, 111
  promazine and, (Cob) 398
  propiomazine and, (Lia) 406
Analgesics, chlorpromazine and, 62–63
Anaphylaxis, promazine and, (Fox) 391
Anatensol, 20
Anatran, 12
Anesthesia,
  droperidol and, 229
  fluanisone and, 227
  fluphenazine and, (Hym) 318
  local or spinal, chlorpromazine and, 67, 110
  mepazine and, (Dav) 327
  perphenazine and, (Alb) 347, (Dob) 350
  promazine and, (Bos) 397
  thiethylperazine and, (Deb) 415
  triflupromazine and, (Dav) 463
Anesthetics,
  activity, chlorpromazine and, 61
Angiocardiography, chlorpromazine and, 154
Angiotensin, chlorpromazine and, 95

Angiotonin, chlorpromazine and, 84
Anisperidone,
  adrenolytic potency, 215
  antiemesis and, 213
  clinical use of, 231
  pharmacological effects of, 216
  potency of, 210, 211, 213
  ptosis and, 216
  structure of, 202
Antazoline, depressor response and, 109
Anthelmintic(s),
  phenothiazines as, 2, 3, 5, 118, 143
  psychotherapeutic activities and, (Min) 438
Anti-amphetamine test, neuroleptic potency and, 210, 214, 215
Anti-apomorphine activity,
  fluphenazine and, (Bur) 311, (Bur) 316
  neuroleptic potency and, 210–213
  trifluoperazine and, (Jan) 438
Anti-arrhythmic activity,
  promazine and, (Kam) 392
  thioridazine and, (Mad) 430
Antibody, production, chlorpromazine and, 69
Anticholinergic effects, Parkinsonism and, (Whi) 440
Anticonvulsant activity,
  methyprylon and, (Fuj) 493
  phenaglycodol and, (Car) 477
  phenothiazine structure and, 120
Antidiabetic compounds, tranquilizers and, 65
Antidiuretic hormone,
  chlorpromazine and, 99, 101, 110–111, 118
  promazine and, (Smi) 393
Antiemetic activity,
  carphenazine and, (Car) 309
  chlorpromazine and, 2, 152, 161
  droperidol and, 229
  fluphenazine and, (Bon) 315, (Cor) 316, (Rao) 312
  haloperidol and, 220
  pipamazine and, (Bla) 363
  prochlorperazine and, (Ber) 379
  promazine and, (Bla) 397, (Ros) 392
  thiethylperazine and, (Bar) 414
  triflupromazine and, (Bel) 462
  trimeprazine and, (Poo) 474
Antigen, schizophrenic serum and, 255
Anti-hallucinatory activity, fluphenazine and (Kru) 314

Antihistaminic activity, 3, 5
  chlorpromazine and, 2
  methdilazine and, (Cra) 330
  mitochondrial swelling and, 75
  phenothiazine structure and, 121
  trimeprazine and, (Gra) 472
Antimicrobial activity, perphenazine and, (Luk) 339
Anti-norepinephrine test, neuroleptic potency and, 210, 214–215
Antioxidants, phenothiazines as, 24
Antipar, 11
Anti-pica, 200
Antisialogogue effect,
  phenothiazines and, (Dob) 448
  prochlorperazine and, (Dob) 368
Antitussive activity,
  phenothiazines and, 5
  trimeprazine and, (Poo) 474
Antiwhealing drugs, (Col) 416
Anxiety,
  acetophenazine and, (Rob) 306
  alcohol-tranquilizer combinations and, 62
  chlorpromazine and, 38
  chlorprothixene and, (Gov) 312
  droperidol and, 230
  floropipamide and, 227
  fluphenazine and, (Bod) 315, (Car) 316, (Hes) 318
  hydroxyphenamate and, (Cah) 483
  pentobarbital and, 62
  perphenazine and, (Ern) 351, (Pre) 358
  phenaglycodol and, (Zuk) 478
  thiopropazate and, (Ric) 419
  thioridazine and, (Blu) 426, (Cot) 427
  trifluoperazine and, (Ern) 448, (Ham) 450, (Phi) 455, (Sai) 456
AP800, 291
Apes,
  motor activity, prothipendyl and, (Bar) 408
Aplasia, prochlorperazine and, (Bha) 373, 379
Apomorphine,
  antagonism, phenothiazine structure and, 120
  emesis,
    chlorpromazine and, 57–58
    inhibition of, 35
    phenothiazine structure and, 116–117
Apprehension, chlorpromazine and, 153
Approach-avoidance conflict, perphenazine and, (Gro) 338

Aprobith, 5
Arousal response,
 chlorpromazine and, 38, 40, 46, 51
 lysergic acid diethylamide-chlorpromazine and, 64
 promazine and, (Wil) 393
Arterial thrombosis, promazine and, (Ham) 395, (Opi) 396
Arthrithis,
 ceruloplasmin and, 252
 chlorpromazine and, 100, 152
Ascidians, chlorpromazine and, 115
Ascites cells, tranquilizers and, 77, 78
Ascorbic acid,
 adrenal, chlorpromazine and, 83, 98–99
 ceruloplasmin and, 251–252
 stress and, 97
Ascorbic acid oxidase, chlorpromazine and, 74
Aspirin,
 activity, chlorpromazine and, 62
Asthma, chlorpromazine and, 152
Ataractics, paper chromatography of, (Vec) 421
Atosil, 7
Atropine,
 chlorpromazine and, 91, 105
 electroencephalographic effects, chlorpromazine and, 51
 tremor and, 57
 tremorine activity and, 66
 yohimbine activity and, 65–66
Atropine-like activity, phenothiazine activity and, 121
Attention span, promazine and, (Das) 398
Audiogenic seizures, chlorpromazine and, 53
Autonomic nervous system, chlorpromazine and, 84–91
Autooxidation, chlorpromazine and, 73
Aventyl, 293
Avomine, 7
Axolotl, regeneration, chlorpromazine and, 78
Azacon, 290
Azacyclonol,
 diethyltriptamine activity and, 66
 proprietary names and use of, 291
Azaphenothiazines, 33
Azoxodon, proprietary name and use of, 285

B

Bananas, amine excretion and, 260
Bantu(s),
 schizophrenic, thioridazine and, (Rom) 432
Barbital,
 activity, chlorpromazine and, 60, 61
Barbiturates,
 activity, chlorpromazine and, 60–61
 body temperature and, 69
 conditioned responses and, 44
 fighting behavior and, 43
 floropipamide and, 227
 liver nonprotein sulfhydryl groups and, 75
 potentiation, phenothiazine structure and, 119, 122–123
 sedative effects of, 34
Barium chloride,
 spasm, chlorpromazine and, 105
Basal ganglia, chlorpromazine and, 74
Behavior, prochlorperazine and, (Kel) 383
Behavioral disorders,
 chlorpromazine and, 155
 fluphenazine and, (Lav) 319
 thioridazine and, (All) 425, (Oet) 431
Behavior rating scales, chlorpromazine and, 153
Bemegride, 283
 proprietary name and use of, 285
Benactyzine,
 mammary glands and, 103
 proprietary names and use of, 294
 tremorine activity and, 66
Benperidol, 208
 adrenolytic potency, 215
 clinical uses, 228–229
 potency of, 210, 211
 trade names for, 201
Benzindopyrin, 297
Benzperidol, trade names for, 201
Benzquinamide, proprietary name and use of, 298
Benztropine,
 droperidol and, 230
 trifluperidol therapy and, 222, 223
Benzylhydrazine, serotonin and, 79
Benzylimidazoline, antihistaminics and, 109
6-Benzylthiouracil, chlorpromazine and, 101
Beri-beri, neuropathy and, 276
Betaine, effect in schizophrenia, 261

Betta splendens, chlorpromazine and, 118
Bile, phenothiazines in, 135, 139
Bile flow, chlorprothixene and, (Ste) 506
Biperiden, proprietary name and use of, 296
Black widow spider,
 poisoning, methocarbamol and, (Jon) 487
Blood,
 metabolism, chlorpromazine and, 76–77
Blood-brain barrier,
 chlorpromazine and, 78
 trifluoperazine and, (Gue) 450
Blood dyscrasias, promazine and, (Bes) 394, (Cou) 394
Blood electrolytes, chlorpromazine and, 72
Blood flow,
 chlorpromazine and, 92, 93
 hepatic, thioridazine and, (Eck) 421
Blood lipids, chlorpromazine and, 72–73
Blood pressure,
 chlorpromazine and, 84, 91, 92, 95
 phenothiazine structure and, 121
Blood sugar,
 chlorpromazine and, 72
 promazine and, (Cit) 391
Blood vessels,
 major, chlorpromazine and, 91–93
Body temperature, chlorpromazine and, 68–70, 77
Body weight, chlorpromazine and, 83
BP 400, 292
BP 401, 290
Bradykinin,
 edema, chlorpromazine and, 109
Brain,
 bioelectric activity, trifluoperazine and, (Lei), 438
 chlorpromazine effect on, 73–74, 80
 nonprotein sulfhydryl groups, tranquilizers and, 80–81
 phenothiazine uptake by, 134, 137, 138
 sulfolipids, trifluoperazine and, (Gle) 437
 syndromes, thioridazine and, (San) 432
Bretylium, norepinephrine and, 263
Bromine, phenothiazines and, 149
2-Bromo-2-ethylbutyrylurea, (But) 491
Bromolysergic acid diethylamide,
 hypothermia and, 69
 visceral serotonin and, 79
Bromosulfophthalein,
 excretion, chlorpromazine and, 75, 106
Bromthymol blue, phenothiazines and, 149

Brucella melitensis,
 toxin, chlorpromazine and, 96
Bruxism, methocarbamol and, (Cha) 486
Bufotenine,
 excretion of, 269
 formation of, 269
 neurotransmitters and, 255
Bulbocapnine,
 activity, chlorpromazine and, 65
 effects of, 41
Burn shock, chlorpromazine and, 97
Butabarbital,
 activity, chlorpromazine and, 60
Butropipazone, 209
 adrenolytic potency, 215
 antiemesis and, 213
 clinical use of, 230
 pharmacological effects of, 216
 potency of, 210, 211
 ptosis and, 216
 structure of, 202
Butyrophenones,
 bibliography, 217
 clinically tested, not available commercially, 202–204
 clinical uses, 217–231
 commercially available, 200–201
 pharmacological activity of, 209–217
 structure-activity relationships, 206–209
Butyrothienones, potency of, 206
Butyrylcholine, tranquilizers and, 63
2-Butyryl-10-[3'-(4-methyl-l-piperazinyl)-propyl]phenothiazine, 22
Butyrylperazine, 22
 chlorpromazine and, 156

C

Calcification, chlorpromazine and, 83
Calcium chloride, tremor and, 57
Calmeran, 291
Candida, chlorpromazine and, 115
Canine practice, promazine and, (Gra) 391
Cannibalism, fluanisone and, 227
Capazine, 15
Capillaries, chlorpromazine and, 92, 95
Captodiamine,
 metabolic effects of, 70
 proprietary names and use of, 296
Caramiphen,
 stretch reflex and, 108
 tremorine activity and, 66

SUBJECT INDEX

Carbachol, chlorpromazine and, 91
Carbohydrates, chlorpromazine and, 80
Carbon, activated, phenothiazines and, 150
Carbon dioxide,
  chlorpromazine metabolism and, 139
  tolerance, chlorpromazine and, 155
Carbonic anhydrase, chlorpromazine and, 77, 82
Carbromal, use of, 285
Cardiac arrhythmias, perphenazine and, (Dob) 337
Cardiac catheterization, chlorpromazine and, 154
Cardiac patients,
  acetophenazine and, (Tor) 307
  ethchlorvynol and, (Bli) 497
Cardiazol, 284
Cardio-inhibitory center, chlorpromazine and, 44
Cardiovascular activity,
  thiaxanthene derivatives and, (Ham) 501
  thioridazine and, (Mad) 424
Cardiovascular disease,
  hydroxyphenamate and, (Gre) 483
  prochlorperazine and, (Smi) 386
Cardiovascular system,
  chlorpromazine and, 91–95
  droperidol and, 230
Carisoprodol, stretch reflex and, 108
Carotid occlusion, chlorpromazine and, 87, 90
Carphenazine, 22
  antiemetic specificity of, (Car) 309
  biology and pharmacology of, 308
  chemical papers, 308
  chemistry of, (Rus) 308
  chronic schizophrenics and, (Bar) 309, (Cac) 309, (Tyc) 310
  clinical evaluation of, (Cla) 309
  clinical papers, 309–310
  electroencephalographic effects of, (Hos) 308
  extrapyramidal regulation and, (Niv) 309
  hepatological studies and, (Tia) 308
  hospitalized patients and, (Kot) 309
  mental defectives and, (Car) 309
  out patients and, (Mer) 309
  schizophrenia and, (Che) 309
  sequential analysis and, (Bel) 309
  side effects of, 308–309
  toxicity of, (Men) 309, (Tis) 308
Casantin, 11

Cat,
  reaction to chlorpromazine, 41, 50–52
  trimeprazine and, (Can) 469
Catalase, chlorpromazine and, 74, 140
Catalepsy, chlorpromazine and, 41
Catalepsy test,
  phenothiazine activity, structure and, 120, 130–131
Cataract surgery, promazine and, (Sha) 403
Catatonia,
  chlorpromazine and, 152
  promazine and, (May) 395
  thioridazine and, (Boi) 426
Catatonics,
  withdrawn, trifluoperazine and, (Sti) 457
Catecholamine(s), *see also* Adrenaline, Epinephrine, etc.
  brain, phenothiazines and, (Vog) 440
  chlorpromazine and, 81, 84–86, 88–89
  degradation of, 257–258
  effects on heart, chlorpromazine and, 85
  faulty adrenergic nerve transmission and, 262–265
  metabolism of, 255–258
  neurotoxin theories and, 258–262
  performance and, 46
  psychopharmacological agents and, 34
Catecholamine-depleting agents, promazine and, (Sto) 393
Catecholamine derivatives, mental disease and, 255–265
Catechol O-methyl transferase, 258
  norepinephrine and, 263, 264
Cathepsin,
  secretion, chlorpromazine and, 104
Cattle, promazine and, (Lan) 392
CB 1522, 12
CB 1678, 16
Centalun, 287
Centractil, 8
Centractyl, 8
Central nervous system,
  chlorpromazine and, 40–57
  clinical applications of phenothiazines, 150–153
  depressants, chlorpromazine and, 60–63
  effects, chemical structure and, (Bar) 435
  localization,
    thiethylperazine and, (Spa) 415
    methyprylon and, (Sch) 495
Central sympathetic suppressants, electron-donating properties of, (Lyo) 435

Cerebellum,
  metabolism, chlorpromazine and, 80
  stimulation, chlorpromazine and, 43
Cerebral circulation, chlorpromazine and, 155
Cerebral cortex,
  metabolism, chlorpromazine and, 80
Cerebral hemodynamics, promazine and, (Ehr) 391
Cerebral metabolism, chlorprothixene and, (Gey) 504
Cerebral palsy,
  chlorpromazine and, 155
  phenaglycodol and, (Kug) 477
Cerebrosides, mental defects and, 275
Cerebrospinal fluid,
  pressure, chlorpromaxine and, 95
Ceric sulfate, phenothiazines and, 138, 149
Ceruloplasmin, mental disease and, 251–252
Cerveau isolé, chlorpromazine and, 51–52
Cervical-lingual-masticator myoclonus, prochlorperazine and, (Eck) 374
Cetyltrimethylammonium bromide, lipid films and, 106
Cevanol, 294
Cevine, chlorpromazine and, 56
Chemical structure, central nervous system effects and, (Bar) 435
Chicken, fluanisone and, 227
Child psychiatry,
  promazine and, (Bov) 397
  thioridazine and, (Maj) 430
  trifluoperazine and, (Fis) 449
Children,
  aggressive, thioridazine and, (Ald) 425
  anxiety in, thioridazine and, (Cot) 427
  autistic, prochlorperazine and, (Fer) 381
  disturbed, promazine and, (Ver) 404
  fluphenazine and, (Tor) 322
  haloperidol and, 220
  hyperemotional, trimeprazine and, (Dou) 472
  hypermotor syndrome, trifluoperazine and, (Gra) 450
  nervous diseases, thoridazine and (Kub) 430
  prochlorperazine and, (Car) 380
  retarded, fluphenazine and, (Wai) 322
Chimpanzees, perphenazine and, (Wal) 341
Chloracizine, 293
Chloral hydrate, fighting behavior and, 43

Chloralose, tremor and, 57
Chlorazisin, 5
Chlordan, chlorpromazine metabolism and, 139–140
Chlorderazin, 6
Chlordiazepoxide,
  cardiac effects, 85
  chlorpromazine and, 156
  conflict-induced fixations and, 46
  convulsant shock and, 34
  mammary glands and, 103
  nalorphine and, 67
  proprietary name and use of, 289
  serotonin and, 65
  toxemias and, 98
  ulcers and, 104
Chlormeprazine, 15
Chlormethazanone, proprietary name and use of, 287
2-Chloro-10-(2″, N^1-acetoxyethyl-N^2,3′-piperazinyl-1′-propyl)phenothiazine, 21
2-Chloro-10-(4″-carboxamido-N,3′-piperidino-1′-propyl)phenothiazine, 17
2-Chloro-10-(2′-dimethylamino)phenothiazine, 4
2-Chloro-10-(3′-diethylamino-1′-propyl)-phenothiazine, 13, *see* Chlorpromazine
2-Chloro-10-(3′-dimethylamino-1′-propyl)-phenothiazine-5-oxide, 5
m-Chlorodiphenylamine, phenothiazine synthesis and, 25
N-(2-Chloroethyl)dibenzylamine, chlorpromazine hypothermia and, 70
Chloroform,
  inhalation, chlorpromazine and, 85
2-Chloro-10-(2″, N^2-hydroxyethyl-N^2,3′-piperazinyl-1′-propyl)phenothiazine, 18
2-Chloro-4-methyl-10-(3′-dimethylamino-2′-propyl)phenothiazine, 10
2-Chloro-10-(1″-methyl-4″-piperazinyl-3′-propyl-1′)phenothiazine, 15
2-Chloro-10-(1′-methyl-2′,2″-piperidinyl-ethyl)phenothiazine, 15
2-Chlorophenothiazine, excretion of, 145
2-Chlorophenothiazine-10-propionic acid, excretion of, 145
2-Chlorophenothiazine sulfoxide, excretion of, 145
Chloroquine, vitamins and, 115
2-Chloro-10-{3′-[4-(3,4,5-trimethoxy-benzoyloxyethyl)-1-piperazinyl]-propyl}phenothiazine, 23

Chlorphenethazin, 4
Chlorpiperazin, 18
Chlorpiprozin, 18
Chlorproethazin, 13
Chlorpromazine,
  adrenergic agents and, 84–86
  adrenolytic activity, 215
  amino acid metabolism and, 80–81
  analgesia and, 111
  antiemetic effects, 213
    drug induced emesis and, 57–59
    motion sickness and, 59–60
    radiation sickness and, 59
  antihistaminic activity of, 108
  anti-inflammatory effects, 109–110
  antishock effects, 96–97
  blocking of sympathetic stimulation and, 86–87
  blood chemistry and, 72–73
  blood metabolism and, 76–77
  blood pressure and, 84
  brain and, 73–74
  carbohydrate metabolism and, 80
  catecholamines and, 81
  central nervous system depressants and, 60–63
  comparative potency of, 130–131
  decompression and, 111
  demethylation of, 139
  effects, environmental temperature and, 136
  electron donor properties of, 150
  enzyme effects, 81–83
  glucuronide metabolites, 141, 143
    duration of excretion, 144
  hallucinogenic agents and, 64–65
  influenza and, 110
  irritable colon syndrome and, (Wol) 388
  lipid films and, 106
  liver metabolism and, 75–76
  local anesthetic activity, 110
  mechanism and site of action, 39–40
  metabolism of, 132–135
    diabetes and, 137
    mitochondria and, 137
  metabolites, small intestine and, 138
  miscellaneous effects, 83–84
    endocrine, 100-102
  moniliasis and, (Kan) 442
  new phenolic metabolites of, 142
  nontherapeutic applications, 155

Chlorpromazine—*continued*
  other drugs and, 65–68, 155–156
  overdosage, 160–161
  oxidized intermediate, activity of, 135
  oxygen consumption and, 70–71
  parasympathetic nervous system and, 90–91
  pharmacology, 2–3, 37–40, 216
    activity of other drugs and, 60–68
    antiemetic effects, 57–60
    autonomic nervous sytem and, 84–91
    body temperature and, 68–70
    cardiovascular effects, 91–95
    central nervous system and, 40–57
    endocrine effects, 95–104
    gastrointestinal and hepatic effects, 104–106
    metabolic effects, 70–84
    miscellaneous effects, 108–112
    neuromuscular effects, 106–108
    toxicity and, 112–119
  pituitary-gonadal effects, 102–103
  potency of, 210, 211
  proprietary names for, 6
  ptosis and, 216
  "red," dehydrogenase and, 81
  renal effects, 110–111
  schizophrenia and, 222–223
  sedative effects of, 34, 38
  semiconductor properties of, 150
  stretch reflex and, 108
  stress effects and, 97–100
  structure, activity and, 116
  sympathomimetic amines and, 63–64
  synthesis of, 26
  test, indican and, 149
  thyroxine effects and, 100–101
  tolerance to, 45–46, 49, 52
  toxicity,
    acute, 112
    chronic, 112–113
    lower organisms, 115–119
    pregnancy, 113–114
    temperature and, 70
    tissue culture, 115
  tryptamines and, 79–80
  tumors and, 77–78
  uptake and excretion of, 134, 139
  vascular reflexes and, 87–90
  withdrawal of, 153
Chlorpromazine index, phenothiazine activity and, 121

Chlorpromazine N-oxide,
  activity of, 136, 144
  excretion of, 144
Chlorpromazine sulfoxide,
  activity of, 135, 136
  dehydrogenase and, 81
  enzymatic formation of, 137
  excretion of, 144–145
  hemolysis and, 76
  metabolic effects of, 70
Chlorpropamide, vitamins and, 115
Chlorprothixene,
  agitated patients and, (Cha) 510
  ambulatory psychiatry and, (Anj) 508
  analysis of, (Awe) 498
  antidiabetic compounds and, 65
  anxiety and, (Gov) 512
  bile flow and, (Ste) 506
  biology and pharmacology of, 503–507
  cerebral metabolism and, (Gey) 504
  chemical papers, 498–502
  clinical experience and (Uck) 517
  clinical papers, 508–518
  comparative evaluation of, (Las) 514
  convulsive seizures and, (Fie) 507
  depressive states and, (Ala) 508, (Dar) 510
  dyskinetic syndrome and, (Die) 507
  ejaculation and, (Dit) 507
  interaction with thiopentone, (Dob) 503
  laboratory evaluation of, (Ma-) 514
  liver function and, (Tes) 508
  lupus erythematosus and, (Hai) 507
  manic-depressives and, (Mad) 514
  metabolic effects of, 70 (All) 503
  monoamine metabolism and, (Gey) 504
  overdosage of, (Plu) 508
  paranoid symptoms and, (Cah) 510
  poisoning and, (Ehl) 507, (Fre) 507
  polyneuritis and, (Har) 507
  premedication and, (Nae) 515
  private practise and, (Dar) 510
  prolonged administration of, 71
  pruritis and, (Ney) 515
  psychiatry and, (Bec) 509, (Kar) 513
  psychotic patients and, (Bar) 509
  reactions, (Ste) 508
  respiration and, 95, (Flo) 504
  schizophrenia and, (Gay) 512, (Kur) 514
  serotonin and, 79
  side effects of, 507–508
  state hospitals and, (Hag) 512
Chlorprothixene—*continued*
  suicide and, (Lie) 507, (Rav) 508
  toxicology of, (Gom) 512
  ulcers and, 104
  uricosuric effect and, (Hea) 504
Chlorprothixene sulfoxide, 70
Cholecystokinin, chlorpromazine and, 105
Cholestasis, prochlorperazine and, (Wei) 379
Cholesterol,
  mental defects and, 275
  serum, trifluoperazine and, (Rei) 443
  synthesis, chlorpromazine and, 83
  turnover, chlorpromazine and, 75
Choline oxidase, chlorpromazine and, 83
Cholinesterase,
  chlorpromazine and, 73
  inhibitors, chlorpromazine and, 65
  serum, chlorpromazine and, 76
Chorea, haloperidol and, 218
Chorea gravidarum, promazine and, (Cam) 397
Chromatography,
  paper,
    ataractics and, (Vec) 421
    methyprylon and, (Dre) 493
    phenothiazines, (Mel) 390, 502
  column, 147
  gas, 147, (Mar) 435
  ion exchange, 147
  paper, 147, (Eag) 435, (Str) 390
  reversed phase, (Str) 390
  thin layer, 147, (Mar) 435
Chronaxie, chlorpromazine and, 56, 90
Cianatil, 11
Circulatory effects,
  prochlorperazine and, (Lan) 376
  thiethylperazine and, (Dob) 415
Citrate,
  synthesis, chlorpromazine and, 74
Climbing test,
  phenothiazine activity, structure and, 120
  schizophrenic serum and, 254
Cloropromazina, 6
Cocaine,
  anesthesia and, 110
  serotonin and, 79
  vagus stimulation and, 63
Coccidioides imitis, chlorpromazine and, 115
Cochlea, electrical response, chlorpromazine and, 56–57

Codeine,
  metabolism,
    diabetes and, 137
    microsomes, and, 138
Coenzyme A, chlorpromazine and, 83
Coffee, amine excretion and, 260
Colchicine,
  treatment, chlorpromazine and, 77
Cold,
  acclimatization, chlorpromazine and, 70
Cold stress,
  chlorpromazine and, 99, 100
  diphosphopyridine nucleotide levels and, 75
Colitis, prothipendyl and, (Cat) 408
Colorimetry, phenothiazines and, 148, (Rya) 390
Combelen, 16
Compazine, 15
Compound 20B, 295
Compulsive rituals, trifluoperazine and, (Alt) 444
Conceptual disorders, chlorpromazine and, 152
Conditioned response,
  blocking,
    drug testing and, 35
    phenothiazine structure and, 116–117, 120, 130–131
  chlorpromazine and, 2–3, 40, 151
  promazine and, (Gar) 391
  with operant conditioning, chlorpromazine and, 47–50
  without operant conditioning, chlorpromazine and, 44–47
Confinement motor activity, trifluoperazine and, (Fow) 437, (Ted) 439
Congenital pellagra, cause of, 275
Contact dermatitis,
  promazine and, (Goo) 395
  thiopropazate and, (Goo) 418
  triflupromazine and, (Goo) 461
Contomin, 6
Conversion hysteria, perphenazine and, (Sha) 346
Convulsions,
  chlorpromazine and, 50, 155
  chlorprothixene and, (Fig) 507
  ethchlorvynol and, (Blu) 497
  promazine and, (Coh) 394, (Han) 395
Convulsive thresholds, chlorpromazine and, 52–53

Copper,
  plasma levels, chlorpromazine and, 72
Copper sulfate,
  emesis, chlorpromazine and, 59
Coramine, 286
Cornea,
  opacity, chlorpromazine and, 159
Corneal reflex, chlorpromazine and, 39
Cortex,
  chlorpromazine in, 141
  pericruciate area, chlorpromazine and, 43
  stimulation, chlorpromazine and, 46
Cortisone,
  edema and, 97
  effects, chlorpromazine and, 83
  inflammation and, 100
  influenza and, 110
Cotard's syndrome, thioridazine and, (Hen) 424
Counter-current distribution, phenothiazines and, 147
Covatin, 296
Covatix, 296
Cretinism, treatment of, 274
Crossed-extensor reflex, tranquilizers and, 43
Cyamepromazine, 11
Cyanide,
  chlorpromazine effects and, 77
  intoxication, chlorpromazine and, 67
2-Cyano-10-(3′-dimethylamino-2′-methyl-1′-propyl)phenothiazine, 11
2-Cyano-10-(4″-hydroxy-N,3′-piperidino-propyl-1″)phenothiazine, 17
Cyanosis, chlorpromazine and, 155
Cyclopropane,
  inhalation, chlorpromazine and, 85
Cystathionuria, effects of, 275
Cytochrome oxidase, chlorpromazine and, 74, 82

D

D-775, 20
Dartal, 10
Dartalan, 21
Dartan, 21
Dartilan, 21
Deaner, 284
Deanol, proprietary names and use of, 284
Deaths, phenothiazines and, 160
Decentan, 18

Decerebrate animals,
  activity, chlorpromazine and, 43–44
Decompression, chlorpromazine and, 111
Defense reaction, phenothiazine structure and, 120
Dehydrobenzperidol, 297
  trade names for, 201
Dehydrogenases,
  phenothiazines and, 81–82, 137–138
  red chlorpromazine and, 140
Deidrobenzperidolo, 201
Delazin, 8
Delirium,
  alcoholic, haloperidol and, 218, 220
  chronic,
    chlorpromazine and, 152
    trifluoperazine and, (Slu) 457
  fluanisone and, 227
Delirium tremens,
  chlorpromazine and, 152
  promazine and, (Dan) 398, (Fig) 399
  trifluoperazine and, (Bar) 445
Delta waves, chlorpromazine and, 50
Delysid, 295
Demethylamitriptyline, proprietary name and use of, 293
Demethylchlorpromazine sulfoxide, excretion of, 145
Demethylimipramine,
  norepinephrine and, 264–265
  proprietary names and use of, 292
  uptake, tissues and, 134
Dental patients, chlorpromazine and, 154
Deoxycortisone,
  hypertension, chlorpromazine and, 94
  shock threshold and, 53
Deparkin, 11
Dependency, ethchlorvynol and, (Sie) 497
Depot action, fluphenazine and, (Bur) 315
Depressants,
  central nervous system, chlorpromazine and, 60–63
Depression,
  chlorprothixene and, (Ala) 508, (Dar) 510
  endogenous, thioridazine and, (Bas) 425, (Bau) 425
  haloperidol and, 221
  norepinephrine and, 264, 265
  thioridazine and, (Flu) 428, (Pet) 431
  trifluperazine and, (Pet) 455
  trifluperidol and, 224
  tryptamine excretion and, 268–269

Dermatology,
  chlorpromazine and, 152, 159
  ethchlorvynol and, (Rei) 497, (Sch) 497
  trifluperazine and, (Kam) 451, 465
  hydroxyphenamate and, (Cah) 483
Dermatoses,
  itching, trimeprazine and, (Cal) 472
  perphenazine and, (Fan) 351, (Rei) 359, (Yon) 362
  trimeprazine and, (And) 471, (Pan) 473
Desipramine, 292
Desmethyl- compounds, see Demethyl-
Desoxyn, 286
Desyphed, 286
Dexedrine, 285
Dexoval, 286
Dextran,
  edema, phenothiazines and, 37
Diabetes, chlorpromazine and, 72
Diarrhea, thiopropazote and, (McH) 419
Diaspasmyl, 5
Diazepam, proprietary name and use of, 289
Diazepoxide, effects of, 225
Dibenzyline, shock and, 96
Dibucaine, anesthesia and, 110
Dibutil, 14
Dichlorisoproterenol, norepinephrine level and, 81
2,4-Dichloro-10-(3'-dimethylamino-1'-propyl)phenothiazine, 5
Dichloropromazine, 5
Didemethylchlorpromazine sulfoxide, excretion of, 145
Diet, catecholamine excretion and, 260, 262
Diethazine,
  proprietary names for, 11
  synthesis of, 29
10-(2'-Diethylaminoethyl)phenazine, 11
10-(2'-Diethylamino-1'-propyl)phenothiazine, 14
Diethyltryptamine, tranquilizers and, 66
Digestive disorders, fluphenazine and, (Wis) 322
Digitalis, chlorpromazine and, 59, 67
Digitoxin, chlorpromazine effects and, 94
Dihydroergotamine,
  antihistaminics and, 109
  chlorpromazine and, 67
3,4-Dihydroxymandelic acid, catecholamines and, 257, 258, 263
3,4-Dihydroxymandelic aldehyde, catecholamines and, 257, 258

3,4-Dihydroxyphenylacetic acid,
  dopamine and, 258, 259
  elimination, chlorpromazine and, 81
3,4-Dihydroxyphenylalanine,
  catecholamine biosynthesis and, 256
  decarboxylation, chlorpromazine and, 79
  metabolites, chlorpromazine and, 81
  uptake, chlorpromazine and, 80
3,4-Dihydroxyphenylglycol, catecholamines and, 257, 258
Dilosyn, 9, 12
Dimapp, 7
Dimethoxanate, 5
3,4-Dimethoxymandelic acid, catecholamines and, 257
3,4-Dimethoxyphenethylamine,
  dopamine and, 259
  excretion of, 260-261
  pharmacological effects of, 261-262
  schizophrenia and, 254
3,4-Dimethoxyphenylacetic acid,
  dopamine and, 259
  excretion of, 261
4-Dimethylaminoazobenzene, chlorpromazine and, 78
10-(2'-Dimethylaminoethyl)phenazine, 4
10-(3'-Dimethylamine-2'-methyl-1'-propyl)-phenothiazine, 10
10α-Dimethylaminopropionyl phenothiazine methobromide, metabolic fate of, 135
10-(2'-Dimethylamino-1'-propyl)phenothiazine, 7
10-(3'-Dimethylamino-1'-propyl)phenothiazine, 8
10-(2',3'-bis-Dimethylamino-1'-propyl)-phenothiazine, 15
N,N-Dimethylaminopropylphenoxazine, metabolic effects of, 70
N,N-Dimethyl-p-phenylene diamine, oxidation, mental disease and, 251
Dimethylphenylpiperazinium iodide, effects, chlorpromazine and, 90
N,N-Dimethylserotonin, see Bufotenine
2-(N,N-Dimethylsulfonamido)-10-(1"-methyl-4",3'-piperazinyl-1'-propyl)-phenothiazine, 20
N,N-Dimethyltryptamine,
  formation of, 269
  neurotransmitters and, 255
Dinezin, 11
2,4-Dinitrophenol,
  chlorpromazine and, 82

2,4-Dinitrophenol—continued
  pyrexia, chlorpromazine and, 69, 71
Diparcol, 11
Diphazin, 5
Diphenhydramine, emesis and, 59-60
Diphenylamine(s), phenothiazine synthesis and, 24-25
Diphenylhydantoin, chlorpromazine and, 67
Diphosphopyridine nucleotide,
  levels, chlorpromazine and, 65, 75
  schizophrenia and, 261
  synthesis, promazine and, (Bur) 390
Dipiperon, 201, 296
  clinical use, 227-228
Diprazin, 7
Diprozin, 7
1,4-Di-1-pyrolidinyl-2-butyne, see Tremorine
Diquel, 17
Discrimination, trifluoperazine and, (Shu) 439
Dislocations, methocarbamol and, (Kan) 487, (Sha) 488, (Tro) 489
Disyncran, 9
Diuresis,
  chlorpromazine and, 101-102, 110-111
  phenothiazines and, 61
Dixyrazine, 23
Dizziness,
  chlorpromazine and, 158-159
  thiopropazate and, (Eli) 417
Docosanylpyridinium bromide, lipid films and, 106
Dodecyl sulfate, lipid films and, 106
Dog,
  body temperature, chlorpromazine and, 69
  chlorpromazine and, 50, 161
  fluanisone and, 227
  neuroleptic classification and, 209-213
  phenothiazine metabolism in, 138
  trimeprazine and, (Can) 469
Dolisina, 11
Dominal, 290, (Bou) 408
Dominil, 290
DOPA, see Dihydroxyphenylalanine
Dopa decarboxylase, norepinephrine and, 263
Dopamine,
  biosynthesis of, 256
  metabolism, 258, 259
    schizophrenia and, 261
  neurotransmission and, 262

Dopamine-β-oxidase, norepinephrine and, 263
Dopa-β-oxidase, localization of, 262
Dorevan, 16
Doriden, 288
Dormison, 284
Dornwal, 287
Doxyfed, 286
Dragendorff reaction, chlorpromazine metabolites and, 144–145
Drinalfa, 286
Driving, thioridazine and, (May) 424
Droperidol,
  adrenolytic potency, 215
  bibliography, 217
  clinical use, 229–230
  duration of action, 213
  pharmacological effects of, 216
  potency of, 208, 210, 211
  speed of action, 213
  toxicity of, 216
  trade names for, 201
Drugs,
  activity, chlorpromazine and, 60–68
  abuse, ethchlorvynol and, (Sch) 497
  immobilization of wild animals and, (Dit) 437
  overdosage, thiopropazate and, (Kay) 418
  resistance,
    inbreeding and, (Plo) 438
    trifluoperazine and, (All) 444
  withdrawal, promazine and, (Rol) 403
Dumping syndrome, thioridazine and motor activity in, (Tob) 422
Dyes,
  phenothiazine, synthesis of, 3
Dyskinesia,
  chlorprothixene and, (Die) 507
  haloperidol and, 220, 221
  methylperidol and, 225
  perphenazine and, (Uhr) 346
  phenothiazine derivatives and, (Fle) 441
  thiopropazate and, (Fle) 417, (Vai) 420
Dysmenorrhea, promoxolane and, (Boi) 481, (Viv) 481
Dystonic reaction,
  perphenazine and, (Bar) 341, (Dav) 350, (Neg) 345
  trifluperazine and, (Dav) 441, (McK) 461

E

Eazaminum, 11
Ectylurea,
  affective behavior and, (Dob) 491
  evaluation of, 42
  jaundice and, (Hoc) 491
  metabolic fate of, (But) 491
  proprietary names and use of, 285
  seizures and spasticity, (Utl) 491
Edathamil disodium, chlorpromazine and, 66
Edema,
  chlorpromazine and, 91–93, 109
  egg white, hypothermia and, 97
Efroxine, 286
Ejaculation,
  chlorprothixene and, (Dit) 507
  thioridazine and, (Cle) 423, (Qur) 424, (Sin) 433
Ektyl, 285
Electrocardiogram,
  abnormalities, thioridazine and, (Kel) 424, (Wen) 424
  chlorpromazine and, 93–94
  phenothiazines and, (Ban) 440
Electroconvulsive therapy, chlorpromazine and, 53, 94
Electrode(s),
  implanted, chlorpromazine and, 55–56
  intracranial, self stimulation by, 37
Electrode dermagrams, chlorpromazine and, 56
Electroencephalogram,
  abnormalities, thiopropazote and, (Hol) 418
  activation, trifluoperazine and, (Lin) 453
  arousal, phenaglycodol and, (Gan) 477
  carphenazine effects and, (Hos) 308
  changes, promazine and, (Rei) 396, (Win) 396
  chlorpromazine and, 40, 46, 155
    encephal isolé and cerveau isolé animals, 51–52
    in humans, 52
    intact animals, 50–51
  dimethoxyphenethylamine and, 261–262
  methyprylon and, (Mar) 494, (Sen) 495
  promazine and, (Sko) 393
  tetanus toxin and, 107
  thioridazine reaction and, (Iti) 422, (Ule) 423

Electroencephalography, methdilazine and, (Bor) 330
Electromyographic activity, involuntary, chlorpromazine and, 56
Electron-donating properties, central sympathetic suppressants and, (Lyo) 435
Electron paramagnetic resonance, chlorpromazine oxidation and, 141
phenothiazines and, (Pie) 436
Electron spin resonance, phenothiazine derivatives and, 140
Electron-withdrawing groups, phenothiazine activity and, 128-129
Electrophoresis, phenothiazines, 147, (Mel) 436, 502, (Mol) 390
Electroshock,
chlorpromazine and, 39, 96, 98, 100, 156
psychopharmacological agents and, 34
threshold,
chlorpromazine and, 53
promazine and, (Ted) 393
trifluoperazine and, (Fre) 449, (Ros) 456
Elevan, 284
Elevol, 284
Emesis, *see also* Nausea, Vomiting
drug induced, chlorpromazine and, 57-59
perphenazine and, (Wea) 341
prochlorperazine and, (Con) 380
Emesis gravidarum,
fluphenazine and, (Pri) 320
thiethylperazine and, (Alw) 414
triflupromazine and, (Bur) 463
Emotional activity, chlorpromazine and, 40
Emotional disorders,
malignant, trifluoperazine and, (Bea) 445
prochlorperazine and, (McF) 384
promazine and, (Gif) 399
thioridazine and, (Bro) 426, (Bar) 425
Emylcamate,
internuncial blocking and, (Mar) 482
subjective reactions under stress and, (Uhr) 482
Encephal isolé, chlorpromazine and, 51-52
Endocrine effects,
chlorpromazine and, 95-103
perphenazine and, (Jar) 339
Endoscopy, triflupromazine and, (Reb) 467
Endotoxins,
effects, chlorpromazine and, 96, 98
Energy metabolism, mental disease and, 273
Enuresis nocturna, thioridazine and, (Bur) 426

Enzymes,
chlorpromazine and, 81-83
promazine and, (Smi) 393
propiomazine and, (Usd) 407
Eosinophils, chlorpromazine and, 77, 98, 99, 106
Ephedrine,
blood pressure and, 91
chlorpromazine and, 84
eosinophils and, 98
tremor and, 57
Epilepsy,
chlorpromazine and, 52, 53, 67-68
ethchlorvynol and, (Car) 497
thioridazine and, (Fra) 428, (Pau) 431
Epileptiform seizures, promazine and, (Voe) 396
Epileptogenic lesions,
secondary, chlorpromazine and, 53
Epinephrine, *see also* Adrenaline
activity, chlorpromazine and, 54, 63, 64, 105, 109, 151
adrenalectomy and, 100
biosynthesis of, 256
blood pressure and, 91
brain, morphine and, 63
chlorpromazine and, 38
chlorpromazine side effects and, 159
degradation of, 257, 258
droperidol and, 230
eosinophils and, 98, 99
heart and, 93
lethal dose, chlorpromazine and, 86
release, phenothiazines and, (Wei) 440
tremor and, 57
Ergotamine, chlorpromazine and, 84
Erythema, methdilazine and, (McK) 330
Erythrocytes,
chicken, schizophrenic serum and, 252-253
Eserine,
activity, chlorpromazine and, 65, 105
chlorpromazine and, 40
Eskazinyl, 18
Esparin, 8
Estrogens,
chlorpromazine and, 78
effects, chlorpromazine and, 102
phenothiazine tests and, 150
Estrus,
chlorpromazine and, 102, 103
phenothiazines and, (Bha) 436
Esucos, 23

Etaperazin, 18
Ethaperazin, 18
Ethchlorvynol, 283, 284
  addiction and, (Ess) 497
  cardiac patients and, (Bli) 497
  convulsions and, (Blu) 497
  dependency, (Sie) 497
  dermatology and, (Rei) 497, (Sch) 497
  drug abuse and, (Sch) 497
  epilepsy and, (Car) 497
  labor and, (Bor) 497
  urologic patients and, (Bar) 497
  withdrawal and, (Ayc) 497
Ether,
  activity, chlorpromazine and, 61
  brain adenosine triphosphate and, 73
Ethinamate, 283
  liver damage, chlorpromazine and, 76
  mammary glands and, 103
  proprietary name and use of, 286
  sleeping time, chlorpromazine and, 60
Ethopropazine, proprietary names for, 14
2-Ethyl-10-(3′-dimethylamino-2′-methyl-1′-propyl)phenothiazine, 17
Ethylemin, 11
Ethylisobutrazine, proprietary names for, 17
Ethylmorphine, chlorpromazine metabolism and, 140
2-Ethylthio-10-(1″-methyl-4″,3′-piperazinyl-1′-propyl)phenothiazine, 20
17α-Ethynyl-estra-$\Delta^{5,10}$enolone, ovulation and, 103
Eutonyl, 287
Exercise, schizophrenia test and, 253
Extrapyramidal symptoms,
  benperidol and, 229
  butyrophenones and, 216, 223
  carphenazine and, (Niv) 309
  chlorpromazine and, 38, 158
  droperidol and, 230
  floropipamide and, 227
  fluanisone and, 226
  fluphenazine and, (Kru) 314
  haloperidol and, 220–221
  methylperidol and, 225
  perphenazine and, (Ayd) 341, (Ler) 344
  plasma copper levels and, 72
  prochlorperazine and, (Dar) 374, (Fre) 374, (Ler) 376
  promazine and, (Ayd) 394
  thiopropazate and, (Vat) 420
  trifluoperazine and, (Ano) 440
  trifluperidol and, 222–224
  triflupromazine and, (Ayd) 461

Eye, phenothiazines and, 138

F

F33, 204
Fargan, 7
Fat,
  hepatic, chlorpromazine and, 75, 76
Fatalities,
  fetal, promazine and, (Ami) 394, (Cli) 394, (Ome) 396
  fluphenazine and, (Ans) 313
  promazine and, (Ear) 394
Fear, chlorpromazine and, 45, 49
Fecal incontinence, promazine and, (Fre) 399
Feces,
  chlorpromazine in, 141
  phenothiazine metabolites and, 136
Fenactil, 6
Fenazil, 7
Fenergan, 7
Fenethazin, 5
Fenethiazin, 4
Fentanyl,
  droperidol and, 229, 230
  fluanisone and, 227
Fentazin, 18
Ferric chloride,
  chlorpromazine metabolites and, 146
  phenothiazines and, 148, 149
Ferric perchlorate, phenothiazines and, 149
Fetal abnormalities, trifluoperazine and, (Sch) 443
Fibroblasts, chlorpromazine and, 78
Fighting behavior,
  acetophenazine and, (Kni) 305
  tranquilizers and, 43
  trifluoperazine and, (Ted) 439
Filter paper,
  impregnated, phenothiazine detection and, 149
Fine-motor performance, promazine and, (Wei) 404
Fish, chlorpromazine and, 115
Flavin adenine dinucleotide, chlorpromazine and, 82
Floropipamide, 209
  adrenolytic potency, 215
  antiemesis and, 213
  clinical use, 227–228
  pharmacological effects of, 216
  potency of, 210, 211

Floropipamide—*continued*
  ptosis and, 216
  trade names for, 201
Floropipton, 209
  structure of, 203
Fluanisone, 209
  adrenolytic potency, 215
  antiemesis and, 213
  clinical use, 226–227
  pharmacological effects of, 216
  potency of, 210, 211
  ptosis and, 216
  trade names for, 200
Fluomazina, 9
Fluorocortisone,
  effects, chlorpromazine and, 96
Fluphenazine,
  acute schizophrenia and, (Ale) 314, (Chi) 316
  adrenolytic potency, 215
  anesthesia and, (Hym) 318
  anti-apomorphine action, (Bur) 311, 316
  anti-emetic activity, (Bon) 315, (Cor) 316, (Rao) 312
  anti-hallucinatory effect, (Kru) 314
  anxiety and, (Bod) 315, (Car) 316, (Hes) 318
  behavior disorders and, (Lav) 319
  biochemistry and pharmacology of, 311–313
  chemistry of, 311
  children and, (Rus) 321, (Tor) 322
  chronic psychotic patients and, (Bar) 315, (Bar) 348
  chronic schizophrenia and, (Fog) 317
  chronically ill and, (Che) 316
  clinical studies of, 314–322
  comparative studies of, (Dar) 316
  depot action and, (Bur) 315
  digestive disorders and, (Wis) 322
  emesis gravidarum and, (Pri) 320, (San) 321
  extrapyramidal symptoms and, (Kru) 314
  fatalities and, (Ans) 313
  general practice and, (Ern) 317
  hospitalized psychotic females and, (Lap) 319
  jaundice and, (Wal) 314
  neurosis and, (Kud) 319
  obstetrics and, (Pri) 321
  Parkinsonism and, (Kru) 314
  pharmacological effects of, 216
  potency of, 210, 211

Fluphenazine—*continued*
  pregnancy and, (Gri) 318, 352
  private practice and, (Mor) 320
  proprietary names for, 20
  psychiatric patients and, (Ayd) 315
  psychotic patients and, (Den) 316, (Hol) 318
  pyridoxine and, (Lav) 319
  rehabilitation and, (Rez) 321
  retarded children and, (Wai) 322
  side effects of, 313–314
  speed of action, 213
  tension and, (Pro) 321
  thiopentone anesthesia and, (Dob) 317
Fluphenazine enanthate, metabolism of, 137
Fluopromazine, 9
Fluorofen, 9
Folic acid,
  requirement, drugs and, 115
Follicle stimulating hormone, chlorpromazine and, 78, 102–103
Food intake,
  chlorpromazine and, 83
  psychotic behavior and, 269–270
Formaldehyde, chlorpromazine metabolism and, 139
FR33, 293
Fractures, methocarbamol and, (Kan) 487
Free fatty acids,
  plasma, tranquilizers and, 98
Free radicals, phenothiazines and, 140–141
Frenactyl, 201
Frenolone, 23
Frenoton, 291
Frenquel, 291
Frog,
  eggs, chlorpromazine and, 78
  pregnancy tests, promazine and, (Fox) 391
Fulmezine, 20

G

Galactorrhea,
  chlorpromazine and, 103
  thioridazine and, (Cas) 423
Galactose,
  incorporation, chlorpromazine and, 74
Galactosemia, treatment of, 274–275
Gallamine triethiodide,
  effects, chlorpromazine and, 107
Gall bladder, phenothiazines and, 105, 106
Gangliosides, mental defects and, 275

Gangrene, promazine and, (Dea) 394, (She) 396
Gas chromatography, *see* Chromatography
Gastric effects,
  chlorpromazine and, 104
  prochlorperazine and, (Cum) 367
  thiopropazate and, (Lic) 419
Gastrointestinal disorders, chlorpromazine and, 152
Gastrointestinal tension, trifluoperazine and, (Ern) 448
Generalized tic, chlorpromazine and, 56
General practice,
  fluphenazine and, (Ern) 317
  thioridazine and, (Neu) 431
Genetics, mental illness and, 250, 274–275
Geriatrics,
  acetophenazine and, (Ham) 306
  methprylon and, (Goo) 493
  prochlorperazine and, (Rot) 386
  promazine and, (Meh) 401
  thoridazine and, (Jac) 429
  trifluoperazine and, (Ham) 450
Gerobit, 286
Gerodyl, 292
Gestation, chlorpromazine and, 102
Glaucoma, thioridazine and, (Joh) 429
Glioblastoma multiforme,
  X-irradiation, tranquilizers and, 59
α-Globulin factor, mental disease and, 252–253
Glomerulonephritis,
  acute, chlorpromazine and, 155
Glucose,
  brain metabolism and, 270
  metabolism,
    chlorpromazine and, 70, 72
    phenothiazine derivatives and, (Arn) 436
  uptake, chlorpromazine and, 80
Glucose-6-phosphate dehydrogenase, phenothiazines and, 82
β-Glucuronidase, phenothiazine metabolites and, 144, 146
Glutamic acid,
  brain metabolism and, 270, 271
  distribution, chlorpromazine and, 82
  transport, schizophrenic serum and, 253
Glutamic acid decarboxylase, chlorpromazine and, 82
Glutamine,
  brain metabolism and, 270
  levels, chlorpromazine and, 80
  synthesis, chlorpromazine and, 82

Glutathione,
  brain, tranquilizers and, 81
  schizophrenia and, 273
Glutethimide, 283
  proprietary name and use of, 288
Glyceraldehyde-3-phosphate dehydrogenase, chlorpromazine and, 82
Glycine,
  uptake, chlorpromazine and, 82
Glycogen,
  brain, chlorpromazine and, 80
  hepatic, chlorpromazine and, 70, 75
Glycolysis,
  chlorpromazine and, 74, 77
  mental disease and, 253
Goat(s), triflupromazine and, (Jha) 461
Gold, chlorpromazine and, 150
Granulocytes, *see also* Agranulocytosis
  depression,
    thioridazine and, (Bac) 423
    trifluoperazine and, (Sim) 457
Granuloma, chlorpromazine and, 78
Gravimetry, phenothiazines and, 147
Growth, chlorpromazine and, 112–113
Growth hormone,
  secretion, chlorpromazine and, 101
Guanethidine,
  norepinephrine and, 263
  sympathomimetic amines and, 63
Guinea pig,
  phenothiazine metabolism in, 136, 137
  reaction to chlorpromazine, 41
Gynecology,
  promazine and, (Gal) 399
  trifluoperazine and, (Bur) 446

H

Haldol, 200
Hallucination,
  benperidol and, 228–229
  chlorpromazine and, 50
  floropipamide and, 227, 228
  fluanisone and, 227
  haloperidol and, 220
  methylperidol and, 225
  trifluoperazine and, (Kru) 452
  urinary indoles and, 268
Hallucinogenic agents, chlorpromazine and, 64–65
Haloanisone, 295
  clinical uses, 226–227
  trade names for, 200

Haloanisone compositum, 200
Halopal, 200
Haloperidid, 299
Haloperidide,
    adrenolytic potency, 215
    antiemesis and, 213
    clinical use of, 230
    duration of action, 213
    pharmacological effects of, 216
    potency of, 208, 210
    structure of, 203
Haloperidol,
    adrenolytic potency, 215
    bibliography, 217–220
    clinical uses, 217–221
    duration of action, 213
    emesis and, 58, 213
    pharmacological effects of, 216
    potency of, 207, 210, 211
    proprietary names and use of, 295
    ptosis and, 215
    recommended dosage, 218
    speed of action, 213
    trade names for, 200
    undesirable effects, 220–221
Halopidol, 200
Handwriting,
    benperidol and, 228
    methylperidol and, 225
Harmaline, serotonin and, 79
Hartnup's disease, cause of, 275
Hay fever, methdilazine and, 331
Headaches,
    tension, chlorpromazine and, 152
Heart,
    arrhythmias, chlorpromazine and, 85, 94
    chlorpromazine and, 93–95
    serotonin, chlorpromazine and, 79
    tissue culture, chlorpromazine and, 115
Heat stress, chlorpromazine and, 97
Hebanil, 6
Hebephrenia, trifluperidol and, 224
HeLa cells,
    chlorpromazine and, 78
    schizophrenic serum and, 253
Hematocrit, chlorpromazine and, 77
Hemineurin, 284
Hemodynamics,
    liver, chlorpromazine and, 76
Hemolysis,
    methocarbamol and, (Tru) 489
    phenothiazines and, 76
Hemophilus pertussis,
    endotoxin, chlorpromazine and, 96

Hemorrhage, chlorpromazine and, 95–97
Heparin, decompression and, 111
Hepatic dysfunction, promazine and, (Wai) 396
Hepatitis,
    cholestatic, trifluoperazine and, (Koh) 442
    viral, chlorpromazine and, 156–157
Hepatolenticular degeneration, 275
Hepatological studies, carphenazine and, (Tia) 308
Heredity, drug-induced parkinsonism and, 158
Hexadecyl sulfate, lipid films and, 106
Hexafluorodiethyl ether, *see* Indoklon
Hexamethonium, blood pressure and, 94
Hexobarbital,
    chlorpromazine and, 52
    metabolism,
        diabetes and, 137
        microsomes and, 138
        potentiation, phenothiazine structure and, 120
    sleeping time, chlorpromazine and, 60
Hexokinase, chlorpromazine and, 83
Hexose-monophosphate shunt, mental disease and, 253
Hibanil, 6
Hiberna, 7
Hibernal, 6
Hibernation,
    artificial, mepazine and, (Mig) 329
Hippocampus,
    stimulation, chlorpromazine and, 55–56
Hirnamin, 13
Hirudineae, perphenazine and, 118
Histamine,
    effects, chlorpromazine and, 99, 102, 104, 105, 108–109
    hypothermia and, 69
    localization in brain, 272–273
    metabolism, 272
        chlorpromazine and, 66, 74, 84
    transport, schizophrenic serum and, 253
Histidine, 272
Holothuriae, tranquilizers and, 118
Homogentisic acid oxidase, chlorpromazine and, 74
Homovanillic acid, 259, 260
    elimination, chlorpromazine and, 81
Horse,
    chlorpromazine and, 161
    promazine and, (Rak) 392

Human,
  basal metabolic rate, chlorpromazine and, 71
  body temperature, chlorpromazine and, 69
  electroencephalographic studies, chlorpromazine and, 52
  phenothiazine distribution and metabolism in, 143–146
  phenothiazine metabolism in, 135, 136, 138
Huntington's chorea,
  perphenazine and, (Con) 350, (Pak) 358
  thiopropazate and, (Ful) 417, (Sou) 420
  thioridazine and, (Ris) 432
  trifluoperazine and, (Coh) 447
Hyaluronidase, capillaries and, 95
Hydergin, chlorpromazine and, 59
Hydrocortisone,
  shock threshold and, 53
  stress and, 97, 99, 100
Hydrogen peroxide, phenothiazines and, 149
Hydromedusae, tranquilizers and, 118
5-Hydroxy-N-acetyltryptamine, 266
Hydroxybutyric acid, formation of, 271
7-Hydroxy-nor-chlorpromazine, 142
7-Hydroxychlorpromazine, excretion of, 141–143
7-Hydroxychlorpromazine sulfoxide, 142, 143
7-Hydroxy-N-demethylchlorpromazine, 142 143
7-Hydroxydidemethylchlorpromazine, 142, 143
10-{3′-[4-(2-Hydroxyethyl-1-piperazinyl]-propyl}-phenothiazine, 19
1-(2-Hydroxyethyl)-4-[10-(2-trifluoromethylthiazinyl)-3-propyl]-homopiperazine, 21
5-Hydroxyindole acetic acid,
  excretion of, 268, (Ros) 390
  formation of, 266, 267
Hydroxyphenamate, 483
  alcoholics and, (Gou) 483
  anxiety and, 483
  cardiovascular disease and, (Gre) 483
  chemistry of, (Bos) 483
  dermatology and, (Cah) 483
  toxicology of, (Bas) 483
3-Hydroxyphenothiazine, formation of, 143
6-Hydroxyskatole, excretion of, 270
17-Hydroxysteroids, chlorpromazine and, 99
5-Hydroxytryptamine,
  brain, central nervous system depressants and, 80
  formation of, 266, 267
5-Hydroxytryptophan,
  decarboxylation, chlorpromazine and, 79
  emesis, chlorpromazine and, 59
  formation of, 266, 267
  head twitch, drug testing and, 37
  uptake, chlorpromazine and, 80
Hydroxyzine,
  alcohol and, 62
  evaluation of, 42
  mammary glands and, 103
  toxemia and, 98
Hyminal, 289
Hyoscine,
  emesis and, 60
  tremor and, 57
Hyperemesis gravidarum, see Emesis gravidarum
Hyperglycemia
  chlorpromazine and, 86
  schizophrenia and, 273
Hyperkinesia,
  choreic, chlorpromazine and, 56
Hyperlipemia,
  essential, chlorpromazine and, 72–73
Hypermotor syndrome,
  chlorpromazine and, 152
  in children, trifluoperazine and, (Gra) 450
Hyperpyrexia, promazine and, (Dow) 394
Hypertension,
  acetabuton and, 231
  chlorpromazine and, 155
Hypnorm, 200
Hypnotic,
  nonbarbiturate, methyprylon and, (Bel) 492
Hypophysectomy, tranquilizers and, 75
Hypotension,
  chlorpromazine and, 94–95, 158–159
  droperidol and, 230
  floropipamide and, 227
  fluanisone and, 226
  haloperidol and, 221
  perphenazine and, (Mid) 345
  promazine and, (Kap) 395
  thioridazine and, (Swa) 424, (Ros) 424
Hypothalamus,
  chlorpromazine and, 38, 95, 102
  metabolism, chlorpromazine and, 80
Hypothermia,
  antagonism of, 69
  chlorpromazine and, 56–57
  phenothiazine activity, structure and, 122–123
Hypoxia, chlorpromazine and, 71
Hysteria, haloperidol and, 221

I

Ibogaine, serotonin and, 79
ID 22, 298
Idiopathic hypercalcemia, 275
4-Imidazole carboxylic acid, 272
4-Imidazolylacetaldehyde, 272
Imipramine,
  anesthesia and, 110
  chlorpromazine and, 156
  electroconvulsive therapy and, 53
  electroencephalography and, 52
  metabolic effects of, 70
  d-methamphetamine and, 63
  norepinephrine levels and, 81, 264–265
  serotonin and, 65, 79, 80
  tumors and, 77–78
Inapsin, 201
Inbreeding, drug resistance and, (Plo) 438
Inclined plane test,
  phenothiazine activity, structure and, 120
Indican, phenothiazine color tests and, 149, (Lev) 435
Indoklon,
  activity,
    chlorpromazine and, 66
    ipronazid and, 66
Indole acetamide, excretion of, 270
Indole-3-acetic acid,
  excretion of, 268
  formation of, 267
Indole pyruvic acid, 267
Indoles,
  chloropromazine and, 151
  mental disease and, 265–270
Indorm, 16
Infantile aumorotic familial idiocy, 275
Inflammation, chlorpromazine and, 100, 109, 110
Influenza,
  infection, anti-inflammatory agents and, 110
Infrared spectra, phenothiazines, 147
Infusoria, chlorpromazine and, 115
Innovan, 201
Innovar, 201
Innovar-vet, 201
Inotropic effects, chlorpromazine and, 85
Inoval, 201
Insomnia,
  haloperidol and, 221
  methyprylon and, (Bil) 492
  propiomazine and, (Kra) 406
Insulin,
  activity, chlorpromazine and, 65, 72, 80, 104
  drug metabolism and, 137
  schizophrenia and, 273
  therapy, chlorpromazine and, 156
Intact animals,
  activity and behavior, chlorpromazine and, 41–43
Intelligence factors, chlorpromazine and, 154
Internal medicine, thioridazine and, (Cuc) 427
Internuncial blocking,
  emylcamate and, (Mar) 482
  methocarbamol and, (Par) 488
Intolerance reaction, prochlorperazine and, (Mas) 376
Intramyocardial lesions, phenothiazines and, 160
Intraocular pressure, chlorpromazine and, 112
Iodic acid, phenothiazines and, 148
Iodine,
  uptake, chlorpromazine and, 101
Iproniazid,
  activity, chlorpromazine and, 65, 81
  depression and, 264
  diethyltryptamine activity and, 66
  evaluation of, 42
  Indoklon activity and, 66
  serotonin and, 65
Iron, chlorpromazine and, 150
Irradiation sickness, see Radiation sickness
Irritable colon,
  chlorpromazine and, (Wol) 388
  phenaglycodol and, (Kai) 477
  promazine and, (Wol) 405
Isocarboxazid, chlorpromazine and, 156
Isomerization,
  geometric, thiaxanthenes and, (Hof) 502
Isophen, 286
Isophenergan, 5
Isoproterenol,
  chlorpromazine and, 84
  heart and, 93
Isotazin, 14
Isothiazin, proprietary names for, 14
Isothazine, 14

J

Jatroneural, 18

SUBJECT INDEX

Jaundice,
  chlorpromazine and, 105-106, 156-157
  ectylurea and, (Hos) 491
  fluphenazine and, (Wal) 314
  neonatal,
    chlorpromazine and, 152
    promazine and, (Sut) 396
  perphenazine and, (Ber) 341
  prochlorperazine and, (Del) 374, 375, 376, (Sol) 378
  promazine and, (Kem) 395, (Zin) 396
JB-516, 78
Jenotone, 15
Jumping box test, butyrophenones and, 209, 210, 213-214

K

Kaolin, phenothiazines and, 150, (Sor) 390
α-Keto acids, chlorpromazine and, 82
α-Ketoglutaric acid, mental illness and, 273
17-Ketosteroids, chlorpromazine and, 99
Kidney, chlorpromazine and, 110-111
Klorpromex, 6
Kö 339, proprietary name and use of, 287
Ks 33, 18

L

Labor,
  chlorpromazine and, 67
  ethchlorvynol and, (Bor) 497
  perphenazine and, (Gre) 352
  premature, methocarbamol and, (Man) 487
  prochlorperazine and, (Kap) 383
  promazine and, (Mar) 401
Lactation,
  chlorpromazine and, 103, 152, 159
  phenothiazines and, (Ben) 436
Lactic acid,
  formation, chlorpromazine and, 80
Lactobacillus leichmannii,
  vitamin requirements, tranquilizers and, 115
Lactogenic hormone, chlorpromazine and, 78
Lacumin, 12
Lantoside C, chlorpromazine and, 59
Largactil, 6
Largaktyl, 6
Largon, 16, (Gli) 406, see Propiomazine
Lateral reticular formation,
  stimulation, chlorpromazine and, 43
Lathyrism, 276

Latibon, 11
Lead poisoning, methocarbamol and, (Luk) 487
Lealgin compositum, 200
Learning, tranquilizers and, 43
Lens,
  opacity, chlorpromazine and, 159
Leptofen, 201
Lergigan, 7
Leucine,
  incorporation, chlorpromazine and, 84
Leucinosis, treatment of, 274
Leucocytes, chlorpromazine and, 77
Leucocytosis, promazine and, (Hat) 395
Leuco-methylene blue, electron energy levels of, 150
Leukemia,
  survival time, chlorpromazine and, 78
Leukemoid reaction, promazine and, (Mic) 396
Levanil, 285
Levomepromazine,
  electroconvulsive therapy and, 53
  inflammation and, 109
  mammary glands and, 103
  metabolic fate of, 135
  prolonged administration of, 71
  proprietary names for, 13
Levorphan,
  activity, chlorpromazine and, 62
Libido disorders, thioridazine and, (Pom) 424
Librium, 289
Limbic system, chlorpromazine and, 38, 40
Lipemia, *see also* Hyperlipemia
  chlorpromazine and, 77
Lipid films,
  penetration, phenothiazines and, 106
Lipid peroxidase, chlorpromazine and, 83
Liranol, 8
Lisergan, 4
Lispamol, 15
Liver,
  function, phenothiazine tests and, 150
  hemodynamics, thioridazine and, (Pla) 422
  metabolism, chlorpromazine and, 75-76, 105-106
  phenothiazine uptake by, 134, 137
Liver disease, ceruloplasmin and, 252
Liver function,
  test, promazine and, (Par) 402
  thioridazine and, (Kev) 424, (Bov) 423
Lobeline,

effects, chlorpromazine and, 90
Local anesthesia, phenothiazine structure and, 121
Locomotor depression, comparative potencies of phenothiazines and, 130–131
Lophosetta maculata,
  melanocyte stimulating hormone, chlorpromazine and, 118
Lorusil, 15
Low-back disorders, methocarbamol and, (Gri) 487, (Mey) 487
Lower organisms, chlorpromazine and, 115–119
Lucidil, 294
Lungs, phenothiazine uptake by, 134, 137, 141
Lupus erythematosus,
  chlorprothixene and, (Hai) 507
  thioridazine and, (Led) 430
Luvatren, 200
Luvatrena, 200
Luvatrene, 200
Lymphocytes, chlorpromazine and, 98, 99
Lyogen, 20
Lysergic acid diethylamide,
  activity, chlorpromazine and, 64
  brain metabolism and, 74, 80
  electroencephalographic effects, chlorpromazine and, 51
  generalization and, 46
  hippocampal-evoked potentials and, 56
  hypothermia and, 69
  leukemia and, 78
  mental illness and, 250
  psychopharmacological drug testing and, 34
  serotonin and, 265
  visceral serotonin and, 79
Lysergide, proprietary name and use of, 295
Lysivane, 14
Lysolecithin,
  hemolysis, chlorpromazine and, 76–77

M

Magnesium chloride, tremor and, 57
Majeptil, 20
Mallorol, 19
Malloryl, 19
Mammary gland, chlorpromazine and, 103
Mania,
  chlorpromazine and, 152
  floropipamide and, 227

Manic depressives,
  ceruloplasmin and, 251
  chlorprothixene and, (Mad) 514
Manic reactions, haloperidol and, 218, 220, 221, 224
Maple syrup urine disease, treatment of, 274
Marophen, 4
Mast cells, chlorpromazine and, 77
Mastocytoma P-815, chlorpromazine and, 77–78
Maternal-fetal effects, propiomazine and, (Ull) 407
MD 5501, 4
Me 4703, 9
Mebubarbital, insect behavior and, 118
Medeprozin, 8
Médiamer, 9
Megacolon, chlorpromazine and, 104
Megaphen, 6
Megimide, 285
Melancholia,
  chlorpromazine and, 152
  floropipamide and, 227
β-Melanocyte stimulating hormone,
  activity, chlorpromazine and, 66, 118
  promazine and, (Sco) 392
Melanophore(s),
  dispersion, phenothiazines and, 101
Melatonin,
  carboline metabolites, behavior and, 270
  formation of, 266, 267
Meleril, 19
Mellaril, 19, (For) 420, *see* Thioridazine
  suicides and, (Gue) 423
Melleretten, 19
Melleril, 19
Membranes,
  chlorpromazine and, 39
  permeability, chlorpromazine and, 75, 78–80, 118
Menopause,
  promoxolone and, (Boi) 481
  thioridazine and, (Cal) 426
  trifluoperazine and, (Coh) 447
Mental defectives,
  carphenazine and, (Car) 309
  chlorpromazine and, 152
  prochlorperazine and, (Rob) 385
  promazine and, (Ber) 397, (Ben) 397
  thioridazine and, (Bad) 425
Mental disease,
  chronic, trifluoperazine and, (All) 444, (Bar) 445, (Che) 316

etiology of, 250
faulty energy metabolism and, 273
6-hydroxyskatole and, 270
neurotoxin theories, 258–262
promazine and, (Azi) 397
theories,
  abnormal protein factors, 251–255
  conclusion, 276
  endogenous amines, 255–273
  faulty energy metabolism, 273
  genetic defects, 274–275
  nutritional disorders, 275–276
Mental patients,
  refractory, trifluoperazine and, (Gun) 450
Mental retardation,
  fluanisone and, 227
  promazine and, (Ese) 399
  trifluoperazine and, (Hei) 450
  triflupromazine and, (Bai) 462
Mepasin, 12
Mepazine,
  activity, (Bru) 326
  agranulocytosis and, (Fel) 325
  anesthesia and, (Dav) 327
  artificial hibernation and, (Mig) 329
  chronic toxicity of, (Koe) 326
  comparative potency of, 130–131
  proprietary names for, 12
  synthesis of, 29
  tests, indican and, 149
Meperidine,
  activity, chlorpromazine and, 62
  blood pressure and, 94
  chlorpromazine and, 55
  effects, chlorpromazine and, 155
  glutathione and, 81
  promazine and, (Cli) 398
  structure, 199
    activity and, 127–128
Mephazine, 5
Mephenesin,
  chlorpromazine and, 67
  decerebrate animals and, 43
  stretch reflex and, 108
  tetanus and, 108
Mephenoxalone,
  neurophysiological actions of, (Gra) 479
  peptic ulcer and, (Gor) 479
  psychogenic syndromes and, (Can) 479
  psychophysiological test performance and, (Mul) 480
  spasticity and, (Tim) 480
  toxicity of, (Yea) 480
Mephentermine,
  pressor effect, chlorpromazine and, 84
Meprobamate,
  alcohol and, 62
  brain metabolism and, 74
  chlorpromazine and, 156
  combination with promazine, (Rob) 402
  convulsant shock and, 34
  diethyltryptamine activity and, 66
  diphosphopyridine nucleotide levels and, 65
  effects of, 225
  estrus and, 103
  evaluation of, 42
  fighting behavior and, 43
  glutathione and, 81
  learning and, 43
  mammary glands and, 103
  metabolic effects of, 70
  nalorphine and, 66–67
  overdosage, 160
  shock and, 97, 98
  thyroxine and, 100
  ulcers and, 104
Mepyramine,
  depressor response and, 109
  hypothermia and, 69
Meratran, 292
Mercuric acetate-perchloric acid, phenothiazine titration and, 147
Mercuric salts, phenothiazines and, 149
Mescaline,
  activity,
    chlorpromazine and, 64–65
    diethyltryptamine and, 66
  blood chemistry and, 64
  drug testing and, 35
  neurotransmitters and, 255, 258, 259
  psychopharmacological drug testing and, 34
Mesodiencephalon,
  stimulation, chlorpromazine and, 55
Metabolism,
  chlorpromazine and, 70–84
  chlorprothixene and, (All) 503
  ectylurea and, (But) 491
  labeled fluphenazine and, (Ebe) 317
  methdilazine and, (Wei) 331
  methocarbamol and, (Cam) 486, (Huf) 487
  methyprylon and, (Ran) 495
  perphenazine and, (Hua) 338, (Sym) 340
  phenothiazines and, (Emm) 389, 437, (Pos) 392
  promazine and, (Ehr) 391

thiethylperazine and, (Zeh) 415
thioridazine and, (Rut) 431, (Zeh) 423
triflupromazine and, (Smi) 460
Metahexamide, vitamins and, 115
Metanephrine, 357
Metaxolone, muscle relaxation and, (Car) 485
Meterazin, 15
Methacholine, blood pressure and, 54
Methamphetamine, 283
   analgesia and, 111
   pressor effect, chlorpromazine and, 84
   proprietary names and use of, 286–287
d-Methamphetamine,
   activity, chlorpromazine and, 63
Methantheline bromide, vitamins and, 115
Methapyrilene, vitamins and, 115
Methaqualone, proprietary names and use of, 289
Methdilazine,
   allergic disorders and, (Gra) 330, (Raw) 331, (Spo) 331
   antihistaminic activity of, (Cra) 330
   electroencephalography and, (Bor) 330
   erythema and, (McK) 330
   metabolic fate of, (Wei) 331
   proprietary names for, 9
   pruritic dermatoses and, (Fro) 330
Methedrinal, 286
Methedrine, 286
Methiomeprazin, 14
Methionine,
   effect in schizophrenia, 261, 269–270
   uptake, chlorpromazine and, 80
Methionine sulfoximine, epileptiform symptoms and, 276
Methocarbamol, 486
   alcoholism and, 487, (Moo) 487
   black widow spider poisoning and, (Jon) 487
   bruxism and, (Cha) 486
   dislocation and fractures and, (Kan) 487, (Sha) 488, (Tro) 489
   equine tetanus and, (Smi) 488
   hemolytic activity of, (Tru) 489
   interneuronal blocking and, (Par) 488
   labor and, 489
   lead poisoning and, (Luk) 487
   low-back disorders and, (Gri) 487, (Mey) 487
   metabolism and, (Cam) 486, (Huf) 487
   muscle spasms and, (Est) 486, 487, (Pop) 488, (Rog) 488
   neuromuscular diseases and, (Odo) 488
   neuromuscular reactions and, (Gri) 486
   opiate withdrawal and, (Zuc) 489
   oral surgery and, (Fei) 486
   orthopedics and, (For) 486, (Lew) 487
   pain and, (Fit) 486
   paralytic ileus and, (Koz) 487
   plasma levels of, (Huf) 487
   potentiation and, (Lan) 487
   premature labor and, (Man) 487
   proprietary names and use of, 288
   spastic states and, (Big) 486
   tetanus and, (Les) 487
Methophenazin, 23
Methopromazine, see also Methoxypromazine
   gall bladder and, 105
   mammary glands and, 103
   pharmacodynamic properties of, (Cou) 333
   proprietary names for, 10
Methotrimeprazine,
   analgetic effect of, 62–63
   morphine abstinence and, 153
   proprietary names for, 13
   tetanus and, 108
Methoxamine,
   pressor effect, chlorpromazine and, 84
5-Methoxy-N-acetylserotonin, formation of, 266, 267
7-Methoxychlorpromazine, 142
7-Methoxychlorpromazine sulfoxide, 142
2-Methoxy-10-(3'-dimethylamino-2'-methyl-1'-propyl)phenothiazine, 13
2-Methoxy-10-(3'-dimethylamino-1'-propyl)phenothiazine, 10
10-Methoxyharmalan, mental illness and, 270
3-Methoxy-4-hydroxymandelic acid,
   catecholamines and, 257, 258, 263
   depression and, 265
3-Methoxy-4-hydroxymandelic aldehyde,
   catecholamines and, 257, 258
3-Methoxy-4-hydroxyphenylacetic acid,
   dopamine and, 258, 259
3-Methoxy-4-hydroxyphenylglycol, catecholamines and, 257
5-Methoxyindole acetic acid, formation of, 266, 267
2-Methoxy-10-[2'-(1-methyl-2-piperidinyl)-ethyl]phenothiazine, 18
4-Methoxyphenethylamine,
   isolation of, 260
   pharmacological effects of, 261–262
Methoxypromazine, 332, see also Methopromazine
   brain amino acid levels and, 80
   chronic schizophrenia and (Apf) 332

metabolic fate of, 135
ocular side effects of, (Apt) 332
pharmacodynamic actions of, (Gra) 333
proprietary names for, 10
urinary elimination of, (All) 332
6-Methoxytryptamine, mental illness and, 270
3-Methoxytyramine, dopamine and, 258–260
Methprylon, 283
  proprietary name and use of, 287
Methylchlorisophenergan, 10
α-Methyldihydroxyphenylalanine, brain serotonin and, 80
α-Methyldopa,
  depression and, 264
  norepinephrine and, 263
Methylene blue, use in medicine, 2
2,3-Methylenedioxyphenothiazine, synthesis of, 31
1-Methylhistamine, 272
10-{2′-Methyl-3′-[4-(2-hydroxyethoxyethyl)-1-piperazinyl]propyl}phenothiazine, 23
1-Methylimidazol-4-yl acetic acid, 272
1-Methyl-d-lysergic acid butanolamide tartrate, hypothermia and, 69
N-Methylmetanephrine, 257, 258
  excretion of, 262
Methylparafynol, 283
  brain serotonin and, 80
  proprietary name and use of, 284
Methylperidide,
  adrenolytic potency, 215
  clinical use of, 230
  pharmacological effects of, 216
  potency of, 208, 210
  structure of, 202
Methylperidol,
  adrenolytic potency, 215
  antiemesis and, 213
  clinical uses, 225–226
  potency of, 207, 210, 211
  trade names for, 200
Methylphenidate, 283
  proprietary names and use of, 289
10-(1′-Methyl-4′-piperazinyl-2′-ethyl)-phenothiazine, 13
10-(1″-Methyl-4″-piperazinyl-3′-propyl-1′)-phenothiazine, 16
2′-Methyl-3″-piperidine-10-propylphenothiazine, inflammation and, 109
10-(1′-Methyl-2′-piperidinylmethyl)phenothiazine, 12
Methylpromazine, 10

10-(1′-Methyl-3′-pyrrolidinomethyl)phenothiazine, 9
2-Methylsulfinyl-10-[2′-(1-methyl-2-piperidinyl)ethyl]phenothiazine, 19
Methyltestosterone, liver and, 106
2-Methylthio-10-(3′-dimethylamino-2′-methyl-1′-propyl)phenothiazine, 14
2-Methylthio-10-[2′-1(1-methyl-2-piperidinyl)ethyl]phenothiazine, 19
N-Methyl transferase, catecholamines and, 258
O-Methyl transferase, serotonin metabolism and, 266
α-Methyltryptamine, serotonin and, 79
α-Methyl tyrosine, sedation and, 264
α-Methyl m-tyrosine, norepinephrine and, 265
Methyprylon, 492
  addiction and, (Ber) 492, (Jen) 494
  anticonvulsant action, (Fuj) 493
  central nervous system and, 495
  electroencephalogram and, (Mar) 494, (Sen) 495
  geriatric psychiatric patients and, (Goo) 493
  insomniac patients and, (Bil) 492
  metabolism of, (Ran) 495
  nonbarbiturate hypnotic and, (Bel) 492
  overdosage of, (Cha) 492, (Wei) 496
  paper chromatography of, (Dre) 493
  placebo and, (Las) 494
  poisoning and, 495
  sedation and, (Bil) 492, (Cas) 492
  surgery and, (Dob) 492
  toxicity of, (Pel) 494, (Jac) 494
Metoxypromazin, 10
Metrazole, 284
  convulsions, prochlorperazine and, (Des) 368
Microorganisms, chlorpromazine and, 115
Microsomes,
  chlorpromazine metabolism and, 137, 138, 140
  drug metabolism by, 146
  thioridazine and, 134
Migraine, prochlorperazine and, (Dal) 381
Milk,
  chlorpromazine in, 114
  ejection, tranquilizers and, 103
Minozinan, 13
Mitochondria,
  brain, chlorpromazine and, 74
  chlorpromazine and, 39
  chlorpromazine metabolism by, 137
  swelling, chlorpromazine and, 75

SUBJECT INDEX

Moditen, 20
Moniliasis, chlorpromazine and, (Kan) 442
Monkey,
   behavior, promazine and, (Lea) 392
   reactions to chlorpromazine, 41, 50
   tranquilization, phenothiazine structure and, 120
Monoamine(s),
   metabolism, chlorprothixene and, (Gey) 504
Monoamine oxidase,
   catecholamines and, 258, 263
   inhibitors,
      brain metabolism and, 74
      head twitch and, 37
      norepinephrine and, 263–265
      schizophrenia and, 261
      serotonin and, 266
   tryptophan metabolism and, 267, 270
Mopazine, 10
Moperone,
   clinical uses, 225–226
   trade names for, 200
Mornidine, 17
Morphine,
   activity, chlorpromazine and, 62, 63
   analgesia and, 111
   blood pressure and, 84
   chlorpromazine and, 54, 55
   conditioned responses and, 44
   droperidol and, 230
   emesis, chlorpromazine and, 58–59
   glutathione and, 81
   liver and, 105
   thiopropazate and, (Sch) 420
   tolerance, chlorpromazine and, 62
   withdrawal signs, chlorpromazine and, 153
Mosquito larvae, phenothiazine and, 24
Motility,
   disturbance, prochlorperazine and, (Chr) 380, (Dia) 368
Motion sickness, chlorpromazine and, 59–60
Motor activity,
   chlorpromazine and, 40, 41
   depression,
      drug testing and, 35
      phenothiazine structure and, 116–117
   prothipendyl and, (Bar) 408
   tranquilizer evaluation and, 42
Motor reflexes, promazine and, (Sil) 393
Mouse,
   body temperature, chlorpromazine and, 68, 69
   fighting behavior, promazine and, (Jan) 392
   phenothiazine metabolism in, 136
   reaction to chlorpromazine, 41
   tranquilizer screening test with, 42
MPMP, 12
Mucopolysaccharides, phenothiazines and, 37
Multergan, 5
Multezin, 5
Muscle,
   relaxation,
      chlorpromazine and, 106–108
      metaxolone and, (Car) 485
      nalorphine and, 107
      psychopharmacological agents and, 35
   spasm,
      methocarbamol and, 487, (Est) 486, (Pop) 488, (Rot) 488
      perphenazine and, (Din) 342
Mycobacterium tuberculosis, chlorpromazine and, 115
Myocardial lesions,
   stress-induced, chlorpromazine and, 97
Myopia, prochlorphenazine and, (Yas) 379

N

Nalorphine,
   challenge, chlorpromazine and, 153
   chlorpromazine and, 66–67
   muscle relaxation and, 107
Narcotics,
   withdrawal, chlorpromazine and, 62, 152
Nastyn, 285
Nausea, *see also* Emesis, Vomiting
   chlorpromazine and, 114
   perphenazine and, (Bel) 348
   postoperative,
      perphenazine and, (Bel) 348, (Cut) 350, (Gra) 352, (Moo) 357
      thiethylperazine and, (Dow) 415, (Nor) 415
      thioridazine and, (Bar) 425
      trifluoperazine and, (Bla) 446, (Bru) 463
   prochlorperazine and, (Sul) 387
   thiethylperazine and, (Bro) 414
   trifluoperazine and, (Pru) 455
Neck-face syndrome, thiopropazate and, (Rob) 419
Neo-Hibernex, 8
Neonatals,
   jaundice, promazine and, (Sut) 396
   pathology, promazine and, (Dam) 398

Neoproma, 10
Neozin, 13
Nerves, chlorpromazine and, 56
Nervous diseases,
 children, thioridazine and, (Kub) 430
Neuractil, 13
Neuriplége, 13
Neurocil, 13
Neuroleptic action, thiethylperazine and, (Boi) 414
Neurolipoidosis, types of, 275
Neurological disorders, promazine and, (Spi) 396
Neurological reactions, prochlorperazine and, (Buc) 373
Neurological toxicity, thioridazine and, (Fur) 423
Neuromuscular diseases, methocarbamol and, (Odo) 488
Neuromuscular reactions,
 chlorpromazine and, 106–108, 158
 methocarbamol and, (Gri) 486
 prochlorperazine and, (Gai) 375
Neuropharmacological actions,
 mephenoxalone and, (Gra) 479
 thioridazine and, (Swi) 422
Neuropsychiatric practice, thioridazine and, (Ric) 432
Neurosis,
 fluphenazine and, (Kud) 319
 haloperidol and, 220
 trifluoperazine and, (Ayd) 445
Neurotoxin theories, mental disease and, 258–262
Newcastle disease virus,
 hemorrhage, chlorpromazine and, 97
Niacin, effect in schizophrenia, 261
Nialamide, chlorpromazine and, 156
Nicotinamide,
 activity, chlorpromazine and, 65, 75
 blood pyridine nucleotides and, 76
 effect in schizophrenia, 261
Nicotinamide-methylpherase, chlorpromazine and, 81
Nicotine,
 chlorpromazine and, 39, 51, 52, 87, 101
 tremor, phenothiazine structure and, 121
Nicotinic acid,
 blood pyridine nucleotides and, 76
 mental disorders and, 276
Nictitating membrane, chlorpromazine and, 87, 90
Nikethamide, 283
 chlorpromazine and, 39, 52

 proprietary name and use of, 286
Nipodal, 9, 15
Nirvan, 13
Nitoman, 294
Nitric acid, phenothiazines and, 148
Nitrites, phenothiazines and, 148
Nitrogen,
 excretion, chlorpromazine and, 83
3-Nitrophenothiazine sulfoxide, synthesis of, 25
Nitrous oxide,
 activity, chlorpromazine and, 61
Nivoman, 9
Noludar, 287
Nométine, 17
Nonbarbiturate hypnotic, methyprylon and, (Bel) 492
Noradrenaline, see also Norepinephrine
 hypothalamic, chlorpromazine and, 54
Norchlorpromazine, activity of, 136, 144
Norepinephrine, see also Noradrenaline
 activity, tranquilizers and, 63
 adrenalectomy and, 100
 affective states and, 264
 biosynthesis of, 256
 blood pressure and, 91, 95
 brain, morphine and, 63
 chlorpromazine, side effects and, 159
 degradation of, 257, 258
 heart and, 93
 neurotransmission and, 262
 permeation, chlorpromazine and, 78–79
 pools of, 262–263
 schizophrenia test and, 253
 tremor and, 57
Normeperidine,
 butyrophenone, properties of, 205
 propiophenone, potency of, 205
Normetanephrine, 257, 258
 depression and, 265
Norodin, 286
Norpramine, 292
Nortriptyline, proprietary name and use of, 293
Nostyn, 285
Notenquil, 12
Notesil, 12
Nothiazine, 12
Novamin, 15
Novomazina, 6
Nozinan, 13
Nuclear magnetic resonance,
 chlorpromazine and, 141
 phenothiazines and, 147

SUBJECT INDEX 603

Nupercaine hydrochloride, lipid films and, 106
Nutinal, 294
Nutritional disorders, mental illness and, 275–276
Nylidrin, chlorpromazine and, 63
Nystagmus, chlorpromazine and, 60

O

Obesity, perphenazine and, (Amd) 341
Oblivon-C, 284
Obstetrics,
  analgesia,
    promazine and, (Cab) 397, (Dav) 398
    propiomazine and, (Gri) 406, (Pow) 406
  chlorpromazine and, 152
  fluphenazine and, (Pri) 321
  promazine and, (Gal) 399
  sedation, promazine and, (Gri) 400
  thiethylperazine and, (Aus) 414
  thioridazine and, (Bac) 425
  trifluopromazine and, (Dav) 463
Octopamine, 256
  norepinephrine and, 264
Octopoda, perphenazine and, 119
Ocular changes, thioridazine and, (Dem) 423
Ocular side effects,
  methoxypromazine and, (Apt) 332
  perphenazine and, (Bur) 312
  promazine and, (Bur) 394
Ocular surgery, perphenazine and, (Nie) 357
Oculogyric crisis, perphenazine and, (Koz) 344
Office patients, trifluoperazine and, (Gea) 449
Old yellow enzyme, chlorpromazine and, 82
Oligophrenia, fluanisone and, 226, 227
Omca, 20
Operant behavior, drug testing and, 35–37
Opiate(s),
  withdrawal, methocarbamol and, (Zuc) 489
Oral moniliasis, chlorpromazine and, (Kan) 442
Oral surgery, methocarbamol and, (Fei) 486
Organic phosphate poisoning, chlorpromazine and, 160
Orphenadrine, thioridazine and, (Man) 430
Orthopedics, methocarbamol, (For) 486, (Lew) 487
Orthostatic hypotension,
  perphenazine and, (Wit) 347
  promazine and, (Wit) 396
Out-patients,
  carphenazine and, (Mer) 309
  promazine and, (Eng) 398
  thioridazine and, (Ana) 425
  triflupromazine and, (Ros) 467
Overdosage,
  chlorprothixene and, (Plu) 508
  methyprylon, (Cha) 492, (Wei) 496
  trifluoperazine and, (Bar) 440
Ovulation,
  inhibition, tranquilizers and, 103
  thioridazine and, (Pur) 422
Oxanamide, 490
  proprietary name and use of, 285
Oxazepam, 299
Oxygen,
  chlorpromazine metabolism and, 137
  consumption, chlorpromazine and, 70–71, 73–74, 82, 100
  lack, schizophrenia and, 273
  toxicity, chlorpromazine and, 93, 111
Oxypertine, 298
  trifluoperazine and, (Cal) 446
Oxytocin, chlorpromazine and, 64, 99

P

Pacatal, 12
  urine and, (For) 389
Pacatol, 12
Pacinol, 20
Pain,
  chlorpromazine and, 67, 152
  methocarbamol and, (Fit) 486
  trifluoperazine and, (Dun) 448
Palladium chloride, phenothiazines and, 149
Palladium lauryl sulfate, phenothiazines and, 149
Panectyl, 10
Pantothenate,
  requirement, drugs and, 115
Paper chromatography, *see* Chromatography
Papilledema, thioridazine and, (Blu) 423
Paralytic ileus, methocarbamol and, (Koz) 487
Paramagnetic resonance, phenothiazines and, 150
Paranoia,
  chlorpromazine and, 152
  trifluperidol and, 222, 223
Paranoid schizophrenia,
  promazine and, (Gon) 400

SUBJECT INDEX

thioridazine and, (Gom) 428
trifluoperazine and, (Gal) 449
Paranoid symptoms, acetophenazine and, (She) 307
Paraperidide,
  adrenolytic potency, 215
  clinical use of, 230
  potency of, 208, 210, 211
  structure of, 202
Parasan, 294
Parasympathetic nervous system, chlorpromazine and, 90–91
Parathiazin, 9
Paratyphoid,
  endotoxin, chlorpromazine and, 96
Parcidol, 14
Pardidol, 14
Parfezin, 14
Pargyline, proprietary name and use of, 287
Parkazin, 11
Parkezin, 11
Parkinofen, 11
Parkinsonism,
  chlorpromazine and, 38, 56, 57, 158
  haloperidol and, 220, 221
Parkinson's disease,
  anticholinergic effects and, (Whi) 440
  fluphenazine and, (Kru) 314
  phenothiazines and, 24
  promazine and, (Eng) 399
  thiopropazate and, (Hea) 418
  thioridazine and, (Str) 424
Parphezein, 14
Parphezin, 14
Parsidol, 14
Parsitan, 14
Parsotil, 14
Parstelin, composition of, 18
Pasaden, 21
Patellar reflex, chlorpromazine and, 44, 84
Patients,
  ambulatory,
    prochlorperazine and, (Lea) 384
    triflupromazine and, (Ree) 467
  disturbed, promazine and, (Faz) 399
  hospitalized, carphenazine and, (Kot) 309
Paxital, 12
Pecazin, 12
Pecking syndrome,
  phenothiazines and, (Bur) 436
  tranquilizers and, 47
Pediatric patients,
  fluphenazine and, (Rus) 321
  thioridazine and, (Ren) 432

trifluoperazine and, (Iba) 451
trimeprazine and, (Sea) 474
Pediatrics,
  chlorpromazine and, 154–155
  thioridazine and, (Bar) 425, (Die) 427
Pellagra, mental disorders and, 275–276
Penicillin,
  activity, chlorpromazine and, 115
Pentamethonium, shock and, 97
Pentazol, 284
Pentobarbital,
  activity,
    chlorpromazine and, 60, 61
    nicotinamide and, 65
  analgesia and, 111
  anxiety and, 62
  conditioned response and, 48
  forced activity and, 42
  promazine and, (Cli) 391
  stretch reflex and, 108
Pentylenetetrazole, 283
  chlorpromazine and, 39, 51–53
  convulsions, tranquilizers and, 34
  effects, chlorpromazine and, 118
  proprietary names and use of, 284
Pepsin,
  secretion, chlorpromazine and, 104
Peptic ulcer,
  acute, thiopropazate and, (McH) 419
  mephenoxalone and, (Gor) 479
Peptone,
  effects, chlorpromazine and, 109
Perazin, 13, 16
Perfenacin, 18
Performance, promazine and, (Dew) 391
Perichlor, 288
Permitil, 20
Pernox, 200
Peroxidase, chlorpromazine and, 77, 140
Perphenan, 18
Perphenazine,
  adrenocorticotropic hormone and, (Kiv) 339
  alcoholism and, (Bar) 348, (Gre) 352, (Sal) 359
  allergic conditions and, (Coh) 349, (Rud) 359
  amblyopia and, (Joh) 344
  anesthesia and, (Alb) 347, (Dob) 350
  antimicrobial properties of, (Luk) 339
  anxiety states and, (Ern) 351, (Pre) 358
  approach-avoidance conflict and, (Gro) 338

SUBJECT INDEX

biology and pharmacology of, 336–341
capillaries and, 95
cardiac arrhythmias and, (Dob) 337
chemical papers, 335–336
chimpanzees and, (Wal) 341
chronic schizophrenia and, (Ann) 347
clinical papers, 347–362
comparative potency of, 130–131
conditioned response and, 49
conversion hysteria and, (Sha) 346
dermatoses and, (Fan) 351, (Rei) 359, (Yon) 362
drug resistant schizophrenics and, (Ill) 354
dyskinesia and, (Uhr) 346
dystonic reaction and, (Adl) 341, (Bar) 341, (Dav) 350, (Neg) 345
emesis and, 58, (Wea) 341
endocrine effects and, (Jar) 339
estrus and, 103
experimental shock and, (McK) 339
extrapyramidal reactions and, (Ayd) 341, (Ler) 344
Huntington's chorea and, (Con) 350, (Pak) 358
hypotensive effect of, (Mid) 345
invertebrates and, 118–119
jaundice and, (Ber) 341
labor and, (Gre) 352
mammary glands and, 103
metabolism and, 143, (Hua) 338, (Sym) 340
muscle spasms and, (Din) 342
nausea or vomiting and, (Bel) 348
normal males and, (Dim) 337
obesity and, (Amd) 341
obstetrics and, (Can) 342
ocular side effects and, (Bur) 342
ocular surgery and, (Nie) 357
oculogyric crisis and, (Koz) 344
orthostatic hypotension and, (Wit) 347
ovulation and, 103
phrenotropic action of, (Pen) 358
poisonings and, (Cil) 342
postoperative nausea or vomiting and, (Bel) 348, (Cut) 350, (Gra) 352, (Moo) 357
premedication with, (Oto) 358
premenstrual tension and, (Kat) 354
prolactin secretion and, (Dan) 337
psychiatry and, (Dzi) 351
psychoses and, (Dre) 357, (Nah) 345
psychotherapy and, (Smi) 360

psychotics and, (Bar) 348
psychotropic action of, (Pen) 358
retinopathy and, (Wee) 346
schizophrenic reactions and, (Cas) 349
shock and, (Rot) 340
side effects of, 341–347
suicidal attempt and, (Cam) 342
surgery and, (Lan) 355
synthesis of, 30
thyroid function and, (Ayd) 347, (Cra) 337, 350
tolerance development and, (Irw) 338
trade names for, 18
trismus and, (Mar) 344
verbal behavior patterns and, (Got) 338
vomiting and, (Bir) 348
Personality tests, chlorpromazine and, 154
Pertofrane, 292
Pervetral, 294
Pervitin, 286
Pethidine, radiation and, 59
Petit mal, chlorpromazine and, 51
Petrichloral, 283
  proprietary name and use of, 288
Petroleum ether,
  inhalation, chlorpromazine and, 85
PF 97, 297
Phagocytosis, chlorpromazine and, 118
Phargan, 7
Pharmacodynamic action,
  methocarbamol and, (Tru) 489
  methopromazine and, (Cou) 333
  methoxypromazine and, (Cra) 333
Pharmacology,
  comparison of chlorpromazine and thioridazine and, (Hal) 422
  prochlorperazine and, (Coo) 367
  promazine and, (Bie) 390
  thioridazine and, (Wei) 423
  trifluoperazine and, (Ted) 439
Phenacemide, shock threshold and, 53
Phenacetin,
  activity, chlorpromazine and, 62
Phenaglycodol,
  anticonvulsant activity, (Car) 477
  anxiety and, (Zuk) 478
  cerebral palsy and, (Kug) 477
  electroencephalographic arousal and, (Gan) 477
  irritable colon and, (Kai) 477
Phenazin, 13, 19
Phencyclidine, proprietary name and use of, 291
Phenergan, 7

Phenetazin, 4
Phenformin, vitamins and, 115
Phenmetrazine, 283
  activity, chlorpromazine and, 63
  proprietary name and use of, 288
Phenobarbital,
  activity, chlorpromazine and, 60
  adaptive metabolism of, 146
  brain adenosine triphosphate and, 73
  brain serotonin and, 80
  diphosphopyridine nucleotide levels and, 65
  edema and, 97, 109
  epilepsy and, 67–68
  epileptogenic lesions and, 53
  mammary glands and, 103
  schizophrenia and, 223
  thyroxine and, 100
Phenoctyl, 16
Phenopropazin, 14
Phenoselenazines, 33
Phenothiazine(s),
  alkylation procedures, 26–28
  analytical methods for, 146–150
  aromatic ring substituents, 31–32
  blood and, (Het) 389
  brain catecholamines and, (Vog) 440
  clinically useful, synthesis of, 28–30
  colorimetric assay of, (Rya) 390
  compounds, uveal pigment and, (Pot) 443
  derivatives,
    cross sensitivities between, (Ger) 399
    dyskinesia and, (Fle) 441
    glucose metabolism and, (Arn) 436
  determination, indican and, (Lev) 435
  electrocardiogram and, (Ban) 440
  electron energy levels of, 150
  electron paramagnetic resonance of, (Pie) 436
  epinephrine release and, (Wei) 440
  estrous cycle and, (Bha) 436
  first use in medicine, 2
  gas chromatography of, (Mar) 435
  lactation and, (Ben) 436
  mental illness and, 250
  metabolism of, 132–134, 139–143
    in man, 143–146
  miscellaneous properties of, 150
  mucopolysaccharides and, 37
  nitrogen substituents, 32–33
  nomenclature of, 24
  paper chromatography of, (Eag) 435
  pecking syndrome and, (Bur) 436

  "pink spot" and, 261
  research, synthesis of, 30–33
  ring substituents in, 128–132
  serotonin antagonism by, (Ted) 439
  sickling and, (Lew) 438
  side chain modifications in, 121–128
  structure-activity relationships, 116–117, 119–132
  summary of clinical applications,
    central nervous system activity, 150–153
    miscellaneous effects, 155–156
    overdosage, 160–161
    pediatric applications, 154–155
    psychometric techniques, 153–154
    side effects, 156–160
    vascular and respiratory effects, 155
    veterinary use, 161
  synthetic methods for, 3–24
    Smiles rearrangement, 25
    thionation and, 24–25
    Ullmann reaction, 26
  thin layer chromatography of, (Coc) 435
  tissue distribution, 134–139
    in man, 143–146
  unsubstituted, metabolism of, 143
  urine color test for, (For) 389
Phenoxazines, 33
Phenoxybenzamine,
  cardiac effects, 85
  leukemia and, 78
  milk ejection and, 103
  norepinephrine and, 263
  stress and, 97
  sympathomimetic amines and, 63
Phenylalanine, catecholamine biosynthesis and, 256
Phenylbutazone,
  adaptive metabolism of, 146
  arthritic response and, 100
Phenylephrine,
  blood pressure and, 91
  chlorpromazine side effects and, 159
  norepinephrine and, 263
  pressor effect, chlorpromazine and, 84
  tremor and, 57
β-Phenylisopropylhydrazine hydrochloride,
  leukemia and, 78
Phenylisopropylhydrazine, serotonin and, 79, 80
Phenylketonuria,
  phenothiazine tests and, 149
  relief of, 274
4-Phenylpiperidin-4-ol,

butyrophenone, properties of, 205
Phenyltoloxamine, proprietary name and use of, 291
Phobex, 294
Phosphatase,
   acid, chlorpromazine and, 82
   alkaline, chlorpromazine and, 82
Phosphate,
   uptake, chlorpromazine and, 74, 78
Phosphocreatine,
   brain, chlorpromazine and, 73
6-Phosphogluconate dehydrogenase, phenothiazines and, 82
Phospholipids,
   brain, chlorpromazine and, 74, 82
Phosphoprotein, antihistaminics and, 75
Phosphoric acid, phenothiazines and, 148
Phosphoric ester poisoning, promazine and, (Fra) 391
Phosphorylation,
   oxidative, chlorpromazine and, 39, 47, 75, 82
Photooxidation, phenothiazines and, 138
Photosensitivity,
   chlorpromazine and, 140, 159
   trifluoperazine and, (Cah) 440, (Gor) 441
   trimeprazine and, (Kno) 471
Phrenotropic action, perphenazine and, (Pen) 358
Physostigmine,
   electroencephalographic effects, chlorpromazine and, 51
   tremorine activity and, 66
Picrotoxin, chlorpromazine and, 52, 53
Pigeon,
   apomorphine and, 58
   reaction to chlorpromazine, 41, 47-48
Pinnal reflex, chlorpromazine and, 39
Pipamazine, 363-364
   emesis and, 58, (Bla) 363
   proprietary names for, 17
Piperacetazine, 22
10-(1'-Piperazinocarbonyl)phenothiazine, 4
Piperazinopropyl side chain, preparation of, 28
Piperidinochlorphenothiazin, 15
Piperonyl, 201
Pipethanate,
   proprietary name and use of, 295
Piplophen, 7
Pipradol, 292
Pipradrol,
   chlorpromazine and, 41

proprietary names and use of, 292
Pitressin,
   blood pressure and, 91
   chlorpromazine and, 111
Pituitary,
   metabolism, chlorpromazine and, 80
Pituitary-gonadal effects, chlorpromazine and, 102-103
Placebo, methyprylon and, (Las) 494
Placidyl, 284
Planarians,
   regeneration, chlorpromazine and, 78
Plasma, methocarbamol levels in, (Huf) 487
Platelets, chlorpromazine and, 77, 79
Plegicil, 12
Plegicin, 12
Plegicyl, 12
Plegomazin, 6
Poisoning,
   chlorprothixene and, (Fre) 507
   methyprylon and, (Rei) 495
   prochlorperazine and, (Jac) 376
   trimeprazine and, (Jac) 471
Polarography, phenothiazines and, 147
Polyneuritis, chlorprothixene and, (Har) 507
Polyvinylpyrrolidone, chlorpromazine and, 109
Porphyria,
   prochlorperazine and, (Kla) 383
   trifluoperazine and, (Lee) 442
Post-alcoholic syndrome,
   promazine and, (Gol) 400
   promoxolane and, (Kis) 481
   triflupromazine and, (Gol) 464
Post-cardiotomy delirium, trifluoperazine and, (Bla) 446
Posterior pituitary hormone, strychnine absorption and, 86
Potassium bromate, phenothiazine titration and, 147
Potassium ferricyanide, phenothiazines and, 149
Potassium iodoplatinate, phenothiazines and, 149
Potentiation,
   methocarbamol and, (Lan) 487
   phosphorus insecticides, phenothiazine derivatives and, (Art) 394
   prochlorperazine and, (Mur) 370
   promazine and, (Vot) 404
   thiethylperazine and, (Boi) 414
   thiopental anesthesia, (Dob) 437

thiopentone anesthesia, (Dob) 363
  fluphenazine and, (Dob) 317
  thiopropazate and, (Dob) 417
Praying mantis,
  aggressive behavior, drugs and, 118
Prazine, 8
Preanesthetic medication,
  promazine and, (Dob) 398
  propiomazine and, (Lea) 406
  trifluoperazine and, (Bas) 445
  triflupromazine and, (Zee) 468
Predelivery regimen, promazine and, (Fit) 399
Prednisolone, stress and, 97
Pregnancy,
  ceruloplasmin and, 252
  chlorpromazine toxicity and, 113–114
  fluphenazine and, (Gri) 318, 352
  thioridazine and, (Mur) 422, (Cag) 426, (Sav) 433
  trifluoperazine and, (Mor) 454, (Pru) 455
Pregnancy tests,
  false positive, promazine and, (Hil) 395
  frog, promazine and, (Fox) 391
  immunological, chlorpromazine and, 152
  male-frog, chlorpromazine and, 152
Preludin, 288
Premedication,
  chlorprothixene and, (Nae) 515
  children, trimeprazine and, (Cop) 472
  surgical patients, chlorpromazine and, 84
  trimeprazine and, (Gil) 472
Premenstrual syndrome,
  perphenazine and, (Kat) 354
  thioridazine and, (Rom) 432
Preoperative sedatives, chlorpromazine and, 67
Private practice,
  chlorprothixene and, (Dar) 510
  promazine and, (Ayd) 397
  psychiatric, fluphenazine and, (Mor) 320
P.R.N., 291
Proazamin, 7
Procaine,
  analgesia and, 111
  anesthesia and, 110
  toxicity of, 115
Procaine esterase, chlorpromazine and, 76
Procalmadiol, insect behavior and, 118
Prochlorpemazin, proprietary names for, 15
Prochlorperazine,
  activity index, 121
  adrenolytic potency, 215
  aged patients and, (Shu) 386
  alcoholism and, (Rog) 386

  ambulatory treatment and, (Lea) 384
  antiemetic action of, 213, (Ber) 379
  antisialagogue effect of, (Dob) 368
  aplasia and, (Bha) 373, (Bha) 379
  autistic child and, (Fer) 381
  autoradiography of, (Cua) 367
  behavior and, (Kel) 383
  biology and pharmacology of, 366–372
  cardiovascular disease and, (Smi) 386
  cervical - lingual - masticator myoclonus and, (Eck) 374
  chemical papers, 365–366
  children and, (Car) 380
  chlorpromazine and, 156
  cholestasis and, (Wei) 379
  chronic schizophrenia and, (Cha) 380, (Raj) 385
  circulatory effects of, (Lan) 376
  clinical papers, 379–388
  comparative study of, 130–131, (Lap) 384
  configuration of, 125–126
  diphosphopyridine nucleotide levels and, 65
  diuresis and, 110
  emesis and, 58, (Con) 380
  emotional disturbances and, (McA) 384
  extrapyramidal symptoms and, (Dar) 374, (Fre) 374, (Ler) 376
  gastric secretion and, (Cum) 367
  geriatric group and, (Rot) 386
  glucose uptake and, 80
  hemolysis and, 76
  intolerance reaction to, (Mas) 376
  irradiation sickness and, (Sol) 386
  jaundice and, (Del) 374–376, (Sol) 378
  labor and delivery, (Kap) 383
  mammary glands and, 103
  mental deficiency and, (Rob) 385
  metrazole induced convulsions and, (Des) 368
  migraine and, (Dal) 381
  motility disturbance and, (Chr) 380, (Dia) 368
  myopia and, (Yas) 379
  nausea or vomiting and, (Sul) 387
  neurological reactions and, (Buc) 373
  neuromuscular reactions and, (Gai) 375
  ovulation and, 103
  poisoning and, (Jac) 376
  porphyria and, (Kla) 383
  potency of, 210, 211
  potentiation and, (Mur) 370
  pregnancy and, 113–114

SUBJECT INDEX

psychotic patients and, (Fri) 382
psychoneurotic patients and, (Vis) 387
seasickness and, (Whe) 387
side effects of, 372–379
structure, activity and, 117
sulfur labeled, (Phi) 370
  metabolism of, (Phi) 370
synergistic action of, (Bra) 380
synthesis of, 28
toxic effects of, (Gol) 375, (Sil) 378
trade names for, 15
trismus and, (Mar) 376
tuberculosis and, (Shu) 386
uptake and excretion of, 139
withdrawal of, 153
Prochlorpremazine, 15
Procyclidine, electroencephalography and, 52
Prodictazin, 14
Profenamin, 14
Progesterone, 102
  ovulation and, 103
Proketazin, 23
Proketazine, 22
Prolixin, 20
Promactil, 6
Promazil, 6
Promazinamid, 7
Promazine,
  acute alcoholism and, (Coh) 398, (Fox) 399
  acute psychiatric syndromes and, (Chi) 398, (Deb) 398
  adenosine, triphosphatase and, (Low) 392
  adrenolytic potency, 215
  aggressiveness in rats and, (Sio) 393
  agitated senile patients and, (Set) 403
  agranulocytosis and, (Chi) 394, (Woo) 396
  alcoholism and, (Bry) 397, (God) 400, (Gor) 391, (San) 392
  amphetamine toxicity and, (Las) 392
  analgesia and, (Cob) 398
  anaphylaxis and, (Fox) 391
  anesthesia and, (Bos) 397
  anti-arrhythmic action of, (Kam) 392
  antidiuretic hormone and, (Smi) 393
  anti-emesis and, 213, (Bla) 397, (Ros) 392
  arousal responses and, (Wil) 393
  attention span and, (Das) 398
  biology and pharmacology of, 390–394
  blood dyscrasias and, (Bes) 394, (Cou) 394
  blood sugar and, (Cit) 391
  canine practice and, (Gra) 391, (Web) 393
  capillaries and, 95
  cataract surgery and, (Sha) 403
  catatonia and, (May) 395
  catecholamine-depleting agents and, (Sto) 393
  cattle and, (Lan) 392
  cerebral hemodynamics and, (Ehr) 391
  chemical papers, 389–390
  chorea gravidarum and, (Cam) 397
  chronic alcoholism and, (Fel) 399
  chronic catatonic schizophrenics and, (Man) 401
  chronic psychoses and, (Agr) 397, (Cre) 398, (Fle) 399, (Har) 400
  chronic schizophrenic patients and, (Bar) 397
  clinical papers, 397–407
  comparative potency of, 130–131
  conditioning and, (Gar) 391
  contact dermatitis and, (Goo) 395
  convulsions and, (Han) 395
  corticotropic hormone-induced psychosis and, (Pla) 402
  delirium tremens and, (Dan) 398, (Fig) 399
  determination of, (Wis) 390
  diphosphopyridine nucleotide synthesis and, (Bur) 390
  disturbed patients and, (Faz) 399
  drug withdrawal and, (Rol) 403
  electroencephalogram and, (Rei) 396, (Sko) 393, (Win) 396
  electroshock seizure threshold and, (Ted) 393
  emotional dysfunction and, (Gif) 399
  enzyme systems and, (Smi) 393
  epileptiform seizures and, (Voe) 396
  evaluation of, 42
  extrapyramidal reactions and, (Ayd) 394
  fatal agranulocytosis and, (Ear) 394
  fecal incontinence and, (Fre) 399
  fetal death and, (Ami) 394, (Cli) 394
  fine-motor performance and, (Wei) 404
  frog pregnancy tests and, (Fox) 391
  gall bladder and, 105
  gangrene and, (Dea) 394, (She) 396
  geriatric patients and, (Meh) 401
  gynecology and obstetrics and, (Gal) 399
  hemolysis and, 76
  hepatic function and, (Kor) 395, (Par) 402, (Wai) 396
  horses and, (Cun) 391, (Rak) 392, 402
  hydroxy derivatives, activity of, 136
  hydroxylation of, 134
  hyperpyrexia and, (Dow) 394
  hypotension and, 95
  irritable colon syndrome and, (Wol) 405

jaundice and, (Zin) 396
labor and, (Mar) 401
leucocytosis and, (Hat) 395
leukemoid reaction and, (Mic) 396
lipid films and, 106
mechanism of action, (Gre) 391
melanocyte stimulating hormone and, (Sco) 392
mental deficiency and, (Bcn) 397, (Ber) 397
mental retardation and, (Ese) 399
mental syndromes and, (Azi) 397
meperidine and, (Bol) 397, (Cli) 398
metabolism and, 70, (Ehr) 391, (Emm) 389, (Opi) 392, (Wal) 393
monkey behavior and, (Lea) 392
motor reflexes and, (Sil) 393
mouse fighting behavior and, (Jan) 392
neonatal jaundice and, (Sut) 396
neonatal pathology and, (Dam) 398
neurological disorders and, (Spi) 396
neuropsychiatric disturbances in children and, (Bov) 397, (Ver) 404
obstetric analgesia and, (Cab) 397, (Dav) 398, (Gri) 400
ocular side effects and, (Bur) 394
orthostatic hypotension and, (Wit) 396
out patients and, (Eng) 398
overdosage of, (Hin) 395
ovulation and, 103
paranoid schizophrenics and, (Gon) 400
Parkinson's disease and, (Eng) 399
pentobarbital anesthesia and, (Cli) 391
performance and, (Dew) 391
pharmacological effects of, 216, 225
phosphoric ester poisoning and, (Fra) 391
post alcoholic syndrome and, (Gol) 400
potency of, 210, 211
potentiating action of, (Vot) 404
pre-anesthetic medication and, (Dob) 398, (Pes) 402
predelivery regimen and, (Fit) 399
private practice and, (Ayd) 397
protozoa and, (Gut) 391
psychiatric hospitalization and, (Eng) 398
psychiatric symptoms and, (Edi) 398
ptosis and, 216
pyloric stenosis and, (Hof) 400
reflex rigidity in decerebrate and, (Ros) 403
rhesus monkey and, (Hos) 392
schizophrenia and, (Aiv) 397, (Cas) 398
senile confusion and, (Rem) 402

serotonin antagonist activity of, (Ted) 393
side effects of, (And) 394, 394–396
spermatic fertility and, (Foo) 391
stress tolerance and, (McG) 401
structure, activity and, 116
suicide and, (Tay) 396
sulfur labeled, (Fed) 391, metabolism of, (Wal) 393
surgery and, (Aco) 397, (Ahn) 397
synthesis of, 28–29
tetanus in animals and, (Lau) 392
thrombosis and, (Roo) 396
test, indican and, 149
tolerance and, (Lag) 392
toxicity of, (Buc) 394, (Pre) 396
trade names for, 8
urine and, (Ebe) 389
uterine contractility and, (Zou) 394
vascular permeability and, (Spe) 393
verbal group participation and, (Fre) 399
veterinary medicine and, (Sch) 392
vitamins and, 115
withdrawal from meprobamate and, (Hol) 400
Promazionon, 8
Promazol, 6
Promethazine,
  capillaries and, 95
  comparative potency of, 130–131
  diphosphopyridine nucleotide levels and, 65
  hemolysis and, 76
  histamine and, 108, 109
  lipid films and, 106
  metabolism of, 135, 143
  pharmacological activity of, 2
  proprietary names for, 7
  radiation and, 59
  structure, activity and, 116
  synthesis of, 28–29
Promilene, 8
Promoxolane,
  dysmenorrhea and, (Boi) 481, (Viv) 481
  menopause and, (Boi) 481
  postalcoholic psychomotor agitation and, (Kis), 481
Promwill, 8
Propaphenin, 6
Propavan, 16
Propazin, 8
Propericiazine, 17
Prophenamin, proprietary names for, 14
Propiomazine,
  double blind study of, (Akr) 406

enzyme systems and, (Usd) 407
insomnia and, (Kra) 406
obstetric analgesia and, (Gli) 406, (Gri) 406, (Pow) 406
preanesthetic medication and, (Lea) 406
proprietary names for, 16
2-Propionyl-10-(2'-dimethylamino-1'-propyl)phenothiazine, 16
2-Propionyl-10-(3'-dimethylamino-1'-propyl)phenothiazine, 16
2-Propionyl-10-{3'-[4-(2-hydroxyethyl)-1-piperazinyl]propyl}phenothiazine, 22
Propionylpromazine, 16
Propitan, 201
2-Propyl-10-{3'-[4-(2-hydroxyethyl)-1-piperazinyl]propyl}phenothiazine, 23
Propylthiouracil, vitamins and, 115
Proquamezin, 15
Protactyl, 8
Protein(s),
    abnormal, mental disease and, 251–255
    synthesis, chlorpromazine and, 80
Prothazin, 7
Prothiaden, 293
Prothipendyl,
    antiemetic action of, (Dem) 409
    clinical activity of, (Car) 408
    colitis and, (Cat) 408
    mammary glands and, 103
    metabolic effects of, 70
    motor activity and, (Bar) 408
    proprietary names for, 290
Protozoa, promazine and, (Gut) 391
Protriptylene, proprietary name and use of, 294
Proveratrine, chlorpromazine and, 56
Prozil, 6
Pruritis,
    anogenital, trimeprazine and, (Lov) 473
    chlorprothixene and, (Ney) 515
    methdilazine and, (Fro) 330
    trimeprazine and, (Arm) 471
Psicoperidol, 201
Psilocybin, mental illness and, 250
Psychiatric disorders,
    acute, promazine and, (Chi) 398, (Deb) 398
Psychiatry,
    ambulant,
        chlorprothixene and, (Anj) 508
        thioridazine and, (Gro) 428
        trifluoperazine and, (Bro) 446
    chlorprothixene and, (Bec) 509, (Kar) 513

fluphenazine and, (Ayd) 315
haloperidol and, 218–220
hospital, trifluoperazine and, (Cas) 447
promazine and, (Edi) 398, (Eng) 398
trifluoperazine and, (Bet) 445
Psychocutaneous disorders, trifluoperazine and, (Ort) 455
Psychogalvanic reflex, chlorpromazine and, 47
Psychogenic syndromes, mephenoxalone and, (Can) 479
Psychometric techniques, chlorpromazine and, 153–155
Psychomotor rating tests, chlorpromazine and, 153
Psychomotor restlessness, thioridazine and, (Flo) 428
Psychoneuroses, trifluoperazine and, (Bra) 446, (God) 449, (May) 454
Psychoneurotic patients,
    ambulatory, thiopropazate and, (Dar) 417
    prochlorperazine and, (Vis) 387
Psychopaths,
    chronic, promazine and, (Agr) 397
Psychopharmacological agents,
    pharmacological evaluation, procedures for, 33–37
Psychophysiological test performance, mephenoxalone and, (Mul) 480
Psychorelaxant effect, thioridazine and, (Pia) 431
Psychosan, 291
Psychoses,
    benperidol and, 228
    chronic,
        fluphenazine and, (Bar) 348
        promazine and, (Cre) 398, (Fle) 399, (Har) 400
        triflupromazine and, (Han) 464
    corticotropic hormone-induced, promazine and, (Pla) 402
    endogenous, thioridazine and, (Sto) 433
    floropipamide and, 227–228
    hallucinatory, trifluperidol and, 224
    methylperidol and, 225
    perphenazine and, (Dre) 357, (Nah) 345
    senile, ceruloplasmin and, 251
Psychosomatic conditions, chlorpromazine, and, 152
Psychotherapeutic activity, anthelmintic activity and, (Min) 438
Psychotherapy,

chlorpromazine and, 151, 152
perphenazine and, (Smi) 360
Psychotics,
   acute and chronic, trifluoperazine and, (Slu) 457
   acutely ill,
      thioridazine and, (Ren) 432
      trifluoperazine and, (Pay) 455
   chlorprothixene and, (Bar) 509
   chronic, fluphenazine and, (Bar) 315, 348
   fluphenazine and, (Den) 316, (Hol) 318, (Lap) 319
   perphenazine and, (Bar) 348
   prochlorperazine and, (Fri) 382
   thioridazine and, (Alo) 425
   trifluoperazine and, (For) 449
Psychotropic action, perphenazine and, (Pen) 358
Psychotropic drugs,
   chemistry of, (Juc) 435
   combined use of, (Gib) 399
Psykoton, 286
Psyquil, 9
Ptosis,
   neuroleptic potency and, 210, 215–216
   tranquilizers and, 34, 40
Puerperal depression, epidemiological study of, (Tod) 458
Pulmonary edema, chlorpromazine and, 86
Purpura,
   allergic, trifluoperazine and, (Ser) 443
Pyloric stenosis, promazine and, (Hof) 400
Pyrathiazine,
   capillaries and, 95
   proprietary names for, 9
   synthesis of, 30
Pyrbenzindol, 297
Pyrethia, 7
Pyrexia,
   dinitrophenol, chlorpromazine and, 69
Pyridine nucleotides,
   blood, chlorpromazine and, 76
Pyridoxal,
   requirement, drugs and, 115
Pyridoxal kinase, chlorpromazine and, 82
Pyridoxine, fluphenazine and, (Lav) 319
Pyrilamine, histamine and, 108
Pyrocatechol disulfonates, influenza and, 110
Pyrrolazote, 9
10-($N,2'$-Pyrrolidino-1'-ethyl)phenothiazine, 9
Pyruvate,
   oxidation, chlorpromazine and, 74
Pyruvic acid, mental illness and, 273

Q

Quantril, 298
Quiactin, 285
Quide, 22

R

R1617, 231
R3264, 203
R4006, 204
R4457, 204
R4749, 201
R7158, 204
Rabbit,
   newborn, drug metabolism by, 138
   phenothiazine metabolism in, 136
Radiation sickness,
   emesis, chlorpromazine and, 59
   prochlorperazine and, (Sol) 386
Radioautography, phenothiazines and, 147
Radium,
   treatment, chlorpromazine and, 77
Rana pipiens,
   melanocyte stimulating hormone, chlorpromazine and, 118
Rana temporaria,
   metamorphosis, drugs and, 118
Randolectil, 22
Rat,
   neuroleptic classification and, 210, 213–214
   phenothiazine metabolism in, 136, 137
Rauwolfia,
   alkaloids, overdosage, 160
Red chlorpromazine, formation of, 140, 141
Reflex rigidity, decerebrate child and, (Ros) 403
Reineckates, phenothiazines and, 149
Repeltin, 10
Reproduction, trifluoperazine and, (Gil) 437
Reserpine,
   activity, chlorpromazine and, 65
   alcohol and, 60
   analgesia and, 111
   brain adenosine triphosphate and, 73
   brain metabolism and, 74
   depression and, 264
   diethyltryptamine activity and, 66
   edema and, 109
   evaluation of, 42
   fighting behavior and, 43
   insect behavior and, 118
   learning and, 43

SUBJECT INDEX

leukemia and, 78
mammary gland and, 103
metabolic effects of, 70
morphine and, 63
nicotinamide and, 65, 75
norepinephrine and, 263
ovulation and, 103
oxygen consumption and, 100
ptosis and, 34
sedative effects of, 34
serotonin and, 65, 79, 80, 265, 266
stress and, 97
tadpole metamorphosis and, 118
thioridazine and, (Reg) 431
toxemias and, 98
yohimbine activity and, 65
Respiration,
  chlorpromazine and, 155
  chlorprothixene and, (Flo) 504
  tranquilizers and, 70, 76, 77, 80, 92, 95
Respiratory center, chlorpromazine and, 54–55
Restless legs syndrome, (Ekb) 381
Retarded children, chlorpromazine and, 155
Reticular formation, chlorpromazine and, 38, 39, 43, 44, 47, 50, 51, 108, 151
Reticulo-endothelial system, chlorpromazine and, 77
Retinopathy,
  perphenazine and, (Wee) 346
  phenothiazines and, 138, 159
  thiopropazate and, (Reb) 419
  thioridazine and, (Hes) 424, (Wee) 424
Reversed phase chromatography, *see* Chromatography
Rhesus monkeys, promazine and, (Hos) 392
Rhinencephalic stimulation, chlorpromazine and, 54
Rhinitis,
  allergic, methdilazine and, (Raw) 331
Riboflavin,
  deficiency, symptoms of, 276
  phenothiazine medication and, 146
Ridazin, 15
Rilatin, 289
Ritalin, 289
Ritalina, 289
Robaxin, 288
Rochipel, 14
Rodipal, 14
Roentgen therapy, thiethylperazine and, (Cod) 414
Rolazote, 9

RP 2987, 11
RP 3015, 4
RP 3276, 8
RP 3277, 7
RP 3356, 14
RP 3828, 15
RP 4270, 9
RP 4560, 6
RP 4632, 10
RP 4909, 13
RP 6140, 15
RP 6484, 17
RP 6549, 10
RP 7044, 13
RP 7204, 11
RP 7843, 20
RP 8030, 5
RP 8909, 17
RP 9153, 17
Rutergan, 4

S

Salicylamide,
  activity, chlorpromazine and, 62
Sanopron, 6
Scale-jiggling test, tranquilizers and, 42
Schizophrenia,
  acute, fluphenazine and, (Ale) 314, (Chi) 316
  adolescent, acetophenazine and, (Dar) 306
  altered metabolism in, 250–251
  ambulatory, acetophenazine and, (Dar) 306
  benperidol and, 228
  catecholamine metabolism in, 258–260
  ceruloplamin and, 251
  chlorpromazine and, 52, 154–156
  chronic,
    carphenazine and, (Cac) 309
    chlorpromazine and, 151–152
    fluphenazine and, (Fog) 317
    methoxypromazine and, (Apf) 332
    perphenazine and, (Ann) 347
    prochlorperazine and, (Cha) 380, (Raj) 385
    promazine and, (Bar) 397
    thioridazine and, (Sal) 432
    trifluoperazine and, (Bar) 445
  floropipamide and, 228
  fluanisone and, 227
  haloperidol and, 220, 223, 224
  mescaline and, 258–259
  methylperidol and, 225

promazine and, (Aiv) 397, (Cas) 398
serotonin metabolism and, 268
trifluoperazine and, (Gar) 449
trifluperidol and, 222–224
Schizophrenic reactions,
chlorprothixene and, (Gay) 512
perphenazine and, (Cas) 349
Schizophrenics,
anergic, trifluoperazine and, (Rez) 455
chlorprothixene and, (Kur) 514
chronic catatonic, promazine and, (Man) 401
drug-resistant,
perphenazine and, (Ill) 354
trifluoperazine and, (All) 444
regressed, thioridazine and, (Udd) 434
thiopropazate and, (Lai) 419
thioridazine and, (Hol) 429
Scopolamine,
stretch reflex and, 108
tremorine activity and, 66
SCTZ, proprietary name and use of, 284
Seasickness,
prochlorperazine and, (Whe) 387
trifluoperazine and, (Don) 448, (Tur) 458
Sea urchin,
eggs, chlorpromazine and, 78, 115
Sebadinine, 56
Secergan, 5
metabolic fate of, 135
Secobarbital,
activity, chlorpromazine and, 60
Secotil, 5
Sedalande, 200
Sedarex, 285
Sedation,
fluanisone and, 226
methyprylon and, (Bil) 492, (Cas) 492
norepinephrine and, 264
Sedavic, 200
Sediston, 8
Seizures,
ectylurea and, (Utl) 491
promazine and, (Kur) 395
Semoxydrine, 287
Senile confusion, promazine and, (Rem) 402
Senile dementia, methylperidol and, 225
Sensitivity,
emotional, thioridazine and, (Bar) 425
Sensory methods, chlorpromazine rating and, 154
Septal activity, chlorpromazine and, 39–40
Sequential analysis, carphenazine and, (Bel) 309

Serenace, 200
Serenase, 200, 295
Serenelfi, 200
Sergetyl, 17
Sernyl, 291
Serotonin,
abnormal metabolites of, 269
accumulation, chlorpromazine and, 65
antagonism,
comparative potencies of phenothiazines and, 130–132, (Ted) 439
promazine and, (Ted) 393
brain, morphine and, 63
chloropromazine and, 38, 77–79, 81, 93, 98, 102
hypothermia and, 69
level, iproniazid and, 66
mental disease and, 265–270
metabolism of, 266–269
methylated derivatives, 261
performance and, 46
psychopharmacological agents and, 34
tadpole metamorphosis and, 118
transport, chlorpromazine and, 78–79
Serum albumin, chlorpromazine and, 72
Serum cholesterol, trifluoperazine and, (Rei) 443
Serum globulin, chlorpromazine and, 72
Serum total protein, chlorpromazine and, 72
Sevinol, 20
Sevinon, 20
Sexual behavior, chlorpromazine and, 43
Sexual dysfunction, thioridazine and, (Sha) 424
Sham rage, chlorpromazine and, 40, 43
Shivering, chlorpromazine and, 155
Shock,
chlorpromazine and, 81, 95–97, 155
droperidol and, 229
experimental, perphenazine and, (Mck) 339
perphenazine and, (Rot) 340
traumatic, droperidol and, 229, 230
Siamese fighting fish, phenothiazine assay and, 120
Sickling, phenothiazines and, (Lew) 438
Side effects,
phenothiazine structure and, (Car) 435
thioridazine and, (Kir) 429, (And) 423, (Ris) 432
trifluoperazine and, (And) 440
Silicotungstic acid, phenothiazine titration and, 147
Silver acetate, phenothiazines and, 149

SUBJECT INDEX 615

Singultus, triflupromazine and, (Bel) 462
Sinogan, 13
Sinophenin, 8
Siqualine, 20
Siquil, 9
SKF 2601, 6
SKF 4648, 9
SKF 4657, 15
SKF 5019, 18
SKF 6270, 14
Skin,
    pigmentation, chlorpromazine and, 159
Skin reactions, thiopropazate and, (Ken) 418
Sleep,
    benperidol and, 228
    chlorpromazine and, 41, 50, 52
Sleep deprivation, chlorpromazine and, 155
Small intestine, chlorpromazine metabolites and, 138
Smiles rearrangement, phenothiazine synthesis and, 25
Smooth muscle, chlorpromazine and, 104–105
Sodium,
    exchange, chlorpromazine and, 78, 83
Sodium persulfate, phenothiazines and, 149
Solusediv, 200
Solypertine, 297
Somnolence, benperidol and, 228
Soprintin, 12
Soprontin, 12
Spamol, 15
Spansule forms, prochlorperazine and, (Fid) 381
Sparine, 8
Spasmolytic activity, phenothiazines and, 5
Spasticity,
    chlorpromazine and, 44
    ectylurea and, (Utl) 491
    mephenoxalone and, (Tim) 480
    methocarbamol and, (Big) 486
Spectrofluorometry,
    phenothiazines and, 147, (Rie) 421
    thioridazine and, (Rag) 421
Spectrophotometry, phenothiazines, 147
Sperm, chlorpromazine and, 102
Spermatic fertility, promazine and, (Foo) 391
Sphingomyelins, mental defects and, 275
Spider, chlorpromazine and, 41
Spinal cord,
    chlorpromazine and, 40
    potentials, chlorpromazine and, 57
    tissue culture, chlorpromazine and, 115
Spiroperidol, 208
    adrenolytic potency, 215

Spiroperidol—*continued*
    duration of action, 213
    potency of, 210, 211
    speed of action, 213
    structure of, 204
Spleen,
    serotonin, chlorpromazine and, 79
    tissue culture, chlorpromazine and, 115
Starazin, 8
Stearylamine, lipid films and, 106
Stelazine, 18
Stémétil, 15
Stemmetil, 15
Sterazin, 8
Stereoisomerism, thioxanthenes and, (Sch) 502
Stereotyped behavior, chlorpromazine and, 42
Stoikon, 294
Stomatology, thioridazine and, (Che) 426
Streptococci, chlorpromazine and, 115
Stress,
    chlorpromazine and, 97–100
    emotional, thiopropazate and, (Mor) 419
    tolerance, promazine and, (McG) 401
Stretch reflex, drugs and, 107–108
Strophanthin, chlorpromazine effects and, 94
Structure,
    antiemetic activity and, (Cer) 414
    side effects and, (Car) 373
    phenothiazines, (Car) 435
Strychnine,
    absorption, chlorpromazine and, 85–86
    chlorpromazine and, 39, 51, 52
    conditioned response and, 46
Suavitil, 294
Subjective reactions, stressed, emylcamate and, (Uhr) 482
Submaxillary gland, chlorpromazine and, 87
Succinate,
    oxidation, chlorpromazine and, 74
Succinic dehydrogenase, chlorpromazine and, 82
Succinic oxidase, schizophrenic serum and, 253
Succinic semialdehyde, formation of, 271
Succinylcholine, chlorpromazine and, 67
Sugar,
    absorption, chlorpromazine and, 104
Suicide,
    chlorprothixene and, (Lie) 507, (Rav) 508
    mellaril and, (Gue) 423
    perphenazine and, (Cam) 432
    phenothiazines and, 160

promazine and, (Tay) 396
thioridazine and, (Ent) 423
Sulfanilic acid,
  diazotized, phenothiazines and, 149
Sulfhydryl groups,
  nonprotein, chlorpromazine and, 75, 80–81
Sulfinyl diphenylamine, phenothiazine synthesis and, 25
Sulfolipids,
  brain, chlorpromazine and, 74
Sulfonylureas, chlorpromazine and, 65
Sulfuric acid, phenothiazines and, 148
Sulfuryl chloride, phenothiazine synthesis and, 25
Surgery,
  childrens, triflupromazine and, (Ori) 466
  chlorpromazine and, 152
  droperidol and, 229–230
  methyprylon and, (Dob) 492
  oral, methocarbamol and, (Fei) 486
  perphenazine and, (Lan) 355
  prochlorperazine and, (Lam) 384
  promazine and, (Aco) 397, (Ahn) 397
Surgical stress, chlorpromazine and, 99
Sustained release studies, trimeprazine and, (Joh) 470
Suvren, 296
Sweating, chlorpromazine and, 86, 91
Sycotrol, 295
Sympathetic stimulation,
  blocking, chlorpromazine and, 86–87
Sympathomimetic amines, chlorpromazine and, 63–64
Syndrox, 287
Synergistic action, prochlorperazine and, (Bra) 380

T

Tacaryl, 9
Tachycardia,
  fluanisone and, 226
  haloperidol and, 221
Tacryl, 9
Talc, phenothiazines and, 150
Talofen, 8
Tanidil, 7
Taraxein, mental disease and, 252
Tarpan, 290
Taste sensitivity, extrapyramidal symptoms and, 158
Taxilan, 13, 16

Temaril, 10
Tematil, 15
Témentil, 15
Temperature,
  environmental, chlorpromazine effects and, 136
  rat toxicity and, (Kep) 392
Temporal discrimination, chlorpromazine and, 48
Tension,
  fluphenazine and, (Pro) 321
  trifluoperazine and, (Ern) 448
Tensofin, 20
Tentone, 10
Teralen, 10
Terfluzin, 18
Testis,
  weight, chlorpromazine and, 113
Tetanus,
  animal, promazine and, (Lav) 392
  chlorpromazine and, 67, 155
  equine, methocarbamol and, (Smi) 488
  methocarbamol and, (Les) 487
  trifluoperazine overdosage and, (Wal) 444
Tetanus toxin,
  effects, chlorpromazine and, 107, 108
Tetrabenazine,
  depression and, 264
  proprietary name and use of, 294
Tetracaine, anesthesia and, 110
Tetrahymena pyriformis,
  permeability, chlorpromazine and, 118
  vitamin requirements, tranquilizers and, 115
Tetrameprozine, 15
Tetraprozin, 15
Thalamic reticular system, chlorpromazine and, 51
Thalamonal, 201
Théralène, 10
Theraplix, 18
Thiamine, neuropathy and, 276
Thiamylal,
  activity, chlorpromazine and, 60
Thiantan, 11
Thiantettin, 11
Thiaxanthene(s),
  analogs of phenothiazines, (Pet) 390
  derivatives, cardiovascular activity, (Ham) 501
  geometric isomerization, (Hof) 502, (Sch) 502
Thiergan, 7

SUBJECT INDEX

Thiethylperazine, 20
  anesthesiology and, (Deb) 415
  antiemetic effects of, (Bar) 414
  circulatory response to, (Dob) 415
  localization in central nervous system, (Spa) 415
  metabolism of, (Zeh) 415
  nausea or vomiting and, (Bro) 414
  neuroleptic action of, (Boi) 414
  obstetrics and, (Aus) 414
  postoperative emesis and, (Dow) 415, (Nor) 415
  potentiation and, (Boi) 414
  roentgen therapy and, (Cod) 414
  tuberculosis and, (Tel) 415
  uptake, tissues and, 134
  vertigo and, (Lum) 415, (Ras) 415
  vestibular function and, (Chi) 414
  vomiting mechanism and, (Bro) 414
Thin-layer chromatography, *see* Chromatography
Thioctic acid, chlorpromazine effects and, 76
Thiodiphenylamine, 24
Thiontan, 11
Thionthan, 11
Thiopental,
  activity, chlorpromazine and, 60
  chlorpromazine and, 55
  thiopropazate and, (Dob) 417
Thioperazine, proprietary names for, 20
Thiopropazate,
  acute peptic ulcer and, (McH) 419
  alcoholism and, (Him) 418
  ambulatory psychoneurotic patients and, (Dar) 417
  anxiety in aged and, (Ric) 419
  combined psychopharmaceutic treatment and (Pen) 419
  contact dermatitis and, (Goo) 418
  diarrhea and, (McH) 419
  dizziness and, (Eli) 417
  drug overdosage and (Kay) 418
  dyskinesias and, (Vai) 420, (Fle) 417
  electroencephalographic abnormalities and, (Hol) 418
  emesis and, 58
  emotional stress and, (Mor) 419
  extrapyramidal syndromes and, (Vat) 420
  gastric secretion and, (Lic) 419
  Huntington's chorea and, (Ful) 417, (Sou) 420
  mode of action of, (Kli) 418

  morphine and, (Sch) 420
  neck-face syndrome and, (Rob) 419
  Parkinsonism and, (Hea) 418
  proprietary names for, 21
  psychiatry and, (Ben) 415
  retinopathy and, (Reb) 419
  schizophrenic patients and, (Lai) 419
  skin reactions and, (Ken) 418
  synthesis of, 30
  thiopental anesthesia and, (Dob) 417
  thiopentone anesthesia and, (Dob) 417
  ulcerative colitis and, (Kir) 418
  urine color test for, (For) 417
Thioproperazine,
  proprietary names for, 20
  thioridazine and, (Sch) 433
Thioridazine,
  adrenolytic potency, 215
  adaptation difficulties and, (Ren) 432
  aged and, (Dar) 427
  aggressive children and, (Ald) 425
  agranulocytosis and, (Sha) 424
  akathisia and, (Fre) 423
  ambulant psychiatry and, (Gro) 428
  amenorrhea and, (Des) 427, (Zuc) 424
  anti-amphetamine test and, 214
  antiarrhythmic activity of, (Mad) 430
  antiemesis and, 213
  anxiety and, (Blu) 426
    in children, (Cot) 427
  Bantu schizophrenics and, (Rom) 432
  behavioral disturbances and, (All) 425, (Oet) 431
  brain syndromes and, (San) 432
  catatonia and, (Boi) 426
  child psychiatry and, (Maj) 430
  children and, (Bun) 426
  chronic schizophrenia and, (Sal) 432
  color test for, (For) 420
  comparative potency of, 130–131
  complications and, (May) 424
  Cotard's syndrome and, (Hen) 424
  depressive states and, (Flu) 428, (Pet) 431
  driving and, (May) 424
  dumping syndrome and motor activity, (Tob) 422
  duration of action, 213
  ejaculation and, (Cle) 423), (Our) 424
  electrocardiographic abnormalities and, (Kel) 424, (Wen) 424
  electroencephalographic reaction and, (Iti) 422, (Ule) 423
  emotional disorders and, (Bro) 426
  emotional sensitivity and, (Bar) 425

endogenous depression and, (Bas) 425, (Bau) 425
endogenous psychoses and, (Sto) 433
enuresis nocturna and, (Bur) 426
epilepsy and (Fra) 428), (Pau) 431
excretion pattern of, (Eid) 420, (Gel) 428
experimental methods and, (May) 422
galactorrhea and, (Cas) 423
general medicine and, (Neu) 431
geriatric patients and, (Jac) 429
glaucoma and, (Joh) 429
granulocyte suppression and, (Bac) 423
hepatic blood flow and, (Eck) 421
Huntington's chorea and, (Ris) 432
hypotension and, (Swa) 424
hypotensive side effects of, (Ros) 424
internal medicine and, (Cuc) 427
libido disorders and, (Pom) 424
liver function and, (Bov) 423, (Keu) 424
liver hemodynamics and, (Pla) 422
lupus erythematosus and, (Led) 430
menopause and, (Cal) 426
mental deficiency and, (Bad) 425
metabolism of, 135, 144, (Pla) 422, (Rut) 421
nervous diseases of children and, (Kub) 430
neurological toxicity of, (Fur) 423
neuropsychiatric practice and, (Ric) 432
obstetrics and, (Bac) 425
ocular changes and, (Dem) 423
orphenadrine and, (Man) 430
out-patients and, (Ana) 425
ovulation and, (Pur) 422
papilledema and, (Blu) 423
paranoid schizophrenia and, (Gom) 428
pediatrics and, (Ren) 432
pediatric psychiatry and, (Bar) 425, (Die) 427
pharmacological effects of, 216
postoperative period and, (Bar) 425
potency of, 210, 211
pregnancy and, (Mur) 422, (Sav) 433
premature ejaculation and, (Sin) 433
premenstrual syndrome and, (Rom) 432
proprietary names for, 19
psychomotor restlessness and, (Flo) 428
psychorelaxant effect of, (Pia) 431
psychotic patients and, (Alo) 425
ptosis and, 216
regressed schizophrenic patients and, (Udd) 434
reserpine and, (Reg) 431
retinopathy and, (Hes) 424, (Wee) 424
schizophrenics and, (Hol) 429
sexual dysfunction and, (Sha) 424
side effects of, (Kir) 429, (Ris) 432
spectrofluorometric determination of, (Rag) 421
speed of action, 213
stomatology and, (Che) 426
suicide and, 161, (Ent) 423
sulfur labeled, (Eid) 420
test, indican and, 149
thioproperazine and, (Sch) 433
traction test and, (Boi) 421
trigeminal neuralgia and, (May) 430
tuberculous patients and, (Gov) 428
uptake tissues and, 134–135
urine tests and, (For) 420, (Nev) 422
visual symptoms and, (Mor) 424
Thioridazine sulfone, excretion of, 135
Thorazine, 6
Thrombocytes,
  serotonin, tranquilizers and, 79
Thrombosis, promazine and, (Roo) 396
Thymidine,
  incorporation, chlorpromazine and, 84
Thymus,
  weight, chlorpromazine and, 99, 103
Thyroid function, perphenazine and, (Ayd) 347, (Cra) 350
Thyroid hormone, cretinism and, 274
Thyrotropin,
  uptake, chlorpromazine and, 101
Thyroxine,
  activity, chlorpromazine and, 71, 100–101
  mitochondria and, 75
Tic nerveux, haloperidol and, 218
Timovan, 290
Tindal, 21
Tissue culture, chlorpromazine toxicity and, 115
Tolbutamide, vitamins and, 115
Tolerance,
  perphenazine and, (Irw) 388
  promazine and, (Lag) 392
Torazina, 6
Torecan, 20
Toxemias,
  bacterial, chlorpromazine and, 98
Toxicity,
  acute, neuroleptic drugs and, 210, 216
  carphenazine and, (Men) 309, (Tis) 308
  chlorprothixene and (Gom) 512
  chronic, mepazine and, (Koe) 326
  hydroxyphenamate and, (Bas) 483
  mephenoxalone and, (Yea) 480

SUBJECT INDEX

methdilazine and, (Wei) 331
methyprylon and, (Pel) 494
prochlorperazine and, (Sil) 378
promazine and, (Buc) 394, (Moo) 396, (Pre) 396
rat, temperature and, (Kep) 392
TPS-23, 19
Traction test, thioridazine and, (Boi) 421
Tradon, 285
Trancin, 20
Trancopal, 287
Tranquilizer(s),
    combinations of, (Tal) 457
    testing of, 151
Transaminases,
    brain, chlorpromazine and, 74
Transergan, 5
Transportation,
    stress, chlorpromazine and, 97
Tranylcypromine,
    chlorpromazine and, 65
    phenothiazines and, 156
    trifluoperazine and, (Buf), 446, (Gro) 450
    in obstetrics, (Pru) 455
Tremor,
    chlorpromazine-induced, abolishment of, 57
    unilateral, triflupromazine and, (Zlo) 462
Tremorine, antagonism of, 66
Tresortil, 288
Tribolium confusum, chlorpromazine and, 118
Trichlorethylene,
    inhalation, chlorpromazine and, 85
Triethyltin, creatine phosphate and, 73
Trifluoperazine,
    acute alcoholism and, (Cos) 447
    acute or chronic psychotics and, (Slu) 457
    acutely ill psychotics and, (Pay) 455
    adrenolytic potency of, 215
    aged and, (Fal) 448
        depressed, (Bro) 446
    alcoholic hallucinosis and, (Bar) 445, 450
    allergic purpura and, (Ser) 443
    allergy and, (San) 456
    ambulatory psychiatry and, (Bro) 446
    amylobarbitone and, (Whi) 458
    anergic schizophrenic patients and, (Rez) 455
    antiemesis and, (Ber) 445, (Cau) 447
    anxiety or tension states and, (Ern) 448, (Ham) 450, 455, (Sai) 456
    apomorphine antagonism and, (Jan) 438
    auditory hallucinations and, (Kru) 452

    bioelectric activity of brain and, (Lei) 438
    biology and pharmacology of, 436–440
    blood-cerebrospinal fluid barrier and, (Gue) 450
    brain sulfolipids and, (Gle) 437
    chemical papers, 435–436
    child psychiatry and, (Fis) 449
    chlorpromazine and, 156
    cholestatic hepatitis and, (Koh) 442
    chronic delirium and, (Slu) 457
    chronic mental disorders and, (All) 444, (Bar) 445
    clinical papers, 444–459
    combinations,
        amitriptyline and, (Che) 447
        chlorpromazine and, (Bar) 445
    comparative potency of, 130–131
    compulsive rituals and, (Alt) 444
    confinement motor activity and, (Fow) 437
    delirium tremens and, (Bar) 445
    depressed patients and, (Pet) 455
    dermatology and, (Kam) 451
    discrimination and, (Shu) 439
    drug-resistant schizophrenics and, (All) 444
    dystonic reaction and, (Dav) 441
    electroencephalographic activation and, (Lin) 453
    electroshock therapy and, (Fre) 449, (Ros) 456
    emesis and, 58
    extrapyramidal effects of, (Ano) 440
    fetal abnormalities and, (Sch) 443
    gastrointestinal tension states and, (Ern) 448
    geriatric patients and, (Ham) 450
    granulocytic depression and, (Sim) 457
    gynecology and, (Bur) 446
    hospital psychiatry and, (Cas) 447
    Huntington's chorea and, (Coh) 447
    hypermotor syndrome in children and, (Gra) 450
    hypothermia and, 69
    malignant emotional disturbances and, (Bea) 445
    mammary glands and, 103
    menopausal syndrome and, (Coh) 447
    mental retardation and, (Hei) 450
    mescaline and, 64
    nausea or vomiting and, (Pru) 455
    neuroses and, (Ayd) 445
    obstetrics and, (Dav) 463
    office patients and, (Gea) 449

overdosage, tetanus and, (Wal) 444
ovulation and, 103
oxypertine and, (Cal) 446
pain and, (Dun) 448
paranoid schizophrenia and, (Gal) 449
pediatrics and, (Iba) 451, (Vez) 458
pharmacology,
    confinement motor activity and, (Ted) 439
    fighting behavior and, (Ted) 439
photosensitivity and, (Cah) 440, (Gor) 441
porphyria and, (Lee) 442
postcardiotomy delirium and, (Bla) 446
postoperative emesis and, (Bla) 446
potency of, 210, 211
preanesthetic medication and, (Bas) 445
pregnancy and, 113–114, (Mor) 454, (Pru) 455
proprietary names for, 18
psychiatry and, (Bet) 445
psychocutaneous disorders and, (Ort) 455
psychotic patients and, (For) 449
refractory patients and, (Erd) 448, (Gun) 450
reproduction and, (Gil) 437
schizophrenia and, 223, (Gar) 449
    chronic, (Bar) 445
seasickness and, (Don) 448, (Tur) 458
serum cholesterol and, (Rei) 443
side effects of, (And) 440, 440–444
suicide attempts and, 161
synthesis of, 29
thymopathies and, (Fer) 448
tranylcypromine and, (Buf) 446, (Kru) 452
uptake and excretion of, 139
withdrawn catatonics and, (Sti) 457
2-Trifluoromethyl-10-(3′-dimethylamino-1′-propyl)phenothiazine, 9
2-Trifluoromethyl-10-(2″,N^1-hydroxyethyl-N^2,3′-piperazinyl-1′-propyl)phenothiazine, 20
2-Trifluoromethyl-10-(4″-methyl-1″,3′-piperazinyl-1′-propyl)phenothiazine, 18
2-Trifluoromethylsulfonylphenothiazine, synthesis of, 31
Trifluorperazine, 18
Trifluperidol,
    adrenolytic potency, 215
    bibliography, 217
    clinical use, 221–224
    optimal dosage, 221
    potency of, 207, 210, 211
    trade names for, 201
Triflupromazine,

acute alcoholism and, (Gru) 464
agranulocytosis and, (Ayd) 461
ambulatory patients and, (Ree) 467
anesthesia and, (Dav) 463
biology and pharmacology of, 460–461
chemical papers, 460
chronic psychoses and, (Han) 464
clinical papers, 462–468
comparative potency of, 130–131
contact dermatitis and, (Goo) 461
dermatology and, (Kam) 465
dystonic reaction and, (McK) 461
effectiveness, controlled study of, (Hee) 464
emesis and, 58
endoscopies and, (Reb) 467
extrapyramidal reactions and, (Ayd) 461
goats and, (Jha) 461
hyperemesis gravidarum and, (Bur) 463
hypotension and, 95
mental retardation and, (Bai) 462
out patients and, (Ros) 467
postalcoholic syndrome and, (Gol) 464
postoperative nausea and, (Bru) 463
preanesthetic medication and, (Zee) 468
proprietary names for, 9
side effects of, 461
singultus and, (Bel) 462
specific test for, 148
surgery in children and, (Ori) 466
synthesis of, 29
test, indican and, 149
unilateral tremor and, (Zlo) 462
Trigeminal neuralgia, thioridazine and, (May) 430
Trihexylphenidyl, droperidol and, 230
Trilafon, 18
Trimeprazine,
    agranulocytosis and, (Bra) 470
    anogenital pruritus and, (Lov) 473
    antiemetic activity of, (Poo) 474
    antihistamine agents and, (Gra) 472
    antitussive activity of, (Poo) 474
    chemical poisonings and, (Jac) 471
    dermatoses and, (And) 471, (Pan) 473
    dogs or cats and, (Can) 469
    hyperemotional child and, (Dov) 472
    hypothermia and, 69
    inflammation and, 109
    isomers, activity of, 121, 124
    itching dermatoses and, (Cal) 472
    pediatric practice and, (Sea) 474
    photosensitivity and, (Kno) 471
    pregnancy and, 113–114
    premedication, (Gil) 472

children, (Cop) 472
proprietary names for, 10
pruritis and, (Arm) 471
sulfur labeled, (Ros) 469
excretion of, (Fla) 469
sustained release studies, (Joh), 470
synthesis of, 30
Tripelennamine, chlorpromazine hypothermia and, 70
Triphenidyl, chlorpromazine side effects and, 158
Triphosphopyridine nucleotide,
reduced, chlorpromazine oxidation and, 137, 138
Trismus, prochlorperazine and, (Mar) 376
Triton, mitochondria and, 75
Trypan Blue,
accumulation, chlorpromazine and, 92
Trypanosoma,
infection, chlorpromazine and, 68
Trypanosoma cruzi, chlorpromazine and, 115
Trypanosoma evansi, chlorpromazine and, 115
Tryptamine,
abnormal metabolites of, 269–270
antagonism, comparative potencies of phenothiazines and, 130–132
chlorpromazine and, 79–80
excretion of, 268, 270
formation of, 266, 267
mental disease and, 265–270
metabolism of, 266–269
methylated derivatives, 261
Tryptophan,
abnormal metabolites of, 269–270
metabolism of, 266–269
Tryptophan hydroxylase, 266
Tuazole, 289
Tubercle bacilli, chlorpromazine and, 115
Tuberculosis,
ceruloplasmin and, 252
chlorpromazine and, 152
prochlorperazine and, (Shu) 386
thiethylperazine and, (Tel) 415
thioridazine and, (Gov) 428
d-Tubocurarine, chlorpromazine and, 107
Tumors, chlorpromazine and, 77–78
Twins, mental illness in, 274
Typhoid,
endotoxin, chlorpromazine and, 96
Tyramine,
norepinephrine and, 262
tranquilizers and, 63
Tyrosine, catecholamine biosynthesis and, 256
Tyrosine hydroxylase,
norepinephrine and, 263
sedation and, 264

U

Ulcerative colitis, thiopropazate and, (Kir) 418
Ulcers, chlorpromazine and, 104
Ulcolind, 200
Ullmann reaction, phenothiazine synthesis and, 26
Ultraviolet absorption,
phenothiazine metabolites and, 136, 138
tranquilizers and, 146, 147
Ultraviolet irradiation, chlorpromazine derivatives and, 140
UML 491, 69
Unconditioned response, comparative phenothiazine potency and, 130–131
Uranyl nitrate, phenothiazines and, 148
Uricosuric effect, chlorprothixene and, (Hea) 504
Urinary antiseptic, phenothiazine and, 3
Urine,
chlorpromazine metabolites in, 141, 142
chlorprothixene tests and, (Mel) 502
methoxypromazine elimination in, (All) 332
phenothiazines in, 135, 139
schizophrenic, fractionation of, 255
thiopropazate color test and, (For) 417
thioridazine and, (For) 420
Urologic patients, ethchlorvynol and, (Bar) 497
Uterus,
contraction,
chlorpromazine and, 86
promazine and, (Zou) 394
Uveal pigment, phenothiazine compounds and, (Pot) 443

V

Valium, 289
Vallergal, 10
Vallergan, 10
Vallergin, 7
Valmid, 286
Vanadium sulfate, phenothiazines and, 149
Vanillic acid, catecholamines and, 257, 258
Vascular effects, chlorpromazine and, 155
Vascular permeability, promazine and, (Spe)

RC
483
G68
v.2

APR 5 1976